HANDBOOK OF
GENETICS

Volume 3
Invertebrates of
Genetic Interest

HANDBOOK OF GENETICS

HANDBOOK OF GENETICS

ROBERT C. KING, EDITOR

Professor of Genetics, Department of Biological Sciences
Northwestern University, Evanston, Illinois

Volume 3
Invertebrates of
Genetic Interest

SPRINGER SCIENCE+BUSINESS MEDIA, LLC

Library of Congress Cataloging in Publication Data

King, Robert C
  Invertebrates of genetic interest.

  (His Handbook of genetics; v. 3)
  Includes bibliographies and index.
  1. Invertebrates—Genetics. I. Title. [DNLM: 1. Genetics. QH430 H236]
QL3629.K56   592'.01'5   75-17802
ISBN 978-1-4615-7147-6   ISBN 978-1-4615-7145-2 (eBook)
DOI 10.1007/978-1-4615-7145-2

©1975 Springer Science+Business Media New York
Originally published by Plenum Press, New York in 1975
Softcover reprint of the hardcover 1st edition 1975

United Kingdom edition published by Springer Science+Business Media, LLC
A Division of Plenum Publishing Company, Ltd.
Davis House (4th Floor), 8 Scrubs Lane, Harlesden, London, NW10 6SE, England

Preface

The purpose of the first four volumes of the *Handbook of Genetics* is to bring together collections of relatively short, authoritative essays or annotated compilations of data on topics of significance to geneticists. Many of the essays will deal with various aspects of the biology of certain species or species groups selected because they are favorite subjects for genetic investigation in nature or the laboratory. Often there will be an encyclopedic amount of information available on such species, with new papers appearing daily. Most of these will be written for specialists in a jargon that is bewildering to a novice, and sometimes even to a veteran geneticist working with evolutionarily distant organisms. For such readers what is needed is a written introduction to the morphology, life cycle, reproductive behavior, and culture methods for the species in question. What are its particular advantages (and disadvantages) for genetic study, and what have we learned from it? Where are the classic papers, the key bibliographies, and how does one get stocks of wild type or mutant strains? Lists giving the symbolism and descriptions for selected mutants that have been retained and are thus available for future studies are provided whenever possible. Genetic and cytological maps, mitotic karyotypes, and haploid DNA values are also included when available.

The chapters in this volume deal with invertebrate species that are favorites of geneticists. Attempts to obtain a chapter dealing with the genetics of *Caenorhabditis elegans* proved unsuccessful. Therefore, the volume begins with a survey of molluscan species that have been studied genetically and then turns to the Insecta, with *Blattella germanica* representing the hemimetabolous species. Next come representatives of certain holometabolous orders (for the Lepidoptera, *Bombyx* and *Ephestia*; for the Coleoptera, *Tribolium*; and for the Hymenoptera, *Apis,*

Habrobracon and *Mormoniella*). The remaining chapters concern dipterans of genetic interest. Among these are species famous for their giant polytene chromosomes (*Rhynchosciara, Sciara, Chironomus,* and *Glyptotendipes*) and species of great importance to human and veterinary medicine (*Anopheles, Aedes, Culex, Musca,* and *Lucilia*). Eleven chapters are devoted to the invertebrate for which the greatest amount of genetic information is available, *Drosophila melanogaster,* and five chapters deal with other species belonging to the same genus.

I am particularly grateful for the splendid assistance provided by Pamela Khipple and Lisa Gross during the preparation of this volume. Volume 4 will cover the vertebrates of genetic interest.

Robert C. King

Evanston
June, 1975

Contributors

Hiromu Akai, National Sericultural Experiment Station, Tokyo, Japan

James T. Arnold, Division of Entomology, Commonwealth Scientific and Industrial Research Organization, Canberra City, Australia

Michael Ashburner, Department of Genetics, University of Cambridge, Cambridge, England

A. Ralph Barr, School of Public Health, University of California, Los Angeles, California

Antonio Brito da Cunha, Departmento de Biologia, Universidade de São Paulo, São Paulo, Brazil

Ernst W. Caspari, Department of Biology, University of Rochester, Rochester, New York

Joseph D. Cassidy, O.P., Department of Biological Sciences, Northwestern University, Evanston, Illinois

Frances E. Clayton, Department of Zoology, University of Arkansas, Fayetteville, Arkansas

Donald G. Cochran, Department of Entomology, Virginia Polytechnic Institute, Blacksburg, Virginia

Mario Coluzzi, Institute of Parasitology, University of Rome, Rome, Italy

Theodosius Dobzhansky, Department of Genetics, University of California, Davis, California

Hiroshi Doira, Kyushu University, Fukuoka, Japan

Geoffrey G. Foster, Division of Entomology, Commonwealth Scientific and Industrial Research Organization, Canberra City, Australia

Natalia Gabrusewycz-Garcia, Onondaga Community College and Department of Anatomy, State University of New York, Syracuse, New York

Frederick J. Gottlieb, Department of Biology, University of Pittsburgh, Pittsburgh, Pennsylvania

Joseph Grossfield, Department of Biology, The City College of The City University of New York, New York, N.Y.

Klaus Hägele, Institute for Genetics, Ruhr-University Bochum, Bochum, West Germany

W. Keith Hartberg, Department of Biology, Southern College, Statesboro, Georgia

Oswald Hess, Institut für Allegmeine Biologie, Universität Düsseldorf, Düsseldorf, West Germany

Robert C. King, Department of Biological Sciences, Northwestern University, Evanston, Illinois

James B. Kitzmiller, Florida Medical Entomology Laboratory, Vero Beach, Florida

Christine Konowalow, Division of Entomology, Commonwealth Scientific and Industrial Research Organization, Canberra City, Australia

Philippe L'Héritier, Department of Genetics, University of Clermont-Ferrand, Clermont-Ferrand, France

Riccardo Milani, Istituto di Zoologia, Universita di Pavia, Pavia, Italy

J. Dawson Mohler, Department of Zoology, The University of Iowa, Iowa City, Iowa

Daigoro Moriwaki, Department of Biology, Faculty of Science, Tokyo Metropolitan University, Tokyo, Japan

James Murray, Department of Biology, University of Virginia, Charlottesville, Virginia

Stephen J. O'Brien, National Cancer Institute, National Institutes of Health, Bethesda, Maryland

William L. Pak, Department of Biological Sciences, Purdue University, Lafayette, Indiana

Crodowaldo Pavan, Department of Zoology, The University of Texas at Austin, Austin, Texas and Departmento de Biologia, Instituto de Bicciencias, Universidade de São Paulo, São Paulo, Brazil

Jeffrey R. Powell, Department of Biology, Yale University, New Haven, Connecticut

Karamjit S. Rai, Department of Biology, University of Notre Dame, Notre Dame, Indiana

Lynn J. Romrell, Department of Pathology, Division of Anatomical Sciences, College of Medicine, University of Florida, Gainesville, Florida

Mary H. Ross, Department of Entomology, Virginia Polytechnic Institute, Blacksburg, Virginia

Walter C. Rothenbuhler, Departments of Entomology, Zoology, and Genetics, Ohio State University, Columbus, Ohio

Patricia Sanders, Office of Medical Genetics, Department of Medicine, Baylor College of Medicine, Houston, Texas

Imogene Schneider, Department of Entomology, Walter Reed Army Institute of Research, Washington, D.C.

Alexander Sokoloff, Department of Biology, California State College, San Bernardino, California

David T. Suzuki, Department of Zoology, The University of British Columbia, Vancouver, B.C., Canada

Yataro Tazima, National Institute of Genetics, Misima, Japan

Lynn H. Throckmorton, Department of Biology, University of Chicago, Chicago, Illinois

Yoshiko N. Tobari, Faculty of Science, Tokyo Metropolitan University, Tokyo, Japan

Ludwig Walter, Institute for Genetics, Ruhr-University, Bochum, Bochum, West Germany

Marshall R. Wheeler, Department of Zoology, University of Texas at Austin, Austin, Texas

Maxwell J. Whitten, Division of Entomology, Commonwealth Scientific and Industrial Research Organization, Canberra City, Australia

Contents

K. The Genus Drosophila

L. Drosophila melanogaster

PART G
MOLLUSCS OF
GENETIC INTEREST

1

The Genetics of the Mollusca

JAMES MURRAY

Introduction

The available information on the genetics of the Mollusca is scattered in a rather disjointed fashion through the literature of malacology, ecology, marine biology, cytology, and even tropical medicine. The different facets of the subject have grown up independently of one another, each with its own internal logic. I have allowed these semiautonomous units to determine the organization of this review, retaining a historical coherence at the expense of a more systematic treatment. I trust that the following disparate subject headings will provide sufficient orientation for the reader.

Reproduction

With something over 80,000 species, the phylum Mollusca encompasses a bewildering diversity of form and function. There is, of course, a basic body plan of "head–foot," soft visceral mass, and enveloping mantle, but the variations on this theme are protean, ranging from minute snails

JAMES MURRAY—Department of Biology, University of Virginia, Charlottesville, Virginia.

TABLE 1.   *An Abbreviated Classification of the Molluscs, Indicating the Relative Position*
of Taxa Mentioned in the Text[a]

Class Monoplacophora	*Neopilina*

Class Amphineura (Chitons and
          solenogasters)
    Order Chitonida	

Class Gastropoda (Snails and slugs)
  Subclass Prosobranchia
    Order Archaeogastropoda
      Family Patellidae
	Patella

Order Mesogastropoda Family Viviparidae	*Campeloma*
Valvatidae	*Valvata*
Littorinidae	*Littorina*
Hydrobiidae	*Potamopyrgus, Oncomelania*
Melaniidae	*Melanoides*
Calyptraeidae	*Calyptraea, Crepidula*
Order Neogastropoda Family Muricidae	*Purpura*

Subclass Opisthobranchia
    Order Cephalaspidea
      Family Actaeonidae
	Actaeonia

Order Anaspidea
    Order Sacoglossa
    Order Notaspidea
  Subclass Nudibranchia
  Subclass Pulmonata
    Order Basommatophora
      Family Lymnaeidae
	Lymnaea

Physidae	*Physa*
Planorbidae	*Planorbis, Biomphalaria, Bulinus*
Ancylidae	
Order Stylommatophora Family Succineidae	*Catinella*
Achatinellidae	*Achatinella*
Partulidae	*Partula*
Achatinidae	*Limicolaria, Rumina*
Arionidae	*Arion*
Philomycidae	*Philomycus*
Zonitidae	
Bulimulidae	*Liguus*
Helicidae	*Cochlicella, Monacha, Hygromia,* *Arianta, Cepaea, Helix*
Fructicicolidae	*Bradybaena*
Class Scaphopoda (Tusk shells)	

TABLE 1. *Continued*

Class Bivalvia or Pelecypoda (Clams,	
mussels, oysters and scallops)	
Order Taxodonta	
Family Arcidae	*Anadara*
Order Anisomyaria	
Family Mytilidae	*Mytilus, Modiolus*
Pectinidae	*Pecten*
Ostreidae	*Crassostrea*
Order Schizodonta	
Family Unionidae	*Unio*
Order Heterodonta	
Family Tridacnidae	*Tridacna*
Veneridae	*Mercenaria*
Order Adapedonta	
Family Myidae	*Mya*
Class Cephalopoda (Squids, cuttlefish,	
octopods and nautili)	
Order Octopoda	

[a] Following Morton (1967), after Thiele (1931–1935).

to giant squids over fifty feet long. The abbreviated classification given in Table 1 will serve to introduce the forms discussed in this article.

Life histories and modes of reproduction in molluscs are as diverse as their body forms. Judging from primitive living forms, molluscan gonads originally opened directly into the pericardial cavity, and the eggs and sperms were swept into the sea through the coelomoducts. Fertilization was external, with the zygote developing first into a trochophore larva and then into a veliger adapted to a planktonic life. Sexes were probably separate.

From this primitive state, a number of trends may be discerned. Most groups of molluscs have developed some method of internal fertilization, and with this advance has come increasing complexity of the genital ducts and glands and the appearance of copulatory organs. In gastropods one can see a progression from forms (e.g., *Patella*) which shed their gametes directly into the water, via those (e.g., *Calyptraea*) with genital ducts consisting only of ciliated grooves in the mantle, to those (e.g., *Helix*) with fully enclosed systems, specialized stimulatory organs, and associated glands for processing eggs and spermatophores. Copulatory organs are of various types. Normally in gastropods a penis is developed from a portion of the foot, but in some forms (e.g., *Campeloma*) it is a modified tentacle. In *Actaeonia* the penis is armed with a spine so that copulation takes place by hypodermic injection directly through the body wall. The cephalopods have perhaps the most bizarre form of sperm transfer, by means of a modified arm, or hectocotylus, which deposits spermatophores within the mantle cavity of the female.

Another trend in molluscs is toward the development of various methods of enhancing the survival of young. The eggs may be supplied with increasing amounts of yolk, and the free-swimming, vulnerable, larval stages may be reduced. Concomitantly, a tendency toward the brooding of eggs or young may develop. These changes are often associated with the colonization of more stringent habitats. In freshwater clams, for example, although fertilization is technically external (in the mantle cavity), the brood is maintained until hatching within the gill chamber. The larva (e.g., the glochidium of *Unio*) may be modified as a parasite of freshwater fishes. Freshwater and land gastropods suppress the larval stages altogether, in extreme cases retaining the eggs within the oviduct until hatching (e.g., *Partula*). Cephalopods also lay large, yolky eggs and care for them with elaborate brooding behavior.

Still another general trend, especially in gastropods, is toward either hermaphroditism or alternating sexuality. In amphineurans, scaphopods, cephalopods, and streptoneuran gastropods the sexes are separate, but the higher gastropods are increasingly committed to hermaphroditism, with (e.g., *Lymnaea*) or without (e.g., *Helix*) self-fertilization. The other method of relaxing the restrictions of sexuality is by means of consecutive or alternating sexuality. In the classic case of *Crepidula* each individual begins life as a male, then becomes a hermaphrodite, and later a female. Mating chains are arranged in stacks with females below and a young male at the summit. Other forms such as *Valvata* undergo rhythmic changes, with alternating episodes of male and female gametogenesis. Parallel developments are found in the pelecypods, *Mercenaria* undergoing protandric sex reversal and oysters showing alternating sexual states.

True parthenogenesis is rare in molluscs but has been convincingly demonstrated in the snails *Potamopyrgus*, *Campeloma*, and *Melanoides*.

For a highly readable introduction to molluscan biology, *Molluscs* by J. E. Morton (1967) may be recommended. Further details may be pursued in Volume V of *Traité de Zoologie*, edited by Grassé (1960 and 1968).

Polymorphism in the Helicidae

The land snails of the family Helicidae exhibit extensive variation in color and in the ornamentation of the shell with longitudinal bands

(Taylor, 1914). The investigation of the genetic basis of this polymorphism had already commenced at the time of the rediscovery of Mendel's laws, and Lang's (1904) paper on *Cepaea hortensis* and *C. nemoralis* provides some of the earliest examples of Mendelian segregation in animals. The breeding of helicids was continued in the early decades of this century by Stelfox (1915, 1918, 1968), Oldham (1934), and Diver (Diver, 1932; Fisher and Diver, 1934). Although much of this work remains unpublished, Cook and King (Cook, 1965, 1967, 1969, 1970; Cook and King, 1966) have provided accounts of the results.

With the development of studies on the control of gene frequencies in natural populations of *Cepaea* (e.g., Cain and Sheppard, 1950, 1954; Lamotte, 1951, 1959; Clarke, 1960; Goodhart, 1962; Cain and Currey, 1963; Murray, 1964), the need for a better understanding of the genetics of land snails became apparent. Over the past 20 years a fairly clear picture of the genetics of *C. nemoralis* and *C. hortensis* has emerged. In addition, some data are available for *Arianta arbustorum, Helix aspersa, Cochlicella acuta, Monacha cantiana,* and *Hygromia striolata.*

Cepaea nemoralis

Both in field studies on gene frequencies and in laboratory breeding *C. nemoralis* has received the greatest attention. It is a fairly large and colorful animal inhabiting much of western Europe and introduced into a number of places in the United States. The shell may be brown, pink, yellow, or white and may bear up to five (or rarely more) longitudinal stripes or bands. The various patterns of bands are conventionally indicated by number from the suture down to the umbilicus. Thus, 12345 represents the full five-banded condition, while 00345 indicates that the two uppermost bands are missing. A colon (as in 00:45) indicates the reduction of a band to an indistinct trace. The known genetic variations affect the color of the shell, the color of the dermal pigment, and the development, color, and modification of the bands. The loci and alleles determining these characters are summarized in Table 2.

The *C, B, I, S,* and *P* loci are associated in one tight linkage group. The resulting "supergene" provides a mechanism whereby natural selection can maintain the linkage disequilibrium often observed in natural populations, i.e., with coupling or repulsion chromosomes present in greater than expected proportions. There is some evidence that recombination frequencies may vary in different lines (Fisher and Diver, 1934; Lamotte, 1954; Cain *et al.,* 1960; Cook and King, 1966; Cook, 1969). The *U, T,* and *R* loci, although unlinked to the supergene, are

TABLE 2. *Loci and Alleles of C. nemoralis*

	Locus		Alleles[a]		References
	C	Ground color of shell	C^B	Brown	Lang (1904, 1908),
			C^{DP}	Dark pink	Stelfox (1918),
			C^{PP}	Pale pink	Lamotte (1951,
			C^{FP}	Faint pink	1954), Cain and
			C^{DY}	Dark yellow	Sheppard (1957),
			C^{PY}	Pale yellow	Cain *et al.* (1960, 1968)
	B	Presence or absence of bands	B^O	Unbanded	Lang (1904, 1908),
			B^B	Banded	Darbishire (1905),
					Lamotte (1951,
					1954), Cain and
					Sheppard (1957)
linked	I	Punctate bands	I^I	Punctate	Lang (1908, 1912),
			I^-	Unmodified	Stelfox (1918),
					Lamotte (1951),
					Cook (1967), Cain *et al.* (1968)
	S	Spreading of band pigment	S^S	Spread bands	Cain *et al.* (1960, 1968)
			S^-	Unmodified	
	P	Pigmentation of bands and lip	P^N	Normal (dark brown) bands and lip	Lang (1904, 1908, 1911), Stelfox
			P^L	Light brown bands and lip[b]	(1918), Lamotte (1951), Murray
			P^A	White lip and normal bands (albolabiate)[b]	(1963), Cook (1967), Cain *et al.* (1968)
			P^T	White lip and transparent bands (hyalozonate)	
	U	Suppression of bands 1, 2, 4, and 5	U^3	Mid-banded (00300)	Lang (1912), Lamotte (1951, 1954), Cain
			U^-	Unmodified	and Sheppard (1957)
	T	Suppression of bands 1 and 2	T^{345}	Bands 1 and 2 suppressed (00345)	Lamotte (1954), Cook (1967)
			T^-	Unmodified	
	D	Dermal pigmentation	D^R	Reddish dermal pigment	Murray (1963), Wolda (1969)
			D^G	Gray dermal pigment	
	Q	Quantity of dermal pigment	Q^M	Medium gray	Cain *et al.* (1968),
			Q^P	Very pale (yellowish)	Wolda (1969)

TABLE 2. *Continued*

Locus		Alleles[a]		References
R	Darkening bands	R^-	Unmodified	Cain *et al.* (1960), Cook
		R^D	Bands gradually darken from apex to lip	(1969)
O	Orange bands	O^-	Unmodified	Cain *et al.* (1960, 1968)
		O^O	Orange bands and lip	

[a] Alleles are listed in order of decreasing dominance.
[b] The dominance relationships of P^L and P^A have not yet been established.

nevertheless associated with its expression, since B^O is epistatic to R, U, and T, and U^3 is epistatic to T. Finally, P^T is epistatic to some alleles at the C locus (Murray, 1963; Cain *et al.*, 1968).

A number of other segregating types are known, which may be assignable to these loci. Yellow-white, pale brown, and faint brown are probably determined by alleles at the C locus (Cain *et al.*, 1968). The 00:45 banding pattern is dominant to 00345 and may be an allele at the T locus (Cook, 1967). Yellow and red body color segregate, with yellow dominant, but it is not clear whether these types are controlled at the D locus (Wolda, 1969).

Still other conditions appear to be under multifactorial control. The width of bands varies such that at one extreme, banded shells may be indistinguishable from the phenotype determined by the B^O allele (Cain *et al.*, 1968; Wolda, 1969); and at the other, extra, or satellite, bands may appear on phenotypes such as 00300 (Cook, 1967; Wolda, 1969). The fusion of adjacent bands (Cain *et al.*, 1960; Wolda, 1969) and shell size are also under polygenic control. Cook (1967) has estimated the heritability of size to be about 60 percent.

Variation in a number of enzymes and other proteins has been demonstrated by electrophoresis in *C. nemoralis* (Manwell and Baker, 1968; Levan and Fredga, 1972; Oxford, 1971, 1973*a,b,c*; Brussard and McCracken, 1974). By analogy with other organisms, it may be assumed that the variation is genetic, although the work of Oxford (1973*a,b*) has shown how difficult it is to draw direct conclusions in the absence of a thorough genetic and physiological study. He has shown three different patterns of inheritance for different groups of esterase bands. The first is a series of bands produced by a locus with five alleles. Since as many as five heavily staining bands may appear in a single individual, Oxford originally interpreted this as the expression of a compound locus resulting from a

TABLE 3. Loci and Alleles of C. hortensis

	Locus		Alleles[a]	References
C	Ground color of shell	C^B	Brown	Lang (1904, 1908),
		C^P	Pink	Murray (1963), Cook
		C^{DY}	Dark yellow	and Murray (1966),
		C^{PY}	Pale yellow	Guerrucci (1971)
B	Presence or absence of bands	B^O	Unbanded	Lang (1904, 1906,
		B^B	Banded	1908), Murray (1963), Guerrucci (1971)
P	Pigmentation of bands	P^N	Normal (dark brown) bands	Boettger (1950), Murray (1963), Cook
		P^L	Light brown bands (lurida)	and Murray (1966)
		P^T	Transparent bands (hyalozonate)	
I	Punctate bands	I^I	Punctate bands	Guerrucci (1971)
		I^-	Unmodified	

linked (bracket spanning C, B, P, I)

[a] Alleles are listed in order of decreasing dominance.

process of duplication. He has now shown, however, that phenocopies can be induced by changes in the diet of the snails, only two alleles being present in any one individual (G. S. Oxford, personal communication). The second pattern is the expression of a classic dimeric enzyme with three alleles at a single locus and triple-banded heterozygotes. The third pattern, originally thought to result from the presence or absence of activity at a single locus, has now been shown to display two active alleles, with no intermediate band in the heterozygote (G. S. Oxford, personal communication). Oxford (1973c) has emphasized that these enzymes in Cepaea are rather different in their physical and chemical properties from the esterases commonly found in vertebrates. Brussard and McCracken (1974) have also performed breeding experiments to show that two variable loci controlling leucine aminopeptidase (LAP II) and phosphoglucomutase (PGM II) display simple Mendelian inheritance, with three and two alleles, respectively.

The cytogenetics of C. nemoralis has recently been clarified by Bantock (1972), who has obtained unusually good preparations of chromosomes. There is a single very large pair, an intermediate pair, and twenty small pairs. Usually each chromosome shows only a single, localized chiasma, although the large pair may have up to four. Variation from population to population in the chiasma frequency in the large pair (Price, 1974) leads to the interesting speculation that this pair may contain the elements of the supergene controlling the visible polymorphism.

Cepaea hortensis

The principal interest in the polymorphism of *C. hortensis* is in the remarkable degree to which it parallels that of *C. nemoralis*. All the known loci of the visible polymorphism in the former (see Table 3) are found in the latter, and all show similar linkage relationships. In addition, homologies may be detected in two of the groups of polymorphic esterases (Oxford, 1973*b*). Indeed, it appears that these homologies extend to the other two species of the genus, *C. sylvatica* and *C. vindobonensis* (Oxford, 1971). An apparent exception was the orange-banded condition in *C. nemoralis* which is phenotypically similar to, but genotypically different from, the *lurida* form in *C. hortensis*. The predicted discovery of the P^L allele in *C. nemoralis* restores the homology (Cook and Murray, 1966; Cook, 1967). Fusion of bands is multifactorially controlled in *C. hortensis* as in *C. nemoralis* (Lang, 1904; Murray, 1963).

    C. hortensis and *C. nemoralis* can be crossed with great difficulty in the laboratory. Lang (1904, 1906, 1908) succeeded in producing some hybrids and showed that segregation and dominance were quite regular with respect to shell color, lip color, and banding pattern. The form of the love dart, the mucous glands, and the shape of the shell were intermediate. Manwell and Baker (1968) have interpreted similarities in the electrophoretic patterns of enzyme variation as evidence for hybridization in nature, but this aspect of the problem requires further study.

Arianta arbustorum

The genetic system of *Arianta arbustorum* (see Table 4) shows some similarities to that of *Cepaea* (Cook and King, 1966). Two of the principal components are closely linked loci determining the color of the shell and the presence or absence of banding, although in the latter case the dominance is reversed and only a single, centrally placed band is developed. Other loci are less easy to relate. In general, *Arianta* is more cryptically colored than *Cepaea*, particularly as a result of the gene for mottling and of the reduced penetrance and expressivity of banding. The gene for transparent bands is probably not homologous with P^T in *Cepaea*. There is a segregation for pale banding *versus* dark banding, which may be another allele at the *B* locus (Cook and King, 1966). An esterase polymorphism has been described by Levan and Fredga (1972).

TABLE 4. *Loci and Alleles of Arianta arbustorum*

		Locus		Alleles[a]	References
linked	C	Ground color of shell	C^D	Brown (dark pigment)	Oldham (1934), Cook and King (1966)
			C^P	Yellow (pale, albino)	
	B	Presence or absence of a central band	B^B	Banded	Cook and King (1966)
			B^-	Unbanded	
	F	Mottling	F^F	Mottled shell	Oldham (1934), Cook and King (1966)
			F^-	Clear shell	
	T	Transparent band	T^-	Nontransparent	Cook and King (1966)
			T^T	Transparent band	
	W	White opaque stripe	W^W	White opaque stripe	Cook and King (1966)
			W^-	Unbanded	

[a] Alleles are listed in order of decreasing dominance.

Components of shell size and shape are multifactorially controlled, with a heritability of about 60 percent (Cook, 1965).

Other Species

Helix aspersa also displays a more restricted range of phenotypes than *Cepaea*. It shares with *Arianta* the crypsis resulting from heavy mottling. A suggestion of the color polymorphism of *Cepaea* remains, however, in the very young individuals, which may be either reddish brown or yellowish brown (Cain, 1971). Cain has shown that this difference depends on a single pair of alleles, with red dominant to yellow. At least one recessive gene (*exalbida* = albino shell and bands) affects both the color of the shell and the pigmentation of the bands (Stelfox, 1915, 1918; Cook, 1969). Cook suggests that by analogy with *Cepaea* this locus may represent two closely linked loci normally found in linkage disequilibrium in natural populations. Another segregation of a recessive, pale-banded condition may represent an additional allele at the *exalbida* locus. Two other loci control the reduction of the five-banded pattern (12345) to the formula 10005 and the delayed pigmentation of the bands *versus* normal pigmentation (Cook, 1969). By means of selection, Stelfox (1968) has shown that differences in shell shape are heritable. Enzyme polymorphisms have been described by Selander and Kaufman (1973*a,b*).

Cochlicella acuta, an elongate helicid, is polymorphic for at least three loci controlling the color and banding of the shell. Lewis (1968) has interpreted the banding as basically pentataeniate as in *Cepaea.* He has shown that the unbanded condition is recessive to 00040 and to the five-banded with all bands fused [indicated as (12345)]. 00040 is recessive to 00340, to (123)(45), and to (12345). It seems likely that these forms represent an allelic series, although the breeding results are not yet conclusive. Discontinuously opaque ostracum (DO) is dominant to continuously opaque ostracum (CO), and amber shell color segregates with colorless shell. Taken together with studies of chromosome frequencies in natural populations, the breeding experiments establish that the loci controlling the principal elements of the polymorphism, i.e., shell color, condition of the ostracum, and type of banding, are tightly linked and function as a supergene (Lewis, 1968).

In both *Monacha cantiana* (Cain, 1971) and *Hygromia striolata* (Cain, 1959a,b) there is segregation for dark and light coloration of the mantle. Cain has suggested in *Monacha* that dark is dominant to light and has shown that mantle color is independent of body color and shell color. Mantle and body color are correlated in *Hygromia,* although the color of the shell is independent.

Asymmetry in Gastropods

Snails, which typically display asymmetrical coiling of the shell and viscera, may be classed as either dextral or sinistral. If the shell is held with the apex upward and the aperture facing the observer, a dextral shell will have the aperture on the right and a sinistral shell will have it on the left. Most species of snails are dextral, but many species and even whole genera (e.g., *Physa*) are sinistral.

It is not uncommon for species that are regularly dextral to produce occasional sinistral individuals and *vice versa.* More rarely, some species are truly amphidromic, producing both dextrals and sinistrals in the same population (e.g., *Partula suturalis*). Usually snails of opposite coil show true mirror-image reversal of the internal organs, but in some cases the shell may be dextral and the soft parts sinistral (e.g., *Planorbis*).

The genetics of coiling was first worked out by Diver and his colleagues in *Lymnaea peregra* (Boycott and Diver, 1923; Diver *et al.,* 1925; Boycott *et al.,* 1930; Diver and Andersson-Kottö, 1938). *L. peregra* is normally dextral, with some populations containing a small proportion of sinistrals. Diver and his co-workers showed that there is a major locus controlling the direction of coiling, with the allele for dextrality (*R*)

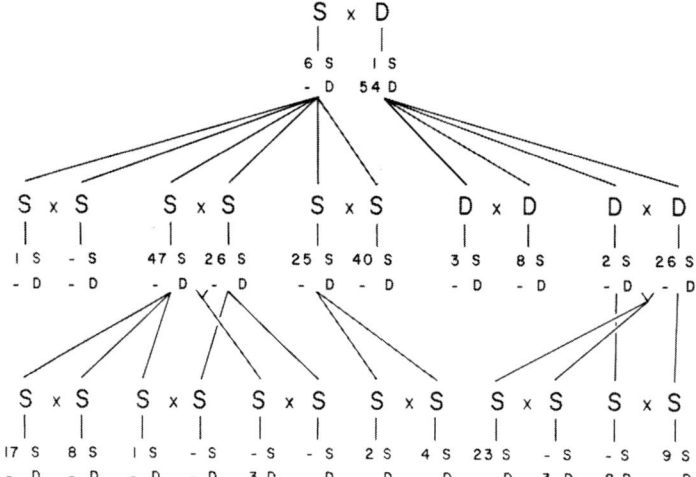

Figure 1. The inheritance of the direction of coiling of the shell in Partula
suturalis. S and D indicate the phenotypes of sinistral and dextral individuals. Lines indicate the parentage of individuals used for breeding. In
three cases in the third generation, individuals used as parents were born
prior to the separation of their parents and, therefore, can only be
assigned to the pair. A fork at the origin of the line indicating parentage
expresses this uncertainty.

dominant to that for sinistrality (r). The trait shows a delayed Mendelian
segregation, since the phenotype of a snail is determined by the genotype
of the maternal parent. Thus, the genetic constitutions of the parents are
displayed in the F_1, dominance is indicated by the phenotypes in the F_2,
and segregation occurs by whole broods in the F_3 (Sturtevant, 1923).

In *L. peregra* a number of other genes are capable of modifying the
sinistral ($r\,r$) type so that mixed broods of sinistral and dextral young are
produced. Both sinistral and dextral types continue to produce mixed
broods of similar compositions. Pure lines may be extracted, giving different proportions of modified young, high proportions being associated
with lowered viability. Dextral lineages also produce sporadic sinistrals,
but these seem to be genetically sinistral (Diver and Andersson-Köttö,
1938). The inheritance of one other character in *L. peregra* has been
studied by Boycott and Diver (1927); albino body is inherited as a simple
Mendelian recessive. Similar results have been obtained with coiling and
color in another species of "*Limnaea*" from Hawaii by Crampton
(1932*b*), although the data have not been published.

The inheritance of coiling in *Partula suturalis* is similar but more
regular (Murray and Clarke, 1966, 1969). Since self-fertilization is less

common and crosses of dextral and sinistral individuals are more easily obtained, direct analysis of delayed segregation is facilitated. Figure 1 shows a typical lineage involving a cross between homozygous dextral and sinistral animals. The dominance of sinistrality is seen in the F_2 and segregation in F_3. Usually all offspring of any individual show one type of coil, but sporadic individuals of opposite coil are produced.

Among the Helicidae there seems to be no good evidence for the genetic determination of the rare cases of sinistrality. Bantock *et al.* (1973) record a mating of two sinistral individuals of *C. hortensis* which produced all dextral offspring (64), but in view of the delayed segregation expected in this case the observation is inconclusive. Bantock *et al.*, however, cite a report by Jeffries (1860) of a 100-percent sinistral race of *Helix aspersa.*

Polymorphism in Other Gastropods

A number of other examples of genetic polymorphism have been investigated in gastropods. The available data vary from anecdotal accounts to reasonably systematic studies.

Because of the difficulty of rearing forms with pelagic larvae, very little work has been done on marine gastropods. Struhsaker (1968) has made a beginning with *Littorina picta.* She has managed to rear larvae derived from smooth and sculptured forms of this species. The extreme forms produce all smooth and all sculptured offspring, respectively, while intermediates produce very variable young. The inference is, therefore, that shell form is multifactorially determined. *Littorina mariae* and *L. obtusata,* which have no pelagic larvae, have recently been successfully bred by Reimchen (1974). He has shown that in *L. mariae* the two principal color morphs, reticulata and citrina, segregate in crosses. The most likely interpretation of the data is that two loci are involved with reticulata determined by the joint occurrence of dominant alleles at both. In *L. obtusata* he has shown segregation of three forms, reticulata, olivacea, and citrina. In *Purpura* (= *Thais*) *lamellosa,* Spight (1972) has shown that the patterns of shell color and banding are genetically controlled.

The remaining studies embrace forms from a number of different families of the Stylommatophora: Partulidae, Achatinidae, Bulimulidae, Philomycidae, Arionidae, and Fructicicolidae.

Two species of *Partula* have been bred by Murray and Clarke (1966, and unpublished). In *P. taeniata,* several shell colors show Mendelian segregation. Brownish purple, light brown, yellow, and white form an allelic series, with dominance descending in that order. Dominance is incomplete in that homozygotes of the alleles for the darker colors are darker than heterozygotes with yellow or white. Pink shell is also dominant to yellow and white but is probably at a different locus. The reflected lip of the shell is usually white, but a single, dominant gene alters the color to pink. Another dominant converts the extreme apex of the shell to dark purple. Three types of banding patterns (frenata, zonata, and lyra, in the terminology of Crampton, 1932a) segregate with the unbanded condition. All are dominant to unbanded and segregate among themselves. The lyra pattern may also be formed by the joint presence of zonata and frenata in the same animal, suggesting that the lyra "allele" is composed of coupled dominants at the two closely linked loci. Indeed, shell color, lip color, spire color, and banding pattern are all so closely linked as to constitute a supergene.

In *P. suturalis,* Murray and Clarke (1966) have shown segregation for Crampton's (1932a) patterns, frenata, bisecta, atra, cestata, strigata, and apex. The indications are that all these patterns are under the control of a single, complex locus or supergene. In some populations, *P. suturalis* is amphidromic (for the genetics of coiling, see above). In both species of *Partula,* components of shell size show high heritability (Murray and Clarke, 1968).

From among the Achatinidae, Barker (1968) has investigated two species of *Limicolaria.* In both *L. flammulata* and *L. aurora,* streaked (U) is dominant to unstreaked (u) shell, and gray (g) is recessive to pink (G^P) in *L. aurora* and to brown (G^B) in *L. flammulata.* The U and G loci are tightly linked with deficiencies of the coupling chromosomes noted by Barker (1968). There may be another locus affecting the depth of pigmentation of the streaks. Owen (1969) has noted a similar polymorphism in *L. martensiana.* In another achatinid, Selander and Kaufman (1973b) have described genetic variation in a number of enzymes. Among European and North African populations, 16 of 25 enzyme loci are variable in *Rumina decollata.* Populations of this species introduced into North America are, however, apparently invariant at all of these loci from South Carolina to California.

The extravagant polymorphism in the bulimulid *Liguus fasciatus* has aroused great interest among shell collectors, but very little is known of the genetics of this species. Pilsbry (1912, 1946) recorded a single brood of eight offspring showing segregation for pink *versus* white spire (4 : 4) and unbanded *versus* banded (6 : 2). Presumably the difficulty in rearing these snails has deterred further work.

Ikeda (1937) has used the genetics of *Philomycus bilineatus* to show that uniparental reproduction in this species is by self-fertilization and not parthenogenesis. Individuals heterozygous for a dominant gene producing three longitudinal black stripes on the mantle give rise to true-breeding striped (A A), heterozygous striped (A a), and true-breeding unstriped (a a) offspring in Mendelian proportions.

Two species of the Arionidae have been investigated. Abeloos (1944, 1945) has described a color polymorphism in *Arion hortensis* depending on three alleles at a single locus. The normal gray-blue (C^B) is dominant to pink (C^r), which is in turn dominant to white (C^O). The genetics of color in *A. ater* is more complex. Williamson (1959) has identified three loci controlling the type of pigment and its location. One determines the kind of melanin, with black (M) dominant to brown (m). A second locus affects the development of lateral longitudinal bands, the presence of bands (U) being dominant to their absence (u). A third locus, with three alleles, determines the extent of the dorsal pigmentation. Full color (F) is dominant to streaked (f^s), which is dominant to white (f). The white condition is epistatic to the U locus since pigment is found only in the tentacles or foot fringe. In addition, full-color individuals can only be scored for banding as juveniles since in adults the pigment spreads uniformly over the whole animal. The F and U loci are very tightly linked; no crossovers occurred in 474 offspring. The M locus segregates independently.

Finally, the polymorphism of *Bradybaena similaris* has been studied by Komai and Emura (1955). There are two principal loci: brown (C^B) is dominant to yellow (C), and banded (S^t) is dominant to unbanded (S). The two loci are closely linked, so closely that absolute linkage disequilibrium is possible. The C^B S^t chromosome has not been found.

Thus, one can observe certain regularities in the polymorphisms of land snails. In general, there is at least one locus with several alleles for different colors, and there is another locus controlling the presence or absence of stripes or bands. These loci are usually tightly linked to form supergenes capable of maintaining linkage disequilibrium. It seems that the better known the genetics of any gastropod becomes, the more complex the supergene polymorphism is found to be.

Genetics of the Pelecypoda

The economic importance of certain species of oysters and clams has stimulated a beginning on genetic studies of bivalves, despite the formidable technical problems involved (Chanley, 1961; Imai and Sakai, 1961; Longwell and Stiles, 1970; Menzel, 1972). Most of the work has combined cytogenetics (for references, see below) and the methods of quantitative genetics.

The American oyster, *Crassostrea virginica,* shows all the characteristics of a highly outbred species (Longwell and Stiles, 1970, 1973). Full-sib crosses fail completely, with reduced fertilization (40 percent *vs.* 87 percent in controls), abnormal cleavage (97 percent *vs.* 30 percent in controls), and no larval setting. Polyspermy and parthenogenesis are increased. Since gamma irradiation reduces these effects, Longwell and Stiles (1973) suggest the existence of a system of incompatibility alleles similar to that found in many plants. The Pacific oyster, *C. gigas,* is less sensitive to inbreeding, as Imai and Sakai (1961) have been able to rear sib-mated lines for three generations.

Estimates of heritability of larval growth rates in *C. virginica* and *C. gigas* vary widely (Lannan, 1972; Longwell and Stiles, 1973) but suggest that these species possess sufficient additive genetic variance for commercial improvement by selection. On the other hand, Longwell and Stiles (1970) have detected nonadditive effects which should favor the development of hybrid commercial stocks. Parental stocks for producing hybrids would probably be obtained by intraspecific selection since most species crosses result in a high degree of developmental abnormality (Davis, 1950; Imai and Sakai, 1961). In contrast with these studies, however, Menzel (1968*b*, 1973) has reported normal development in crosses of several species of *Crassostrea* and normal meiosis in hybrids of *C. virginica* and *C. gigas* reared to adulthood. Interspecific hybrids between the clams *Mercenaria mercenaria* and *M. campechiensis* combine the desirable qualities of both species (Chestnut *et al.,* 1957; Haven and Andrews, 1957; Menzel, 1972), if indeed they are good species (Haven and Andrews, 1957; Menzel, 1968*b*).

The genetics of shell marking in *M. mercenaria* has been studied by Chanley (1961), who reared both F_2 and backcross progenies to show that white and brown clams differ at a single locus. The so-called *notata* "subspecies," with reddish brown zigzag lines, is the heterozygote. Chanley also showed, by means of selection experiments, that genetic variation in growth rate is quite marked in *Mercenaria.*

Genetic variation in the electrophoretic mobility of enzymes and other proteins has been described for a number of species of clams. Milkman and Beaty (1970) surveyed populations of *Mytilus edulis* and *Modiolus demissus* and detected three allozymes of leucine aminopeptidase (Lap) in each species. Different populations differed in gene frequencies, as did young and adults from single populations. Koehn and Mitton (1972) have shown that, although the Lap allozymes are different in the two species, they nevertheless vary in a parallel fashion from population to population. *Mercenaria mercenaria* and *Pecten irradians* also have a three-allele Lap system, while *Mya arenaria* has two Lap loci with three alleles each. Malate dehydrogenase (Mdh) is also polymorphic in *Mytilus* and *Modiolus* (Koehn and Mitton, 1972); and "tetrazolium" oxidase, in *Modiolus* (Koehn *et al.,* 1973). Mitton and Koehn (1973) have investigated the relationship between Lap and aminopeptidase (Ap) in *Mytilus edulis.* They have found consistent nonrandom associations of the various alleles, with changes in the degree of association with increasing age.

Gooch and Schopf (1972), Levinton (1973), and Ayala *et al.* (1973) have surveyed enzymes in bivalves to assess the effect of environmental variability on genetic variability. These studies have detected a wealth of genetic variation (e.g., 25 polymorphic loci out of 30 surveyed in *Tridacna maxima* by Ayala *et al.*), but the relation between the two does not appear to be a simple one.

Schaal and Anderson (1974) have begun an electrophoretic study of variation in the American oyster, *Crassostrea virginica.* They have reported 13 polymorphic loci out of a total of 31 coding for 25 enzyme systems.

One of the two hemoglobins in the arcid clam *Anadara trapezia* occurs in two allelic forms (Nicol and O'Gower, 1967). A cline in gene frequency is correlated with the effects of currents on the east coast of Australia (O'Gower and Nicol, 1968).

Cytogenetics

Reports of chromosome counts for a variety of molluscan species may be found in the literature, dating back as far as the nineteenth century. Many of the older accounts [for references, see Makino (1951)] are, however, of doubtful accuracy since they antedate the introduction of modern squash techniques. The recent and more reliable literature on molluscan cytogenetics has been well reviewed by Patterson (1969). Her work incorporates and extends earlier important reviews by Perrot (1938), Burch (1960a, 1965), Inaba (1961), Patterson (1967), and Menzel (1968a).

Chromosome numbers are known for at least some members of four molluscan classes. The range of reported numbers (see Table 5) is $n = 6$ for one species of the Amphineura, $n = 10–23$ for the Pelecypoda, $n = 28$ for two species of the Cephalopoda, and $n = 5–44$ (excluding polyploids) among the Gastropoda. There are as yet no reports for the class Scaphopoda. Only the class Gastropoda is anything like well surveyed.

TABLE 5.   Chromosome Numbers Known for the Orders of Molluscs

Group	Haploid number	References[a]
Class Amphineura		
Order Chitonida	6	Dolph and Humphrey (1970)
Class Gastropoda		
Subclass Prosobranchia		
Order Archaeogastropoda	9–21	
Order Mesogastropoda	7–60[b]	
Order Neogastropoda	13–36	
Subclass Opisthobranchia		
Order Cephalaspidea	17–18	
Order Anaspidea	17	
Order Sacoglossa	7–17	
Order Notaspidea	12	
Order Nudibranchia	13	
Sublcass Pulmonata		
Order Basommatophora	15–72[b]	
Order Stylommatophora	5–44	
Class Bivalvia (Pelecypoda)		
Order Anisomyaria	10–14	Ahmed and Sparks (1970)
Order Heterodonta	12–23	
Order Adapedonta	17	
Class Cephalopoda		
Order Octopoda	28	

[a] After Patterson (1969) with additions as indicated.
[b] Counts including species believed to be polyploid.

Those groups of molluscs which are well enough known to warrant a generalization show a remarkable degree of conservatism. For example, 44 species of nudibranchs, representing 16 different families, all have a haploid number $n = 13$ (Patterson, 1969). With only a few exceptions, change of chromosome number appears to have taken place by means of the addition or subtraction of single pairs (Husted and Burch, 1946; Burch, 1965). Families rarely vary more than ± 2 bivalents from the basic number of the group.

Although favorable preconditions exist, such as extensive hermaphroditism and even occasional parthenogenesis (Boycott, 1919; Rhein, 1935; Mattox, 1937; Jacob, 1954; van der Schalie, 1965), polyploidy seems to be rather rare. Apart from sporadic polyploid individuals (Natarajan and Burch, 1966), polyploid species have been detected in four families of gastropods: Hydrobiidae (Rhein, 1935; Sanderson, 1940), Melaniidae (Jacob, 1954), Ancylidae (Burch et al., 1960; Burch, 1967a), and in two different subfamilies of the Planorbidae (Burch, 1960c,d, 1965, 1967a,b) including the medically important *Bulinus* discussed below. In every case polyploidy is expressed at the lower taxonomic levels and does not appear to have contributed to the evolution of higher categories.

Burch (1965) has remarked on the general tendency among the gastropods for the more specialized (evolutionarily advanced?) species to have higher chromosome numbers. This regularity argues against the popular theory that freshwater pulmonates (Basommatophora), which have a modal number $n = 18$, are derived from land pulmonates (Stylommatophora), which tend to have higher numbers. There are some notable exceptions, however, since *Catinella rotundata* among the Succineidae has the lowest number ($n = 5$) recorded for any mollusc (Burch, 1964).

The interpretation of chromosome numbers as an indicator of evolutionary status must be viewed with caution. Burch (1965) has pointed out that *Achatinella,* considered by Pilsbry (1900) to be among the most primitive of the Stylommatophora, also has the low chromosome number of $n = 20$. On the other hand, *Partula,* placed in an equivalent position by Pilsbry, has $n = 29$ (Scvortzoff, 1966), higher than most of the supposedly advanced Helicidae. Butot and Kiauta (Butot and Kiauta, 1969; Kiauta and Butot, 1969) have also suggested that there have been evolutionary trends toward lower numbers in the Helicidae and the Zonitidae.

When cytological details can be discerned, the chromosomes of molluscs are seen to be elongate with median, submedian, or terminal centromeres (Burch, 1960a). There has been disagreement over the occurrence and extent of chromosomal sex determination in molluscs with separate sexes (Jacob, 1959b; Nishikawa, 1962). Nevertheless, XY or XO mechanisms have been described for species from the Hydrobiidae (Burch, 1960b; Patterson, 1963), the Viviparidae (Patterson, 1965), and the Melaniidae (Jacob, 1959a,b). The sex chromosomes may be heterochromatic (Jacob, 1959b).

Supernumerary chromosomes have been noted in a number of species [see Patterson (1969) for references]. Evans (1960) has described a particularly notable example in *Helix pomatia* in which up to six additional chromosomes are present. They are smaller than the normal chromosomes but behave regularly during meiosis.

Finally, a most unusual example of intraspecific variation in chromosome number has been described in *Purpura* (= *Thais*) *lapillus* by Staiger (1954, 1955). On the coast of Brittany this muricid snail is represented by two "races," with $n = 13$ and $n = 18$. The 13-chromosome race has 8 acrocentrics and 5 metacentrics, whereas the 18-chromosome race has only acrocentrics. Studies of pairing in intermediate populations show that each of the metacentrics is represented by 2 acrocentrics in the other race. About 1 percent of the animals are heterozygous for translocations, usually involving the metacentrics, so that multivalents are formed at meiosis. The differences in chromosome structure are correlated with the habitats of the populations. The 13-chromosome race inhabits rocky coasts with heavy surf while the 18-chromosome race is found in sheltered bays. Only the 13-chromosome race has been reported in North America.

Genetics of Vectors of Schistosomiasis

The most pressing practical problems in molluscan genetics are to be found in the study of the vectors of schistosomiasis. The solution of the grave public health problems posed by this group of diseases may perhaps be found in the understanding and manipulation of the genetics of the vector species. These are *Biomphalaria* (= *Australorbis*) *glabrata* for *Schistosoma mansoni*, *Bulinus* spp. for *Schistosoma haematobium*, and *Oncomelania hupensis* ssp. for *Schistosoma japonicum*. *Biomphalaria* and *Bulinus* belong to the family Planorbidae while *Oncomelania* is in the Hydrobiidae.

A number of genetic markers are available for the study of *Biomphalaria glabrata*. The recessive gene for albinism (*c*) characterized by Newton (1954) has been used to demonstrate the precedence of cross-fertilization over self-fertilization (Newton, 1953; Paraense, 1955), to test for reproductive isolation between putative species (Paraense and Deslandes, 1955; Barbosa *et al.*, 1956), to test the genetic compatibility of allopatric populations within species (Paraense, 1956, 1959; Richards, 1962), and to investigate susceptibility to *Schistosoma mansoni* (Newton, 1955; Richards, 1970). Richards (1967) has described another allele at this locus, blackeye (c^b), which has dark eyes but no collar or body pigment and which may be used in crosses ($C\,c \times c^b\,c$) to determine that reciprocal cross-fertilization has occurred. Pearl formation, antler tentacles, and everted preputium (with swollen tentacles) are inherited as simple recessives (Richards, 1970, 1972, 1973*c*).

By means of selection and transfer from strain to strain, a number of other characters in *Biomphalaria* have been shown to be inherited, although most are variable in penetrance and expressivity. They include presence of "apertural lamellae" associated with a tendency to aestivation (Richards, 1968), tentacle and eye malformations (Richards, 1969*a*), mantle pigmentation (Richards, 1969*b*), and pulmonary occlusion, head bulb, scalariform shell, polyembryony, and hemolymph pigmentation (Richards, 1970, 1971). Mantle pigmentation may be selected in strains to the point where it will segregate for at least one generation, with spotted dominant to unspotted. Head bulb and scalariform shell are sublethal.

The series of body-color alleles at the *C* locus in *B. glabrata* is also found in *B. straminea*. The latter species may be selected for mantle spotting as well, even the albinos sometimes showing this trait, a condition not found so far in *B. glabrata* (Richards, 1973*b*).

The susceptibility of *B. glabrata* to *S. mansoni* infection varies with age and strain. Juvenile susceptibility is multifactorially controlled (Newton, 1953; Richards, 1970; Richards and Merritt, 1972). Snails which are susceptible as juveniles may be either susceptible or resistant as adults, depending on a single locus, with resistance being dominant (Richards, 1970, 1973*a*).

Similar work has been begun by Davis and Ruff (1973) with *Oncomelania hupensis*. In crosses between geographical subspecies, body pigmentation and shell ornamentation are determined by two unlinked loci, with pigmented body dominant to albino and ribbed shell dominant to smooth. Susceptibility to *S. japonicum* seems to be multifactorially controlled [Davis and Ruff (1973); but see Chi *et al.* (1971)].

In *Bulinus,* the problem of susceptibility to *S. haematobium* is complicated by the confused and difficult taxonomy of the group. Many of the species are virtually impossible to identify by means of gross morphology. Burch (Burch, 1960*d*, 1967*b*; Burch and Lindsay, 1970) has begun to unravel the tangle by showing that populations with similar morphological characters may have different chromosome numbers, forming a polyploid series ($2n = 36$, $4n = 72$, $6n = 108$, $8n = 144$). Diploid species (*tropicus* species group) are resistant to infection, although in at least one instance an experimental infection has been achieved (Lo *et al.*, 1970). On the other hand, tetraploids (*truncatus* species group) are regularly susceptible, as is an octoploid species from Ethiopia (Lo, 1972). At least one genetic marker, a simple recessive gene for albinism, has been employed to follow the results of crosses between species (Wu, 1972, 1973).

A number of studies of the electrophoretic variation in the vectors of schistosomiasis have been undertaken (Wright *et al.*, 1966; Coles, 1969; Malek and File, 1971; Wium-Andersen, 1973), but the goal has usually been the identification of species in these difficult groups. Consequently genetic variation within species has generally been regarded only as a nuisance. Much more could be made of these characters as markers in genetic studies of these organisms.

The pioneering work that has been begun in the search for genetic answers to the problem of controlling schistosomiasis is being followed up actively in a number of laboratories around the world at the present time.

Acknowledgments

For their generous help in the preparation of this digest, I should like to thank Dr. J. B. Burch, Professor A. J. Cain, Professor B. C. Clarke, Dr. L. M. Cook, Dr. G. M. Davis, Dr. A. C. Longwell, and Dr. C. S. Richards. (Decisions on the inclusion and interpretation of material are, however, my own.)

Literature Cited

Abeloos, M., 1944 Allélomorphes multiples conditionnant la pigmentation et l'albinisme chez *Arion hortensis* de Fér. *C. R. Hebd. Séances Acad. Sci. Ser. D Sci. Nat.* **218**:884–885.

Abeloos, M., 1945 Sur la génétique de gastéropode *Arion hortensis* de Fér. *C. R. Séances Soc. Biol.* **139**:13–14.

Ahmed, M. and A. K. Sparks, 1970 Chromosome number, structure and autosomal polymorphism in the marine mussels *Mytilus edulis* and *Mytilus californianus*. *Biol. Bull.* **138**:1–13.

Ayala, F. J., D. Hedgecock, G. S. Zumwalt and J. W. Valentine, 1973 Genetic variation in *Tridacna maxima,* an ecological analog of some unsuccessful evolutionary lineages. *Evolution* **27**:177–191.

Bantock, C. R., 1972 Localisation of chiasmata in *Cepaea nemoralis* L. *Heredity* **29**:213–221.

Bantock, C. R., K. Noble and M. Ratsey, 1973 Sinistrality in *Cepaea hortensis*. *Heredity* **30**:397–398.

Barbosa, F. S., M. V. Coelho and E. Carneiro, 1956 Cross-breeding of *Australorbis glabratus* and *Biomphalaria boissyi*. *Trans. R. Soc. Trop. Med. Hyg.* **50**:296–297.

Barker, J. F., 1968 Polymorphism in West African snails. *Heredity* **23**:81–98.

Boettger, C. R., 1950 Analyse einer bemerkenswerten Population der Schnirkelschnecke *Cepaea hortensis* Müller. *Abh. Braunschw. Wiss. Ges.* **2**:1–12.

Boycott, A. E., 1919 Parthenogenesis in *Paludestrina jenkinsi*. *J. Conchol.* **16**:54.

Boycott, A. E. and C. Diver, 1923 On the inheritance of sinistrality in *Limnaea peregra*. *Proc. R. Soc. Lond. Ser. B Biol. Sci.* **95**:207–213.

Boycott, A. E. and C. Diver, 1927 The origin of an albino mutation in *Limnaea peregra*. *Nature (Lond.)* **119**:9.

Boycott, A. E., C. Diver, S. L. Garstang and F. M. Turner, 1930 The inheritance of sinistrality in *Limnaea peregra* (Mollusca, Pulmonata). *Philos. Trans. R. Soc. Lond. Ser. B Biol. Sci.* **219**:51–131.

Brussard, P. F. and G. F. McCracken, 1974 Allozymic variation in a North American colony of *Cepaea nemoralis*. *Heredity* **33**:98–101.

Burch, J. B., 1960a Chromosome studies of aquatic pulmonate snails. *Nucleus* **3**:177–208.

Burch, J. B., 1960b Chromosomes of *Pomatiopsis* and *Oncomelania*. *Am. Malacol. Union Annu. Rep. Bull.* 1959 **26**:15–16.

Burch, J. B., 1960c Chromosomes of *Gyraulus circumstriatus,* a freshwater snail. *Nature (Lond.)* **186**:497–498.

Burch, J. B., 1960*d* Chromosome numbers of schistosome vector snails. *Z. Tropenmed. Parasitol.* **11**:449–452.

Burch, J. B., 1964 Chromosomes of the succineid snail *Catinella rotundata*. *Occas. Pap. Mus. Zool. Univ. Mich.* **638**:1–8.

Burch, J. B., 1965 Chromosome numbers and systematics in euthyneuran snails. *Proc. First Europ. Malacol. Congr.* **1962**:215–241.

Burch, J. B., 1967*a* Cytological relationships of Pacific gastropods. *Venus, Jap. J. Malacol.* **25**:118–135.

Burch, J. B., 1967*b* Some species of the genus *Bulinus* in Ethiopia, possible intermediate hosts of schistosomiasis haematobia. *Ethiop. Med. J.* **5**:245–257.

Burch, J. B. and G. K. Lindsay, 1970 An immuno-cytological study of *Bulinus* s.s. (Basommatophora: Planorbidae). *Malacol. Rev.* **3**:1–18.

Burch, J. B., P. F. Basch and L. L. Bush, 1960 Chromosome numbers in ancylid snails. *Revta Port. Zool. Biol. Ger.* **2**:199–204.

Butot, L. J. M. and B. Kiauta, 1969 Cytotaxonomic observations in the stylommatophoran family Helicidae, with considerations on the affinities within the family. *Malacologia* **9**:261–262.

Cain, A. J., 1959*a* An undescribed polymorphism in *Hygromia striolata* (C. Pfeiffer). *J. Conchol.* **24**:319–322.

Cain, A. J., 1959*b* Inheritance of mantle colour in *Hygromia striolata*. *J. Conchol.* **24**:352–353.

Cain, A. J., 1971 Undescribed polymorphisms in two British snails. *J. Conchol.* **26**:410–416.

Cain, A. J. and J. D. Currey, 1963 Area effects in *Cepaea*. *Philos. Trans. R. Soc. Lond. Ser. B Biol. Sci.* **246**:1–81.

Cain, A. J. and P. M. Sheppard, 1950 Selection in the polymorphic land snail *Cepaea nemoralis*. *Heredity* **4**:275–294.

Cain, A. J. and P. M. Sheppard, 1954 Natural selection in *Cepaea*. *Genetics* **39**:89–116.

Cain, A. J. and P. M. Sheppard, 1957 Some breeding experiments with *Cepaea nemoralis* (L.). *J. Genet.* **55**:195–199.

Cain, A. J., J. M. B. King and P. M. Sheppard, 1960 New data on the genetics of polymorphism in the snail *Cepaea nemoralis* L. *Genetics* **45**:393–411.

Cain, A. J., P. M. Sheppard and J. M. B. King, 1968 The genetics of some morphs and varieties of *Cepaea nemoralis* (L.). *Philos. Trans. R. Soc. Lond. Ser. B Biol. Sci.* **253**:383–396.

Chanley, P. E., 1961 Inheritance of shell markings and growth in the hard clam, *Venus mercenaria*. *Proc. Natl. Shellfish. Assoc.* **50**:163–169.

Chestnut, A. F., W. E. Fahy and H. J. Porter, 1957 Growth of young *Venus mercenaria, Venus campechiensis,* and their hybrids. *Proc. Natl. Shellfish. Assoc.* **47**:50–56.

Chi, L. W., E. D. Wagner and N. Wold, 1971 Susceptibility of *Oncomelania* hybrid snails to various geographic strains of *Schistosoma japonicum*. *Am. J. Trop. Med. Hyg.* **20**:89–94.

Clarke, B., 1960 Divergent effects of natural selection on two closely-related polymorphic snails. *Heredity* **14**:423–443.

Coles, G. C., 1969 Isoenzymes of snail livers. I. Hydrolysing enzymes and peroxidases. *Comp. Biochem. Physiol.* **29**:403–411.

Cook, L. M., 1965 Inheritance of shell size in the snail *Arianta arbustorum*. *Evolution* **19**:86–94.

Cook, L. M., 1967 The genetics of *Cepaea nemoralis. Heredity* **22**:397–410.

Cook, L. M., 1969 Results of breeding experiments of Diver and Stelfox on *Helix aspersa. Proc. Malacol. Soc. Lond.* **38**:351–358.

Cook, L. M., 1970 Genetical studies on *Helix aspersa* and other helicid snails: A review of work by A. W. Stelfox. *Ir. Nat. J.* **16**:249–252.

Cook, L. M. and J. M. B. King, 1966 Some data on the genetics of shell-character polymorphism in the snail *Arianta arbustorum. Genetics* **53**:415–425.

Cook, L. M. and J. Murray, 1966 New information on the inheritance of polymorphic characters in *Cepaea hortensis. J. Hered.* **57**:245–247.

Crampton, H. E., 1932*a* Studies on the variation, distribution and evolution of the genus *Partula.* The species inhabiting Moorea. *Publ. Carnegie Instn.* **410**:1–335.

Crampton, H. E., 1932*b* The genetic direction of the inheritance of coil in a species of *Limnaea* from the Hawaiian Islands. *Proc. 6th Interntl. Congr. Genet.* **2**:238–239.

Darbishire, A. D., 1905 Professor Lang's breeding experiments with *Helix hortensis* and *H. nemoralis*; an abstract and review. *J. Conchol.* **11**:193–200.

Davis, G. M. and M. D. Ruff, 1973 *Oncomelania hupensis* (Gastropoda: Hydrobiidae). Hybridization, genetics and transmission of *Schistosoma japonicum. Malacol. Rev.* **6**:181–197.

Davis, H. C., 1950 On interspecific hybridization in *Ostrea. Science (Wash., D.C.)* **111**:522.

Diver, C., 1932 Mollusca genetics. *Proc. 6th Interntl. Congr. Genet.* **2**:236–238.

Diver, C. and I. Andersson-Kottö, 1938 Sinistrality in *Limnaea peregra* (Mollusca, Pulmonata): The problem of mixed broods. *J. Genet.* **35**:447–525.

Diver, C., A. E. Boycott and S. Garstang, 1925 The inheritance of inverse symmetry in *Limnaea peregra. J. Genet.* **15**:113–200.

Dolph, C. I. and D. G. Humphrey, 1970 Chromosomes of the chiton, *Katherina tunicata. Trans. Am. Microsc. Soc.* **89**:229–232.

Evans, H. J., 1960 Supernumerary chromosomes in wild populations of the snail *Helix pomatia* L. *Heredity* **15**:129–138.

Fisher, R. A. and C. Diver, 1934 Crossing-over in the land snail *Cepaea nemoralis,* L. *Nature (Lond.)* **133**:834.

Gooch, J. L. and T. J. M. Schopf, 1972 Genetic variability in the deep sea: Relation to environmental variability. *Evolution* **26**:545–552.

Goodhart, C., 1962 Variation in a colony of the snail *Cepaea nemoralis* (L.). *J. Anim. Ecol.* **31**:207–237.

Grassé, P.-P., editor, 1960 and 1968 *Traité de Zoologie,* Tome V, Fasc. 2 & 3, Masson & Cie., Paris.

Guerrucci, M.-A., 1971 Étude de la transmission de quelques caractères de la pigmentation chez *Cepaea hortensis. Archs. Zool. Exp. Gén.* **112**:211–219.

Haven, D. and J. D. Andrews, 1957 Survival and growth of *Venus mercenaria, Venus campechiensis,* and their hybrids in suspended trays and on natural bottoms. *Proc. Natl. Shellfish. Assoc.* **47**:43–49.

Husted, L. and P. R. Burch, 1946 The chromosomes of polygyrid snails. *Am. Nat.* **80**:410–429.

Ikeda, K., 1937 Cytogenetic studies on the self-fertilization of *Philomycus bilineatus* Benson. *J. Sci. Hiroshima Univ. Sct. B, Div. 1 (Zool.)* **5**:67–123.

Imai, T. and S. Sakai, 1961 Study of breeding of Japanese oyster, *Crassostrea gigas. Tohoku J. Agric. Res.* **12**:125–171.

Inaba, A., 1961   Cytotaxonomy of the euthyneuran gastropods. *Venus, Jap. J. Malacol.* **21**:402–413.

Jacob, J., 1954   Parthenogenesis and allopolyploidy in the melaniid snails (Gastropoda-Prosobranchia). *Curr. Sci. (Bangalore)* **23**:56–58.

Jacob, J., 1959*a*   The chromosomes of six melaniid snails (Gastropoda: Prosobranchia). *Cytologia (Tokyo)* **24**:487–497.

Jacob, J., 1959*b*   Sex chromosomes in melaniid snails. 1. *Paludomus tanschaurica* (Gmelin) (Prosobranchia: Gastropoda). *J. Zool. Soc. India* **11**:17–25.

Jeffries, J. G., 1860   On the origin of species. *Ann. Mag. Nat. Hist.* **IV**:152.

Kiauta, B. and I. J. M. Butot, 1969   Contribution to the knowledge of the cyto-taxonomic conditions in the stylommatophoran superfamily Zonitacea. *Malacologia* **9**:269–270.

Koehn, R. K. and J. B. Mitton, 1972   Population genetics of marine pelecypods. 1. Eco-logical heterogeneity and evolutionary strategy at an enzyme locus. *Am. Nat.* **106**:47–56.

Koehn, R. K., F. J. Turano and J. B. Mitton, 1973   Population genetics of marine pelecypods. II. Genetic differences in microhabitats of *Modiolus demissus. Evolution* **27**:100–105.

Komai, T. and S. Emura, 1955   A study of population genetics of the polymorphic land snail *Bradybaena similaris. Evolution* **9**:400–418.

Lamotte, M., 1951   Recherches sur la structure génétique des populations naturelles de *Cepaea nemoralis* (L.). *Bull. Biol. Fr. Belg. Suppl.* **35**:1–239.

Lamotte, M., 1954   Sur le déterminisme génétique du polymorphisme, chez *Cepaea nemoralis* L. *C. R. Hebd. Séances Acad. Sci. Ser. D Sci. Nat.* **239**:365–367.

Lamotte, M., 1959   Polymorphism of natural populations of *Cepaea nemoralis. Cold Spring Harbor Symp. Quant. Biol.* **24**:65–86.

Lang, A., 1904   Ueber Vorversuche zu Untersuchungen über die Varietätenbildung von *Helix hortensis* Müller und *Helix nemoralis* L. *Denkschr. Med.-Naturwiss. Ges. (Jena)* **11**:439–506.

Lang, A., 1906   Ueber die Mendelschen Gesetze, Art- und Varietätenbildung, Mutation und Variation, insbesondere bei unsern Hain- und Gartenschnecken. *Verh. Schweiz. Naturforsch. Ges.* **88**:209–254.

Lang, A., 1908   Ueber die Bastarde von *Helix hortensis* Müller und *Helix nemoralis* L. *Festschr. Univ. Jena*: 1–120.

Lang, A., 1911   Fortgesetzte Vererbungsstudien. *Z. Indukt. Abstammungs.-Vererbungsl.* **5**:97–138.

Lang, A., 1912   Vererbungswissenschaftliche Miszellen. *Z. Indukt. Abstammungs.-Vererbungsl.* **8**:233–283.

Lannan, J. E., 1972   Estimating heritability and predicting response to selection for the Pacific oyster, *Crassostrea gigas. Proc. Natl. Shellfish. Assoc.* **62**:62–66.

Levan, G. and K. Fredga, 1972   Isozyme polymorphism in three species of land snails near Lund, Sweden. *Hereditas* **71**:245–252.

Levinton, J., 1973   Genetic variation in a gradient of environmental variability: Marine Bivalvia (Mollusca). *Science (Wash., D.C.)* **180**:75–76.

Lewis, G., 1968   Polymorphism in the shell characters of certain helicid molluscs, particu-larly the genus *Cochlicella*. D. Phil. Thesis, Oxford University, Oxford, England.

Lo, C. T., 1972   Compatibility and host–parasite relationships between species of the genus *Bulinus* (Basommatophora: Planorbidae) and an Egyptian strain of *Schistosoma haematobium* (Trematoda: Digenea). *Malacologia* **11**:225–280.

Lo, C. T., J. B. Burch and C. H. J. Schutte, 1970   Infection of diploid *Bulinus* s.s. with *Schistosoma haematobium*. *Malacol. Rev.* **3**:121–126.

Longwell, A. C. and S. S. Stiles, 1970   The genetic system and breeding potential of the commercial American oyster. *Endeavour* **29**:94–99.

Longwell, A. C. and S. S. Stiles, 1973   Oyster genetics and the probable future role of genetics in aquaculture. *Malacol. Rev.* **6**:151–177.

Makino, S., 1951   *An Atlas of the Chromosome Numbers in Animals*, Iowa State College Press, Ames, Iowa.

Malek, E. A. and S. K. File, 1971   Electrophoretic studies on the digestive gland esterases of some biomphalarid and lymnaeid snails. *Bull. WHO* **45**:819–825.

Manwell, C. and C. M. A. Baker, 1968   Genetic variation of isocitrate, malate and 6-phosphogluconate dehydrogenases in snails of the genus *Cepaea*—Introgressive hybridization, polymorphism and pollution? *Comp. Biochem. Physiol.* **26**:195–209.

Mattox, N. T., 1937   Oogenesis of *Campeloma rufum*, a parthenogenetic snail. *Z. Zellforsch. Mikrosk. Anat.* **27**:455–464.

Menzel, R. W., 1968*a*   Chromosome numbers in nine families of marine pelecypod mollusks. *Nautilus* **82**:45–58.

Menzel, R. W., 1968*b*   Cytotaxonomy of species of clams (*Mercenaria*) and oysters (*Crassostrea*). *Proc. Symp. Mollusca Mar. Biol. Assoc. India* **1**:75–84.

Menzel, R. W., 1972   The role of genetics in molluscan mariculture. *Am. Malacol. Union Annu. Rep. Bull. 1971* **37**:13–15.

Menzel, R. W., 1973   Hybridization in oysters (*Crassostrea*). *Malacol. Rev.* **6**:179.

Milkman, R. and L. D. Beaty, 1970   Large-scale electrophoretic studies of allelic variation in *Mytilus edulis*. *Biol. Bull.* **139**:430.

Mitton, J. B. and R. K. Koehn, 1973   Population genetics of marine pelecypods. III. Epistasis between functionally related isoenzymes of *Mytilus edulis*. Appendix by T. Prout. *Genetics* **73**:487–496.

Morton, J. E., 1967   *Molluscs*, fourth (rev.) edition, Hutchinson, London.

Murray, J., 1963   The inheritance of some characters in *Cepaea hortensis* and *Cepaea nemoralis* (Gastropoda). *Genetics* **48**:605–615.

Murray, J., 1964   Multiple mating and effective population size in *Cepaea nemoralis*. *Evolution* **18**:283–291.

Murray, J. and B. Clarke, 1966   The inheritance of polymorphic shell characters in *Partula* (Gastropoda). *Genetics* **54**:1261–1277.

Murray, J. and B. Clarke, 1968   Inheritance of shell size in *Partula*. *Heredity* **23**:189–198.

Murray, J. and B. Clarke, 1969   The inheritance of sinistrality in *Partula suturalis* (Gastropoda, Stylommatophora). *ASB Bull.* **16**:61.

Natarajan, R. and J. B. Burch, 1966   Chromosomes of some Archaeopulmonata (Mollusca: Basommatophora). *Cytologia (Tokyo)* **31**:109–116.

Newton, W. L., 1953   The inheritance of susceptibility to infection with *Schistosoma mansoni* in *Australorbis glabratus*. *Exp. Parasitol.* **2**:242–257.

Newton, W. L., 1954   Albinism in *Australorbis glabratus*. *Proc. Helminthol. Soc. Wash.* **21**:72–74.

Newton, W. L., 1955   The establishment of a strain of *Australorbis glabratus* which combines albinism and high susceptibility to infection with *Schistosoma mansoni*. *J. Parasitol.* **41**:526–528.

Nicol, P. I. and A. K. O'Gower, 1967   Haemoglobin variation in *Anadara trapezia* (Deshayes). *Nature (Lond.)* **216**:684.

Nishikawa, S., 1962 A comparative study of the chromosomes in marine gastropods, with some remarks on cytotaxonomy and phylogeny. *J. Shimonoseki Coll. Fish.* **11**:539–576.

O'Gower, A. K. and P. I. Nicol, 1968 A latitudinal cline of haemoglobins in a bivalve mollusc. *Heredity* **23**:485–492.

Oldham, C., 1934 Some albinistic varieties of *Arianta arbustorum* (L.). *Proc. Malacol. Soc. Lond.* **21**:103–108.

Owen, D. F., 1969 Ecological aspects of polymorphism in an African land snail, *Limicolaria martensiana. J. Zool. (Lond.)* **159**:79–96.

Oxford, G. S. 1971 The properties, genetics and ecogenetics of esterases in *Cepaea* (Mollusca, Helicidae). Ph. D. Thesis, University of Liverpool, England.

Oxford, G. S., 1973*a* The genetics of *Cepaea* esterases. I. *Cepaea nemoralis. Heredity* **30**:127–139.

Oxford, G. S., 1973*b* Molecular weight relationships of the esterases in *Cepaea nemoralis* and *Cepaea hortensis* (Mollusca: Helicidae) and their implications. *Biochem. Genet.* **8**:365–382.

Oxford, G. S., 1973*c* The biochemical properties of esterases in *Cepaea* (Mollusca: Helicidae). *Comp. Biochem. Physiol.* **45B**:529–538.

Paraense, W. L., 1955 Self and cross-fertilization in *Australorbis glabratus. Mem. Inst. Oswaldo Cruz (Rio de J.)* **53**:285–291.

Paraense, W. L., 1956 A genetic approach to the systematics of planorbid molluscs. *Evolution* **10**:403–407.

Paraense, W. L., 1959 One-sided reproductive isolation between geographically remote populations of a planorbid snail. *Am. Nat.* **93**:93–101.

Paraense, W. L. and N. Deslandes, 1955 Reproductive isolation between *Australorbis glabratus* and *A. nigricans. Mem. Inst. Oswaldo Cruz (Rio de J.)* **53**:325–327.

Patterson, C. M., 1963 Cytological studies of *Pomatiopsis* snails. *Am. Malacol. Union Annu. Rep. Bull. 1963* **30**:13–14.

Patterson, C. M., 1965 The chromosomes of *Tulotoma angulata* (Streptoneura: Viviparidae). *Malacologia* **2**:259–265.

Patterson, C. M., 1967 Chromosome numbers and systematics in streptoneuran snails. *Malacologia* **5**:111–125.

Patterson, C. M., 1969 Chromosomes of molluscs. *Proc. Symp. Mollusca Mar. Biol. Assoc. India* **2**:635–686.

Perrot, M., 1938 Étude de cytologie comparée chez les gastéropodes pulmonés. *Revue Suisse Zool.* **45**:487–566.

Pilsbry, H. A., 1900 On the zoölogical position of *Partula* and *Achatinella. Proc. Acad. Nat. Sci. Philad.* **52**:561–567.

Pilsbry, H. A., 1912 A study of the variation and zoogeography of *Liguus* in Florida. *J. Acad. Nat. Sci. Philad. (2nd Ser.)* **15**:427–472.

Pilsbry, H. A., 1946 *Land Mollusca of North America (north of Mexico)*, Academy of Natural Sciences of Philadelphia, Philadelphia, Pa.

Price, D. J., 1974 Variation in chiasma frequency in *Cepaea nemoralis. Heredity* **32**:211–217.

Reimchen, T. E. 1974 Studies on the biology and colour polymorphism of two sibling species of marine gastropod (*Littorina*). Ph.D. Thesis, University of Liverpool, England.

Rhein, A., 1935 Diploide Parthenogenese bei *Hydrobia jenkinsi* Smith (Prosobranchia). *Naturwissenschaften* **23**:100.

Richards, C. S., 1962   Genetic crossing of pigmented Caribbean strains with an albino
     Venezuelan strain of *Australorbis glabratus*. *Am. J. Trop. Med. Hyg.* **11**:216–219.

Richards, C. S., 1967   Genetic studies on *Biomphalaria glabrata* (Basommatophora:
     Planorbidae), a third pigmentation allele. *Malacologia* **5**:335–340.

Richards, C. S., 1968   Aestivation of *Biomphalaria glabrata* (Basommatophora: Planor-
     bidae). Genetic studies. *Malacologia* **7**:109–116.

Richards, C. S., 1969*a*   Genetic studies on *Biomphalaria glabrata*: Tentacle and eye
     variations. *Malacologia* **9**:327–338.

Richards, C. S., 1969*b*   Genetic studies on *Biomphalaria glabrata*: Mantle pigmentation.
     Malacologia **9**:339–348.

Richards, C. S., 1970   Genetics of a molluscan vector of schistosomiasis. *Nature (Lond.)*
     227:806–810.

Richards, C. S., 1971   *Biomphalaria glabrata* genetics: Spire formation as a sublethal
     character. *J. Invertebr. Pathol.* **17**:53–58.

Richards, C. S., 1972   *Biomphalaria glabrata* genetics: Pearl formation. *J. Invertebr.
     Pathol.* **20**:37–40.

Richards, C. S., 1973*a*   Susceptibility of adult *Biomphalaria glabrata* to *Schistosoma
     mansoni* infection. *Am. J. Trop. Med. Hyg.* **22**:748–756.

Richards, C. S., 1973*b*   Pigmentation variations in *Biomphalaria glabrata* and other
     Planorbidae. *Malacol. Rev.* **6**:49–51.

Richards, C. S., 1973*c*   Genetics of *Biomphalaria glabrata* (Gastropoda: Planorbidae).
     Malacol. Rev. **6**:199–202.

Richards, C. S. and J. W. Merritt, Jr., 1972   Genetic factors in the susceptibility of ju-
     venile *Biomphalaria glabrata* to *Schistosoma mansoni* infection. *Am. J. Trop. Med.
     Hyg.* **21**:425–434.

Sanderson, A. R., 1940   Maturation in the parthenogenetic snail *Potamopyrgus jenkinsi*
     Smith, and in the snail *Peringia ulvae* (Pennant). *Proc. Zool. Soc. Lond. A*
     110:11–15.

Schaal, B. A. and W. W. Anderson, 1974   An outline of techniques for starch gel elec-
     trophoresis of enzymes from the American oyster *Crassostrea virginica* Gmelin.
     Georgia Marine Science Center Technical Report **74–3**:1–18.

Scvortzoff, E., 1966   Chromosome numbers of the land snails of the genus *Partula* that
     inhabit the island of Moorea. M. A. Thesis, University of Virginia, Charlottesville,
     Va.

Selander, R. K. and D. W. Kaufman, 1973*a*   Genic variability and strategies of adaptation
     in animals. *Proc. Natl. Acad. Sci. USA* **70**:1875–1877.

Selander, R. K. and D. W. Kaufman, 1973*b*   Self-fertilization and genetic population
     structure in a colonizing land snail. *Proc. Natl. Acad. Sci. USA* **70**:1186–1190.

Spight, T. M., 1972   Patterns of change in adjacent populations of an intertidal snail,
     Thais lamellosa. Ph. D. Thesis, University of Washington, Seattle, Wash.

Staiger, H., 1954   Der Chromosomendimorphismus beim Prosobranchier *Purpura
     lapillus* in Beziehung zur Ökologie der Art. *Chromosoma (Berl.)* **6**:419–478.

Staiger, H., 1955   Reziproke Translokationen in natürlichen Populationen von *Purpura
     lapillus* (Prosobranchia). *Chromosoma (Berl.)* **7**:181–197.

Stelfox, A. W., 1915   A cross between typical *Helix aspersa* and var. *exalbida*: Its results
     and lessons. *J. Conchol.* **14**:293–295.

Stelfox, A. W., 1918   Researches into the hereditary characters of some of our British
     Mollusca. Part II. *Helix aspersa* Müll. and *H. nemoralis* L. *J. Conchol.* **15**:268–275.

Stelfox, A. W., 1968   On the inheritance of scalariformity in *Helix aspersa. J. Conchol.* **26**:329–332.

Struhsaker, J. W., 1968   Selection mechanisms associated with intraspecific shell variation in *Littorina picta* (Prosobranchia: Mesogastropoda). *Evolution* **22**:459–480.

Sturtevant, A. H., 1923   Inheritance of direction of coiling in *Limnaea. Science (Wash., D.C.)* **58**:269–270.

Taylor, J. W., 1914   *Monograph of the Land and Freshwater Mollusca of the British Isles,* Taylor Brothers, Leeds, England.

Thiele, J., 1931–1935   *Handbuch der systematischer Weichtierkunde,* Gustav Fischer, Jena.

van der Schalie, H., 1965   Observations on the sex of *Campeloma* (Gastropoda: Viviparidae). *Occ. Pap. Mus. Zool. Univ. Mich.* **641**:1–15.

Williamson, M., 1959   Studies on the colour and genetics of the black slug. *Proc. R. Phys. Soc. Edinb.* **27**:87–93.

Wium-Andersen, G., 1973   Electrophoretic studies on esterases of some African *Biomphalaria* spp. (Planorbidae). *Malacologia* **12**:115–122.

Wright, C. A., S. K. File and G. C. Ross, 1966   Studies on the enzyme systems of planorbid snails. *Ann. Trop. Med. Parasitol.* **60**:522–525.

Wolda, H., 1969   Genetics of polymorphism in the land snail, *Cepaea nemoralis. Genetica (The Hague)* **40**:475–502.

Wu, S.-K., 1972   Breeding experiments in the *Bulinus tropicus/natalensis* complex. *Malacol. Rev.* **5**:13–14.

Wu, S.-K., 1973   Cross-breeding experiments with the African snail genus *Bulinus* (Gastropoda: Planorbidae). *Malacol. Rev.* **6**:203.

PART H
INSECTS OF
GENETIC INTEREST

2

The German Cockroach, *Blattella germanica*

Mary H. Ross and Donald G. Cochran

Introduction

There are approximately 4000 described species of cockroaches (Cornwell, 1968). The vast majority are creatures of the wild and have little or no contact with people. On a worldwide basis, about 30 species are of importance as pests noxious to man (Rehn, 1945). Of them, the German cockroach, *Blattella germanica* L., is probably the most important. It is believed to have originated in northeast Africa, from where it made early entry into Europe and Asia Minor. Subsequently, it was spread by man to virtually every corner of the earth. Its introduction into the New World is presumed to be from Europe rather than from Africa (Rehn, 1945).

Cockroaches have a life cycle consisting of egg, nymph, and adult. Groups of eggs are normally enclosed in a discrete ootheca. These egg capsules may be deposited, carried externally before deposition, or carried internally by the female. In the German cockroach, the egg case is carried externally until it is nearly ready to hatch. Nymphs are wingless and

Mary H. Ross and Donald G. Cochran—Department of Entomology, Virginia Polytechnic Institute, Blacksburg, Virginia.

grow by a series of molts. Finally, the winged adults appear, mate, and produce eggs to complete the life cycle. The German cockroach has 3–4 generations per year; other species vary from a few weeks to several years. *B. germanica* can be reared easily in the laboratory by providing shelter, food (commercial dog biscuits), and water. Cultures must be cleaned regularly to suppress odor and disease.

Genetic studies of *B. germanica* were initiated as part of a broad investigation of insecticide resistance, an important phenomena in this species but not in most other cockroaches. Within five years, about 30 mutants were isolated, and 5 of the 12 linkage groups were tentatively identified. This material was summarized in a World Health Organization publication (Cochran and Ross, 1967a). Subsequently, the scope of the genetic research widened. Cytogenetic investigations, particularly those leading to the identification of wild-type chromosomes (Cochran and Ross, 1967b, 1969), opened new avenues of research (Ross and Cochran, 1971; Cochran and Ross, 1974). Recently, the background of genetic and cytogenetic information and the availability of the requisite genetic stocks led to consideration of genetic-control measures (Ross and Cochran, 1973).

Although the genetics of *B. germanica* is of interest with respect to possible genetic control and in the elucidation of resistance problems, it is of equal importance from the viewpoint of basic science. This species belongs to one of the most ancient insect orders, in contrast to other insects studied intensively by geneticists. To our knowledge, the latter are confined to the most advanced group of orders. *B. germanica* is unique among such species in its low taxonomic position, generalized morphology, and incomplete metamorphosis. For these reasons, it is not surprising that two mutations are reminiscent of characteristics found in ancestral insects (Ross, 1964, 1966a,b).

In this chapter we have attempted to bring out some of the differences and similarities between the genetics of the cockroach and that of other insects, as well as to update the earlier review (Cochran and Ross, 1967a). The section on formal genetics is largely condensed from published reports (Cochran, 1973a,b; McDonald *et al.*, 1969; Ross, 1971a,b, 1972, 1973a,b,c, 1974; Ross and Cochran, 1967, 1968a,b, 1969a,b, 1970, 1971). On the other hand, unreported findings from recently completed experiments using chromosome translocations are also included, particularly in later sections and in the linkage map (Figure 1). These data will be presented in full in separate publications.

All genetic stocks described herein are maintained in our laboratory and most are available upon request.

Genetic and Phenotypic Diversity

If marked phenotypic differences characterized geographically separated populations of *B. germanica,* it is probable that some enterprising entomologist would have described subspecies. Certainly we have seen comparatively little variation among stocks collected from different areas of the United States, as well as from Mexico, Brazil, Kenya, Thailand, and Germany. Crosses between such stocks show no evidence of incipient reproductive isolation, suggesting some degree of genetic, as well as phenotypic, uniformity. Nevertheless, interpopulation differences, though minimal, might be analyzed profitably. There are some signs of diversity, in that: (1) a marked polymorph, *or,* occurs in Virginia and Florida stocks, but has not appeared in any other strain, (2) a Brazilian stock carries a new wing-vein mutation and a recurrence of *crs,* and (3) a stock from Thailand is apparently homozygous for *Bbp.*

Rough calculations of mutation load, following an admittedly subjective method (VandeHey, 1969), give estimates of 0.02–0.04 mutants per cockroach—quite different from estimates of 0.5–1.5 for *Drosophila* or 0.5–3.0 for mosquitoes (Craig and Hickey, 1967). Perhaps this explains why it has taken fifteen years of continuous search, aided by large-scale sib-mating projects, to isolate 60 mutant stocks!

B. germanica, insofar as is known, shows complete reproductive isolation from other *Blattella* species (Roth, 1970). Like many other cockroaches, it seems to possess a highly successful adaptive system. The antiquity of the *Blattaria* is such that its species may have developed their evolutionary specialities at some very early time. If so, one wonders if such species are evolutionary end points.

Formal Genetics

Mutations

Mutants are listed in Table 1. The table is divided into two sections: visible mutants and physiological traits. Chromosomal mutations are noted separately under "Cytogenetics" and in Table 3, except those with phenotypic effects, i.e., $T(2;11)Cu$ and the prowing traits. References include the first formal description and later studies which have added substantially to knowledge of the mutant, principally those establishing linkage relationships. Reference to the earlier review (Cochran and Ross, 1967*a*) is made only where these notes still represent the sole published

TABLE 1. *Alphabetized List of Mutants of Blattella germanica (as of January, 1974)*

Symbol[a]	Name	Linkage	References[b]
VISIBLE MUTANTS			
ab	Appressed bristles	—	
ba	Balloon wing	2	Cochran and Ross (1961)
bb	Bent bristles	—	
Bbp	Broad-banded pronotum	10	Ross and Cochran (1965), Ross (1972, 1973b)
bk	Broken-band pronotum	—	
Bl	Black body	6	Ross and Cochran (1966, 1968a), Ross (1971b)
Bl^e	Elo black body	6	Ross (1973c)
bu	Bulge eye	10	Ross (1971a, 1972)
ci	Cubitus interruptus	—	Ross (1973a)
Ck	Crooked antenna	—	
crs	Crossveinless	6	Ross and Cochran (1970), Ross (1971b)
ct	Curved tarsi	—	Cochran and Ross (1967a)
Cu [= T(2; 11) Cu]	Curly wing	7, 12	Ross and Cochran (1966, 1968a), Cochran and Ross (1969), McDonald et al. (1969)
cv	Curved wing	10	Ross and Cochran (1967, 1969a), Ross (1972, 1973b)
de	Dent wing	—	
dfl	Deformed leg	10	Ross (1972)
di	Divergent wing	—	
dp	Downturned pronotum	—	
dtw	Downturned wing	—	Ross and Cochran (1970)
el	Elevated wing	—	Cochran and Ross (1967a)
fc	Fused cerci	—	
fs	Fused antennae	11	Ross and Cochran (1965, 1970), Ross (1971a)
ft	Fused tarsi	—	Cochran and Ross (1967a)
fv	Forked vannal vein	—	
g	Green eye	—	
gl	Glassy wing	5	Ross and Cochran (1966), Ross (1973c)
hd	Hooded pronotum	9	Ross and Cochran (1968a)
M	Mottled	—	Cochran and Ross (1967a)
N	Notch wing	—	
na	Narrow abdomen	5	Ross (1973c)
np	Notch pronotum	6	Ross (1973a)
Ob	Odd body	10	Ross (1974)
oc	Ocelliless	—[c]	Ross and Cochran (1965)
or	Orange body	4	Ross and Cochran (1962, 1966)

TABLE 1. Continued

Symbol[a]	Name	Linkage	References[b]
p	Pearl eye	—	
Pb	Pale body	11	Ross and Cochran (1965), Ross (1971a)
pe	Peppery	—	
pld	Pallid eye	6	Ross and Cochran (1967, 1968a), Ross (1971b), Cochran (1973a)
pp	Pale purple eye	—	
Pw [= T(9; 10) Pw]	Prowing	3, 8	Ross (1964), Ross and Cochran (1965), Cochran and Ross (1969)
T(9;10) Pw^b	Bubbly prowing	3, 8	Cochran and Ross (1969)
T(9;10) Pw^e	Elo prowing	3, 8	
Df(9) Pw	Deficiency prowing	8	Ross and Cochran (1971)
r	Red eye	3	Ross and Cochran (1965, 1966, 1969b)
rm	Radius-media fused	—	
ro	Rosy eye (rose eye in later studies)	3	Ross and Cochran (1966, 1967, 1969b)
rp	Round pronotum	—	
ru	Ruby eye	8	Ross and Cochran (1967, 1968b, 1971)
sh	Shriveled wing	—	Ross (1973a)
st	Notched sternite	8	Ross and Cochran (1965), Ross (1966a,b), Ross and Cochran (1968b, 1971)
sty	Stumpy	8	
tf	Tent forewing	—	
tn	Truncated antenna	1	Ross and Cochran (1965)
var	Variegated eye	—	Ross and Cochran (1968a)
ww	Wrinkled wing	—	
y	Yellow body	10	Ross and Cochran (1966, 1969a), Ross (1972, 1973b)

PHYSIOLOGICAL TRAITS

Symbol[a]	Name	Linkage	References[b]
r-Cyclo	Cyclodiene resistance	7	McDonald et al. (1969)
r-DDT	DDT resistance	2	Cochran and Ross (1962a,b)
r-Mal	Malathion resistance	—	Cochran (1973b)
r-Pyreth	Pyrethrins resistance	6	Cochran (1973a)

[a] Chromosome mutations are not included, except those with phenotypic effects, i.e., Cu and Pw.
[b] References are in chronological order, starting with the original descriptions and followed by later studies, primarily those which serve to establish linkage relationships of the particular mutant.
[c] Recent backcrosses (Ross, unpublished) failed to confirm linkage of oc with the group-2 marker, ba, as postulated originally.

TABLE 2.   *Notes on Undescribed Mutants of Blattella germanica*

Mutant[a]	Phenotype and other data	Origin
Appressed bristles (*ab*)	One or more leg bristles lie flat against the leg	Spontaneous in *ru* stock
Bent bristles *(bb)*	Leg bristles bent sharply	Spontaneous in *tn* stock
Broken-band pronotum *(bk)*	Dark bands on pronotum split into two sections, adult trait	Two strains, one from linkage of *Bbp* and *fs*, one from *rp* stock
Crooked antenna *(Ck)*	Antennae crooked; autosomal dominant with reduced penetrance and variable expression (R. A. Barlow, unpublished)	Thailand strain, following radiation
Dent wing *(de)*	Slight dent near tip of forewing	Spontaneous in malathion-R strain
Divergent wing *(di)*	Wings extend away from body	From linkage studies of *ro* and *cv*
Downturned pronotum (*dp*)	Pronotum downturned, lacking line of breakage seen in *hd*	From linkage studies of *bu* and *hd*
Fused cerci *(fc)*	Fusion of several segments of the cerci	Wabash strain
Forked vannal vein *(fv)*	One or more vannal veins of forewing branch	Holder strain
Green eye *(g)*	Eye green; inheritable but appears only in *pld* homozygotes	*pld* stock, spontaneous
Notch wing *(N)*	Notches and blisters in forewing; dominant with reduced penetrance and highly variable expression	Holder strain following exposure to apholate
Pearl eye *(p)*	Eye colorless	Spontaneous in *var* stock
Peppery *(pe)*	Body covered with a fine mottling	Holder strain after exposure to apholate
Pale purple eye *(pp)*	Nymphal eyes with purple tint which darkens in adults	Spontaneous in brown strain
Radius-media fused (*rm*)	Fusion of the radial and medial veins of the hindwing in the proximal third of the wing	Brazil strain, spontaneous
Round pronotum *(rp)*	Pronotum small and round; adult trait	From linkage crosses of *ru* and *cv*

[a] Pale purple eye (*pp*) was discovered by Mrs. Nancy F. Boles, our laboratory technician. Other mutants were isolated by M. H. Ross.

TABLE 2. Continued

Mutant[a]	Phenotype and other data	Origin
Stumpy *(sty)*	Body broad, legs thick, males with shorter wings than females, most females sterile; linkage-group 8 (Ross, unpublished)	Brazil strain following radiation
Tent forewing *(tf)*	Forewings curved downward on each side of longitudinal axis	Wabash strain
Wrinkled wing *(ww)*	Surface of forewing rough	Linkage studies of *fs* and *Bbp*

description of the particular mutant. Undescribed mutants are listed again in Table 2 so as to provide brief descriptions of phenotype and origin.

Certain mutants and their interactions are of particular interest. For example, odd body *(Ob)* profoundly disturbs the development, pigmentation, and external structure of diverse body parts. It seems remarkable that many of the heterozygotes survive and reproduce. Stumpy *(sty)* is an autosomal mutant, yet wing length is markedly different in males and females. Wild-type wings in this species show little, if any, sexual dimorphism in length.

Interactions discovered in the study of body and eye colors have implications regarding metabolic pathways. In the light body colors, *or* is epistatic to *y*, and both are epistatic to *Pb*; in the eye colors, *pld* is epistatic to *ru* and *r*, and *ru* is nearly, if not completely, epistatic to *r*. Such reactions could indicate blocks in single metabolic pathways. Conversely, the double homozygote of *or* and *Bl* is phenotypically distinct, as are the double homozygotes of *ro* with *pld* and *ru*. Of the new eye colors, *p* and *pp* (Table 2), we only know that *p* is not allelic to either *pld* or *ro*, and *pp* is a recessive characterized by reduced viability. Peculiarly, there is no evidence to date of multiple alleles other than the possibility that *Bl^e* is an allele of *Bl*. It could also be a recurrence of the *Bl* gene, closely linked with a recessive lethal. Perhaps the prowing *(Pw)* traits should be categorized as allelic, but we have hesitated to do so since these are associated with chromosome breakage.

Interesting data have been obtained from various mutants affecting reproductivity. Ovaries of T(2;11)*Cu* females remain immature unless mating occurs. This reveals a stimulatory capability of normal males which is usually hidden, since yolk deposition takes place in the eggs of wild-type virgin females. Other mutants influence oothecal size (mean number of eggs per ootheca). Matings of hybrid males result in reduced numbers of eggs, suggesting a loss of stimulatory ability. Conversely, hybrid females tend to form large oothecae. This phenomenon was noted first in studies of *Pb*, and later in work with Df(9)*Pw* and several translocations. Matings of *Pb*/+ males also resulted in a high frequency of unfertilized eggs. A sperm characteristic, such as reduced numbers or activity of sperm, might conceivably account for both the reduced stimulatory capability and unfertilized eggs. To date, mutants exhibiting a sex difference in oothecal size have two traits in common: homozygotes are lethal, and there is some type of dominance, either phenotypic or, in the case of interchanges, semisterility.

Reference to discussions of the possible evolutionary significance of the *st* and *Pw* mutations was made previously (Cochran and Ross, 1967*a*). However, the paper noting the apparent rudimentary abdominal legs in *st* embryos was not cited (Ross, 1966*b*). We have also discovered a prowing phenotype associated with a deficiency and two more prowing-type translocations. We suggest these breakages inactivate a locus, possibly a complex one. If so, the normal allele(s) act to suppress formation of the winglike pronotal extension.

Linkage

A provisional summary of linkage relationships is given in Figure 1. The estimates are from first oothecae only, thus assuring similarity of age. Unless the group shows a marked sex differential in recombination, recombination is averaged for the sexes. T(2;11)*Cu* is indicated as a marker for group 12 on the basis of elimination. *Cu* segregates independently from markers for all autosomal groups except group 7. Thus, it is assumed tentatively to mark the one remaining, and otherwise unidentified, group. All available estimates of map distances between genetic loci and chromosome breakpoints are included, except those for T(4;8;10). Linkage of T(4;8;10) is estimated at 0.3 percent with *ro* (group 3) and 9.1 percent with *y* (group 10). These data are omitted from Figure 1 because more study is needed to determine their significance in this ring-of-six. They may represent distances to the margins of an asynaptic area of unusually large magnitude.

Recombination appears to be influenced by age. Data from second oothecae are meager, yet these show a consistent tendency toward reduced crossing over. In one case, a reduction in older females was statistically

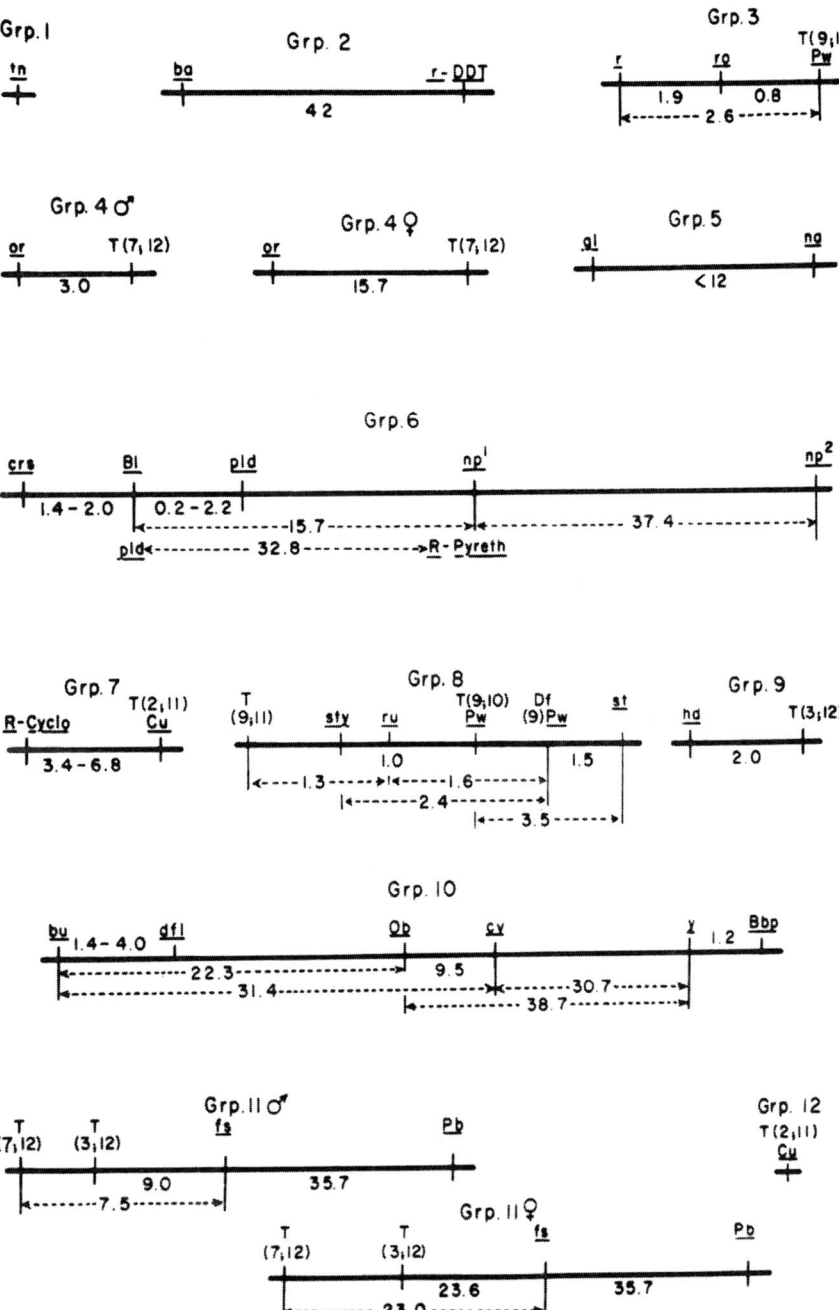

Figure 1. Tentative linkage map for Blattella germanica. Map estimates are average values for the sexes, except in groups 4 and 11, in which sex differences are unusually large (see text).

significant, but the data were disturbed by a viability loss of one of the mutants.

Linkage estimates using simple genetic markers and, in some cases, chromosome mutations, suggest either equality or relatively minor sex differences in crossing over. In the longest linkage groups, 6 and 10, recombination is lower in males, but the difference is generally less than 7 percent for map distances of 33–38. The difference holds true for all segments of group 10, large and small, and is almost certainly a characteristic of the entire group 10 chromosome. Comparisons in group 8 are more difficult for two reasons: (1) close juxtaposition of genetic loci and chromosome breakpoints (see page 58 and Figure 3A), and (2) partial or complete sterility of *sty* and *st* females, respectively. There was a marked tendency for higher crossing over in males in linkage of Df(9)*Pw* with *ru*. On the other hand, in linkage of Df(9)*Pw* with *sty*, meager data for males gave an estimate of 3.3 percent, as opposed to 2.2 percent for females. In *sty* linkage with T(9;10)*Pw*, males averaged 0.9 and females 1.0 percent. These group 8 linkage data, considered in total, do not provide sufficient evidence of a sex differential in crossing over, yet the existence of small differences cannot be ruled out. In group 11, no sex differential was apparent in linkage of *fs* and *Pb,* but it should be noted that lethal effects occurred in the backcrosses using hybrid males. Likewise, group 3 data did not suggest marked sex differences, yet comparisons were hardly adequate. Linkage was close and there was a scarcity of data on male crossing over.

Experiments using T(7;12) and T(3;12) provide the only crossover data for groups 4 and 9, respectively, as well as adding to that of group 11, another of the sparsely marked groups (Figure 1). In the linkage of T(7;12) with *or* (group 4) and *fs* (group 11) and in that of T(3;12) with *fs*, sex differences in recombination occurred which are out of proportion to those found in other groups. Crossing over in females exceeded that of males by 12–15 percent. We do not know whether map distances estimated for males, which suggest rather close linkage (3–9 percent), or the larger estimates based on female recombination are most comparable to the other data. Therefore, separate maps for the sexes are given for groups 4 and 11, i.e., those showing pronounced sex differences (Figure 1). It seems strange that no indication of a sex differential was apparent in the linkage of the group 11 markers, *fs* and *Pb*, although, as noted already, these were complicated by lethal effects. Certainly these data provide grounds for questioning whether large sex differences are normally typical of groups 4 and 11.

In the above discussion, we did not mention a possible sex differential in linkage of the group 9 marker, *hd,* with T(3;12). The difference was not statistically significant, probably due to a lack of counts for males. Nevertheless, an estimate of 2.0 for males and a mere 0.1 for females may indicate a group with higher crossing over in males, but here also it should be kept in mind that the data involve a translocation.

One occurrence of a pronounced sex difference in recombination occurred in crosses which did not involve a translocation. An unidentified factor, present in one set of *Ob* crosses (group 10), apparently increased recombination in different, but adjacent, crossover regions in males and females. The alteration acted in the same direction as that normally present in one region, creating the largest sex difference known thus far, i.e., 26 percent; in the adjacent segment, it reversed the usual situation, causing male crossing over to exceed that of the females.

The unknown factor in the *Ob* studies could be explained if it caused a localization of chiasmata in different portions of the chromosome in males and females. Such differences are normal for many species (White, 1973). Possibly this gives a clue concerning the nature of the extreme sex differences in recombination encountered in the linkage of certain translocations. If, in a specific autosome, male chiasmata were localized in a region close to a breakpoint, there should be a suppressive effect on male crossing over. Meanwhile, localization of chiasmata in a more-distant region in females could result in little or no suppressive effect from the translocation. This is purely conjectural but, in case the idea has merit, it seems worth noting that recombination estimates for females would provide the best comparisons to other linkage data. In some species, factors such as the position of a locus in respect to a breakpoint or its location in a translocated or nontranslocated arm apparently affect recombination, but it is difficult to visualize how these would result in sex differences.

Double crossing over has been studied only in groups 6 and 10. In group 6, interference was complete over a distance of approximately 4 crossover units. Surprisingly, interference also appeared to be complete in studies using the *bu, Ob,* and *cv* loci, covering a distance of 31 in the left half of group 10 (Figure 1). When three-point crosses included the central loci and *y,* at the far right, coincidence values were close to 1. Such contrasts could arise if the centromere lies to the right of *cv,* providing the group 10 chromosome usually has no more than one chiasma per chromosome arm.

In the largest groups, 6, 8, and 10, five or more markers have been found, but questions remain regarding various gene sequences. In group 6, *R-Pyreth* could lie either to the left or right of *Bl,* and the position of the *np* loci is indicated tentatively from F_2 data. In group 8, new data for *sty* and T(9;11) do not change gene sequences postulated earlier (Ross and Cochran, 1971). However, they are responsible for some minor revisions of map estimates (Figure 1). In group 10, gene sequences have been established definitively through three-point data.

A synthesis of information derived from the study of chromosome 12 breakpoints in T(3;12) and T(7;12) and linkage data for *fs* suggests the sequence depicted for group 11 in Figure 1. The basis for this hypothetical arrangement is discussed in the section covering linkage group–chromosome correlations.

One other basic aspect of linkage studies needs to be noted, namely, the extent to which different tests agree. Data for group 10 provide the best opportunities for comparison. These show good agreement (Ross, 1974). Crossing over in females seems to vary slightly more than in males, but such differences are not statistically significant. Possibly crossing over in females is more readily influenced by environmental and/or genetical factors. In group 8, only one set of data does not agree well with other estimates. In backcrosses of *ru* and Df(9)*Pw,* crossing over was higher in the presence of a third mutant, *ro,* than in the simple *ru*–Df(9)*Pw* test crosses. Estimates of map distances based on the latter conformed closely to expectations based on other group 8 data. Lastly, in group 6, recombination of *Bl* with *pld* was less than expected in crosses involving *crs.*

Some further linkage information is discussed in the section covering linkage group–chromosome correlations in cases where map distances have been estimated for particular chromosome regions.

Cytogenetics

Descriptions of meiosis and chromosome number in *B. germanica* have been available for many years. Therefore, this material will be treated rather briefly, placing emphasis on only a few points of interest. The more detailed portions of this section will deal with recent research, particularly that concerning certain chromosomal aberrations.

Meiosis and Sex Determination

Meiosis in *B. germanica* is quite typical (Stevens, 1905). Among its interesting features is an unpaired X chromosome in males which separates precociously at anaphase I. In this stage, as throughout meiosis, the sex chromosome is small, positively heterochromatic, and easily

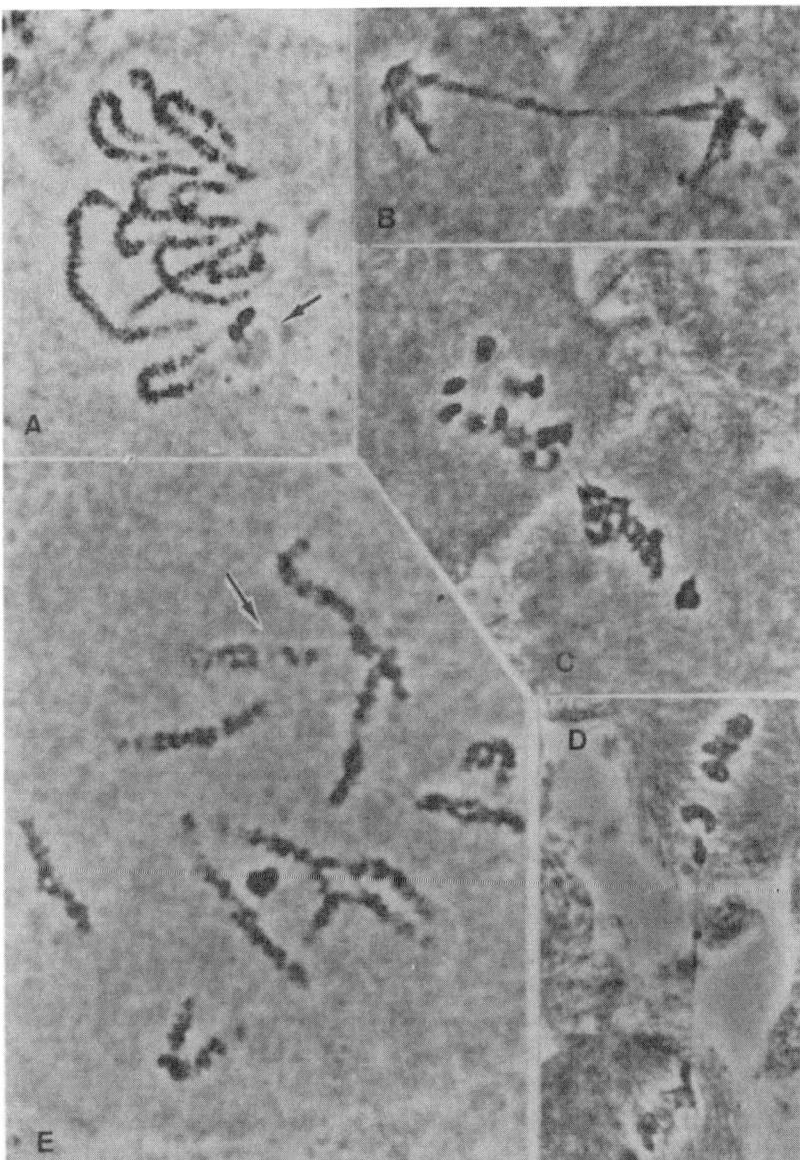

Figure 2. Meiotic cells from nymphal testes: *(A) Fingerlike extensions of the X chromosome into the nucleolus at mid to late pachynema; (B) difficulty in final separation of chromosomes at telophase I; (C) attachments between the metaphase plates of two daughter cells late in the second meiotic division; (D) metaphase-II chromosomes pulled to cell margins with attenuated chromatin material in the intercellular region; (E) chromosome 3 (arrow) showing characteristic light-staining internal areas and, at left, a diffuse terminal region. The cell also shows a typical translocation configuration.*

identified. It is associated with a single nucleolus up to the time of early diplonema, when this nucleolus disappears. During the period of their association, the X chromosome is often seen to extend two fingerlike projections into the substance of the nucleolus (Figure 2A). At the second meiotic division the X chromosome divides, as do the autosomes, and there is no precocious movement. However, the paired X often lines up at the end of the second-meiotic-metaphase plate.

Other points of interest include the apparent absence of a premetaphase stretch reported for another cockroach species (Lewis and John, 1957). We have not seen any evidence suggesting the existence of this phenomenon in the German cockroach. Additionally, in some cells there appears to be an unusual amount of difficulty in the final separation of chromosomes in wild-type cockroaches at telophase I (Figure 2B). This situation also occurs in certain mutant stocks, where it might more readily be explained, and is accompanied by a very extensive ability of the chromosomes to undergo attentuation. In some instances, the connection between chromatin masses is maintained late into second meiotic division, when the metaphase plates of the two daughter cells are still attached (Figure 2C). Frequently in this circumstance, the chromosome mass of each daughter cell, or part thereof, is pulled to the edge of its corresponding cell (Figure 2D). How long this type of connection is retained is not known, but it could easily cause severe problems in spermiogenesis unless the connection is finally broken.

Another observation frequently made concerning first-meiotic-division chromosomes is their ability to form nonhomologous attachments. It is not unusual to see several point attachments among the chromosomes of a given cell. The heterochromatic X chromosome is usually involved, but connections between autosome pairs are not uncommon. Presumably, these are attachments between heterochromatic regions. In the *ru* mutant stock an apparent association of this type occurs between the X chromosome and one specific autosome pair. The X is attached to one end of the autosomes. This connection remains intact until diplonema-diakinesis, at which time it ruptures. Thereafter, there is no connection, and the chromosomes proceed through the rest of meiosis in a normal fashion. The significance of this association is unknown as *ru* is a simple recessive eye color.

As in other blattids, sex determination in this species is XO, with the male being the heterogametic sex (Suomalainen, 1946). In such organisms, sexual dimorphism is probably dependent on a balance between female-determining genes on the X chromosome and male-determining genes on the autosomes (White, 1973). Some support for this contention comes from study of the only sex-linked mutant yet discovered in this species. The mutant, *tn,* has a pleiotropic effect on colleterial glands of females (Ross and Cochran, 1965), and in first instar *tn* male nymphs there is often a partial expression of a female trait on the ninth sternite (Ross and F. L. Campbell, unpublished). Also, genetic findings suggest there are interactions between the X chromosome and the autosomes. For example, autosomes show sex differences in recombination frequency, and an autosomal mutant, *sty,* causes sexual dimorphism in wing length. It is interesting that the *sty* female is closer to wild type, since in *Drosophila* the males of such mutants are more nearly normal in phenotype (Smith and Lucchesi, 1969).

No sound statement with respect to dosage compensation is possible at present. However, certain results from study of the sex-linked mutant, *tn,* may have a bearing on this question. The mutant reduces the number of and affects the ability to properly form new antennal segments, particularly in the third and fourth instars (Ross and F. L. Campbell, unpublished). Expression of the trait is most severe in *tn* males, suggesting that dosage compensators, if present, may not affect this mutant allele. Contrarily, study of the wild-type allele has not shown sex differences in the numbers of new segments added during normal nymphal development. Thus, these very limited observations seem to favor a dosage-compensation mechanism.

Karyotype

All available data for *B. germanica* agree that $2n = 23$ in males, and, where measured, $2n = 24$ in females (Cochran and Ross, 1967b; Cohen and Roth, 1970; Stevens, 1905; Suomalainen, 1946; Wassilieff, 1907). Insofar as known, this appears to be the most characteristic chromosome number for the genus *Blattella* (Cochran and Ross, 1967b; Cohen and Roth, 1970). However, these same authors demonstrated that various other chromosome numbers occur frequently in other cockroach genera, and to a limited extent in *Blattella.*

The autosomes of *B. germanica* are either metacentric or submetacentric (Cohen and Roth, 1970). This finding agrees with an earlier report of primarily metacentric chromosomes (Suomalainen, 1946). Based on the mitotic chromosomes depicted by Cohen and Roth (1970; their Figure 58) our estimate is that three autosome pairs are submetacentric, with the remaining eight pairs being metacentric. The X chromosomes are either submetacentric or possibly acrocentric. This

figure also shows a gradation in chromosome size, with one outstandingly
large autosome pair that is definitely submetacentric. The length differences appear to be similar to those of the meiotic chromosomes
(Cochran and Ross, 1969), and a correlation on this basis might be
possible. Comparisons of centromere position would be helpful, but, unfortunately, meiotic centromeres have proven very difficult to detect.

A system for identifying meiotic chromosomes from testes by total-
length measurements has been developed (Cochran and Ross, 1969). To
achieve consistency, measurements were made at mid to late pachynema
using only cells in which the longest autosome pair had a length of 12–14
microns. By this method, each chromosome pair was distinguishable individually with a high degree of reliability. Accordingly, the chromosome
pairs were numbered from 1 to 12, beginning with the smallest (the unpaired X chromosome) as 1. The size of the autosomes ranged from an
average of 5.2 microns for the smallest (2) to 12.9 for the largest (12). The
X chromosome is dotlike and measured 2.5 microns.

As experience was gained with the meiotic chromosomes, it became
evident that some of them have characteristics which aid in their identification (Cochran, unpublished). For example, chromosome pair 3 has two
prominent internal regions which barely take strain, as well as a terminal
region that is very diffuse (Figure 2E). In addition, pairs 2 and 7 have an
indistinct terminal region at one end of the chromosome. In the case of
pair 7 the very tip of this region has a rather distinct pair of telomeres.
These features, together with the dotlike X and the very long chromosome
12, make it possible to identify 5 of the 12 pairs by inspection. Distinguishing features of other autosomes will undoubtedly be discovered as
detailed studies of different translocations are conducted. Hopefully, it will
soon be possible to replace our published illustration of the meiotic chromosomes (Cochran and Ross, 1969) with a more precise chromosome
map. Quinacrine or related staining techniques may also prove useful in
this regard.

Chiasma Frequency

Only rather preliminary data can be given in this section. However,
they are the first such attempts for this species, and may be useful for that
reason. The calculations are based upon observations of testicular cells at
diplonema. Since the X chromosome is unpaired under these circumstances only autosomes are considered. Examples of bivalent pairs with
one or two chiasmata were frequently found. Bivalents with more than
one chiasma per arm were rare but did occur. The average number of

chiasmata for the eleven autosomes was 14.3, or 1.3 per bivalent. The extremes found were all 11 as rods on the one hand, but a maximum of 6 as rings on the other. Calculations derived from these data reveal a total genetic length for the autosomes of about 700 crossover units. On the average, this turns out to be 60–65 units per bivalent. From genetic data, linkage group 10 has a total length of about 65 units (Figure 1). It is one of the best-established linkage groups, and current data may be fairly indicative of its extent. While both of these calculated crossover distances may have to be refined, they appear to be in at least general agreement.

The number of multivalents in tetraploid meiotic cells can also be instructive with respect to chiasma frequencies (White, 1973). We have often observed tetraploidy in both wild-type and translocation chromosome preparations, but have not yet studied them in a systematic manner.

Chromosome Rearrangements

More than 20 translocation stocks are currently available in *B. germanica*. All except two were isolated following exposure to ionizing radiation. Four stocks have been tested for the existence of a viable homozygote with completely negative results. Thus, all aberrants are maintained as heterozygotes $(T/+)$ with backcrossing to wild type at each generation. One stock has a stable ring-of-six, involving three chromosome pairs. Genetic and cytogenetic analyses of the translocations are far from complete, yet it is evident that each has its own unique attributes. The only other type of chromosome mutation found thus far is a terminal deficiency involving about one-third of the total length of chromosome 9 [Df(9)Pw]. It is viable as a heterozygote, and the breakpoint, as well as the phenotypic expression, is approximately the same as the Pw translocations (see Table 1, Pw).

The length measurement system for identifying individual chromosomes has been used in two ways to determine which chromosomes are involved in the translocations: (1) The normal chromosomes are measured, and those of the translocation identified by elimination, and (2) the chromosomes in the cross configuration are measured directly. The latter measurements also serve to distinguish the translocated from the intact chromosomes in the cross configuration. The lengths of the exchanged segments can be estimated by measuring from the end of the translocated chromosome to the approximate breakpoint, i.e., the small area of nonalignment at the center of the translocation figure. By this means it is possible to determine the approximate location of breakpoints in each chromosome involved in a translocation. These breakpoints have been referred to earlier in connection with the linkage maps.

Table 3 summarizes the current status of chromosome identification in 20 translocation stocks, none of which has phenotypic effects. The T(2;11)*Cu* and T(9;10)*Pw* translocations were listed in Table 1. Although many identifications are incomplete, measurements have been sufficient to narrow the possibilities in most stocks. Analysis of these data with regard to involvement of individual autosomes gave the following results:

No. 12—5	No. 7 or 8—1	No. 5—2
No. 11—3	No. 7 —1	No. 4—2
No. 10—4	No. 6 or 7—1	No. 3—1
No. 9—5(8)	No. 6 —2	No. 2—1
No. 8—2	No. 5 or 6—1	

The most frequent breakage occurred in the longer autosomes (9–12). However, those of medium length do not seem to break more frequently than the short autosomes. Chromosomes 9 and 12 have the largest number of breaks. In addition, chromosome 9 has one small region, the segment involved in the prowing traits, which seems to be especially frangible. If all occurrences of prowing-type breakage in this chromosome were counted in the above list, the total would be 8 rather than 5.

Typical pachytene cross configurations occur in all but one or two stocks. This probably means that exchanged segments generally represent relatively large portions of the chromosomes. With those unusual cases, the autosome pairs lined up more like an end-to-end association, suggesting very small exchanged parts. Possibly breakage occurs most frequently in the region of the centromere, as in *Drosophila* and *Zea mays* (Jancey and Walden, 1972). Of course, the higher frequency of breakage in the longer autosomes by itself would increase the chances for larger interchanges, particularly if breakage does tend to occur toward the center of the chromosome.

Rings-of-four [or six in T(4;8;10)] occur in the majority of diplotene-diakenesis cells in most of the stocks studied. This indicates at least one chiasma in each of the four (or six) arms. However, a few interchanges show a marked tendency to break up into chains and even into bivalents. Such events appear to be influenced, in part, by the lengths of the pairing arms, and these in turn may be influenced by the sizes of the autosomes involved. For example, in T(2;11)*Cu,* which involves the smallest autosome, there is one very short arm. In this stock about 17 percent of the diplotene cells have a chain-of-four, as opposed to about 1

TABLE 3.   *Summary of Chromosome Identification in Translocation Stocks of B. germanica*[a]

Laboratory reference No.	Chromosome identification[b]	Laboratory reference No.	Chromosome identification[b]
2c	T(9;11)	2d	1 Large, 1 medium
2b	T(4;8;10)	2e	6 and 8 ?
7c	T(7;12)	2f	1 Medium, 1 large
7d	T(3;12)	2g	No data
7h	T(6;9)	2i	9 and 10 ?
9b	T(11;12)	7f	No data
1a	T(5;7 or 8)	7g	9 and 10 ?
1c	1 large, 1 medium	7i	1 Large, 1 small
1d	T(4;5 or 6)	9a	T(6 or 7;12)
2a	T(5 ?;12)	19	Both large ?

[a] All translocations currently in stock are listed, except those with phenotypic effects [i.e., T(2;11) *Cu* and the T(9;10) *Pw* traits, which are listed in Table 1].
[b] In certain translocations where chromosome identifications are incomplete, the relative sizes of the chromosomes have been noted.

percent in T(9;10)*Pw*, in which all four arms are more nearly equal. It is probable that the frequency of breakup may also be related to other autosome peculiarities, such as chiasma frequency and localization. Thus, the frequency of ring breakup is considerably higher in T(7;12) than in T(3;12), even though T(7;12) involves a longer autosome and longer pairing segments. There is little evidence from this species to support the contention that chromosomes regularly break up into bivalents in interchanges showing semisterility (White, 1973).

Data are also available on the translocations with reference to size of oothecae and mortality. This information was tabulated for 16 of the 20 stocks lacking phenotypic effects (Ross and Cochran, 1973). The data were gathered from egg cases produced during 5–8 generations of crossing heterozygous (T/+) males and females to a wild-type stock. The stocks fell into categories on the basis of oothecal size (mean number of eggs per ootheca): (1) those in which T/+ females produced unusually large oothecae, but matings of T/+ males resulted in a reduction in egg deposition, (2) stocks which consistently averaged 2 or 3 more eggs than wild type, although the differences were seldom significant, and (3) those with mean oothecal size nearly identical with the wild type. Two additional stocks gave a preliminary indication of reduced oothecal size, but further data failed to confirm a significant difference. The sex difference in oothecal size (category 1) raises an intriguing question. What is the relationship between the apparent loss of stimulatory capability of T/+ males, with resultant small oothecae, and heightened fecundity of T/+ females? As noted previously, a similar situation occurs in *Pb*. Those interchanges showing a small elevation in number of eggs for both sexes may possess a slight heterotic effect (category 2).

Description of mortality estimates was also facilitated by grouping the translocations (Ross and Cochran, 1973). Thus, 8 interchanges showed average mortalities of 50 percent or above for both sexes. The highest mortality was associated with the ring-of-six. We have begun detailed study of this stock and find the 1973 data need revision. Mortality is now estimated at 68–70 percent and chromosome identification is T(4;8;10), rather than T(4;9;10). The high mortality is undoubtedly a reflection of the involvement of three autosomes in a stable ring-of-six translocation. A second group of 5 stocks was characterized by mortalities of about 50 percent in one sex, but with the opposite sex giving mortalities in the range of 40–45 percent. In 2 of these cases the higher mortality was associated with the T/+ male matings; in the other 3 stocks, the situation was reversed. Lastly, three interchanges had low mortalities in both sexes. The most marked reduction in mortality occurred with interchange 19, with averages of 28 and 35 percent for females and males, respectively. It may or may not be significant that this is one of the few translocations in which the size of the exchanged pieces is comparatively small.

Additional studies of certain translocations, including T(2;11)*Cu* and T(9;10)*Pw,* support the contention that lower mortalities associated with translocation stocks arise from a favoring of alternate over adjacent disjunction at metaphase I. Similarly, when mortalities approximating 50 percent are obtained there is a random disjunction. Cytological data on T(9;10)*Pw* showed that 64 percent of metaphase-I cells from testes undergo alternate disjunction, while the corresponding number for T(2;11)*Cu* is 50 percent. Clearly, chromosomal meiotic drive favoring alternate disjunction is associated with *Pw* but not *Cu*. Hatch data on these two stocks are in close agreement with the cytological information. It remains to be seen whether high mortalities are associated with meiotic drive favoring adjacent disjunction, although this is probably the case. Another interesting point from our data is that meiotic drive may be under separate control in males and females in some stocks. On the other hand, for stocks like *Pw* this is apparently not the case since hatch data are nearly identical from crosses of T/+ males and females.

We have assumed that mortality estimates are characteristic for each translocation since they show little change from one generation to the next. However, an exception seems to occur with T(4;8;10). Repeated use of T(4;8;10) progeny from matings with the highest-percent hatch seems to raise the average hatch in later generations. This suggests the possibility that the frequency of alternate *vs.* adjacent disjunction at metaphase I may have been altered by selection. This and other factors influencing disjunction frequencies deserve close attention, not only because of their scientific interest, but also because there is considerable interest in using translocations in genetic-control programs.

One further point must be made relative to mortalities. The mortality estimates described above are based on productive oothecae only. Such estimates gauged actual lethal effects by the translocations as accurately as possible. However, excluded from these data were a number of oothecae which did not hatch progeny, although they contained fully developed, viable embryos (also excluded were those embryos which died in earlier embryonic stages). It appeared as though the combined effort of the living embryos was not sufficient to open the egg case. Normally the embryos all hatch more or less simultaneously and force open the keel of the egg case. The greater the lethality associated with a translocation, the higher the frequency of such unproductive oothecae. In recent crosses of T(9;11) × T(3;12), 11 of 13 matings were unproductive. This finding could be an important bonus for genetic-control programs involving this species.

An additional characteristic peculiar to most of the translocations is an end-to-end association of certain chromatid pairs at prophase II. This association is related to disjunction at metaphase I. Apparently, terminalized chiasmata persist through anaphase I, when adjacent disjunction occurs. Cytologically this can be visualized by the ring structures at anaphase I being pulled apart in their lateral arms, but not at their ends. This observation seems to argue in favor of the separation of chiasmata by mechanical tension, rather than the specific chemical action proposed by White (1973). In most translocation stocks these end-to-end associations at prophase II are consistent enough to allow their use as an additional stage in the meiotic cycle to count alternate *vs.* adjacent disjunction-type cells. Presumably, these connections rupture prior to spermiogenesis. If they did not, this behavior would be expected to significantly lower the number of mature spermatozoa resulting from adjacent disjunction-type cells. The agreement between cytological counts of alternate *vs.* adjacent disjunction with hatch data, presented above, appears to rule out such a possibility.

In spite of the paucity of detailed information on many of the translocations, it is evident that they show a unique range of characteristics, both cytological and biological. Continued study of these aberrations should

TABLE 4. Linkage Group—Chromosome
Correlations

Linkage group	Chromosome
1	1 (X chromosome)
2	4, 5, or 8
3	10
4	7
5	4, 5, or 8
6	6
7	2 or 11
8	9
9	3
10	4 or 8
11	12
12	2 or 11

add immeasurably to our understanding of genetic mechanisms in *B. germanica.*

Linkage Group–Chromosome Correlations and the Location of Genetic Loci

Cytologic and linkage analyses of T(9;10)*Pw*, T(2;11)*Cu*, T(9;11), T(7;12), T(3;12), T(4;8;10), and T(6;9), as well as Df(9)*Pw*, have resulted in the correlations listed in Table 4. In the linkage of T(2;11)*Cu* with *R-Cyclo*, it is not known whether this group 7 trait is on chromosome 2 or 11. Likewise, linkage group 10 is known to lie on one of the chromosomes in T(4;8;10), but it could be either 4 or 8, since neither has been correlated with a linkage group. However, this narrows the possibilities for the two groups, 2 and 5, which have not yet shown linkage with any translocation. One should be on chromosome 5; the other, on either 4 or 8—whichever does *not* carry group 10. The translocations needed to solve this problem and to complete this phase of genetic study are on hand.

It was not surprising to find that linkage group 9, containing only one marker, is on a small autosome (3). More noteworthy is the discovery that neither of the genetically longest linkage groups, 6 or 10, is on one of the longest autosomes. Another peculiarity of the correlations is the small total map distance of group 8 (Figure 1) since it is carried by one of the relatively long autosomes (9). In fact, the entire linkage map apparently lies within the central third of the chromosome.

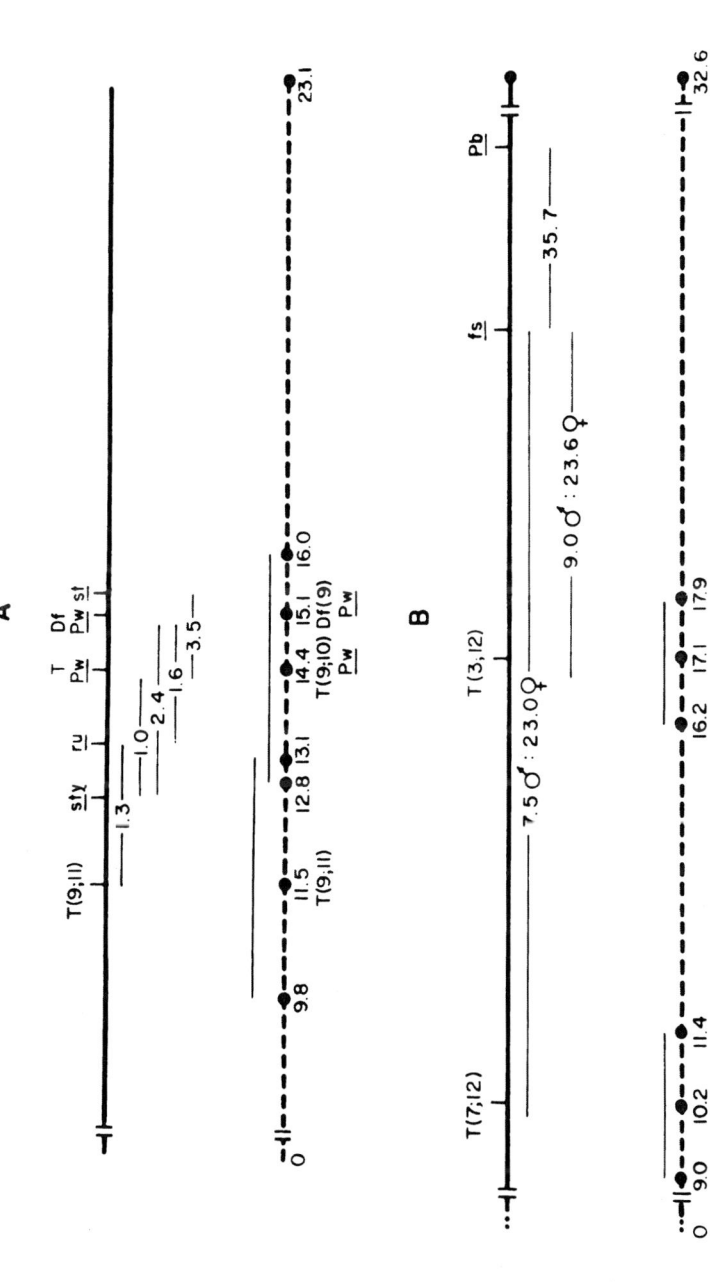

Figure 3. Diagrammatic representation of two chromosomes and their respective linkage groups. The solid lines and associated values represent linkage maps. The dotted lines indicate the chromosomes with distances in micrometer-scale units as measured from the left. The extent of asynaptic areas associated with translocations are shown by short solid lines, and the approximate location of breakpoints are indicated at the mid-point of these areas. (A) Chromosome 9 (linkage group 8); (B) chromosome 12, linkage group 11.

The identification of two breakpoints in chromosome 9 and the available linkage data provide sufficient information for the tentative assignment of genetic loci to specific chromosome regions (Figure 3A). Also, these data permit a comparison of the map distance with the actual chromosome length lying between the T(9;11) and Df(9)*Pw* breakpoints. Projecting this ratio to estimate the total length of chromosome 9 gives *ca.* 20 crossover units. It seems reasonable to assume this extremely low estimate indicates a paucity of chiasmata in this particular chromosome region. The centromere lies close to, if not within, this segment. Chiasma interference in the centromeric region is a well-known phenomenon. Nevertheless, it should be kept in mind that we are only beginning to learn something of the genetic makeup of specific autosomes. Until chiasma frequencies are determined for specific chromosomes, we cannot rule out the possibility that the chromosome 9 data indicate an autosome with an unusually low chiasma frequency, rather than a specific region of little crossing over. The three marker genes, *ru, sty,* and *st,* show close linkage, so there is, at least, evidence that the results are not due entirely to a suppressive effect of the translocations, T(9;11) or T(9;10)*Pw.*

Recently completed experiments with T(3;12) and T(7;12) were productive of three linkage group–chromosome correlations. These data also make possible a first attempt to map chromosome 12 (Figure 3B). The latter requires some explanation. The two ends of chromosome 12 are distinguishable cytologically (Cochran, unpublished). Positioning the breakpoints in relation to the same end places T(3;12) centrad to that of T(7;12). In linkage studies with *fs,* the map distances estimated to each breakpoint were extremely close in both males and females. This observation suggested the breakpoints would be very close. Actually, the breakpoints are separated by about 7 chromosome-measurement units. As in chromosome 9, we seem again to be dealing with a region of very little crossing over, perhaps due to proximity of the centromere. The chromosome is submetacentric, and the centromere could lie close to T(7;12). Crossing over is more frequent in other portions of group 12, as indicated by distant linkage between *fs* and *Pb,* estimated at 35.7 percent. Also, in females, estimates of 23.0 and 23.6 percent for *fs* with T(7;12) and T(3;12), respectively, indicate frequent crossing over in the segment between *fs* and T(3;12) (Figure 3B). The lower crossing over in males for this segment presents a second problem, as noted previously. The mapping of *fs* and *Pb* to the right of T(3;12) in Figure 3B is very tentative. Linkage data for *Pb* and T(3;12) indicate a sequence of T(3;12)—*fs—Pb.* The total map distance for this area is estimated at 43–44 or 59, depending on whether calculations are for males or females, respectively. It seems more likely the region to the right would allow the frequency of crossing over requisite to such large map distances. To the left, about half of the segment is occupied by the region of little to no crossing over encompassed between the two breakpoints. This leaves only about one-fourth of the chromosome, which appears rather small for the frequency of crossing over indicated by the map distances. Conversely, a minimum estimate of 128 for the total linkage map, based on Figure 3B, seems reasonable (59 crossover units per 15 chromosome-measurement units). Chromosome 12 is the longest of the karyotype. Chiasma frequencies in specific autosomes have not been determined, but we have noticed as many as 3 in chromosome 12.

Concluding Remarks

Questions, rather than answers, may serve best to focus attention on some of the more intriguing aspects of the genetic studies of *B. germanica*. For example, is the low mutation load a reflection of extreme canalization of developmental systems, or is there an unusual degree of genetic homozygosity? Does this species retain remnants of genetic systems close to those of ancestral insects, as suggested by the *st* and *Pw* traits? Why is it so difficult to find markers for certain groups? One of the most poorly known groups is on the second-longest autosome, while the best established and longest linkage groups lie on short or middle-sized autosomes. These observations bring up another problem. Are the large sex differences in recombination genuine characteristics of groups 4 and 11 or are they artifacts introduced by the use of translocations? This phenomenon is limited to the very groups in which there is a scarcity of mutant markers. We advanced a theory based on a difference of chiasma localization in males and females, but genetic markers are needed to test this hypothesis. Unfortunately, it has been much easier to obtain chromosome breakpoints than mutant markers for these groups.

Two developments worth noting are the continuation of good agreement between different linkage studies and the integrity of the linkage groups as revealed by the translocations. In the past, we have attributed the former to the work being carried out in the same laboratory and to the collection of linkage data from first oothecae, thus eliminating possible differences due to aging. A third factor may also be important. Close agreement of two-point and three-point data, as in group 10, could arise from a lack of double crossing over, possibly in entire chromosome arms. It was in group 10 that interference was complete over 31 crossover units. The overall chiasma frequency of 1.3 suggests that two crossover events per chromosome arm are rare in most autosomes. The second development, the integrity of the linkage groups, was unexpected. Several groups have one marker only, and others consist of a few closely spaced loci. We had thought intermediate markers would eventually be found, and the groups would need revision accordingly. Instead, the correlation of linkage groups with specific autosomes indicates most, and probably all, are on different chromosomes. Only two of the poorly marked groups, 2 and 5, remain to be correlated. The possible autosomes have been narrowed to chromosome 5 and either 4 or 8, whichever proves not to bear group 10.

The wealth of characteristics, cytological and biological, wherein the translocations differ deserves emphasis. These stocks vary in the autosomes affected, size of exchanged pieces, breakup of the translocation configuration in meiosis, fecundity (eggs per ootheca), and mortality. Apparently the latter arise from differing frequencies of alternate *vs.* adjacent disjunction. Certain stocks show sex differences in some of these features. The range of characteristics is, to our knowledge, unique among insects, but then, where else are there identifiable breakpoints in 11 autosomes of varying length?

The progress made to date in our attempt to establish *B. germanica* as a genetically useful animal stems from a combination of genetic and cytologic data. Cytologic findings have unraveled genetic problems and *vice versa*. We have only begun to utilize the translocations in genetic experiments, but already there are a multitude of opportunities for continued research.

Literature Cited

Cochran, D. G., 1973a   Inheritance and linkage of pyrethrins resistance in the German cockroach. *J. Econ. Entomol.* **66**:27–30.

Cochran, D. G., 1973b   Inheritance of malathion resistance in the German cockroach. *Entomol. Exp. Appl.* **16**:83–90.

Cochran, D. G. and M. H. Ross, 1961   Balloon-wing, a new mutation in *Blattella germanica* (L.). *Virginia J. Sci.* **12**(N.S.):10–17.

Cochran, D. G. and M. H. Ross, 1962a   Inheritance of resistance to DDT in *Blattella germanica*. *J. Econ. Entomol.* **55**:88–89.

Cochran, D. G. and M. H. Ross, 1962b   Inheritance of DDT resistance in a European strain of *Blattella germanica* (L.). *Bull. WHO* **27**:257–261.

Cochran, D. G. and M. H. Ross, 1967a   Cockroach genetics. In *Genetics of Insect Vectors of Disease*, edited by J. W. Wright and R. Pal, pp. 403–415, Elsevier, Amsterdam.

Cochran, D. G. and M. H. Ross, 1967*b* Preliminary studies of the chromosomes of twelve cockroach species (Blattaria: Blattidae, Blatellidae, Blaberidae). *Ann. Entomol. Soc. Am.* **60**:1265–1272.

Cochran, D. G. and M. H. Ross, 1969 Chromosome identification in the German cockroach. *J. Hered.* **60**:87–92.

Cochran, D. G. and M. H. Ross, 1974 Cytology and genetics of T(9:11) in the German cockroach, and its relationship to other chromosome 9 traits. *Can. J. Genet. Cytol.* **16**:639–649.

Cohen, S. and L. M. Roth, 1970 Chromosome numbers of the Blattaria. *Ann. Entomol. Soc. Am.* **63**:1520–1547.

Cornwell, P. B., 1968 *The Cockroach,* Vol. I, Hutchinson, London.

Craig, G. B. and W. A. Hickey, 1967 Genetics of *Aedes aegypti.* In *Genetics of Insect Vectors of Disease,* edited by J. W. Wright and R. Pal, pp. 67–131, Elsevier, Amsterdam.

Jancey, R. D. and D. B. Walden, 1972 Analysis of pattern in distribution of breakage points in the chromosomes of *Zea mays* L. and *D. melanogaster* Meigen. *Can. J. Genet. Cytol.* **15**:429–442.

Lewis, K. R. and B. John, 1957 Studies on *Periplaneta americana.* II. Interchange heterozygosity in isolated populations. *Heredity* **11**:11–22.

McDonald, I. C., M. H. Ross and D. G. Cochran, 1969 Genetics and linkage of aldrin resistance in the German cockroach. *Bull. WHO* **40**:745–752.

Rehn, J. A. G., 1945 Man's uninvited fellow traveler—The cockroach. *Sci. Monthly* **61**:265–276.

Ross, M. H., 1964 Pronotal wings in *Blattella germanica* (L.) and their possible evolutionary significance. *Am. Mid. Nat.* **71**:161–180.

Ross, M. H., 1966*a* Notched sternite: A mutant of *Blattella germanica,* with possible implications for the homology and evolution of ventral abdominal structures. *Ann. Entomol. Soc. Am.* **59**:473–484.

Ross, M. H., 1966*b* Embryonic appendages of the notched sternite mutant of *Blattella germanica. Ann. Entomol. Soc. Am.* **59**:1160–1162.

Ross, M. H., 1971*a* Genetic variability in the German cockroach. VII. Studies of pale-body and bulge-eye. *J. Hered.* **62**:110–116.

Ross, M. H., 1971*b* Three-point data for linkage group VI of the German cockroach. *Ann. Entomol. Soc. Am.* **64**:1178–1180.

Ross, M. H., 1972 Genetic variability in the German cockroach. VIII. Studies of deformed-leg and broad-banded pronotum. *J. Hered.* **63**:26–32.

Ross, M. H., 1973*a* The notch-pronotum, shriveled-wing and cubitus interruptus mutants of the German cockroach. *Ann. Entomol. Soc. Am.* **66**:112–116.

Ross, M. H., 1973*b* Additional data for linkage group X of the German cockroach. *J. Hered.* **64**:44–45.

Ross, M. H., 1973*c* Genetic variability in the German cockroach. IX. Genetics of narrow abdomen and Elo black-body. *J. Hered.* **64**:143–146.

Ross, M. H., 1974 The genetics and linkage of odd-body, a mutant of the German cockroach. *Ann. Entomol. Soc. Am.* **67**:416–420.

Ross, M. H. and D. G. Cochran, 1962 A body colour mutation in the German cockroach. *Nature (Lond.)* **195**:518–519.

Ross, M. H. and D. G. Cochran, 1965 A preliminary report on genetic variability in the German cockroach, *Blattella germanica. Ann. Entomol. Soc. Am.* **58**:368–375.

Ross, M. H. and D. G. Cochran, 1966　Genetic variability in the German cockroach. I. Additional genetic data and the establishment of tentative linkage groups. *J. Hered.* **57**:221–226.

Ross, M. H. and D. G. Cochran, 1967　Genetic variability in the German cockroach. II. A description of new mutants and linkage tests. *J. Hered.* **58**:274–278.

Ross, M. H. and D. G. Cochran, 1968*a*　Genetic variability in the German cockroach. III. Eye color traits and linkage data for the curly, hooded and pallid mutants. *J. Hered.* **59**:105–110.

Ross, M. H. and D. G. Cochran, 1968*b*　Genetic variability in the German cockroach. IV. Linkage studies with markers for groups III and VIII. *J. Hered.* **59**:318–320.

Ross, M. H. and D. G. Cochran, 1969*a*　Genetic variability in the German cockroach. V. Studies of the yellow and curved mutants. *J. Hered.* **60**:361–364.

Ross, M. H. and D. G. Cochran, 1969*b*　Red-rose linkage in the German cockroach. *Ann. Entomol. Soc. Am.* **62**:665–666.

Ross, M. H. and D. G. Cochran, 1970　Genetic variability in the German cockroach. VI. Studies of fused-antennae, crossveinless and downturned-wing. *J. Hered.* **61**:123–128.

Ross, M. H. and D. G. Cochran, 1971　Cytology and genetics of a pronotal-wing trait in the German cockroach. *Can. J. Genet. Cytol.* **13**:522–535.

Ross, M. H. and D. G. Cochran, 1973　German cockroach genetics and its possible use in control measures. *Patna J. Med.* **47**:325–337.

Roth, L. M., 1970　Interspecific mating in Blattaria. *Ann. Entomol. Soc. Am.* **63**:1282–1285.

Smith, P. D. and J. C. Lucchesi, 1969　The role of sexuality in dosage compensation in *Drosophila. Genetics* **61**:607–618.

Stevens, N. M., 1905　Studies in spermatogenesis with special reference to the "accessory chromosome." *Carnegie Inst. Wash. Publ.* **36**:1–75.

Suomalainen, E., 1946　Die Chromosomenverhaltnisse in der Spermatogenese einiger Blattarien. *Ann. Acad. Sci. Fenn.* **4**:1–60.

VandeHey, R. C., 1969　Incidence of genetic mutations in *Culex pipiens. Mosquito News* **29**:183–189.

Wassilieff, A., 1907　Die Spermatogenese von *Blatta germanica. Arch. Mikroscop. Anat.* **70**:1–42.

White, M. J. D., 1973　*Animal Cytology and Evolution,* third edition, Cambridge University Press, Cambridge.

3

The Domesticated
Silkmoth, *Bombyx mori*

Yataro Tazima, Hiroshi Doira,

and Hiromu Akai

Introduction

The domesticated silkmoth, *Bombyx mori* L., is one of the organisms whose genetics has been most intensively studied. It is classified as belonging to the order Lepidoptera, the suborder Heteroneura, and the family Bombycidae (Latreille, 1802; Imms, 1957). This moth lacks certain of the special conveniences of *Drosophila melanogaster* for formal genetics. For example, its haploid chromosome number is 28, in contrast to 4 for the fruit fly. However, because of its relatively great size, it is far more suitable for the study of physiological, biochemical, and developmental problems. Furthermore, with the advances in our knowledge of the mechanism of silk production, the silkmoth has become recognized as an excellent experimental animal for studies in molecular biology.

In 1964 Tazima published *The Genetics of the Silkworm,* in which he gave a general account of the achievements made with this particular organism. In that book he described 81 loci, distributed among 19 linkage

Yataro Tazima—National Institute of Genetics, Misima, Japan. Hiroshi Doira—Kyushu University, Fukuoka, Japan. Hiromu Akai—National Sericultural Experiment Station, Tokyo, Japan.

groups. Ten years have passed, and 27 new loci have been discovered, and genetic maps are now available for three more linkage groups. At the present time there are 108 gene loci distributed among 22 linkage groups. There are still 6 linkage groups left unknown, but already they are each represented by an independent marker gene. Up-to-date linkage maps and lists of mutants are given in Figure 4 and Table 5, respectively.

During the past ten years investigations on biochemical and physiological traits have been enthusiastically carried forward, and a considerable number of biochemical genetic markers has become available. The study of silk production has made steady progress in the light of recent advances in molecular biology, and marked progress has also been made in the study of insect hormones. These topics are briefly reviewed in this article, and we have also provided brief explanations of the life cycle, rearing methods, artificial and semisynthetic diets, and the methods of artificial hatching, with the hope that these will all be helpful for the reader who is not well aquainted with this insect.

The Life Cycle

There are in the silkworm at least three different types of voltinism. Fertilized silkworm eggs laid in the autumn normally enter diapause after about two days of embryonic development. Such embryos will complete their development only if they have been exposed to a temperature of around 0°C for several months. Some races of *B. mori* have one generation per year and are called "univoltine." In such strains every generation enters embryonic diapause. Other races are bivoltine or multivoltine. In these, there are two or more uninterrupted generations during the summer, before the winter generation of diapause eggs is produced. The serosal cells of such diapause eggs are characterized by pigment deposits. Silkworm races indigenous to temperate regions are either univoltine or bivoltine, while those of subtropical regions usually exhibit multivoltine behavior. The moths of univoltine and bivoltine races lay diapausing eggs when they are incubated at high temperature (> 25°C) and long day length (>16 hours). Under natural conditions these eggs estivate, hibernate, and hatch out the following spring. However, if desired, eggs can be induced to hatch within two weeks by applying hydrochloric acid. Eggs which pass through diapause or are subjected to the HCl treatment hatch in 11–14 days when incubated at 23–25°C. The nondiapausing eggs laid by moths of multivoltine races or bivoltine races incubated at low temperature (<18°C) and in dark conditions complete embryonic development in 10–11 days.

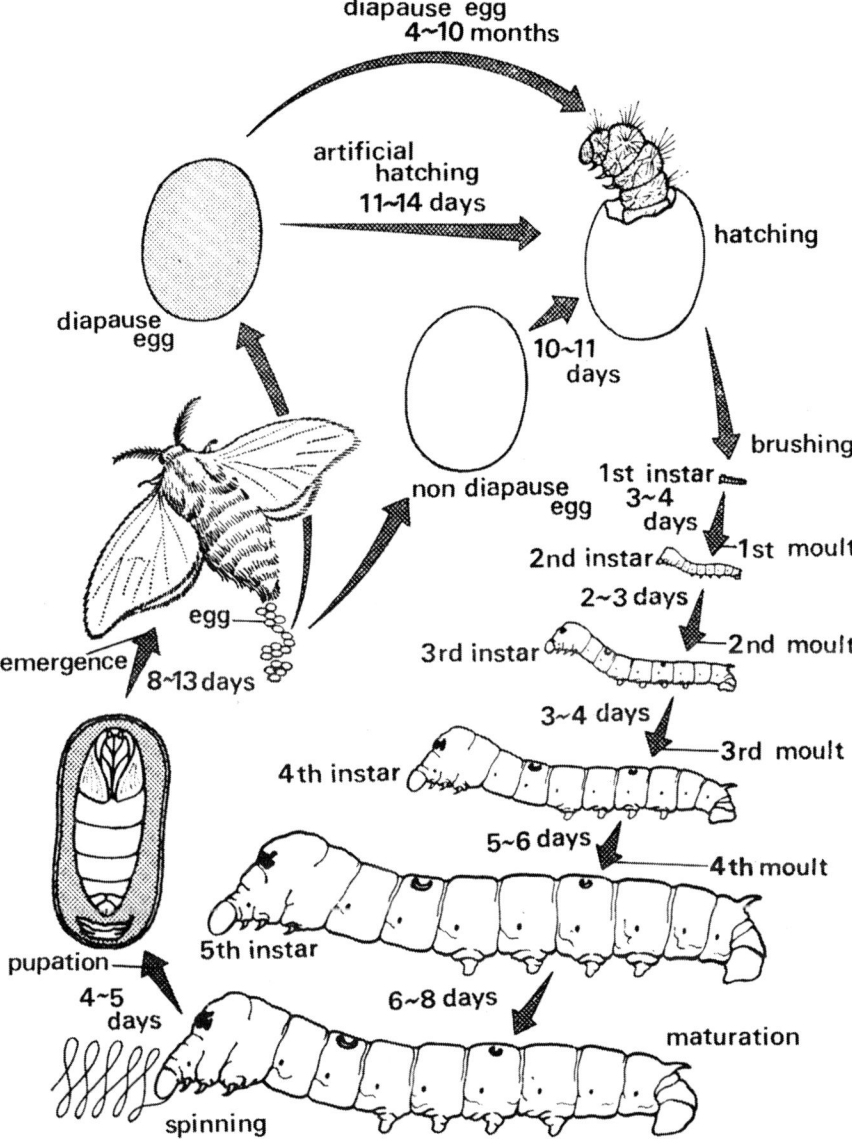

Figure 1. Life cycle of B. mori cultured at 24 ± 1°C. Adapted from Mori (1970a).

The life cycle of *B. mori* is diagramed in Figure 1. The newly hatched larvae are black, about 3 mm long, and are often called gisan (ants) by the Japanese. These tiny gisan grow very quickly, feeding solely on mulberry leaves. They will also grow on an artificial diet, but a fairly large proportion of mulberry-leaf powder is needed in the formula. The

TABLE 1. *Duration, Growth Rates, and Amount of Mulberry Leaves Supplied to Larvae*

| | Duration,[a] days | | | | |
Instar	Feeding	Molt	Total	Relative increase in body weight,[b] times	Leaves supplied,[c] g
1st	3.0	1.0	4.0	10–15	70
2nd	2.5	1.0	3.5	75–100	240
3rd	3.0	1.0	4.0	350–500	1,090
4th	4.0	1.5	5.5	1,800–2,200	5,000
5th	8.0	—	8.0	8,000–10,000	35,000
Total	20.5	4.5	25.0	10,000	41,400

[a] Duration for rearing Japanese bivoltine breeds at 25°C.
[b] The ranges shown are for seven commercial breeds.
[c] The amount refers to weight of leaves per 1000 hybrid larvae from the cross J 122 × C 122.

durations of each instar and the rates of increase in body weight are shown in Table 1.

When larvae are fully grown and ready to spin cocoons, they are called "ripe" or "mature." They stop eating and become very restless, raising their heads in search of an appropriate substratum for cocoon spinning. In the mature larva, the silk glands are so large that they make up about 40 percent of the body weight. The larvae are next transferred to a spinning nest, which is usually made of straw or cardboard. This transfer is called jôzoku (mounting) by the Japanese. It takes a larva 4 or 5 days after mounting to pupate, and another 8–13 days pass before the moths emerge. This emergence usually takes place in the morning.

The male and female moths (Figure 2) mate soon after emergence. When one wishes to cross moths from two different strains, the moths must be separated before the adults emerge to ensure the virginity of the female. Different sexes are identified either by the genital imaginal buds of the larvae or the pupae, or by utilizing sex-limited serosal color or larval markings. The latter is possible only in special translocation strains (Tazima, 1941; Hasimoto, 1948b; Tazima *et al.*, 1951; Sturunnikov and Gulamova, 1969). As to the duration of copulation, periods of 2–3 hours are enough to ensure good fertility. A male moth can mate with two or three females, but its ability to copulate deteriorates very quickly. If males are kept in a refrigerator at 10°C when not mating, their sexual ability can be preserved for a week.

The female moth starts to lay eggs shortly after separation from the male and continues oviposition overnight until almost all eggs are deposited. From 350 to 650 eggs are laid by one mother, with an average of about 500. Eggs are not covered with pigment when deposited, but they have a light or dark yellow tint, depending on the coloration of the yolk. Diapausing wild-type eggs gradually develop the final dark color as pigment granules are formed in the serosal cells, a process that is completed 5–7 days after deposition. In contrast, nondiapausing eggs do not form pigment. Storage for at least three months at low temperatures (2–5°C) is necessary to break the dormancy of diapausing eggs and to induce subsequent development at warm incubation temperatures. The length of the incubation period prior to hatching is 11–14 days at 23–25°C. The whole life cycle of the silkworm takes about 45–50 days at the optimum

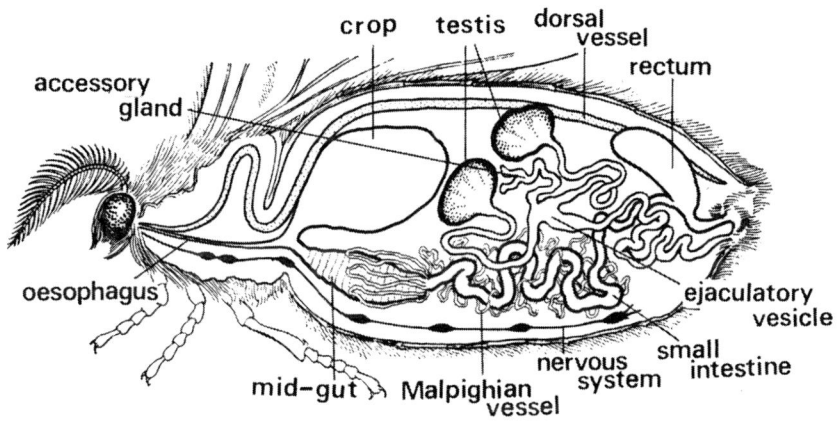

A

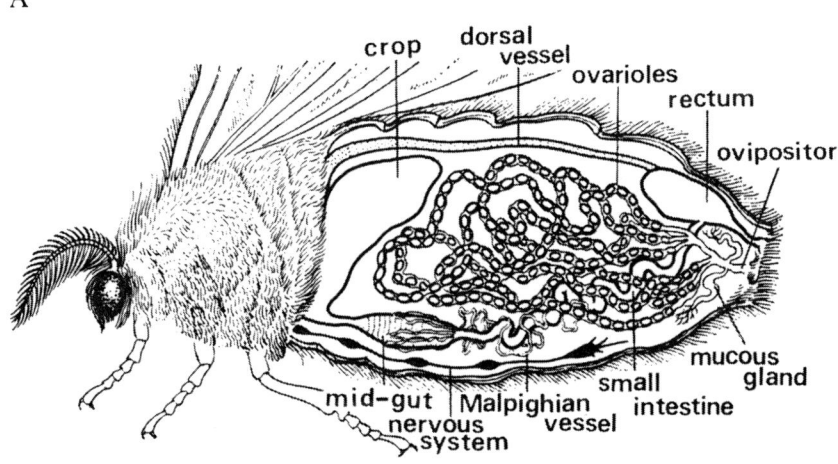

B

Figure 2. The internal organs of adult male (A) and female (B) of B. mori. Adapted from Mori (1970a).

temperature of 25°C. A collection of 60 color slides is available illustrating the various stages in the life cycle of the silkmoth (Mori, 1970b).

Artificial and Semisynthetic Diets

Since the initial success in rearing silkworms on an artificial diet in 1960, efforts have been made by many workers to find suitable dietary compositions, not only for practical rearing, but also for several experimental purposes. At present it is possible to foster normal growth and to produce cocoons of almost normal size and weight from larvae grown upon artificial diets which contain mulberry-leaf powder as one of the essential components. An example of such an artificial diet is shown in Table 2. This diet contains approximately 50 percent dried-mulberry-leaf powder. It is possible, however, to decrease the proportion of leaf powder. Furthermore, a semisynthetic diet has been devised which can be used for culturing silkworms through all larval stages; its composition is given in Table 3. Larval growth is more-or-less retarded, but it should be appreciated that natural substances, such as mulberry powder and soybean meal, are replaced by pure amino acids in this formulation.

*TABLE 2.   An Example of an
Artificial Diet for Bombyx[a]*

Substance	Dry diet, g
Dried-mulberry-leaf powder	50
Potato starch	20
Soybean meal	20
Mineral	1
Ascorbic acid	2
Citric acid	0.5
Cellulose powder	8
Agar	12
Total	113.5
Vitamin B mixture[b]	Added
Antiseptic[c]	Added
Distilled water	300 ml

[a] See Ito (1969) for details.
[b] Vitamins (μg/g of the dry diet): biotin, 2; choline chloride, 1500; folic acid, 2; inositol, 2000; niacin, 100; Ca-pantothenate, 150; pyridoxine-HCl, 30; riboflavin, 20; and thiamine, 20.
[c] Sorbic acid, 0.3 g or propionic acid, 1.0 g.

TABLE 3. Semisynthetic Diet for Bombyx[a]

Substance	Dry diet, g
Agar	15.0
Potato starch	5.0
Sucrose	15.0
Amino acid mixture[b]	20.0
Soybean oil, refined	3.0
β-Sitosterol	0.5
Salt mixture	4.0
Ascorbic acid	2.0
Cellulose powder	35.2
Morin = pentahydroxyflavone	0.3
Total	100.0
Vitamin B mixture[c]	Added
Antiseptic	Added
Distilled water	300 ml

[a] See Ito and Arai (1966) for further details.
[b] Amino acids (parts by weight): arginine–HCl, 6.0; histidine–HCl, 2.5; isoleucine, 5.5; leucine, 8.5; lysine–HCl, 6.0; methionine, 2.5; phenylalanine, 5.5; proline, 4.0; threonine, 5.0; tryptophan, 4.0; valine, 6.0; alanine, 7.0; aspartate, 12.0; cystine, 2.5; glutamate, 12.0; glycine, 4.5; hydroxyproline, 1.0; serine, 3.5; tyrosine, 2.0.
[c] Identical to the formulation shown in the footnote *b* of Table 2.

As to artificial diets, two kinds of rearing systems have been investigated, one with diets containing an antiseptic and the other by "aseptic rearing" with diets containing only small amounts of an antiseptic. So far, the latter system seems more promising for small-scale culture. Erlenmeyer flasks are usually used for this purpose. The components of the diet, previously ground and mixed thoroughly, are transferred with water containing the vitamins and antiseptic to a Petri dish. The dish is heated to approximately 95°C in a water bath for 10 minutes and then cooled, whereupon the medium becomes a gel. The gel is cut into slices and placed in sterilized flasks, which are plugged with cotton and autoclaved for 20 minutes at 10 psi pressure. The silkworm eggs, disinfected beforehand by immersion in 2-percent formalin for 15 minutes and rinsed in sterile water, are placed on slices of the medium in sterile flasks, which are then incubated at 25°C. As soon as the larvae hatch, they start feeding. Since silkworms grow very quickly, enough space and nutrient must be supplied. For large-scale culture, special methods have been devised (Shimizu and Ito, 1973).

TABLE 4.   *Artificial Hatching Method and the Time Interval between Oviposition and the Start of the Next Rearing*

Method	Interval between oviposition and rearing, days	Duration of cold storage, days
Ordinary	12	—
Acid treatment followed by cold storage	30	20
Acid treatment following cold storage	52–72	40–60

Artificial Hatching Methods

An appropriate method for inducing hatching can be applied depending on the time interval scheduled between oviposition and the start of the next rearing (See Table 4).

Hydrochloric Acid Treatment

Eggs that have been kept at 25°C for 20–25 hours after oviposition are soaked in warm hydrochloric acid. The standardized conditions are (1) hydrochloric acid at a specific gravity of 1.075 at 15°C, (2) the acid bath maintained at 46°C, and (3) treatment for 4–8 minutes, depending on the *Bombyx* strain, the temperature, and the age of the eggs. After soaking, eggs are washed with water to remove the acid and are dried in air at 25°C. The eggs hatch about 11 days after treatment when incubated at 25°C. If desired, the hatching time can be prolonged 20 days more by storing the eggs at 5°C one day after the acid treatment. Cold storage longer than 3 weeks is injurious to the embryo.

Acid Treatment after Cold Storage

The time interval between the deposition and the start of the next rearing can be prolonged far longer, if eggs are refrigerated first and then treated with hydrochloric acid. In this method eggs are transferred from 25°C to 5°C 42–50 hours after oviposition and are kept in cold storage for 40–60 days. Then they are allowed to return to room temperature for 3 hours and are subsequently treated with hydrochloric acid. The standard conditions for acid treatment are a specific gravity of 1.10 at 15°C, the temperature of the acid bath at 48°C, and treatment for 5–10 minutes.

The Production of Silk Substance

Once they have attained maturity, *Bombyx* larvae produce in their silk glands large amounts of various silk proteins (fibroin and three kinds of sericin). The silk gland is a large, tubular gland which folds upon itself posteriorly (see Figure 3). The gland is divided into anterior, middle, and posterior divisions. The main fibrous component of silk fibroin is produced in the posterior division of the gland, while the gelatinous component, sericin, which coats the fibroin, is secreted in the middle division. The fibroin has a very simple sequence of amino acids. Taken together, glycine, alanine, and serine make up 86 percent of the amino acids of fibroin, and 60 percent of each fibroin molecule consists largely of

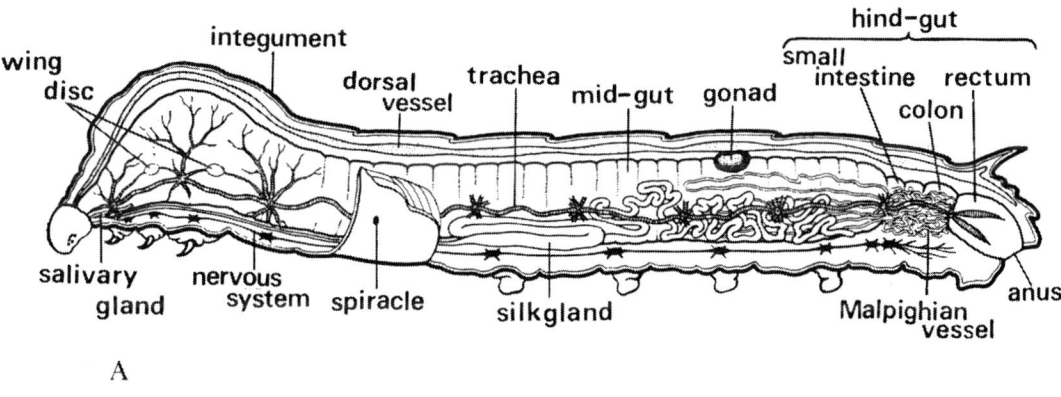

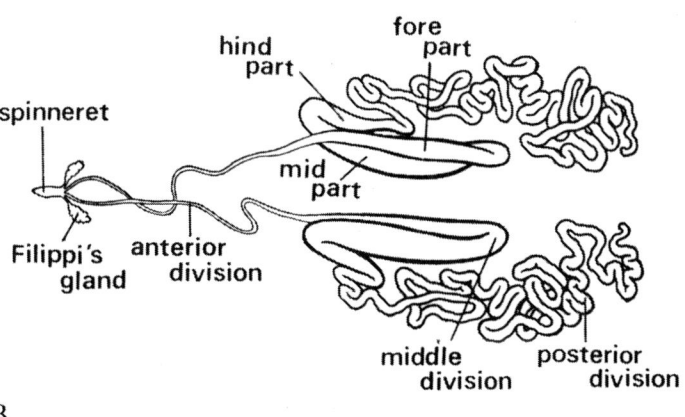

Figure 3. (A) Internal organs of larva of B. mori. (B) The silk gland of the silkworm. Adapted from Mori (1970a).

a repeating hexapeptide sequence, Gly-Ala-Gly-Ala-Gly-Ser (Lucas and Rudall, 1968). Granular endoplasmic reticulum, Golgi apparatus, and fibroin globules are conspicuous in cells of the posterior silk gland that are actively synthesizing this silk protein (Akai, 1963). The fibroin molecules stored in Golgi vacuoles have been observed under the electron microscope. They are helical bundles of about 130 Å in diameter and are composed of 5–7 threads, each 20–30 Å thick (Akai, 1971). Those organelles necessary for the biosynthesis of fibroin are rapidly organized in the cell at an earlier stage of the fifth instar so that synthesis of fibroin proceeds at the maximum rate later in the same instar (Morimoto *et al.,* 1968). By this time the mRNA necessary for the production of fibroin is synthesized and accumulated in the cell, comprising about 1 percent of the cellular RNA (Suzuki and Brown, 1972). Recently the fibroin mRNAs from *B. mori* (Suzuki *et al.,* 1972; Suzuki and Suzuki, 1974) and *B. mandarina* have been isolated and their nucleotide sequences have been partially determined (Suzuki, 1974).

Matsuzaki (1966) observed a correlation between the amino acid composition of fibroin and the extent of acylation of each tRNA in an *in vitro* system that contained tRNA and aminoacyl-tRNA synthetases obtained from the posterior silk gland of late-fifth-instar larvae. Kawakami and Shimura (1973) reported preparing Gly-tRNAs from the posterior silk gland of fifth-instar larvae. They isolated three fractions (tRNA$_1^{Gly}$, tRNA$_{2-1}^{Gly}$, and tRNA$_{2-2}^{Gly}$) which were 70–90 percent pure. They also separated Ala-tRNAs into 6 fractions, 4 of which were 70–90 percent pure. These three isoaccepting tRNA^{Gly}s were tested for their *in vitro* ribosome-binding activity in the presence of artificially synthesized triplets. The tRNA$_1^{Gly}$ responded to GGA and GGG, and both tRNA$_{2-1}^{Gly}$ and tRNA$_{2-2}^{Gly}$ responded to GGU and GGC.

DNA contents of the silk gland cells have been measured with special reference to the polyploidization which takes place in their nuclei. Gillot and Daillie (1968) found that the DNA content of the silk gland increased from the end of the second instar to the end of the fifth instar (from 0.4 μg per gland to 150 μg per gland). Also, Morimoto *et al.* (1968) and Tashiro *et al.* (1968) measured an increase in the DNA content of the posterior silk glands from 1.5 μg per gland at the beginning of the fourth instar to 100 μg per gland at the middle of the fifth instar. A preliminary study by Feulgen microspectrophotometry has revealed that a single, posterior silk gland cell nucleus on the sixth day of the fifth instar has 400,000 times as much DNA as a spermatogonium (Nakanishi *et al.,* 1969).

From recent studies it seems quite clear that the increase in DNA in silk gland cells during the last week of larval life is accomplished by multiple cycles of uniform replication of all sequences in the *B. mori* genome. Neither the fibroin genes, nor any other detectable DNA fraction, fails to replicate, is under-replicated, or is specifically amplified during periods of DNA synthesis by silk gland cells (Gage, 1974a,b; Gage *et al.*, 1972).

Hormones

Much progress has been made in the purification of insect hormones, and a great deal is known concerning the mechanism of their actions.

The Brain Hormone

The brain hormone plays an important role in molting and metamorphosis through controlling the activity of the prothoracic gland. Since the brain hormone was extracted from *B. mori* by Kobayashi and Kirimura (1958), the purification of the hormone has been continued by several investigators. The hormone was shown to be a protein by Ichikawa and Ishizaki (1963). Recently, the hormone has been purified from an extract of brains of *Bombyx* pupae (Kobayashi and Yamazaki, 1966; Yamazaki and Kobayashi, 1969). Only 0.02 μg of this purified hormone is required to cause adult development in a test abdomen. The hormone is inactivated by treatment with trypsin, pronase, and subtilysin, but it is not inactivated by chymotrypsin or sialidase. Its molecular weight was estimated by gel filtration on Sephadex G-100 to be about 20,000. A highly purified preparation was made by means of zone electrophoresis on acrylamide gels. This hormone may be a glycoprotein.

The Prothoracic Gland and Ecdysone

Since the endocrinological studies of Fukuda (1940) and the chemical studies of Butenandt and Karlson (1954) on the *Bombyx* molting hormone were first published, it has generally been believed that the prothoracic glands are responsible for ecdysone synthesis. Karson and Hoffmeister (1963) have shown that ecdysone is derived from dietary cholesterol. Ultrastructural observations of the prothoracic gland cells in the silkworm have revealed a close correlation between mitochondrial transformations and the cyclical release of ecdysone. Observations support the conclusion that both mitochondrial enzymes and those bound to the agranular endoplasmic reticulum are involved in the conversion of cholesterol to ecdysone (Beaulaton, 1968). Recent studies in which isolated prothoracic glands of *Bombyx* were cultured in an improved medium have proved conclusively that the prothoracic gland is the site where the molting hormone is synthesized (Chino *et al.*, 1974). The product secreted into the medium behaved similarly to free ecdysone during thin-layer chromatography, and chemical analysis revealed that the hormone was identical to α-ecdysone.

Juvenile Hormone

The successful identification and synthesis of the juvenile hormone (JH) of *Hyalophora cecropia* moth (Röller *et al.*, 1967; Dahm *et al.*, 1967) has prompted the use of JH as a new insecticide. On the other hand, JH has been administered to *B. mori* in hope of inducing increased silk production (Akai *et al.*, 1971; Chang *et al.*, 1972; Niimura *et al.*, 1972). A single injection of JH during the early half of the fifth instar prolongs the duration of the feeding period, of RNA synthesis, and of fibroin synthesis. The cocoon shell weight increases about 30 percent as compared with that of controls (Akai *et al.*, 1973). Also, a single injection of large amount of JH induces dauer larvae, which are inhibited from undergoing the larva to pupa metamorphosis. Moreover, the injection of JH into allatectomized larvae suppresses the deposition of the black pigment which causes the larval markings (Kiguchi, 1972).

The Diapause Hormone

Silkmoths lay either pigmented diapause eggs or unpigmented nondiapause eggs. The diapause hormone (DH) is responsible for the determination of embryonic diapause and pigmentation of the egg; DH is secreted from the subesophageal ganglion under the control of the brain during the pupal stage (Hasegawa, 1957). The hormone also plays an important role in the accumulation of 3-hydroxykynurenine and glycogen in developing oocytes (Yamashita *et al.*, 1972). Two diapause hormones were recently extracted from the heads of 2 million adult *Bombyx* males (Isobe *et al.*, 1973). One of the hormones is a protein with a molecular weight between 2000 and 4000.

Gametogenesis and Crossing Over

Studies of gametogenesis in both sexes of *Bombyx* have shown that sister germ cells are joined by canals (Nakanishi *et al.*, 1965). Since intercellular connections of this type result from an arrested cleavage furrow (King and Akai, 1971a; Danilova, 1974), it follows that both male and female gametocytes undergo a specialized type of mitotic division prior to meiosis that involves incomplete cytokinesis. In the male a cycle of six divisions occurs, and it results in a cluster of 64 interconnected, sister spermatocytes. In the female only three divisions occur, and these generate a cluster of eight cells. The sister spermatocytes go through the stages of meiotic prophase in synchrony, and all eventually complete the meiotic divisions. These haploid cells contain 0.52×10^{-12} g DNA (Rasch, 1974). However, in the female only one of the eight sister germ cells undergoes the meiotic nuclear divisions. The other seven become highly endopolyploid nurse cells. These transfer their cytoplasm to the oocyte which grows at their expense (Miya *et al.*, 1969).

Synapsis of homologous chromosomes is an essential prerequisite for normal meiotic crossing over. Synapsis is accomplished through the construction of a synaptonemal complex. Sado (1963) reported that spermatocytes in synaptic stages of meiosis are first seen in silkworms during the fourth instar. King and Akai (1971b) made ultrastructural studies of such spermatocytes; synaptonemal complexes were observed and a model was advanced to explain the three dimensional packing of the DNA of the tetrads into this organelle. In *B. mori* crossing over occurs only in males, which are the homogametic sex (Tanaka, 1914). Presumably crossing over cannot occur until the fourth instar, when synaptonemal complexes first appear. In the female synaptonemal complexes have been reported in oocytes during the fifth larval instar (Miya *et al.*, 1970). Since crossing over does not occur in females, it is probable that certain of the enzyme systems required for the molecular events that result in an exchange between DNA duplexes [see Whitehouse's review (1970)] are missing in oocyte nuclei.

Genetical Approaches to Biochemical and Physiological Traits

Recent studies on the genetic control of biochemical and physiological traits have taken advantage of fairly numerous genes affecting (1) the nonenzymic proteins of the hemolymph, (2) the hemocytes, (3) the enzymes of various tissues, and (4) the behavior of the embryo with respect to diapause. The list of *Bombyx* genes is given in Table 5. Linkage maps are given in Figure 4.

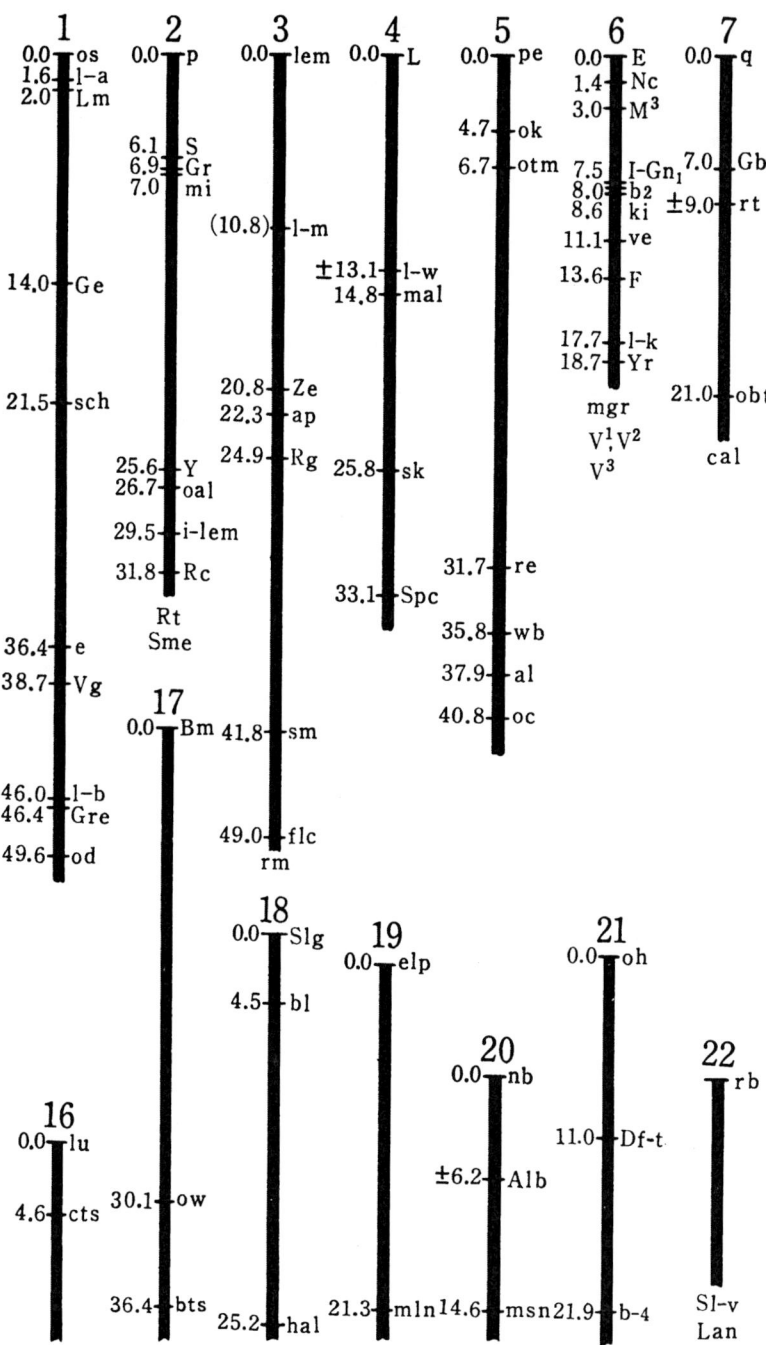

Figure 4. The linkage maps of B. mori. Females are ZW and males are ZZ. The Z chro-

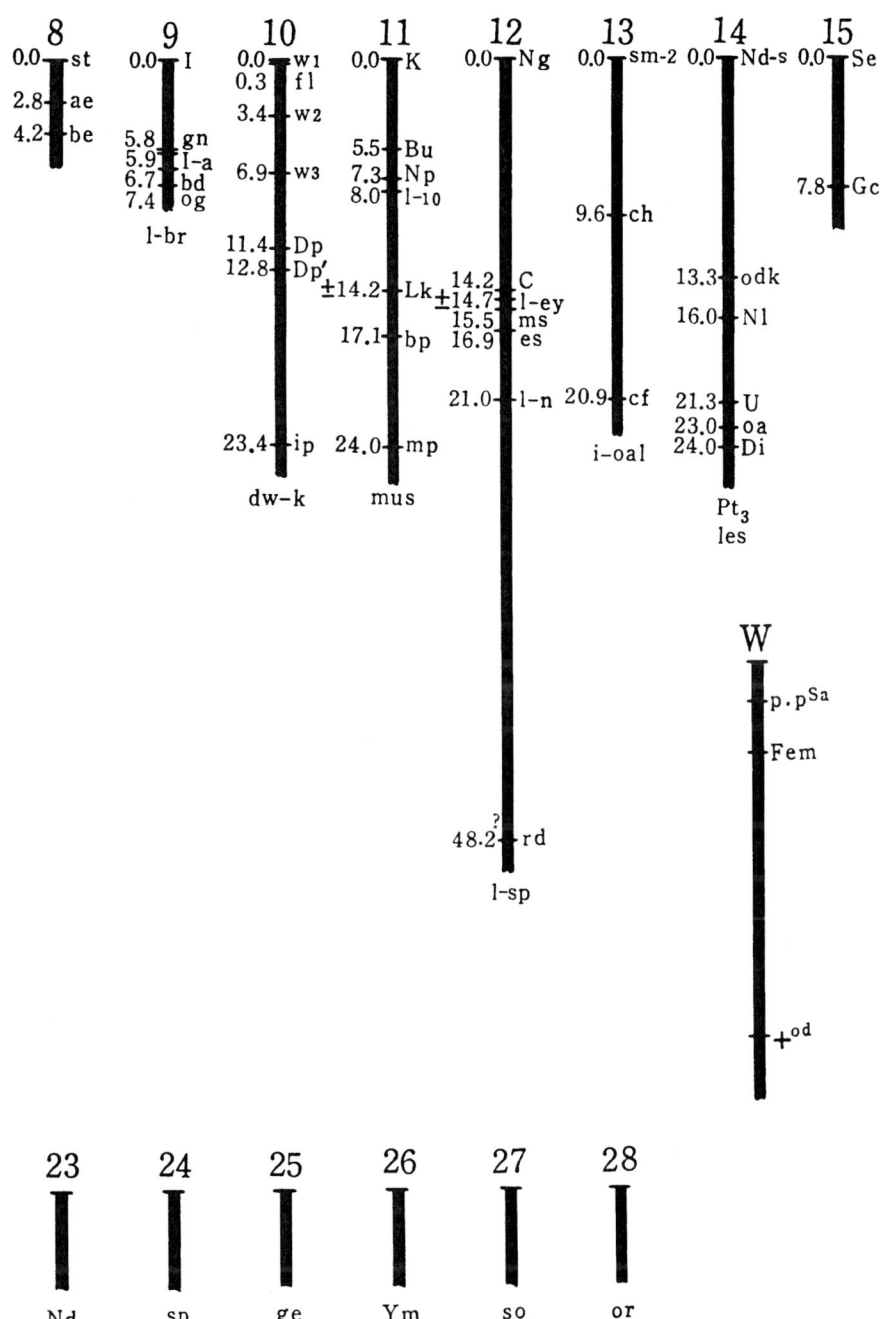

mosome is number 1. For a discussion of sex determination see Tazima (1964, Chapter 5).

TABLE 5. List of *Bombyx* Genes[a]

Gene[b] symbol	Locus[c]	Name of gene	Phenotypic expression[a]	Authority
EGG				
b_1	6–8.0	Brown egg 1	Serosa cells brown, inherited maternally; compound eye black	Toyama (1912, 1913), Nagashima (1956)
b_2	6–8.0	Brown egg 2	Serosa cells brown, inherited maternally; compound eye black	Uda (1923)
b_3	10–6.9	Brown egg 3	Serosa cells light brown; larval skin weakly translucent; compound eye black.	Tazima (1958)
b_4	21–21.9	Brown egg 4	Serosa cells reddish brown; compound eye of the moth black but faintly reddish	Nakajima (1956), Doira *et al.* (1974*a*)
bo	—	Ordinary brown	Serosa cells light brown, inherited ordinarily; compound eye black.	Tanaka (1924*a*)
coc	5–31.7	Cocoa	Serosa cells reddish brown; larval head cocoa colored; compound eye deep red	Tanaka (1952), Chikushi *et al.* (1972)
Dp	10–11.4	Dilute purple	Serosa cells light purple; compound eye black	Chikushi (1959*b*)
Dp'	10–12.8	Dilute purple 2	Like *Dp*, but located separately	
E-Gr[L]	2–?	Epistatic gene to *Gr[L]*	Suppresses inhibitory action of *I-Gr[L]*	Takasaki (1947*c*)
Ees₁	—	Egg esterase 1	Five kinds of isozymes are known in eggs; *Ees₁* and *Ees₂* are identified as	
Ees₂	—	Egg esterase 2	cholinesterases; *Ees₃*, *Ees₄*, and *Ees₅* as	Yoshitake and Akiyama (1965*a*)
Ees₃	—	Egg esterase 3	aliesterases	
Ees₄	—	Egg esterase 4		
Ees₅	—	Egg esterase 5		
elp	19–0.0	Ellipsoid egg	Egg shape ellipsoidal; no dimple on egg surface	Hasimoto (1961)

Fc	—	Ferric chloride positive	Egg shell is dyed with FeCl$_3$	Shimizu and Horiuchi (1959)
Ge	1–14.0	Giant egg	Egg size large, longitudinal wrinkles on egg surface	Aruga (1943e)
Gr	2–6.9	Gray egg	Egg shape ellipsoidal; shells opaque in heterozygote, but transparent in homozygote	Toyama (1910), Tanaka (1919)
Gr^{16}	2–6.9	E-16 gray egg	Egg shell highly opaque; longitudinal wrinkles on egg surface	Takasaki (1947c)
Gr^{B}	2–6.9	Egg resembling bird's eye	Egg laid by heterozygote is gray at the periphery, but transparent in the center; homozygote infertile	Takasaki (1947c)
Gr^{col}	2–6.9	Collapsing egg	Eggs collapse soon after deposition; recessive to normal	Sado and Chikushi (1958)
Gr^{L}	2–6.9	Light gray egg	Egg shell faintly opaque, slightly wrinkled	Takasaki (1947c)
Gr^{X-1}	2–6.9	Gray egg X-1	Chorion grayish, expression variable	⎫ Takasaki (1958)
Gr^{X-2}	2–6.9	Gray egg X-2	Phenotype similar to *Gr^{X-1}*	⎬
Gre	1–46.4	Green egg shell	Egg shell tinged yellowish green	Aruga (1943f)
I-Gr^{L}	2–?	Inhibitor of light gray egg	Expression of *Gr^{L}* is inhibited; lethal when homozygous	Takasaki (1947c)
ip	10–23.4	Inhibited purple egg	Serosa cells faintly purple	Chikushi (1959b)
ki	6–8.6	Kidney	Egg kidney shaped; only ectodermal tissues develop during embryogenesis	Suzuki (1932), Takasaki et al. (1957)

[a] In this list the silkworm genes are classified into groups according to the different developmental stages and physiological traits they affect. Wild-type genes are not listed, with some exceptions. The grouping is rather arbitrary. Lethals that manifest their action in the embryonic stage are classified under the Egg heading, but those accompanied by retarded growth in larval stages are dealt with under the Physiological heading. Illustrations for many of the mutants can be found in Tazima (1964) and Chikushi (1972).

[b] Dominant or recessive genes are symbolized by capital or lower case letters, respectively. Mutants which have been lost are indicated by an asterisk to the left of the gene symbol.

[c] The first Arabic number gives the linkage group and those following the hyphen give the locus.

[d] COV = crossover value.

TABLE 5. Continued

Gene[b] symbol	Locus[c]	Name of gene	Phenotypic expression[a]	Authority
ki[c]	6–8.6	Kidney of Chikushi	Phenotype similar to ki	Doira et al. (1973b)
*l-10	11–8.0	Lethal 10	Homozygote lethal in embryo	Shimodaira (1947a)
l-72	—	Lethal 72	Homozygote lethal in embryo	Takasaki (1947c)
*l-a	1–1.6	Lethal a	Lethal in embryo	Tanaka (1941)
*l-b	1–46.0	Lethal b	Lethal in embryo	
*l-be	—	Brown egg lethal	Homozygote lethal in embryo	Nishikawa (1925)
*l-bk	—	Blastokinesis lethal	Homozygote lethal in embryo	
*l-bl	—	Bluish egg lethal	Homozygote lethal in embryo	Umeya (1927)
l-br	9–?	Lethal brown	Homozygote lethal showing brown pigmentation in serosa	Otsuki (1956), Chikushi et al. (1971b)
*l-d	—	Dark-spotted egg lethal	Homozygote lethal in embryo	Nishikawa (1925)
*l-db	—	Dark-spotted egg lethal b	Homozygote lethal in embryo	Nishikawa (1930)
l-ey	12–14.7 (±)	Early lethal	No pigmentation in serosa; lethal	Hasimoto (1960)
*l-hb	—	Hibernating egg lethal	Homozygote dies during hibernation	Umeya (1927)
l-k	6–17.7	Lethal k	Homozygote lethal in embryo	Hasimoto (1934b)
*l-m	3–10.8	Lethal m	Homozygote lethal in embryo; locus determined by crossing over between Ze and l-m	Hasimoto (1940)
*l-mn	—	Monster lethal	Lethal due to malformation of embryo	Nishikawa (1930)
l-n	12–21.0	Noncolored egg lethal	Serosa of homozygote colorless; dies before blastokinesis	Hirobe et al. (1952), Ooi (1968)
*l-r	—	Red egg lethal	Homozygote lethal in embryo	Nishikawa (1925)
*l-rb	—	Red egg lethal b	Homozygote lethal in embryo	Nishikawa (1930)
*l-sa	1–?	Sex-linked lethal a	Lethal in embryo	Nishikawa (1932)
*l-sb	1–?	Sex-linked lethal b	Lethal in embryo	
*l-sc	1–?	Sex-linked lethal c	Lethal in embryo	Nishikawa (1934)
*l-sd	1–?	Sex-linked lethal d	Lethal in embryo	

Symbol	Name	Map	Phenotype	Reference
l-sp	Lethal-spindle egg	12-?	Lethal in embryo	Hirobe (1952), Ooi (1962)
l-w	Lethal white-rot egg	4-13.1 (±)	Pigments aggregate in serosa cells; lethal in embryo	Nakayama (1958)
mgr	Mottled gray	6-?	Egg shell mottled gray	Sado (1957), Doira et al. (1971)
oew	White-egg translucent	10-6.9	Serosa colorless; larval skin highly translucent	Tanaka and Matsuno (1929), Chikushi (1957)
os^l	Sex-linked opaque lethal	1-0.0	Lethal in embryo	Tanaka (1933)
ove	Translucent-white egg	—	Serosa colorless; larval skin highly translucent	Sakata (1941)
pe	Pink-eyed white egg	5-0.0	Pigments in serosa cells light orange; compound eye pink	Uda (1928)
pe^l	White lethal egg	5-0.0	Homozygous egg colored yellow and lethal	Otsuki (1968)
rd	Clumpy	12-48.2	Egg shape irregular and highly variable; map position determined by crossing over between C and rd (34.0 COV)	Kei (1937)
re	Red	5-31.7	Pigments in serosa cells red; compound eye deep red; hatchability variable	Uda (1928)
Se	White-sided egg	15-0.0	Eggs laid by homozygote gray with wrinkles; eggs from heterozygote gray on the periphery of egg shell	Kei (1943)
sm	Small egg	3-41.8	Egg size extremely small and almost spherical; egg sterile	Hayashi (1937), Chikushi and Doira (1970)
sm-2	Small egg 2	13-0.0	Phenotype similar to *sm*	Otsuki (1965), Doira et al. (1974c)

TABLE 5. *Continued*

Gene[b] symbol	Locus[c]	Name of gene	Phenotypic expression[a]	Authority
Sme	2–?	Dominant small egg	Egg small, but fertile; lethal in embryo when homozygous	Takasaki (1947c)
sp	24–?	Spindle shaped	Egg shell attenuated at both ends; no hollowing on egg surface	Toyama (1912)
spm	—	Spanish brown	Egg dark yellow; compound eye black; semidominant	Nagashima et al. (1957)
w_1	10–0.0	White egg 1	No pigments in serosa cells, inherited maternally; compound eye white	Toyama (1910), Suzuki (1939)
w_2	10–3.4	White egg 2	Freshly laid eggs yellowish white, gradually becoming red tinted; compound eye white	Suzuki (1939)
w_3	10–6.9	White egg 3	Serosa cells light yellowish brown; larval skin weakly translucent; compound eye black	Suzuki (1943)
w^{ol}	10–6.9	Aojuku white-egg translucent	Serosa cells colorless; larval skin translucent; compound eye white; lethal when reared under 23°C	Nakano (1931), Kikkawa (1947)
w^{ox}	10–6.9	New white-egg translucent	Almost similar to w^{ol}	Tsujita (1960)
LARVA				
*Ac	3–?	Abnormal corselet	Fissure along dorsal median line of first and second thoracic segments, lethal when homozygous	Aruga (1943a)
ae	8–2.8	Digestive juice amylase-negative	Amylase activity in digestive juice distinctly weak	Matsumura (1933)
al	5–37.9	Albino	Body and head cuticle light brown; second instar larvae unable to eat leaves and starve to death	Tanaka (1952), Doira et al. (1973a)

Symbol	Name	Description		Reference
al^2	Albino 2	Like al, but the time of death variable	5–37.9	Doira et al. (1973a)
Alb^F	Albumin F	Albumin of hemolymph rapidly migrating during electrophoresis	20–6.2 (±)	Gamo (1968)
Alb^S	Albumin S	Albumin of hemolymph slowly migrating during electrophoresis	20–6.2 (±)	} Gamo (1968)
ap	Apodal	Thoracic legs degenerate; female moth less fertile; male fertile, but must be held in appropriate mating position by experimenter to achieve copulation	3–22.3	Hirobe (1944)
Aph_1	Alkaline phosphatase 1	Alkaline phosphatase isozyme of mid-gut characterized by fast electrophoretic mobility	—	Yoshitake (1964), Yoshitake et al. (1966)
Aph_2	Alkaline phosphatase 2	Alkaline phosphatase isozyme of mid-gut with slow mobility. Linked with Aph_1 with COV of ca. 31 percent	—	}
*A_S	Abnormal segment	First to fourth abdominal segments constricted; lethal when homozygous	—	Aruga (1943b)
*Bb	Brown body color	Body color of larva brown; lethal when homozygous	—	Shimodaira (1928)
bd	Dilute black	Larval trunk gray from first through sixth segment; female moth sterile	9–6.7	Sasaki (1941)
bd'	New dilute black	Similar to bd except for good fertility in female	9–6.7	Sakate and Nakasone (1962)
be	Body fluid amylase	Amylase activity in hemolymph distinctly weak	8–4.2	Matsumura (1933), Tazima et al. (1960)
Bes^A	Blood esterase A	The most rapidly moving isozyme of esterase in hemolymph	—	Eguchi et al. (1965)
Bes^B	Blood esterase B	Rapidly moving isozyme of esterase in hemolymph	—	}
Bes^C	Blood esterase C	Slowly moving isozyme of esterase in hemolymph	—	}
Bes^O	Blood esterase O	Isozyme band of esterase in hemolymph lacking	—	}

TABLE 5. Continued

Gene[b] symbol	Locus[c]	Name of gene	Phenotypic expression[a]	Authority
bl	18–4.5	Blind	Eye spot on the second segment completely black	Hirobe (1951), Chikushi (1960b)
Bph^A	—	Blood acid phosphatase A	The most slowly moving isozyme of acid phosphatase in hemolymph	Yoshitake and Akiyama (1964)
Bph^B	—	Blood acid phosphatase B	Slowly moving isozyme of acid phosphatase in hemolymph	
Bph^C	—	Blood acid phosphatase C	Rapidly moving isozyme of acid phosphatase in hemolymph	
Bph^D	—	Blood acid phosphatase D	The most rapidly moving isozyme of acid phosphatase in hemolymph	
Bph^O	—	Blood acid phosphatase O	Acid phosphatase activity in hemolymph lacking	
*Br	—	Brown	Black pigment of larval skin turned to brown	Aruga (1939b)
Bs	—	Brown spot	Pairs of brown spots appear on each segment just after molting due to excretes of exuvial gland	Yukimura (1949)
bts	17–36.4	Brown head and tail spot	Head cuticle and outside of thoracic legs reddish brown	Chikushi (1948, 1960a)
Bu	11–5.5	Burnt	Scars on dorsal midline from fifth to eighth segment; dorsal vessel widened; homozygote lethal in embryo	Aruga (1939a)
cal	7–?	Susceptibility to muscardines	Susceptible to white muscardine disease	Aratake (1961)
ch	13–9.6	Chocolate	Head cuticle and trunk of newly hatched larva reddish brown; markings of grown larva reddish brown	Toyama (1909), Suzuki (1942)

Symbol	Position	Name	Description	Reference
co	—	Constricted	Segment constricted in central part due to annular concentration of pigments	Tanaka (1919)
*cp	—	Compressed	All segments of larva wide and short, zigzag alimentary canal	Asano (1947)
*Ct	—	Dominant constricted	Segments of larva wide and short	Ogawa (1949)
cts	16-4.6	Cheek and tail spots	Head cuticle and anal plate pigmented light brown	Tanaka (1935), Hasimoto (1965)
dep	—	Depressed	Second thoracic segment depressed; section behind eyespots dark brown; semilethal	Tanaka (1952)
Di	14-24.0	Dirty	Larval markings with numerous spots and lines of dark pigment	Chikushi (1949)
e	1-36.4	Elongate	Fourth and fifth segments elongated, intersegmental membrane fully stretched	Tanaka (1923)
e^l	1-36.4	Elongate lethal	Lethal in larva; associated with e	Kogure (1935)
E	6-0.0	Plain extra-legs	Rudimentary crescents and extra abdominal legs on fourth and fifth segments; star spots present	Sasaki (1930)
E^{ca}	6-0.0	Additional crescents	Additional crescents on sixth segment; star spots absent; homozygous embryo lacking abdominal legs; lethal	Suzuki (1929)
E^{cd}	6-0.0	Cd-double crescents	Extra-crescents on fourth segment; homozygotes lack abdominal legs and die as embryos	Sakaguchi et al. (1972)
E^{ct}	6-0.0	Ct-triple crescents	Additional crescents on fourth and sixth segments; supernumerary legs on fourth and sixth segments; homozygote lethal	Sakaguchi et al. (1972)

TABLE 5. Continued

Gene[b] symbol	Locus[c]	Name of gene	Phenotypic expression[a]	Authority
E^D	6–0.0	Double crescents	Extra-crescents on fourth segment; supernumerary legs seldom present on fourth and fifth segments; third and fourth segments frequently fused	Hasimoto (1941a)
E^{Dc}	6–0.0	Dc-double crescents	Additional crescents on fourth segment; homozygote semilethal	Tsujita and Sakaguchi (1959b)
E^{Dl}	6–0.0	Extra-crescents and degenerated abdominal legs	In homozygote extra-crescents on sixth segments; star spots lacking; first abdominal legs rudimentary	Gamo (1965)
E^{Ds}	6–0.0	Double stars	Extra star spots on seventh segments; homozygote lethal	Takasaki (1947b)
E^{El}	6–0.0	Extra-crescents and extra-legs	Additional crescents on fourth segment; small abdominal legs on fourth and fifth segments; homozygote lethal	Sasaki (1932)
E^{Gd}	6–0.0	Deformed gonad	Additional crescents on fourth segment; supernumerary legs on fourth and fifth segments; gonads abnormal	Sakata (1938)
E^H	6–0.0	H-extra-crescents	Extra-crescents on fourth segment but often incomplete; semilethal	Hasimoto (1941a)
E^{Kh}	6–0.0	Kh-extra-crescents	Extra-crescents on fourth segment; extra-thoracic legs on fourth segment and extra-abdominal legs on fifth segment	Tanaka (1926), Doira et al. (1973b)
E^{Kp}	6–0.0	Kp-supernumerary legs	In homozygote crescents on fifth and sixth segments, extra legs on fifth segments; heterozygote lacks extra-crescent	Hasimoto (1930, 1941a)

Gene	Name	Map	Description	Reference
E^M	E-mustache	6–0.0	Eye spot mustachelike; crescents absent; thorax elongated at beginning of molt; wings abnormal; homozygote lethal	Fujieda (1970)
E^{Mc}	Multicrescents	6–0.0	Extra-crescents on sixth segment, but no star spots; small extra-legs on fifth segment; homozygote lethal	Tsujita (1952)
E^{Ms}	New multistar	6–0.0	Additional star spots on seventh segment and rarely on ninth segment; homozygotes with supernumerary legs on tenth and eleventh segments, die as embryos	
E^{Mu}	Mu-supernumerary legs	6–0.0	Additional star spots on ninth segment; extra-legs on tenth segment	Hasimoto (1957)
E^N	New additional crescents	6–0.0	Extra-crescents on sixth segment; star spots lacking; homozygote lethal	Itikawa (1943)
E^{Nc}	No crescent, supernumerary legs	6–0.0	Crescents absent in homozygote, extra-legs on fifth segment	Sasaki (1940)
E^{Np}	Np supernumerary	6–0.0	Additional crescents on sixth and seventh segments; star spots absent; extra-legs rarely on fourth segment	Itikawa (1948)
E^{Ns}	New no star	6–0.0	Star spots absent	Tsujita and Sakaguchi (1959b)
E^{Sw}	Extra crescents and short wings	6–0.0	Additional crescents on fourth segment; small abdominal legs on fourth and fifth segments; hind wings stunted	Sasaki and Kawano (1963)
E^T	Tanaka's double crescents and supernumerary legs	6–0.0	Additional crescents on fourth segment; in homozygote supernumerary legs on fourth and fifth segments; homozygous female sterile	Chikushi (1970)
E^{Tc}	Triple crescents	6–0.0	Crescents on fourth, fifth, and sixth segments; star spot absent; abdominal legs entirely missing	Tsujita and Sakaguchi (1959a)

TABLE 5. Continued

Gene[b] symbol	Name of gene	Locus[c]	Phenotypic expression[a]	Authority
E-od	Enhancer of od-mottled	—	Expression of od^m changed to normal	Hatamura (1939)
es	Extra spiracles	12–16.9	A pair of small spiracles on twelfth segments	Fukuda (1951), Hashiguchi and Ooi (1955)
ge	Geometrid	25–?	Elongated body shape like geometrid	Tanaka (1936)
Gl	Glossy	—	Larval skin of third instar lustrous; homozygote lethal	Tanaka (1952)
gn	Gooseneck	9–5.8	Larval body slender, constricted between the segments	Doira et al. (1974b)
hal	Hare lip	18–25.2	First thoracic segment fused with second segment at a longitudinal line	Chikushi (1960b), Tanaka and Miyashita (1964)
i-lem	Inhibitor of lem	2–29.5	Manifestation of lem inhibited	Chikushi (1961)
i-oal	oal inhibitor	13–?	Manifestation of oal inhibited	Takasaki (1940)
I-a	Dominant chocolate	9–5.9	Body color of newly hatched larva chocolate but head cuticle black	Endo (1940), Hasimoto (1948a)
I-cr	Crescent suppressor	—	Manifestation of crescent marking of $+^p$ suppressed	Tazima (1943a)
Ies^A	Integument esterase A	—	Rapidly moving esterase isozyme of integument	Eguchi and Yoshitake (1966)
Ies^B	Integument esterase B	—	Slowly moving esterase isozyme of integument	
Ies^C	Integument esterase C	—	Most slowly moving esterase isozyme of integument	
Ies^O	Integument esterase O	—	Esterase isozyme of integument lacking	
K	Knobbed	11–0.0	Knobs appearing on the dorsal side of second, third, fifth, and eighth segments	Toyama (1912), Aruga (1939a)

Symbol	Name	Map	Description	Reference
kmt	Knob of Malpighian tubule	—	Knobs appearing on Malpighian tubule	Ono (1942)
L	Multilunar	4–0.0	A pair of large yellowish brown markings on dorsal side of each segment, mostly from fifth to eighth segments	Toyama (1912), Tanaka and Matsuno (1927)
L^c	Caltrop-type multilunar	4–0.0	Similar marking to *L* until fourth instar, then changing to caltroplike pattern in fifth instar; homozygote lethal	Nagashima *et al.* (1971)
lem	Lemon	3–0.0	Skin of grown larva is lemon yellow; dark brown marking on anal plate	Nozaki (1917), Ogura (1922)
lem^l	Lemon lethal	3–0.0	Body and head cuticle yellow just after first ecdysis; unable to chew mulberry leaves and starves to death	Suzuki (1950), Tsujita (1955)
les	Light eye spot	14–?	Triangular black spots on both sides of eye spot lacking	Tanaka (1952), Chikushi (1959a)
ma	Mustache a	—	Mustachelike brown markings on first segment	Sakata (1943)
mal	Malformation	4–14.8	Monster, larval body twisted mostly around eighth segment	Omura (1949), Takasaki (1957)
mb	Mustache b	—	Mustachelike brown markings on first segment	Sakata (1943)
mi	Mildewed stripe	2–7.0	Striped marking with gray spots on each segment and mildewedlike mottling on both subdorsal spots	Chikushi and Sakamoto (1967), Chikushi *et al.* (1972)
ms	Multistars	12–15.5	Pairs of star spots on dorsal side of sixth through tenth segments	Tanaka (1927, 1969)
mse	Segment monster	—	Posterior segments malformed	Umeya (1949)
mse_2	Segment monster 2	—	Second segment twisted; forewing lacking	Hirobe and Ooi (1954)
msn	New multistar	20–14.6	Light-colored star spots on sixth and seventh segments	Chikushi (1953), Tanaka (1963)

TABLE 5. Continued

Gene[b] symbol	Locus[c]	Name of gene	Phenotypic expression[d]	Authority
mus	11–?	Susceptibility to muscardine	Highly susceptible to white muscardine fungus disease	Takasaki (1959)
nb	20–0.0	Narrow breast	Thorax narrow; abdomen stout; whole body spindle shaped	Chikushi (1953)
Nc	6–1.4	No crescents	No crescents, light star spots, light eye spots; lethal in embryo when homozygous	Itikawa (1944)
Nl	14–16.0	No lunule	Crescents lacking but eye spots present; spontaneous deficiency; COV between *odk* and *Nl* is 2.7	Tanaka (1925a), Chikushi (1959a)
Nl₁	14–18.5	No lunule 1	Similar to *Nl*; x-ray induced; lethal in embryo when homozygous; deficiency; COV between *odk* and *Nl₁* is 5.2	Tsujita (1959)
Nl₂	14–20.5	No lunule 2	Similar to *Nl*; x-ray induced; lethal in embryo; deficiency, COV between *odk* and *Nl₂* is 7.2	
*o-5	—	Translucent E 5	Larval skin highly translucent; growth retarded	Tanaka and Matsuno (1929)
*o-21	—	Oily 21	After second molt skin becomes translucent; homozygote lethal in late larval stage	Nakayama (1954)
o-106	10–?	Translucent C 106	Larval skin weakly translucent	Watanabe (1961)
*o-115	—	Translucent J 115	Larval skin moderately translucent; mortality very high in late larval stage	Takasaki (1943)
oa	14–23.0	Aojuku translucent	Larval skin moderately translucent; semilethal	Tanaka and Matsuno (1929), Chikushi (1959a)

oa^2	14–23.0	Aojuku translucent 2	Similar to *oa*	Chikushi *et al.* (1972)
oa^v	14–23.0	Variegated *oa*	Mottled skin with translucent and opaque	Chikushi *et al.* (1972)
oal	2–26.7	*oal* mottled translucent	Mottled skin with translucent and opaque; mortality high	Takasaki (1940)
*obl	—	Black translucent	Weakly translucent; larval body color dark	Kei (1942)
obt	7–21.0	Mottled translucent B 8	Mottled translucent with a number of small opaque dots scattered	Hasimoto (1934*a*)
oc	5–40.8	Chinese translucent	Moderately translucent; viability good	Tanaka and Matsuno (1929), Yokoyama (1939)
od	1–49.6	Distinct translucent	Highly translucent; semilethal at first molt; development retarded in younger larval stage	Tanaka (1925*b*)
od^m	1–49.6	*od* mottled translucent	Mottled skin with translucent and opaque; dominant to *od*; mutable gene	Hatamura (1939)
odk	14–13.3	Translucent E 15	Mottled skin with a number of translucent and small opaque dots	Hasimoto (1941*c*)
og	9–7.4	Giallo Ascoli translucent	Translucency of extremely high degree; mortality very high in pupa; female almost infertile	Sasaki (1938)
og^t	9–7.4	*og* of Tanaka	Skin highly translucent; viability low; homozygotes mostly die in pupal stage; almost infertile (= *ot*)	Tanaka and Matsuno (1929), Chikushi and Kihara (1973)
oh	21–0.0	Hoarfrost translucent	Mottled translucent with a number of indistinct fine opaque dots	Doira *et al.* (1974*a*)
*oi	—	Marché translucent	Highly translucent; growth retarded; all die before fourth instar	Tanaka and Matsuno (1929)
ok	5–4.7	Kinshiryu translucent	Translucency of high degree; mortality high in young larval stage	Tanaka and Matsuno (1929), Yokoyama (1939)

TABLE 5. Continued

Gene[b] symbol	Locus[c]	Name of gene	Phenotypic expression[a]	Authority
om	10–6.9	Matamukashi translucent	Weakly translucent skin, distinct in young larvae, but indistinguishable in grown larva; viability low	Tanaka and Matsuno (1929), Chikushi et al. (1964)
oml	10–6.9	Melamine-induced oily skin and white egg	Skin weakly translucent; compound eye black; F_1 with w_3 or oew exhibits white egg and oily skin	Doira et al. (1963)
or	28–?	or translucent	Skin highly translucent	Tanaka (1948)
os	1–0.0	Sex-linked translucent	Skin weakly translucent	Tanaka (1917)
otm	5–6.7	Tanaka's mottled translucent	Mottled translucent with a number of fine opaque dots	Tanaka and Chiang (1939), Chikushi (1966)
ow	17–30.1	Waxy translucent	Moderately translucent	Tanaka and Matsuno (1929), Chikushi (1960a)
p	2–0.0	Plain	A rudimentary pattern of normal marking develops but it lacks black pigments	Toyama (1906), Tanaka (1913)
p¹	2–0.0	Lightest normal	Eye spots faintly dark; crescents and star spots uncolored	Tanaka (1916)
p²	2–0.0	Light normal	Eye spots black but crescents and star spots almost uncolored	
p³(+P)	2–0.0	Standard normal	Normal larval marking with eyespots on the second, crescents on the fifth, and star spots on the eighth segments	
p⁴	2–0.0	Dark normal	Eye spots, crescents, and star spots deep black	
p^B	2–0.0	Black	Whole body black with gray wavy markings along dorsal and subdorsal lines	Kawaguchi (1933)

$*p^D$	Dorsal spot	Dark triangular spots on dorsal side from third to eighth abdominal segments	2–0.0	Shimodaira (1947b)
p^G	Ventral striped	Light-colored striped marking on the dorsal side; ventral stripe deep black	2–0.0	Takasaki (1947c)
$*p^L$	Light crescent	Crescents pale in heterozygote and vestigial in homozygote	2–0.0	Chikushi (1938)
p^M	Moricaud	Larval marking consisting of numerous dark spots and lines on grayish skin; frontal markings on the head	2–0.0	Tanaka (1913)
p^S	Striped	Body black with white stripe on posterior margin of each segment; center line on the ventral side black	2–0.0	Toyama (1909), Tanaka (1913)
p^{Sa}	Sable	Lightly pigmented striped marking; crescents extremely light colored; homozygote lethal; deficiency and inversion	2–0.0	Tazima (1938)
p^{Sa-2}	Sable 2	Almost similar to p^{Sa}; skin between thoracic legs light black; chitinized parts of thoracic legs deep black; deficiency	2–0.0	Tazima (1943b)
p^{St}	Pale striped	Light-colored striped marking	2–0.0	Takasaki (1947a)
p^{Sw}	Whitish striped	Heterozygote with plain light-colored stripes, dorsal side of thorax nearly white; homozygote similar to p^S	2–0.0	Tanaka (1952)
Pl	Eye spotted	Markings other than eye spots lacking	—	Takasaki (1947c)
Pl_3^F	Blood protein 3 F	Third band of hemolymph protein moves rapidly on gel electrophoresis	14–?	Kawaguchi et al. (1970)
Pl_3^S	Blood protein 3 S	Third band of hemolymph protein moves slowly on gel electrophoresis	14–?	Kawaguchi et al. (1970)
q	Quail	Quail-like pattern of black spots and lines on light reddish purple skin	7–0.0	Toyama (1909), Hasimoto (1934a)

TABLE 5. Continued

Gene[b] symbol	Name of gene	Locus[c]	Phenotypic expression[a]	Authority
rb	Red hemolymph	22–?	Larval skin reddish; hemolymph turns red in the air	Inagami and Akagi (1954), Doira *et al.* (1973*c*)
Rs	Reddish skin	—	Skin of mature larva deep red	Suda and Kawaguchi (1922), Tanaka (1943)
S	New striped	2–6.1	Larval marking like p^S but deeper black; spontaneous	Tanaka (1933)
S²	Striped 2	2–6.1	Larval marking like p^S; x-ray induced	Takasaki (1947*a*)
S^d	Dilute striped	2–6.1	Larval marking light striped	Tanaka (1933)
*S^w	White thorax striped	2–6.1	Larval marking like p^S in homozygote, but much lighter in heterozygote	Chikushi (1938)
*sb	Short bristle	—	Bristles of newly hatched larva short	Harizuka (1947*b*)
sch	Sex-linked chocolate	1–21.5	Head cuticle of newly hatched larva dark brown; body color reddish brown	Mano and Itagaki (1965)
Ses^A	Silk gland esterase A	—	Rapidly moving esterase isozyme of silk gland	Yoshitake *et al.* (1965)
Ses^B	Silk gland esterase B	—	Slowly moving esterase isozyme of silk gland	
Ses^O	Silk gland esterase O	—	Esterase isozyme of silk gland lacking	
sk	Stick	4–25.8	Body shape slender, and texture hard like a stick	Tanaka and Matsuno (1927)
*Sl	Supernumerary legs	—	Supernumerary legs on fifth segments, crescents incomplete	Aruga (1943*d*)
Sl-v	V-supernumerary legs	22–?	Supernumerary legs of variable size on fifth segment; homozygotes with supernumerary legs on tenth segment; die as embryos	Doira *et al.* (1973*c*)

so	27-?	Sooty	Larval skin sooty black; usually accompanied by black pupal case	Tanaka (1943)
Spc	4-33.1	Speckled	Dark brown small spots scattered on both sides of larval body; female sterile.	Tazima and Ohta (1952)
st	8-0.0	Stony	Each segment tight in the middle, but bulgy in the intersegmental portion; larval body hard to the touch	Tanaka (1919), Tazima et al. (1960)
*Swl	—	Swollen	Larval body bloated; many black small spots scattered all over skin	Takasaki (1947c)
*Tb	—	Transparent back	Dorsal side of mature larva transparent; silk glands situated on the dorsal side of the mid-gut	Aruga (1940)
ts	3-?	Tail spot	Light brown tail spots on anal plate	Chikushi (1948)
ty	—	Hemolymph tyrosinase	Lowered tyrosinase (phenol oxidase) activity in hemolymph	Sakaguchi (1957)
U	14-21.3	Ursa	Dorsal and lateral sides of larva covered with dark brown pigments	Hasimoto (1941c)
*U^{Br}	14-21.3	Brown ursa	Ground color of Ursa marking reddish brown; lethal in fourth molt when homozygous	Tsujita (1946)
Y	2-25.6	Yellow blood	Hemolymph yellow colored; abdominal legs yellow	Toyama (1906), Tanaka (1913)
Y^a	2-25.6	Mandarina yellow	Hemolymph and abdominal legs light yellow, especially in grown larvae	Kawaguchi (1934)
Y^d	2-25.6	Pale yellow blood	Hemolymph colored light yellow in fifth instar larvae	Nakajima (1963)
Ym	26-?	Yellow molting	Skin just after ecdysis covered with yellowish powder due to yellow crystals secreted from Malpighian vessel	Shimizu (1936)

TABLE 5. Continued

Gene[b] symbol	Locus[c]	Name of gene	Phenotypic expression[a]	Authority
Ze	3–20.8	Zebra	Narrow black bands on anterior portion of each larval segment; head cuticle dark brown in both sides	Toyama (1906), Ogura (1922)
Ze^f	3–20.8	Zebra faded	Outlines of zebra markings indistinct	Hirobe (1951)
COCOON				
Acp	—	Absorbent of carotenoid pigment	Modifier of I and I^s	Nakajima (1963)
C	12–14.2	Golden yellow	Cocoon golden yellow outside, nearly white inside	Uda (1919), Ogura (1931a), Tanaka (1969)
C^i	12–14.2	Inner layer yellow	Inner layer of cocoon yellow	Uda (1919), Kei (1943)
C^{st}	12–14.2	Straw color	Cocoon faintly yellow; presumably identical with C^d of Nakajima	Harizuka et al. (1960), Nakajima (1963)
Cb	6–?	Cinnamon buff	Cocoon color; presumably identical with F	Harizuka (1953)
F	6–13.6	Flesh	Cocoon reddish yellow or salmon in outer layer but white in inner layer	Cleghorn (1918), Ogura (1931b)
Fl	—	Flossy	Cocoon loosely composed; cottonlike appearance	Takasaki (1947c)
flc	3–49.0	Flimsy cocoon	Cocoon shell very thin	Doira (1973)
Ga	—	Green a	Cocoon light green when in combination with Gb	Hasimoto (1941b)
Gb	7–7.0	Green b	Cocoon light green when in combination with Ga	Hasimoto (1941b)
Gc	15–7.8	Green c	Cocoon light green	Kei (1937)

Symbol	Map	Name	Description	Reference
Grc	—	Green cocoon	Cocoon dark green, inner layer white; egg shell tinged with deep yellow	Takasaki (1947c)
ha	—	Perforated a	One end of cocoon elongated and open at tip	Kobari (1932b)
Hb	—	Perforated b	One end of cocoon elongated and open at tip	
Hc	—	Perforated c	One end of cocoon elongated and open at tip	
I	9–0.0	Yellow inhibitor	Completely suppresses Y, hence it produces a dominant white cocoon	Coutagne (1902), Kellog (1908), Sasaki (1938)
I^s	9–0.0	Sooty plain yellow inhibitor	Completely suppresses Y, but recessive to I	Tanaka (1924b), Nakajima (1971)
$I\text{-}Gn_1$	6–7.5	Green inhibitor 1	Inhibits permeability of two kinds of yellowish brown fluorescent pigments through middle part of silk gland	Fujimoto et al. (1962)
Nd	23–?	Naked	Cocoon layer only contains sericin, frequently unable to form cocoon; middle and posterior divisions of silk glands degenerated	Nakano (1951b)
Nd^H	23–?	Naked of Hasimoto	Similar to Nd	Hasimoto (1956)
*Ndb	—	Naked b	Silk glands degenerate; about 50 percent of larvae spin cocoons, the rest pupate without spinning	Nakano (1951b)
$Nd\text{-}s$	14–0.0	Sericin cocoon	Cocoon filament contains only sericin	Horiuchi et al. (1963)
Pk	—	Pink cocoon	Cocoon pink; coexistence with Y and F is needed for the manifestation of Pk	Tanaka (1919), Harizuka (1953)
Rc	2–31.8	Rusty	Outer layer of cocoon yellowish brown, inner layer white	Kei (1943)
Sc	—	Soft	Cocoon layers loose in texture	Akiyama (1921), Takasaki (1947c)

TABLE 5. Continued

Gene[b] symbol	Locus[c]	Name of gene	Phenotypic expression[a]	Authority
Yf	—	Yellow fluorescent	Cocoon shell shows a yellow fluorescence under UV light	Kobari (1932a), Adachi (1936)
Ymc	—	Mandarina yellow cocoon	Cocoon faintly yellow in combination with Y[a]	Kawaguchi (1934)
Yr	6–18.7	Yellowish brown	Cocoon yellowish brown	Tanaka (1955), Hasimoto (1956)
PUPA				
bp	11–17.1	Black pupa	Pupal skin tinged with black, temperature dependent	Gamo (1923), Harizuka (1942)
cf	13–20.9	Crayfish	Forewings and hindwings of pupa swollen and protruding laterally from body	Suzuki (1942)
Cw	—	Curled wing	Forewings curled at margin; incompletely dominant	Suzuki (1947, 1952), Takasaki (1960)
fl	10–0.3	Wingless (Flügellos)	Forewings and hindwings lacking in pupae and moths	Katsuki (1935), Harizuka (1948), Ueda et al. (1959)
Wp	—	White-winged pupa	Wings of pupa very light colored, often nearly white; incompletely dominant	Harizuka (1947a)
IMAGO				
Bm	17–0.0	Black moth	Scales both on body and wings dark	Kosminsky and Schragina (1933), Hirobe (1947a)

cd	Constricted vagina d	—	When combined with cv, vestibulum connected with oviduct constricted and incapable of passing eggs	Suzuki and Omura (1951b)
cv	Constricted vagina v	—	Female incapable of oviposition when combined with cd	
fs	Female sterile	—	Females highly sterile due to reversed orientation of eggs in the ovarioles	Fujimoto (1943)
lu	Lustrous	16–0.0	Compound eye black, but extremely lustrous	Uda (1930), Hirobe (1958)
mln	Melanism	19–21.3	Head cuticle and tail spots of larva pigmented dark brown; moth black	Hasimoto (1961)
mp	Micropterous	11–24.0	Wings about 80 percent of normal in size	Hirobe (1947b), Ooi et al. (1953)
Ng	No glue	12–0.0	Eggs nonadhesive due to poor development of mucous glands in female	Tanaka (1919), Muroga (1953)
peg	Piled egg	—	Peculiar ovipositing habit of moth	Hirobe (1960)
rv	Degenerated radius	—	Veins degenerated; usually radius, sometimes media, cubitus and anal veins absent	Hashida (1934)
slo	Oligospermy	—	Low fertility in male due to failure to produce eupyrene sperm; fertility good in female	Suzuki and Omura (1951a)
slp	Degenerated penis muscle	—	One or two pairs of three copulatory muscles degenerated; male usually sterile	Umeya (1926)
sls	Abnormal spermatophore	—	Movement of sperm into ductus seminalis prevented due to abnormality at cervical region of spermatophore; female sterile	Umeya and Omura (1950)
Sui	Short wing	—	Wings of moths short	Takasaki (1947c)

TABLE 5. Continued

Gene[b] symbol	Name of gene	Locus[c]	Phenotypic expression[a]	Authority
ve	Varnished eye	6–11.1	Compound eye small in size, but lustrous	Doira (1970, and unpublished)
Vg	Vestigial	1–38.7	Wings degenerate; degree variable; lethal in hemizygous state	Tazima (1944)
wb	White-banded wing	5–35.8	Wings dark brown at outer margin and proximally, leaving a wide white band in between	Kanbe and Nara (1959)
Wm	Wild melanism	—	Body and wing color of moths dark brown	Hirobe (1947a)
Ws	Wild wing spot	—	Black spot on apex of anterior wing of moth	Hirobe (1967a)
ya	Yellow antenna	—	Antenna of moth yellow. Color variable, appearing sometimes only on one side or on a part of the antenna	Takasaki (1947c)
PHYSIOLOGICAL				
d	Dwarf	—	Body size reduced to 75 percent of normal	Suda and Hashida (1931)
Df	Dominant dwarf	—	Larval development retarded, homozygous lethal in larva	Aruga (1943c)
Df-t	Tsujita's dwarf	21–11.0	Larval growth retarded; homozygous lethal in embryo	Doira et al. (1972, 1974a)
dw	Lethal dwarf	—	Growth delayed 3 days in the first instar; skin transparent; homozygous lethal in larva	Morohoshi (1943)
dw-k	Dwarf-k	10–?	Body size very small; larval development retarded; viable, but females infertile	Doira et al. (1974d)

H_1	—	Autosomal hibernating 1	Controlling voltinism to hibernation	Nagatomo (1942)
H_2	—	Autosomal hibernating 2	Controlling voltinism to hibernation	
H_3	—	Autosomal hibernating 3	Controlling voltinism to hibernation	
Hs	1–?	Sex-linked univoltine	Controlling voltinism to hibernation	
Hs^m	1–?	Sex-linked multivoltine	Controlling voltinism to multivoltine	
Lan	22–?	Tsujita's lanky	Body shape slender; larval development slightly retarded; homozygous lethal in embryo	Doira et al. (1973c)
$*Lk$	11–14.2 (±)	Lanky	Phenotype similar to Lan	Umeya and Asano (1956), Asano and Itikawa (1958)
Lm	1–2.0	Late maturity	Larval maturity defered	Nagatomo (1926), Morohoshi (1957)
Lm^e	1–2.0	Early maturity	Larval maturity promoted	Morohoshi (1957), Takasaki (1957)
m^2	—	Dimolting	Larvae mature after 2 molts; apt to produce trimolters	Oota et al. (1957)
M^3	6–3.0	Trimolting	Larvae mature after 3 molts	Toyama (1912), Ogura (1931b)
$+^M$	6–3.0	Tetramolting	Larvae mature after 4 molts	
M^5	6–3.0	Pentamolting	Larvae mature after 5 molts; recessive to normal	Takase (1919), Ogura (1931b)
me	6–3.0	E 7 trimolting	Recessive trimolting	Tskasaki and Mitarai (1949)
mo	—	Hereditary mosaic	Mosaics and gynandromorphs formed due to double fertilization	Goldschmidt and Katsuki (1927, 1928a,b, 1931)

TABLE 5. Continued

Gene[b] symbol	Locus[c]	Name of gene	Phenotypic expression[a]	Authority
nm	—	Non-molting	Homozygotes survive about two weeks without molting; a few pass through first molt and develop normally	Umeya and Karasawa (1930)
Np	11–7.3	Non-preference	Unable to discriminate mulberry leaves from others; lethal when homozygous	Tazima (1954)
pnd	—	Pigmented non-diapausing egg	Egg pigmented normally, but embryo nonhibernating	Katsumata (1968)
Rg	3–24.9	Retarded growth	Larval growth distinctly retarded; homozygous lethal in embryo	Chikushi et al. (1971a)
rh	—	Retarded hatching	Due to decreased amount of inhibiting substance, embryos in pigmented eggs develop and hatch	Muroga (1948)
rm	3–?	Retarded molting	Development of larva retarded; perhaps due to abnormality in protein components of body fluid	Tsujita and Sakurai (1965)
rt	7–9.0 (±)	Recessive trimolting	Simple recessive to ordinary tetramolting character	Asano (1948), Hirobe (1954)
Rt	2–?	Retarding	Heterozygote small, and retarded in development	Tanaka (1959)
Slg	18–0.0	Slow growing	Larval development retarded by about one week as compared to normal; homozygous lethal	Tanaka and Miyashita (1960, 1964)

V^1	Univoltine	6–?	Univoltine, caused by enhanced production of hibernating substance	Morohoshi and Mezaki (1956)
$V^2(+^v)$	Bivoltine	6–?	Bivoltine, caused by standard production of hibernating substance	
V^3	Multivoltine	6–?	Multivoltine, caused by reduced production of hibernating substance	
vo	Vomiting habit	—	Larvae vomits gastric juice on feeding during fifth instar	Nakano (1951a)

Hemolymph Proteins

The hemolymph proteins of the silkworm undergo a complex sequence of changes which are synchronized to the morphological alterations which take place during metamorphosis (Doira, 1968). Heritable changes in the nonenzymic proteins have also been reported. An albumin fraction migrating more rapidly than other proteins to the anode on polyacrylamide gel electrophoresis is controlled by a pair of codominant alleles, Alb^F and Alb^S. The Alb alleles are linked to the nb gene (20-0.0)* with a crossover value of 6.2 percent (Gamo, 1968). A protein, which shows solubilities characteristic of an albumin and migrates next to the Alb zone, is controlled by the codominant Pt_3^F and Pt_3^S alleles. Kawaguchi *et al.* (1970) have shown that the Pt_3 alleles are located on the 14th chromosome, 46.0 crossover units away from the U locus (21.3).

Measurements of the total hemolymph protein level in *Bombyx* pupae have a diagnostic value in understanding the intricacies of the female reproductive cycle. Females homozygous for the small-egg mutants (*sm*, 3-41.8 or *sm-2*, 13-0.0) produce oocytes that lack protein yolk spheres (Otsuki, 1965). In such cases the vitellogenic, female-specific protein (FP) and some non-sex-limited proteins of pupal hemolymph are accumulated in enormous quantities in the hemolymph rather than undergoing the normal decrease to trace amounts. A similar increase occurs in genetically normal females that have been ovariectomized. Therefore, the small-egg genes do not seem to regulate the synthesis of vitellogenic hemolymph proteins, but rather control the transfer of the proteins from the hemolymph into the ovaries (Doira and Kawaguchi, 1972, 1974; Kawaguchi and Doira, 1973, 1974).

Hemocytes

The blood cells of the silkworm are classified into five types: proleucocytes, plasmatocytes, granular cells, spherule cells, and oenocytoids. Among 301 silkworm races examined, 26 strains lacked spherule cells in the hemolymph of all larvae tested, whereas spherule cells (Sph) normally make up 10–30 percent of the hemocyte population at the early stages of each larval instar. Twenty five strains segregated both Sph-plus (Sph$^+$) and Sph-minus (Sph$^-$) larvae; in 249 strains all of the larvae examined had Sph in the larval hemolymph. F_1 individuals arising from a cross between Sph$^+$ moths and those from Sph$^-$ strains (such as Shisen-tri-

---

* For an explanation of this notation see footnote *c* to Table 5.

molter, Daizo, or Ringetsu) lacked spherule cells. F_2 progeny showed a 3 :
1 ratio of Sph$^-$ to Sph$^+$ larvae. In the backcross between F_1 and Sph$^-$
moths spherule cells were absent from the hemolymph of all larvae
examined, whereas in the progeny of the backcross between F_1 and Sph$^+$
moths, segregation took place with a ratio of 1 Sph$^+$: 1 Sph$^-$. These
results show that the Sph$^-$ character is controlled by a dominant gene. In
contrast to the above, mating experiments using Sph$^-$ moths from the H-5
minor strain revealed that the absence of spherule cells was inherited as a
recessive character (Nittono, 1960). Nittono *et al.* (1964) observed in
Sph$^-$ larvae from the Rosa strain abnormally shaped hemocytes unlike
those seen in silkmoths or other lepidopteran insects. The presence or
absence of abnormal hemocytes is inherited along with the recessive Sph$^-$
character. Silkworm races which lack spherule cells produce less silk and
have a shortened larval life. The physiological role of the spherule cells
and the relationship between the dominant and recessive genes that control their absence need to be clarified.

Enzymes

Analyses of naturally occurring polymorphisms of various enzymes
have been mainly performed by means of agar gel electrophoresis.
Linkage studies of the genes specifying these enzymes have not yet been
successful, except for the pioneering studies on the amylase genes of the
hemolymph and digestive juices by Matsumura [see review by Tazima
(1964)].

Esterases of the hemolymph have the properties of both
cholinesterases and aliesterases. Three types of hemolymph esterases are
found: A, B, and C; they are controlled by codominant alleles, Bes^A,
Bes^B, and Bes^C, respectively. Larvae homozygous for the Bes^O allele lack
esterase activity (Eguchi *et al.*, 1965).

The esterase activity of the silk gland is very high at the anterior
portion of the middle division when compared to other parts of the gland.
Two types of silk gland esterases, A and B, are controlled codominantly
by the Ses^A and Ses^B alleles. An inactive allele Ses^O is also known for this
locus. The A and B esterases can be subdivided into A^D, A^S, B^D, and B^S
isozymes through the quantitative analysis of enzyme activities of their
bands. Activities of A^D or B^D are almost twice as high as those of A^S or
B^S. It is assumed that the A^D and B^D enzymes are controlled by duplicated genes, Ses^{AA} or Ses^{BB}. This may have occurred by unequal crossing
over (Yoshitake *et al.*, 1965).

Four allelic genes, Ies^O, Ies^A, Ies^B, and Ies^C, exist at a locus which controls the production of the esterase isozymes, A, B, and C in the larval integument. Compound types have also been observed, and these may show two bands which correspond to A and B or to A and C. Each band is the same width as that characteristic of the single A, B, or C bands seen in silkworms homozygous for Ies^A, Ies^B, or Ies^C. Such compound types are thought to represent the products of the genes Ies^{AB} or Ies^{AC}, and these may be the result of a duplication of each ancestral gene (Eguchi and Yoshitake, 1966).

Esterases in the egg are classified into five groups of active bands: I, II, III, IV, and V. These are controlled by genes Ees_1, Ees_2, Ees_3, Ees_4, and Ees_5, respectively, which are located at separate loci. These Ees genes may belong to the same linkage group (Yoshitake and Akiyama, 1965a).

Esterase zymograms of hemolymph and extracts of different tissues from 360 individual larvae were compared one by one. Eighty different strains, as well as the offspring of crosses between strains which showed varied esterase types, were tested. Esterase bands in the integument, trachea, and Malpighian tubules were found to be controlled by the same gene, Ies. On the contrary, the esterase types found in the hemolymph, silk gland, and mid-gut differ from one another and from those of the integument or tracheal cells. It seems that the types of isozymes are related to the ontogenic origin of the tissues from which the enzyme extracts were obtained (Eguchi and Yoshitake, 1967).

Alkaline phosphatases of mid-gut tissues can be resolved into active bands, F and S, where F is a soluble enzyme and S is a membrane-bound one. Among 328 strains examined, larvae from 5 lacked the F isozyme and those from 42 strains lacked the S isozyme. However, none of the strains contained silkworms that lacked both isozymes. The F and S bands are controlled by the Aph_1 and Aph_2 genes, respectively. These are located on the same chromosome, and their recombination value is 31 percent (Yoshitake, 1964; Yoshitake et al., 1966). The S form is synthesized in the microsomes of mid-gut cells and is transferred to the lumen, where it is transformed to the alkaline phosphatase of the digestive fluid (Eguchi et al., 1972).

The acid phosphatase isozymes of larval hemolymph are controlled by the codominant alleles Bph^O, Bph^A, Bph^B, Bph^C, and Bph^D. Bph alleles are located on an unknown autosome, independent of the Aph genes (Yoshitake and Akiyama, 1964). Substrate-specificity experiments reveal that when p-nitrophenyl phosphate (NPP) is used as a substrate, instead of the α-naphthyl phosphate generally employed in the demonstration of Bph isozymes, different bands are formed that are specific for NPP. The NPPases also show polymorphism on zymograms, and these enzymes are controlled by separate genes from *Bph* (Yoshitake and Akiyama, 1965*b*).

Phenol oxidase activities in larval hemolymph are also genetically controlled. The mutant characterized by a low tyrosinase (phenol oxidase) activity, *ty*, accumulates the proenzyme in excessive quantities. Individuals heterozygous for the wild-type gene and *ty* show enzyme activities intermediate to those of their parents. The proenzyme may be activated by subjecting the hemolymph to heat (55°C for 5 minutes), low temperature (0°C for 1–3 hours), acetone, chloroform, ethyl ether, or ethyl alcohol. The activity of the tyrosinase of the *ty* mutant after activation of the proenzyme is comparable to that of wild type (Sakaguchi, 1957). According to Hashiguchi and Yoshitake (1966), the phenol oxidase in larval hemolymph is present as a proenzyme which is activated by incubation of hemolymph at 5°C. However, larvae from some strains are unable to activate the proenzyme. Mating experiments between A type (capable of strong activation) and C type (very weak activation) revealed that F_1 individuals show an (B type) activity intermediate to the parental types. The F_2 progeny showed a segregation of 1 A : 2 B : 1 C.

Comparative studies of naturally occurring polymorphic forms of proteins, which have accumulated in the species during the long history of its evolution, have provided detailed insights as to the problem of species differentiation. The nearest relative of *B. mori* is *B. (Theophila) mandarina*, which inhabits China, Korea, and Japan. Yoshitake (1966, 1968) compared the esterases and phosphatases of *B. mandarina* with those of *B. mori*. Most of the esterase and phosphatase isozymes observed in the domesticated silkworm are also present in the wild silkworm. The gene systems controlling these isozymes in the two species of *Bombyx* are recognized with a few exceptions to show a close relationship, although the frequencies of the allelic forms of the genes are distinctly different. The allele specifying the absence of the Aph_1 isozyme could not be found in *B. mandarina*. Only the C type of integument esterase was found in common in *B. mori* and *B. mandarina*. In the wild silkworm Ies^A or Ies^B were not observed, whereas the Ies^D and Ies^E alleles, which are never found in the domesticated silkworm, occurred in high frequencies. The Bes^D allele can be found only in the wild species. The differentiation into new species may involve chances like this where certain alleles are fixed and others lost with time in the population. Duplicated genes, such as Ies^{AB}, Ies^{AC}, Ses^{AA}, and Ses^{BB}, which are widely distributed among domesticated silkworm strains, have not been found in the wild silkworm. During the evolutionary differentiation of *B. mori* and *B. mandarina*, duplication of genes may have played an important role. Such gene duplications may also cause an increase in quantitative characters of economic value. Artificial selection, then, during the long history of sericulture for the improvement of an economic character may have promoted the accumulation of duplicated genes in domesticated races of *B. mori.*

Embryonic Diapause

Voltinism in the silkworm is maternally inherited [see review by Tazima (1964)]. As described earlier, silkmoths lay either pigmented diapause eggs or unpigmented non-diapause eggs. The diapause hormone is thought to be responsible for the determination of embryonic diapause and the pigmentation of the egg. When individuals heterozygous for the wild-type and the *l-n* gene are mated *inter se,* pigmented and nonpigmented eggs are laid in the same batch in a 3 : 1 ratio. The embryos within pigmented eggs enter diapause and are viable, whereas embryos within unpigmented eggs do not enter diapause but continue to develop until blastokinesis and then die (Hirobe *et al.,* 1952). The *l-n* gene expresses itself in serosal cells and yolk nuclei at a very early stage of development, but it acts considerably later in embryos. It is assumed that in the pigmented eggs, yolk nuclei provide some substance which causes diapause of the embryo, whereas in the *l-n/l-n* eggs the substance is not synthesized, thus preventing the embryos from entering diapause (Takei and Nagashima, 1970). Kai and Hasegawa (1973) have isolated an esterase isozyme (esterase A) in eggs that is responsible for the lysis of yolk cells. This lysis in turn signals the termination of embryonic diapause.

A type of voltinism that is not maternally inherited has been reported by Katsumata (1968). Moths of an Indonesian, multivoltine silkworm strain lay pigmented, non-diapause eggs when they are incubated as embryos at 25°C. Mating experiments have revealed that the character (pigmented and non-diapause egg) is under the control of a single, recessive, autosomal gene, *pnd.* F_1 eggs from crosses between moths from *pnd* and uni- or bivoltine strains are pigmented and diapausing, irrespective of the strain of the mother moth. This demonstrates that voltinism is not always maternally inherited. In backcrosses between F_1 and *pnd* moths, segregation takes place in single batches of eggs in the ratio of 1 : 1 in both reciprocal crosses. In F_2 eggs, about 25 percent of the eggs laid by a single F_1 female moth show the pigmented and non-diapause character and 75 percent show the pigmented and diapause character.

Yoshitake and Hashiguchi (1969) have proposed that two processes interact to determine embryonic diapause in silkworms. One, the

TABLE 6. *Bombyx Stock Centers in Japan*

City	Institution	Scientist in charge
Fukuoka	Institute of Silkworm Genetics, Kyushu University	H. Chikushi
Misima	National Institute of Genetics	Y. Tazima
Tokyo	National Sericultural Experiment Station	T. Fukuda
Tokyo	Faculty of Agriculture, University of Tokyo	N. Yoshitake

"brain–subesophageal ganglion–diapause hormone" system (A), is controlled by multiple genes and is inherited maternally. The other (B) is controlled by the normal allele of the *pnd* gene and comes into action after fertilization of the eggs through some unknown mechanism. According to this hypothesis all of the uni-, bi-, and multivoltine strains used so far in the studies of voltinism are normal with respect to the B process, whereas *pnd* is normal with respect to the A process. The proper functioning of the A and B processes together leads to embryonic diapause. The artificial hatching of eggs by HCl treatment may destroy the B process.

Bombyx Stock Centers in Japan

Further information concerning the availability of various strains of silkworms can be obtained by writing to the scientist in charge of the four stock centers listed in Table 6.

Literature Cited*

Adachi, M., 1936   On the fluorescence of cocoons. I. Genetical studies on the fluorescence of green and white cocoons in Japanese bivoltine silkworms. *Bull. Sericult. Exp. Stn. Shizuoka* **2**:1–65. (J)

Akai, H., 1963   Electron microscopical observation on the fibroin formation in the silk gland of the silkworm, *Bombyx mori. Bull. Sericult. Exp. Stn. Tokyo* **18**:271–277. (J, ER)

Akai, H., 1971   Ultrastructure of fibroin in the silk gland of larval *Bombyx mori. Exp. Cell. Res.* **69**:219–223.

Akai, H., K. Kiguchi and K. Mori, 1971   Increased accumulation of silk protein accompanying JH-induced prolongation of larval life in *Bombyx mori* L. (Lepidoptera: Bombycidae). *Appl. Entomol. Zool.* **6**:218–220. (J, ER)

* Abbreviations: (C) in Chinese, (J) in Japanese, (J, ER) in Japanese with an English resumé, (J, GR) in Japanese with a German resumé, and (R) in Russian. The journals *Sakura-kaishi, Sangyo-shinpo,* and *Toa-seni-soran* have ceased publication.

Akai, H., K. Kiguchi and K. Mori, 1973 The influence of juvenile hormone on the growth and metamorphosis of *Bombyx* larvae. *Bull. Sericult. Exp. Stn. Tokyo* **25**:287–305. (J, ER)

Akiyama, T., 1921 Inheritance of certain cocoon character in the silkworm. *Res. Bull. Ueda Sericult. Coll.* **8**:47–50. (J)

Aratake, Y., 1961 Genetical analyses of the infection with muscardines of *Bombyx mori* L. I. Infection with the white muscardine. *Bull. Sericult. Exp. Stn. Tokyo* **17**:155–165. (J, ER)

Aruga, H., 1939a Genetical studies on mutants obtained from silkworms treated with X-rays. I. A dominant mutant "burnt" and its linkage. *Bull. Sericult. Exp. Stn. Tokyo* **9**:295–304. (J, ER)

Aruga, H., 1939b Genetical studies on mutants obtained from silkworms treated with X-rays. IV. A new additional marking mutation, *brown (Br). Bull. Sericult. Exp. Stn. Tokyo* **9**:345–352. (J, ER)

Aruga, H., 1940 Genetical studies on mutants obtained from silkworms treated with X-rays. V. A gene mutant, transparent back (*Tb*), and some chromosomal mutations. *Bull. Sericult. Exp. Stn. Tokyo* **9**:495–520. (J, ER)

Aruga, H., 1943a Genetical studies on mutants obtained from silkworms treated with X-rays. VI. A dominant mutant "abnormal corselet." *Bull. Sericult. Exp. Stn. Tokyo* **11**:467–477. (J)

Aruga, H., 1943b Genetical studies on mutants obtained from silkworms treated with X-rays. VII. A dominant mutant "abnormal segment." *Bull. Sericult. Exp. Stn. Tokyo* **11**:479–488. (J)

Aruga, H., 1943c Genetical studies on mutants obtained from silkworms treated with X-rays. VIII. A dominant mutant "dwarf." *Bull. Sericult. Exp. Stn. Tokyo* **11**:489–493. (J)

Aruga, H., 1943d Genetical studies on mutants obtained from silkworms treated with X-rays. IX. A dominant mutant "supernumerary legs." *Bull. Sericult. Exp. Stn. Tokyo* **11**:495–498. (J)

Aruga, H., 1943e A new sex-linked mutation in the silkworm. *Bull Sericult. Exp. Stn. Tokyo* **11**:499–507. (J)

Aruga, H., 1943f A new sex-linked gene in the silkworm. *Bull. Sericult. Exp. Stn. Tokyo* **11**:509–512. (J)

Asano, K., 1947 Inheritance of the compressed segments in silkworm. *Jap. J. Genet.* **22**:88–92. (J, ER)

Asano, K., 1948 On a recessive trimoulter in the silkworm. *J. Sericult. Sci. Jap.* **17**:9–12. (J)

Asano, K. and S. Itikawa, 1958 Linkage analysis of the "lanky" mutant in the silkworm. *Acta Sericol. Tokyo* **27**:24–25. (J)

Beaulaton, J. A., 1968 Modifications ultrastructurales des cellules sécrétrices de la glande prothoracique de Vers à soie an cours des deux derniers âges larvaires. 1. Le chondriome, et ses relations avec le réticulum agranulaire. *J. Cell Biol.* **39**:501–525.

Butenandt, A. and P. Karlson, 1954 Über die Isolierung eines Metamorphose-Hormones der Insecten in kristallisierter Form. *Z. Naturforsch.* **9b**:389–391.

Chang, C. F., S. Murakoshi and S. Tamura, 1972 Giant cocoon formation in the silkworm *Bombyx mori* L., topically treated with methylenedioxyphenyl derivatives. *Agric. Biol. Chem.* **36**:692–694.

Chikushi, H., 1938 Induced mutations by heat-shock in the silkworm. *J. Sericult. Sci. Jap.* **9**:144–165. (J)

Chikushi, H., 1948   Linkage data. *Silkworm Inf. Serv.* **3**:4. (J)

Chikushi, H., 1949   Inheritance of the *dirty marking* gene of the silkworm, and its interaction to some other markings. *Jap. J. Genet.* **24**:144–149. (J, ER)

Chikushi, H., 1953   On the estimation of recombination values between two characters, *multistar* and *narrow breast*, in the silkworm. *J. Sericult. Sci. Jap.* **22**:1–4. (J, ER)

Chikushi, H., 1957   Linkage data. *Rep. Res. Grantees Minist. Educ., Agric.*: 233–234. (J)

Chikushi, H., 1959*a*   Contributions to genetics of *Bombyx*, with special reference to mechanisms of manifestation of characteristics: 1 and 2. *Sci. Bull. Fac. Agric. Kyushu Univ.* **17**:171–187, 189–196. (J, ER)

Chikushi, H., 1959*b*   On white egg colour loci in the 10th linkage group of the silkworm. *J. Sericult. Sci. Jap.* **28**:184. (J)

Chikushi, H., 1960*a*   A new linkage group of the silkworm. *J. Sericult. Sci. Jap.* **29**:278. (J)

Chikushi, H., 1960*b*   A new linkage between hare-lip (*hal*) and blind (*bl*) in the silkworm. *Proc. 13th Meet. Jap. Soc. Sericult. Kyushu*: 32–33. (J)

Chikushi, H., 1961   Genetical studies of the inhibitor of lemon (*i-lem*) in the silkworm. *J. Sericult. Sci. Jap.* **30**:253–254. (J)

Chikushi, H., 1966   Further studies on the *otm-of* linkage group in the silkworm. *J. Sericult. Sci. Jap.* **35**:228. (J)

Chikushi, H., 1970   Inheritance of the "Tanaka's double crescent and supernumerary leg" in the silkworm. *Proc. Sericult. Sci. Kyushu* **1**:7. (J)

Chikushi, H., 1972   *Genes and Genetical Stocks of the Silkworm*, Keigaku Publishing Co., Tokyo.

Chikushi, H. and H. Doira, 1970   The third linkage map of silkworm, *Bombyx mori*. *J. Sericult. Sci. Jap.* **39**:319–320. (J, ER)

Chikushi, H. and H. Kihara, 1973   Studies of the translucent mutants on the 9th chromosome of *Bombyx mori*. *Proc. 43rd Meet. Jap. Soc. Sericult. Sci.*: 58. (J)

Chikushi, H. and H. Sakamoto, 1967   Linkage studies of the "mildewed-stripe" in the silkworm. *J. Sericult. Sci. Jap.* **36**:257. (J)

Chikushi, H., H. Sakamoto and H. Kihara, 1964   Linkage studies of the *om* gene in the silkworm. *Proc. 18th Meet. Jap. Soc. Sericult. Kyushu*: 2–3. (J)

Chikushi, H., H. Doira and B. Sakaguchi, 1971*a*   Genetical studies of the deletion, "Retarded growth," in the third chromosome of *Bombyx mori*. *Jap. J. Genet.* **46**:301–307.

Chikushi, H., H. Doira and K. Morita, 1971*b*   Inheritance of lethal-brown in *Bombyx mori*. *Proc. Sericult. Sci. Kyushu* **2**:76. (J)

Chikushi, H., B. Sakaguchi, H. Doira and H. Sakamoto, 1972   Contributions to genetics of *Bombyx*. 5. *Sci. Bull. Fac. Agric. Kyushu Univ.* **26**:47–59. (J, ER)

Chino, H., S. Sakurai, T. Ohtaki, N. Ikekawa, H. Miyazaki, M. Ishibashi and H. Abuki, 1974   Biosynthesis of α-ecdysone by prothoracic glands *in vitro*. *Science (Wash., D.C.)* **183**:529–530.

Cleghorn, M. L., 1918   First report on the inheritance of visible and invisible characters in silkworms. *Proc. Zool. Soc. Lond. Parts I and II*: 133–146.

Coutagne, G., 1902   Recherches expérimentales sur l'hérédité chez les vers à soie. *Bull. Sci. Fr. Belg.* **37**:1–194.

Dahm, K. H., B. M. Trost and H. Roller, 1967   The juvenile hormone. V. Synthesis of the racemic juvenile hormone. *J. Am. Chem. Soc.* **89**:5292–5294.

Danilova, L. V., 1974   The ultrastructure of contractile rings in silkworm spermatogenic cells. *Tsitologiya* **15**:5–10. (R, ER)

Doira, H., 1968   Developmental and sexual differences of blood proteins in the silkworm, *Bombyx mori*. *Sci. Bull. Fac. Agric. Kyushu Univ.* **23**:205–214. (J, ER)

Doira, H., 1970   Inheritance of the "varnished eye" mutant in *Bombyx mori*. *Proc. Sericult. Sci. Kyushu* **1**:4. (J)

Doira, H., 1973   Genetical studies of the flimsy cocoon of *Bombyx mori*. *J. Sericult. Sci. Jap.* **42**:425–435.

Doira, H. and Y. Kawaguchi, 1972   Changes in haemolymph and egg protein by the castration and implantation of the ovary in *Bombyx mori*. *J. Fac. Agric. Kyushu Univ.* **17**:119–127.

Doira, H. and Y. Kawaguchi, 1974   Protein pattern of mosaic eggs for normal and small egg character in *Bombyx mori*. *J. Fac. Agric. Kyushu Univ.* **18**:201–206.

Doira, H., H. Chikushi and M. Nakayama, 1963   Genetical studies of the melamine-induced translucent mutant, *oml*. *Proc. 17th Meet. Jap. Soc. Seric. Kyushu*: 20–21. (J)

Doira, H., H. Chikushi and H. Kihara, 1971   Linkage analyses of the "mottled grey" and the "small egg-2" mutants in *Bombyx mori*. *Proc. Sericult. Sci. Kyushu* **2**:75. (J)

Doira, H., M. Tsujita and H. Chikushi, 1972   Inheritance of Tsujita's dwarf mutation in *Bombyx mori*. *Proc. Sericult. Sci. Kyushu* **3**:76. (J)

Doira, H., H. Chikushi and H. Kihara, 1973a   Genetical studies of the albino mutants in *Bombyx mori*. *J. Sericult. Sci. Jap.* **42**:411–416. (J, ER)

Doira, H., H. Chikushi and H. Kihara, 1973b   Inheritance of the "Kh-extra crescents" and the "kidney of Chikushi" mutations in *Bombyx mori*. *Proc. Sericult. Sci. Kyushu* **4**:74. (J)

Doira, H., H. Chikushi and M. Tsujita, 1973c   A new linkage group in *Bombyx mori*. *Proc. 45th Meet. Jap. Soc. Genet.*: 61. (J)

Doira, H., H. Chikushi and H. Kihara, 1974a   Linkage studies of *Bombyx mori*: Discovery and establishment of the *oh–Df–t–b–4* linkage group, the twenty-first chromosome. *J. Sericult. Sci. Jap.* **43**:74–80. (J, ER)

Doira, H., M. Tsujita and H. Kihara, 1974b   Genetical studies of the "gooseneck" mutant in *Bombyx mori*. *J. Sericult. Sci. Jap.* **43**:337–339 (J, ER)

Doira, H., H. Kihara and H. Chikushi, 1974c   Genetical studies of the "small egg-2" mutant in *Bombyx mori*. *J. Sericult. Sci. Jap.* **43**:369–372. (J, ER)

Doira, H., H. Chikushi and H. Kihara, 1974d   Inheritance of the dwarf-k mutant in *Bombyx mori*. *Proc. Sericult. Sci. Kyushu* **5**:97. (J).

Eguchi, M. and N. Yoshitake, 1966   Genetic studies on isozymes of the integument esterase in the silkworm, *Bombyx mori* L. *Jap. J. Genet.* **41**:267–273.

Eguchi, M. and N. Yoshitake, 1967   Comparative studies on esterase zymograms among various tissues in the silkworm, *Bombyx mori* L. *Appl. Entomol. Zool.* **2**:163–167.

Eguchi, M., N. Yoshitake and H. Kai, 1965   Types and inheritance of blood esterase in the silkworm, *Bombyx mori* L. *Jap. J. Genet.* **40**:15–19.

Eguchi, M., M. Sawaki and Y. Suzuki, 1972   Multiple forms of midgut alkaline phosphatase in the silkworm: New band formation and the relationship between the midgut and digestive fluid enzymes. *Insect Biochem.* **2**:297–304.

Endo, S., 1940   Inheritance of dominant chocolate. *Bot. Zool.* **8**:1439–1444. (J)

Fujieda, T., 1970   A new mutant of the *E* locus on the sixth chromosome of the silkworm. *Proc. 40th Meet. Jap. Soc. Sericult. Sci.*: 60. (J)

Fujimoto, N., 1943   On a cause of sterility in a special strain of the silkworm. *J. Sericult. Sci. Jap.* **14**:283–293. (J)

Fujimoto, N., N. Yoshitake and O. Yamashita, 1962   On the green inhibitor-1 mutation in the silkworm, *Bombyx mori. J. Sericult. Sci. Jap.* **31**:239–244. (J, ER)

Fukuda, S., 1940   Induction of pupation in silkworm by transplanting the prothoracic gland. *Proc. Imp. Acad. Tokyo* **16**:414–416.

Fukuda, S., 1951   On the number of segments of the silkworm larva. *J. Sericult. Sci. Jap.* **20**:180–181. (J)

Gage, L. P., 1974a   Polyploidization of the silk gland in *Bombyx mori. J. Mol. Biol.* **86**:97–108.

Gage, L. P., 1974b   The *Bombyx mori* genome: Analysis by DNA reassociation kinetics. *Chromosoma (Berl.)* **45**:27–42.

Gage, L. P., Y. Suzuki and D. D. Brown, 1972   Specific hybridization of the silk fibroin genes in *Bombyx mori*. In *Molecular Genetics and Developmental Biology,* edited by M. Sussman, p. 127, Prentice-Hall, Englewood Cliffs, N.J.

Gamo, T., 1923   Studies on the black pupa appeared in a silkworm race, Kairyo-matamukashi. *Sakura-kaishi* **13**:14–15. (J)

Gamo, T., Jr., 1965   A new extra-crescent gene (E^{Dl}) causing degeneration of abdominal legs in the silkworm. *Jap. J. Genet.* **40**:219–226. (J, ER)

Gamo, T., Jr., 1968   The inheritance of electrophoretic patterns of blood albumin in the silkworm, *Bombyx mori* L. *Jap. J. Genet.* **43**:271–277.

Gillot, S. and J. Daillie, 1968   Rapport entre la mue et la synthèse d'ADN dans la glande séricigène du Ver à soie. *C. R. Acad. Sci. Paris, Sér.* D Sci. Nat. **266**:2295–2298.

Goldschmidt, R. and K. Katsuki, 1927   Erblicher Gynandromorphismus und somatische Mosaikbildung bei *Bombyx mori* L. *Biol. Zentralbl.* **47**:45–54.

Goldschmidt, R. and K. Katsuki, 1928a   Zweite Mitteilung über erblichen Gynandromorphismus bei *Bombyx mori* L. *Biol. Zentralbl.* **48**:43–49.

Goldschmidt, R. and K. Katsuki, 1928b   Zytologie des erblichen Gynandromorphismus von *Bombyx mori* L. *Biol. Zentralbl.* **48**:685–699.

Goldschmidt, R. and K. Katsuki, 1931   Vierte Mitteilung über erblichen Gynandromorphismus und somatische Mosaikbildung bei *Bombyx mori* L. *Biol. Zentralbl.* **51**:58–74.

Harizuka, M., 1942   Genetical studies on the black pupa of *Bombyx mori. J. Sericult. Sci. Jap.* **13**:4–8. (J)

Harizuka, M., 1947a   Genetical and physiological studies on the black pupa of the silkworm. *Bull. Sericult. Exp. Stn. Tokyo* **12**:531–593. (J, ER)

Harizuka, M., 1947b   Stock list. *Silkworm Inf. Serv.* **1**:5. (J)

Harizuka, M., 1948   Linkage between wingless and white egg-2 of the silkworm. *J. Sericult. Sci. Jap.* **17**:6–8. (J)

Harizuka, M., 1953   Physiological genetics of the carotenoids in *Bombyx mori*, with special reference to the pink cocoon. *Bull. Sericult. Exp. Stn. Tokyo* **14**:141–156. (J, ER)

Harizuka, M., S. Ueda and T. Hirao, 1960   Physiogenetic studies on carotenoids in the silkworm, *Bombyx mori* L. (2) On the origin of pigments and the conditions of development of cocoon colour in pink-, and flesh-coloured strains. *Bull. Sericult. Exp. Stn. Tokyo* **16**:1–34. (J, ER)

Hasegawa, K., 1957 The diapause hormone of the silkworm, *Bombyx mori. Nature (Lond.)* **179**:1300–1301.

Hashida, K., 1934 On an abnormal type of vein in the silkworm moth. *J. Sericult. Sci. Jap.* **5**:168–169. (J)

Hashiguchi, H. and H. Ooi, 1955 Linkage studies of an "extra spiracle." *Acta Sericol. Tokyo* **11**:1–3. (J)

Hashiguchi, T. and N. Yoshitake, 1966 Racial differences on the phenoloxidase activity of the blood in the silkworm, *Bombyx mori* L. *J. Sericult. Sci. Jap.* **35**:387–392. (J, ER)

Hasimoto, H., 1930 Hereditary superfluous legs in the silkworm. *Jap. J. Genet.* **6**:45–54. (J)

Hasimoto, H., 1934a Linkage studies in the silkworm. I. Quail and mottled translucent. *Bull. Sericult. Exp. Stn. Tokyo* **8**:465–472. (J, ER)

Hasimoto, H., 1934b Linkage studies in the silkworm. II. Supernumerary and a lethal. *Bull. Sericult. Exp. Stn. Tokyo* **8**:473–479. (J, ER)

Hasimoto, H., 1940 A new lethal which belongs to the third linkage group of silkworm. *J. Sericult. Sci. Jap.* **11**:34–35. (J)

Hasimoto, H., 1941a Linkage studies in the silkworm. III. *Kp* multiple alleles. *Bull. Sericult. Exp. Stn. Tokyo* **10**:327–346. (J, ER)

Hasimoto, H., 1941b Linkage studies in the silkworm. IV. Inheritance of the green cocoons. *Bull. Sericult. Exp. Stn. Tokyo* **10**:347–358. (J, ER)

Hasimoto, H., 1941c Linkage studies in the silkworm V. Linkage between *dk* translucent and a new dominant colour pattern gene. *Bull. Sericult. Exp. Stn. Tokyo* **10**:359–363. (J, ER)

Hasimoto, H., 1948a Linkage between dominant white and dominant chocolate *J. Sericult. Sci. Jap.* **16**:60–61. (J)

Hasimoto, H., 1948b Sex-limited zebra, an X-ray mutation in the silkworm. *J. Sericult. Sci. Jap.* **16**:62–64. (J)

Hasimoto, H., 1956 Genetical studies on the naked pupa and the dilute yellow cocoon genes. *Rep. Res. Grantees Minist. Educ., Agric.*: 215. (J)

Hasimoto, H., 1957 A new supernumerary-leg gene (E^{Mu}) obtained by the heat parthenogenesis in the silkworm. *J. Sericult. Sci. Jap.* **26**:256. (J)

Hasimoto, H., 1960 A newly established linkage group in the silkworm. *Rep. Res. Grantees Minist. Educ., Agric.*: 247–248. (J)

Hasimoto, H., 1961 Genetic study of melanism of silkworm larva. *J. Sericult. Sci. Jap.* **30**:389–391. (J)

Hasimoto, H., 1965 Austausch zwischen glänzende Augen und Wange-Schwanz-Flecken Gene beim Seidenspinner, *Bombyx mori. J. Sericult. Sci. Jap.* **34**:285–286. (J, GR)

Hatamura, M., 1939 Genetical studies of the d-mottled silkworm. *Bull. Sericult. Exp. Stn. Tokyo* **9**:353–375. (J, ER)

Hayashi, T., 1937 Morphological studies on abnormally shaped eggs in *Bombyx mori.* I. *Sci. Bull. Fac. Agric. Kyushu Univ.* **7**:359–372. (J, ER)

Hirobe, T., 1944 A new recessive mutant "apodal" in *Bombyx mori. Jap. J. Genet.* **20**:78. (J)

Hirobe, T., 1947a Mutants and linkage data. *Silkworm Inf. Serv.* **1**:4. (J)

Hirobe, T., 1947b On a mutant "micropteral" in the silkworm. *Jap. J. Genet.* **22**:9. (J)

Hirobe, T., 1951 Mutants discovered. *Silkworm Inf. Serv.* **4**:56. (J)

Hirobe, T., 1952 On lethal spindle egg in the silkworm. *J. Sericult. Sci. Jap.* **21**:122. (J)

Hirobe, T., 1954 Inheritance of a recessive trimoulting gene in the silkworm. *J. Sericult. Sci. Jap.* **23**:199–200. (J)

Hirobe, T., 1958 Linkage studies in the silkworm; on the linkage between *cts* and *lu*. *Rep. Res. Grantees Minist. Educ., Agric.*: 202–203. (J)

Hirobe, T., 1960 Linkage studies in the silkworm. *Rep. Res. Grantees Minist. Educ., Agric.*: 247. (J)

Hirobe, T. and H. Ooi, 1954 On a new heritable, deformed silkworm and environmental conditions. *Jap. J. Genet.* **29**:156. (J)

Hirobe, T., T. Takatsu and H. Ooi, 1952 On a new linkage of the silkworm between lethal non-hibernated (*l-n*), no-glue (*Ng*) and yellow cocoon (*C*). *Jap. J. Genet.* **27**:231. (J)

Horiuchi, Y., C. Namishima, K. Nakamura and N. Yasue, 1963 On the sericin-cocoon mutant discovered in a Burmese race of the silkworm. *J. Sericult. Sci. Jap.* **32**:195–196. (J)

Ichikawa, M. and H. Ishizaki, 1963 Protein nature of the brain hormone of insects. *Nature (Lond.)* **198**:308–309.

Imms, A. D., 1957 *A General Textbook of Entomology* (revised by O. W. Richards and R. G. Davies), ninth edition, Methuen, London.

Inagami, K. and M. Akagi, 1954 Chemical and genetical studies on the formation of the pigment in the silkworm. I. Inheritance of the mutant "Aka-aka." *J. Sericult. Sci. Jap.* **23**:225–227. (J, ER)

Isobe, M., K. Hasegawa and T. Goto, 1973 Isolation of the diapause hormone from the silkworm, *Bombyx mori. J. Insect Physiol.* **19**:1221–1239.

Itikawa, N., 1943 Genetical and embryological studies of a dominant mutant, "new additional crescent," of the silkworm, *Bombyx mori* L., *Jap. J. Genet.* **19**:182–188. (J)

Itikawa, N., 1944 A new mutant *Nc* belonging to the eighth linkage group. *Toa-seni-soran* **15**:182–188. (J)

Itikawa, N., 1948 New mutants. *Silkworm Inf. Serv.* **3**:3. (J)

Ito, T., 1969 Germfree rearing of the silkworm, *Bombyx mori* L. in *Technology in Germfree and Gnotobiotic Life Research,* edited by M. Miyakawa and B. S. Wostmann, pp. 67–73, Academic Press, Tokyo.

Ito, T., and N. Arai, 1966 Nutrition of the silkworm, *Bombyx mori.* XI. Requirements for aspartic and glutamic acids. *J. Insect Physiol.* **12**:861–869.

Kai, H. and K. Hasegawa, 1973 An esterase in relation to yolk cell lysis at diapause termination in the silkworm, *Bombyx mori. J. Insect Physiol.* **19**:799–810.

Kanbe, R. and S. Nara, 1959 Genetical studies of a new mutant, white banded black (*wb*) wing, in silkworm. *J. Sericult. Sci. Jap.* **28**:37–39. (J)

Karlson, P. and H. Hoffmeister, 1963 Zur Biogenese des Ecdysons. I. Umwandlung von Cholesterin in Ecdysone. *Hoppe Seyler's Z. Physiol. Chem.* **331**:298–300.

Katsuki, K., 1935 Weitere Versuche über erbliche Mosaikbildung und Gynandromorphismus bei *Bombyx mori* L. *Biol. Zentralbl.* **55**:361–383.

Katsumata, F., 1968 Non-maternal inheritance in voltinism, observed in the crossing experiments between Indonesian polyvoltine and Japanese bivoltine races of the silkworm, *Bombyx mori* L. *J. Sericult. Sci. Jap.* **37**:453–461. (J)

Kawaguchi, E., 1933 "Black," eine mutation der Körperfarbe beim Seidenspinner (*Bombyx mori* L.). *Jap. J. Genet.* **8**:97–107. (J, GR)

Kawaguchi, E., 1934 Die Faktoren-Analyse bei den Bastarden zwischen *Bombyx mori* var. *mandarina* M. und *Bombyx mori* L. *Jap. J. Genet.* **9**:154–156.

Kawaguchi, Y. and H. Doira, 1973 Gene-controlled incorporation of haemolymph protein into the ovaries of *Bombyx mori. J. Insect Physiol.* **19**:2083–2096.

Kawaguchi, Y. and H. Doira, 1974 Incorporation and synthesis of protein by the ovaries of *Bombyx mori. J. Fac. Agric. Kyushu Univ.* **18**:139–147.

Kawaguchi, Y., H. Doira and H. Chikushi, 1970 Genetical studies on the haemolymph protein of the silkworm. *Proc. Sericult. Sci. Kyushu* **1**:51. (J)

Kawakami, M. and K. Shimura, 1973 Fractionation of glycine-, alanine- and serine-transfer ribonucleic acids from the silkglands of silkworms. *J. Biochem.* **74**:33–40.

Kei, O. S., 1937 Genetic studies on the Cantonese silkworm, *Bombyx mori. Res. Rep. Liao Chung Kai Agric. Indust. Sch. Canton* **5**:1–80. (C)

Kei, O. S., 1942 Inheritance of the 'black translucent' in *Bombyx mori. Jap. J. Genet.* **18**:147–149. (J)

Kei, O. S., 1943 Studies on the inheritance of cocoon colour and egg shape in the silkworm. Doctorate thesis, Kyushu University, Fukuoka. (J)

Kellog, V. L., 1908 Inheritance in silkworms: I. *Stanford Univ. Pub. Univ. Ser.* **I**:1–80.

Kiguchi, K., 1972 Hormonal control of the coloration of larval body and the pigmentation of larval markings in *Bombyx mori.* 1. Endocrine organs affecting the coloration of larval body and the pigmentation of markings. *J. Sericult. Sci. Jap.* **41**:407–412. (J, ER)

Kikkawa, H., 1947 Linkage data. *Silkworm Inf. Serv.* **1**:7. (J)

King, R. C. and H. Akai, 1971*a* Spermatogenesis in *Bombyx mori.* I. The canal system joining sister spermatocytes. *J. Morphol.* **134**:47–56.

King, R. C. and H. Akai, 1971*b* Spermatogenesis in *Bombyx mori.* II. The ultrastructure of synapsed bivalents. *J. Morphol.* **134**:181–194.

Kobari, K., 1932*a* Studies on discernment of cocoon quality by means of ultraviolet light, in the silkworm. I. Inheritance of fluorescence of cocoon shell. *Bull. Katakura Sericult. Exp. Stn.* **1**:1–35. (J)

Kobari, K., 1932*b* Studies on perforated cocoons in the silkworm. I. Selection and inheritance. *Bull. Katakura Sericult. Exp. Stn.* **1**:45–59. (J)

Kobayashi, M. and J. Kirimura, 1958 The brain hormone in the silkworm, *Bombyx mori* L. *Nature (Lond.)* **181**:1217.

Kobayashi, M. and M. Yamazaki, 1966 The protenic brain hormone in an insect, *Bombyx mori* L. (Lepidoptera: Bombycidae). *Appl. Entomol. Zool.* **1**:53–60. (J, ER)

Kogure, M., 1935 A new sex-linked lethal. *J. Sericult. Sci. Jap.* **6**:184–193. (J)

Kosminsky, P. A. and B. Schragina, 1933 Beiträge zur Genetik des Seidenspinners. X. Zusammenhang zwischen neutralen Merkmalen und der Lebensfähigkeit. *Zool. Zhur. Moscow* **12**:26–58. (R, GR)

Latreille, P. A., 1802 *Histoire Naturelle, Ge'nerale et Particuliere des Crustace's et des Insectes.* Dufart, Paris.

Lucas, F. and K. M. Rudall, 1968 Extracellular fibrous proteins: The silks. In *Comprehensive Biochemistry,* edited by M. Florkin and E. H. Stotz, Chapter 7, 26B, pp. 475–558, Elsevier, Amsterdam.

Mano, Y. and M. Itagaki, 1965 The locus of the sex-linked chocolate. I. Recombination value between *sch* and *od. J. Sericult. Sci. Jap.* **34**:216. (J)

Matsumura, S., 1933 Four genetic types of amylase activity in the silkworm. *J. Sericult. Sci. Jap.* **4**:168–170. (J)

Matsuzaki, K., 1966 Fractionation of amino acid-specific s-RNA from silkgland by methylated albumin column chromatography. *Biochim. Biophys. Acta* **114**:222–226.

Miya, K., M. Kurihara and I. Tanimura, 1969 Electron microscope studies on the oogenesis of the silkworm, *Bombyx mori* L. I. Fine structure of the oocyte and nurse cells in the early developmental stages. *J. Fac. Agric. Iwate Univ.* **9**:221–237.

Miya, K., M. Kurihara and I. Tanimura, 1970 Electron microscope studies on the oogenesis of the silkworm, *Bombyx mori* L. III. Fine structure of the ovary in the early fifth instar. *J. Fac. Agric. Iwate Univ.* **10**:59–83.

Mori, T., editor, 1970*a* *The Silkworm,* Sanseido, Chiyoda-ku, Tokyo.

Mori, T., 1970*b* Sixty color slides illustrating the life cycle, genetics and endocrinology of *Bombyx mori,* photographs by R. Yoshida, Toyo Kyozai Kenkyusho Co., Hinoshi, Tokyo.

Morimoto, T., S. Matsuura, S. Nagata and Y. Tashiro, 1968 Studies on the posterior silk gland of the silkworm, *Bombyx mori.* III. Ultrastructural changes of posterior silk gland cells in the fourth larval instar. *J. Cell Biol.* **38**:604–614.

Morohoshi, S., 1943 Über eine erblich neue Zwergseidenraupe. *Jap. J. Genet.* **19**:75–78. (J, GR)

Morohoshi, S., 1957 *Physiological Studies on Moultinism and Voltinism in Bombyx mori: A New Hormonal Antagonistic Balance Theory on the Growth,* Japan Society for the Promotion of Science, Ueno Park, Tokyo.

Morohoshi, S. and M. Mezaki, 1956 Studies on the voltinism in the silkworm, *Bombyx mori.* III. The relation between voltinism and superfluous abdominal legs. (*Kp*). *J. Sericult. Sci. Jap.* **25**:228. (J)

Muroga, H., 1948 Inheritance of voltinism in the silkworm. V. The linkage group to which the *uh* (*rh*) gene belongs. *J. Sericult. Sci. Jap.* **16**:86–87. (J)

Muroga, H., 1953 Studies on linkage in silkworm, *Bombyx mori* L. V. The chromosome bearing the gene *Ng. J. Sericult. Sci. Jap.* **22**:51. (J)

Nagashima, E., 1956 Studies on the brown egg mutation in the silkworm, *Bombyx mori.* I. On the brown egg 1 (*b-1*) and brown egg 2 (*b-2*) genes. *J. Sericult. Sci. Jap.* **25**:423–429. (J, ER)

Nagashima, E., S. Tanaka and T. Miyashita, 1957 Studies on the brown egg mutation in the silkworm, *Bombyx mori.* III. Relation between the brown egg and the white egg genes. *J. Sericult. Sci. Jap.* **26**:252–253. (J)

Nagashima, E., H. Kataoka and R. Takei, 1971 Studies on the caltrop gene appearing by spontaneous mutation in the silkworm, *Bombyx mori* L. *J. Sericult. Sci. Jap.* **40**:97–100. (J)

Nagatomo, T., 1926 On the sex-linked inheritance of quantitative characters in the silkworm *Bombyx mori. J. Sci. Agric. Soc. Tokyo* **281**:155–180. (J)

Nagatomo, T., 1942 Inheritance of the voltinism in the silkworm, *Bombyx mori. J. Sericult. Sci. Jap.* **13**:114–115. (J)

Nakajima, M., 1956 Linkage studies on the sooty plain white (*a*) and the peony (*b₃*) genes. *Rep. Res. Grantees Minist. Educ., Agric.*: 215–216. (J)

Nakajima, M., 1963 Physiological studies on the function of genes concerning catotenoid permeability in the silkworm. *Bull. Fac. Agric. Tokyo Univ. Agr. Technol.* **8**:1–80. (J, ER)

Nakajima, M., 1971 Allelic relation between the sooty plain white *a* and the yellow inhibitor *I* genes in *Bombyx mori. J. Sericult. Sci. Jap.* **40**:107–110. (J, ER)

Nakanishi, Y. H., I. Iwasaki and H. Kato, 1965 Cytological studies on the radiosensitivity of spermatogonia of the silkworm. *Jap. J. Genet.* **40 (Suppl.)**:49–67.

Nakanishi, Y., H. Kato and S. Utsumi, 1969   Polytene chromosomes in silk gland cells of the silkworm, *Bombyx mori. Experientia (Basel)* **25**:384–385.

Nakano, Y., 1931   Genetical studies of the Aojuku white egg-translucent gene. *J. Sericult. Sci. Jap.* **2**:140–153. (J)

Nakano, Y., 1951*a*   Physiological, anatomical and genetical studies of the "excreter" silkworm. *J. Sericult. Sci. Jap.* **20**:169–179. (J)

Nakano, Y., 1951*b*   Physiological, anatomical and genetical studies on the "naked" silkworm pupa. *J. Sericult. Sci. Jap.* **20**:232–248. (J)

Nakayama, M., 1954   A lethal translucent occurring in the C21 strain. *Acta Sericol. Tokyo* **12**:1–4. (J)

Nakayama, M., 1958   Linkage studies of the "lethal white-rot egg" gene in the silkworm. *Acta Sericol. Tokyo* **25**:1–6. (J)

Niimura, M., S. Aomori, K. Mori and M. Matsui, 1972   Utilization of a synthetic compound with juvenile hormone activity for silkworm rearing. *Agric. Biol. Chem.* **36**:889–892.

Nishikawa, H., 1925   Studies on lethals in the silkworm (A preliminary note). *Sangyo-shinpo* **33**:964–971. (J)

Nishikawa, H., 1930   On lethal factors in the silkworm (*Bombyx mori* L.). *Rep. Sericult. Exp. Stn. Chosen* **2**:179–291. (J)

Nishikawa, H., 1932   On the second sex-linked lethal factor in the silkworm (*Bombyx mori* L.). *Rep. Sericult. Exp. Stn. Chosen* **3**:1–38. (J)

Nishikawa, H., 1934   On two new sex-linked lethal factors in the silkworm (*Bombyx mori* L.). *Jap. J. Genet.* **9**:150–153. (J)

Nittono, Y., 1960   Studies on the blood cells in the silkworm, *Bombyx mori* L. *Bull. Sericult. Exp. Stn. Tokyo* **16**:171–266. (J, ER)

Nittono, Y., S. Tomabechi and N. Onodera, 1964   A strange type of hemocyte found in a strain of the silkworm, *Bombyx mori* L. *J. Sericult. Sci. Jap.* **33**:46–48. (J, ER)

Nozaki, K., 1917   A new case of Mendelian inheritance in the silkworm. *Sangyo-shinpo* **25**:85–90. (J)

Ogawa, S., 1949   Studies on a mutant constricted in the silkworm. *J. Sericult. Sci. Jap.* **18**:181–183. (J)

Ogura, S., 1922   Linkage phenomena between the zebra-factor and others in the silkworm. *Jap. J. Genet.* **1**:195–217. (J)

Ogura, S., 1931*a*   Erblichkeitsstudien am Seidenspinner *Bombyx mori* L. I. Genetische Untersuchung der Kokonfarbe. *Z. indukt. Abstammungs.-Vererbungsl.* **58**:122–156.

Ogura, S., 1931*b*   Erblichkeitsstudien am Seidenspinner *Bombyx mori* L. II. Uber die Koppelung zwischen dem Häutungsfaktor und dem Faktor *F. Z. indukt. Abstammungs.-Vererbungsl.* **58**:403–421.

Omura, S., 1949   Hereditary abdominal malformation of the silkworm. *Jap. J. Genet.* **25**:71–72. (J)

Ono, M., 1942   Über die Malpighischen Gefässe des Seidenspinners mit Knötchen an ihren Distalschenkeln. I. Mitteilung. *Bull. Kagoshima Agric. Coll.* **14**:161–169. (J, GR)

Ooi, H., 1962   Genetical and embryological studies on a mutant, lethal spindle-shaped egg, in *Bombyx mori* L. *Bull. Sericult. Exp. Stn. Tokyo* **18**:35–48. (J, ER)

Ooi, H., 1968   Developmental and genetical studies on the expression of some abnormal characters in the silkworm, *Bombyx mori* L. *Bull. Sericult. Exp. Stn. Tokyo* **23**:35–80 (J, ER)

Ooi, H., T. Hirobe, K. Nakamaki, I. Minagawa, M. Yasuda and Y. Yamashita, 1953 On the loci of some mutations in the silkworm. *Acta Sericol. Tokyo* **4**:24–25. (J)

Oota, S., A. Watanabe and H. Tokunaga, 1957 Genetical study on a spontaneous mutant, two molter, in the silkworm, *Bombyx mori*. *J. Sericult. Sci. Jap.* **26**:77–81. (J)

Otsuki, Y., 1956 Development of the embryo homozygous for lethal-brown. *Proc. 10th Meet. Jap. Soc. Sericult. Kyushu*: 1. (J)

Otsuki, Y., 1965 Studies on the yolk formation in the silkworm, *Bombyx mori* L. *Bull. Fac. Text. Fib., Kyoto Univ. Indust. Arts Text. Fib.* **4**:314–344. (J, ER)

Otsuki, Y., 1968 On the locus of "White lethal egg" gene in the silkworm. *J. Sericult. Sci. Jap.* **37**:95–101. (J, ER)

Rasch, E. M., 1974 The DNA content of sperm and hemocyte nuclei of the silkworm, *Bombyx mori* L. *Chromosoma (Berl.)* **45**:1–26.

Röller, H., H. Dahm, C. C. Sweeley and B. M. Trost, 1967 The structure of the juvenile hormone. *Angew. Chem.* **6**:179–180.

Sado, T., 1957 Inheritance of "mottled-grey." (A preliminary note). *Proc. 11th Meet. Jap. Soc. Sericult. Sci. Kyushu*: 16–17. (J)

Sado, T., 1963 Spermatogenesis of the silkworm and its bearing on radiation-induced sterility. I., II. *J. Fac. Agric. Kyushu Univ.* **12**:359–386, 387–404.

Sado, T. and H. Chikushi, 1958 Genetical studies on the abnormal egg shells in *Bombyx mori*. *Sci. Bull. Fac. Agric. Kyushu Univ.* **16**:499–518. (J, ER)

Sakaguchi, B., 1957 Genetic determination of tyrosinase and protyrosinase in blood of silkworm, *Bombyx mori*. L. *Annu. Rep. Natl. Inst. Genet. Jap.* **8**:16–18.

Sakaguchi, B., H. Doira, H. Kihara and H. Chikushi, 1972 Group of analogous genes with E^{ca} on the *E* pseudoallele of silkworm, *Bombyx mori*. *Proc. Sericult. Sci. Kyushu* **3**:78. (J)

Sakata, T., 1938 Genetical studies on deformed gonads in the silkworm. *J. Sericult. Sci. Jap.* **9**:284. (J)

Sakata, T., 1941 Genetical study of an artificially induced translucent mutation. *J. Sericult. Sci. Jap.* **12**:228–229. (J)

Sakata, T., 1943 Inheritance of an artificially induced mutant "moustache" in the silkworm. *J. Sericult. Sci. Jap.* **14**:206–207. (J)

Sakate, S. and S. Nakasone, 1962 A new case of dilute black, a larval character of the silkworm, *Bombyx mori*. *J. Sericult. Sci. Jap.* **36**:366.

Sasaki, S., 1930 Genetical studies of a mutant, supernumerary legs in the silkworm. *J. Sericult. Sci. Jap.* **1**:87–102. (J)

Sasaki, S., 1932 Relation between an "extra-crescents and legs" mutant and a "plain extra-legs" mutant. *J. Sericult. Sci. Jap.* **3**:1–15. (J)

Sasaki, S., 1938 Linkage studies between the dominant white cocoon and the translucent mutants of a silkworm. (A preliminary note). *Jap. J. Genet.* **13**:285–288. (J, ER)

Sasaki, S., 1940 Inheritance of a new mutant "no-crescent supernumerary legs" in the silkworm. *J. Sericult. Sci. Jap.* **11**:1–13. (J)

Sasaki, S., 1941 A new silkworm mutant, "dilute black," and its linkage. *J. Sericult. Sci. Jap.* **12**:32–42. (J)

Sasaki, S. and Y. Kawano, 1963 Genetical studies of "extra crescents and short wing" (E^{sw}) in the silkworm. *J. Sericult. Sci. Jap.* **32**:198. (J)

Shimizu, M. and T. Ito, 1973 Studies on the large scale culture of silkworms on artificial diets. *Tech. Bull. Sericult. Exp. Stn. Tokyo* **96**:1–165. (J)

Shimizu, S., 1936   On yellow moulters in the silkworm. *J. Sericult. Sci. Jap.* **7**:167–170. (J)

Shimizu, S. and Y. Horiuchi, 1959   Stainability of the silkworm egg-shell with ferric chloride. *J. Sericult. Sci. Jap.* **28**:277–280. (J)

Shimodaira, M., 1928   Studies on the third case of lethal gene which accompanies morphological characteristics in the silkworm. *Sanshi-gakuho* **10** (12):1–10. (J)

Shimodaira, M., 1947a   Studies on the linkage of the silkworm. II. Inheritance of lethal factor (*1-10*). *Jap. J. Genet.* **22**:84–86. (J)

Shimodaira, M., 1947b   Studies on the linkage in the silkworm. III. Inheritance of "haimonkata" type. *J. Sericult. Sci. Jap.* **22**:87–88. (J)

Sturunnikov, V. A. and L. M. Gulamova, 1969   Artificial sex control in the silkworm (*Bombyx mori* L.). I. The origin of sex-labelled silkworm strains. *Genetika (Moscow)* **5**:52–71. (R, ER)

Suda, J. and K. Hashida, 1931   Characteristics and inheritance of a dwarf in the silkworm. *J. Sericult. Sci. Jap.* **2**:1–16. (J)

Suda, K. and E. Kawaguchi, 1922   Inheritance of reddish skin. *Sangyo-shinpo* **30** (346):33–35. (J)

Suzuki, K., 1929   Genetical studies on a "double crescents" in the silkworm. *Jap. J. Genet.* **4**:144. (J)

Suzuki, K., 1932   On the inheritance and abnormal development of embryos in a mutant strain, "kidney-shaped". *J. Sericult. Sci. Jap.* **3**:316–326. (J)

Suzuki, K., 1939   On the linkage between two different white-egg genes in *Bombyx mori*. *Jap. J. Genet.* **15**:183–193. (J, ER)

Suzuki, K., 1942   A new mutant in the silkworm, "cray-fish pupa," and its linkage. *Jap. J. Genet.* **18**:26–33. (J)

Suzuki, K., 1943   Genetical studies on egg and eye colours of *Bombyx mori*. *Bull. Sericult. Exp. Stn. Tokyo* **11**:125–196. (J)

Suzuki, K., 1947   List of genes. *Silkworm Inf. Serv.* **1**:2. (J)

Suzuki, K., 1950   On the inheritance of yellow silkworm which appears after the first moult. *Jap. J. Genet.* **25**:95–99. (J, ER)

Suzuki, K., 1952   Inheritance of a pupal character "curl wing" in the silkworm. *Papers Coord. Comm. Res. Genet. Tokyo.* **III**:117–129. (J, ER)

Suzuki, K. and S. Omura, 1951a   Inheritance of non-fertilization phenomena in the silkworm. II. On oligospermy. *Bull. Sericult. Exp. Stn. Tokyo* **13**:347–366. (J, ER)

Suzuki, K. and S. Omura, 1951b   Inheritance of non-fertilization phenomena in the silkworm. III. On the vaginal constriction. *Bull. Sericult. Exp. Stn. Tokyo* **13**:367–385. (J, ER)

Suzuki, Y., 1974   Differentiation of the silk gland. A model system for the study of differential gene action. In *Results and Problems in Cell Differentiation,* edited by W. Beermann, J. Reinert and H. Ursprung. Springer-Verlag, New York, (in press).

Suzuki, Y. and D. D. Brown, 1972   Isolation and identification of the messenger RNA for silk fibroin from *Bombyx mori*. *J. Mol. Biol.* **63**:409–429.

Suzuki, Y. and E. Suzuki, 1974   Quantitative measurements of fibroin messenger RNA synthesis in the posterior silk gland of normal and mutant *Bombyx mori*. *J. Mol. Biol.* **88**:393–408.

Suzuki, Y., L. P. Gage and D. D. Brown, 1972   The genes for silk fibroin in *Bombyx mori*. *J. Mol. Biol.* **70**:637–649.

Takasaki, T., 1940 Studies on the second linkage group in the silkworm, *Bombyx mori* L. I. A new factor, mottled (*oα*), closely linked with *Y* and a factor that inhibits mottling. *Bull. Sericult. Exp. Stn. Tokyo* **9**:521–555. (J, ER)

Takasaki, T., 1943 A new lethal translucent which occurred in the J 115 (N) strain of the silkworm. *J. Sericult. Sci. Jap.* **14**:48–57. (J)

Takasaki, T., 1947*a* On the second chromosome of the silkworm and its linkage map, with special reference to the problem of spindle-fibre attachment. *Bull. Sericult. Exp. Stn. Tokyo* **12**:595–607. (J, ER)

Takasaki, T., 1947*b* On *Kp*-multiple allelic series, with special reference to a new mutant *C₇*. *J. Sericult. Sci. Jap.* **16**:42–43. (J)

Takasaki, T., 1947*c* New mutants. *Silkworm Inf. Serv.* **2**:4. (J)

Takasaki, T., 1957 Determination of the gene locus of "malformation" and "late maturity". *Rep. Res. Grantees Minist. Educ., Agric.*: 239–242. (J)

Takasaki, T., 1958 Loci of grey egg genes and their functional relationship. *Rep. Res. Grantees Minist. Educ., Agric.*: 198–199. (J)

Takasaki, T., 1959 Susceptible genes to muscardine. *Rep. Res. Grantees Minist. Educ., Agric.*: 213. (J)

Takasaki, T., 1960 Further studies on locus specificity of gene action and multiple allelism in the silkworm. *Rep. Res. Grantees Minist. Educ., Agric.*: 244. (J)

Takasaki, T. and T. Mitarai, 1949 Recessive and hypo- and hyper-dominant trimoulters. *Sanshi-gijutsu-shiryo* **6**:8. (J)

Takasaki, T., K. Maruyama and H. Ueno, 1957 On the locus of "kidney" gene (*ki*) in *Bombyx mori*. *Proc. 11th Meet. Jap. Soc. Sericult. Kyushu*: 9–10. (J)

Takase, K., 1919 Studies of "penta-moulter" strain of the silkworm. *Sangyo-shinpo* **27** (312):256–262. (J)

Takei, R. and E. Nagashima, 1970 Development of embryo in the non-hibernating lethal egg of the silkworm. *J. Sericult. Sci. Jap.* **39**:267–272. (J, ER)

Tanaka, Y., 1913 Gametic coupling and repulsion in the silkworm, *Bombyx mori*. *J. Coll. Agric. Sapporo* **5**:115–148.

Tanaka, Y., 1914 Sexual dimorphism of gametic series in the reduplication. *Trans. Sapporo Nat. Hist. Soc.* **5**:61–64.

Tanaka, Y., 1916 Genetic studies in the silkworm. *J. Coll. Agric. Sapporo* **7**:129–255.

Tanaka, Y., 1917 Sex-linked inheritance in the silkworm. *Sanshi-kaiho* **26** (311):5–8. (J)

Tanaka, Y., 1919 *Lectures on Silkworm Genetics,* Meibundo Ltd., Tokyo. (J)

Tanaka, Y., 1923 Inheritance of "elongate." (A preliminary note). *Sanshi-kaiho* **32**:21–23. (J)

Tanaka, Y., 1924*a* Maternal inheritance in *Bombyx mori* L. *Genetics* **9**:479–486.

Tanaka, Y., 1924*b* Further studies on the inheritance of cocoon colour in *Bombyx mori*. *Sangyo-shinpo* **32**:92–96. (J)

Tanaka, Y., 1925*a* "No-lunule," a lethal factor in the silkworm. *Sci. Bull. Fac. Agric. Kyushu Univ.* **1**:210–242. (J, ER)

Tanaka, Y., 1925*b* Mutation of the somatic cells in animals. *Bull. Jap. Assoc. Adv. Sci.* **1**:275–285. (J)

Tanaka, Y., 1926 Studies on some mutants manifesting superfluous legs. *Zool. Mag.* **38**:26–27. (J)

Tanaka, Y., 1927 Genetic behaviour of a mutant "multi-stars" in the silkworm. *Sangyo-shinpo* **35**:184–190. (J)

Tanaka, Y., 1933   Multiple-allelomorphic series in *Bombyx mori*. *Trans. Tottori Soc. Agric. Sci.* **4**:195–199.

Tanaka, Y., 1935   Inheritance of the "cheek and tail" spots in *Bombyx mori*. *Bull. Sericult. Silk Industry Ueda* **8**:127–129. (J)

Tanaka, Y., 1936   A mutant "geometrid" of the silkworm. *J. Sericult. Sci. Jap.* **7**:265. (J)

Tanaka, Y., 1941   Chromosome map of *Bombyx mori*. *Bull. Jap. Assoc. Adv. Sci.* **16**:111–112. (J)

Tanaka, Y., 1943   *Animal Thremmatology and Genetics*, Yokendo, Tokyo. (J)

Tanaka, Y., 1948   Stock list. *Silkworm Inf. Serv.* **3**:24. (J)

Tanaka, Y., 1952   *Silkworm Genetics*, Shôkabô, Tokyo. (J)

Tanaka, Y., 1953   Genetics of the silkworm, *Bombyx mori*. *Adv. Genet.* **5**:239–317.

Tanaka, Y., 1955   Linkage between a light brown cocoon and a tri-moulting gene in the silkworm. *J. Sericult. Sci. Jap.* **24**:216. (J)

Tanaka, Y., 1959   Linkage analysis of "retarding" in the silkworm. *Rep. Res. Grantees Minist. Educ., Agric.*: 219. (J)

Tanaka, Y., 1963   Inheritance of the new multistar marking *msn* in the silkworm. *Rep. Silk Sci. Res. Inst.* **11**:29–31. (J)

Tanaka, Y., 1969   Revision of the genetical map of chromosome 12 in the silkworm. *Rep. Silk Sci. Res. Inst.* **17**:15–19. (J)

Tanaka, Y. and T. Chiang, 1939   Influence of temperature on the function of genes. I. On the t-mottled translucent. *J. Sericult. Sci. Jap.* **10**:77–80. (J)

Tanaka, Y. and S. Matsuno, 1927   "Stick" and "multilunar," a fourth linkage group in the silkworm. *J. Dept. Agric. Kyushu Univ.* **1**:266–274.

Tanaka, Y. and S. Matsuno, 1929   Genetical studies on non-sex-linked translucent mutants in the silkworm. *Bull. Sericult. Exp. Stn. Tokyo* **7**:305–425. (J)

Tanaka, Y. and T. Miyashita, 1960   Linkage of the number of multilunar spots and the rate of development (I). *Rep. Silk Sci. Res. Inst.* **8**:1–12. (J)

Tanaka, Y. and T. Miyashita, 1964   A genetical map of the chromosome 18 of the silkworm. *Rep. Silk Sci. Res. Inst.* **12**:46–51. (J)

Tashiro, Y., T. Morimoto, S. Matsuura and S. Nagata, 1968   Studies on the posterior silk gland cells and biosynthesis of fibroin during the fifth larval instar. *J. Cell Biol.* **38**:574–588.

Tazima, Y., 1938   Sable, a new mutant type of *Bombyx mori*, induced by X-rays. *Jap. J. Genet.* **14**:117–128. (J, ER)

Tazima, Y., 1941   A simple method of sex discrimination by means of larval marking in *Bombyx mori*. *J. Sericult. Sci. Jap.* **12**:184–188. (J)

Tazima, Y., 1943a   Cytogenetical improvement of autosexing method with use of larval marking. (A supplementary note). *J. Sericult. Sci. Jap.* **14**:69–75. (J)

Tazima, Y., 1943b   Studies on chromosome aberrations in the silkworm. I. Attachment of two second chromosomes and some related problems. *Bull. Sericult. Exp. Stn. Tokyo* **11**:525–604. (J)

Tazima, Y., 1944   Studies on chromosome aberrations in the silkworm. II. Translocations involving second and W-chromosomes. *Bull. Sericult. Exp. Stn. Tokyo* **12**:109–181. (J)

Tazima, Y., 1954   Alteration of food selecting character by artificial mutation in the silkworm. *Bull. Interntl. Silk Assoc.* **20**:27–29.

Tazima, Y., 1958   Inheritance of a new mutant "brown-3" of the silkworm. *Annu. Rep. Natl. Inst. Genet. Jap.* **8**:9–10.

Tazima, Y., 1964   *The Genetics of the Silkworm,* Logos Press, London.

Tazima, Y. and N. Ohta, 1952   On a new gene locus determined on the fourth chromosome of the silkworm. *Jap. J. Genet.* **27**:228. (J)

Tazima, Y., C. Harada and N. Ohta, 1951   On a sex discriminating method by colouring genes of silkworm eggs. I. Induction of translocation between the W and the tenth chromosomes. *Jap. J. Breed.* **1**:47–50. (J, ER)

Tazima, Y., T. Ozawa, E. Inagaki and T. Kobayashi, 1960   Genetic maps of the eighth linkage group of the silkworm. *Annu. Rep. Natl. Inst. Genet. Jap.* **10**:17–18.

Toyama, K., 1906   Studies on the hybridology of insects. I. On some silkworm crosses with special reference to Mendel's laws of heredity. *Bull. Coll. Agric. Tokyo Univ.* **7**:259–393.

Toyama, K., 1909   Studies on the hybridology of insects. II. A sport of the silkworm, *Bombyx mori* L. and its hereditary behaviour. *J. Coll. Agric. Tokyo Imp. Univ.* **2**:85–103.

Toyama, K., 1910   Inheritance of certain traits in the silkworm. *Sangyo-shinpo* **18** (206):7–13. (J)

Toyama, K., 1912   On certain characteristics of the silkworm which are apparently non-Mendelian. *Biol. Zentralbl.* **32**:593–607.

Toyama, K., 1913   Maternal inheritance of Mendelism (First contribution). *J. Genet.* **2**:351–404.

Tsujita, M., 1946   Inheritance of *brown ursa,* a new mutant of the silkworm. *Jap. J. Genet.* **21**:32. (J)

Tsujita, M., 1952   Studies on the so-called multiple-allelic series in the silkworm. *Annu. Rep. Natl. Inst. Genet. Jap.* **2**:14–17.

Tsujita, M., 1955   On the relation of the "lethal yellow" gene to the "lemon" gene in *Bombyx mori,* with special reference to the maternal inheritance of "lethal yellow." *Jap. J. Genet.* **30**:107–117. (J, ER)

Tsujita, M., 1959   On lethal Nl_1 and Nl_2 embryos of the silkworm. *Annu. Rep. Natl. Inst. Genet. Jap.* **9**:13–15.

Tsujita, M., 1960   Genetic and biochemical studies on the new white-egg mutant in the silkworm. *Annu. Rep. Natl. Inst. Genet. Jap.* **10**:13–15.

Tsujita, M. and B. Sakaguchi, 1959a   On the *E*-region composed of several functionally related genes. *Annu. Rep. Natl. Inst. Genet. Jap.* **9**:10–11.

Tsujita, M. and B. Sakaguchi, 1959b   Functional relation among several genes composing complex loci. On the *E*-complex loci in silkworm. In *Recent Advances in Experimental Morphology,* edited by K. Takewaki, M. Harizuka and M. Fukaya, pp. 283–291, Yokendo, Tokyo. (J)

Tsujita, M. and S. Sakurai, 1965   *rm* gene on the 3rd chromosome in the silkworm. *Jap. J. Genet.* **40**:422–423. (J)

Uda, H., 1919   On the relation between blood colour and cocoon colour in the silkworm, with special reference to Mendel's law of heredity. *Genetics* **4**:395–416.

Uda, H., 1923   On "maternal inheritance." *Genetics* **8**:322–335.

Uda, H., 1928   Genetical studies on the compound eye colour in the silkworm moth. *Bull. Mie Agric. Coll.* **1**:1–30. (J)

Uda, H., 1930   Genetical studies on the compound eye colour in the silkworm moth. *Jap. J. Genet.* **5**:111–113. (J)

Ueda, S., T. Hirao and M. Harizuka, 1959   On the recombination value between "wingless" and "white-1." *Acta Sericol., Tokyo* **28**:6–8. (J)

Umeya, Y., 1926   On the degeneration of the male copulatory organs of the silkworm. (*Bombyx mori*). *J. Coll. Agric. Tokyo Imp. Univ.* **9**:57–84.

Umeya, Y., 1927   Studies on dead eggs of the silkworm, *Bombyx mori* L. I. Hibernating eggs. *Bull. Agric. Sci. Soc. Tokyo* **299**:458–486. (J)

Umeya, Y., 1949   Influence of environment on the inheritance of segment monster. *Zool. Mag. Jap.* **58**:94–95. (J)

Umeya, Y. and K. Asano, 1956   Inheritance of new mutant, lanky (*Lk*) of the silkworm, *Bombyx mori. J. Sericult. Sci. Jap.* **25**:338–340. (J, ER)

Umeya, Y. and I. Karasawa, 1930   Preliminary note on the inhibitory gene of development in the silkworm. *Jap. J. Genet.* **6**:188–194. (J)

Umeya, Y. and S. Omura, 1950   Studies on the sterility in the silkworm. I. On the abnormal spermatophore. *Bull. Sericult. Exp. Stn. Tokyo* **13**:63–78. (J, ER)

Watanabe, H., 1961   Studies on the pleiotropic effects of a mutant gene at *o-106* locus in the silkworm, *Bombyx mori. J. Sericult. Sci. Jap.* **30**:456–462. (J, ER)

Whitehouse, H. L. K., 1970   The mechanism of genetic recombination. *Biol. Rev.* **45**:265–315.

Yamashita, O., K. Hasegawa and M. Seki, 1972   Effect of the diapause hormone on trehalase activity in pupal ovaries of the silkworm, *Bombyx mori* L. *Gen. Comp. Endocrinol.* **18**:515–523.

Yamazaki, M. and M. Kobayashi, 1969   Purification of the protenic brain hormone of the silkworm, *Bombyx mori. J. Insect Physiol.* **15**:1981–1990.

Yokoyama, T., 1939   Linkage phenomena between non-sex-linked translucent genes, *oc* and *ok*, and egg-colour genes, *p* and *r. J. Sericult. Sci. Jap.* **10**:18–24. (J)

Yoshitake, N., 1964   Genetical studies on the alkaline-phosphatase in the mid-gut of the silkworm, *Bombyx mori* L. *J. Sericult. Sci. Jap.* **33**:28–33. (J, ER)

Yoshitake, N., 1966   Difference in the multiple forms of several enzymes between wild and domesticated silkworms. *Jap. J. Genet.* **41**:259–267. (J, ER)

Yoshitake, N., 1968   Esterase and phosphatase polymorphism in natural population of wild silkworm, *Theophila mandarina* L. *J. Sericult. Sci. Jap.* **37**:195–200. (J)

Yoshitake, N. and M. Akiyama, 1964   Genetical studies on the acid-phosphatase in the blood of the silkworm, *Bombyx mori* L. *Jap. J. Genet.* **39**:26–30.

Yoshitake, N. and M. Akiyama, 1965a   Genetic aspects on the esterase activities of the egg in the silkworm, *Bombyx mori* L. *J. Sericult. Sci. Jap.* **34**:327–332. (J, ER)

Yoshitake, N. and M. Akiyama, 1965b   Substrate specificity and isozymes of acid-phosphatase in the blood of silkworm, *Bombyx mori* L. *Jap. J. Appl. Entomol. Zool.* **9**:115–120.

Yoshitake, N. and T. Hashiguchi, 1969   On the diapause of Indonesian polyvoltine silkworm *Bombyx mori* L. *Jap. J. Appl. Entomol. Zool.* **13**:206–207. (J)

Yoshitake, N., M. Eguchi and Y. Tsuchiya, 1965   Distribution of the silkgland esterase types in various strains of the silkworm, *Bombyx mori* L. *J. Sericult. Sci. Jap.* **35**:331–335. (J, ER)

Yoshitake, N., M. Eguchi and M. Akiyama, 1966   Genic control on the alkaline phosphatase of the mid-gut in the silkworm, *Bombyx mori* L. *J. Sericult. Sci. Jap.* **35**:1–7. (J, ER)

Yukimura, A., 1949   Inheritance of brown spot which appears on the larval epidermis immediately after 4th moulting. *J. Sericult. Sci. Jap.* **18**:152–156. (J)

4

The Mediterranean Meal Moth, *Ephestia kühniella*

ERNST W. CASPARI AND FREDERICK J. GOTTLIEB

Introduction

The Mediterranean meal moth was first described by Zeller in 1879 under the name *Ephestia kühniella*. Heinrich (1956), in his review of the subfamily *Phycitinae,* excluded the organism from the genus *Ephestia* and renamed it *Anagasta kühniella.* This name is now generally used in the entomological literature, but in the genetic literature the old name, *Ephestia,* with or without the species designation, is maintained. A recent taxonomic investigation, however, re-establishes the generic name *Ephestia* and uses *Anagasta* as subgenus (Roesler, 1973).

Ephestia is a pest in flour mills. It lives on ground cereals and, by spinning dense webs, may clog the ducts in the mills. It was originally described by Zeller from a flour mill in Halle, Germany, which received part of its wheat from America. Since the presence of the larvae in mills is rather obvious and disturbing, it may be assumed that it did not invade the mills long before it was described. Its original home area and habitat are unknown.

Ephestia was first used in genetic research by Whiting (1919).

ERNST W. CASPARI—Department of Biology, University of Rochester, Rochester, New York. FREDERICK J. GOTTLIEB—Department of Biology, University of Pittsburgh. Pittsburgh, Pennsylvania.

Whiting, however, gave it up after a few years in favor of its parasite *Bracon hebetor* (*Habrobracon juglandis*). It was taken up again by Kühn and Henke (1929) as an object for the study of developmental genetics. They chose *Ephestia* primarily because of its possession of a well-defined, but not too complex, wing pattern. Pattern formation may be regarded as a special case of organization, i.e., the orderly arrangement of differentiated cells with respect to each other. The color patterns of insects represent a relatively simple instance of this fundamental developmental phenomenon since they are two-dimensional rather than three-dimensional, as is the organization in the vertebrate embryo. In the course of time, *Ephestia* has also shown itself to be a good object for problems of biochemical genetics, starting out with eye-color mutants (Caspari, 1933) and proceeding later in a variety of directions. As a result of the concentration on developmental problems, the mutants described in *Ephestia* mostly affect the adult patterns on the forewing, eye pigmentation, and, more recently, the development of particular proteins. In *Ephestia,* the normal development of many structures, particularly the wing and the eye, has been thoroughly investigated.

Life Cycle

The length of the life cycle is dependent on temperature, crowding, food, and genotype. For wild-type strains raised on corn meal, development requires 50 days at 24°C, from egg laying to the appearance of the first adults in a culture, and 80–85 days at 18°C. The female starts laying eggs within 24 hours after copulation, and it deposits all its eggs within 3 days. The eggs hatch within 5–6 days at 24°C and 9 days at 18°C. Larval development proceeds in instars, divided by molts. The number of molts is either four or five, depending mainly on the temperature and other seasonal factors. In some cultures, larvae with both four and five molts are found; in others, all larvae undergo five molts. The last molt occurs about 30 days after egg laying at 24°C. The last instar may be divided into the feeding stage and the prepupal stage. The progression to the prepupal stage is marked by noticeable changes: the animals stop feeding, they move out of the food, they become very active, and the pink ommochrome pigment of the hypodermis cells disappears. The feeding stage of the last larval instar lasts about 9 days at 24°C, while the prepupal stage is more variable, from 4–7 days. Pupal development takes 12 days. The adults usually hatch from the pupal case in the late afternoon and evening (Moriarty, 1959). They frequently copulate during the same night. The animals stay *in copula* for several hours. They are firmly attached to each other during copulation, and if they are separated by force, the male genitalia remain attached to the female. Frequently, the animals cannot separate after copulation, a major reason for sterility. The adults do not feed since their mid-gut has been reduced to a solid strand of epithelium (Blaustein, 1935). The adult life span is highly variable since the animals die shortly after egg laying, viz., copulation, but they can survive considerably longer when they do not reproduce. Summaries of the life cycle of *Ephestia* can be found in Kühn and Henke (1929).

For developmental investigations, it is important to identify time sequences starting at definite points in development. Embryonic development has been described by Sehl (1931). The early larval instars have not been well investigated. The larvae live in the food, spinning tunnels, and are sensitive to manipulation. The instars are best identified by the size of the head capsule. The last (fifth or sixth) instar has been studied, starting with the time of the last larval molt. Animals before the last molt stay quietly in their tunnels and can be recognized by the fact that their heads have already withdrawn from the old head capsules, so that the head capsule appears sharply set off from the body. After the molt, the larvae have the same size, but they possess larger head capsules, which are at first white, turning gradually brown in the course of 2–3 hours. Last-instar larvae can be timed by isolating, from a culture about 30 days old, larvae belonging, as judged by their head capsules, to the next to the last instar. They are kept in Petri dishes, with little food, so that they can be readily observed, and they are scored at intervals (daily or more frequently) for animals which have molted. The molted larvae are isolated and fed and will develop synchronously through the next 9 days. They grow considerably during the last instar.

The first sign of the prepupal stage is that the caterpillars stop feeding and start moving out of the food. They subsequently lose their hypodermal pigmentation, spin a tough cocoon, the hemolymph assumes a greenish color, and the head tissue withdraws from the head capsule. In order to distinguish stages of the prepupa, Kühn and Piepho (1936) have used stages of withdrawal of pigment from the ommatidia: in the prepupa, the pigment of the larval ommatidia migrates from the ommatidia along the optic nerve to the brain, where it disappears. This method of timing works well in wild-type strains but cannot be applied to animals from mutant strains characterized by the absence of ommatidial pigment, such as *a, wa, alb.* In these strains, the ingrowth of tracheae into the wing imaginal discs can be used for staging. Wing discs can easily be observed in animals immersed in water through the skin of the meso- and meta-thorax. (Larvae can survive immersion in water for an hour or more.)

Pupae can be timed by isolating fully grown larvae and prepupae and checking them at intervals for pupation. Immediately after the pupal molt, the pupae appear green like the prepupae, but the cuticle becomes tanned within a few hours after pupation. Time is a reliable criterion for developmental stages in the pupa since variation is low in inbred strains kept at constant temperature. Timing in the pupa can be supplemented by observation of the progress of eye pigmentation in the first half of pupal development, and by observation of the wing pigmentation in the last days. At 24°C, adults eclose on the thirteenth day after the pupal molt.

Culture Methods

One of the great advantages of *Ephestia* for research is that it can be easily and cheaply raised. Cultures derived from single females may be reared in round crystallizing dishes (4½ inches in diameter) closed by a glass plate as a cover, or in plastic refrigerator boxes, 5¼ × 2¾ × 2½ inches having fitted plastic tops with overhanging edges. Mass cultures can be maintained in the same types of containers if relatively few larvae are involved, or in larger boxes of a similar type when the number of animals desired is large.

Some cotton wool or a piece of filter paper is placed at the bottom of the culture jar since females usually deposit their eggs there; one or several freshly hatched pairs can be transferred to the box. The adults usually sit quietly and can be handled individually in small vials, 1 cm in diameter and 6 cm high. If after 3 days few or no eggs have been laid, the culture may be discarded. It is advantageous to wait with feeding until the young larvae start to hatch in order to be sure that the culture is viable.

The foods used are either coarse whole wheat meal, prepared by grinding up wheat grains purchased from a feed store by means of a Waring blender or a hand mill, or commercial granulated corn meal, either white or yellow. A mixture of wheat and corn meal is very good food. Wheat or corn flour is insufficient. A semisynthetic diet for *Ephestia* has been described by Fraenkel and Blewett (1946a,b). It contains about 80 percent carbohydrate (glucose), and requirements for cholesterol and linoleic acid have been demonstrated.

The imagoes usually sit quietly at the walls and on the covers of the jars and can be removed by forceps without anesthesia. Adults can be easily anesthesized with ether, but they are rather resistant to anesthesia with CO_2. Virgins for crosses are obtained by removing all animals in the morning and checking in the late afternoon for freshly hatched females. They should be mated to virgin males the same day. A healthy female lays 100–200 eggs.

After feeding the larvae, no care of the cultures is necessary unless they are overcrowded. In this case, larvae may be removed with a light forceps and transferred to fresh food. A good single mating can produce 150–200 offspring, while in inbred and mutant strains lower numbers, 50–100 progeny, are often obtained. *Ephestia* is rather tolerant of inbreeding. They can be propagated by brother–sister mating through 100 or more generations. Under continued inbreeding, no morphological abnormalities arise, but fecundity or fertility may become reduced; either difficulties in copulation may arise, or the animals lay eggs which develop into embryos which cannot hatch. These periods of impaired reproduction can usually be overcome by careful selection of fully fertile animals. The mutant genes *a* and *wa* have been made "isogenic" with an inbred wild-type strain BII by outcrossing for 84 and 36 generations, respectively, and recovering the mutant homozygotes in F_2.

Migration of larvae presents a minor cross-culture contamination problem. This can be prevented by taping around the box lid with masking tape or by setting the culture boxes on top of inverted, disposable, Petri dish bottoms in a tray containing mineral oil 2–4 mm deep.

Parasites of *Ephestia*

Ephestia has a number of parasites. These are unusually well investigated because of the hope of using them for pest control. Some of them may become highly damaging in cultures. The following should be mentioned: *Bacillus thuringensis* is a spore-forming bacterium which may kill insects as larvae. It is regarded by some authors as synonymous with *B. cereus*. Since it is a spore-former, it can be controlled by repeated heat sterilization of food and culture dishes (Heimpel, 1967). *Mattesia dispora* is a gregarine living in the hemolymph of larvae. It is not dangerous when present in low numbers, but it may become pathogenic and lethal (Leibenguth, 1970). *Tyroglyphus casei* is a mite which can do much damage by eating eggs of *Ephestia*. It also attaches itself to adults, decreasing their ability to copulate. It can be controlled by keeping the incubator rooms clean, keeping the humidity low, and by carefully checking the eggs before addition of food. *Trichogramma minutum* is a hymenopteran insect which attacks the eggs of *Ephestia,* and it has been used in the control of the moths. It has not been found in the laboratory. *Habrobracon* (*Bracon*) spp. and *Nemeritis canescens* are hymenopterans

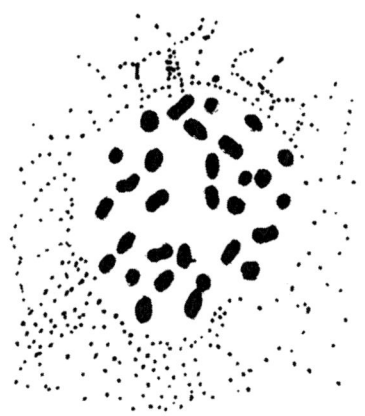

Figure 1. Spermatocyte I metaphase from larval testis. Preparation by E. M. Eicher. Air-dried preparation stained with Giemsa (2400 ×).

whose larvae are parasites on *Ephestia* larvae and kill them. Most of these parasites are easily controlled. Only *B. thuringensis* and *Tyroglyphus* may become so entrenched that they interfere with the culture of *Ephestia*. Mycoplasmalike organisms have been observed in electron micrographs of the larval and adult testis sheath. They produce no pathological effects (Gottlieb, 1972).

Cytology

The chromosomes of *Ephestia* have been studied by Traut and Mosbacher (1968) and Traut and Rathjens (1973). The haploid number of chromosomes, as seen in meiotic metaphase, is 30. Somatic cell divisions from the wing bud show 60 chromosomes per cell in males and females with a certain amount of variation. The individual metaphase chromosomes are all small, round or oval, and they possess a diffuse centromere. The different chromosomes cannot be distinguished morphologically (Figure 1). They can, however, be distinguished in the pachytene nuclei of primary oocytes and in nurse cell nuclei, where they are elongated and show differential banding patterns when stained with a fluorescent Feulgen stain (Traut and Rathjens, 1973).

The female is the heterogametic sex. The male is ZZ, while the female carries, in addition to one Z chromosome, a W chromosome, which is distinguished in pachytene cells by its uniform fluorescence. Heterogamety of the female has been confirmed by the existence of three sex-linked genes, *dz, df-1,* and *ls.* Several translocations involving the W chromosome and autosomes have been described (Rathjens, 1974).

The interphase nuclei are large and show a clear pattern of chromocenters, mostly close to the nuclear membrane. The number of chromocenters has been described as 30, suggesting somatic pairing of homologous chromosomes in interphase. Different degrees of polyploidy occur in larval and adult tissues; the number of chromocenters in polyploid cells is increased (Henke and Pohley, 1952). The nuclei of spinning gland cells are highly polyploid and have a bizarre, branched shape. A circular piece of sex chromatin which becomes a large and conspicuous structure in polyploid cells is found in female interphase nuclei. The sex chromatin has been shown to represent the W chromosome. In translocations involving the W chromosome and an autosome, the sex chromatin appears fragmented in highly polyploid cells, apparently because of opposing tendencies of the autosomal and W-chromosomal parts of the same translocation chromosome (Traut and Rathjens, 1973, Rathjens, 1974).

Synaptonemal complexes are found in gonial cells. Moses (1968) has included in his Table I a personal communication from G. F. Meyer reporting the presence of synaptonemal complexes in both male and female *Pieris, Ephestia,* and *Galleria.* One of us (F. J. Gottlieb, unpublished) has also observed synaptonemal complexes in the nuclei of primary spermatocytes in larval *Ephestia* testes.

Formal Genetics

A number of mutant genes in *Ephestia* has been described, but no systematic linkage studies have been carried out. The large number of chromosomes, making linkage between any two genes rather unlikely, has been a discouraging factor. The three sex-linked genes, *dz, df-1,* and *ls,* are obviously linked. Autosomal linkage has been found for the genes *b* and *bch* (=*t*) (Kühn and Berg, 1955), *a* and the protein loci *abp* (Eicher and Caspari, 1968) and *ubp* (Hauptman, 1974), and the enzyme-determining loci *Est-1* and *Est-2* (Jelnes, 1971). According to G. F. Meyer [unpublished; see Moses (1968)] *Ephestia* spermatocytes show chiasmata, while oocytes do not; but recombination between *a* and *ubp* occurs in both sexes (Hauptman 1974).

A list of the mutations described in *Ephestia* is presented in Table 1. Genes described in the literature whose monogenic nature appears doubtful have been omitted.

TABLE 1. *Mutations of Ephestia kühniella*

Symbol[a]	Name[b]	Phenotypic effects	References
a	Red	Lack of tryptophan pyrrolase activity; therefore, absence of ommochrome pigments and storage of tryptophan	Kühn and Henke (1930), Caspari (1933, 1946), Egelhaaf (1958, 1963)
abp	a-Band protein	Presence of a protein in adults	Eicher and Caspari (1968)
Adh	Alcohol dehydrogenase (ADH)	Number of ADH allozymes, 0–2	Imberski (1972)
alb	Oculis albis	Cream-colored eyes; ommochromes and colored pteridines missing; scales on hind wings oval (Figure 2B)	Kühn (1966), Caspari and Eicher (1975)
An	Ala nigra	Black wings with white symmetrical bands (similar to Figure 4C)	Cotter (unpublished)
as	Antennae short	Antennae reduced in number and length of segments	Cotter (1960)
b	Black	Black wings with white symmetrical bands; background scales replaced by black pattern scales (Figure 4C)	Whiting (1919), Kühn and Henke (1929)
br	Brown	Brown eyes, red testis; ommin missing; presence of an orange ommochrome; probably allelic to rt	Kühn and Egelhaaf (1959a)
Ch	Charcoal	Wings dark, without pattern; all scales with dark tip; allelic to ml (Figure 4G)	Yearich (1970)
cy	Curly	Forewings curved upward throughout distal two-thirds of their length	Gottlieb and Yearich (unpublished)
*d	Dark	Dark central area	Whiting (1919)
*df-1 (originally df)	Dark field-1	Shadow spots fused to form a band; area posterior to the "shadow band" dark; sex-linked recessive (like Figure 4D)	Kühn and Henke (1935)

df-2 (originally df$_1$)	Dark field-2	Phenotype identical with df-1 (Figure 4D); autosomal recessive	Kühn (1942)
dh	Eye-pigment intensifier	Modifier of red eye pigments in aa adults	W. Maier (unpublished)
*dia	Diminutio aetatis, colorationis et fertilitatis	Reduced adult life span and fertility; wing pigmentation light	Strohl and Köhler (1935)
dz	Dark central field	Central area dark, symmetry system reduced in size; sex-linked (Figure 4E)	Kühn (1939b)
Est-1	Esterase-1	Two allozymes of Esterase-1 (present in gut only); identical with Est-A	Leibenguth (1972), Jelnes (1971)
Est-2	Esterase-2	Three allozymes of Esterase-2 (present in all organs); identical with Est-B	Leibenguth (1972, 1973a), Jelnes (1971)
gl	Glass wing	Loss of scales on the wing	Hanser (1955)
he	Light	Wings light, pigmentation inhibited; chitin soft, inelastic (Figure 4B)	Kühn (1939a), Richards (1958)
Hu	Light outer area	Proximal and distal outer areas which are continuous with the white zone of the symmetrical band	Seeger (1955)
kfl	Short wings	Wings small; rate of cell divisions in wing disc of last instar larva and prepupa reduced	Şengün (1940), Muth (1961)
ls	Lethal of Schwartz	Sex-linked recessive lethal	Schwartz (1937)
ml	Lack of pattern	Forewing covered by white pattern scales exclusively	Kühn (1939c)
*Mo	Mosaic	Mosaicism of wing pattern, probably due to somatic non-disjunction; female sterile	Kühn (1960)
om	Ommochromes	Absence of ommochromes in the Malpighian tubules	Wolfram (1948)
P-3,4	Protein 3,4	Allozymes of a hemolymph protein	Egelhaaf (1965)

[a] Mutations marked with an asterisk have to our knowledge been lost.
[b] Names originally given in German have been translated into English. Latin names have been kept.

TABLE 1. Continued

Symbol[a]	Name[b]	Phenotypic effects	References
P-2r	Protein 2r	Amount of protein represented by band 2	K. Cölln (unpublished)
P-IV	Protein IV	Allozymes of hemolymph protein IV	Chatard (1969)
P-III-1a°	Protein III-1a	Absence of larval hemolymph protein III-1a	
Pgm	Phosphoglucomutase (PGM)	Allozymes of PGM	Jelnes (1971)
rt	Red testis	Testis pigment red, as opposed to brown in the dominant allele Rt; ommin missing	Caspari (1943)
*S	Sooty	Dark proximal and distal outer areas	Whiting (1919)
scl	Scaleless	Wing scales partly or completely lost	Caspari (unpublished)
Sy	Symmetry field	Central area reduced in size; symmetrical bands close to each other, enlarged; homozygous lethal	
*Syb	Symmetry field broad	Central area enlarged, symmetrical bands further removed from each other; maternal effect in reciprocal F_1s	Kühn and Henke (1936)
t	Transparent (identical with bch)	Isoxanthopterin and 2-amino-4-OH-pteridin accumulated, other pteridines reduced; aa; tt eyes light, transparent	Kühn et al. (1935), Hadorn and Kühn (1953)
tpb	Timing of "pupation band" II-4	Controls the timing of the appearance and disappearance of a particular protein II-4 around the time of pupation	Chatard (1969)
ubp	Upper band protein	Presence of a protein	Hauptman (1974)
Us	Undifferentiated symmetry system	Symmetrical bands missing, outer areas darker than in wild type (Figure 4F); probably allelic to Ch and ml	Schwartz (1944)
*vd	Darkened	Morphology and pigmentation of scales disturbed	Kühn (1944)
wa	White eyes	All ommochrome and pteridine pigments missing; precursor granules absent	Kühn and Schwartz (1942), Hanser (1948)

Eye-Color Mutants

The eyes of *Ephestia* contain both ommochrome and pteridine pigments [see review by Ziegler (1961)]. The ommochrome pigments are derived from tryptophan via kynurenine and 3-hydroxykynurenine. In wild-type *Ephestia* eyes, three ommochromes can be distinguished by paper chromatography: xanthommatin, a red ommatin, and the slow-moving purple ommin. Ommochrome pigments are found in the larval ommatidia and the larval hypodermis (starting in the late embryo, and disappearing in the prepupa), in the adult testis (starting in the last larval instar), in the adult eye, and in some parts of the brain (starting in the pupa). Ommochromes are carried in (1) retinula cells of the eye (starting in the early pupa in the dorso-caudal part of the eye and spreading gradually over the eye), and (2) accessory pigment cells of the eye (appearing all over the eye in 5- to 6-day-old pupae (24°C) (Muth, 1965). The red pigments of the *Ephestia* eye are two pteridines, pterorhodin and erythropterin, formed *in vitro* from dihydroekapterin via ekapterin (Viscontini and Stierlin, 1962). In addition, a number of colorless, fluorescent pteridines have been found by paper chromatography (Hadorn and Kühn, 1953; Kühn and Egelhaaf, 1959b). The red pteridines, as seen in *a a* animals, appear all through the eye on the ninth day after pupation. At the same time, a yellow pigment of uncertain nature appears in the primary pigment cells.

Both ommochrome and pteridine pigments are deposited on granules which contain protein and RNA, "carrier" or "precursor" granules (Hanser, 1948; Caspari, 1955; Horstmann, 1971). Mutant genes may affect ommochromes, in all or some of the organs in which they occur, or pteridines, or both.

Most eye-color mutants affect the synthesis of ommochromes and pteridines in some or all of the pigmented organs. The mechanism of action is well investigated for *a*: the *a a* homozygote is lacking tryptophan pyrrolase activity (Egelhaaf, 1958). Consequently, the products of the reaction, kynurenine and the ommochrome pigments, are missing, and substrate tryptophan is stored (Caspari, 1946). In *wa*, the precursor or carrier granules of the pigments are missing (Hanser, 1948). Other mutant genes affecting ommochrome and pteridine pigments are listed in Table 1.

Mutants Affecting the Wing and Its Pattern

The surfaces of the wings of *Ephestia* are made up of two types of cells, epithelial cells, and scale cells. The development of the wing

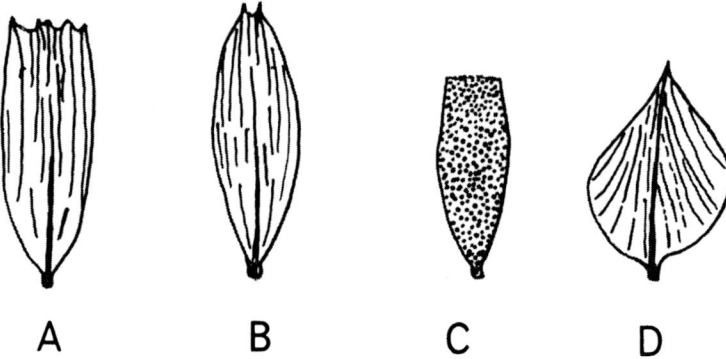

Figure 2. Scales from the hindwing of Ephestia (165 ×): (A) wild type, strain NCR; (B) alb, (C) mutant scale, ES1, induced by x rays [after Pohley (1955)]; (D) mutant scale "leaf" [after Caspari et al. (1965)]. The scales on the hindwing are devoid of pigment, except for ES1.

imaginal disc in the larva and the differentiation of the adult wing and the scales in the pupa have been described at the microscopic and the electron microscopic levels. The scales are derived from stem cells which can first be distinguished from the epithelial cells immediately after pupation. These stem cells in the early pupa undergo two differential cell divisions, giving rise to the scale cell, the socket cell, and an aborting cell (Stossberg, 1938). The subsequent differentiation of the scale has been described by Kühn (1948), Paweletz and Schlote (1964), and Overton (1966).

The scales on the hindwing are colorless and of similar size and shape (Figure 2A), except for scales located on the veins and at the base of the wing. The scales of the hindwing have been used in somatic-mutation studies, as will be described later. The underside of the forewing does not show a color pattern either, except for slight continuation of the bands on the upper surface on the anterior distal tip of the wing. The upper side of the forewing is covered by scales that show different pigmentation and morphology and which are arranged to form a color pattern. This pattern was first described by Kühn and Henke (1929), and the extensive early investigations on this subject have been reviewed by Henke (1935) and Caspari (1941).

On the forewing of *Ephestia,* Kühn and Henke (1932) distinguished eight types of scales, which differ from each other in pigmentation, size, and shape. The scales cover each other like shingles, so that the visible color pattern is made up of the tips of the longer scale types. Scales of the shorter types contribute little to the color pattern. The different types of scales are not always clearly distinct from each other, and they vary in different inbred strains. It appears, therefore, preferable, in the context of this review, to distinguish only three types of pattern scales: dark pattern scales, light pattern scales, and gray scales forming the background. These types differ not only in pigmentation, but also in their shapes and in the structure of the chitin. In a particular scale type, a particular combination of color, shape, and structure is always maintained. The three main types of scales forming the surface pattern of the wing are represented in Figure 3.

The wild-type wing color pattern of *Ephestia* is illustrated in Figure 4A. Kühn and Henke (1929) have divided it into four pattern systems: (1) the symmetry system [This system consists of two bands running across the wing from the anterior to the posterior margin. Each band consists of three zones, a central white zone, and a proximal, and a distal black zone. Both bands run across the wing in an antero-posterior direction, and are broader on the main longitudinal veins. The bands divide the wing into a central area, enclosed by the bands and proximal and distal outer areas.], (2) the discoidal elements or central spots [These are two dark spots located in the central area on the only crossvein of the wing.], (3) the shadow spots [Four ill-defined spots are seen in the central area. They may be fused into a continuous dark band running from the middle of the

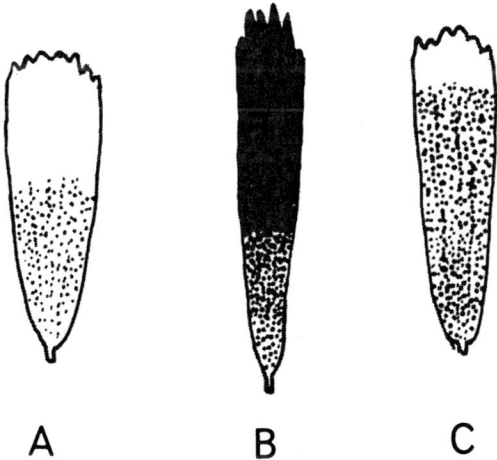

A　　　　B　　　　C

Figure 3. Scales from the forewing of Ephestia (165 ×): (A) white pattern scale [Type VIII of Kühn and Henke (1932)], (B) black pattern scale [Type IV of Kühn and Henke (1932)], and (C) background scale [Type II of Kühn and Henke (1932)].

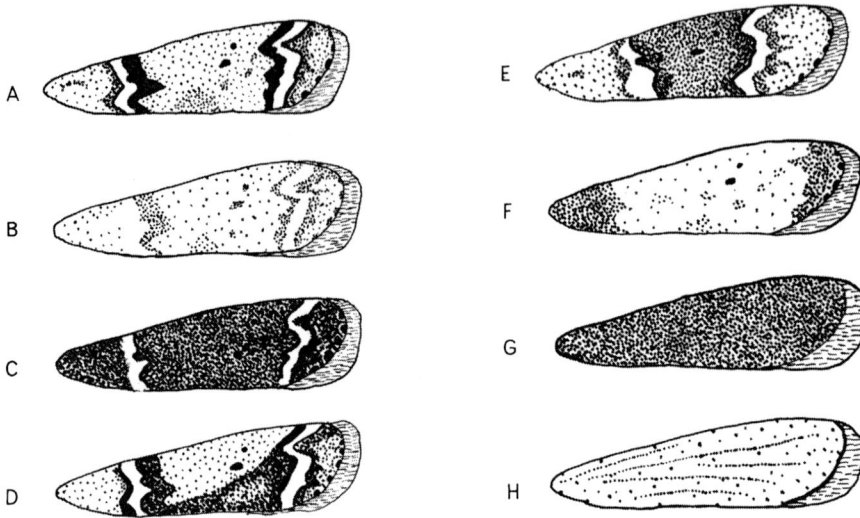

Figure 4. Mutants influencing the pattern of the forewing of Ephestia (5 ×): (A) Wild type, (B) he he; (C) b b, (D) df-2 df-2, (E) dz, (F) Us Us, (G) Ch, (H) ml ml. F and G After Yearich (1970).

dark component of the distal symmetrical band to the posterior margin of the proximal symmetrical band.], and (4) marginal spots.[Dark spots, 5 or 6 in number, are located at the distal margin of the wing between the longitudinal veins.]

The systems just described are developmental entities insofar as the different components of one system have identical sensitive periods against heat and cold shocks and vary concomitantly under the influence of genes and of environmental factors (Feldotto, 1933). Certain mutants affect single components of the wing pattern.

The developmental nature of the pattern systems is unknown, except for the symmetry system (1). This is determined early in the pupal period by a "determination stream," a process which originates at the underside of the forewing and passes over the anterior and posterior margin of the upper side on the second day of pupal life. The course of the "spreading process" has been studied by Kühn and von Engelhardt (1933) by means of localized burns on the wing surface applied at different times of pupal development. The results, illustrated in Figure 5, indicate that the "spreading process" determines the position of the white zone of the symmetry system. Early cauterization, on the first and part of the second day of pupal life at 18°C inhibits the "determination stream" from passing across the killed cells, so that the white zone of the symmetry system is located central from the wound (Figure 5B). Burns on the third and part of the second pupal day result in a smaller symmetry system, independent of the location of the burn (Figure 5C and D). This is interpreted to mean that the "determination stream" is stopped by the injury wherever it happens to be; the white band of the symmetry system appears at the places where the stream has been stopped. Burns inflicted later than pupal day 3 kill the affected cells, but they do not affect the wing pattern otherwise, indicating that at this time the wing pattern has been determined. The spread of the determination stream is affected by genes (*dz, Sy, Syb*) which affect the position of the symmetrical bands and reduce or increase the central area. The area over which the determination stream has passed is not different in color from the outer areas in the wild type, but several mutant genes (*d, dz, Hu, S, Us*) affect the pigmentation of central area and outer areas differently, indicating a physiological difference between the areas. The nature of the spreading process is unknown. It does not involve movement of cells, but it may be due to diffusion of a specific substance or the transmission of an excited state from cell to cell.

Other mutants affect the differentiation of the scales (*gl, he, vd, scl*) or replace, in the color pattern, one type of scale by another (*b, ml, Ch*). Other mutants affecting the wing are included in Table 1.

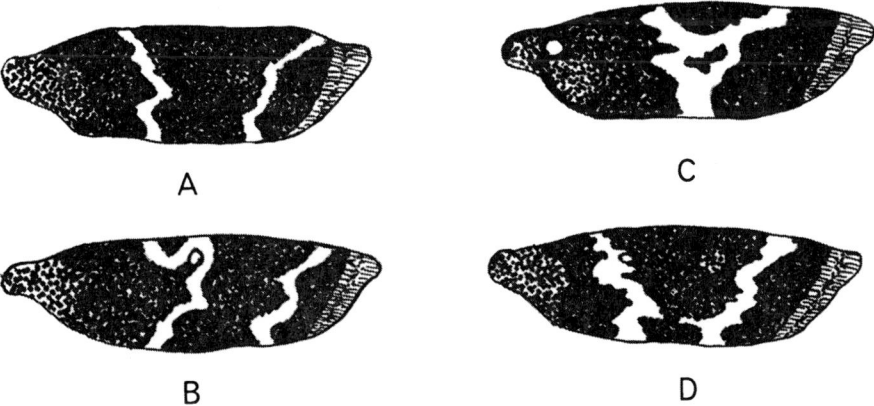

A   C

B   D

Figure 5. Effects of cauterization in the early pupa on the wing pattern of b b Ephestia (9 ✕): (A) Control (not cauterized), (B) cauterized on first pupal day, (C) and (D) cauterized on third pupal day. The wings were removed from late pupae, and show, therefore, a different shape from the fully expanded wings in Figure 4. Redrawn after Kühn and von Engelhardt (1933).

Genes Affecting Proteins

The protein patterns of the hemolymph and of the fat body have been investigated by means of electrophoresis by Egelhaaf (1965), Chatard (1969), and Cölln (1970). In both laboratories, the patterns for last-instar larvae, prepupae, pupae, and adults have been described for a number of strains. In the course of these developmental investigations, genetic variation was found both between and within strains. Some of these differences have been genetically investigated by Egelhaaf and by Chatard. Unfortunately, the protein bands observed by these two authors cannot be identified with each other because of differences in technique. The function of the proteins found in these investigations is usually not known. Proteins with enzymatic activities have been identified and genetically investigated by Chatard (1969), Jelnes (1971), Imberski (1972), and Leibenguth (1972). The genetic polymorphisms described are included in Table 1. Imberski and Gertson (1974) described the changes in the histone fractions occurring during metamorphosis.

The three alleles at the *Est-2* locus differ not only in their electrophoretic mobilities, but also in their sensitivities to temperature and urea. The enzyme activity changes in development, reaching a peak in the 5-day-old pupa. In heterozygotes for two alleles, the activities of the two enzymes are often different and characteristic for specific organs. Thus, in the $Est\text{-}2^M/Est\text{-}2^F$ heterozygous larva, the amounts of enzyme corresponding to the two alleles are equal in the testis, but twice as much M enzyme than F enzyme is found in fat body and hemolymph. Similar results were found for the other two types of heterozygotes. These results suggest that the different alleles may show a type of allelic interaction such that the activity of one allele may be reduced as compared to that of the other allele, and that the occurrence and degree of this interaction depends on the type of cell involved (Leibenguth, 1973*a,b*).

Mutation and Transformation

Some of the mutations described have been induced by radiation and EMS. But no systematic investigations of germinal mutation have been carried out. *Ephestia* is, however, an excellent organism for the study of somatic mutations. The method for the study of somatic mutations uses the scales of the hindwing, which can be easily scored under a low-power microscope (250✕). After irradiation with x rays, aberrant scales are found on the wing. These are either single or occur in longitudinally arrayed clusters, reflecting the direction of growth of the wing (Henke and

Pohley, 1952; Pohley, 1955). Irradiation early in the last-larval instar induces relatively low numbers of large clusters. Irradiation of late last-instar larvae generates large numbers of small clusters, and even single aberrant scales are induced. The aberrant scales are interpreted as somatic mutations. In the early last-larval instar, the imaginal disc consists of few cells and individual mutated cells will undergo several divisions, producing large clusters of mutant cells. In the late last-larval instar, the mutated cells undergo few or no divisions before differentiation. A large number of morphological scale types induced by radiation can be distinguished. Some of these are induced exclusively in the heterogametic female and are considered sex-linked recessive mutations. Since a single hindwing contains 6000 scales, this system is a sensitive system for mutation studies. Events occurring with a frequency of 10^{-5} can be observed easily, and a sensitivity of 10^{-6} or less can be readily attained. The sensitivity approaches that of microbial systems. In practice, treated wings are scored for the appearance of one particular sex-linked mutation (Figure 2C). The method has been used to investigate x-ray induced mutations at low dosages and for the comparison of the mutagenic effect of radiations of different wavelengths (Löbbecke and Müller, 1960; Müller *et al.*, 1966). Nitrogen mustard induces mutations similar to those induced by ionizing radiations (Löbbecke, 1967). 5-Bromodeoxyuridine (BDU), on the other hand, induces types of phenotypically very different scale abnormalities (Caspari *et al.*, 1965) (Figure 2D). These are regarded as mutations because it has been shown that (1) BDU is incorporated into nuclei of cells of the wing bud, (2) induction of aberrant scales is inhibited by thymidine, and (3) in heterozygotes for *alb,* the characteristic scale morphology may be induced by BDU (Caspari and Eicher, 1975).

A similar technique has been used for studies of induction of genetic changes by DNA (Caspari and Nawa, 1965). In this case, the *ml* mutant was used. DNA isolated from wild-type *Ephestia* was injected into last-instar *ml ml* larvae, and their wings scored for black pattern scales on the uniformly light background of white pattern scales. While this procedure leads to the production of isolated dark scales, their genetic nature is doubtful and cannot be further investigated. Nawa and Yamada (1968) used, therefore, the mutant *a*. Eggs and last-instar larvae of an *aa* strain were treated with wild-type DNA, and the treated animals and their progeny were scored for eye color. Few treated animals had dark eyes, and some of them did not transmit this trait to their progeny, suggesting somatic changes involving kynurenine formation. In backcrosses of treated animals to untreated *aa*, more black-eyed animals appeared in the first and second generations. At first, the dark eyes showed an irregular, atypical type of transmission, but by the third generation all strains showed regular Mendelian segregation, suggestive of incorporation of the gene *a* into the chromosomes. The wild-type character is transmitted unchanged through many generations. These results have been confirmed and extended to the mutant gene *alb* by H. S. Friedman and E. M. Young (unpublished). The results indicate that the injected DNA may be taken up by somatic as well as germ cells, that it can reproduce and become transmitted to progeny cells, and that it becomes associated with the chromosomes.

Population Genetics

A method for studying laboratory populations of *Ephestia* has been described by Cotter (1963) and applied to the gene *a*, introduced by generations of backcrosses to an inbred wild-type strain. In these populations, *a* was rapidly lost, according to an estimated selection coefficient of $s = 0.35$. The extinction of *a* cannot be explained by the reduced viability of *a a* animals only, but it depends primarily on reduction in the mating efficiency of the *a a* males in crowded populations. Experiments involving the alleles *Rt* and *rt* have been reported. *Rt* and *rt* are polymorphic in natural populations. In his laboratory populations, Cotter (1973) observed the establishment of polymorphism at $q_{rt} \sim 0.6$. Caspari (1950) concluded that the polymorphism is maintained by heterosis since *Rt rt* animals combine the increased viability of *rt rt* and the higher mating activity of *Rt Rt*. Cotter (1973), however, found that in his cultures the mating activity of heterozygote males *Rt rt* was lower than that of either homozygote.

General Remarks

The last review of the genetics of *Ephestia* was published in 1971 in Robinson (1971) (his pp. 314–349). An *Ephestia News Letter* is being prepared by Gottlieb at the University of Pittsburgh, the first issue of which appeared in March, 1973. A forthcoming issue will contain a complete bibliography of all work on *Ephestia*. Copies can be obtained by writing to Dr. Frederick J. Gottlieb, Department of Biology, University of Pittsburgh, Pittsburgh, Pennsylvania 15260.

Acknowledgment

We want to thank Professor Albrecht Egelhaaf for reading the manuscript and making many valuable suggestions.

Literature Cited

Blaustein, W., 1935   Histologische Untersuchungen über die Metamorphose der Mehlmotte *Ephestia kühniella* Zeller. *Z. Morph. Oekol. Tiere* **30**:333–354.

Caspari, E., 1933   Über die Wirkung eines pleiotropen Gens bei der Mehlmotte *Ephestia kühniella* Zeller. *Wilhelm Roux' Arch. Entwicklungsmech. Org.* **130**:353–381.

Caspari, E., 1941   The morphology and development of the wing pattern of Lepidoptera. *Quart. Rev. Biol.* **16**:249–273.

Caspari, E., 1943   Genes affecting testis color in *Ephestia kühniella* Z. *Genetics* **28**:286–294.

Caspari, E., 1946   On the effects of the gene *a* on the chemical composition of *Ephestia kühniella* Zeller. *Genetics* **31**:454–474.

Caspari, E., 1950   On the selective value of the alleles *Rt* and *rt* in *Ephestia kühniella*. *Am. Nat.* **84**:367–380.

Caspari, E., 1955   On the pigment formation in the testis sheath of *Rt* and *rt Ephestia kühniella* Zeller. *Biol. Zentralbl.* **74**:585–602.

Caspari, E. W. and E. M. Eicher, 1975   Induction of somatic mutations by 5-bromodeoxyuridine in the wing-scale system of *Ephestia kühniella* Z. In: *Problems of Experimental Biology;* volume in memory of B. L. Astaurov. Edited by D. K. Belayev and O. G. Stroeva (in press).

Caspari, E. and S. Nawa, 1965   A method to demonstrate transformation in *Ephestia*. *Z. Naturforsch.* **20b**:281–284.

Caspari, E., W. Muth and H. J. Pohley, 1965   Effects of DNA base analogues on the scales of the wing of *Ephestia*. *Genetics* **51**:771–794.

Chatard, P. M., 1969   A study of the development and genetics of proteins in the Mediterranean flour moth, *Ephestia kühniella*. Ph.D. Thesis, University of Rochester, Rochester, N.Y.

Cölln, K., 1970   Untersuchungen zur Ontogenese der Hämolympheproteine von *Ephestia kühniella* Z. *Verh. Deutsch. Zool. Ges.* **63**:121–127.

Cotter, W. B., 1960   A new developmental mutant in *Ephestia kühniella* affecting antennal morphology. *Rec. Genet. Soc. Am.* **29**:54.

Cotter, W. B., 1963   Population genetic studies of alleles at the *a* locus in *Ephestia kühniella* Z. *Evolution* **17**:233–248.

Cotter, W. B., 1973   On male reproductive behavior and sustained polymorphism of the *rt* locus in laboratory populations of *Ephestia kühniella*. *Evolution* **28**:109–123.

Egelhaaf, A., 1958   Nachweis eines genabhängigen L-Tryptophanoxydase-systems bei *Ephestia kühniella*. *Z. Naturforsch.* **13b**:275–279.

Egelhaaf, A., 1963   Über das Wirkungsmuster des *a*-locus von *Ephestia kühniella* Z. *Z. Vererbungsl.* **94**:349–384.

Egelhaaf, A., 1965   Zur Genetik stadienspezifischer Proteine bei *Ephestia kühniella*. *Z. Vererbungsl.* **97**:150–156.

Eicher, E. M. and E. W. Caspari, 1968   Genic control of the disappearance of a protein in *Ephestia*. *Genetics* **60**:175.

Feldotto, W., 1933   Sensible Perioden des Flügelmusters bei *Ephestia kühniella* Zeller. *Wilhelm Roux' Arch. Entwicklungsmech. Org.* **128**:249–341.

Fraenkel, G. and M. Blewett, 1946a   The dietetics of the caterpillars of three Ephestia species, *E. kühniella*, *E. elutella* and *E. cautella* and of a closely related species, *Plodia interpunctella*. *J. Exp. Biol.* **22**:162–171.

Fraenkel, G. and M. Blewett, 1946*b*   Linoleic acid, vitamin E and other fat-soluble substances in the nutrition of certain insects, *Ephestia kühniella, E. elutella, E. cautella* and *Plodia interpunctella* (Lep.) *J. Exp. Biol.* **22**:172–190.

Gottlieb, F. J., 1972   A cytoplasmic symbiont in *Ephestia kühniella* Zeller. Location and morphology. *J. Invertebr. Pathol.* **20**:351–355.

Hadorn, E. and A. Kühn, 1953   Chromatographische und fluorometrische Untersuchungen zur biochemischen Polyphänie von Augenfarbgenen bei *Ephestia kühniella*. *Z. Naturforsch.* **8b**:582–589.

Hanser, G., 1948   Über die Histogenese der Augenpigmentgranula bei verschiedenen Rassen von *Ephestia kühniella* Z. und *Ptychopoda seriata* Schrk. *Z. Indukt. Abstammungs.-Vererbungsl.* **82**:74–97.

Hanser, G., 1955   Eine neue glassflügelige Mutante (*gl*) von *Ephestia kühniella*. *Z. Naturforsch.* **10b**:161–166.

Hauptman, A., 1974   The relationship between the eye color gene *a* and the protein pattern in *Ephestia kühniella*. Senior Thesis, University of Rochester, Rochester, N.Y.

Heimpel, A. M., 1967   *Bacillus thuringensis. Annu. Rev. Entomol.* **21**:287–322.

Heinrich, C., 1956   *American Moths of the Subfamily Phycitinae. Anagasta kühniella. U. S. Natl. Museum Bull.* **207**:299–302.

Henke, K., 1935   Entwicklung und Bau tierischer Zeichnungsmuster. *Verh. Deutsch. Zool. Ges., Zool. Anz. Suppl.* **8**:176–224.

Henke, K. and H. J. Pohley, 1952   Differentielle Zellteilungen und Polyploidie bei der Schuppenbildung der Mehlmotte *Ephestia kühniella* Z. *Z. Naturforsch.* **7b**:65–79.

Horstmann, G., 1971   Über die Pigmentgranulogenese im Auge von *Ephestia kühniella* Z. *Z. Naturforsch.* **26b**:484–485.

Imberski, R. B., 1972   Genetic control of alcohol dehydrogenase in *Ephestia kühniella*. *Genetics* **71** (*Suppl.*):s27.

Imberski, R. B. and P. N. Gertson, 1974   Changes in basic proteins during metamorphosis of the moth *Ephestia kühniella. Insect Biochem.* **4**:341–344.

Jelnes, J. E., 1971   The genetics of three isoenzyme systems in *Ephestia kühniella* Z. *Hereditas* **69**:138–140.

Kühn, A., 1939*a*   Über die Mutation *he* (gehemmte Ausfärbung) bei *Ephestia kühniella* Z. *Z. Indukt. Abstammungs.-Vererbungsl.* **77**:337–385.

Kühn, A., 1939*b*   Über eine geschlechtsgekoppelte Mutation des Zeichnungsmusters (*dz*) bei *Ephestia kühniella* Z. *Biol. Zentralbl.* **59**:347–357.

Kühn, A., 1939*c*   Vollständige Unterdrückung des Zeichnungsmusters durch eine Mutation der Mehlmotte *Ephestia kühniella* Z. *Naturwissenshaften* **27**:597.

Kühn, A., 1942   Über eine zu *df*₁ isophäne Mutation bei *Ephestia kühniella* Z. *Biol. Zentralbl.* **62**:550–554.

Kühn, A., 1944   Über eine Schuppenformbildung und Schuppenpigmentierung beeinflussende Mutation (*vd*) von *Ephestia kühniella* Z. *Biol. Zentralbl.* **64**:81–97.

Kühn, A., 1948   Über die Determination der Form-, Struktur- und Pigmentbildung der Schuppen bei *Ephestia kühniella* Z. *Wilhelm Roux' Arch. Entwicklungsmech. Org.* **143**:408–487.

Kühn, A., 1960   Genetisch bedingte Mosaikbildungen bei *Ephestia kühniella* Z. *Vererbungsl.* **91**:1–26.

Kühn, A., 1966   Über die Mutation *alb* (oculis albis) bei *Ephestia kühniella*. Z. *Vererbungsl.* **98**:91–96.

Kühn, A., and B. Berg, 1955   Zur genetischen Analyse der Mutation biochemica von *Ephestia kühniella. Z. Indukt. Abstammungs.-Vererbungsl.* **87**:25–35.

Kühn, A. and A. Egelhaaf, 1959a Über die Mutation *br* (braunäugig) bei *Ephestia kühniella. Z. Vererbungsl.* **90**:244–250.

Kühn, A. and A. Egelhaaf, 1959b Der rote Augenfarbstoff von Ephestia und Ptychopoda ein Pterinpigment. *Z. Naturforsch.* **14b**:654–659.

Kühn, A. and M. von Engelhardt, 1933 Über die Determination des Symmetrie-systems auf dem Vorderflügel von *Ephestia kühniella* Zeller. *Wilhelm Roux' Arch. Entwicklungsmech. Org.* **130**:660–703.

Kühn, A. and K. Henke, 1929 Genetische und entwicklungsphysiologische Untersuchungen an der Mehlmotte *Ephestia kühniella* Zeller, I–VII. *Abh. Ges. Wiss. Göttingen, Math.-Phys. Kl., N.F.* **15,1**:1–121.

Kühn, A. and K. Henke, 1930 Eine Mutation der Augenfarbe und der Entwicklungsgeschwindigkeit bei der Mehlmotte *Ephestia kühniella* Z. *Wilhelm Roux' Arch. Entwicklungsmech. Org.* **122**:204–212.

Kühn, A. and K. Henke, 1932 Genetische und entwicklungsphysiologische Untersuchungen an der Mehlmotte *Ephestia kühniella* Zeller, VIII–XII. *Abh. Ges. Wiss. Göttingen, Math.-Phys. Kl., N. F.* **15,2**:127–219.

Kühn, A. and K. Henke, 1935 Über einen Fall von geschlechtsgekoppelter Vererbung mit wechselnder Merkmalsausprägung bei der Mehlmotte *Ephestia kühniella* Zeller. *Nachr. Ges. Wiss. Göttingen, Math.-Phys. Kl., N. F. Nachr. Biol.* **1**(14):247–259.

Kühn, A. and K. Henke, 1936 Genetische und entwicklungsphysiologische Untersuchungen an der Mehlmotte *Ephestia kühniella* Zeller, XIII–XIV. *Abh. Ges. Wiss. Göttingen, Math.-Phys. Kl., N. F.* **15,3**:225–272.

Kühn, A. and H. Piepho, 1936 Über hormonale Wirkungen bei den Verpuppung der Schmetterlinge. *Nachr. Ges. Wiss. Göttingen, Math.-Phys. Kl., N. F. Nachr. Biol.* **2**(9):141–154.

Kühn, A. and V. Schwartz, 1942 Über eine weissäugige Mutante (*wa*) von *Ephestia kühniella. Biol. Zentralbl.* **62**:226–230.

Kühn, A., E. Caspari and E. Plagge, 1935 Über hormonale Genwirkungen bei *Ephestia kühniella* Z. *Nachr. Ges. Wiss. Göttingen, Math.-Phys. Kl., N. F. Nachr. Biol.* **2**(1):1–29.

Leibenguth, F., 1970 Veränderungen der Haemolymphe ausgewachsener *Ephestia* Raupen nach Infektion mit *Mattesia dispora. Z. Parasitenk.* **33**:235–245.

Leibenguth, F., 1972 Polymorphismus und Aktivitätsregulation der Esterase-2 bei *Ephestia kühniella. Mol. Gen. Genet.* **116**:166–176.

Leibenguth, F., 1973a Esterase-2 in *Ephestia kühniella.* I. Genetics and characterization. *Biochem. Genet.* **10**:219–229.

Leibenguth, F., 1973b Esterase-2 in *Ephestia kühniella.* II. Tissue-specific patterns. *Biochem. Genet.* **10**:231–242.

Löbbecke, E. A., 1967 Die Auslösung von somatischen Mutationen bei *Ephestia* durch Injection von Senfgas-Lösungen. *Mol. Gen. Genet.* **99**:115–125.

Löbbecke, E. A. and I. Müller, 1960 Das somatische Mutantenspektrum von *Ephestia kühniella* Z. bei verschiedenen Dosen weicher 10 kV und mittelharter 100 kV Röntgenstrahlen, sowie der harten 60 Co Strahlung. *Z. Vererbungsl.* **91**:338–349.

Moriarty, F., 1959 The 24-hour rhythm of emergence of *Ephestia kühniella* Zeller from the pupa. *J. Insect Physiol.* **3**:357–366.

Moses, M. H., 1968 Synaptinemal Complex. *Annu. Rev. Genet.* **2**:363–412.

Müller, I., S. Pentz and C. Harte, 1966 Die Abhängigkeit des somatischen Mutantenspektrums von *Ephestia kühniella* Z. vom Entwicklungsstadium der bestrahlten Tiere. *Z. Vererbungsl.* **97**:353–360.

Muth, F. W., 1961   Untersuchungen zur Wirkungsweise der Mutante *kfl* bei der Mehl-motte *Ephestia kühniella* Z. *Wilhelm Roux' Arch. Entwicklungsmech. Org.* **153**:370–418.

Muth, W., 1965   The effect of 5-fluorouracil on the eye pigmentary system in *Ephestia kühniella. Exp. Cell Res.* **37**:54–64.

Nawa, S. and M. Yamada, 1968   Hereditary change of an eye color mutant induced by DNA in *Ephestia. Genetics* **68**:573–584.

Overton, J., 1966   Microtubules and microfibrils in morphogenesis of the scale cells of *Ephestia kühniella. J. Cell Biol.* **29**:293–305.

Paweletz, N. and F. W. Schlote, 1964   Die Entwicklung der Schmetterlingsschuppe bei *Ephestia kühniella* Zeller. *Z. Zellforsch.* **63**:840–870.

Pohley, H. J., 1955   Über die somatische Mutabilität bei *Ephestia kühniella. Biol. Zentralbl.* **74**:474–480.

Rathjens, B., 1974   Zur Funktion des W-Chromatins bei *Ephestia kühniella* (Lepidoptera). Isolierung und Charakterisierung von W-Chromatin-Mutanten. *Chromosoma (Berl.)* **47**:21–44.

Richards, A. G., 1958   The pupal cuticle of several genetic stocks of the moth, *Ephestia kühniella. Z. Z. Naturforsch.* **13b**:813–816.

Robinson, R., 1971   *Lepidoptera Genetics.* Pergamon Press, Oxford.

Roesler, R. V., 1973   Die trifinen Acrobasiina der Phycitinae (Lepidoptera, Pyralidae). In *Microlepidoptera Palaearctica*, G. Fromme, Vienna.

Schwartz, V., 1937   Über einen geschlechtsgebundenen Letalfaktor bei *Ephestia kühniella* Z. *Biol. Zentralbl.* **57**:347–354.

Schwartz, V., 1944   Eine neue Mutation des Zeichnungsmusters (*Us*) bei *Ephestia kühniella. Biol. Zentralbl.* **64**:316–324.

Seeger, H., 1955   Genetische Untersuchungen an der neuen Mutation "helles Umfeld" (*Hu*) der Mehlmotte *Ephestia kühniella* Zeller. *Z. Vererbungsl.* **86**:545–573.

Sehl, A., 1931   Furchung und Bildung der Keimanlage bei der Mehlmotte *Ephestia kühniella* Zeller, nebst einer allgemeinen Übersicht über den Verlauf der Embryonalentwicklung. *Z. Morph. Oekol. Tiere* **20**:533–598.

Şengün, A., 1940   Eine neue Mutation "kurzflügelig" (*kfl*) bei der Mehlmotte *Ephestia kühniella* Zeller. *Biol. Zentralbl.* **60**:23–34.

Stossberg, M., 1938   Die Zellvorgänge bei der Entwicklung der Flügelschuppen von *Ephestia kühniella* Z. *Z. Morph. Oekol. Tiere* **34**:173–206.

Strohl, J. and W. Köhler, 1935   Die Wirkung eines pleiotropen Gens auf Färbung, Lebensdauer und Fortpflanzungsfähigkeit bei der Mehlmotte *Ephestia kühniella. Nachr. Ges. Wiss. Göttingen, Math.-Phys. Kl., N. F. Nachr. Biol.* **2**:31–55.

Traut, W. and C. Mosbacher, 1968   Geschlechtschromatin bei Lepidopteren. *Chromosoma (Berl.)* **25**:343–356.

Traut, W. and B. Rathjens, 1973   Das W-Chromosom von *Ephestia kühniella* (Lepidoptera) und die Ableitung des Geschlechtschromatins. *Chromosoma (Berl.)* **41**:437–446.

Viscontini, M. and H. Stierlin, 1962   Fluoreszierende Stoffe aus *Ephestia kühniella* Zeller. (3. Mitteilung). Isolierung und Strukturen von Erythropterin, Ekapterin und Lepidopterin. *Helvet. Chim. Acta* **45**:2479–2487.

Whiting, P. W., 1919   Genetic studies on the Mediterranean flour-moth *Ephestia kühniella* Zeller. *J. Exp. Zool.* **28**:413–441.

Wolfram, R., 1948   Die Ommochrom-Menge in den Malpighischen Gefässen bestimmende Allele der Mehlmotte *Ephestia kühniella. Z. Naturforsch.* **3b**:291–293.

Yearich, M. S., 1970 Genetic investigation of a dominant pattern mutant (*Ch*) in *Ephestia kühniella* Z. M. S. Thesis, University of Pittsburgh, Pittsburgh, Pa.

Zeller, H., 1879 *Ephestia kühniella* n. sp. *Stettiner Entomologische Zeitschr.* **40**:466.

Ziegler, I., 1961 Genetic aspects of ommochrome and pterin pigments. *Adv. Genet.* **10**:349–403.

5

The Flour Beetles, *Tribolium castaneum* and *Tribolium confusum*

Alexander Sokoloff

Introduction

Flour beetles of the genus *Tribolium* and related genera of the Tenebrionidae constitute important primary and secondary pests in all kinds of cereal products. *Tribolium castaneum* (hereafter referred to as CS) and *T. confusum* (CF) have received considerable attention from ecologists. Hence, from the point of view of population dynamics, they are probably among the best "ecologically documented" species of insects in existence.

Most of the genetic information for flour beetles has been obtained in the last 15 years. At the present time there are about 125 mutations described in CS, about 75 in CF, and about 75 in other Tenebrionidae and in other families of beetles (chiefly in Dermestidae and Silvanidae). These have been described and illustrated in my monographs (Sokoloff, 1966, 1975), which should be consulted for details. These two references also provide maps for those mutants whose linkage relationships have been established. Because of space limitations I have restricted this

Alexander Sokoloff—Department of Biology, California State College, San Bernardino, California.

chapter to a general summary of the types of mutations available, some notable discoveries in the basic genetics of *Tribolium*, and general conclusions regarding the usefulness of flour beetles in genetic research.

Technical Advantages and Disadvantages in Using *Tribolium* in Genetics

The technical advantages and disadvantages in using *Tribolium* in genetics have been listed in Sokoloff (1966). The main advantages are in the ease in preparation of the rearing medium, their small size, the ease in extracting all the stages of the life cycle from the medium, the ease in identifying the sex from the pupa onward, their short developmental period compared with their long expectation of life, and the ease in identifying morphological changes in the larva, pupa, and adult. Of greatest importance is the fact that flour beetles respond readily to selection for quantitative traits controlling behavior or body size.

When one compares the biological attributes of different species of beetles amenable to rearing in the laboratory, it is clear that flour beetles offer distinct advantages over other tenebrionid species, and within the genus probably CS is the most useful one from the technical standpoint, with CF not too far behind. The availability of genetic material has made it possible to initiate extensive studies on ecological genetics as well as population genetics.

The main disadvantages lie in the propensity of these beetles toward cannibalism; their sensitivity to protozoan parasites; their tendency toward "conditioning" of the medium by the accumulation of wastes and/or quinones secreted from the odoriferous glands, which may affect productivity of adult beetles or may produce teratological specimens if the quinones come in contact with immature stages at critical periods of their development; and the need for a continuous watch to detect the presence of predatory mites. This latter problem is no longer serious since there are effective acaricides available [see Sokoloff (1975)].

Karyotype

Extensive studies by Smith (1950, 1951, 1952*a,b*, 1953, 1960*a*, 1962) on the karyotypes of beetles in 191 species, 127 genera, 66 families, and 51 superfamilies have led him to conclude that the primitive number of chromosomes in Coleoptera is 10 pairs (9 pairs of autosomes, an X about the size of the autosomes, and a minute Y). Both sex chromosomes are V-shaped, and they associate during maturation divisions at two terminal contact points in the form of a "parachute." There are 27 species included in *Tribolium*, but only five have been studied cytologically. CS has the primitive chromosome number. CF, with only eight pairs of autosomes (a large X, and a large Y), is a derived species in which one of the autosome pairs became associated with the X and Y. [A third species, *T. destructor*, was subsequently derived from a CF-like ancestor. For details, see Smith (1952*a*).]

T. madens, in addition to the primitive number, has three pairs of supernumeraries capable of forming bivalents in the spermatocyte (Smith, 1956, 1960*b*). *T. audax*, a sibling species of *T. madens*, has an identical karyotype (Halstead, 1969).

For illustrations of karyotypes in various species of *Tribolium*, see Smith (1952*a,b*) or Sokoloff (1972). The lack of polytene chromosomes in beetles in general will make cytogenetic studies extremely difficult with present techniques.

Mutants

The normal appearance of adult CS is a beetle approximately 2 mm in length and 1 mm in width, weighing a little more than 2 mg. Its normal body color is chestnut. The compound eyes are black. CF is of the same color, a little larger, but there is considerable overlap. [For illustrations including scanning electron micrographs of the beetle, see Sokoloff (1972).]

Heritable variations have been noted in color and shape of the eyes; shape of antennae, legs, elytra, and other appendages; body size; increase in bristle number; body color; developmental rate; and modifications of the biochemical pathway in the production of end products such as quinones in the reservoirs of the stink glands or riboflavin in the Malpighian tubules or in the ability to utilize foods (e.g., the corn-oil-sensitive mutant). Some mutants are paedomorphic, the trait in the larva or pupa being retained in the adult, while others are homeotic, producing structures not normally borne on the body segments of present-day insects (e.g., wings on prothorax) or having appendages of a body segment modified to resemble other appendages (e.g., labial palps or antennae modified into leglike appendages).

In regard to their mode of inheritance, the mutants known in *Tribolium* are as varied as those in other insects. There are sex-linked dominant, semidominant, and recessive visibles and recessive lethals. Among autosomal genes there are dominants, dominants with recessive lethal effects, semidominants, recessives, incomplete recessives, and recessive lethals. Viability may be good to poor; expressivity may be uniform or variable; and penetrance may be complete, penetrance may be poor, or the gene may have pleiotropic effects.

A summary of available mutants has been made (Sokoloff, 1966, 1975). Most of the mutant stocks and useful combinations are available at the Tribolium Stock Center, California State College, San Bernardino, California 92407. Information on new mutants is available in the *Tribolium Information Bulletin* (*TIB*). *TIB*-16 is available on subscription basis. *TIB*-17 is available free of charge to investigators. It includes stock lists, research and technical notes, a current bibliography, and an alphabetical and geographical directory. It is edited by the author at the California State College, San Bernardino.

Notable Contributions from Basic Genetic Studies of *Tribolium*

Estimates of Mutation Rate

There have been few attempts to determine or increase the mutation rate in *Tribolium*. Irradiation studies sometimes have yielded visible mutations, but the high spontaneous rate in controls suggests the few mutants found in irradiated material were spontaneous, and not induced. Feeding *N*-methyl-*N*-nitroso-*N*-nitroguanidine to male flour beetles had an adverse effect on fertility but no sex-linked lethals were induced. A few visible mutants were found, but their low frequencies "suggest the possibility of either low penetrance or environmental origin" (Bell *et al.*, 1966). The investigators concluded that this chemical did not have as large a mutagenic effect as diethysulfate has in *Drosophila*. Lerner and Inouye (1967) applied Cavalli-Sforza's (1962) method for estimating spontaneous mutation rate for sex-linked lethals in both CS and CF by the regression of the sex ratio of live-born offspring on the age of the maternal grandfather at the time of the mother's birth. Although 150,000 pupae were examined, there was no significant regression, and estimates of the mutation rate were not possible.

Bartlett (1962), using high selection, random selection, and X rays to intensify changes in gene frequency, estimated the mutation rate of genes controlling body weight of CS to be between 1.7×10^{-3} and 2×10^{-5} mutations/r/locus.

Sokoloff (1959) and Sokoloff and Shrode (1960) estimated the forward mutation (+ to p) for the pearl locus from somatic mutations. In CS this frequency was of the order of 1 : 10,000. In *Latheticus oryzae*, another tenebrionid, based on a smaller sample, this value was 1 : 12,500.

Time of Action of Genes in *Tribolium*

In *Tribolium,* the larva, although certainly different in detail from the adult, has some similarities: the head has antennae, eyes, and mouth parts, and the prothoracic, mesothoracic, and metathoracic segments each bear a pair of legs subdivided into similar podomeres (coxa, trochanter, femur, tibia, and tarsus). The tergites and sternites of the abdomen bear some similarities as well. It is, therefore, possible to determine fairly precisely when various genes begin to act.

Many genes affecting the eye color and morphology of the adult already exert their effect as soon as the larva emerges from the egg. Some genes (for example, those affecting the antennae) exert their effect only in the adult. The *reduced gin traps* gene is an example of one that affects only pupal traits.

Factors Affecting Penetrance and Expressivity

There are a number of genes in *Tribolium* which exhibit incomplete penetrance. For some genes, a change in temperature improves penetrance. Thus, the tarsal irregular (*ti*) gene was 71 percent penetrant at room temperature, 97 percent penetrant at 32.8°C, and completely so at 37.8°C (Krause, 1963). The scar (*sc*) gene became fully penetrant at 35°C. In addition, temperature may alter the dominance relationships: *sc* became partially dominant at 35°C (Eddleman 1965*a,b*). In other cases, temperature failed to improve penetrance. Thus, the mottled (*mt*) mutant was reared at 25 and 35°C. Although the expression of *mt* was modified from "bloodspot" to brown or black, there was no change in the frequency of beetles that exhibited the trait (Schmitz and Englert, 1967).

Genetic background is also important in increasing penetrance of a trait. This is particularly true for phenodeviants, i.e., traits such as the white-leg character in CS which appear at low incidence in a "closed population"* but whose incidence increases following selection (Dawson, 1965*b*).

Multiple Alleles

The discovery of multiple alleles, of the position effect, and, later, of pseudoalleles in complex loci in fruit flies and other organisms has been of importance in the analysis of structure and function of the gene. As shown in the next section, pseudoalleles have not yet been demonstrated in

---

* A closed population is one in which no immigration or emigration is possible, as in the case of stocks which are never outcrossed.

Tribolium, but multiple alleles are known both in CS and CF. Owing to space limitations, only a few of the most extensive and striking allelic series will be mentioned [for other series, refer to Sokoloff (1966, 1975)].

Among the sex-linked genes affecting the normally black eye color in CF is eyespot, (*es*), a recessive which produces a red eye readily identifiable in the pupa or callow beetle. In aged beetles the eye becomes so dark as to be mistaken for the black eye in the + beetle. A recessive allele es^{lt} produces a uniform, lighter red eye. In CS the red (*r*) locus includes four alleles: +, *r*, r^H, and r^D. The *r* and r^H alleles are similar, producing a dark red eye in both sexes. The color may lighten on inbreeding, but outcrosses will re-establish the dark red eye. The r^D allele is sex-influenced, being darker in the female. In CF the red locus has 3 alleles: + is black, *r* is dark red, and r^u is light red.

Among the autosomal genes the Short antenna (*Sa*) locus in linkage group VII is the most extensive. There are four dominants with recessive lethal effects (*Sa, Sa-1, Sa-2, Sa-3*) and four semidominant or overlapping wild-type (*sa, sa-1, sa-2, sa-3*). That *Sa* and *sa* are allelic can be recognized by the fact that *Sa/sa* × *sa/sa* crosses produce only *Sa*-like and *sa*-like beetles. If any wild-type beetles were obtained, then a complex locus might be demonstrated (Sokoloff *et al.,* 1963). Dawson and Sokoloff (1964) obtained a few normal individuals in crosses of *Sa-3/sa* × *sa/sa* and suggested the possibility of having found such a complex locus in *Tribolium.* However, they lacked marker genes on both sides of the *sa* locus to distinguish between the possibility that the few normal individuals resulted from a rare crossover event rather than from a backmutation (either from *Sa* to + or *sa* to +).

The genotypes at the black locus in CS or CF are: +/+, producing a chestnut or red rust; +/*b*, producing a bronze; and *b/b*, which gives a black body color (Miller, 1944; Sokoloff *et al.,* 1960; Stanley and Slatis, 1955). Some alleles of this semidominant black are recessives (+/+ × *b/b* produces a red rust rather than a bronze heterozygote).

Body-color mutants are among the most frequently found aberrations, probably because they are immediately obvious to the naked eye.

Pseudoallelism

Using two alleles of pearl, *p* and p^{Pk}, Dewees and Bell (1967) tried to show the presence of pseudoallelism in *Tribolium.* They crossed $p +/p^{Pk}$ i × $p^{Pk} +/p^{Pk} +$ in mass matings. They examined 36,654 progeny. All of the beetles proved to have pink eyes (p^{Pk} is dominant to *p*), and thus they failed to establish the presence of pseudoallelism. At a similar level of resolution, Chovnick (1961), after crossing two garnet alleles, g_1 and g_2 in *Drosophila*, obtained two wild-type flies among 68,000 examined, indicating a crossover frequency of about 0.003 percent.

Recombination

Effect of Sex. Sokoloff (1964) found that recombination between any given pair of genes in linkage group VII, whether in coupling or repulsion, is not significantly different within a sex, but is significantly different between sexes. The recombination values may differ only slightly (but significantly) between the sexes or they may differ considerably, with the result that the values in the male may approach 50 percent, giving the erroneous impression that the genes are not linked, while the values obtained from females clearly indicate that these genes are linked. This phenomenon was not observed in data derived from linkage group IV. Sokoloff advanced the hypothesis that the difference in recombination, reflected in the crossover values in the two sexes in *T. castaneum*, results from a difference in the distribution of a single chiasma.

Johnson (1966) found that recombination is increased in the male sex for linkage group VII and in the female for linkage group IV genes. Dawson (1972a) established that hazel (*h*) and Bar eye (*Be*) are located on one chromosome arm and cut (*ct*) and juvenile urogomphi (*ju*) are on the other of chromosome IV. The centromere, on the basis of interference values, is located between *Be* and *ct*. Furthermore, Dawson (1972b) has resolved the apparent discrepancy between the results of Sokoloff (1964) and those of Johnson (1966) for linkage-group-IV recombination values. His data support Sokoloff's conclusions that for this linkage group no differences in the two sexes are observable for genes far apart (25–30 units); however, when this region is subdivided into smaller regions, crossover values were higher in males for one region and in females for another (Dawson, 1972b).

Dewees (1967) found unequal recombination values for males and females, but these were not affected by the *cis* or *trans* position of the genes within a given sex. He suggested that the unequal recombination values may result from a differential segregation of chromosomes in one sex (probably the female), with the result that the recombinant chromosome is incorporated more often in the polar body during second-division segregation, resulting in a lower number of recombinant progeny.

The phenomenon which brings about a difference in recombination in the two sexes is apparently widespread. Dunn and Bennett (1967) have surveyed the literature on the subject and have concluded that this phenomenon is present both in plants and in animals. Their survey also pointed out that crossing over occurs in both sexes in the majority of animals. There is some tendency for crossover values in females to exceed those in males. They found that, as in *Tribolium,* in the house mouse marked sex-differences can occur in opposite directions in different chromosomes.

Effect of *Cis* or *Trans* Arrangements.   Englert and Bell (1963) reported unequal rates of recombination between the two sexes for linkage group VIII only in the coupling or *cis* phase (female values exceeding those of the male), while the repulsion or *trans* phase showed equal recombinations in the two sexes. Dewees (1967), following recombination of genes in linkage group V, found that the pattern of recombination of *cis* and *trans* phases was the same within a sex, i.e., recombination was greater in the male than the female regardless of *cis* or *trans* arrangement.

To remove sex as the confounding factor from the linkage phase, Englert (1969a,b) investigated recombination rates of the sex-linked recessive marker genes pygmy (*py*) and red (*r*) in the female in single-pair matings. The pooled data gave a recombination rate for the *cis* phase of about 11 percent and for the *trans* phase of about 7.3 percent, a significant difference.

Effect of Age and Temperature.   Age has no apparent effect on the rate of recombination, but a highly significant difference has been found between the linkage phases at two temperatures. At 25°C the recombination values were 23.2 ± 3.0 percent for the *cis* and 5.8 ± 1.5 percent for the *trans* phase, indicating that temperature affects the rate of recombination for the *cis* linkage phase (essentially doubling it), but does not affect the *trans* phase (the values remaining the same at both temperatures).

Close Linkage of Genes with Similar Functions

A number of genes affecting the same character and producing the same phenotype have been found to be closely linked. In CS, the paddle (*pd*) and serrate (*ser*), genes which affect the antennae, are less than one crossover unit apart on the X chromosome (Dawson, 1965a). Several eye-color mutants are closely linked. On the X chromosome, ring (*rg*) and rose (*rs*) are 3.2 units apart. On chromosome II, pearl (*p*) and ivory (*i*) are only 0.03 units apart, and on chromosome V, ruby (*rb*) and maroon (*m*) show 1.5 percent recombination in males and 0.12 percent in females (Dewees and Bell, 1967). Several paedomorphic mutants (juvenile urogomphi, elongated juvenile urogomphi, and reduced juvenile urogomophi), although located near each other on the same linkage group and producing a similar phenotypic effect, are not allelic (Sokoloff, 1962, 1963); and two biochemical mutants (melanotic stink glands and mottled), though closely linked and producing the same phenotype, are not allelic in the usual sense of the word (Schmitz and Englert, 1967).

In CF, the genes pearl (p) and riboflavinless pearl (p^r) are further examples of closely linked genes (Weber and Roberts, 1967), and indeed these genes may be homologous to p and i in CS (Roberts and Juriloff, 1968).

Dawson (1965a) has suggested that *ser* and *pd* represent a gene duplication that has persisted without much change. Dewees and Bell (1967) have proposed that the three pairs of genes they investigated may represent a breakup of a primitive gene system. Finally, Dawson (1971) has suggested that the sex-linked recessive, blob (bb), which does not show dosage compensation, represents an intermediate stage in the process of chromosome evolution; namely, that bb is a duplication of the pd (or *ser*) region which has been shifted to another location by a chromosomal aberration. Selection for modifiers to equalize gene dosage in males and females has not been completed.

Intra-locus Heterosis

The discovery of the sex-linked Modifier–suppressor (M^r) of the red gene (r) established the existence of a very unusual interaction of genes. Hemizygous r males or homozygous r/r females have a light red eye. $r\,M^r$ males and $r\,M^r/r\,M^r$ females have a dark red eye. $r\,M^r/r\,M^+$ females have a fully pigmented, normal black eye. Thus, neither M^r/M^r nor M^+/M^+ can block the effect of r/r, but M^r/M^+ can (Sokoloff, 1965). This is the best evidence available for the existence of a true *intra*-locus heterosis.

Paedomorphic and Homeotic Mutants

Paedomorphic mutations are those that retain juvenile (larval or pupal) traits in the adult. For example, in CS the urogomphi are retained in adult juvenile urogomphi (ju), reduced juvenile urogomphi (rju), and elongated juvenile urogomphi (eju) mutants.

Homeotic mutations are those which produce allotypic structures. The alate prothorax mutation (apt) in CS and in CF produces wings in the prothoracic segment which normally is free of wings. Antennapedia (ap) in CS modifies antennae into legs; labiopedia in CS and CF transforms the labial palps into legs, and maxillopedia (mxp) in CS changes the maxillary palps, and sometimes the labial palps, into leglike structures. Other homeotic mutants may produce serial homology of structures: in CF, pointed abdominal segments (*pas*) accomplished this serial homology of all the abdominal sternites, while in CS, partially pointed abdominal segments (*ppas*) affects only the second apparent abdominal segment. Other mutants produce a duplication of structures: in CS the extra urogomphi (*Eu*) mutant and the multiurogomphi (*Mu*) mutant produce either double urogomphi or an extra aedeagus. (The effects in the female are not as prominent.)

Homeotic mutants such as the alate prothorax mutant and the labiopedia mutant have been particularly useful in providing support to the hypothesis advanced by Smith (1952*a*) that the X and Y in CF were formed by a translocation of an autosome to the primitive X and Y (Sokoloff, *et al.,* 1967; Dawson, 1968). The paedomorphic and homeotic mutations *Eu* and *Mu* have been useful in providing markers to identify homologous structures in the reproductive organs of the two sexes (Sokoloff and Hoy, 1968).

Morphogenesis

Mutants have provided some insight on the manner in which different beetle structures such as genitalia or antennae are formed. In *Tribolium,* wings, legs, and genitalia form in the larva from poorly defined primordia. In the pupa these appendages are everted and elaborated further to attain the typical appearance present in the adult. In the mutation emasculated (*em*), the structures leading to the formation of the aedeagus fail to evert, with the result that only a sclerotized, ball-like structure forms, or, at best, only various lengths of the partly everted tip of the aedeagus may be observed from this sclerotized ball-like structure (Sokoloff, 1966).

In the case of the antennae, I have concluded that genes affecting these appendages begin to exert their effect at the distal end first, and later they affect more proximal portions. If the effect is constant, then fusion of all adjacent segments is produced. If the effect is sporadic, then blocks of fused adjacent segments may be separated by normal antennameres (Sokoloff, 1966). Dawson (1966) has proposed an alternative hypothesis.

Mosaics

Mosaics Due to Somatic Mutation. Mosaics are organisms bearing cells of two different genotypes. In *Tribolium* the most frequent mosaics, as indicated above, are those involving the pearl gene. In +/*p* heterozygotes, it is not uncommon for some beetles to have one eye black and the other either partly or completely pearl. These mosaics arise by somatic mutation: in the $+/p$ cell there may be a mutation from $+$ to p with the result that the descendants of this p/p cell will be pearl. If the event occurs at the first cleavage, one eye will be black and the other will be pearl. If the event occurs later, smaller and smaller areas of the compound eye will lack black pigment. Cases in which a single ommatidium exhibits a pearl phenotype have been found.

Mosaics Resulting from Double Fertilization. Slatis discovered a male CS beetle whose body exhibited a sharp color demarcation along the midline. The right half of the body was pigmented as in the wild type, and the left half of the body was pigmented as in a bronze $(b/+)$ beetle. The color of the appendages corresponded to the color of that side of the body. The male was mated to a normal female and they produced 42 $+/+$ and 50 $b/+$ progeny, indicating that the testes were probably $b/+$ in genotype, although other possibilities exist. Slatis *et al.* (1969) believe that this bilateral mosaic condition is most probably explained by a double fertilization, when two separate sperms enter an egg and fertilize two nuclei. Each half of the beetle is then formed from the descendants of one of the original zygotes. In the egg, the two nuclei could arise by the accidental inclusion of two nuclei within one cell during oogenesis, or they might be the egg pronucleus and a haploid polar body nucleus. At the present time there are no data to distinguish between the two possibilities. Other more complex suggestions for mosaics are less likely.

Biochemical Mutants

Although body-color and eye-color mutants are available in *Tribolium,* the biochemical changes involved have not been worked out. The main difficulty with body-color mutants lies in the fact that black, jet, and sooty are probably modifications of melanin pigments, while eye colors probably are ommochromes. Both types of pigment are difficult to analyze biochemically.

There has been some effort in determining the biochemical changes in the pathway of three mutants: melanotic stink glands (*msg*) discovered in CS and CF; riboflavinless pearl (p^r); and corn oil sensitive (*cos*).

The msg^+ beetles normally store in the reservoirs of their stink glands a yellowish, quinone-containing liquid which is not visible through the exoskeleton. In *msg* the contents of the reservoirs are modified into a visible, solid black mass (Sokoloff, 1966). Analysis of the contents of the reservoirs of normal and mutant CF beetles reveals that young beetles contain only ½₀ of the 2-methyl and 2-ethyl-1,4-benzoquinones present in normal beetles; on aging, the quinones in *msg* mutants completely disappear. Ladisch and Ladisch (1967) have confirmed the great reduction of quinones in *msg.* The black mass in the reservoirs is a polymeric substance of high molecular weight (Engelhardt *et al.*, 1965).

Weber and Roberts (1966, 1967) have found that in one of the pearl (*p*) eye mutants, p^r, there is a block in the production of riboflavin, with the result that this substance is absent from the Malpighian tubules, while in the normal allele or other pearl mutants riboflavin is found in greatest concentration (4–10 times the concentration found in the body) in these excretory organs.

The corn oil sensitive mutant (*cos*) is an autosomal recessive whose growth and viability are affected by the presence of corn oil in the diet. The effect, due to an alteration in lipid metabolism, is inversely proportional to the concentration of corn oil in the diet (Costantino *et al.*, 1966).

Conclusions

The availability of mutant material has made it possible to obtain fundamental information on the genetics of representatives of the Coleoptera. The linkage studies have identified homologous genes in *T. castaneum* and *T. confusum,* and have also identified the autosome which, in the evolution of *T. confusum* from a primitive species like *T. castaneum,* became translocated to the X and Y chromosomes. These studies have also revealed a number of closely linked genes which affect traits in a similar fashion. These represent primitive gene systems in the process of breaking up. Other studies have shown that recombination in the two sexes is not equal. Homeotic and paedomorphic mutants have been used successfully to identify homologous chromosomes in species which can no longer hybridize and homologous structures in the genitalia of the two sexes within a given species. One of the mutants in *T. castaneum* provides the best available evidence for *intra*-locus heterosis.

In other work, it has been found that *Tribolium* beetles respond very well to selection for quantitative traits (body weight, running through a maze, flying ability, etc.). The availability of homologous mutants in CS and CF has opened up the possibility of carrying out studies of comparative population genetics as well as in the new field of ecological genetics.

Literature Cited

Bell, A. E., L. Brzostowski and R. D. Brock, 1966   Response of *Tribolium castaneum* to adult feeding of n-methyl-n-nitroso-n-nitroguanidine. *Tribolium Inf. Bull.* **5:**13.

Bartlett, A. C., 1962   Section on new mutants. *Tribolium Inf. Bull.* **5:**13.

Cavalli-Sforza, L. L., 1962   Un metodo per la stima della frequenza di mutazione nell'uomo: Risultati preliminari. *Atti Assoc. Genet. Ital.* **6:**151–162.

Chovnick, A., 1961   The garnet locus in *Drosophila melanogaster*. I. Pseudoallelism. *Genetics* **46:**493–507.

Costantino, R. F., A. E. Bell and J. C. Rogler, 1966   Genetic control of lipid metabolism in *Tribolium*. *Nature (Lond.)* **210:**221–222.

Dawson, P. S., 1965a   "Serrate": A sex-linked recessive gene in the flour beetle, *Tribolium castaneum*. *Can. J. Genet. Cytol.* **7:**559–562.

Dawson, P. S., 1965b   The while leg character in *Tribolium castaneum*. *Tribolium Inf. Bull.* **8:**70–72.

Dawson, P. S., 1966   Insect antennal development and the serrate gene in *Tribolium castaneum*. *J. Theor. Biol.* **12:**133–139.

Dawson, P. S., 1968   Genetic evidence for an hypothesis concerning evolution in *Tribolium*. *J. Hered.* **59:**188–190.

Dawson, P. S., 1971   The blob mutant of *Tribolium castaneum*. *Can. J. Genet. Cytol.* **13:**801–810.

Dawson, P. S., 1972a   Linkage group IV of *Tribolium castaneum*. *Can. J. Genet. Cytol.* **14:**675–680.

Dawson, P. S., 1972b   Sex and crossing over in linkage group IV of *Tribolium castaneum*. *Genetics* **72:**525–530.

Dawson, P. S. and A. Sokoloff, 1964   A multiple allelic series in *Tribolium castaneum*. *Am. Nat.* **98:**455–457.

Dewees, A., 1967   Sex differences in recombination values for linkage group V of *T. castaneum*. *Tribolium Inf. Bull.* **10:**89–90.

Dewees, A. and A. E. Bell, 1967   Close linkage of eye color genes in *Tribolium castaneum*. *Genetics* **56:**633–640.

Dunn, L. C. and D. Bennett, 1967   Sex differences in recombination of linked genes in animals. *Genet. Res.* **9:**211–220.

Eddleman, H., 1965a   Effect of temperature on penetrance of the scar mutant of *Tribolium castaneum*. *Genetics* **52:**441.

Eddleman, H., 1965b   Scar: A temperature sensitive mutation in *Tribolium castaneum* Herbst. *Ind. Acad. Sci. Proc.* **74:**398–401.

Engelhardt, M., H. Rapoport and A. Sokoloff, 1965   Comparison of the content of the odoriferous gland reservoirs in normal and mutant *Tribolium confusum*. *Science (Wash., D.C.)* **150:**632–633.

Englert, D. C., 1969a   The influence of linkage phase on recombination rates in *Tribolium*. *Genetics* **61:**16.

Englert, D. C., 1969b   Linkage phase differences in recombination rates for linkage group I in *Tribolium castaneum*. *Tribolium Inf. Bull.* **11:**78–79.

Englert, D. C. and A. E. Bell, 1963   "Antennapedia" and "squint," recessive marker genes for linkage group VIII in *Tribolium castaneum*. *Can. J. Genet. Cytol.* **5:**467–471.

Halstead, D. G. H., 1969   A new species of *Tribolium* from North America previously confused with *Tribolium madens* (Charp.) (Coleoptera: Tenebrionidae). *J. Stored Prod. Res.* **4**:295–304.

Johnson, G. R., 1966   Recombination differences with reciprocal crosses in *Tribolium castaneum. Genetics* **56**:633–640.

Krause, E., 1963   Effect of temperature on penetrance of the *ti* mutant. *Tribolium Inf. Bull.* **6**:44.

Ladisch, R. K. and S. K. Ladisch, 1967   Quinoid secretions in *Tribolium confusum. Tribolium Inf. Bull.* **10**:108–111.

Lerner, I. M. and N. Inouye, 1967   Regression of the sex ratio on maternal grandfather's age. *Tribolium Inf. Bull.* **10**:113.

Miller, L. W., 1944   Investigations of the flour beetles of the genus *Tribolium.* A color strain of *T. castaneum* (Hbst). *J. Dept. Agric. Victoria* **42**:469–471.

Roberts, C. W. and D. Juriloff, 1968   Evidence for gene homology of two pearl-eyed genes in the *Tribolium castaneum* and *Tribolium confusum. Can. J. Genet. Cytol.* **10**:139–142.

Schmitz, T. H. and D. C. Englert, 1967   The "mottled" mutation in *Tribolium castaneum. Can. J. Genet. Cytol.* **9**:335–341.

Slatis, H. M., H. Fakhrai and R. A. Bancroft, 1969   One beetle with two genotypes (*Tribolium castaneum* (Herbst.) (Coleoptera, Tenebrionidae). *J. Stored Prod. Res.* **5**:181–182.

Smith, S. G., 1950   The cytotaxonomy of Coleoptera. *Can. Entomol.* **82**:58–68.

Smith, S. G., 1951   Evolutionary changes in the sex chromosomes of Coleoptera. *Genetica (The Hague)* **25**:522–524.

Smith, S. G., 1952a   The evolution of heterochromatin in the genus *Tribolium* (Tenebrionidae:Coleoptera). *Chromosoma (Berl.)* **4**:585–610.

Smith, S. G., 1952b   The cytology of some tenebrionoid beetles (Coleoptera). *J. Morphol.* **91**:325–364.

Smith, S. G., 1953   Chromosome numbers of Coleoptera. *Heredity* 7:31–48.

Smith, S. G., 1956   The status of supernumerary chromosomes in *Diabrotica* after a lapse of 50 years. *J. Hered.* **47**:157–164.

Smith, S. G., 1960a   Cytogenetics of insects. *Annu. Rev. Entomol.* **5**:69–84.

Smith, S. G., 1960b   Chromosome numbers of Coleoptera. II. *Can. J. Genet. Cytol.* **2**:66–88.

Smith, S. G., 1962   Cytogenetic pathways in beetle speciation. *Can. Entomol.* **94**:941–955.

Sokoloff, A., 1959   The nature of the "pearl" mutation in *Tribolium castaneum* and *Latheticus oryzae* (Tenebrionidae). *Anat. Rec.* **134**:641–642.

Sokoloff, A., 1962   Linkage studies in *Tribolium castaneum* Herbst. V. The genetics of Bar eye, microcephalic, and Microphthalmic and their relationships to black, jet, pearl and sooty. *Can. J. Genet. Cytol.* **4**:409–425.

Sokoloff, A., 1963   Further linkage results for *Tribolium castaneum. Genetics* **48**:910–911.

Sokoloff, A., 1964   Sex and crossing over in *Tribolium castaneum. Genetics* **50**:491–496.

Sokoloff, A., 1965   An unusual modifier-suppressor system in *Tribolium castaneum. Am. Nat.* **99**:143–151.

Sokoloff, A., 1966   *The Genetics of Tribolium and Related Species,* Academic Press, New York.

Sokoloff, A., 1972   *The Biology of Tribolium with Special Emphasis on Genetic Aspects,* Vol. 1, Clarendon Press, Oxford.

Sokoloff, A., 1975   *The Biology of Tribolium with Special Emphasis on Genetic Aspects,* Vols. 2 and 3, Clarendon Press, Oxford.

Sokoloff, A. and M. A. Hoy, 1968   Mutations as possible aids for establishing genitalic homologies in the sexes in *Tribolium castaneum. Entomol. Soc. Am. Ann.* **61**:550–553.

Sokoloff, A. and R. R. Shrode, 1960   Linkage studies in *Latheticus oryzae* Waterh. *I.* Recombination between "red" and "truncated elytra." *Can. J. Genet. Cytol.* **2**:418–428.

Sokoloff, A., H. M. Slatis and J. Stanley, 1960   The black mutation in *Tribolium castaneum. J. Hered.* **52**:131–135.

Sokoloff, A., P. S. Dawson and D. C. Englert, 1963   Linkage studies in *Tribolium castaneum* Herbst. VIII. Short antenna, a dominant marker for the seventh linkage group. *Can. J. Genet. Cytol.* **5**:299–306.

Sokoloff, A., M. Ackermann and L. F. Overton, 1967   Linkage studies in *Tribolium confusum* Duval. II. The map position of three homeotic mutants. *Can. J. Genet. Cytol.* **9**:490–502.

Stanley, J. and H. M. Slatis, 1955   Studies from the autotrephon. IV. A black mutation of *T. confusum* compared with the normal reddish-brown strain. *Ecology* **36**:473–485.

Weber, J. and C. W. Roberts, 1966   The genetics of a riboflavinless, pearl-eyed trait in *Tribolium confusum. Can. J. Genet. Cytol.* **8**:796–806.

Weber, J. and C. W. Roberts, 1967   Riboflavin accumulation in p^r, p^s, and wild-type genotypes of *Tribolium confusum. Can. J. Genet. Cytol.* **9**:565–568.

6

The Honey Bee,
Apis mellifera

Walter C. Rothenbuhler

The Colony

Social life of the honey bee has evolved to such an extent that an individual apart from its colony is not capable of reproduction or even of normal survival. The individual is important only for its contribution to the colony, and the colony has become the primary unit of natural selection. An ongoing natural colony is composed of a queen, 7,000 to 70,000 worker bees, and zero to a few thousand drones. The colony's nest is built of waxen combs which in nature are attached to the ceiling and walls of some cavity such as a hollow tree or between the walls of a house. Open-air colonies seldom if ever survive. In modern beekeeping, combs are built inside individual wooden frames and all are housed inside a hive. Pollen and honey are stored and young bees are reared in the combs.

When the colony's population increases greatly in late spring or early summer, and when food is available from blooming plants, swarming, which constitutes the reproduction of the colony, may occur. A dozen to two dozen queen cells may be built to rear a like number of young queens. When some of these cells are sealed (and the larvae are transforming to pupae), the old queen and approximately half of the worker bees will

Walter C. Rothenbuhler—Departments of Entomology, Zoology, and Genetics, Ohio State University, Columbus, Ohio.

leave the nest and seek a new nesting place where new combs will be built, broods reared, and food stored. As soon as young queens emerge in the parental nest, one or more "after swarms" may be cast. When swarming is finished, the young queens fight among themselves until only one remains alive. She or the worker bees will destroy any remaining queen cells, and she will be the queen of the colony.

The Individuals

The individuals of the colony have unique origins and functions. Both queens and workers are females, developed from fertilized eggs, and characterized by the diploid number of chromosomes (32). They develop their very different morphologies and behaviors in response to environmental differences in rearing (Weaver, 1966). Drones are males developed from unfertilized eggs, and characterized by the haploid number of chromosomes (16). High degrees of endopolyploidy are found in tissues of both sexes and castes (Risler, 1954; Merriam and Ris, 1954). Developmental times from deposition of the egg to emergence of the adult is approximately 15–16 days for the queen and 20–21 days for the worker. The developmental time for drones is usually given as 24 days.

Queens live 1–3 years, deposit fertilized and unfertilized eggs in worker cells (smaller) and drone cells (larger), respectively, and produce pheromones essential to colony life (Butler, 1967). Egg production may exceed 1600 in one day. A queen mates in flight with six to ten drones before oviposition begins (Taber and Wendel, 1958).

Workers live about 6 weeks in the summer, but they live much longer during the winter (perhaps 4–6 months). Under certain conditions, "laying workers" may produce unfertilized eggs which usually become drones (see the following section). The normal functions of workers are brood care and nursing, comb building, nest maintenance and defense, and foraging for pollen, nectar, water, and propolis; the latter is a sticky substance collected from plants and used to seal cracks and joints in the walls of the hive.

Drones live probably for about 6 weeks and function only to fertilize a queen. A drone mates only once, in flight, and usually at some distance from the colony in a drone congregation area (Ruttner, 1966).

Cytology and Genetics

Meiosis in queens proceeds in the usual way, resulting in gametes with 16 chromosomes. The egg is capable of development regardless of fertilization, but it normally develops into a male if unfertilized. Occasionally an unfertilized egg develops into a female (Mackensen, 1943; Tucker, 1958). The first meiotic division in drones is abortive, producing a cytoplasmic bud. The second meiotic division is equational, but cytokinesis is unequal, and only one sperm is formed from each primary spermatocyte.

In the process of fertilization it is normal for several sperms to enter the bee's egg. Normally the accessory sperm degenerate, but in certain gynandromorph-producing strains, accessory sperm give rise to the male tissue, whereas the zygote gives rise to the female tissue of the sex mosaic. Dozens to hundreds of gynandromorphs can be found in colonies of some strains (Drescher, 1965; Rothenbuhler, 1958a). As a consequence of gynandromorph origin and production, a drone's genotype can be multiplied indefinitely by sperm-producing gynandromorphs which arise from a single-drone mating (Tucker and Laidlaw, 1966).

Sex determination follows the *Habrobracon* system, by which individuals that are hemizygous (haploid) or homozygous for the sex allele (or chromosome segment) become males and those that are heterozygous become females (Kerr, 1974). Diploid males if left in the colony are eaten when they are very small larvae by the worker bees (Woyke, 1963).

A list of mutations in the honey bee is given in Table 1 [further information can be found in Rothenbuhler *et al.* (1968b) and Kerr (1974)]. At present, a stock center for mutations is maintained by Dr. Harry H. Laidlaw, at the University of California, Davis, California, 95616, and, for inbred lines and other stocks, by the United States Department of Agriculture Bee Breeding Laboratory, at Louisiana State University, Baton Rouge, Louisiana, 70803. The mutants droopy (D), schwarzsüchtig (S), rudimental wing (Rw), lethal (l), and white eye of Michailoff ($-$) are among those no longer maintained. The hairless (h) and chartreuse (ch) loci are linked with about 4.1 percent crossing over; pearl (pe) and cream (cr) are linked with 0.33 percent crossing over. No linkage of the sex locus with other loci has been found in those cases where checked (Rothenbuhler *et al.*, 1968b). Analysis of segregation of alleles in impaternate worker progeny of heterozygous unmated queens has shown that ch segregates as if it were 38.8 crossover units from its centromere and ivory (i) segregates as if it were 3.6 units from its centromere (Tucker, 1958).

Apis mellifera, derived presumably from stock originating in southeastern Asia, has spread by natural means over much of Europe and Africa and part of Asia. A great deal of geographic variation has been developed, and some 25 geographic races are recognized (Rothenbuhler *et*

TABLE 1. List of Mutations. (Modified and Expanded from Rothenbuhler et al., 1968b and Kerr, 1974.)

Symbol	Name of mutation	Type of mutation
ac	Brown	Abdominal color
bk	Brick	Eye color
bl	Black	Body color
c	Cordovan	Body color
ch	Chartreuse	Eye color
ch¹	Chartreuse-1	Eye color
ch²	Chartreuse-2	Eye color
ch^B	Benson green	Eye color
ch^c	Cherry	Eye color
ch^r	Red	Eye color
cr	Cream	Eye color
D	Droopy	Wings
e	Eyeless	Eye morphology
Est^F, Est^S	Esterase isozymes	Esterase electrophoretic mobility
g	Garnet	Eye color
h	Hairless	Body hair
i	Ivory	Eye color
i^u	Umber	Eye color
l	Lethal	Viability
la	Laranja (orange)	Eye color
m	Modifier	Chartreuse-1 eye color
p	Pink	Eye color
pe	Pearl	Eye color
$P\text{-}3^F, P\text{-}3^S$	Protein-3 isozymes	Protein-3 electrophoretic mobility
r	Removing	Behavior
Rw	Rudimental wing	Wings
s	Snow	Eye color
s^t	Tan	Eye color
S	Schwarzsüchtig (black hairless)	Body hair
sh	Short	Wings
tr	Truncate	Wings
u	Uncapping	Behavior
wr	Wrinkled	Wings
—	White or ivory [of Michailoff (1931)]	Eye color
X^1–X^N	Sex alleles	Sex determination

al., 1968*b*). These races provide vast stores of morphological and, perhaps more importantly, behavioral variation with respect to stinging, foraging, brood rearing, dancing, etc. Ruttner (1967), after wide experience with various races, has concluded that very specific local adaptations (ecotypes) exist within the geographic races. Such differences have developed in response to local nectar and pollen-flow conditions. It should be pointed out that many countries (including the U. S.) have restrictions on importation of bees. Tremendous variability exists, nevertheless, within the bees already in the U. S. The same is true in Brazil (personal observation), and, presumably, great variation also exists in other countries to which bees have been extensively imported.

A number of breeding programs have been carried out successfully. For instance, bees have been developed which show no symptoms of American foulbrood disease following enormous dosages of the pathogen *Bacillus larvae* [reviewed in Rothenbuhler (1958*b*)]. Lines have been developed for high and low collection of pollen from alfalfa (*Medicago sativa*). In the fifth generation of selection, 85 percent of pollen collected by the high line came from alfalfa, whereas only 18 percent came from alfalfa in the low one (Nye and Mackensen, 1968). Even greater differences in stinging behavior have characterized certain strains and races of bees [reviewed in Rothenbuhler *et al.* (1968*b*)]. Inbreeding depression has usually been found in the honey bee, and hybrid vigor in oviposition, honey production, and certain morphological characters has been demonstrated (Cale and Gowen, 1956; Roberts, 1961).

Culture of Bees

It is of course impossible in the space available to provide essential directions for maintaining bees. An excellent beginner's book is *Starting Right with Bees* (Editorial staff of *Gleanings in Bee Culture*, 1971). Three other more advanced works are Grout (1963), Root (1966), and Eckert and Shaw (1960). Equally important if available to the beginner is preliminary instruction, guidance, and help from a local beekeeper. They are usually anxious to assist a new beekeeper and can help to avoid many pitfalls and numerous stings.

There are two easy ways to acquire bees: buy colonies locally which are already established or buy package bees to be established in hives. A third way is to "hive" swarms reported to the police department of any sizeable town. The keeping of at least two colonies is recommended to the beginner because of the value of comparing one with the other.

From a single selected colony it is possible to raise dozens or even hundreds of queens and thousands of drones with a reasonable expenditure of labor and materials. Of course it is in the nature of a colony to rear tens of thousands of worker bees. In general, one can test a bee-mating extensively in whatever way is desired, but the number of matings that can be tested is somewhat restricted. Queen and drone rearing are described in differing detail by Cale (1963), Laidlaw and Eckert (1950), and Mackensen and Tucker (1970).

For genetic studies on bees, instrumental insemination is necessary. Fortunately, this technique, first demonstrated by Watson (1928), has now been greatly improved by the work of Nolan, Laidlaw, Mackensen, Roberts, and others (Mackensen and Tucker, 1970). A queen may be inseminated with semen from one or several drones. If kept confined, drones no older than 3 weeks of age are generally used.

For genetic studies of whole-colony behavior, it is necessary that worker bees of a colony be genetically alike. This result can be achieved by an inbred queen–single drone mating technique which capitalizes on male haploidy (Rothenbuhler, 1960). Lines homozygous for the different genetic elements in question can be crossed and F_1 queens produced. The hybrid queen's sons, which are genetically her gametes, can be tested by backcrossing them individually to queens of the parental homozygous lines. Worker bees within each resulting colony are expected to be genetically and phenotypically similar, but worker bees of different colonies will fall into a number of phenotypically different classes, depending on the genetic differences between the original lines.

Small colonies consisting of a few dozen to a few hundred bees, usually in a glass-sided observation hive, have been used by several investigators to study specific problems. Keeping such units warm and free of robber bees necessitates special measures. One method involves use of thermostatically controlled, heated, walk-in-size observation-hive shelters made of plywood, from which each colony may fly into a walk-in-size plastic-screen cage (Rothenbuhler et al., 1968a). Bees will forage in these cages for dry pollen in dishes and for sugar syrup. Such units provide the isolation necessary for some types of disease research.

Investigators must be aware of some bee diseases (Gochnauer, 1963). Normally bees are free of disease, but if they contract certain diseases like American foulbrood, they can be a menace to all other bee colonies in the area. This and some other diseases may interfere seriously with a research program.

Colonies ordinarily do not interact one with another, but under certain conditions may do so. When nectar is not available in the field, colonies will attempt to steal honey from each other. This robbing is prevented by proper beekeeping techniques. If colonies are within a few inches or a few feet of each other, drifting of bees from one colony to another will occur. Therefore, it must *not* be assumed that all bees within a colony are progeny of that queen. Drifting of workers will be minimized if hives are placed at least 15 feet apart and are located amidst some prominent landmarks such as trees, bushes, stones, posts, or flowers. Drones probably drift to a much greater extent than workers.

Conclusion

In spite of a few complications encountered in their care and maintenance, honey bees are fascinating, valuable creatures for research. Their haplo-diploid origin brings certain advantages. Above and beyond research opportunities presented by insects living solitary lives, honey bees present to the investigator a great profusion of behavior patterns (and behavioral variation) associated with their highly evolved social life. Behavior genetics, genetics of disease resistance, and genetic-environmental control of morphogenesis are challenging, accessible areas for investigation in this species.

Literature Cited

Butler, C. G., 1967 Insect pheromones. *Biol. Rev.* **42**:42–87.

Cale, G. H., Jr., 1963 The production of queens, package bees, and royal jelly. In *The Hive and the Honey Bee,* edited by R. A. Grout, pp. 437–462, Dadant & Sons, Hamilton, Illinois.

Cale, G. H., Jr. and J. W. Gowen, 1956 Heterosis in the honey bee (*Apis mellifera* L.). *Genetics* **41**:292–303.

Drescher, W., 1965 Der Einfluss von Umweltbedingungen auf die Bildung von Gynandromorphen bei der Honigbiene *Apis mellifica* L. *Insectes Sociaux* **12**:201–218.

Eckert, J. E. and F. R. Shaw, 1960 *Beekeeping,* Macmillan, New York.

Editorial staff of *Gleanings in Bee Culture,* 1971 *Starting Right With Bees,* 15th edition, A. I. Root Co., Medina, Ohio.

Gochnauer, T. A., 1963 Diseases and enemies of the honey bee. In *The Hive and the Honey Bee,* Edited by R. A. Grout, pp. 477–516, Dadant & Sons, Hamilton, Illinois.

Grout, R. A., editor, 1963 *The Hive and the Honey Bee,* Dadant & Sons, Hamilton, Illinois.

Kerr, W. E., 1974 Advances in cytology and genetics of bees. *Annu. Rev. Entomol.* **19**:253–268.

Laidlaw, H. H., Jr. and J. E. Eckert, 1950 *Queen Rearing,* Dadant & Sons, Hamilton, Illinois.

Mackensen, O., 1943 The occurrence of parthenogenetic females in some strains of honey bees. *J. Econ. Entomol.* **36**:465–467.

Mackensen, O. and K. W. Tucker, 1970 *Instrumental Insemination of Queen Bees,* Agricultural Handbook No. 390, U. S. Government Printing Office, Washington, D. C.

Merriam, R. W. and H. Ris, 1954 Size and DNA content of nuclei in various tissues of male, female, and worker honey bees. *Chromosoma (Berl.)* **6**:522–538.

Michailoff, A. S., 1931 Über die Vererbung der Weissäugigkeit bei der Honigbiene (*Apis mellifera*). *Z. Induk. Abstammungs-Vererbungsl.* **59**:190–202.

Nye, W. P. and O. Mackensen, 1968 Selective breeding of honeybees for alfalfa pollen collection: Fifth generation and backcrosses. *J. Apic. Res.* **7**:21–27.

Risler, H., 1954 Die somatische Polyploidie in der Entwicklung der Honigbiene (*Apis mellifica* L.) und die Weiderherstellung der Diploidie bei den Drohnen. *Z. Zellforsch. Mikrosk. Anat.* **41**:1–78.

Roberts, W. C., 1961 Heterosis in the honey bee as shown by morphological characters in inbred and hybrid bees. *Ann. Entomol. Soc. Am.* **54**:878–882.

Root, A. I., 1966 *The ABC and XYZ of Bee Culture,* 33rd edition, A. I. Root Co., Medina, Ohio.

Rothenbuhler, W. C., 1958a Progress and problems in the analyses of gynandromorphic honey bees. *Proc. Tenth Interntl. Congr. Entomol.* **2**:867–874.

Rothenbuhler, W. C., 1958b Genetics and breeding of the honey bee. *Annu. Rev. Entomol.* **3**:161–180.

Rothenbuhler, W. C., 1960 A technique for studying genetics of colony behavior in honey bees. *Am. Bee J.* **100**:176, 198.

Rothenbuhler, W. C., V. C. Thompson and J. J. McDermott, 1968a Control of the environment of honeybee observation colonies by use of hive-shelters and flight-cages. *J. Apic. Res.* **7**:151–155.

Rothenbuhler, W. C., J. M. Kulinčević and W. E. Kerr, 1968b Bee genetics. *Annu. Rev. Genet.* **2**:413–438.

Ruttner, F., 1966 The life and flight activity of drones. *Bee World* **47**:93–100.

Ruttner, F., 1967 Methods of breeding the honey bee: Intraracial selection or hybrid breeding. In *Proceedings of the 21st Interntl. Beekeeping Congress,* pp. 222–226, Apimondia Publishing House, Bucharest I, Str. Pitar Mos 20.

Taber, S., III, and J. Wendel, 1958 Concerning the number of times queen bees mate. *J. Econ. Entomol.* **51**:786–789.

Tucker, K. W., 1958 Automictic parthenogenesis in the honey bee. *Genetics* **43**:299–316.

Tucker, K. W. and H. H. Laidlaw, 1966 The potential for multiplying a clone of honey bee sperm by androgenesis. *J. Hered.* **57**:213–214.

Watson, L. R. 1928 Controlled mating in honeybees. *Q. Rev. Biol.* **3**:377–390.

Weaver, N., 1966 Physiology of caste determination. *Annu. Rev. Entomol.* **11**:79–102.

Woyke, J., 1963 What happens to diploid drone larvae in a honeybee colony? *J. Apic. Res.* **2**:73–75.

7

The Parasitoid Wasps, *Habrobracon* and *Mormoniella*

JOSEPH D. CASSIDY, O.P.

The problem of sex determination is nowhere of greater interest than in the Hymenoptera. The occurrence of parthenogenesis as well as sexual reproduction adds interest, especially in view of the fact that considerable variation obtains.
—*P. W. Whiting, 1918*

Introduction

The importance of the parasitoid Hymenoptera derives from the regulatory effect they exert on host insect populations (Matthews, 1974). Although it has been estimated that one hundred thousand species exist (Salt, 1961), geneticists during the last 55 years have studied only a few Ichneumonoid, Braconid, and Chalcidoid wasps (A. R. Whiting, 1961*a*, 1967; Baldwin, 1961, 1969; P. E. King and Fordy, 1970; Saul *et al.*, 1965; Schmieder, 1933; P. W. Whiting, 1940, 1950). These wasps sting and paralyze the larvae or pupae of host insects and then lay eggs upon them. Since only the larval stage of the wasp feeds upon the host, the term parasitoid is used to distinguish it from the true parasitic insects, which spend their entire life cycle upon their host (Doutt, 1959; Evans and Eberhard, 1970; Askew, 1971).

JOSEPH D. CASSIDY, O. P.—Department of Biological Sciences, Northwestern University, Evanston, Illinois.

The greatest attention has been given to *Habrobracon juglandis* Ashmead and *Mormoniella vitripennis* Walker. The first wasp oviposits on the surface of paralyzed larvae of certain moth species, while the second uses the pupae of muscoid flies as hosts. Like many other Hymenoptera, these wasps undergo parthenogenesis to generate haploid males.

Sexual reproduction in metazoa generally involves the generation of both sexes from fertilized eggs. However, in bees and wasps, parthenogenetic reproduction occurs in which males are normally fatherless, having developed from unfertilized eggs. These eggs have undergone a reduction in chromosome number as if in preparation for fertilization, and the males developing from such unfertilized eggs have a reduced set of chromosomes. If fertilized, the eggs will normally develop into females. Recessive genes, which may be masked in the diploid parent, will express themselves in her haploid sons. The Whitings and their colleagues have exploited this unique reproductive behavior to genetically analyze the genome of the haploid male.

Habrobracon and *Mormoniella* have provided the majority of the genetic reports available for wasps. Mutants and wild-type individuals from both species are readily cultured in the laboratory, produce large numbers of offspring, and are comparable with *Drosophila melanogaster* in size and generation time. The aim of this introductory survey is to help new investigators gain entrance to the original literature on these species. The reader should consult the comprehensive reviews of Doutt (1959), Grosch (1962a, 1974), Saul *et al.* (1965, 1967), La Chance (1967), La Chance *et al.* (1968), R. H. Smith and von Borstel (1971, 1972), Askew (1971), and Matthews (1974). Emphasis will be given to the papers published after the excellent reviews of A. R. Whiting (1961a, 1965, 1967).

The Braconid, *Habrobracon*

The first laboratory culture was generated from a single female that P. W. Whiting found parasitizing a culture of the Mediterranean flour moth in 1918. Three names for this Braconid wasp are found in the recent literature: *Habrobracon juglandis* Ashmead, *Bracon hebetor* Say, and *Microbracon hebetor* Muesebeck [see Lin (1965) for an account of the taxonomic problem]. P. W. Whiting immediately recognized the importance of an easily cultured wasp for the study of the problem of sex determination in Hymenoptera. Studies on this wasp were carried out by P. W. Whiting and his students with great enthusiasm, and a wide variety of behavioral, cytological, physiological, and biochemical problems, in addition to sex determination, were pursued.

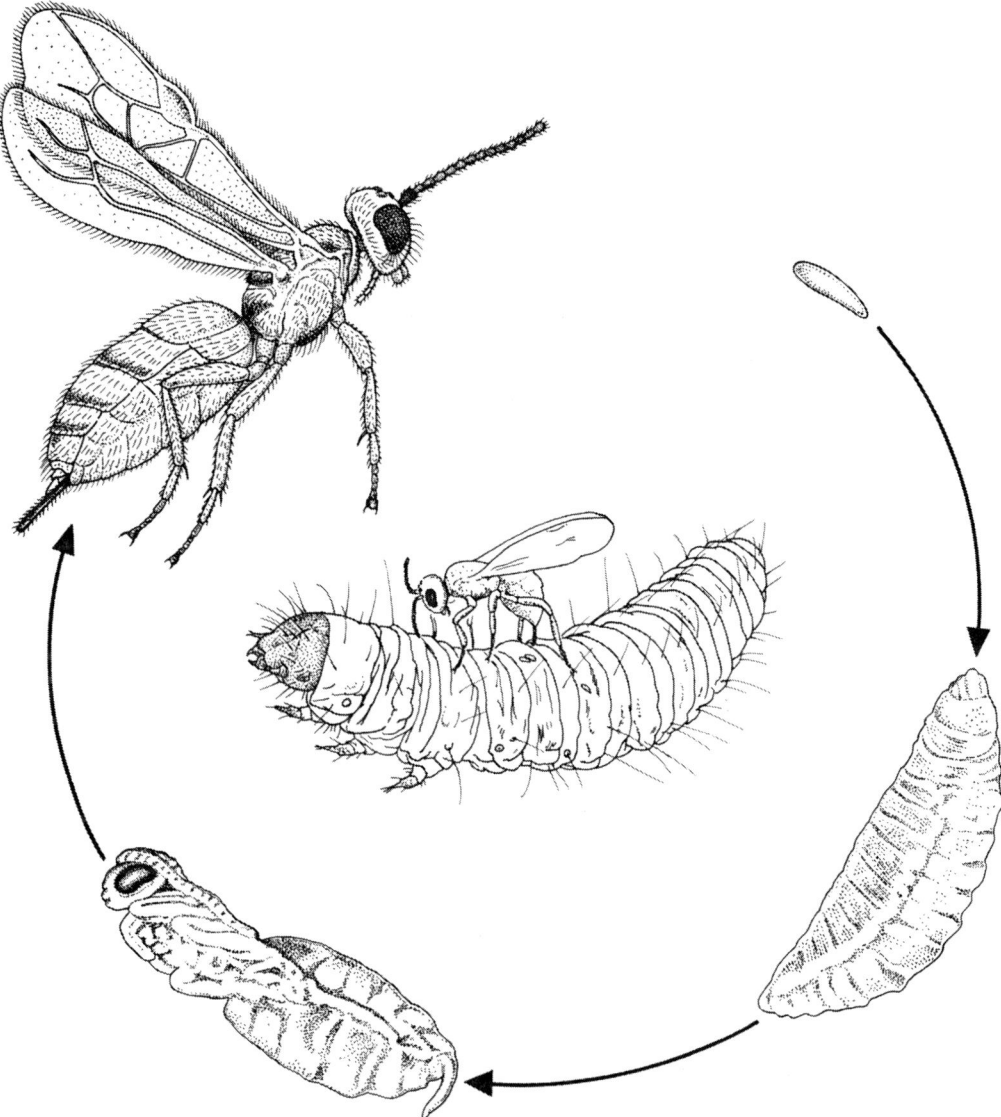

Figure 1. The life cycle of Habrobracon juglandis. The paralyzed Ephestia kühniella larva shown in the center of the drawing is 11 mm long.

In a volume no longer in print, Martin (1947) surveyed the first 30 years of research and has listed various experimental advantages of *Habrobracon*. In a subsequent review, A. R. Whiting (1961a) has discussed the genetics of sex determination, the occurrence of gynanders and other genetic mosaics, the specific effects of temperature, radiations, and chemical mutagens, and has provided lists of mutations, linkage data, and the early publications.

Habrobracon Stock Centers

Wild-type and mutant stocks of *Habrobracon juglandis* may be obtained from several laboratories in the United States. The names of the scientists in charge and the addresses of some of the laboratories are: Dr. A. M. Clark, Department of Biological Sciences, University of Delaware, Newark, Delaware 19711; Dr. D. S. Grosch, Genetics Department, North Carolina State University, Raleigh, North Carolina 27608; and Dr. G. S. Van Pelt, Zoology Department, University of North Carolina at Greensboro, Greensboro, North Carolina 27412. Detailed information reported for 42 mutations and 8 linkage groups is given by P. W. Whiting and Novitski (1964). Since the termination of federal financial support for the stock-keeping center at the University of Delaware, nearly half of the wild-type and mutant stocks of *Habrobracon* have been lost. The stocks of *H. juglandis* and *H. serinopae* still available for teaching and research purposes have been distributed among the American investigators listed above.

Wild-type and temperature-sensitive mutants of *H. serinopae* Ramakriska (=*Bracon serinopae* Cherian) may be obtained from Dr. A. C. Hoffmann, Department of Biology, Millersville State College, Millersville, Pennsylvania 17551, and Dr. R. H. Smith, Biology Division, Oak Ridge National Laboratory, Oak Ridge, Tennessee 37830. The host, *Ephestia kühniella* Zeller (=*Anagasta kühniella* Heinrich), is propagated in small boxes of corn meal. It may be obtained from Dr. E. W. Caspari, Department of Biology, University of Rochester, Rochester, New York 14627, Dr. F. J. Gottlieb, Department of Biology, University of Pittsburgh, Pittsburgh, Pennsylvania 15260, and from our laboratory at the Department of Biological Sciences, Northwestern University, Evanston, Illinois 60201. The use of alternative hosts, the larvae of *Plodia interpunctella* Hubner and *Galleria mellonella* L., has been evaluated by Beard (1972). Conditions for rearing both the parasitoid and the common host are given by R. H. Smith and von Borstel (1971). Additional experimental centers using *Habrobracon* are directed by Dr. R. C. von Borstel, Department of Genetics, University of Alberta, Edmonton, Alberta, Canada, and by Dr. F. Leibenguth, Zoological Institute of the University of Tübingen, Tübingen, West Germany.

Wild type stocks of *H. juglandis* (*#1, Whiting #33,* and *Raleigh*) are currently available. Mutant genes can be obtained in a variety of stocks:

black body (*8bl, 35bl, 73bl, 92bl, 109bl*), cantaloupe eyes (*c, c³*), ebony body (*e*), eyeless (*el*), gynoid sex mosaic (*gy*), honey body (*ho*), ivory eyes (*o⁻ⁱ*), lemon body (*le*), long antennae (*l*), notched wings (*no*), orange eyes (*o⁻*), oval eyes (*ov*), pin head (*ph*), pink eyes (*p*), small wings (*sw*), temperature sensitive lethal (*ts31*), and white eyes (*wh, 74wh*). Approximately 12 multiple-mutant stocks are accessible for laboratory experiments and classroom demonstrations.

The larger Indian species, *H. serinopae,* invites wider investigation, since it is relatively disease-free, has a shorter developmental cycle, longer adult life span, smaller cells, and greater fecundity (Clark and Smith, 1967). Our recent comparative studies with the scanning electron microscope (Cassidy and Clark, unpublished) distinguished *H. serinopae* from *H. juglandis* by size and protrusions from the surface of the ommatidia and dorsal ocelli. Stocks available to geneticists include wild type (New Delhi), plum eyes (*pl*), and a new series of temperature-sensitive lethal mutations (*tsl-9, tsl-5, tsl-11, tsl-rs, tsl-1, tsl-6, tsl-2, tsl-4, tsl-ble*), listed from the earliest to the latest lethal phase of expression during the developmental cycle (R. H. Smith, 1974).

The Life Cycle of *Habrobracon juglandis*

Newly emerged adult wasps sting host larvae of moths and cereal-infesting caterpillars, paralyzing them, and the adult feeds upon the body fluids exuding from the wound. After feeding, the females oviposit upon the host as shown in Figure 1. In wasps reared at 30°C the embryonic period lasts 28–30 hours, the larval period 79–89 hours, and the pupal period 104–124 hours. Therefore, the total time spent in preadult stages is between 9 and 10 days. When fresh host caterpillars are supplied in the laboratory, the female lives for approximately 28 days (Samis *et al.,* 1973). Not feeding upon the host as an adult, the male emerges, mates, and dies within a few days. Figure 1 presents illustrations of egg, fourth-instar larva, pupa, and adult female. In the adult stage, *H. juglandis* is 2.5–3.0 mm in length.

Accounts of various stages of preadult development have been provided by a number of workers (i.e., Genieys, 1925; Henschen, 1928; Glover, 1934; Speicher, 1936; Inaba, 1939; Grosch, 1952; Nelson and Farstad, 1953; Amy, 1955; Erdman, 1961; Clark, 1963). Embryogenesis has been staged by Amy (1961) and Grosch (1969). Grosch (1948) has presented criteria which allow one to classify larvae into the appropriate instars. Developmental events of the prepupal and pupal stages have been established and timed by Van Pelt (1970).

Arrhenotokous parthenogenesis (haplo-diploidy) is common among the Hymenoptera. Since fertilized eggs develop into diploid females and unfertilized ones into haploid males, arrhenotoky is both a form of reproduction and sex determination. That males are not invariably haploid in all Hymenoptera was shown by the studies of P. W. Whiting on *Habrobracon*. In 1933 he proposed the multiple-allele theory of sex determination. His later studies utilizing marker genes showed that the maternal and paternal sets of chromosomes of females are not entirely alike, and that a locus with a variety of sex alleles exists in this species. A complete summary of the evidence for the complementary action of sex alleles in *Habrobracon* followed (P. W. Whiting, 1943). Wasps heterozygous for any two alleles develop into females. Haploid males ($n = 10$) are, of course, hemizygous for a given allele, whereas diploid males are homozygous. Bacci (1965) has continued the analysis of the sex alleles, which he considers to be differential chromosome segments as proposed by Whiting. The role upon the sex ratio of environmental factors such as humidity changes, age, and experimentally delayed mating and oviposition has been studied by Rotary and Gerling (1973). In our laboratory, females of *H. serinopae* mated to unrelated males produce diploid daughters and haploid males in a $3:7$ ratio; for mated *H. juglandis* females the ratio is $2:1$. Reinert and King (1971) have shown that the sex ratio varies with the host: parasite ratio.

Developmental Patterns

That environmental manipulations might unmask subtle expressions of the genome during development was appreciated by Dunning (1931), P. W. Whiting and Anderson (1932), Greb (1933), Speicher (1934), and A. R. Whiting (1934). Genieys' experiments (1925) demonstrated that cold treatment of eggs produced black-body adults, a variation transmitted through the third generation. In 1930, accidental heat treatment produced "shot veins" (*sv*), the first wing mutation, and A. R. Whiting induced with x-ray the kidney eye mutation, highly lethal at 30°C, while of excellent viability and fertility at 25°C (P. W. Whiting, 1932*a*). Her discovery of the first temperature-sensitive lethal mutation opened the way to a field of contemporary research—identifying genes active in the developmental sequence of complex eukaryotes (see Chapter 23 by Suzuki in this volume).

Notched wings (*no*) is a recessive temperature-sensitive allele in *H. juglandis* investigated by Clark and Baird (1974). The size of the wing is dependent upon the temperature at which development occurs. When the mutant is reared at 35°C, the wings are phenotypically indistinguishable from wild type reared at the same temperature. Progressive decrease in wing size is correlated with rearing the mutant at lower temperatures (30°, 25°, 18°C).

Utilizing *H. serinopae,* R. H. Smith (1971, 1974) and R. H. Smith and von Borstel (1971) systematically detected the timing of expression of nine developmental genes. First to be achieved was the precise timetable of developmental events at 28°C. Next, techniques were perfected for isolating and analyzing conditional lethal mutations, expressed at 35°C. Now, the temperature-sensitive patterns and lethal phases characterizing this series of mutant strains, induced by ethyl methanesulfonate, will permit in-depth genetic dissection of haploid and diploid embryonic, larval, and pupal development.

Genetic mosaicism has been observed in humans, mice, sea urchins, fruit flies, moths, and honey bees (Stern, 1968; see Chapter 6 by Rothenbuhler in this volume). Developmental problems studied with mosaic individuals include selection in mixed cell populations, patterns of tissue morphogenesis, cell lineage relationships, primordial cell pool sizes, and sexual differentiation (Nesbitt and Gartler, 1971). In the hymenopterous haplo-diploid systems, direct analysis of genetic mosaics is simplified, unencumbered by elaborate technique or experimental equipment. A complete introduction to the early work on *Habrobracon* gynandromorphs, gynandroids, and intersexes has been given by von Borstel and Smith (1960). The discovery and interpretation of mosaic diploid males was the key which resulted in the proposal of the complementary sex-allele mechanism for *Habrobracon* sex determination (P. W. Whiting *et al.,* 1934). Mosaic ocelli, eye pigments, antennae, legs, and heads are useful in tracing temporal aspects of gene action during development and the cytogenetic basis of behavior whenever mosaicism leads to variations in behavioral patterns, as in *Apis mellifera.*

The use of reproductive reactions in sex-mosaic progeny by P. W. Whiting (1921, 1928, 1932*b,c*) has been extended greatly by new interpretations of the behavior of *Habrobracon* mosaics associated with the ebony locus. In the first of a series of important studies, Clark *et al.* (1968) discovered that the recessive mutant, ebony body color, increases the frequency of mosaicism among fertilized eggs. The same mosaic and androgenetic progeny are not produced by unmated ebony females. The diverse types of unusual progeny were interpreted by assuming that the ebony mutant acts to delay the migration of the female pronucleus. Such a delay would allow precocious cleavage of the egg or sperm pronucleus or delay might allow the sperm and egg pronuclei to divide, and some of the products to fuse subsequently. Hence, diploid and haploid clones of cells would be generated. The developmental behavior of imaginal discs containing both haploid and diploid cells was analyzed (Clark *et al.*, 1971). Studies on the mating behavior of wasps with mosaic heads suggested that the brain was a mosaic of haploid and diploid cells. This finding makes possible the experimental use of individuals with two or more genomes for developmental neurobiology and localization of the site of sex activity. In the latest work, genetic crosses of mutants, *e* and *ho*, and *no* and *sw*, gave new approaches to follow the origin and development of haplo-diploid mosaic patterns in antennae, legs, and wings (Clark *et al.*, 1973; Clark and Baird, 1974).

Oogenesis and Mutagenesis

Several aspects of the female reproductive system and venom apparatus were reported by Henschen (1928), Bender (1943), Piek (1966), and Beard (1972). The microscopic anatomy of a single ovariole was detailed as the basis for the study of the response of meiotic and mitotic cells to radiations (A. R. Whiting, 1945a). Normal oogenesis has been described by Cassidy and King (1969, 1972), giving accounts of: (1) the mitotic behavior of oogonia and the 5 cystocyte divisions; (2) an analysis of the formation of ring canals connecting ovarian cystocytes; (3) the production of synaptonemal complexes by pro-oocytes; (4) the development of an egg chamber; (5) the ultrastructural details of the transfer of cytoplasmic organelles to the oocyte by the nurse cells; and (6) the genesis and distribution of accessory nuclei and protein yolk spheres in the ooplasm. Oogenesis can be divided into 9 timed and readily recognizable stages (R. C. King and Cassidy, 1973). Criteria include: (1) the mitotic behavior of the follicle cells; (2) the cytoplasmic and nucleocytoplasmic growth of the nurse cells, follicle cells, and oocyte; (3) the endomitotic DNA replications that accompany nuclear growth in the nurse and follicle cells; (4) the activity of the oolema during development; and (5) the migratory and secretory activities of the follicle cells.

At the suggestion of Herman Muller, even before his own epochal study was published, early haplo-diploid experiments demonstrated radiation mutagenesis in *Habrobracon* (P. W. Whiting, 1929). The following decades of radiation genetics have been reviewed by A. R. Whiting (1961a), von Borstel and St. Amand (1963), and Grosch (1962a, 1974). A. R. Whiting's classic papers (1945a,b) gave the first adequate experimental design and interpretation of differential radiosensitivity in germ cells at different stages of differentiation. The uterus contains the large, differentiated, meiotic metaphase I oocytes, many times more sensitive to ionizing radiation than the nearby oocytes from the same ovariole in late prophase I. It was reported, also, that embryonic mortality was the result of chromosomal aberrations induced in the maternal chromosomes.

The "transitional zone" is a region of rapid differentiation near the distal end of the ovariole, found to be radiosensitive by Grosch and Sullivan (1952). R. C. King and Cassidy (1973) called attention to the vulnerability of the rapidly dividing follicular epithelium enveloping the early-developing chambers. They postulated that radiation damage during the follicle cell cycle could explain the radiosensitivity of the "transitional-zone" egg chambers. Recent experiments (R. Przybelski and Cassidy, unpublished) have confirmed this observation. The rationale and techniques to plan radiation experiments during oogenesis have been outlined by A. R. Whiting et al. (1968).

Radiation effects have been demonstrated upon fecundity (La Chance, 1959), developmental stages (Amy, 1955; von Borstel and Rekemeyer, 1959; Erdman, 1961; Clark and Mitchell, 1951; Grosch, 1970), metamorphosis, and life span of male and female adults (Clark and Smith, 1968; Baird and Clark, 1971). The *Habrobracon* females subjected to space-flight irradiation showed a significant increase in longevity (von Borstel et al., 1970). Subsequent to the NASA Biosatellite II program, Grosch (1970) has interpreted the radiation effects upon *H. juglandis* genes and chromosomes, while von Borstel (1971) has considered the sensitivity and unexpected radioresistance of developing ova in the same space flight.

Mutagens, Lethal Mutations, and Senescence

Complete reviews have discussed the experiments on responses to ionizing radiations (Grosch, 1962a, 1974), chemical mutagens (La Chance, 1967), temperature, diet, and age (A. R. Whiting, 1961b; Clark and Rockstein, 1964; Rockstein and Miquel, 1973). Specific criteria for five classes of radiation-induced mutations are given by A. R. Whiting et al. (1968). Interest has centered upon dominant lethal genetic changes detected among the altered progeny after the parental males had been irradiated. Heidenthal (1945) and Heidenthal et al. (1972) quantified the distinctions between dominant and recessive lethal and visible mutation rates. A dominant lethal mutation results in the death of a zygote even though contributed from only one of the gametes (Grosch, 1974). Mutagen-induced dominant lethality, the basis of the "sterile male" principle applied in insect control, can be easily distinguished from germ cell inactivation in *Habrobracon* (R. H. Smith and von Borstel, 1971). This reliable test has been used for a variety of chemical mutagens, e.g., ethyl methanesulfonate (Löbbecke and von Borstel, 1962; La Chance and Leverich, 1969; Hoffman and Grosch, 1971; Mizianty and Venit, 1971), apholate (Valcovic and Grosch, 1968), and mitomycin c (R. H. Smith, 1969; Mizianty and Venit, 1971). La Chance and Leverich (1968) screened eight chemosterilants inducing dominant lethal mutations. Tepa and its analogs led to sperm inactivation. Tretamine and metepa caused complete sterility without sperm inactivation.

The haplo-diploid genetic system of these parasitoids presents advantages uniquely useful for aging studies (Clark and Rockstein, 1964). Clark's series of experiments on the genetic components of senescence (Clark, 1963; Clark *et al.,* 1963; Clark and Smith, 1968; Baird and Clark, 1971) will not be discussed here since they have been so well analyzed in the review by Rockstein and Miquel (1973). Comparative studies involving both *H. juglandis* and *H. serinopae* showed no correlation between fecundity and life span (Clark and Smith, 1967). In contrast, Heidenthal *et al.* (1972) reported that fecundity is correlated with longevity in the progeny of irradiated *H. juglandis* males. They showed that, in a genetically heterogeneous population of F_1 mothers, freedom from carrying lethals is associated with greater fecundity and longer life. Heterozygosity for lethals, or translocations leading to low hatchability, is correlated with lower egg production and shorter life span, supporting the viewpoint that newly arisen lethals induced by radiation are harmful to heterozygotes.

Molecules, Chromosomes, and Experimental Populations

Molecular fractionation of gene products has focused upon characterization of eye-color mutants (Beadle *et al.,* 1938; Leibenguth, 1967, 1970, 1971; Van Pelt, 1970), uric acid metabolism (Lin, 1965; R. E. Smith, 1968), and control of xanthine dehydrogenase activity (Keller, 1970). In the Biosatellite II experiments, at all radiation levels the activity of this enzyme was depressed in the male flight animals, compared with that in the ground controls (von Borstel *et al.,* 1970). Nucleic acid analogs (and antagonists) and antimetabolites have been tested for alteration of reproductive performance (Grosch and Valcovic, 1967; R. H. Smith, 1969; Hoffman and Grosch, 1971; Grosch, 1968; Cassidy, 1967; Cassidy and Grosch, 1973; Kratsas and Grosch, 1974). Ovipositional data reflect six modes of action in this experimental system. Hence, it has been possible to diagnose cytological damage to oogonial or follicle cells and to partition somatic debility, failure of vitellogenesis, compensatory oviposition, and resorption of mature oocytes (Grosch, 1959, 1962*b*, 1963, 1971). Hoffman (1972) has delineated genetic-repair mechanisms.

The ten chromosomes of the haploid male are small and distinguishable only by relative size and V-, L-, J-, and rod-like morphology (Torvik-Greb, 1935). Diploid *Habrobracon* have each of these chromosomes in duplicate. Lin (1965) found species differences in his karyotypic analysiss of l *H. juglandis* and *H. serinopae*. Thus far, the chromosomes have not been mapped with techniques of molecular cytology, and the genetical and cytological data remain to be integrated.

Few population geneticists have investigated *Habrobracon* Mendelian populations, with the exception of the late Professor Kojima and his students. Dyson (1966) studied natural selection of two independent alleles for 20 generations and evaluated the selective effects at the level of fitness component traits. Dalebroux and Kojima (1967) reported a striking increase of genetic variance in body weight after gamma irradiation of females with homozygous or heterozygous genetic backgrounds. However, no significant increase was detected among the male progeny of heterozygous females. Both studies proposed a genetic model based on the absence of nonallelic interactions.

A variety of genetic methods for regulating insect population size have been detailed by R. H. Smith and von Borstel (1972). The most promising techniques proposed are based upon radiation and chemically-induced dominant, recessive, and conditionally lethal mutations developed by *Habrobracon* geneticists. Kojima (1971) designed a stochastic model to predict the outcome of applying the "sterile male" principle to collapse economically destructive insect populations. A unique component was a parameter for genetic improvement of pest populations from natural selection whenever control measures are elected. Reinert and King (1971) held environmental parameters constant and varied the densities of *H. juglandis* in founder populations. Population-to-population equilibrium was not sought, but rather the optimum ratio of parasite-to-host density for most efficient control of the destructive meal moth, *Plodia*. The sex ratio of surviving hosts in a parasitized colony depended upon the density of female parasitoids. A significantly larger number of female larvae were parasitized in preference to male.

Least is known about the comparative aspects of natural *vs.* laboratory *Habrobracon* populations. In addition to fluctuations in experimental populations as functions of the known variables of temperature, humidity, and superparasitism, Lum and Flaherty (1973) demonstrated the effect of continuous light on oocyte maturation, another component of fitness. Earlier experiments (Clark, 1963) showed that fecundity and longevity were altered significantly by access to honey as an alternate diet to Lepidopteran hosts. Laboratory population data are useful in deriving cautious estimates of complex parasitoid–host interactions in nature, recalling that environmental conditions play an important role in parasitoid distribution and population size (Matthews, 1974).

The Chalcidoid, *Mormoniella*

Challenged by his discovery of new opportunities to advance the genetics of Hymenoptera, P. W. Whiting began research on *Mormoniella* in 1948. *Mormoniella vitripennis* Walker is also referred to in the scientific literature by the names *Nasonia brevicornis* Ashmead and *Nasonia vitripennis* Walker. This Chalcidoid wasp has certain advantages over *Habrobracon:* it produces a larger number of offspring, has fewer and larger chromosomes, and possesses a larval diapause stage which permits the investigator to experimentally manipulate the length of the life cycle. Numerous spontaneous and radiation-induced mutations are available for teaching and research purposes (Saul *et al.*, 1965). The wasp is suited ideally for classroom demonstrations of parthenogenesis, host detection and other interesting parasitoid–host relationships, and the differential response of haploid and diploid organisms to environmental factors (P. W. Whiting, 1955). The complex gregarious behavior of the wasps offers an inviting system for the genetic analysis of insect communication (Barash and Ryder, 1972). The *Mormoniella* literature, which is quite extensive, has been reviewed ably in monographs by A. R. Whiting (1965, 1967). As a cosmopolitan ectoparasitoid, the species has some economic potential for the control of destructive Dipterans. This organism's well-studied behavior, physiology, and organization of germinal and somatic tissues have established a foundation for many new experiments.

Stock Centers for *Mormoniella*

Collections of most of the known wild-type and mutant strains of *M. vitripennis* may be obtained from Dr. G. B. Saul, Biology Department, Middlebury College, Middlebury, Vermont 05753; Dr. D. T. Ray, Zoology Department, Howard University, Washington, D. C. 20001; and from Dr. P. E. King, University College of Swansea, Glamorgan, United Kingdom. Protocols for experiments utilizing *Calliphora* and *Lucilia* species as hosts have been described by P. W. Whiting (1955). Another

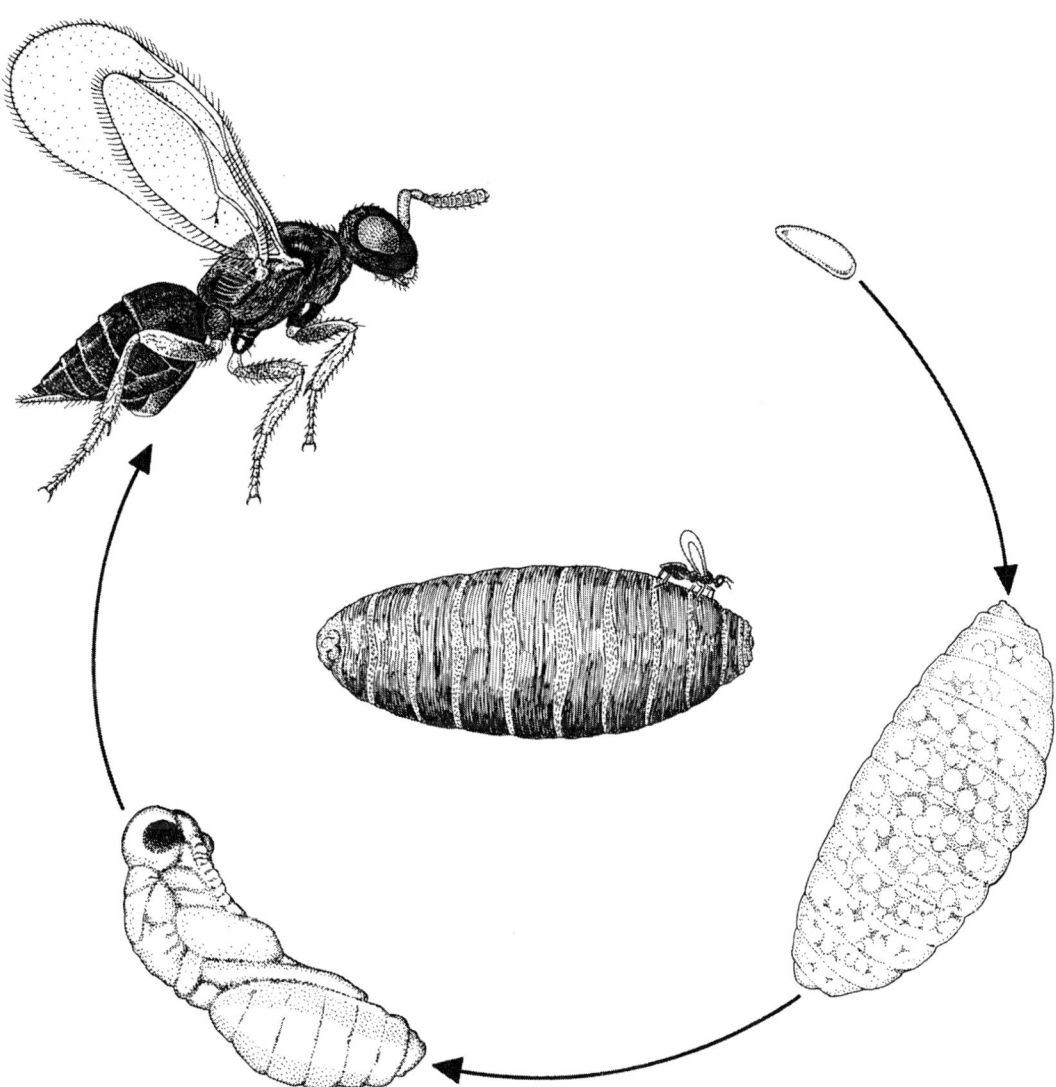

Figure 2. The life cycle of Mormoniella vitripennis. The Sarcophaga bullata shown in the center of the drawing is 12 mm long.

convenient host is the flesh fly, *Sarcophaga bullata* (P. W. Whiting and Bush, 1959), and pupae of this species are produced commercially by the Carolina Biological Supply Company, Elon College, North Carolina 27244.

The *Mormoniella* stock center at Middlebury College is maintained utilizing grant funds from the National Science Foundation. Nearly 200 single mutations and multiple-mutant combination stocks have been investigated. Examples of the several classes of visible mutations include purple body color (*pu*), orange eye color (*or*), and scarlet R-locus allele (*Rst*). Stocks producing fertile, diploid males are also available. Professor Saul has prepared an introductory guide and a bibliography of the *Mormoniella* literature covering the years through 1973, and will supply these to interested workers.

The Life Cycle of *Mormoniella*

The temporal sequence of the major developmental stages at 25°C of the commonly used Ithaca wild strain has been detailed by Schneiderman and Horwitz (1958) and Firtel and Saul (1967). Figure 2 illustrates the major events in the life cycle under laboratory conditions. The adult female drills into the host puparium, feeds on host fluids, and oviposits. In nature, *Mormoniella* females may parasitize pupae of *Musca domestica* and many other Dipteran hosts (Chabora, 1970b). When the female pierces the *Sarcophaga* puparium with her ovipositor, a continuous tube is formed between the underlying pupal skin and the outer puparium, facilitating the extraction of body fluids from the host. Eggs are oviposited on the underlying pupa through other punctures in the hard puparium. At 25°C, the embryonic period takes 28–30 hours. For the next 126–130 hours, *Mormoniella* larvae feed upon the outside of the host pupa. There are 3 larval instars and a prepupal stage (Foster, 1967). The pupal molt and the terminal events of metamorphosis occur about 108 hours later. After eclosion on the twelfth day, the adults gnaw a hole through the puparium, emerge, and mate. Males and females average 2 and 2.5 mm in length, respectively; the sex ratio is 2:3. The adult life span of wild-strain females is 30–37 days. Males, which cannot pierce the host puparium and feed, live only a few days after mating. Embryogenesis has been analyzed by Azab *et al.* (1967) and Gerling (1967). The adult life span varies with the host (Saunders *et al.*, 1970) and the developmental temperature (Clark and Kidwell, 1967; Samis *et al.*, 1973).

The functional anatomy of the male reproductive system has been described by Sanger and King (1971). They found that sperm are deposited at the opening of the spermathecal duct of the female and that no spermatophore is produced. B. R. Speicher has staged spermatogenesis during pupal development; these results are to be found in A. R. Whiting's 1967 review. The distribution of carbohydrates, proteins, lipids, and nucleic acids in the female germplasm has been localized cytochemically, and the ovaries, spermatheca, and accessory glands have been examined at the light and electron microscopic levels (Ratcliffe and King, 1967; P. E. King and Ratcliffe, 1969). Sixteen cystocytes give rise to the new egg chambers. The development of the oocyte was divided into five stages, and the probable functions of its organelles and trophocytes were detailed by P. E. King and Richards (1969). Richards and King (1967) and Richards (1968) have discussed the origin of membrane systems during oogenesis, and the steps in transfer of protein yolk precursors were outlined by P. E. King *et al.* (1972). Recent information is available, also, on cytology and sex-ratio determination (Wylie, 1966; Gershenson, 1968), oviposition (Chabora, 1967; Wylie, 1970, 1973), fertilization (Wylie, 1972a), and larval competition (Wylie, 1971, 1972b).

The Karyotype and Chromosomal Variation

Johnson and Ray (1972) have published the haploid karyotype ($n = 5$) from mitotic figures in the testes of 6-day-old pupae as a necessary step toward correlation of the five linkage groups with the chromosomes. The arm ratios and classification sizes of four metacentric chromosomes and a submetacentric chromosome were used for identification; three of the metacentric chromosomes showed secondary constrictions, suggesting the possibility of satellite chromosomes. Earlier, Foster (1967) found secondary constrictions in larval brain, metaphase figures. During the third instar, the haploid male complement consisted of 5 V-shaped chromosomes, 3 metacentrics, and 2 submetacentrics. One of the submetacentrics had two secondary constrictions near the end of the longer arm. One of the metacentrics had a secondary constriction near the end of one arm, while the other arm terminated in a satellite connected to the main body of the chromosome by a thin, heterochromatic strand. Brain-cell chromosomes of n and $2n$ males and $2n$ and $3n$ females varied characteristically by their metacentric and submetacentric nature, by the presence of satellites and secondary constrictions on one or more of their respective chromosomes, and by their total length. Resolution of the nonheterochromatic centromere regions, secondary constrictions, and satellite chromosomes with the differential interference and scanning electron microscopes would be rewarding.

Polyploidy, exceptional in the Hymenoptera, was found in 3 spontaneous mutations to diploid males and triploid females by P. W. Whiting (1960). The $4n$ females, normal in appearance and identified by genetic markers, were used by Macy and Whiting (1969) to interpret the meiotic behavior, fertility, and phenotypic differences in tetraploids. When $2n$ males were mated to $2n$ females, fertile $3n$ females resulted, giving rise to n and $2n$ eggs, and inviable aneuploids. Fertilized by sperm from $2n$ males, these eggs produced 3n and 4n daughters in unequal ratio. Variation from expected frequencies, confirmed cytologically, was consistent with the theory of preferential segregation (Conner, 1966) based upon aberrant meiotic divisions in the euploid eggs of 3n females. Macy and Whiting (1969) also reported that experimental stocks on the diploid–tetraploid level can be maintained for many stable generations by mating 4n females to their 2n brothers.

Clark and Cole (1967) have used the karyotypic differences of *Mormoniella* to approach the problem of natural *vs.* radiation-induced aging. Comparisons of adult life spans of n and 2n males and 2n and 3n females reflected the influence of specific genes rather than the number of sets of chromosomes. These radiation experiments revealed that 2n males were more resistant than n males, while the 2n and 3n females were equal in sensitivity, suggesting the interpretation that injuries leading to natural aging differ from those leading to radiation-induced decrease in life span.

The *R* Locus, Genes, and Phenes

One of the most complex genetic regions, the *R* locus, is located in a short chromosomal segment. The first x-radiation-induced visible mutations, oyster and scarlet, complementary for eye color, exposed this complex locus. The series of multiple alleles have been compared to the sex-locus alleles of *Habrobracon* by P. W. Whiting (1951). Mutations governing inviability and sterility have been traced to the same locus, the subject of an extensive review by A. R. Whiting (1965). Roozen and Conner (1969) measured recombination frequencies between *R*-locus eye-color alternative alleles and non-*R* markers linked on either side of the complex locus. They concluded that radiation-induced chromosome abnormalities may account for the apparent absence of recombination between three mutant factors. Analysis of *R*-locus linkage relationships has been continued by Roozen and Conner (1970). All identified *R*-locus mutant characters involve either eye color or eye color associated with viability or fertility changes (A. R. Whiting, 1967).

Conner and Roozen (1967) distinguished the gene action of two *R*-locus, dahlia eye-color mutations, and P. W. Whiting (1966) analyzed the genetic fine structure of 13 distinct, black-eyed classes of wasps. The reader is referred to Saul (1972) and Saul *et al.* (1965, 1967) for detailed information concerning the mapping of 47 mutants and 5 linkage groups.

The physiological genetics experiments of Miner and Kennington (1968) showed that pupae of 5 different strains of *Mormoniella* subjected to anoxia differed in their resistance to oxygen-depleted conditions. Earlier,

Ferschel and Wolsky (1956), Rohner and Wolsky (1957), and Rohner (1959) demonstrated a posterior-to-anterior polarity in pupal pigment development, and a direct parallel between respiration and ommochrome synthesis. Saul (1960) separated two eye pigment systems in pupal stages and adult *Mormoniella*. The components of the phenol oxidase system involved in melanin formation have been identified by Firtel and Saul (1967), and activation was shown to be similar to that of *Drosophila* and *Musca*.

The lastest published work on the problem of cross incompatibility confirms that the unidentified cytoplasmic "factor" is maternally inherited, acts at the time of fertilization, and, that although the sperm enters the egg, it does not contribute paternal chromosomes (Ryan and Saul, 1968).

Gregarious Populations

Since the last review of this literature (A. R. Whiting, 1967), behavioral studies have received the greatest attention. Examples include new results on the organization of the antennal sense organs (Slifer, 1969), characterization of the male and female sense receptors (Miller, 1972), and differentiation in behavior of the sexes (Barras, 1969). New diapause studies have included aspects of maternal origin (Saunders, 1966) and the role of the host (Saunders *et al.*, 1970), temperature (Saunders, 1973), and photoperiod (Saunders, 1968, 1969) in diapause induction. Another discovery by P. W. Whiting (1968) has made possible the investigation of diapause resistance.

Significant contributions have been made toward understanding aspects of the parasitoid–host interaction. Legner (1967) and Legner and Gerling (1967) observed the effects of host densities and host feeding on longevity and fecundity, while Holmes (1972) tested the effects of previously parasitized hosts. Male detection of parasitized hosts (P. E. King *et al.*, 1969), wasp preference (Takahashi and Pimentel, 1967), and host selection (G. J. C. Smith, 1969) and discrimination (P. E. King and Rafai, 1970) were investigated. A single population cage makes it possible to observe many of the patterns of gregarious behavior.

During the past decade, a large amount of work has been done with the population dynamics. Velthuis *et al.* (1965) studied the reproductive capacity and the influence of size and age of the females. Using *Calliphora* as the host, a maximum of 60 eggs was oviposited into one host puparium, recognized by females as fully parasitized. Changes occurred in sex ratio of the progeny in relation to female age and density. Ages of females and offspring entering diapause were related quantitatively. When *Musca* was used as the host, Wylie (1965) noted that mature progeny decreased with increasing parasite-to-host ratios, and he ascribed this to lowered fecundity and superparasitism. Larger housefly puparia were more easily discovered and selected for drilling and oviposition (Wylie, 1967). A scramble type of larval competition, involving little direct interaction among the developing larvae, led to the reproductive success of early hatching and more rapidly developing parasitoid larvae (Wylie, 1971).

Another series of important experiments by Pimentel and his associates investigated the components of fitness of parasitism (Pimentel and Al-Hafidh, 1965; Pimentel, 1966; Pimentel and Stone, 1968). Population models of the genetics of *Mormoniella* interacting with *Phaenicia* or *Musca* have been developed by Walker (1967), Rabinovich (1969), and G. J. C. Smith (1969). A general model of genetic feedback as a mechanism for population regulation can be illustrated by the predictable oscillations in the numbers of competing parasitoids and both of these hosts (Pimentel, 1968). It was pointed out that there was a persistent alteration of dominance of first the blowfly and then the housefly during 160 weeks of selection. In another multicelled-cage experiment, intraspecific selection on the dominant species and interspecific selection on the sparse species favored the sparse species. Interactions of the wasp with geographically distinct strains of the blowfly (Chabora, 1970*a*) and housefly (Chabora, 1970*b*) and the influence of genetic variability within host populations upon parasitoid fecundity, growth, and longevity (Chabora, 1970*c*, 1972; Chabora and Pimentel, 1970) support the validity of Pimentel's general theory.

Additional Species

Genetic information is available for a number of other parasitoids, many of economic significance. Braconids include *B. tachordiae* (Glover, 1934), *B. cephi* (Nelson and Farstad, 1953), *B. greeni* (Angalet, 1964), *B. mellitor* (Adams *et al.*, 1969), *B. politiventris* (McKnight, 1971), *B. iranicus* (Fisher, 1972), *Habrobracon lineatellae* (Laing and Caltagirone, 1969), *Apanteles thompsoni* (P. E. King *et al.*, 1969), and *Agathis gibbosa* (Odebiyi and Oatman, 1972). Species of Chalcoid wasps have been studied, including *Pteromalis puparum* (P. W. Whiting, 1940; P. E. King *et al.*, 1968), *Pachycrepoideus dubius* (P. W. Whiting, 1954), *Dahlbominus fuscipennis* (Wilkes, 1965; Baldwin, 1961, 1969), *Mellitobia chalybii* (Kerschner, 1946; Schmieder and Whiting, 1947), *Brachymeria intermedia* (Doane, 1971), *Muscidifurax raptor* (Chabora and Chabora, 1971), and *Spalangia cameroni* (Wylie, 1972*a,b*). Ichneumenoids used in current investigations include *Pimpla turionellae* (Meng, 1968, 1969; Wolf and

Krause, 1971; Went and Krause, 1973), *Ophion luteus* (P. E. King and Fordy, 1970), and *Nemeritis canescens* (Salt, 1968, 1971; Rotheram, 1973).

Problems and Perspectives

As indicated above, these experimental systems permit critical analyses of complex loci, gene action and interaction, parthenogenetic development, genetic dissection of mosaicism and behavior, diapause induction and termination, host detection, parasitism, and the interdependence of interacting populations. In Hymenoptera, the ultrastructure and cytochemistry of accessory nuclei during oogenesis have been observed (P. King and Richards, 1968; P. King and Fordy, 1970; Cassidy and R. King, 1972). The molecular biology of this system is needed to show whether this is a Hymenopteran variation of gene amplification.

The C value, determined from sperm, is 0.16 pg for *H. juglandis* (Rasch *et al.,* 1975). DNA values were determined also, for nuclei of adult hemocytes, and found to be 2C for *both* males and females. DNA values for hemocytes from adult male and female *H. serinopae* were indistinguishable from those of *H. juglandis* (0.30–0.33 pg). Values for hemocytes for *both* male and female *M. vitripennis* fall between 0.72 and 0.74 pg per nucleus, whereas sperm contain 0.33–0.34 pg.

Wasp ovarioles offer excellent experimental systems for studying vitellogenesis (P. King *et al.,* 1972; Kratsas and Grosch, 1974) as well as the disruption of mitosis and meiosis (Grosch, 1974). Questions concerning hormonal control of oogenesis, also, can be investigated in the absence of influences from obligate fertilization.

Microorganisms undergoing fission were localized in developing egg chambers of *H. juglandis* by Cassidy and King (1972, their Figures 2 and 3a). In subsequent studies, similar microorganisms were found in various cells making up the ovaries of *H. serinopae, Bombus terrestris, Apis mellifera, Vespula maculata,* and *Mormoniella vitripennis.* Such inclusions are not restricted to the Hymenoptera since they have been seen in *Drosophila* [see Figure VI-4 in R. C. King's (1970) monograph; and Ehrman and Kernaghan (1971)] and *Culex* (see Chapter 14 by Barr in this volume). Numerous mycoplasma-like cytoplasmic inclusions of comparable dimension and ultrastructure were detected in the larval and adult testes of the Braconid host *Ephestia kühniella* [Gottlieb (1972), and see Chapter 4 by Caspari and Gottlieb in this volume]. It is likely that the symbionts are transmitted through the germ line. Once isolated and successfully cultured outside of the host, it may be possible to determine precisely what advantages they provide their host, and some progress along this line has been made with *Mormoniella* (G. B. Saul, private communication) in current investigations of the problem of cross incompatability. Whether these prokaryotes are essential to eukaryotic parasitoid–host interactions remains to be investigated with antibiotics. Another subtle interaction was tested by Leibenguth (1972), who timed the stages of the schizogregarine *Mattesia dispora* taken up by *Habrobracon* larvae from infected *Ephestia* hosts. The developmental cycle paralleled that of *Habrobracon,* requiring only one third of the time in *Ephestia.* The exciting discoveries of Salt (1968, 1971) invite research attention to the giant teratoid cells demonstrated in many species of several families of Hymenoptera. By definition, teratocytes are not specifically involved in trophic functions, but confer upon the parasitoid larva a means of resistance against the hemocytic defense reactions of the host.

There has been success in the culturing of somatic cell lines derived from some Dipteran species (for example, see Chapter 32 by Schneider in this volume). It would be an obvious advantage for a wide variety of studies to have available haploid and diploid somatic cell lines from the same species. It is, therefore, likely that attempts will be made soon to culture cells from the Hymenoptera, and since *Habrobracon* and *Mormoniella* are available in many laboratories, they are recommended candidates for such studies.

Acknowledgments

This chapter is dedicated to the pioneer investigators of the genetics of Hymenopterans, Professors Anna R. and Phineas W. Whiting. The original reprint collection at the Research Library of the Marine Biological Laboratory at Woods Hole, Massachusetts, was of great aid in the preparation of this contribution. Appreciation is expressed to Francisco Drury, CSC, Pamela Khipple, and Karen Slusser for their able assistance in gathering the hundreds of primary sources, to E. John Pfiffner for final inking of the illustrations, and to Drs. A. M. Clark, D. S. Grosch, G. B. Saul II, and R. C. von Borstel for their helpful comments on an early draft of the manuscript.

Literature Cited

Adams, C. H., W. H. Cross and H. C. Mitchell, 1969   Biology of *Bracon mellitor,* a parasite of the boll weevil. *J. Econ. Entomol.* **62:**889–896.

Amy, R. L., 1955   A comparative study of the effects of β-rays, γ-rays, and X-rays on development of *Habrobracon. Radiat. Res.* **3:**166–181.

Amy, R. L., 1961 The embryology of *Habrobracon juglandis* (Ashmead). *J. Morphol.* **109**:199–217.

Angalet, G. W., 1964 *Bracon greeni* (Hymenoptera: Braconidae) a potential parasite of the boll weevil. *Indian J. Entomol.* **26**:447–452.

Askew, R. R., 1971 *Parasitic Insects,* Heinemann Educational Books, London.

Azab, A. K., M. F. S. Tawfik and K. T. Awadallah, 1967 Morphology of the early stages of *Nasonia vitripennis* (Walker) (Hymenoptera: Pteromalidae). *Bull. Soc. Entomol. Egypte* **51**:457–467.

Bacci, G., 1965 *Sex Determination,* Pergamon Press, Oxford.

Baird, M. B. and A. M. Clark, 1971 X-ray induced life shortening mutations in *Habrobracon*: A genetic approach to senescence and duration of life. *Exp. Gerontol.* **6**:1–8.

Baldwin, W. F., 1961 Latent radiation damage and synchronous cell division in the epidermis of an insect. III. Spontaneous reversal of effects leading to delay during mitosis. *Radiat. Res.* **14**:426–431.

Baldwin, W. F., 1969 Congenital body malformations and eye color mutations in progeny from irradiated female wasps (*Dahlbominus*). *Radiat. Res.* **38**:569–578.

Barash, D. P. and C. A. Ryder, 1972 Ethology laboratory: Reproductive behavior of *Mormoniella vitripennis*. *Am. Biol. Teacher* **34**:14–18.

Barass, R., 1969 Preening and abdomen dipping by male *Mormoniella vitripennis* (Walker) (Hymenoptera: Pteromalidae) after courtship. *Behavior* **35**:304–312.

Beadle, G. W., R. L. Anderson and J. Maxwell, 1938 A comparison of the diffusible substances concerned with eye color development in *Drosophila, Ephestia* and *Habrobracon*. *Proc. Natl. Acad. Sci. USA* **24**:80–85.

Beard, R. L., 1972 Effectiveness of paralyzing venom and its relation to host discrimination by braconid wasps. *Ann. Entomol. Soc. Am.* **65**:90–93.

Bender, J. C., 1943 Anatomy and histology of the female reproductive organs of *Habrobracon juglandis* (Ashmead). *Ann. Entomol. Soc. Am.* **36**:537–545.

Cassidy, J. D., 1967 Base analogue incorporation in the female germ plasm of *Microbracon hebetor* Say. *J. Insect Physiol.* **13**:487–493.

Cassidy, J. D. and D. S. Grosch, 1973 Quantitative effects of purine analog ingestion on reproduction of *Habrobracon juglandis*. *J. Econ. Entomol.* **66**:319–324.

Cassidy, J. D. and R. C. King, 1969 The dilatable ring canals of the ovarian cystocytes of *Habrobracon juglandis*. *Biol. Bull.* (*Woods Hole*) **137**:429–437.

Cassidy, J. D. and R. C. King, 1972 Ovarian development in *Habrobracon juglandis* (Ashmead). (Hymenoptera: Braconidae). 1. The origin and differentiation of the oocyte-nurse cell complex. *Biol. Bull.* (*Woods Hole*) **143**:483–505.

Chabora, P. C., 1967 Hereditary behavior variation in oviposition patterns in the parasite *Nasonia vitripennis* (Hymenoptera: Pteromalidae). *Can Entomol.* **99**:763–765.

Chabora, P. C., 1970a Studies of parasite–host interaction using geographical strains of the blow fly *Phaenicia sericata* and its parasite *Nasonia vitripennis*. *Ann. Entomol. Soc. Am.* **63**:495–501.

Chabora, P. C., 1970b Studies in parasite–host interaction. II. Reproductive and developmental response of parasite *Nasonia vitripennis* (Hymenoptera: Pteromalidae) to strains of house fly host, *Musca domestica*. *Ann. Entomol. Soc. Am.* **63**:1632–1636.

Chabora, P. C., 1970c Studies in parasite–host interactions. III. Host race effect on the life table and population growth statistics of the parasite *Nasonia vitripennis*. *Ann. Entomol. Soc. Am.* **63**:1637–1642.

Chabora, P. C., 1972   Studies in parasite–host interaction. IV. Modification of parasite, *Nasonia vitripennis,* responses to control and selected host, *Musca domestica,* populations. *Ann. Entomol. Soc. Am.* **65:**323–328.

Chabora, P. C. and A. H. Chabora, 1971   Effects of an interpopulation hybrid host on parasite population dynamics. *Ann. Entomol. Soc. Am.* **64:**558–562.

Chabora, P. C. and D. Pimentel, 1970   Patterns of evolution in parasite–host systems. *Ann. Entomol. Soc. Am.* **63:**479–486.

Clark, A. M., 1963   The influence of diet upon the adult life span of two species of *Bracon. Ann. Entomol. Soc. Am.* **56:**616–619.

Clark, A. M. and M. B. Baird, 1974   Genetic mosaicism in the wings of *Habrobracon juglandis. Biol. Bull. (Woods Hole)* **146:**176–185.

Clark, A. M. and K. W. Cole, 1967   The effects of ionizing radiation on the longevity of ploidy types in the wasp *Mormoniella vitripennis. Exp. Gerontol.* **2:**89–95.

Clark, A. M. and R. N. Kidwell, 1967   Effects of developmental temperature on the adult life span of *Mormoniella vitripennis* females. *Exp. Gerontol.* **2:**79–84.

Clark, A. M. and C. J. Mitchell, 1951   Radiosensitivity of haploid and diploid *Habrobracon* during pupal development. *J. Exp. Zool.* **117:**489–498.

Clark, A. M. and M. Rockstein, 1964   Aging in insects. In *The Physiology of Insecta,* Vol. 1, edited by M. Rockstein, pp. 227–281, Academic Press, New York.

Clark, A. M. and R. E. Smith, 1967   Egg production and adult life span in two species of *Bracon* (Hymenoptera: Braconidae) *Ann. Entomol. Soc. Am.* **60:**903–905.

Clark, A. M. and R. E. Smith, 1968   The modification of adult life span in *Bracon hebetor* (Hymenoptera: Braconidae) by irradiation in nitrogen. *Ann. Entomol. Soc. Am.* **61:**541–542.

Clark, A. M., H. A. Bertrand and R. E. Smith, 1963   Life span differences between haploid and diploid males of *Habrobracon serinopae* after exposure as adults to X-rays. *Am. Nat.* **9:**203–208.

Clark, A. M., A. B. Gould and M. F. Potts, 1968   Mosaicism in *Habrobracon juglandis* associated with the *ebony* locus. *Genetics* **58:**415–422.

Clark, A. M., A. B. Gould and S. F. Graham, 1971   Patterns of development among mosaics in *Habrobracon juglandis. Dev. Biol.* **25:**133–148.

Clark, A. M., R. M. Petters and P. J. Bryant, 1973   Patterns of genetic mosaicism in the antennae and legs of *Habrobracon juglandis. Dev. Biol.* **32:**432–445.

Conner, G. W., 1966   Preferential segregation in *Mormoniella. Genetics* **54:**1041–1048.

Conner, G. W. and K. J. Roozen, 1967   Functional differences between two phenotypically identical alleles in *Mormoniella. Genetics* **56:**551–552.

Dalebroux, M. A. and K. I. Kojima, 1967   An analysis of radiation-induced variation on body-weight of *Habrobracon juglandis. Genetics* **55:**315–328.

Doane, C. C., 1971   A high rate of parasitization by *Brachymeria intermedia* (Hymenoptera: Chalcididae) on the gypsy moth. *Ann. Entomol. Soc. Am.* **64:**753–754.

Doutt, R. L., 1959   The biology of parasitic Hymenoptera. *Annu. Rev. Entomol.* **4:**111–182.

Dunning, W. F., 1931   A study of the effect of X-ray radiation on occurrence of abnormal individuals, mutation rate viability, and fertility of the parasitic wasp, *Habrobracon juglandis* (Ashmead). *Genetics* **16:**505–531.

Dyson, J. G., 1966   Natural selection of the two mutant genes *honey* and *orange* in laboratory populations of *Habrobracon juglandis. Diss. Abstr.* **26:**4183.

Ehrman, L. and R. P. Kernaghan, 1971 Microorganismal basis of infectious hybrid male sterility in *Drosophila paulistorum*. *J. Hered.* **62**:67–71.

Erdman, H. E., 1961 Analyses of the differential radiosensitivity of developing tissues in *Habrobracon juglandis* (Ashmead) to ionizing radiation. *Int. J. Radiat. Biol.* **3**:183–204.

Evans, H. E. and M. J. W. Eberhard, 1970 *The Wasps*, University of Michigan Press, Ann Arbor, Mich.

Ferschel, M. J. B., Sr., and A. Wolsky, 1956 Observations on the pigment development in pupae of *Mormoniella vitripennis* (Walker). *Anat. Rec.* **125**:599–600.

Firtel, R. A. and G. B. Saul II, 1967 Characteristics of phenol oxidases in *Mormoniella vitripennis* (Walker). *J. Insect Physiol.* **13**:1197–1206.

Fisher, M., 1972 A new species of *Habrobracon* from Iran (Hymenoptera: Braconidae). *Entomophaga* **17**:89–91.

Foster, G., 1967 Brain karyotypes of the parasitic wasp *Mormoniella vitripennis* (Walker). Thesis, Department of Biological Sciences, University of Delaware, Newark, Del.

Genieys, P., 1925 *Habrobracon brevicornis* (Wesmael). The effect of the environment and the variation which it produces. *Ann. Entomol. Soc. Am.* **18**:143–202.

Gerling, D., 1967 The eggs of the pupal parasites of *Musca domestica* L. *Israel J. Entomol.* **2**:11–13.

Gershenson, S. M., 1968 Chromosomes and determination of sex in *Mormoniella vitripennis* (Walk.). *Tsitol. Genet.* **2**:3–13 (Russian with English summary).

Glover, P. M., 1934 The developmental stages of *Bracon tachordiae*, Cam. (Hym.). *Bull. Entomol. Res.* **25**:521–539.

Gottlieb, F. J., 1972 A cytoplasmic symbiont in *Ephestia kühniella* Zeller. Location and morphology. *J. Invertebr. Pathol.* **20**:351–355.

Greb, R. J., 1933 Effects of temperature on production of mosaics in *Habrobracon*. *Biol. Bull. (Woods Hole)* **65**:179–186.

Grosch, D. S., 1948 Growth in *Habrobracon*. *Growth* **12**:243–254.

Grosch, D. S., 1952 The spinning glands of impaternate (male) *Habrobracon* larvae: Morphology and cytology. *J. Morphol.* **91**:221–236.

Grosch, D. S., 1959 The effects of feeding antimitotic substances to adult female *Habrobracon* (*Microbracon hebetor* (Say); Hymenoptera: Braconidae). *Ann. Entomol. Soc. Am.* **52**:294–298.

Grosch, D. S., 1962*a* Entomological aspects of radiation as related to genetics and physiology. *Annu. Rev. Entomol.* **7**:81–106.

Grosch, D. S., 1962*b* Distribution of zinc-65 in the wasp, *Habrobracon*, and its effects on reproduction. *Nature (Lond.)* **195**:356–358.

Grosch, D. S., 1963 Insect fecundity and fertility: Chemically induced decrease. *Science (Wash., D.C.)* **141**:732–733.

Grosch, D. S., 1968 Reproductive performance of female Braconids compared after brief and protracted exposures to ionizing radiation. *Isotopes and Radiation in Entomology*, edited by E. Doyle, pp. 201–208. International Atomic Energy Agency, Vienna (Unipub., Inc., New York).

Grosch, D. S., 1969 The visible sequence of events in unhatched *Habrobracon* embryos. *Radiat. Res.* **39**:495–496.

Grosch, D. S., 1970 Egg production and embryo lethality for *Habrobracon* from biosatellite II and associated postflight vibration experiments. *Mutat. Res.* **9**:91–108.

Grosch, D. S., 1971   The response of the female arthropod's reproductive system to radiation and chemical agents. Symposium on *Sterility Principle for Insect Control or Eradication,* edited by H. Erdman, pp. 217–227. International Atomic Energy Agency, Vienna (Unipub., Inc., New York).

Grosch, D. S., 1974   Environmental aspects: Radiations. In *The Physiology of Insecta,* second edition, Vol. 2, edited by M. Rockstein, pp. 85–126, Academic Press, New York.

Grosch, D. S. and R. L. Sullivan, 1952   The effect of ingested radiophosphorus on egg production and embryo survival in the wasp *Habrobracon. Biol. Bull. (Woods Hole)* **102:**128–140.

Grosch, D. S. and L. R. Valcovic, 1967   Chlorinated hydrocarbon insecticides (DDT and dieldrin) are not mutagenic in *Bracon hebetor* tests. *J. Econ. Entomol.* **60:**1177–1179.

Heidenthal, G., 1945   The occurrence of X-ray induced dominant lethal mutation in *Habrobracon. Genetics* **30:**197–205.

Heidenthal, G., W. Nelson and L. Clark, 1972   Fecundity and longevity of F_1 females of *Habrobracon* from sperm X-rayed with 3000 R. *Genetics* **71:**349–365.

Henschen, W., 1928   Uber die Entwicklung der Geschlechtsdrüsen von *Habrobracon juglandis* Ash. *Z. Morphol. Oekol. Tiere* **13:**144–178.

Hoffman, A. C., 1972   A characterization of repair mechanisms operating subsequent to genetic damage induced by ethyl methanesulfonate and gamma radiation in *Bracon hebetor. Mutat. Res.* **16:**175–188.

Hoffman, A. C. and D. S. Grosch, 1971   The effects of ethyl methanesulfonate on the fecundity and fertility of *Bracon* (Habrobracon) females. *Pest. Biochem. Physiol.* **1:**319–326.

Holmes, H. B., 1972   Genetic evidence for fewer progeny and a higher percent males when *Nasonia vitripennis* oviposits in previously parasitized hosts. *Entomophaga* **17:**79–88.

Inaba, F., 1939   Diploid males and triploid females of the parasitic wasp, *Habrobracon pectinophorae* Watanabe. *Cytologia (Tokyo)* **9:**517–523.

Johnson, C. D. and D. T. Ray, 1972   Chromosome identification in *Mormoniella. J. Hered.* **63:**217–218.

Keller, E. C., 1970   Xanthine dehydrogenase activity in parental and F_1 *Drosophila* and *Habrobracon* under conditions of hypogravity. *BioScience* **20:**1045–1049.

Kerschner, J., 1946   Dominant lethals induced by X-rays in sperm of the wasp *Melittobia* Sp. (C). *Anat. Rec.* **96:**556.

King, P. E. and M. R. Fordy, 1970   The formation of "accessory nuclei" in the developing oocytes of the parasitoid hymentopterans *Ophion lutens* (L.) and *Apanteles glomeratus* (L.) *Z. Zellforsch. Mikrosk. Anat.* **109:**158–170.

King, P. E. and J. Rafai, 1970   Host discrimination in a gregarious parasitoid *Nasonia vitripennis* (Walker) (Hymenoptera: Pteromalidae). *J. Exp. Biol.* **53:**245–254.

King, P. E. and N. A. Ratcliffe, 1969   The structure and possible mode of functioning of the female reproductive system of *Nasonia vitripennis* (Hymenoptera: Pteromalidae). *J. Zool. (Lond.)* **157:**319–344.

King, P. E. and J. G. Richards, 1968   Accessory nuclei and annulate lamellae in Hymenopteran oocytes. *Nature (Lond.)* **218:**488.

King, P. E. and J. G. Richards, 1969   Oogenesis in *Nasonia vitripennis.* (Walker) (Hymenoptera: Pteromalidae). *Proc. R. Entomol. Soc. Lond. Ser. A, Gen. Entomol.* **44:**143–157.

King, P. E., J. G. Richards and M. J. W. Copland, 1968   The structure of the chorion and its possible significance during oviposition in *Nasonia vitripennis* (Walker) (Hymenoptera: Pteromalidae) and other Chalcids. *Proc. R. Entomol. Soc. Lond. Ser. A, Gen. Entomol.* **43**:13–20.

King, P. E., R. R. Askew and C. Sanger, 1969   The detection of parasitised hosts by males of *Nasonia vitripennis* (Walker) (Hymenoptera: Pteromalidae) and some possible implications. *Proc. R. Entomol. Soc. Lond. Ser. A, Gen. Entomol.* **44**:85–90.

King, P. E., J. Rafai and J. G. Richards, 1972   Formation of protein yolk in eggs of a parasitoid Hymenopteran, *Nasonia vitripennis* (Walker). (Pteromalidae—Hym.). *Z. Zellforsch. Mikrosk. Anat.* **123**:330–336.

King, R. C., 1970   *Ovarian Development in Drosophila melanogaster,* p. 158, Academic Press, New York.

King, R. C. and J. D. Cassidy, 1973   Ovarian development in *Habrobracon juglandis*. II. Observations on growth and differentiation of component cells of egg chamber and their bearing upon interpretation of radiosensitivity data from *Habrobracon* and *Drosophila*. *Interntl. J. Insect Morphol. Embryol.* **2**:117–136.

Kojima, K. I., 1971   Stochastic models for efficient control of insect populations by sterile insect release methods. In *Symposium on Sterility Principle for Insect Control or Eradication,* edited by H. Erdman, pp. 477–488. International Atomic Energy Agency, Vienna (Unipub., Inc., New York).

Kratsas, R. G. and D. S. Grosch, 1974   Contrasts in cell type sensitivity to alanosine demonstrated by altered patterns of *Bracon hebetor* oviposition, hatchability, and egg morphology. *J. Econ. Entomol.* **67**:577–583.

La Chance, L. E., 1959   The effect of chelation and X-rays on fecundity and induced dominant lethals in *Habrobracon*. *Radiat. Res.* **11**:218–228.

La Chance, L. E., 1967   The induction of dominant lethal mutations in insects by ionizing radiation and chemicals—as related to the sterile-male technique of insect control. In *Genetics of Insect Vectors of Disease,* edited by J. Wright and R. Pal, pp. 617–650, Elsevier, Amsterdam.

La Chance, L. E. and A. P. Leverich, 1968   Chemosterilant studies on *Bracon* sperm. I. Sperm inactivation and dominant lethal mutations. *Ann. Entomol. Soc. Am.* **61**:164–173.

La Chance, L. E. and A. P. Leverich, 1969   Chemosterilant studies on *Bracon* sperm. II. Studies of selected compounds for induction of dominant lethal mutations or sperm inactivation. *Ann. Entomol. Soc. Am.* **62**:790–796.

La Chance, L. E., D. T. North and W. Klassen, 1968   Cytogenetic and cellular basis of chemically induced sterility in insects. In *Principles of Insect Chemosterilization,* edited by G. C. Labricque and C. N. Smith, pp. 100–157, Appleton-Century-Crofts, New York.

Laing, D. R. and L. E. Caltagirone, 1969   Biology of *Habrobracon lineatellae* (Hymenoptera: Braconidae). *Can. Entomol.* **101**:135–142.

Legner, E. F., 1967   Behavior changes the reproduction of *Spalangia cameroni, S. endius, Muscidifurax raptor,* and *Nasonia vitripennis* (Hymenoptera: Pteromalidae) at increasing fly host densities. *Ann. Entomol. Soc. Am.* **60**:819–826.

Legner, E. F. and D. Gerling, 1967   Host-feeding and oviposition on *Musca domestica* by *Spalangia cameroni, Nasonia vitripennis,* and *Muscidifurax raptor* (Hymenoptera: Pteromalidae) influences their longevity and fecundity. *Ann. Entomol. Soc. Am.* **60**:678–691.

Leibenguth, F., 1967   Regulation of tryptophan metabolism in the parasitic wasp, *Habrobracon juglandis*. *Experientia (Basel)* **23**:1069–1074.

Leibenguth, F., 1970   Concerning non-darkening of mutant *Habrobracon* (*Bracon hebetor*) eyes as consequence of a new chromogen-reducing mechanism in insect larvae. *Experientia (Basel)* **26**:659–660.

Leibenguth, F., 1971   Zur Pleiotropie des *wh-*und *el-*Locus bei *Habrobracon juglandis*. *Z. Naturforsch. Sect. B* **26**:53–60.

Leibenguth, F., 1972   Die Entwicklung von *Mattesia dispora* in *Habrobracon juglandis*. *Z. Parasitenk.* **38**:162–173.

Lin, J. C. H., 1965   The genetic and physiological diversification of two related species of parasitic wasps, *Habrobracon juglandis* Ashmead and *Habrobracon serinopae* Ramkr. Ph.D. Dissertation, North Carolina State University, Raleigh, N. C.

Löbbecke, E. A. and R. C. von Borstel, 1962   Mutational response of *Habrobracon* oocytes in metaphase and prophase to ethyl methanesulfonate and nitrogen mustard. *Genetics* **47**:853–864.

Lum, P. T. M. and B. R. Flaherty, 1973   Influence of continuous light on oocyte maturation in *Bracon hebetor*. *Ann. Entomol. Soc. Am.* **66**:355–357.

McKnight, M. E., 1971   Biology and habits of *Bracon politiventris* (Hymenoptera: Braconidae). *Ann. Entomol. Soc. Am.* **64**:620–624.

Macy, R. M. and P. W. Whiting, 1969   Tetraploid females in *Mormoniella*. *Genetics* **61**:619–630.

Martin, A., 1947   *An Introduction to the Genetics of Habrobracon juglandis* (Ashmead), Hobson Book Press, New York.

Matthews, R. W., 1974   Biology of Braconidae. *Annu. Rev. Entomol.* **19**:15–59.

Meng, C., 1968   Strukturwandel und histochemische Befunde insbesondere am Oosom während der Oogenese und nach der Ablage des Eies von *Pimpla turionellae* L. (Hymenoptera, Ichneumonidae). *Wilhem Roux' Arch. Entwichlungsmech. Org.* **161**:162–208.

Meng, C., 1969   Autoradiographische Untersuchungen am Oosom in der Oocyte von *Pimpla turionellae* L. (Hymenoptera). *Wilhem Roux' Arch. Entwicklungsmech. Org.* **165**:35–52.

Miller, M. C., 1972   Scanning electron microscope studies of the flagellar sense receptors of *Peridesmia discus* and *Nasonia vitripennis* (Hymenoptera: Pteromalidae). *Ann. Entomol. Soc. Am.* **65**:1119–1124.

Miner, G. D. and G. S. Kennington, 1968   Genetic aspects of anaerobic metabolism in *Mormoniella vitripennis*. *Physiol. Zool.* **41**:220–227.

Mizianty, T. J. and B. Venit, 1971   Effects of ethyl methanesulphonate and mitomycin-C upon duration of adult life span in *Bracon serinopae* (Hymenoptera: Braconidae). *Ann. Entomol. Soc. Am.* **64**:777–779.

Nelson, W. A. and C. W. Farstad, 1953   Biology of *Bracon cephi* (Gahan) (Hymenoptera: Braconidae), an important native parasite of the wheat stem sawfly, *Cephus cinctus* Noct. (Hymenoptera: Cephidae), in western Canada. *Can. Entomol.* **85**:103–107.

Nesbitt, M. and S. Gartler, 1971   The applications of genetic mosaicism to developmental problems. *Annu. Rev. Genet.* **5**:143–162.

Odebiyi, J. A. and E. R. Oatman, 1972   Biology of *Agathis gibbosa* (Hymenoptera: Braconidae), a primary parasite of the potato tuberworm. *Ann. Entomol. Soc. Am.* **65**:1104–1114.

Piek, T., 1966 Site of action of venom of *Microbracon hebetor* Say (Braconidae: Hymenoptera). *J. Insect Physiol.* **12**:561–568.

Pimentel, D., 1966 Wasp parasite (*Nasonia vitripennis*) survival on its house fly host (*Musca domestica*) reared on various foods. *Ann. Entomol. Soc. Am.* **59**:1031–1038.

Pimentel, D., 1968 Population regulation and genetic feedback. *Science (Wash., D.C.)* **159**:1432–1437.

Pimentel, D. and R. Al-Hafidh, 1965 Ecological control of a parasite population by genetic evolution in the parasite–host system. *Ann. Entomol. Soc. Am.* **58**:1–6.

Pimentel, D. and P. A. Stone, 1968 Evolution and population ecology of parasite–host systems. *Can. Entomol.* **100**:655–662.

Rabinovich, J. E., 1969 The applicability of some population growth models to a single species laboratory population. *Ann. Entomol. Soc. Am.* **62**:437–442.

Rasch, E. M., J. D. Cassidy, and R. C. King, 1975 Estimates of genome size in haploid-diploid species of parasitoid wasps. *J. Histochem. Cytochem.* **23**:317.

Ratcliffe, N. A. and P. E. King, 1967 The "venom" system of *Nasonia vitripennis* (Walker) (Hymenoptera: Pteromalidae). *Proc. R. Entomol. Soc. Lond. Ser. A, Gen. Entomol.* **42**:49–61.

Reinert, J. A. and E. W. King, 1971 Action of *Bracon hebetor* Say as a parasite of *Plodia interpunctella* at controlled densities. *Ann. Entomol. Soc. Am.* **64**:1335–1340.

Richards, J. G., 1968 The structure and formation of the egg membranes in *Nasonia vitripennis* (Walker) (Hymenoptera: Pteromalidae). *J. Microscop.* **89**:43–53.

Richards, J. G. and P. E. King, 1967 Chorion and vitelline membranes and their role in resorbing eggs of the Hymenoptera. *Nature (Lond.)* **214**:601–602.

Rockstein, M. and J. Miquel, 1973 Aging in insects. In *The Physiology of Insecta*, second edition, Vol. 1, edited by M. Rockstein, pp. 371–478, Academic Press, New York.

Rohner, M. C., 1959 The influence of depression of respiratory metabolism by carbon monoxide on the pigment development in the insect eye. *Z. Vererbungsl.* **90**:257–262.

Rohner, M. C., Sr., and A. Wolsky, 1957 The effect of carbon monoxide on the eye pigment development of *Mormoniella* and *Drosophila*. *Anat. Rec.* **128**:609.

Roozen, K. J. and G. W. Conner, 1969 Genetic analysis of the *R* locus in *Mormoniella*. *J. Hered.* **60**:269–271.

Roozen, K. J. and G. W. Conner, 1970 Linkage relationships in bifactorial *R* locus mutants in *Mormoniella*. *Genetics* **64**:s54–55.

Rotary, N. and D. Gerling, 1973 The influence of some external factors upon the sex ratio of *Bracon hebetor* Say (Hymenoptera: Braconidae). *Env. Entomol.* **2**:134–138.

Rotheram, S., 1973 The surface of the egg of a parasitic insect. 1. The surface of the egg and first-instar larva of *Nemeritis* (Hym.: Ichneumonidae). *Proc. R. Soc. Lond. Ser. B, Biol. Sci.* **183**:179–194.

Ryan, S. L. and G. B. Saul, 1968 Post-fertilization effects of incompatibility factors in *Mormoniella*. *Mol. Gen. Genet.* **103**:29–36.

Salt, G., 1961 Competition among insect parasitoids. Symposium on *Mechanisms in Biological Competition*, edited by F. L. Milthorpe, pp. 96–119, Academic Press, New York.

Salt, G., 1968 The resistance of insect parasitoids to the defense reactions of their hosts. *Biol. Rev.* **43**:200–232.

Salt, G., 1971 Teratocytes as a means of resistance to cellular defense reactions. *Nature (Lond.)* **232**:639.

Samis, H. V., M. B. Baird and F. A. Lints, 1973   Life span and temperature: Insects. *In Biology Data Book,* second edition, Vol. 2, edited by P. L. Altman and D. S. Dittmer, p. 873, Federation of the American Society of Experimental Biology, Washington, D.C.

Sanger, C. and P. E. King, 1971   Structure and function of the male genitalia in *Nasonia vitripennis* (Walker) (Hymenoptera: Pteromalidae). *Entomologist* **104:**136–149.

Saul, G., 1960   The occurrence of fluorescent substances in the parasitic wasp *Mormoniella vitripennis* (Walker). *Rev. Suisse Zool.* **67:**270–281.

Saul, G. B., 1972   Linkage maps of *Mormoniella.* In *Biology Data Handbook,* second edition, Vol. 1, edited by P. L. Altman and D. S. Dittmer, pp. 48–49, Federation of the American Society of Experimental Biology, Washington, D.C.

Saul, G. B., P. W. Whiting, S. W. Saul and C. A. Heidner, 1965   Wild type and mutant stocks of *Mormoniella. Genetics* **52:**1317–1327.

Saul, G. B., S. W. Saul and S. Becker, 1967   Linkage in *Mormoniella. Genetics* **57:**369–384.

Saunders, D. S., 1966   Larval diapause of maternal origin. II. The effect of photoperiod and temperature on *Nasonia vitripennis. J. Insect Physiol.* **12:**569–581.

Saunders, D. S., 1968   Photoperiodism and time measurement in the parasitic wasp, *Nasonia vitripennis. J. Insect Physiol.* **14:**433–450.

Saunders, D. S., 1969   Diapause and photoperiodism in the parasitic wasp *Nasonia vitripennis,* with special reference to the nature of the photoperiodic clock. In *Dormancy and Survival,* edited by H. W. Woolhouse, pp. 301–329, Academic Press, New York.

Saunders, D. S., 1973   Thermoperiodic control of diapause in an insect: Theory of internal coincidence. *Science (Wash., D.C.)* **181:**358–360.

Saunders, D. S., D. Sutton and R. A. Jarvis, 1970   The effect of host species on diapause induction in *Nasonia vitripennis. J. Insect Physiol.* **16:**405–416.

Schmieder, R. G., 1933   The polymorphic forms of *Melittobia chalybii* Ashmead and the determining factors in their production. *Biol. Bull. (Woods Hole)* **65:**338–354.

Schmieder, R. G. and P. W. Whiting, 1947   Reproductive economy in the chalcidoid wasp *Melittobia. Genetics* **32:**29–37.

Schneiderman, H. A. and J. Horwitz, 1958   The induction and termination of facultative diapause in the chalcidoid wasps *Mormoniella vitripennis* (Walker) and *Tritneptis klugii* (Ratzeburg). *J. Exp. Biol.* **35:**520–551.

Slifer, E. H., 1969   Sense organs on the antennae of a parasitic wasp, *Nasonia vitripennis* (Hymenoptera: Pteromalidae). *Biol. Bull. (Woods Hole)* **136:**253–263.

Smith, G. J. C., 1969   Host selection and oviposition behavior of *Nasonia vitripennis* (Hymenoptera: Pteromalidae) on two host species. *Can. Entomol.* **101:**533–538.

Smith, R. E., 1968   Urate accumulation and life span in two species of *Habrobracon. Diss. Abstr.* **28:**4358B.

Smith, R. H., 1969   Induction of mutations in *Habrobracon* sperm with mitomycin c. *Mutat. Res.* **7:**231–234.

Smith, R. H., 1971   Induced conditional lethal mutations for the control of insect populations. Symposium on *Sterility Principle for Insect Control or Eradication,* edited by H. Erdman, pp. 453–465, International Atomic Energy Agency, Vienna (Unipub., Inc., New York).

Smith, R. H., 1974   Temperature-sensitive mutations in *Habrobracon. Genet. Res.* **23:**63–74.

Smith, R. H. and R. C. von Borstel, 1971   Inducing mutations with chemicals in

Habrobracon. In *Chemical Mutagens Principles and Methods for their Detection,* Vol. 2, edited by A. Hollaender, pp. 445–460, Plenum Press, New York.

Smith, R. H. and R. C. von Borstel, 1972 Genetic control of insect populations. *Science (Wash., D.C.)* **178**:1164–1174.

Speicher, B. R., 1934 The temperature effective period in development of "eyeless" in *Habrobracon. Am. Nat.* **68**:70–71.

Speicher, B. R., 1936 Oogenesis, fertilization and early cleavage in *Habrobracon. J. Morphol.* **59**:401–421.

Stern, C., 1968 *Genetic Mosaics and Other Essays,* Harvard University Press, Cambridge, Mass.

Takahashi, F. and D. Pimentel, 1967 Wasp preference for black-, brown-, and hybrid-type pupae of the house fly. *Ann. Entomol. Soc. Am.* **60**:623–625.

Torvik-Greb, M., 1935 The chromosomes of *Habrobracon. Biol. Bull. (Woods Hole)* **68**:25–34.

Valcovic, L. R. and D. S. Grosch, 1968 Apholate-induced sterility in *Bracon hebetor. J. Econ. Entomol.* **61**:1514–1517.

Van Pelt, G. S., 1970 A study of eye color mutants of *Habrobracon. Diss. Abstr.* **30**:4928-B.

Velthuis, H. H., F. F. Velthuis-Kluppell and G. A. H. Bossink, 1965 Some aspects of the biology and population dynamics of *Nasonia vitripennis* Walker (Hymenoptera: Pteromalidae). *Entomol. Exp. Appl.* **8**:205–227.

von Borstel, R. C., 1971 Mutational and physiological responses of *Habrobracon* in biosatellite II. In *The Experiments of Biosatellite II,* edited by J. E. Saunders, pp. 17–39, NASA, Washington, D.C.

von Borstel, R. C. and M. L. Rekemeyer, 1959 Radiation-induced and genetically contrived dominant lethality in *Habrobracon* and *Drosophila. Genetics* **44**:1053–1074.

von Borstel, R. C. and W. St. Amand, 1963 Stage sensitivity to X-radiation during meiosis and mitosis in the egg of the wasp *Habrobracon.* In *Repair from Genetic Damage and Differential Radiosensitivity in Germ Cells,* edited by F. Sobels, pp. 87–100, Pergamon Press, New York.

von Borstel, R. C. and P. A. Smith, 1960 Haploid intersexes in the wasp *Habrobracon. Heredity* **15**:29–34.

von Borstel, R. C., R. H. Smith, A. R. Whiting and D. S. Grosch, 1970 Biological responses of *Habrobracon* to spaceflight. In *Life Sciences and Space Research* VIII, edited by W. Vishniac and F. G. Favorite, pp. 6–11, North-Holland, Amsterdam.

Walker, I., 1967 Effect of population density on the viability and fecundity in *Nasonia vitripennis* (Walker) (Hymenoptera: Pteromalidae). *Ecology* **48**:294–301.

Went, D. F. and G. Krause, 1973 Normal development of mechanically activated, unlaid eggs of an endoparasitic Hymenopteran. *Nature (Lond.)* **244**:454–455.

Whiting, A. R., 1934 Eye colours in the parasitic wasp *Habrobracon* and their behaviour in multiple recessives and in mosaics. *J. Genet.* **29**:99–107.

Whiting, A. R., 1945a Effects of X-rays on hatchability and on chromosomes of *Habrobracon* eggs treated in first meiotic prophase and metaphase. *Am. Nat.* **79**:193–227.

Whiting, A. R., 1945b Dominant lethality and correlated chromosome effects in *Habrobracon* eggs X-rayed in diplotene and in late metaphase I. *Biol. Bull. (Woods Hole)* **89**:61–71.

Whiting, A. R., 1961a Genetics of *Habrobracon. Adv. Genet.* **10**:295–348.

Whiting, A. R., 1961*b* Temperature effects on lethal mutation rates of *Habrobracon* oocytes X-irradiated in first meiotic metaphase. *Genetics* **46**:811–816.

Whiting, A. R., 1965 The complex locus R in *Mormoniella vitripennis* (Walker). *Adv. Genet.* **13**:341–358.

Whiting, A. R., 1967 The biology of the parasitic wasp *Mormoniella vitripennis* (= *Nasonia brevicornis*) (Walker). *Quart. Rev. Biol.* **42**:333–406.

Whiting, A. R., R. H. Smith and R. C. von Borstel, 1968 Methods for radiation studies during oögenesis in *Habrobracon juglandis* (Ashmead). In *Effects of Radiation on Meiotic Systems,* edited by C. N. Welsh, pp. 201–208, International Atomic Energy Agency, Vienna (Unipub., Inc., New York).

Whiting, P. W., 1918 Sex determination and biology of a parasitic wasp *Habrobracon brevicornis* (Wesmeal). *Biol. Bull. (Woods Hole)* **34**:250–256.

Whiting, P. W., 1921 Rearing meal moths and parasitic wasps for experimental purposes. *J. Hered.* **12**:255–261.

Whiting, P. W., 1928 Mosaicism and mutation in *Habrobracon. Biol. Bull. (Woods Hole)* **54**:289–307.

Whiting, P. W., 1929 X-rays and parasitic wasps. *J. Hered.* **20**:268–276.

Whiting, P. W., 1932*a* Mutants in *Habrobracon. Genetics* **17**:1–30.

Whiting, P. W., 1932*b* Diploid mosaics in *Habrobracon. Am. Nat.* **66**:75–81.

Whiting, P. W., 1932*c* Reproductive reactions of sex mosaics of a parasitic wasp *Habrobracon juglandis. J. Comp. Psychol.* **14**:345–363.

Whiting, P. W., 1934 Mutants in *Habrobracon.* II. *Genetics* **19**:268–291.

Whiting, P. W., 1940 Sex-linkage in *Pteromalus. Am. Nat.* **74**:377–379.

Whiting, P. W., 1943 Multiple alleles in complementary sex-determination of *Habrobracon. Genetics* **28**:365–382.

Whiting, P. W., 1950 Linkage in *Mormoniella. Genetics* **35**:699.

Whiting, P. W., 1951 Multiple complementary alleles in *Habrobracon* and *Mormoniella. J. Genet.* **50**:206–214.

Whiting, P. W., 1954 Comparable mutant eye colors in *Mormoniella* and *Pachycrepoideus* (Hymenoptera: Pteromalidae). *Evolution* **8**:135–147.

Whiting, P. W., 1955 A parasitic wasp and its host for genetics instruction and for biology courses. *Carolina Tips* **18**:13–16.

Whiting, P. W., 1960 Polyploidy in *Mormoniella. Genetics* **45**:949–970.

Whiting, P. W., 1966 "Black" eye colors of *Mormoniella. Genetics* **54**:639–655.

Whiting, P. W., 1968 A diapause resistant stock of *Mormoniella. Carolina Tips* **31**:9.

Whiting, P. W. and R. L. Anderson, 1932 Temperature and other factors concerned in male biparentalism in *Habrobracon. Am. Nat.* **66**:420–432.

Whiting, P. W. and D. J. Bush, 1959 Maintaining stocks in *Mormoniella. Proc. Pa. Acad. Sci.* **33**:248–251.

Whiting, P. W. and E. Novitski, 1964 Linkage groups: Invertebrates. Parasitic Wasp. In *Biology Data Book,* edited by P. L. Altman and D. S. Dittmer, pp. 29–31, Federation of the American Society of Experimental Biology, Washington, D.C.

Whiting, P. W., R. J. Greb and B. R. Speicher, 1934 A new type of sex integrade. *Biol. Bull. (Woods Hole)* **66**:152–165.

Wilkes, A., 1965 Sperm transfer and utilization by the arrhenotokous wasp *Dahlbominus fuscipennis* (Zett.) (Hymenoptera: Eulophidae). *Can. Entomol.* **9**:647–657.

Wolf, R. and G. Krause, 1971 Die Ooplasmabewegungen während der Furchung von

Pimpla turionellae L. (Hymenoptera), eine Zeitrafferfilmanalyse. *Wilhem Roux'* *Arch. Entwicklungsmech. Org.* **167**:266–287.

Wylie, H. G., 1965   Some effects that reduce the reproductive rate of *Nasonia vitripennis* (Walk.) at high adult population densities. *Can. Entomol.* **97**:970–977.

Wylie, H. G., 1966   Some mechanisms that affect the sex ratio of *Nasonia vitripennis* (Walk.) (Hymenoptera: Pteromalidae) reared from superparasitized housefly pupae. *Can. Entomol.* **98**:645–653.

Wylie, H. G., 1967   Some effects of host size on *Nasonia vitripennis* and *Muscidifurax raptor* (Hymenoptera: Pteromalidae). *Can. Entomol.* **99**:742–748.

Wylie, H. G., 1970   Oviposition restraint of *Nasonia vitripennis* (Hymenoptera: Pteromalidae) on hosts parasitized by other hymenopterous species. *Can. Entomol.* **102**:886–894.

Wylie, H. G., 1971   Observations in intraspecific larval competition in three hymenopterous parasites of fly puparia. *Can. Entomol.* **103**:137–142.

Wylie, H. G., 1972a   Oviposition restraint of *Spalangia cameroni* (Hymenoptera: Pteromalidae) on parasitized housefly pupae. *Can. Entomol.* **104**:209–214.

Wylie, H. G., 1972b   Larval competition among three hymenopterous parasite species on multiparasitized housefly (Diptera) pupae.*Can. Entomol.* **104**:1181–1190.

Wylie, H. G., 1973   Control of egg fertilization by *Nasonia vitripennis* (Hymenoptera: Pteromalidae) when laying on parasitized housefly pupae. *Can. Entomol.* **105**:709–718.

PART I
LOWER DIPTERA
WITH GIANT
CHROMOSOMES

8

Rhynchosciara

CRODOWALDO PAVAN,

ANTONIO BRITO DA CUNHA, AND

PATRICIA SANDERS

Introduction

Species of the family Sciaridae are somewhat primitive dipterans which have long been known to be excellent experimental material for cytogenetic and developmental studies. They demonstrate certain rather "unorthodox" biological characteristics, such as a peculiar type of sex determination, elimination of specific chromosomes by some cells during development, and exhibition of large puffs in their polytene chromosomes, which produce RNA and in some cases "metabolic DNA" (DNA puffs). One of the most interesting and valuable characteristics of species in the genus *Rhynchosciara* is that large numbers of individuals descended from a single female have gregarious habits and develop synchronously as a group from zygote to adult. Combined with their developmental synchrony, these individuals are all of the same chronological age and, due to their peculiar method of sex determination, are all of the same sex. Prob-

CRODOWALDO PAVAN—Department of Zoology, The University of Texas at Austin, Austin, Texas, and Departmento de Biologia, Instituto de Biociencias, Universidade de São Paulo, São Paulo, Brazil. ANTONIO BRITO DA CUNHA—Departmento de Biologia, Instituto de Biociencias, Universidade de São Paulo, São Paulo, Brazil. PATRICIA SANDERS—Department of Zoology, The University of Texas at Austin, Austin, Texas.

lems involving developmental synchrony and sex determination inherent in other organisms, particularly in other dipterans, are thereby naturally eliminated in species of *Rhynchosciara,* rendering them amenable to developmental studies where relatively large numbers are required. Their having exceptionally well-developed polytene chromosomes in several tissues makes it possible to examine comparatively in these several tissues the activities manifested in the polytene chromosomes for most of the period of larval development, which in most species of *Rhynchosciara* lasts for 40–50 days.

In addition to these normal features, there are in some species of Sciaridae infections of several tissues by microsporidians (protozoans), gregarines (protozoans), and viruses which result in some very interesting consequences. Infected cells develop into unicellular tumors via an enormous hypertrophy of the cytoplasm, nucleus, and chromosomes. In fact, the chromosomes of some infected salivary gland cells of *Rhynchosciara* become enlarged to such an extent as to be visible to the unaided eye. This chromosomal enlargement is due primarily to two events: an increase in polyteny (extra duplicative cycles of the chromonemata) and an accelerated RNA synthesis rate. Viral infections have been found to induce the enlargement and hyperactivity of the chromosomes found in other infections, plus alterations in the basic structure of the chromosomes, especially visualized cytologically as constrictions, i.e., areas probably representing fewer replicative events.

It is the intention of this chapter to examine somewhat closely the biology of two species of sciarids, *Rhynchosciara angelae* and *Rhynchosciara hollaenderi,* the two most-studied species of *Rhynchosciara.* A brief summation of the "unorthodox" biological idiosyncrasies of sciarids will first be given to better appreciate the characteristics of the two species to be discussed.

The Biological Peculiarities of Sciaridae

Sex Determination

Basically, all species of Sciaridae thus far studied have a similar type of sex determination; sex is determined by the selective elimination of specific chromosomes during embryonic development (see Scheme 1 below). If the limited chromosomes are excluded from consideration, it is found that all sciarid zygotes contain six autosomes and three X chromosomes. The formation of the zygote results from the contribution by the egg of three autosomes and one X chromosome and by the sperm of three

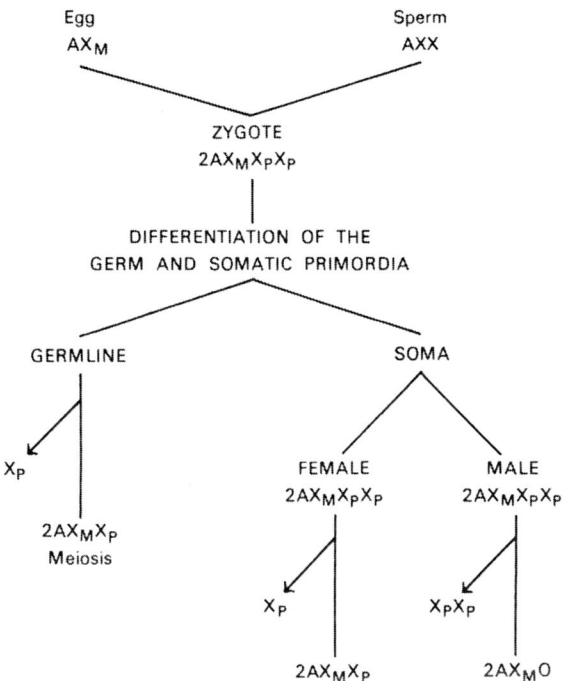

Scheme 1: The limited chromosomes have been eliminated from consideration. X_M and X_P designate the maternally and paternally derived X chromosomes, respectively.

autosomes and two X chromosomes, yielding six autosomes and three X chromosomes. During differentiation of the primordial germline in both male and female embryos, there is a selective loss of one paternal X chromosome. At the initiation of somatic cell differentiation, the cells of the female eliminate one paternal X chromosome, whereas in the male embryo both paternal X chromosomes are eliminated. Hence, the somatic cells of the female are 2AXX, and those of the male are 2AXO. Scheme 1 summarizes what generally occurs in the germ and somatic primordia.

To further complicate an already complicated system, there are species, such as *Sciara coprophila,* which have some strains in which all progeny produced by one female are of only one sex. This is the result of two types of females, based on their X chromosomes, XX (male producers) and XX′ (female producers) (see Scheme 2).

Since the female producers of *S. coprophila* theoretically yield these two types of females in equal proportions, the sex ratio should be equally balanced. However, exceptions exist in some strains of *S. coprophila* and other species of *Sciara,* making the problem of sex determination extremely difficult to clearly define. White (1954) suggested that these

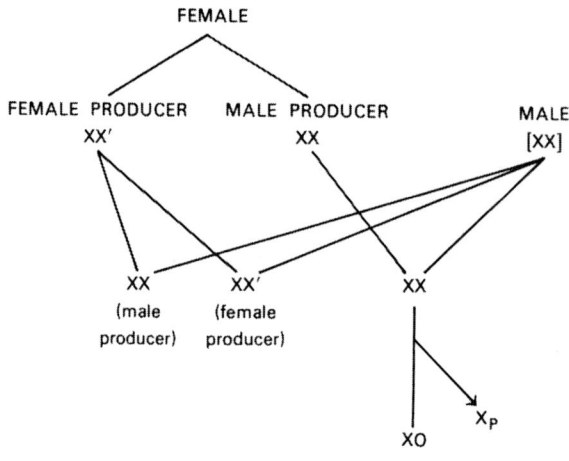

Scheme 2

variations might perhaps be due to a series of different X chromosomes in the population: "It is possible that the two alleles (X and X′) postulated by Metz are not the only ones and that in actuality a series of alleles of varying potency (X′, X″, X‴, etc.) exists." As will be discussed below, this might partially explain the sex-determination mechanisms in *S. ocellaris* and perhaps other species as well (de Souza and Pavan, 1972, and unpublished).

Crossing over occurs only in the females of Sciaridae species. In the females, the picture is not so simple as it at first appears; for, while there is crossing over between homologous autosomes and between homologous X chromosomes, there appear to be great restrictions on crossing-over events occurring between X and X′ chromosomes (Metz and Schmuck, 1931; Crouse, 1943). Perhaps this is due to some lack of homology between these two types of X chromosome or, perhaps, to some other mechanism which restricts such occurrences; the problem is still open. Based on what happens in other organisms, it can be concluded that the 2AXX′ female should be considered heterogametic, i.e., 2AXY. Thus, in *S. coprophila,* one observes that 2AXO males obligatorily exist with 2AXX and 2AXY females (Pavan and da Cunha, 1969a). The males, although somatically 2AXO, are monogametic, i.e., producing only one type of sperm, AXX (see Figure 1 and Scheme 2).

Females of *R. angelae* and *R. hollaenderi,* as in the case of *S. coprophila,* produce unisexual progeny. Morgante (1972) found, by contrast, that bisexual groups may occur in nature; however, on further examination, he was able to conclude that these groups were mixtures of the progeny of different females.

Both these species of *Rhynchosciara* are quite similar to *S. coprophila* in their pattern of chromosomal elimination during development and spermatogenesis (Basile, 1966, 1970; Casartelli, 1970). They, too, have limited chromosomes and, as stated, produce unisexual progeny; on the other hand, their method of sex determination does not

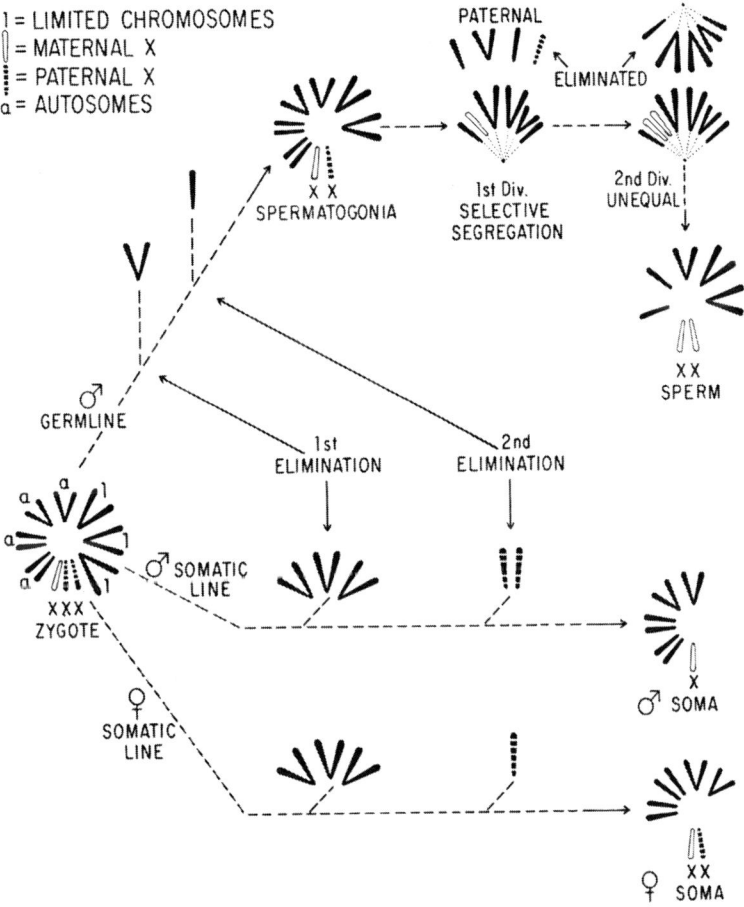

Figure 1. Diagram of chromosomal elimination during development and spermatogenesis of S. coprophila modified from the original of Metz (1938). Oögenesis is not represented because it follows the normal rules for the majority of organisms, i.e., the egg has half the number of chromosomes of the oögonia. From Pavan and da Cunha, Annual Review of Genetics 3:425–450, 1969, with permission of Annual Reviews, Inc.

follow the Metz rule for *S. coprophila.* Some unknown factors involved in the sex determination of these species render them different from *S. coprophila.* In laboratory cultures of *R. angelae* and *R. hollaenderi* it has often been observed that a preponderance in number of one sex may occur on occasion; no conclusion for this variability in the sex ratio has as yet been reached.

A strain of *S. ocellaris,* collected at Oak Ridge National Laboratory in 1965 and since maintained in our laboratory, has three types of female: one which produces bisexual progeny and the others which produce unisexual progeny. Although attempts have been made to select strains which would constantly produce unisexual or bisexual groups, thus far none have been successful (Perondini, 1968; de Souza and Pavan, 1972, and unpublished). Crouse (1939) also found bisexual- and unisexual-group-producing strains of *S. ocellaris.*

The females of bisexual groups in the Oak Ridge strain of *S. ocellaris* produced sex ratios in which the frequency of females varied from practically zero to one hundred percent. Even by careful selection of crosses, strains could not be obtained which would produce progeny with sex ratios close to 50 percent. Mating females and males from groups in which the sex ratios were around 50 percent produced a great variability in sex ratios in the next generation. The conclusion of de Souza and Pavan (1972, and unpublished) is that in *S. ocellaris,* sex determination is dependent on the type of X chromosomes involved in the crosses. They have data which indicate that elimination of either one or two X chromosomes during embryonic development depends on the genetic constitution of the X chromosomes involved and is independent of the genotype of the female which produced the eggs, hence it does not appear to be a maternal effect. Their data further show that there are probably several types of X chromosomes and that some X chromosomes frequently mutate during ontogeny. An X chromosome in a zygote expected to produce a female can mutate during ontogeny and instead allow production of a male, yielding at a rate of about 1 percent a so-called "exceptional male" in an expected female progeny. The crossing of this exceptional male, i.e., that one which was expected to be female, with any kind of female produces unisexual male progeny. The "transformed" X chromosome cannot be maintained in the culture because the male progeny do not transmit it to the next generation. As shown by Metz and co-workers (Metz, 1938; Crouse, 1943), the entire set of paternal chromosomes is eliminated during spermatogenesis (Figure 1). The mature sperm contain, mandatorily, only those chromosomes descended from the female parent. This exceptional male with a transformed X chromosome occurs in a high enough frequency in our cultures to be easily obtained from the progeny resulting from crosses which normally produce only females. These findings complicate still further the problem of sex determination in sciarids since to date it has been assumed that sex determination in these insects usually depends on the genotype of the females [Metz (1938); see also White (1954) p. 244]. However, as was mentioned, in the Oak Ridge strain of *S. ocellaris* there is instead the dependence on the genetic constitution of the X chromosome. On the other hand, several cases of exceptional females among unisexual male progeny were obtained, but it was impossible to predict the sex ratio of their progeny.

Elimination of Chromosomes

Introduction. During very early embryonic development and spermatogenesis, sciarids selectively eliminate or segregate specific chromosomes during cell division (Metz, 1938). Cell division and chromosome behavior are so complicated in sciarids that a summary of only the most salient features of these processes will be given, especially those regarding the differentiated homologous chromosomes.

It is generally the case that all zygotes of any particular sciarid species contain a set number of chromosomes, with variances in this number largely dependent on the existence of so-called "limited chromosomes." These limited chromosomes exist only in the germline of some species and are preferentially eliminated during somatic cell differentiation very early in embryonic development (Figure 1). Furthermore, their number may vary within a species as well as between different species, as was demonstrated by Metz (1938), or be entirely absent, as in *S. ocellaris* and *S. reynoldsi* (Metz and Lawrence, 1938). There is good evidence that the limited chromosomes have no detectable influence on sex determination but that they possibly perform some function vital to the development of the germline cells (Metz, 1938; Crouse, 1943).

Chromosomal Behavior in *S. coprophila*. To give an overview of the behavior of the chromosomes in Sciaridae, the data of Metz and co-workers in *S. coprophila* will be used as a typical case of what happens with minor, specific variations in other sciarids (Figure 1). The zygote of this species has twelve chromosomes: three pairs of autosomes (A, B, and C), three X chromosomes, and three limited, or L, chromosomes. The derivation of these chromosomes is as follows: one of each (A, B, C, X, and L; 5 chromosomes) from the egg and one of each plus an extra X and L (A, B, C, X, X, L, and L; 7 chromosomes) from the sperm.

During early cleavage there is the selective elimination of chromosomes from certain cells. In the soma primordia of the female four chromosomes are eliminated, the three L chromosomes and one paternal

X chromosome, leaving eight chromosomes (2A, 2B, 2C, 2X) in somatic cells. The males lose a total of five chromosomes, the three L chromosomes and two paternal X chromosomes, leaving seven chromosomes (2A, 2B, 2C, X) in the somatic cells. In the germline of both sexes there is the elimination of one of the L chromosomes and one of the paternal X chromosomes.

Nothing particularly extraordinary occurs in oogenesis, i.e., there is the usual synapsis and crossing over. Each mature ovum has five chromosomes (A, B, C, X, and L), or half the number present in the oogonia. Spermatogenesis in few ways resembles that of other organisms, for it is both peculiar and unique. During the first meiotic division there is the selective segregation of chromosomes, and of the two resulting cells only one is functional. The entire maternal complement and the L chromosomes are retained in the functional cell, whereas four of the paternal set (A, B, C, and X) are eliminated through a polar-body-like cell. Meiosis II is also rather special in that it gives origin to two cells with non-disjunction of the X chromosomes. The consequence of this is that the spermatid has seven chromosomes (A, B, C, X, X, and 2L) and the second "polar body" has five chromosomes (A, B, C, L and L) (as seen in Figure 1). As is the case in oögenesis, the "polar body" of spermatogenesis degenerates.

Chromosomal Behavior in Other Organisms. The phenomenon of chromosomal elimination is not a recent observation. Boveri (1887, 1892) described chromosomal diminution and partial elimination during somatic cell differentiation in *Ascaris megalocephala*. Recently, determination of DNA content in differentiated somatic cells and germline cells in *Ascaris lumbricoides* (Tobler *et al.*, 1972) and *Parascaris equorum* (Moritz, 1970) revealed decreases of 27 percent and 80 percent, respectively, in total DNA content in the somatic cells, corresponding to selective elimination of chromatin from these cells. S. Beermann (1966) described similar chromosomal diminution and partial elimination during cytodifferentiation in *Cyclops furcifer*. Chromosomal elimination has been described, as mentioned, in *Sciara* (Du Bois, 1932; Metz, 1934; Crouse, 1947), and also in *Miastor* (Wilson, 1925; White, 1954), *Rhynchosciara* (Basile, 1966, 1970), Cecidomyidae (White, 1950; Bauer and Beermann, 1952; Beermann, 1956; Geyer-Duszyńska, 1959; Bantock, 1961; Kunz *et al.*, 1970), and in Ciliata (Ammermann, 1971). Recently, it has been found that during development of certain somatic tissues in some species of marsupials, the female loses an X chromosome while the male loses the Y chromosome (Sharman, 1970). Elimination or reduction of parts of or whole chromosomes, induced by such treatments as cold shock, have been observed in some animals and plants [see Evans (1956) for review; Pelc (1972), Malvaldi and Viola-Magni (1972), Viola-

Magni (1965), and others]. Thus, elimination of chromatin is not restricted to a few, similar organisms, but is scattered throughout the eukaryotes. The question is: How are the chromosomes to be eliminated delineated from those which are to be retained? It could be due to a differential activity between the sets marked for elimination and for retention. It could be due to a differential constitution, i.e., there may be some qualitative difference between the two. This qualitative difference could either be a "permanent" situation phylogenetic in origin or a "temporary" situation ontogenetic in origin, necessitating some alterations in every generation. There is evidence to support the differential activity and/or differential constitution. Nuclear and chromosomal differentiation is so poorly understood that such observations as a "stable" DNA content from tissue to tissue do not preclude a generalized instead of exceptional occurrence of differentiation through diminution or amplification of specific genetic material. Indeed, a stable content of DNA speaks only of quantitative differences and nothing of qualitative. There are many data being accumulated in such widely separated organisms as ciliates, insects, plants, and vertebrates which support the idea that qualitative differentiation may occur.*

Chromosomal Behavior in *Rhynchosciara*. Comparison of chromosomal activity during spermatogenesis and oögenesis of *Rhynchosciara* reveals a differential activity which may somehow account for the very precise elimination of the paternal complement. The chromosomes of the oögonia are metabolically active during oögenesis only in the early development of the gonad, they then become metabolically inactive after follicle formation, remaining so until after zygote formation. The nurse cell and follicular cells of each follicle provide the mRNA necessary for yolk formation (Basile, 1966, 1969). In sharp contrast to this, the spermatogonia are metabolically active throughout spermatogenesis, reaching such high activity during the growth phase of the spermatocytes as to resemble the chromosomes of gland cells (Casartelli, 1970; Basile, 1970). This phase of hyperactivity lasts for about 20

---

* *For insects see:* Pavan and co-workers (Pavan and Breuer, 1952, 1955; Pavan, 1958, 1959, 1965*a,b*; Pavan and da Cunha, 1968, 1969*a,b*), Crouse and Keyl (1968), Crouse (1968), Gall (1968, 1969), Pardue *et al.* (1970), Eckhardt and Gall (1971), Bayreuther (1952, 1956, 1957), Lima-de-Faria and co-workers (Lima-de-Faria, 1959, 1962; Lima-de-Faria and Moses, 1966; Lima-de-Faria and Jaworska, 1968; Lima-de-Faria *et al.*, 1969), Bier *et al.* (1967), and Dickson *et al.* (1971). *For vertebrates see:* Greig-Holmes and Shaw (1971), Mendelsohn *et al.* (1973), Turpin and Lejeune (1965), Pelc (1972, and earlier papers), Viola-Magni (1965), Malvaldi and Viola-Magni (1972), Miller (1964, 1966), Brown and Dawid (1968 and other works), and Sharman, (1970). *For plants see:* Siegel *et al.* (1973), Evans (1956), Avanzi *et al.* (1970), and Nagl (1972). *For ciliates see:* Ammermann (1971), Alonso and Perez-Silva (1966*a,b*), and Gil *et al.* (1972).

days in *R. angelae,* with an intense synthesis of RNA and considerable accumulation of cytoplasmic materials (Basile, 1966, 1970). Pavan and da
Cunha (1969a) suggested that possibly something akin to the DNA puffs
of the salivary gland chromosomes may occur in the spermatocyte chromosomes, resulting in their alteration. This differentiation would provide
for the elimination process. These changes could be in the heterochromatin, which is apparently the region responsible for selective segregation
of the chromosomes of *S. coprophila,* as shown by Crouse (1960). DNA
puffs are such common events in Sciaridae during active phases of cell
physiology that there may be chromosomal differentiation resulting from
an extra increase in DNA in specific loci in the spermatocytes as in
salivary gland chromosomes (Breuer and Pavan, 1955; Ficq and Pavan,
1957; Rudkin and Corlette, 1957; Swift, 1962; Gabrusewycz-Garcia,
1964; Perondini, 1968). The DNA puff in the nucleolar organizer region
(NOR) of the oöcytes of amphibia and the unstable redundancy of the
genes in the bobbed loci of *Drosophila melanogaster* (Ritossa, 1968; Ritossa and Scala, 1969) lend some support to the supposition that a
structural differentiation of the chromosome may occur during germline
development. Crouse (1960, 1969) suggested that by passage through the
male germline a chromosome acquires an "imprint" which will delineate
it from the chromosomes of maternal origin in the embryo. Pavan and da
Cunha (1969a) speculated, as mentioned above, that this chromosomal
differentiation (Crouse's imprinting) was caused by the high activity of the
chromosomes during spermatogenesis. This would imply some regulating
mechanism (it could be a protein regulator, but it is more probably a nucleic acid change) which would be determined by the sex of the germline
through which it passed. Brown and Chandra (1973) recently proposed a
model to explain inactivation of one X chromosome in mammalians. This
model, based on the location of a "sensitive" site and a "receptor" site on
the same or different chromosomes, could account for the data on mammalian cytogenetics. In Sciaridae the situation seems to be more complicated than in mammalians since one must consider cases in which only the
L chromosomes are selectively eliminated (first elimination), others in
which one or two of the three X chromosomes are eliminated (second
elimination), and still others in which the entire set of paternal chromosomes are eliminated (meiosis I) (Figure 1). Furthermore, in *S.
ocellaris,* as was discussed above, there is the added complication of the
differentiated X chromosome (X′) which would have a behavior different
from that of the undifferentiated X (X). Exceptional males in an expected
female-descendent progeny produce only male progeny, regardless of the
female type to which they are crossed. When these various eliminations
are considered as a whole, the picture looks extremely complicated.

However, the understanding of a single elimination event would perhaps provide a basis for the understanding of others, then eventually the total picture of chromosomal behavior in different organisms.

The Species of *Rhynchosciara*

Nomenclature

The genus *Rhynchosciara* of the Sciaridae family was established by Rübsaamen in 1894, although species which are now included within this genus had already been described in 1821 as *Sciara* by Wiedemann (for example, the species described as *Sciara americana* by Wiedemann is now considered *Rhynchosciara americana*). Breuer (1969), in her excellent review of the genus *Rhynchosciara,* lists ten described and confirmed species, one undescribed species, and four which were described in the last century but which could not be examined and hence could not be affirmed as to the validity of their identification. There are presently at least eleven valid species of *Rhynchosciara.* The first *Rhynchosciara* species described were identified through use of adult specimens collected in nature, preserved, and kept in museum collections. Nonato and Pavan (1951) described *R. angelae,* which was collected in nature as larvae. Dreyfus *et al.* (1951) described for the first time the biology of the flies and made various studies on *R. angelae.* Since then, several species have been collected in nature as larvae, and their behavior and chromosomes have been studied. Breuer (1969), in her review of the genus, concluded that *R. angelae* Nonato and Pavan 1951 is identical to *R. americana* Wiedemann 1821. Although the opinion of Breuer is greatly respected, new data raise some doubts as to her interpretation. Since many papers have already been published using the name *R. angelae,* it seems more appropriate to maintain this name for the present rather than to rename the species, then perhaps later to have to return to the original nomenclature should *R. americana* and *R. angelae* prove to be different species.

Collection

Species of *Rhynchosciara* have been collected in many places in the Americas, from Argentina to Mexico. Some species are common in southern Brazil, in lowlands near the coast of São Paulo and Rio de Janeiro. Other species have been collected at altitudes exceeding 2000 m in Monte Verde and Itatiaia between São Paulo and Minas Gerais (Morgante, 1972). In nature, *Rhynchosciara* can be collected in either the egg, larval, pupal, or adult stage.

R. milleri Pavan and Breuer 1955 has been found near the coast in the state of São Paulo, Brazil and has also been collected in San Remo, La Merced County, Peru, at altitudes ranging from 1500 to 2000 m by Dr. Misael Guevara and members of his laboratory at the University of San Marcos, Lima, Peru. In July, 1972, one of us (Pavan) with Professor Pedro Nuñez (Universidade Nacional del Ecuador) found several thousand adults of an unidentified species of *Rhynchosciara* in inflorescences of *Bacharis polyanta,* a Compositae common around Quito, Ecuador.

Morgante (1972) made a systematic collection of *Rhynchosciara* in several different sites on the coast of the state of São Paulo, Brazil, between 1970 and 1972. He found that the most common species there is *R. angelae,* which occurs in highest frequencies during the period between September and January (December being the month in which his data showed the greatest number of groups collected) and lowest frequencies during the period from February to June. The most convenient sources of *Rhynchosciara* are the banana plantations along the coast of São Paulo and Rio de Janeiro. Several groups have also been collected in the forested regions and in areas cleared for agricultural purposes. Groups of *Rhynchosciara* are common where species of *Tradescantia* or *Ipomoea* (sweet potato) are found. In Morgante's study, the concentration of larvae varied from only a few to over 900 groups per area examined, each group consisting of 100–500 individuals. Both bisexual and unisexual groups have been found in nature, with the bisexual groups usually containing more larvae than the unisexual. Since females of *R. angelae* which are raised in the laboratory always produce unisexual progeny and since the bisexual groups are usually larger, Morgante attributed their bisexuality to a simple mixing of groups derived from different females.

Laboratory Culture

Species of *Rhynchosciara* can survive on many different types of food; however, two types of food are most commonly employed for the laboratory culture of *R. angelae* and *R. hollaenderi*. *R. angelae* thrives best on a medium composed primarily of the leaves of the sweet potato, *Ipomoea batata,* as described by Lara *et al.* (1965) and Morgante *et al.* (1970). For *R. hollaenderi* the preferred food is based on the commerically available Purina CSMA Fly Larval Media (Ralston-Purina Company), in a recipe which was developed around 1969 by Eckhardt while working with Mattingly and Ogle (1969) at the Biology Division of the Oak Ridge National Laboratory [see also Papaconstantinou *et al.* (1972)]. A complete description of the preparation of these two culture media is given below and is based on published and unpublished work of individuals mentioned above as well as on the experience gained in our laboratories. While *R. angelae* larvae do not breed well on a Purina "Fly Chow" diet, *R. hollaenderi* larvae survive excellently on either "Fly Chow" or sweet potato diets. With the exception of the type of food used, all techniques for the successful culturing of both species are identical.

Adult flies can be collected in nature or obtained from puparia of laboratory cultures. These adults are placed in "mating chambers," which in our laboratory are plastic or wooden boxes, 15 × 15 × 30 cm, covered with a thin glass or plastic plate. The bottom of the box is covered with a fairly shallow layer of moist sand or soil. Moisture is of vital importance because the flies are detrimentally affected by low humidity. Damp osmunda (purchased in any plant nursery) is placed at one end of the box as a substrate in which the females can oviposit their eggs. A one-to-one sex ratio of flies is mixed in the chambers; eggs are collected when all flies are dead. These eggs, which are in clusters of up to two thousand, are kept on Petri dishes with a thin layer of 2–2.5 percent agar until hatching. Should fungi, bacteria, or nematodes appear, the eggs must be transferred to new agar plates.

Embryogenesis requires 10–12 days at 20–22°C. The day before the larvae are due to hatch, the eggs acquire a dark coloration, due to the pigmentation of the larval head and mouthparts. All the larvae of a group normally hatch simultaneously, with a less than 1 percent failure to hatch in good cultures. Each group of larvae should be transferred to new agar plates immediately upon hatching. Since larvae still have yolk stored in their intestines after hatching, no food is necessary for several hours, but food should be given when the yolk disappears. Fermented food should not be put in direct contact with eggs which are ready to hatch because it appears that doing so causes the death of large numbers of newly hatched larvae. Newly hatched larvae often do not find food unless it is in their path of travel; thus, best results are obtained when the food is scattered in a 1- to 2-cm-radius circle around the hatching group.

Larval groups are most sensitive to adverse conditions during the first ten days of life. It is, therefore, advisable to take great care in preventing poor culture conditions from occurring (such as contaminations by fungi, bacteria, or nematodes).

Larvae may be kept on 100- × 25-mm plastic Petri dishes with a thin layer of 2–2.5 percent agar to maintain sufficient moisture until 10–15 days of age, but to ensure maximum growth of the group, they should be transferred to larger containers which also have a layer of agar. Such containers may be 150- × 25-mm plastic petri dishes (Mattingly and Ogle, 1969) or 150- × 65-mm aluminum dishes with plastic covers, which are easily found in variety stores. In our laboratory the aluminum dishes are preferred since they can be sterilized and reused.

Bacterial contaminations can be eliminated by the selective use of antibiotics (see below). Bad fungal infections are rare and can be prevented by frequent transfer of the larvae to new, sterilized plates and, if necessary, by the daily replacement of all food. Nematodes often appear on the eggs; they can be done away with by placing a drop of 3 percent H_2O_2 on the affected group of eggs and allowing them to dry (method suggested by S. Ogle). The frequency with which the food should be changed depends on the health, size, and age of the cultures; however, for best results, it should be replaced at least twice a week. Cultures should always be transferred to clean dishes upon any sign of nematodes, bacteria, fungi, or large amounts of excrement. In heavy infestations of nematodes, the larvae should be isolated from as much food as possible and then washed thoroughly in running tap water. This is most easily accomplished by using a regular tea strainer, and for very young larvae, a tea strainer lined with a single layer of nylon mesh (old hose is excellent for this purpose). It is not uncommon in large cultures for a few larvae to die; the dead larvae should be removed to avoid infections of the cultures. Although larvae may be maintained on these dishes until eclosion of the adults, it is preferable to remove them when forming their incipient net and to place them on a dish containing only a small square of blotting paper on the top of a thin layer of moist sand or soil.

The flies should be placed in mating chambers immediately after eclosion. No food is necessary since the adults do not eat; however, there should be a small vial containing a dilute sucrose solution with a bibulous paper wick from which the flies can get water. Although the water is not essential, it has been found that the adults consume it when present and that it prolongs the life of the unmated flies when mating is delayed.

One may place 40–100 flies in the mating chambers in sex ratios dependent on the proportions of flies available. Females normally will lay their eggs within cavities formed by the fibers of the osmunda or beneath the osmunda on the moist sand. Adults, which live from 5 to 7 days, are left in the chambers until all are dead. The eggs are then collected, and the process described is repeated for this generation of eggs.

As has been mentioned, the bottoms of the Petri and aluminum dishes are covered with a thin layer of 2–2.5 percent agar to maintain the humidity. To reduce the incidence of bacterial and fungal contamination, it is recommended that the agar should contain an antibiotic and a mold inhibitor. In our laboratory, 227 μg of methyl-p-hydroxybenzoate ("Tegosept") and 110 μg oxytetracycline (Terramycin; Pfizer) per gram of agar solution are routinely added to the agar immediately before pouring into the plates or dishes.

Rhynchosciara females produce unisexual progenies; theoretically, the cultures of the two sexes should occur with equal frequency in the laboratory. However, for some reason yet to be determined, the cultures sometimes are predominantly composed of flies of only one sex. Should groups of a single sex emerge out of phase with groups of the other sex, problems may arise since they may not survive long enough to be mated with flies which eclose later. To avoid this problem, it is convenient to mix male and female larvae when they are 20–30 days of age and allot these groups for breeding purposes only. If the age difference between the groups being mixed is no more than one week, the larvae will synchronize their development and all will pupate and eclose simultaneously. An alternative to mixing larvae is to put the newly eclosed adults at 4°C, at which temperature they have been found to survive for several days.

Sex of the larvae may be determined in several ways. The males are smaller and more active than the females. When disturbed, the males move rapidly in their gregarious cluster, while the females move rather sluggishly or calmly about. Larvae may also be sexed by dissection of the gonads after 20 days of larval development (Basile, 1966). Cytological preparations will reveal whether the gonad is an ovary or a testis; however, the testis is larger than the ovary, and by comparing the sizes of the gonads of larvae of similar age, sex can be determined by size differences. The gonads are located in the last quarter of the larva in the area of the fat body, approximately at the same level as the insertion of the Malpighian tubules. Both are spindle-shaped, with the ovary being thinner relative to length than the testis. By 30 days of age the testis is as much as 3–5 times the length of the ovary. The larvae being tested should be placed living in a drop of 3 : 1 (ethanol : glacial acetic acid) fixative, then very carefully dissected on a longitudinal axis. If the fat bodies are gently teased away from the carcass, the gonads can be found suspended on thin fibers. The 3 : 1 fixative renders the normally translucent gonads opaque and thus easily visualized.

Preparation of Food

Sweet Potato Food. Leaves of the sweet potato (*Ipomoea batata*) are collected after tuber harvest, dried, powdered, and stored at room temperature in large plastic bags. The powder can be stored in this form for months to years and used when necessary. The food is prepared by putting several pounds of the powder into plastic bags, then water is added until the powder is thoroughly wetted. This is then fermented (using the microorganisms described below) by incubation at room temperature, or for best results at 32–35°C, for 2–10 days. Excess moisture after fermentation is removed by the addition of fresh, dry powder. The fermented food to be given to the larvae should be distinctly moist but never wet. Once fermented, the food can be stored at 4°C for several months. Morgante *et al.* (1970) isolated microorganisms from larvae collected in nature. These were cultured in the laboratory and used for fermentation of the food. Dr. M. Miranda of the Institute of Biophysics, University of Rio de Janeiro, also isolated microorganisms which have been used for fermentation. This food is used to raise *R. angelae, R. hollaenderi, R. milleri,* and *R. baschanti.* An undescribed species which was collected at Monte Verde, Minas Gerais, Brazil, does not thrive on this medium.

Fly Chow. This food is prepared from a commercial base which is easily available and gives excellent results in the breeding of *R. hollaenderi.* The following recipe was kindly supplied by Ms. S. Ogle of the Biology Division at Oak Ridge National Laboratory (Oak Ridge, Tennessee): 350g Fly chow (Purina CSMA medium), 750 ml water, 240 mg Terramycin (Pfizer), 5 ml Tegosept (10 percent solution in 95 percent ethanol, and 17g brewers' yeast. The water is warmed to 40°C; the yeast, mold inhibitor (Tegosept), and Terramycin are added and stirred thoroughly. The Purina medium is then added and the mixture is fermented for 6 hours at 37°C. If the food is too wet, a bit of dry fly medium may be mixed to obtain the desired moisture. Food which is not used within 24 hours should be discarded.

The Biology of *Rhynchosciara*

Introduction

R. angelae and *R. hollaenderi* are the two most-studied species of *Rhynchosciara*; therefore, their biology will be examined and compared.

Adults of *R. hollaenderi* are generally smaller than those of *R. angelae.* Nonato and Pavan (1951) obtained the following measurements for the adults of *R. angelae*: females have a body length of 7–10 mm and a wingspread of 7–12 mm; males have a body length of 6–8 mm and a wingspread of 6–10 mm. Breuer (1969) obtained the following corresponding measurements for *R. hollaenderi* (described as *Rhynchosciara* species in her paper): females have a body length of 6–7 mm and a wingspread of 7–8 mm; males have a body length of 5–6 mm and a wingspread of 6.5–7 mm. It should be noted, however, that these measurements were taken from flies raised in the laboratory, which frequently are smaller than those captured in nature. No data are currently available on adult flies of *R. hollaenderi* collected in nature. There are some differences in the head and genitalia of the two species; otherwise, the adults of the two are so similar as to be difficult to distinguish. The biology and behavior of the two species are quite similar, as will be seen below.

Development

The gonads of adult *Rhynchosciara* emerging from their puparia are already mature. In the ovaries, all the eggs are at an identical stage of development; oogenesis is almost complete, with no new eggs being produced after eclosion (Basile, 1969). The female may be fertilized soon after eclosing from the puparium, in many cases while they are still brownish, an intermediate body color which lasts 1–2 hours before they attain the black color characteristic of known species of *Rhynchosciara*. In the male, spermatogenesis is also almost complete before eclosion, and in the testes only spermatozoid cells and some gland cells are found (Basile, 1970).

After fertilization, the females oviposit all their eggs in a single operation. The eggs remain attached to one another by a type of glue which covers the surface of each egg. Females undisturbed during oviposition will yield groups of eggs totaling 500–1500 individuals. The number of eggs produced by any one female is largely dependent on the conditions in which she lived as a larva. Females raised in poor conditions often produce 500 or fewer eggs. With optimum conditions during development, each female will produce 1000–1500 eggs. A female will on very rare occasions lay several small groups of eggs; on the other hand, it is not at all unusual to find either in nature or in the laboratory two or more females which have oviposited in the same location, giving origin to a very large group of mixed larvae.

Eggs are fertilized during passage down the oviduct and are all laid in a single process lasting 20–60 minutes; consequently the maximum difference in the ages of the first and last eggs to be fertilized in any one group is no more than about one hour. The fertilized eggs develop synchronously, and the larvae hatch practically simultaneously after 8–10 days. These larvae have a gregarious behavior and develop synchronously as a group for 45–50 days. During the entire larval stage, all the larvae of a group have the same chronological and physiological age, are in the same stage of development, and have the same sex; thus, a group of these larvae behave in many ways as though it were a single organism instead of hundreds of individuals. Analysis of a few larvae from such a group is sufficient to determine the stage of development and sex of the entire group. Periodic sampling of individuals permits an accurate study of the developmental changes of the entire group. Throughout larval development, all the larvae remain in direct contact with one another, move together, feed on the same food, and are subject to the same environmental conditions. Though one or two larvae are often found isolated from the group, they are usually found to be sick and die within a few days. All the individuals of a healthy group of larvae are performing the same function at the same time; such behavior raises intriguing questions concerning the genetic basis of behavior and could possibly be a valuable source for studies in behavioral genetics.

There are three larval molts and one pupal molt in *R. angelae* and *R. hollaenderi*. In *R. angelae* maintained at 20–22°C the first larval molt occurs between days 6 and 7, the second between days 12 and 13, the third between days 20 and 21 (Guaraciaba and Toledo, 1967; Morgante and Guevara, 1969; Morgante, 1972; Terra, 1972). The molts in *R. hollaenderi* roughly correspond to those of *R. angelae* (Mattingly and Parker, 1968). The entire larval development may be altered by various environmental factors, e.g., temperature, food, and humidity. Larvae cultured at 15°C have a larval life of over twice the length of those raised at 20–22°C. Poorly fermented food and too high or low humidity may appreciably alter the developmental time.

The fourth instar, which occurs in the interval between day 20 or 21 and the pupal molt, is the longest instar, during which important developmental changes in larval life occur. This instar lasts 30–35 days in both species of *Rhynchosciara* considered. On approximately the 28th to 30th day of the fourth instar (48–50 days of age), the larvae cease eating, leave their food, move sluggishly about, and eventually stop and initiate a temporary "net" (a mucopolysaccharide web) which loosely covers the entire group. This common, temporary cocoon is often disrupted and abandoned by the larvae who begin moving again before reinitiating pupation. Pupation may be delayed by disrupting the net of the temporary cocoon. If a group is divided in half, and one half is repeatedly disrupted while the other is allowed to proceed normally, pupation of the disrupted group may be delayed well past the time that the undisturbed group has eclosed. The delayed group may finally go into pupation and produce normal adults. Although it is known that pupation is regulated by hormones, in the case of *Rhynchosciara* there appears to be some correlation between the cessation of larval movement and the release of hormone.

Early in the elaboration of the definitive puparial net, the larvae become packed together without evident order. Two or three days after movement cessation, the larvae adopt a U shape and begin production of dividing walls which give origin to individual cells for each pupa. Two or three days after this, the larvae straighten and become distended within their individual cells. The puparium usually looks strikingly similar to the honeycombs of bees, with the pupae arranged parallel to one another.

Eclosion, as with the rest of development, is synchronous. When an imago is ready to emerge, it begins to move, which seems to arouse neighboring imagoes and eventually the entire puparium. Though synchrony of eclosion is also susceptible to the environmental conditions, generally, it appears that most of the imagoes emerge within the space of a few hours.

Terra (1972) analyzed the biochemical composition of the hemolymph and cocoon net of *R. angelae* (which was classified by that author as *R. americana*; see previous argument concerning nomenclature). He found that toward the end of cocoon formation the dry part of the net is composed primarily of protein (38 percent), calcium carbonate (43.5 percent), and carbohydrate (10.6 percent). The net was found to be formed by activity of the salivary glands in probable combination with the Malpighian tubules and intestine. The net is a special kind of silk secreted by the salivary gland and an excrementlike material rich in $CaCO_3$ which is deposited within this silk net. The Malpighian tubules are rich in $CaCO_3$ during the major portion of larval life, particularly near pupation. This calcium carbonate is then secreted at the beginning of metamorphosis. Terra concluded that the $CaCO_3$ of the net originates in the Malpighian tubules. Part of the protein of the net is derived from material previously present in the hemolymph, while the carbohydrate constituents of the net probably originate in the fat bodies.

At least one mutant is known in each of the species of *Rhynchosciara* considered here. The mutant "limão" (lemon) of *R. angelae* was found by Basile *et al.* (1970) to be a sex-linked recessive allele. Interestingly, a similar lemon mutant occurs in *R. hollaenderi*; however, by contrast, this mutant appears not to be recessive, since heterozygotes are intermediate in coloration; sex linkage has not been established. Crouse (1943) mentioned a yellow mutant in *S. reynoldsi*; Crouse and Smith-Stocking (1938), Davidheiser (1943), and Perondini (private communication) have observed a similar mutant in *S. ocellaris*; both mutants are sex-linked and recessive.

Chromosomes of *Rhynchosciara*

As in other aspects of the biology of *R. angelae* and *R. hollaenderi*, the shape of the mitotic chromosomes is identical in the two species and the shape, banding, and puffing patterns of the polytene chromosomes are nearly so. Both *R. angelae* and *R. hollaenderi* have four polytene chromosomes, designated A, B, C, and X, which correspond to the eight female or seven male mitotic chromosomes of the diploid somatic tissues (Dreyfus *et al.*, 1951).

The map of the polytene chromosomes (Figure 2), made originally for *R. angelae,* can be used to identify and examine the chromosomes of *R. hollaenderi* (Figures 3 and 4). The main differences in the polytene chromosomes of the two species are as follows: Chromosome A of

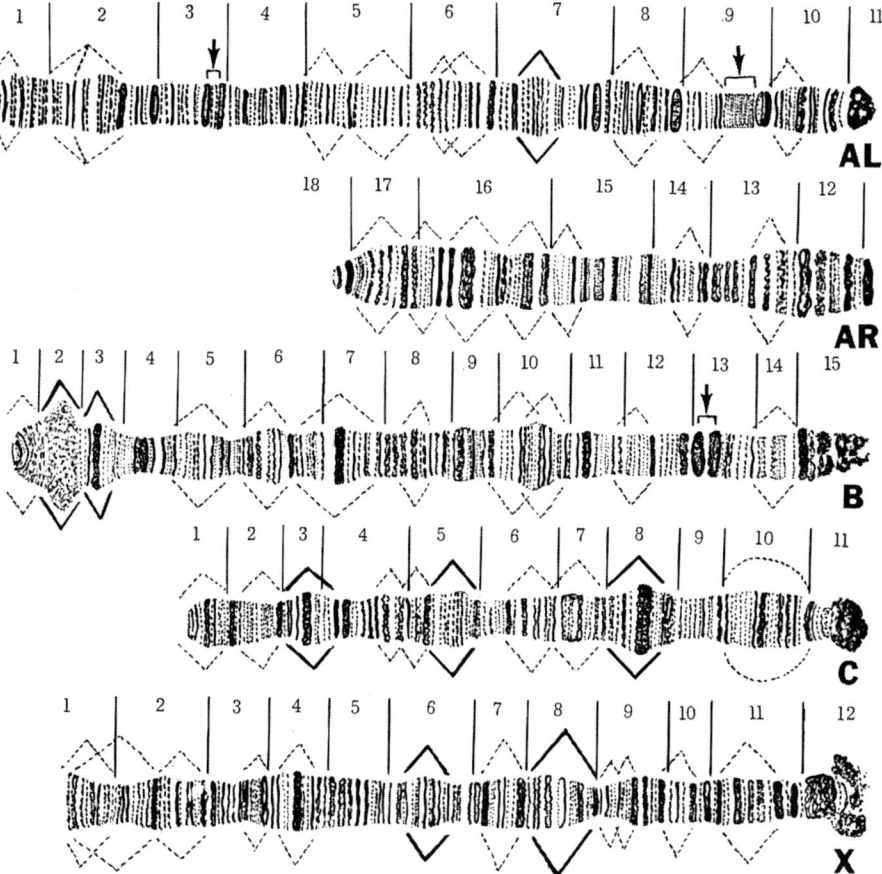

Figure 2. Camera lucida drawings of salivary gland polytene chromosomes of R. angelae adapted from the original drawings of M. E. Breuer (1967). The division of the chromosomes into several sections is also from her original maps. The vertical lines represent points of division. The figure also shows sites of puffing (angular lines along the chromosome) as well as approximate sizes of the puffs described by Guaraciaba and Toledo (1968). The broken angles represent sites of the RNA puffs; the unbroken angles (section 7 of chromosome A; 2 and 3 of chromosome B; 3, 5, and 8 of chromosome C; and 6 and 8 of chromosome X) represent sites of the DNA puffs described by Guevara (1971) (see Figures 7–10). The arrows in chromosomes A and B indicate landmarks of these chromosomes, typical in both R. angelae and R. hollaenderi.

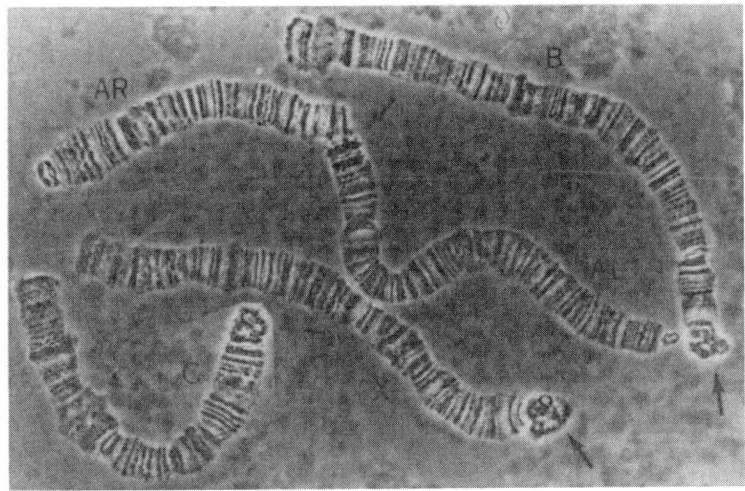

Figure 3. Photomicrograph of a chromosomal complement of the salivary glands of fourth-instar R. hollaenderi larvae. Note landmarks of each chromosome and similarities with those corresponding to complement of R. angelae (as described in text). Arrows indicate centromeric heterochromatin. Ectopic pairing between bands of sections 3 and 7 of chromosome X is common but not present in this case (see Figure 6).

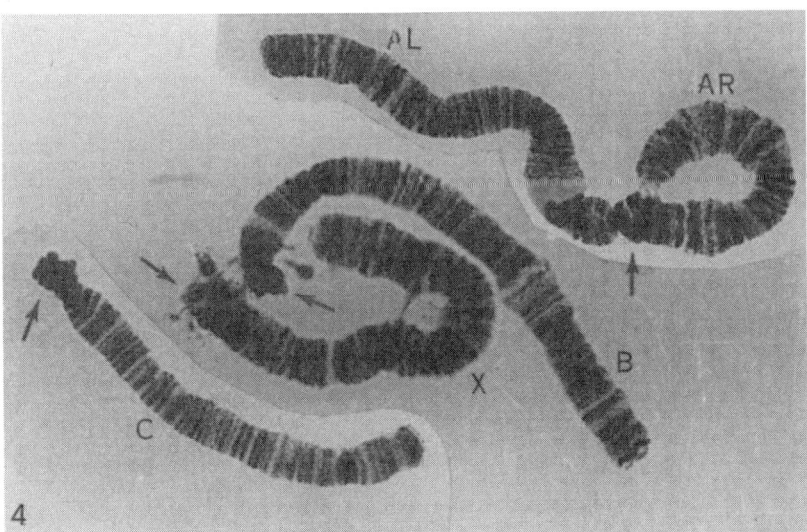

Figure 4. Photomicrograph of a chromosomal complement of the salivary glands of fourth-instar R. angelae larvae. Note landmarks of each chromosome and similarities with those corresponding to complement of R. hollaenderi (as described in text). Note, also, the ectopic pairing between bands of sections 3 and 7 of chromosome X and between the tip and the centromeric heterochromatin of chromosome A. Arrows indicate centromeric heterochromatin.

R. hollaenderi has a centromeric constriction which segregates the AR arm from the AL arm (Figure 3). Chromosome B of *R. hollaenderi* has ectopic pairing between the heterochromatic bands of regions 13 and 15 with greater frequency than in *R. angelae*. Section 1, the telomeric tip of chromosome B in *R. hollaenderi,* also has a thick heterochromatic band which may be fragmented into several spherical granules (Figures 5b and c). A puff in the tip of chromosome B of *R. hollaenderi* is so characteristic of this species that it is the best means of distinguishing the two species chromosomally. Chromosome C is quite similar in the two species, with *R. hollaenderi* having a thick heterochromatic band in the telomeric region (Section 1) (Figures 3 and 4). Chromosome X has great similarity in the two species (Figures 3, 4, and 6). In summation, the evident differences between the polytene chromosomes of *R. angelae* and *R. hollaenderi* are the presence of a centromeric constriction of chromosome A and the thick heterochromatic bands in the telomeric regions of AR, chromosome B, and chromosome C in *R. hollaenderi* (Figures 3 and 4).

Two chromosomal inversions are known in the chromosomes of *R. hollaenderi,* one in chromosome C (Simões, 1967, 1970; Mattingly and Parker, 1968) and one in chromosome B (Pavan, unpublished). The inversion in chromosome C was present in strains which were originally

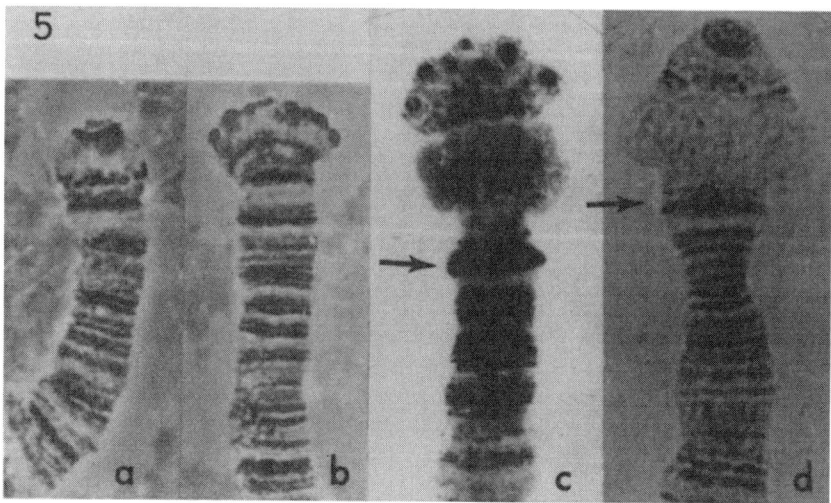

Figure 5. Photomicrograph of the tip of chromosome B (sections 1–6) of R. angelae (a and d) and R. hollaenderi (b and c). Here a and b are from larvae of the fourth instar; c and d are from prepupae with DNA puff B_2. The granular tip, shown in b and c, is typical of chromosome B of R. hollaenderi. Arrows in c and d indicate DNA puff B_3 which has a large accumulation in R. hollaenderi but little in R. angelae.

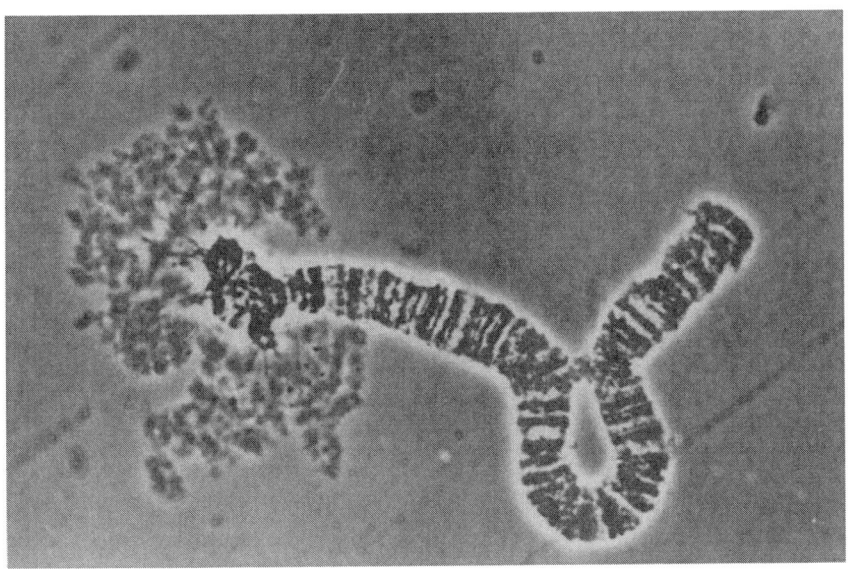

Figure 6. Photomicrograph of chromosome X of R. hollaenderi, showing a well-developed nucleolus with DNA fibers irradiating from the nucleolar organizer region. Note, also, the ectopic pairing between bands of sections 3 and 7.

collected from nature in 1965 and has been maintained since in laboratory strains. Extensive analyses of many strains of *R. angelae* have never revealed the existence of inversions.

Polytene chromosomes are found in many larval tissues, with their polyteny varying from 8 or 16 strands to 16,000. The degree of polyteny depends on the organ under consideration, the age of the larva, and the environmental conditions to which the larva was subjected. Larvae raised at 15–17°C generally attain greater larval sizes than those raised at 20–22°C, with the sizes of the chromosomes and, consequently, of their puffs, correspondingly larger. Table 1 tentatively summarizes estimations of the variations in degree of polyteny as determined by size comparisons in several larval tissues.

Each salivary gland of *R. angelae* and *R. hollaenderi* is about 2 cm long. Pavan (1965*a*) defined three sections for *R. angelae* glands: S_1 corresponds to the proximal quarter of the gland, where two opposing rows of rather thick cells form a crescent envelopment around the lumen of the gland; S_2 includes the middle half of the gland, has a lumen which is greater in diameter than in the other two regions, and is surrounded by a layer of flat cells; S_3 corresponds to the distal quarter of the gland and has a double row of cells surrounding the lumen in an alternating pattern dis-

TABLE 1.   *Variations in Degree of Polyteny*

Tissue	Degree of Polyteny
Fat bodies	8–64 strands
Muscle cells	8–128 (possibly 256)
Anterior mid-gut (large cells)	512–1,024
Malpighian tubules	
proximal	512–1,024
distal	128–512
Salivary glands[a]	
S_1	8–16,000
S_2	4–8,000
S_3	4–8,000

[a] See text for explanation of the salivary gland nomenclature.

tribution. Proximal to the S_1 region there is a layer of relatively small cells enveloping the excretory tube which have chromosomes with a low degree of polyteny. The polytene chromosomes of S_1 are the largest of normal *Rhynchosciara* larvae and among the largest known in Diptera. Although no direct measurements have been made of the degree of polyteny in *Rhynchosciara*, comparison of these with those of known size—4096 in *Sciara coprophila* (Swift, 1962) and approximately 16,000 in *Chironomus* (Edström, 1964)—have shown that the polytene chromosomes of S_1 may reach about 16,000 strands. S_2 and S_3 have a lower level of polyteny, about 4–8000. It is of interest to note that while differences in strand number between the three sections exist, no differences in puffing pattern have been found. There is, however, a gradient of puff development starting in S_3 and progressing through S_2 to S_1. Thus, puffing progresses as a wave from S_3 to S_2 to S_1, with S_3 normally remaining in a slightly more advanced stage of puff development than the two proximal sections.

Chromocenters formed by pericentromeric heterochromatin attachments are exhibited only in cells which have a low degree of polyteny, such as salivary glands of young larvae and the Malpighian tubules, intestine, and other tissues of mature larvae. A chromocenter is usually absent in the salivary gland chromosomes of fourth-instar larvae, with individual chromosomes being separate. Two or three chromosomes are sometimes linked by pericentric heterochromatin; however, the association is generally quite weak.

For the beginner, the best method to distinguish the four chromosomes is by making a cytological preparation of a small section of the S_1 region of the salivary gland. The cells should be separated in the fixative prior to squashing, but care should be taken to maintain the integrity of individual nuclei. In this way, the chromosomal set of a single nucleus may be compared and identified. Chromosome A is the longest of the four chromosomes, has a heterochromatic region located in the mid-portion of the chromosome (section 11 of Figure 2), and is divided into 18 sections (Breuer, 1967). The landmarks of chromosome A are the thick heterochromatic bands of sections 10, 11, and 12, the characteristic banding pattern of the two chromosomal tips, a lightly staining region associated with a thick band at the base of section 9 (arrow, Figure 2), and the two thick bands at the base of section 3 (arrow, Figure 2). The two arms of this chromosome have different lengths, AR being shorter than AL. Chromosome B is divided into 15 sections, has a typical heterochromatic base (section 15), a characteristic banding pattern at the distal tip, and two thick heterochromatic bands at the distal end of section 13 (arrow, Figure 2). Frequently, these two thick bands of region 13 may pair ectopically with section 15 or with the basal heterochromatin of other chromosomes. Chromosome C is the shortest of the set, has 11 sections, and may be distinguished by the banding pattern of the distal end and by the basal heterochromatin (Figure 2). Chromosome X is of the same size as chromosome B but can be easily distinguished by its basal heterochromatin, which represents a NOR and is sometimes banded; the X chromosome has 12 sections (Figure 2). The nucleolus of *Rhynchosciara* is well defined in the cells of the intestine and Malpighian tubules of young larvae, but becomes disperse in cells with higher polyteny. The basal tip of the heterochromatin of this chromosome is frequently spread. The two thick bands of the base of section 11 are also good landmarks for distinguishing between chromosomes X, B, and C. Ectopic pairing between some bands of section 3 and bands of section 7 occurs at a very high frequency.

The chromosomes are most easily identified when puffs are developed. Detailed studies of the puffs in *R. angelae* started with the work of Breuer and Pavan (1952, 1955) and Pavan and Breuer (1955). Subsequently, Guaraciaba and Toledo (1968) made a detailed study of the most conspicuous puffs of the S_1 section of the salivary glands of *R. angelae* during development. They described 18 large puffs in chromosome A, 11 in chromosome B, 10 in chromosome C, and 12 in chromosome X (Figures 7–10). Smaller puffs exist by the hundreds but were not considered by the authors. Guevara (1971) made a detailed comparative study of the puffs which occur in the polytene chromosomes from the salivary glands, Malpighian tubules, and intestine during larval development of *R. angelae*. Part of the results of that study are shown, courtesy of the author, in Figures 7–10. In addition to the hundreds of RNA puffs which occur in the chromosomes of those tissues during development, Guevara (1971) and Guevara and Basile (1973) described in detail ten DNA puffs which occur only in the chromosomes of the salivary glands. No DNA puffs were detectable in tissues other than the salivary glands. They described 1 DNA puff in chromosome A, 3 in chromosome B, 4 in chromosome C, and 2 in chromosome X (see Figures 2, 7–10). As shown by Breuer and Pavan (1955) and Pavan (1959), DNA puffs may result from the extra DNA synthesis either before or during puff expansion with concomitant intense RNA synthesis. In all cases the RNA is released from the chromosomes; however, the DNA is maintained in the puffed regions, giving rise to a thick band after puff regression. Of the ten DNA puffs which Guevara (1971) described, only two (B_3 and C_3) show an accumulation of DNA before puff expansion, while DNA accumulation in the other eight puffs occurs at different periods during puff expansion. All the DNA puffs occur in late fourth-instar larvae.

Genic and Chromosomal Activity

Introduction. Genic and chromosomal activity in polytene chromosomes are morphologically manifested as puffs at specific chromosomal loci. Puffing is common in cells with polytene chromosomes and has been known to occur since Balbiani described it in 1881. It was not until 1952 that the meaning of these events was discerned through the detailed study of their behavior during development in two independent investigations, in *Chironomus* (Beermann, 1952) and in *Rhynchosciara* (Breuer and Pavan, 1952, 1955). Since these initial studies, the literature and research done on the subject has been enormous. No attempt is made here to give anything more than a brief description of observations made in *Rhynchosciara*. [For reviews and references on genic activity in polytene chromosomes see Pavan and da Cunha (1969a), Ashburner (1970), and Beermann (1972).]

Puffing in *R. angelae* and *R. hollaenderi* is of two distinct types: RNA and DNA puffing. The RNA puffs apparently involve only uncoiling of DNA fibers and intensification of RNA synthesis. The size of the puffs is variable and depends on the degree of physiological activity as well as the amount of DNA in the puffed region, i.e., a small band cannot independently produce a large puff. Differential staining showed that RNA exists in the interband (Pavan and Breuer, 1955); however, no puff has yet been shown to occur in these regions. Pavan (1959) showed that puffs result from the uncoiling of DNA in a single band or group of adjacent bands.

DNA puffs are special types of puffs first described by Breuer and Pavan (1954, 1955) and Pavan and Breuer (1955) in *R. angelae*. In these

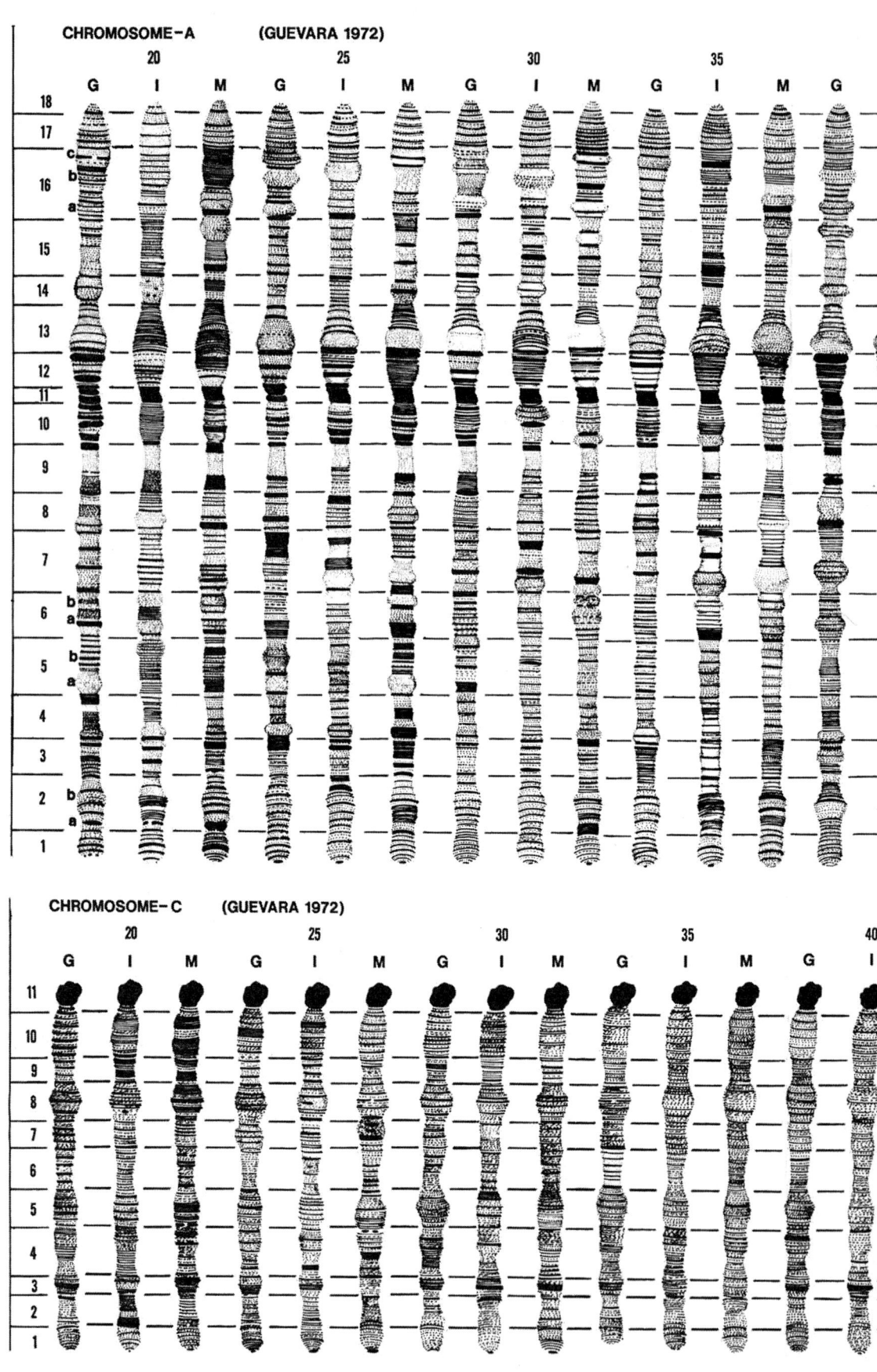

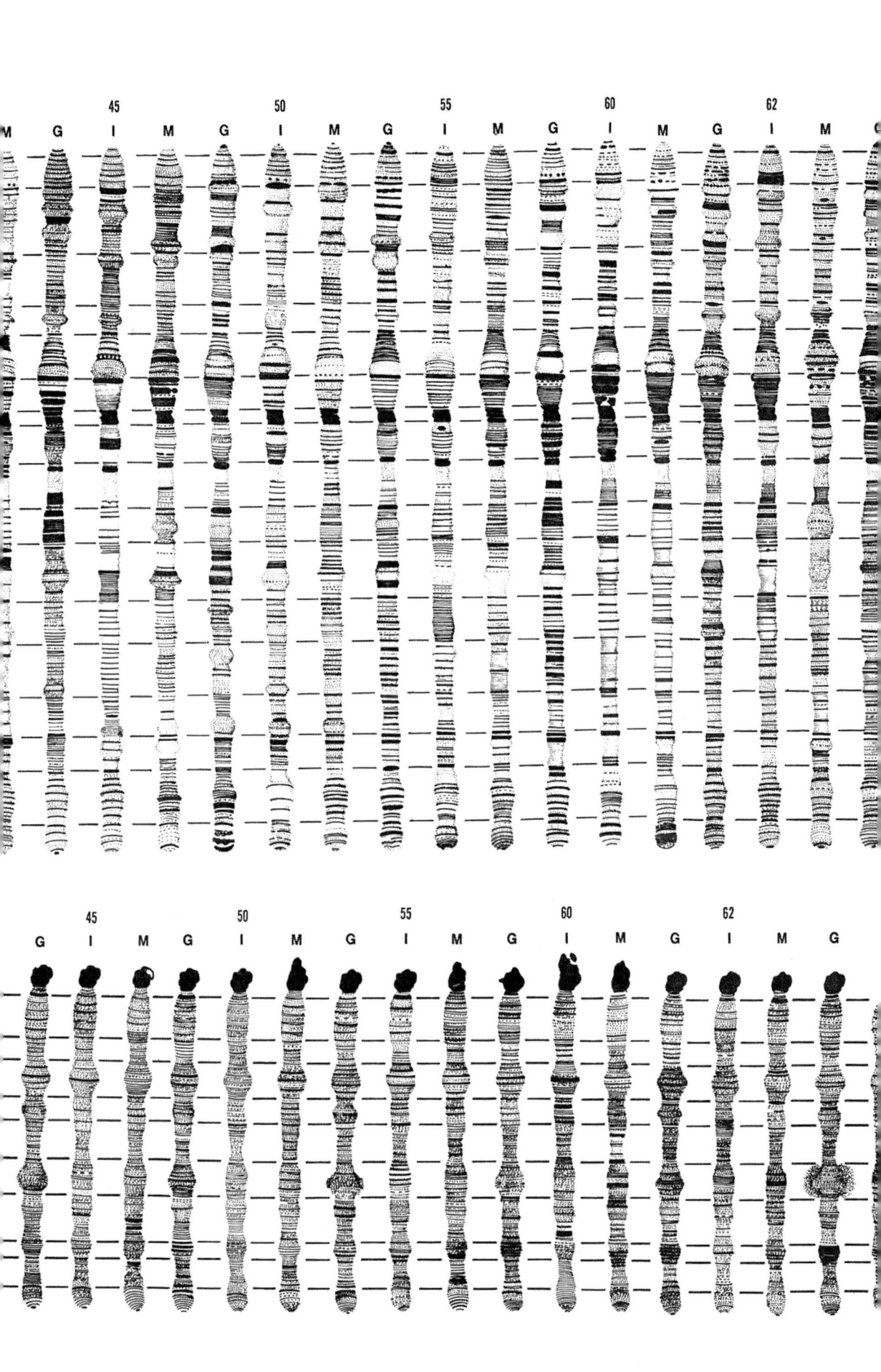

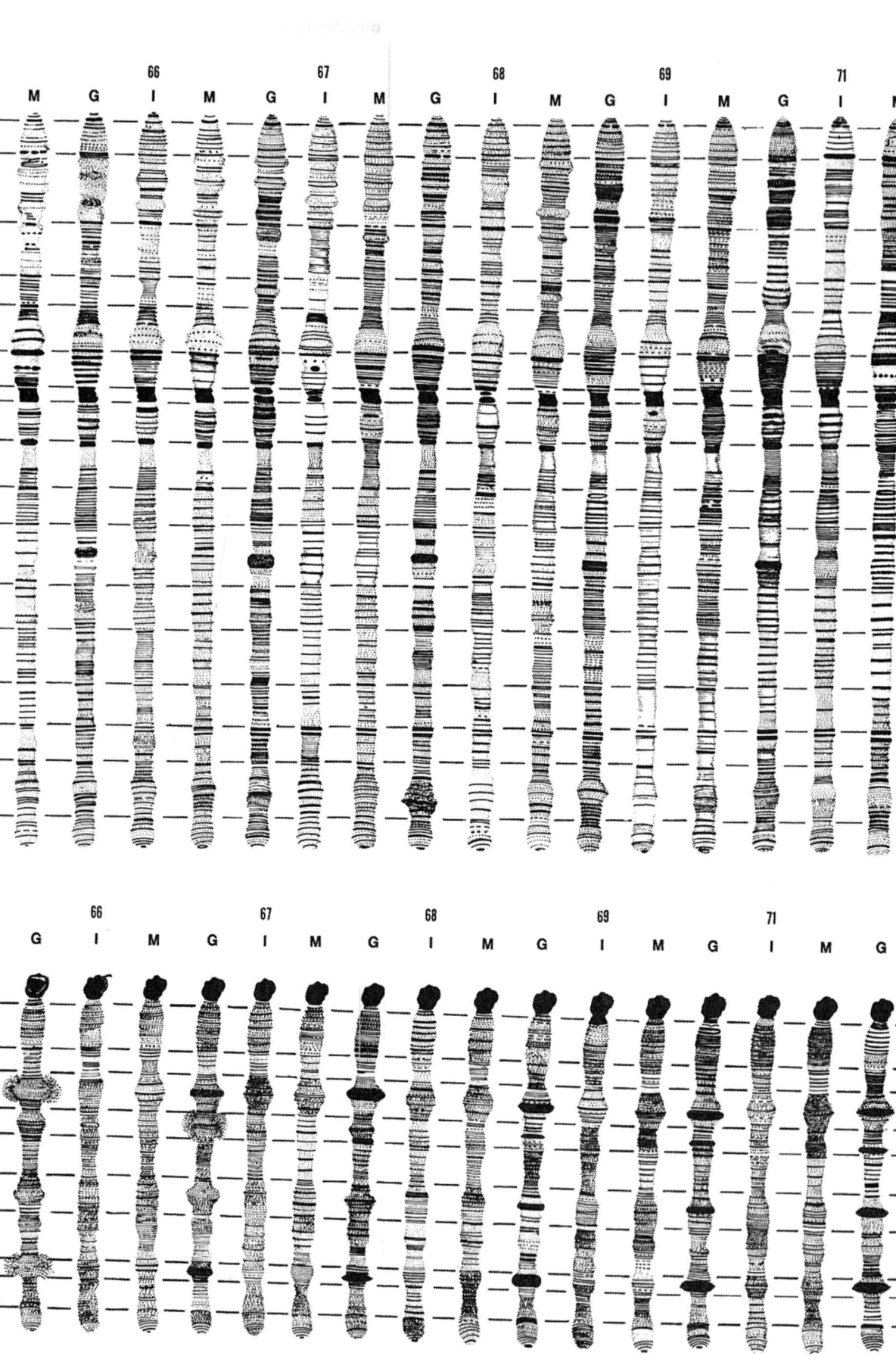

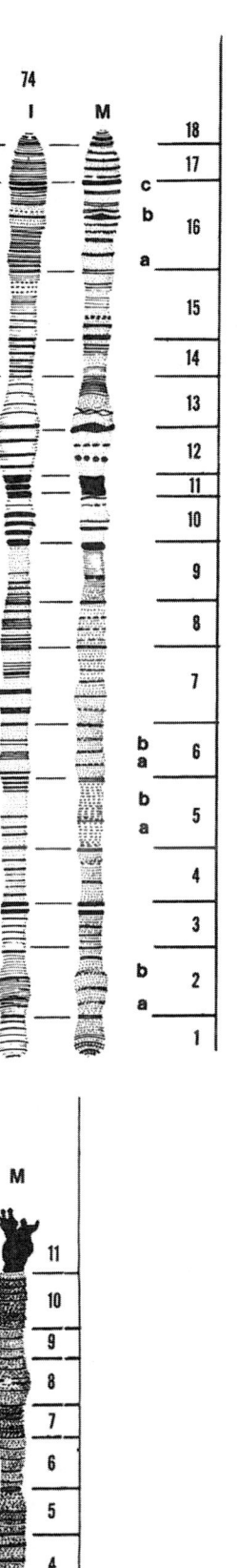

74

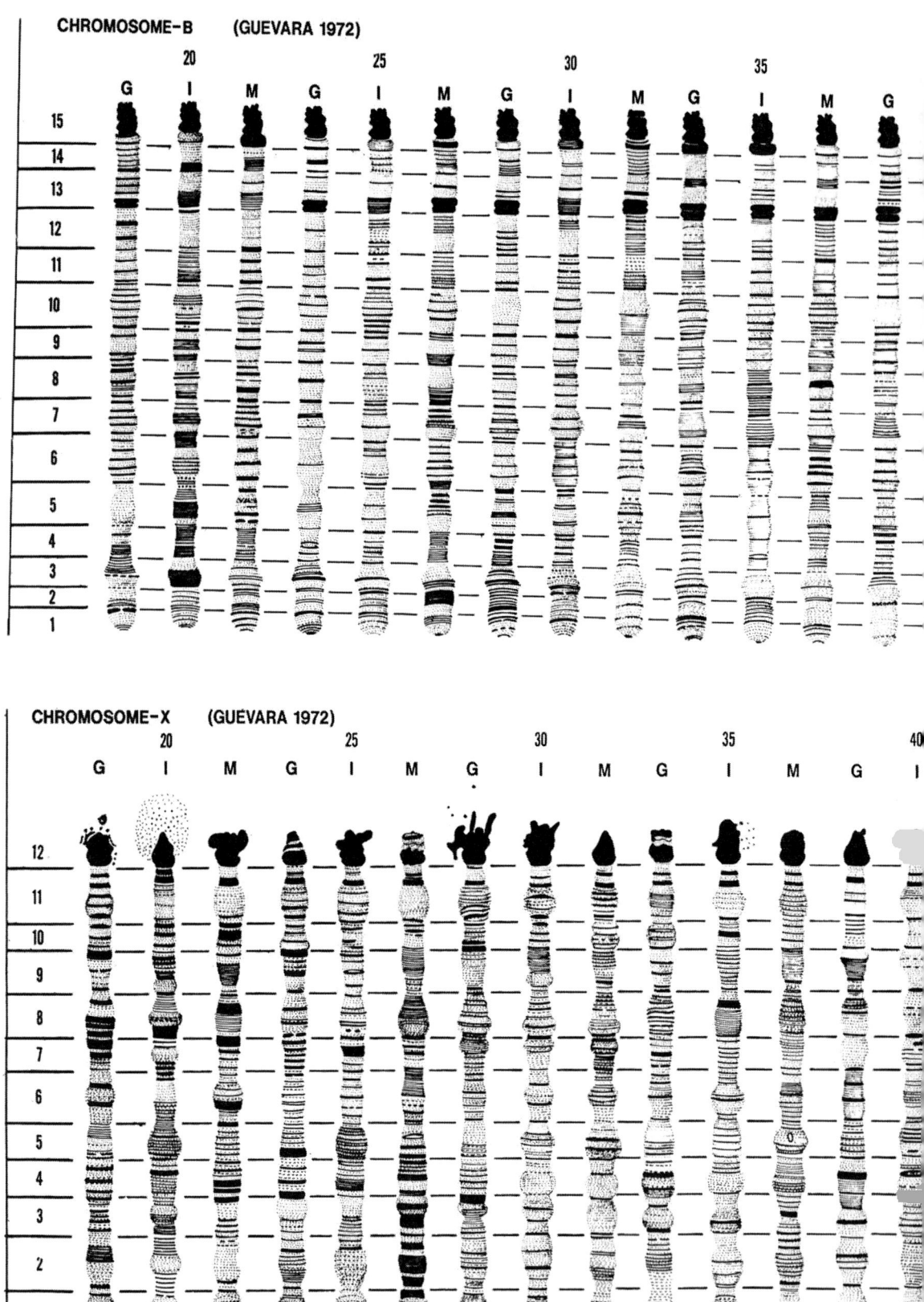

Figures 7-10. Camera lucida drawings of the polytene chromosomes of the salivary glands (G), intestine (I), and Mal... represent the ages in days of the larvae from which the chromosomes were derived. Chromosome B is divided into 15 se...

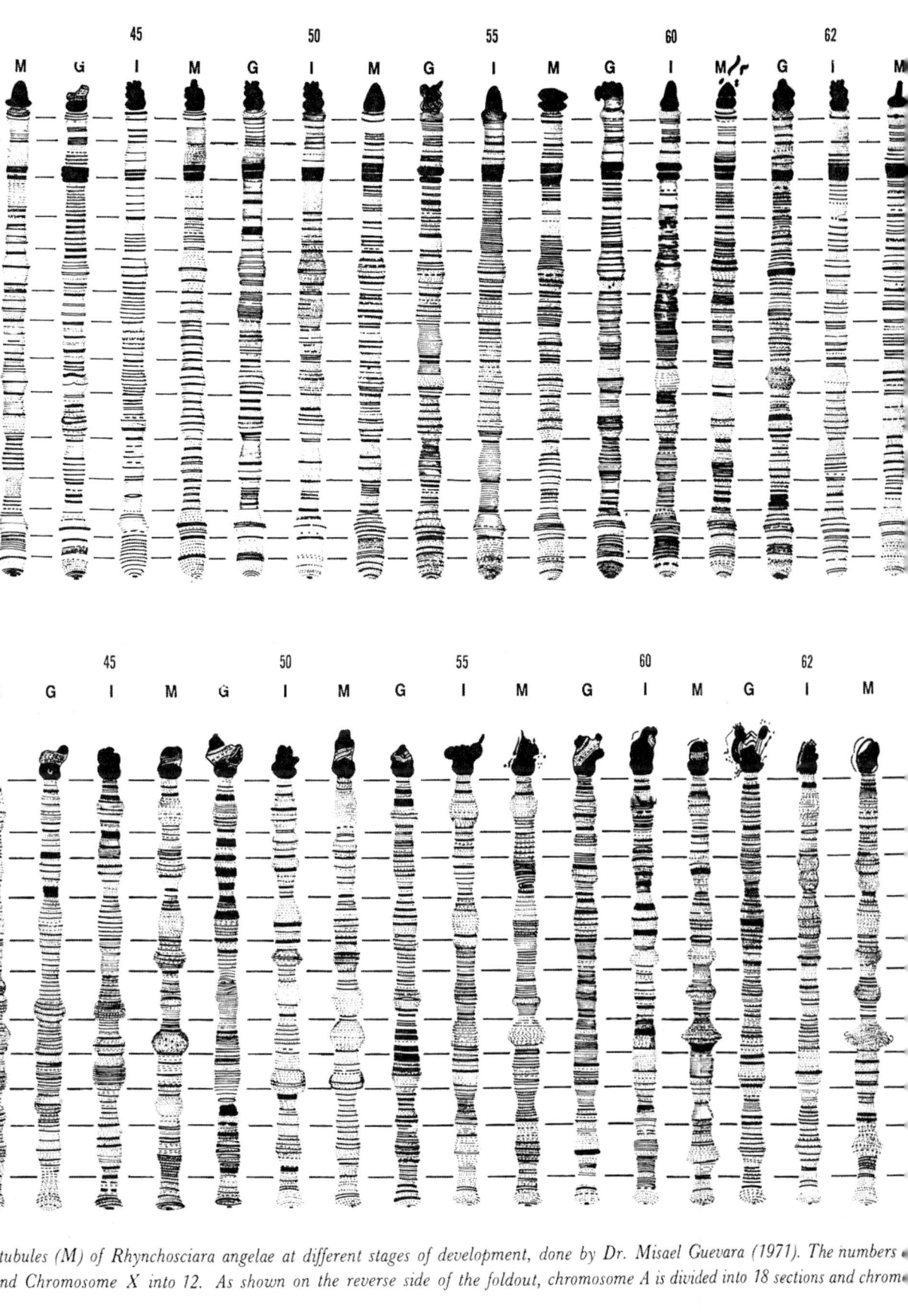

tubules (M) of *Rhynchosciara angelae* at different stages of development, done by Dr. Misael Guevara (1971). The numbers
nd Chromosome X into 12. As shown on the reverse side of the foldout, chromosome A is divided into 18 sections and chrom

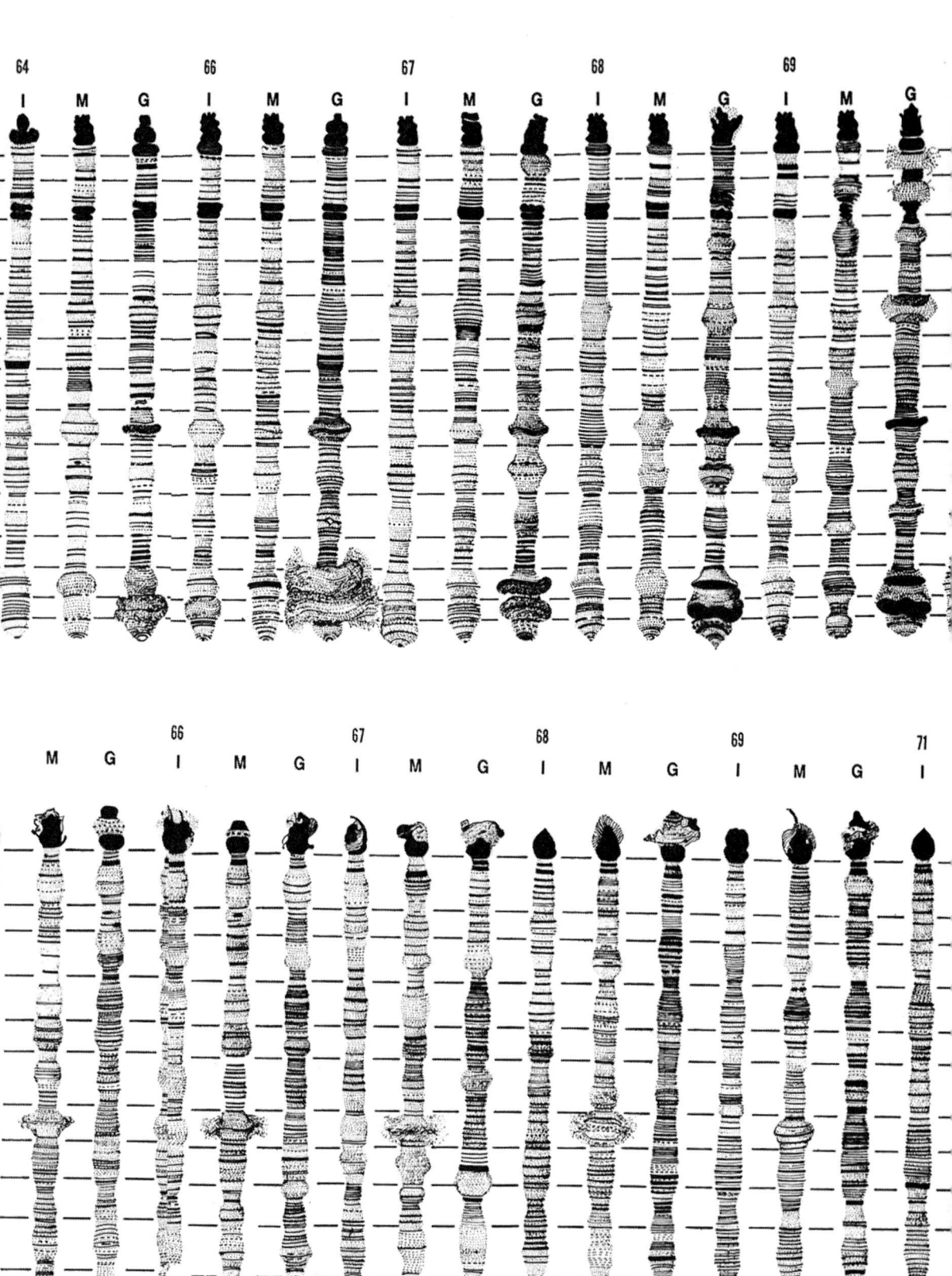

he figures (20-74)
11.

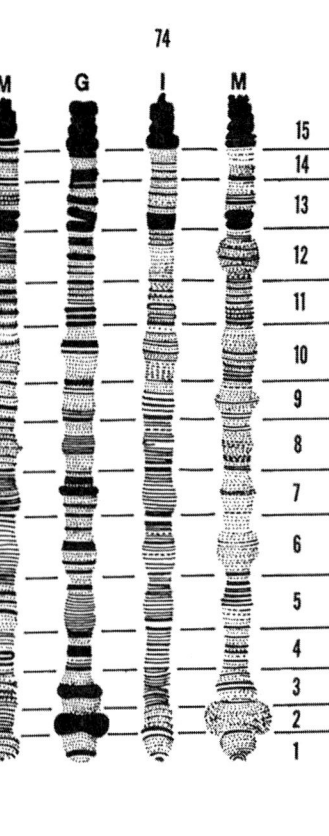

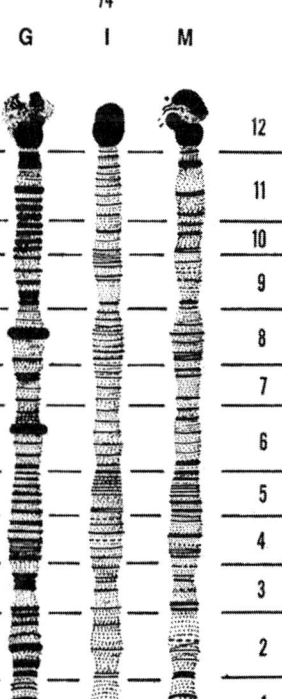

puffs there is an intense synthesis of RNA plus the extra synthesis of DNA before and/or during development of the puff. That this is, indeed, synthesis of DNA above the endomitotic events of the other bands and *not* simply the asynchronous replication of replicons has been confirmed not only by differential staining (Breuer and Pavan, 1954, 1955; Pavan and Breuer, 1955), but also autoradiography (Ficq and Pavan, 1957; Pavan, 1959, 1965*a*) and microspectrophotometry (Rudkin and Corlette, 1957). Guevara (1971) and Guevara and Basile (1973) found at least ten puffs in the salivary gland chromosomes; none, however, was detected in the polytene chromosomes of other tissues (Figures 2, 7–10). Similar observations of DNA puffs have since been made in other sciarids (Swift, 1962; Gabrusewycz-Garcia, 1964; Pavan and Perondini, 1967; Crouse and Keyl, 1968; Crouse, 1968; Perondini and Dessen, 1969; Pavan and da Cunha, 1969*b*; da Cunha *et al.*, 1969*a*), in *Sarcophaga* (Whitten, 1965), in ciliates (Alonso and Perez-Silva, 1966*a,b*; Gil *et al.*, 1972), and in some plants (Avanzi *et al.*, 1970).

Puffing Behavior, RNA Puffs. Puffing was interpreted by Breuer and Pavan (1952, 1955) and Beermann (1952) as genes operating in differentiation and has been defined by many authors as morphological manifestations of genic activity. The sizes of puffs vary from very small to very large and often are tissue and developmental-stage specific. Theoretically, it should be possible to relate a particular, tissue-specific puff with a specific cellular product. Although there have been good correlations between the appearance of specific puffs and the appearance of specific cell products, there has yet to be any direct proof that a product is derived from the RNA produced in a specific puff. There have been several attempts to correlate the puffs with specific products. Beermann (1961), Grossbach (1968, 1969), Baudisch and Panitz (1968), and Helmsing and Berendes (1971) found some degree of correlation between puffing activity and cellular products in *Chironomus, Acricotopus,* and *Drosophila.* Conversely, the studies of da Cunha *et al.* (1969*b*, 1972) in species of *Bradysia* show that there may be a very high production of protein in cells which exhibit no signs of puffs in their polytene chromosomes. Wobus *et al.* (1970, 1971) utilized the electrophoretic techniques described by Grossbach and showed that there are no detectable changes in the protein pattern during salivary gland development, regardless of the stage of activity of the large puffs in *Chironomus thummi.* Toledo *et al.* (1973, and unpublished), in examining the electrophoretic migration characteristics of 20 different isozymes and the soluble proteins of the salivary glands of *R. hollaenderi,* found that there was tissue- and stage-specific variation of only one of the isozymes and no variation in the soluble proteins. Although the variations had a temporal relationship with the activity of certain puffs in the salivary gland chromosomes, no direct correlation between these changes and a specific puff could be made with any degree of confidence since there are many puffs which are active during the time of the variation. The suggestion was made that perhaps some of the puffs have functions other than the production of protein.

Comparison of RNA puffing patterns of a single tissue during development or of several tissues with development has revealed that there is temporal and tissue-specific variation of puffing patterns. There are puffs which are common to all tissues and to all stages, probably representing functions held in common by all cell types. There are puffs which occur in only one tissue and which do not vary with development, probably representing functions necessary for that particular differentiated system. There are still other puffs which are not only tissue specific, but also stage specific, probably representing functions which are specialized (Guevara and Basile, 1973).

Puffing Behavior, DNA Puffs. DNA puffs were interpreted by Breuer and Pavan (1955) and Pavan (1959, 1965a) as being amplification of certain genes when these genes are required in excess of the amount present. Pavan (1959) called the amplification products "metabolic DNA" and defined this type of DNA as "any DNA which is produced by multiplication of chromosome loci, either in excess or independent of the process of genome multiplication," and then added, "metabolic DNA, after being synthesized, in some cases may stay on the chromosome, in others may be released from it" (Pavan, 1965a). By this definition, any DNA which is synthesized above or independent of the amount of DNA present in a specific locus is to be considered metabolic DNA. The amplified nucleolar genes in oocytes of a number of organisms and in polytene chromosomes of some dipterans are examples of metabolic DNA.

There is considerable evidence that the DNA amplified in the DNA puffs of sciarids has no relation with the amplification of the nucleolar genes. It was believed by some for a time that nucleolar genes are the only ones amplified. Recent data based on *in situ* hybridization studies of ribosomal RNA (rRNA) have localized the ribosomal cistrons in the bases of the chromosomes X and C of *R. hollaenderi* (Pardue et al., 1970) and X, C, and B in *R. angelae* (Pardue, personal communication). Hybridization using rRNA was never detected in the bands of the DNA puffs. Similar results in regard to the DNA puffs and ribosomal cistrons have been made in *S. coprophila* (Gerbi, 1971). Jones, Bishop, and da Cunha (1973) annealed polyribouri dylic acid [poly(U)] labeled with tritium to chromosomes from *Rhynchosciara* salivary glands to detect the distribution of AT-rich DNA. A clear pattern of binding was observed to several locations corresponding with structural features of the salivary gland polytene chromosomes. Strong binding also occurred to the cytoplasm of certain testicular cells in *Rhynchosciara*. These findings were interpreted in terms of the distribution of structural and metabolic sequences in polyadenylic acid. Meneghini and Cordeiro (1972), studying the rate of thymidine incorporation into DNA, found that this rate reached a maximum with the formation of the DNA puffs, and that this rate was paralleled by the increase in activity of thymidine kinase. Lara and Hollander (1967) and Armelin *et al.* (1969), in studying the patterns of RNA synthesis in several stages of *R. angelae* salivary glands, found that rRNA synthesis is considerably diminished during the period of the DNA puffs, even though there is an increase in the rate of protein synthesis (Bianchi, 1972). Evidence has been collected for the existence of amplification of genes by the analysis of the hybridization characteristics of certain classes of nuclear RNA with salivary gland DNA of different stages and DNA of different tissues (Meneghini *et al.*, 1971) and by the reinitiation of synthesis of certain classes of nuclear RNA after treatment with actinomycin D (Meneghini *et al.*, 1968). Armelin and Marques (1972a,b) analyzed the transcription and processing of RNA in salivary glands of *R. angelae* at different stages and found some evidence of gene amplification at the time of the appearance of the DNA puffs; however, they were unable to more than correlate the two observations. Bradshaw and Papaconstantinou (1970a) used H^3-BUdR to differentiate newly synthesized DNA in *R. hollaenderi*. They found, on CsCl isopycnic centrifugation, heterodispersion of the DNA of salivary glands at the time of DNA puffing, but not in salivary gland DNA of young larvae or fat body DNA (these tissues do not exhibit DNA puffs). The same authors in an abstract (Bradshaw and Papaconstantinou, 1970b) stated that this DNA hybridized to the DNA-puff region of the chromosomes. Cordeiro and Meneghini (1972, and personal communication) found heterodispersion of the H^3-BUdR-labeled salivary gland DNA of *R. angelae* larvae with and without the DNA puffs. Balsamo *et al.* (1973), in examining the genomic complexity of *R. angelae* salivary gland DNA, obtained results which indicate that a small part of the DNA which reanneals at an "intermediate" rate may be puff DNA. They further found that the salivary gland DNA which anneals at a rapid rate may not be replicated during much of the larval life cycle. Since this DNA is apparently that which bands as a light satellite in isopycnic centrifugation, it is probably analogous with the satellite in *R. hollaenderi* isolated by Eckhardt and Gall (1971), who found this DNA to be underreplicated and localized in the centric heterochromatin of all the chromosomes. Papaconstantinou *et al.* (1972) found a light, dAT-rich satellite which is synthesized in late male larval life. They believe this satellite to be probably mitochondrial in origin.

Ample evidence exists for gene amplification in the salivary glands of *Rhynchosciara* and other sciarids; however, almost none exists in regard to the possible function of the genes amplified. Probably they are amplified as a result of a need for more template by the cell. Sauaia *et al.* (1971) were able to inhibit the development of the DNA puffs in *Bradysia hygida* with hydroxyurea, without interruption in larval development. They suggested that, at least in this sciarid, the DNA puffs are not essential for development of the larvae. Although this may be true, it does not preclude the possibility that the products of these puffs are essential for the further normal development and function of the salivary glands. Microsporidian (see below) and viral infections (tipula iridescent virus or TIV) and irradiation of the neurosecretory glands may change the normal development of the salivary glands, in many cases permitting the permanence of glands or parts of glands until the adult stage, with no signs of lysis. In the cells which are not lysed, no DNA puffs are detected (Pavan *et al.*, 1971*b*).

Changes in Puffing Behavior. Alterations in puffing behavior have been observed in a variety of circumstances: development; exogenous hormone induction; physical, chemical, and biological stimuli; *in vitro* culture; infections; and others. The variation in puffing patterns during development has been attributed to the direct action of specific hormones or to the fluctuations in balance of different hormones. Metamorphosis is under the direct control of hormones, and, since the salivary glands of insects are part of the metamorphic events, they also are under the control of these hormones.

The hormone ecdysone has been found to induce precocious metamorphosis and premature development of certain puffing behavior. Crouse (1968) found that the DNA puffs of *S. coprophila* are associated with the injection of ecdysone. Stocker *et al.* (1972, and unpublished results) has detected premature induction of the prepupal puffing pattern, including DNA puffs, in salivary glands of mid-fourth-instar larvae of *R. hollaenderi* by the injection of high doses of ecdysterone (β-ecdysone). However, in the prematurely induced animals there appears to be some differences in both the puffing pattern and in the amounts of DNA laid down at the sites of gene amplification. Ecdysterone also induces an abrupt acceleration of DNA synthesis along the salivary gland chromosomes. These changes occur until 12–24 hours after injection of hormone, thus differing in timing from the puffing changes observed in other dipterans, in which the ecdysone-induced puffing changes have been examined in detail.

Alterations in puffing patterns, especially of the DNA puffs, have been observed in *R. angelae* larvae whose brains were extirpated (Amabis and Cabral, 1970). These authors found that the DNA puffs were inhibited by this treatment. Simões and Cestari (1969), in *in-vitro*-cultured salivary glands of *R. angelae,* found that the DNA puffs were either inhibited or, if present when culture began, regressed or failed to develop further. Amabis and Simões (1971) implanted the salivary glands of young larvae into older larvae and found an induction of the host puffing pattern in the implant. Implantation of salivary glands in which the puffing has begun, results in either the inhibition of puff development or, if the puff had already begun to develop, the failure of the puff to expand further.

In the salivary gland chromosomes of larvae infected with the microsporidian, the DNA puffs fail to develop. These cells, it should be recalled, often survive metamorphosis, indicating that they did not synthesize the materials necessary for the lysis of the cell. There are RNA puffs seen in these infections, especially in the heterochromatic regions where puffing is not usually seen to occur. Heterochromatic puffing has been observed in various stress conditions, e.g., *in vitro* culture, and viral and protozoan infections. Sanders and Pavan (1972) interpreted the development of some of these heterochromatic puffs as possibly being responses of genes to stress conditions.

Infections in *Rhynchosciara*

Species of Sciaridae are commonly called "fungus gnats" because they derive their main foodstuffs from rotting plant materials and fungi. With the environment in which they exist replete with a variety of microorganisms, they are in constant contact with possible sources of infection. There are several types of infections which affect species of Sciaridae and which are amenable to cytological, developmental, and pathological examination. Among the most interesting of infections are microsporidians, gregarines, and viruses. These cause the induction of unicellular tumors due to the enormous hypertrophy of cytoplasm, nuclei, and chromosomes, i.e., greatly intensified synthesis. The host–parasite interaction of microsporidian and polyhedrosis virus infections will be considered below; the gregarine infections will not be discussed since they have as yet been studied only in *Trichosia pubescens* (Diptera, Sciaridae) but not in *Rhynchosciara* (da Cunha *et al.,* 1968).

Microsporidian Infection. Microsporidians are obligatory cytoplasmic parasites which belong to the phylum Protozoa, subphylum Plasmodroma, class Sporozoa, subclass Cnidosporia, and order Microsporidia. Though reports of microsporidian infections have been made in fish (Summerfelt, 1964; Lom and Corliss, 1967), crabs (Sprague, 1965), and rodents (Lainson *et al.,* 1964; Weiser, 1965), most typically they are found to parasitize insects, among which are several dipterans (Kudo, 1924; Thomson, 1960; Burnett and King, 1962; Kramer, 1964; Diaz and Pavan, 1965; Pavan and Basile, 1966*a,b*; Pavan *et al.,* 1969).

Insects infected by microsporidians with an accompanying host-cell enlargement have been described in papers dating back to the mid-nineteenth century [for references, see Kudo (1924) and Debaisieux and Gastaldi (1919)]. Unfortunately, in the majority of papers published on such infections, emphasis has been given to the biology of the parasite, with little information reflecting on cytological and developmental changes in the host cell. In the paper of Debaisieux and Gastaldi (1919) describing microsporidian infections of Simulidae, there is a beautiful drawing of microsporidian-induced giantism of a salivary gland polytene chromosome, but little attention was given to this paper in the past. Recent work on microsporidian infections of *R. angelae* and *S. ocellaris* have broached the subject from the host point-of-view, especially on the effects of the microorganism on the developmental and physiological behavior of affected cells, as well as on alterations of structure and function of various subcellular parts (Diaz and Pavan, 1965; da Cunha and Pavan, 1969; Pavan *et al.,* 1969, 1971*a,b*; Jurand *et al.,* 1967; Roberts *et al.,* 1967).

The host–parasite relationship in microsporidian infections of *Rhynchosciara* and *Sciara* are of special interest since the presence of the parasite appears only slightly detrimental to the host organism studied as a whole. Indeed, there may be the existence of an endosymbiotic relationship (mutualism) within the context of the individual cells because the infected cells, in many instances, survive longer than the uninfected cells of the same tissue (Pavan *et al.,* 1969). In infected larvae the uninfected cells go through histolysis during metamorphosis, as in the normal salivary gland. The infected cells do not lyse and can be found in adults as isolated bodies at times attached to some gland secretion. The nuclei of these cells are remarkably well-preserved (Figures 11 and 12) and the chromosomes are active in DNA and RNA synthesis.

It may be that the increased longevity of the infected cell may be due to a shift to a new pattern of development induced by the presence of the parasite. Pavan *et al.* (1971*c*), elaborating on this point, defined the behavior of the infected cell as a microcosm within the host which follows a separate and distinct developmental pattern of its own, with no evident relationship to the other cells of the same tissue. There are no apparent indications of products being eliminated by the infected cell which have any effect on the host as a whole or on adjacent cells. Salivary cells which are neighbors to infected cells go through the normal developmental processes, and puffs which occur in the polytene chromosomes at specific stages of development are normal. i.e., exhibit a puffing pattern similar to

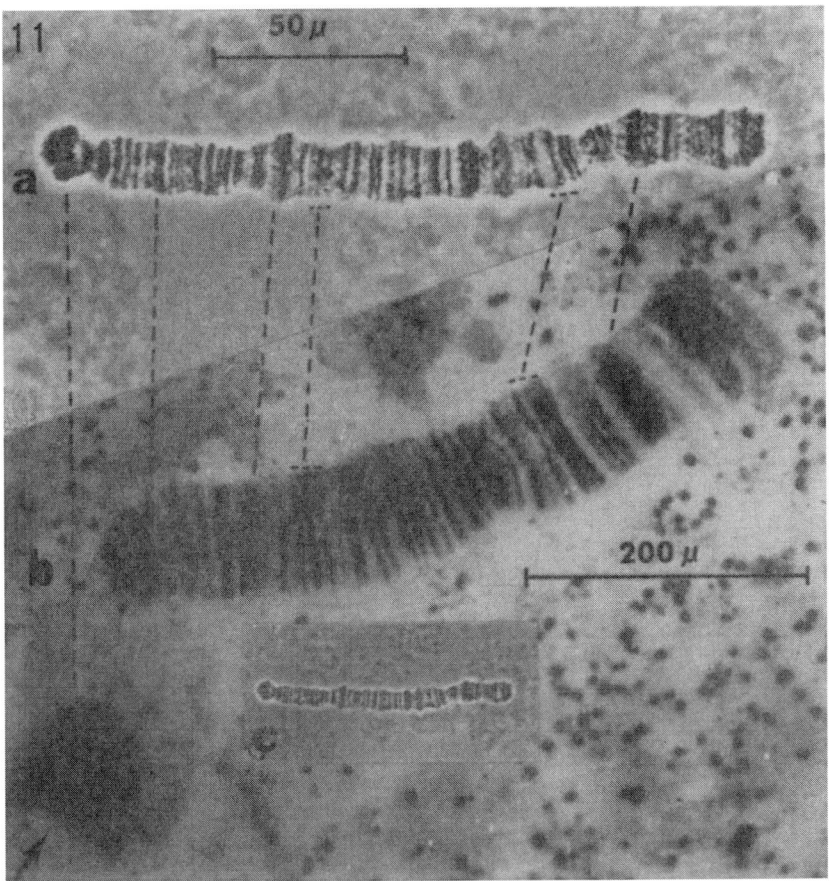

Figure 11. Photomicrographs of chromosome C of R. angelae. Here a and c are the same chromosome; a was enlarged for comparison with chromosome of b, which is from a microsporidian-infected salivary gland cell. The main difference between the uninfected and infected cells, besides the size, is the puffed heterochromatin (indicated by the arrow). Part b and c have the same magnification; the 200-μm scale is valid for these two figures. Black granular objects in the background of part b are spores and other life-cycle forms of microsporidia. From Diaz and Pavan, Proceedings of the National Academy of Sciences, USA 54: 1321–1327, 1965.

that of chromosomes of other uninfected cells of the same tissue or in uninfected larvae of the same age. The puffing behavior of the infected cells is completely altered. Although puffs seen in uninfected cells may be present in the infected cells, the time relationships between different puffs is atypical (Pavan *et al.*, 1971c). The most prominent puffs of the uninfected cells frequently do not appear in infected cells. The most striking case of this is the complete lack of DNA puffs in infected cells. A cell which formerly was part of a balanced system, on infection, becomes a

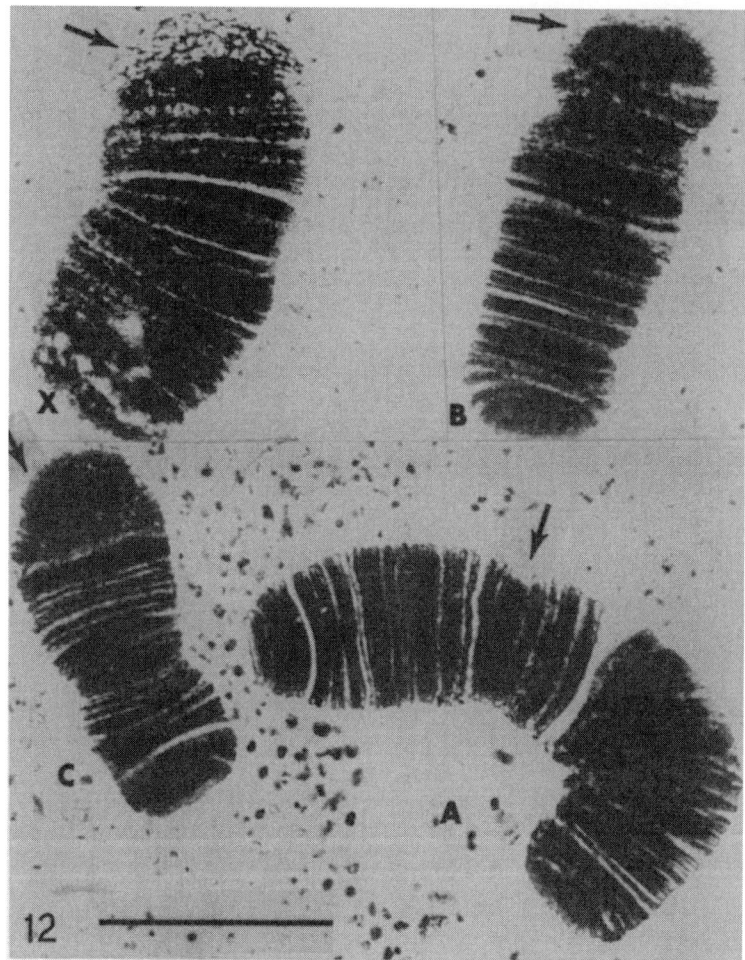

Figure 12. Supergiant chromosomes from a salivary gland cell infected by microsporidia which were recovered from an adult of R. angelae. These chromosomes are enlarged due to an increase in amount of DNA associated with hyperactivity. Chromosome X in normal cells has a volume approximately equal to chromosome B (see Figure 4). In this case, chromosome X is larger than the infected chromosome B due to greater RNA synthesis but not to greater DNA content. Arrows indicate centromeric heterochromatin. Insert is a human karyotype at the same magnification, showing the differences in sizes of the two chromosome sets. Bar at lower left represents 100 μm.

separate entity (a unicellular tumor) which utilizes the organism for its maintenance without any apparent contribution to it and is subject to its own regulating system.

Several larval tissues are affected by the microsporidia, including salivary glands, parietal muscles, visceral muscle connecting the intestinal caeca with the mid-gut, various parts of the intestine, cells of the wall of

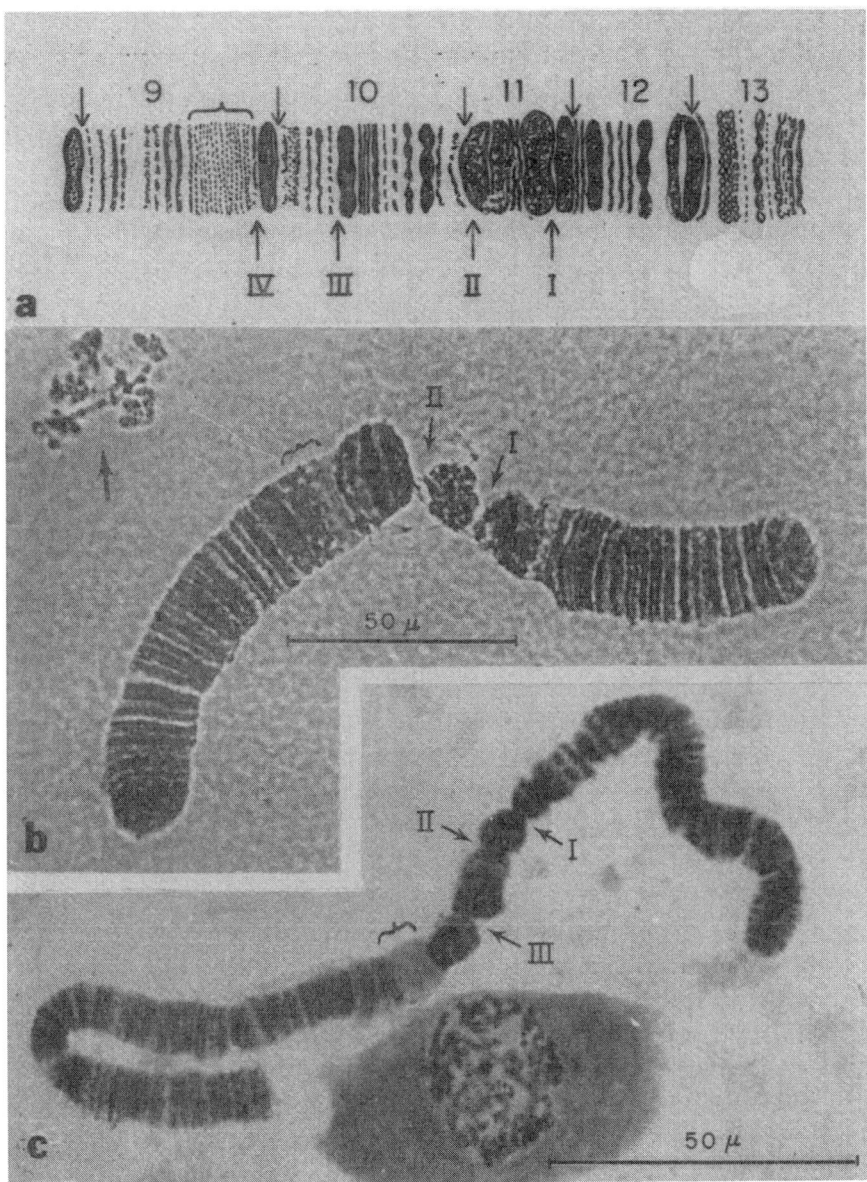

Figure 13. Part a is a camera lucida drawing of sections 9–13 of chromosome A (arrows above) of a normal salivary gland cell of R. angelae [modified after Pavan and Breuer (1952)]. The arrows below (I–IV) indicate sites of constrictions induced by viral (RPV) infection. Part b is a hypertrophied chromosome of a caecal cell, showing constrictions I and II. Above left of part b, the broad arrow indicates a nucleus of an uninfected cell of the same caeca. Part c is a hypertrophied chromosome A of a caecal cell, showing constrictions I, II, and III, viral induced. Below the chromosome of part c is an uninfected cell of the same caeca. The wavy brackets indicate a landmark of section 9. From Diaz and Pavan (1965).

the tracheal tubules, and three or four other glands. Unicellular tumors may develop in any of these susceptible tissues. There is another type of behavior exhibited by infected cells, such as in fat bodies, which is a fusion of several cells, behaving, with the included microorganisms, as a unit. This syncytial unit of fused infected cells is somewhat analogous to that observed in infected striated muscle which is naturally syncytial. The chromosomes in these syncytial tumors become greatly enlarged due to increased polyteny (see later discussion), permitting a detailed analysis of the induced changes in the morphology and physiology of the host polytene chromosomes as a whole or in specific bands. The behavior of the chromosomes and other cellular parts of different infected tissues will be discussed in detail below.

Recent work by Pavan *et al.* (1969) in *S. ocellaris* and by Wertz (1970) and Muñoz de Hoyos (1972) in *R. angelae* and *R. hollaenderi* has disclosed that these three species of sciarids are all subject to a double infection by microsporidians. One of the infecting species belongs to the genus *Thelohania* and has oval spores; the other belongs to the genus *Octosporea* and has elongated spores. The two species always occur together. No cultures of *Rhynchosciara* infected by only one of the species could be obtained. The reason for this apparent necessity for double infection is still to be determined. Octosporean infections are most common in intestinal cells and are the first infection to be manifested; thelohanian infections are more common in cells of the parietal and visceral muscles, salivary glands, fat bodies, and other tissues.

Spores of both species of microsporidia can be kept in the laboratory either as a suspension in distilled water or as a dry mixture with dry food and soil. If kept at 4°C, the spores maintain their viability for several months. To infect the larvae, the spores are mixed with prepared food and then fed to the larvae shortly after hatching. Larvae older than one week become resistant to the infection. Infected cells are easily distinguished under the dissecting microscope by their size and whitish color. Muscle, salivary glands, and fat bodies, when heavily infected, are visible to the naked eye through the transparent skin of the larvae, appearing as whitish bodies within the body cavity. The microsporidia develop in the cytoplasm, and the infected cell increases in size and becomes opaque in appearance. The parietal muscle, which is composed of syncytial fibers, upon infection increases in size and becomes similar in appearance to fat bodies. Although the uninfected fat bodies are formed by discrete cells, the boundaries between the individual cells are not easily discernible. When infected, the fat bodies lose their individual integrity and often fuse, forming a syncytium. In the other affected tissues, it is common to find only a few infected cells scattered among the normal ones. For instance, in the salivary glands of *R. angelae,* which have about 300 cells, there can be found 1–20 isolated infected cells or clusters of several infected cells in various regions of the gland. The infected cells of any particular tissue frequently have different sizes, which would indicate that they are in differential stages of infection. The sizes attained by infected cells depend on the tissue as well as developmental stage. The infected salivary gland cells become the largest; however, the cells of other glands and visceral muscle also were found to reach large sizes.

The chromosomes of the infected cells begin to exhibit increasing polyteny soon after the microsporidian initiates its development in the cytoplasm. The increase in chromosomal size is probably due to stepped-up synthesis of DNA, resulting in a higher degree of polyteny and uncoiling of the condensed portion of the chromonemata for intense synthesis of RNA. Roberts *et al.* (1967), by microspectrophotometrically measuring the DNA content in the chromosomes of infected salivary gland cells of *R. angelae,* found that it follows the geometric series of 2 : 4 : 8 : 16 : 32 times the DNA content of uninfected cells of the same tissue. Furthermore, it was found that chromosomes of different infected cells may occasionally vary in size but not in DNA content because of high metabolic activity of the chromosome. It was observed (Pavan and Basile, 1966*b*) that the chromosomes of these cells may begin a generalized puffing with the X chromosome initiating the process before the autosomes which also eventually exhibit this behavior. This situation corresponds to the transition between the polytene stage and the pompon stage described by Pavan and Basile (1966*b*). The homologous chromonemata in the polytene state give rise to a banded structure and are perfectly synapsed along the entire length of the chromonemata. In the pompon stage, on the other hand, the chromonemata are isolated and attached only at the heterochromatic regions, and the chromosome appears to be one gigantic puff. Occasionally the heterochromatic regions may be divided into several small blocks. Although the banded nature of the chromosomes may be lost and the homologous chromonemata may be separated from one another, there is still a union at the heterochromatic regions and a maintenance of chromosomal individuality, i.e., each chromosome remains distinguishable due to differential sizes and shapes. The gigantic chromosomes of the infected cells exhibit no signs of degeneration for at least 50 days after the infection starts. Another reaction to the presence of the microsporidian is seen in the cells of the fat bodies, in which cases of increased polyteny with an associated polyploidy can be detected. As yet there have been no cases of diploid cells infected with the microsporidian.

As has been stated, the enlargement of the polytene chromosomes in all the tissues mentioned is due to an increase in the polyteny and to hyperactivity of RNA synthesis. There is no alteration in the basic banding pattern of the chromosomes (Figure 11) (Diaz and Pavan, 1965; Roberts *et al.*, 1967). The puffing, which can be limited to isolated bands or which can include the entire chromosome, was interpreted by those authors as being localized as well as generalized puffs, a physiological and not a basic structural change in the chromosomes. There might be changes in the heterochromatic regions of the chromosomes which may replicate less than the euchromatic regions; as yet, this has not been tested in infected cells.

Disruption in the cytoplasm of the infected cells as a result of the microsporidia has been reported by Jurand *et al.* (1967) in *S. ocellaris* and in *R. angelae* (Pavan *et al.*, 1971c). Comparison of normal and microsporidian-infected cells has revealed subcellular disorganization, especially in the immediate vicinity of the developing protozoa. Differentiated cytoplasm so evident in uninfected cells is detectably diminished in those cells with microsporidia, regardless of the enlargement and hyperfunction of the nucleus. The degree of decrease in differentiated cytoplasm is in proportion to the extent of the infection. The only subcellular organelles which appear not greatly affected by the infection are the mitochondria, though they are smaller and more numerous in the infected than in the uninfected cells. Microsporidia do not contain any mitochondria; thus, they probably rely on the host cell for mitochondrial functions. Examination of subcellular elements characteristic of the different tissues (such as myofilaments of muscles) or of all tissues (such as endoplasmic reticulum and Golgi complexes) in normal and infected tissues has revealed that, for the most part, the majority of them are severely altered or eliminated, whereas the mitochondria are almost unchanged. It is interesting to recall that even with great cytoplasmic disruption, there is hyperactivity in the nuclei with serial doubling of DNA. The extreme alterations of the infected-cell cytoplasm can be reconciled with the nuclear hyperactivity and increased longevity of the cells by the proposal of a mutualistic association between the host cell and the microsporidian. The mechanisms involved in such an association are not clear.

Viral Infection. Insects are susceptible to many viruses, among which are a group which form proteinaceous inclusion bodies or crystals and are designated granulosis or polyhedrosis viruses. Granulosis and polyhedrosis viruses, by conventional classification of insect viruses, were considered to be unrelated; however, biochemical and serological analyses of the two prompted the conclusion by Bellet (1969) that they probably are genetically related. Polyhedroses occur in several species of lepidopterous and hymenopterous larvae, but few instances of such infections are known in Diptera (Smith, 1967). Nuclear polyhedrosis in Diptera has been described in *Tipula paludosa* (Rennie, 1923; Smith and Xeros, 1953), *Culex tarsalis* (Kellen *et al.,* 1963; Smith, 1967), *Anopheles subpictus* (Dasgupta and Ray, 1954, 1957; Smith, 1967), and *R. angelae* (Diaz and Pavan, 1965; Pavan and Basile, 1966*b*; Pavan and da Cunha, 1968; Pavan *et al.,* 1971*a*; da Cunha *et al.,* 1972).

R. angelae larvae have been collected in nature or obtained in laboratory cultures infected with a nuclear polyhedrosis virus, called Rhynchosciara polyhedrosis virus (RPV) (Pavan *et al.,* 1971*a*). RPV is a DNA virus, develops in the nuclei of mid-gut and caecal epithelial cells, and is occluded in groups of hundreds in proteinaceous polyhedral inclusion bodies (reaching sizes of 20 μm along the edges and 30 μm apex to apex). Electron microscopic examination of segments of RPV unit membrane destined to form viral envelopes has revealed that probably they originate *de novo* within the infected nuclei without any direct participation of the nuclear membrane (Stoltz *et al.,* 1973). They induce gross cytoplasmic, nuclear, and chromosomal changes in the host cell. The most obvious reactions of the infected cells to the virus are: increase in nuclear size, enlargement of the chromosomes, production of DNA fibers in the nucleoplasm (virogenic stroma), and appearance of a large number of polyhedral crystals (Pavan *et al.,* 1971*a*; da Cunha *et al.,* 1972). Of the enlarged nuclei, some show obvious presence of the virus in a Feulgen-positive nucleoplasm and then degenerate without crystal production; other affected cells exhibit nuclear and chromosomal enlargement with no indication of virus or crystals in a Feulgen-negative nucleoplasm and without degeneration of the host chromosomes. The frequency of the latter type decreases with progress of the disease; it is possible that they represent the early stages of the infection. However, there is no strong evidence to support this.

As in microsporidian infections, the larvae are susceptible to RPV infection only in the first week after hatching. Larvae have been collected in nature which were infected with RPV. The infection can be induced by feeding newly hatched larvae prepared food which has been mixed with triturated carcasses of freshly killed larvae or dried larvae that have been stored at 4°C. Infected larvae are usually smaller and paler than their uninfected sibs. They may survive most of the larval phase; usually, however, they do not pupate. Susceptible tissues include the intestinal caeca and the posterior part of the mid-gut just anterior to the Malpighian tubules. The cells of these tissues are polytene, hence they do not divide; therefore, all DNA multiplication and cellular substances remain in a single giant cell, producing a unicellular instead of a multicellular tumor as in, for example, mammalian tumors. No appreciable interaction between infected and uninfected cells is observed since they are found adjacent in both tissues. The number and size of infected cells vary with development of the infection.

There is undoubtedly viral interference of the control of DNA multiplication of the cells of susceptible tissues and induction of enlarged chromosomes (Figure 13). Though the majority of enlarged chromosomes are active in RNA synthesis, there does not seem to be the intense synthesis of RNA in these infections, as was observed in microsporidian infections. There are, however, some cells which manifest accelerated RNA synthesis in the formation of specific puffs, particularly in the heterochromatin of some or of all four chromosomes. There are also cases of heightened synthesis of micronucleoli production. Most of the heterochromatic puffs are never observed in normal cases. Sanders and Pavan (1972) suggested that these are specific reactions to stress conditions. The interference in DNA multiplication is twofold, there being stimulated synthesis of some chromosomal material as well as inhibition or asynchrony in others. There are four regions of chromosome A which behave as though multiplication is either inhibited or occurs out of phase in relation to the rest of the chromosome, producing constrictions (Figure 13). These regions are either heterochromatic or associated with heterochromatic bands sometime during development and are specific and constant for all individuals of an infected group of larvae. There may be variation between strains of virus which cause various combinations of constrictions (Pavan *et al.*, 1971*c*). Chromosomal breakages in mammalian mitotic cells may be an analogous situation to that in *Rhynchosciara*; however, the breakages in mammalian systems appear to be random and nonuniform, whereas those in *Rhynchosciara* are specific and constant. Several authors have shown that asynchrony and/or differential rates of synthesis in euchromatin and heterochromatin occur during development of normal polytene chromosomes (Müller *et al.*, 1937; Hinton, 1942; Pavan, 1946; Berendes and Keyl, 1967; Rudkin, 1965, 1969). Perhaps during the abnormal enlargement of the polytene chromosomes in virus-infected cells, the asynchrony and/or differential rate of synthesis is specifically manifested in the four regions mentioned, thus producing the constrictions (Sanders and Pavan, 1972). Morgante *et al.* (1974) studied the patterns of DNA synthesis in cells of *Rhynchosciara angelae* infected by RPV. Four patterns of DNA synthesis, in relation to the host chromosomes and the virus, were disclosed by means of tritiated thymidine incorporation in the infected nuclei. The patterns are: (1) incorporation mainly in the chromosomes, (2) incorporation in the chromosomes and in the nucleoplasm, (3) incorporation only in the nucleoplasm, and (4) incorporation mainly in the chromosomes in dissociation. They found indications of a succession 1→2 and 3→4. The succession of patterns indicates that the virus induces first the increase of synthesis of host cell DNA and RNA. The bulk of the synthesis of viral DNA is evident only after the host cell DNA and RNA machinery is amplified.

The RPV-induced unicellular tumor is of special interest since the pathologic agent interferes directly with the genetic material and the chromosome structure of the host cell. The size and the banding pattern of the chromosomes of the infected cells permit detailed analysis of the effects of the virus. Comparison of the banding pattern between the infected and normal situations revealed that there is no appreciable difference between them. The chromosomal enlargement in virus-infected cells is due primarily to an increase in polyteny, often without too great increase in other metabolic activities.

Acknowledgments

We are very grateful to Prof. J. J. Biesele for his contribution of the human karyotype; to Dr. M. Guevara for his original maps of the polytene chromosomes of *R. angelae*; to Drs. R. Basile, A. N. Cestari, J. S. Morgante, L. C. G. Simões, and S. A. Toledo Filho for reading of and suggestions to the manuscript; to M. Cordeiro, S. Ogle, Dr. M. L. Pardue, Dr. A. L. P. Perondini, Dr. D. Steffensen, and Dr. A. J. Stocker for personal communication of unpublished results; and to Lane DeCamp for editorial aid and typing of the manuscript.

The research on *Rhynchosciara* was sponsored by grants from the National Institute of Health (Public Health Grants GM-15769, GM-17590-03, GM-19331-01, and No. 5 TO 1 GM 00337), Conselho Nacional de Pesquisas, and Fundação de Amparo à Pesquisa do Estado de São Paulo.

Literature Cited

Alonso, P. and J. Perez-Silva, 1966a   Giant chromosomes in Protozoa. *Nature (Lond.)* **205**:213–214.

Alonso, P. and J. Perez-Silva, 1966b   Formación de puffs en los cromosomas politénico de ciliados oxtríquidos. *Bol. R. Soc. Esp. Hist. Natl. Secc. Biol.* **64**:361–362.

Amabis, J. M. and D. Cabral, 1970   RNA and DNA puffs in polytene chromosomes of *Rhynchosciara*: Inhibition by extirpation of the prothorax. *Science (Wash., D.C.)* **169**:692–694.

Amabis, J. M. and L. C. G. Simões, 1971   Puff induction and regression in *Rhynchosciara angelae* by the method of salivary gland implantation. *Genetica (The Hague)* **42**:404–413.

Ammermann, D., 1971 Morphology and development of the macronuclei of ciliates *Stylonychia mytilus* and *Euplotes aediculatus*. *Chromosoma (Berl.)* **33**:209–238.

Armelin, H. A. and N. Marques, 1972*a* Transcription and processing of ribonucleic acid in *Rhynchosciara* salivary glands. I. Rapidly labeled ribonucleic acid. *Biochemistry* **11**:3663–3671.

Armelin, H. A. and N. Marques, 1972*b* Transcription and processing of ribonucleic acid in *Rhynchosciara* salivary glands. II. Hybridization of nuclear and cytoplasmic ribonucleic acid with nuclear deoxyribonucleic acid. Indication of deoxyribonucleic acid amplification. *Biochemistry* **11**:3672–3679.

Armelin, H. A., R. Meneghini and F. J. S. Lara, 1969 Pattern of RNA synthesis in salivary gland of *R. angelae* larvae during development. *Genetics* **61** suppl. 1:351–360.

Ashburner, M., 1970 Function and structure of polytene chromosomes during insect development. *Adv. Insect Physiol.* **7**:1–95.

Avanzi, S., P. G. Cionini and F. D'Amato, 1970 Cytochemical and autoradiographic analyses on the embryo suspensor cells of *Phaseolus coccineus*. *Caryologia* **23**:605–638.

Balsamo, J., J. M. Hierro, M. L. Birnstiel and F. J. S. Lara, 1973 *Rhynchosciara angelae* salivary gland DNA: Kinetic complexity and transcription of repetitive sequences. In *Gene Expression and Its Regulation*. pp. 101–122, Plenum Press, New York.

Bantock, C., 1961 Chromosome elimination in Cecidomyidae. *Nature (Lond.)* **190**:466–467.

Basile, R., 1966 Estudo da espermatogênese e da ovogênese em *Rhynchosciara angelae* e da sintese de acidos nucleicos e de proteinas no ovario. Ph.D. Dissertation, Universidade de São Paulo, São Paulo.

Basile, R., 1969 Nucleic acid synthesis in nurse cells of *Rhynchosciara angelae* Nonato et Pavan 1951. *Genetics Suppl.* **61**(1):261–273.

Basile, R., 1970 Spermatogenesis in *Rhynchosciara angelae* Nonato et Pavan 1951. *Rev. Bras. Biol.* **30**:29–38.

Basile, R., S. A. Toledo, A. B. da Cunha, J. S. Morgante and J. Marques, 1970 Analises de mutação que afeta a pigmentação de larvas de *Rhynchosciara angelae* Nonato et Pavan 1951 (Diptera, Sciaridae). *Rev. Bras. Biol.* **30**:471–475.

Bauer, H. and W. Beermann, 1952 Die Polytänie der Riesenchromosomen. *Chromosoma (Berl.)* **4**:630–648.

Baudisch, W. and R. Panitz, 1968 Kontrolle eines biochemischen Merkmals in den Speicheldrüsen von *Acricotopus lucidus* durch einen Balbiani Ring. *Exp. Cell Res.* **49**:470–476.

Bayreuther, K., 1952 Extra-chromosomale Feulgen-positive Körper (Nuklein-körper) in der Oögeneses des Tipuliden. *Naturwissenschaften* **39**:71.

Bayreuther, K., 1956 Die Oögenese der Tipuliden. *Chromosoma (Berl.)* **7**:508–557.

Bayreuther, K., 1957 Extra-chromosomales DNS-hältiges Material in der Oögenese der Flöhe. *Z. Naturforsch. Sect. B* **126**:458–461.

Beermann, S., 1966 A quantitative study of chromatin diminution in embryonic mitoses of *Cyclops furcifer*. *Genetics* **54**:567–576.

Beermann, W., 1952 Chromomerenkonstanz und spezifische Modifikationen der Chromosomenstruktur in der Entwicklung und Organdifferenzierung von *Chironomus tentans*. *Chromosoma (Berl.)* **5**:139–198.

Beermann, W., 1956 Nuclear differentiation and functional morphology of chromosomes. *Cold Spring Harbor Symp. Quant. Biol.* **21**:217–232.

Beermann, W., 1961 Ein Balbiani-Ring als Lokus einer Speicheldrüsenmutation. *Chromosoma (Berl.)* **12**:1–25.

Beermann, W., 1965 Gene action at the level of the chromosome. In *Heritage from Mendel*, edited by R. A. Brink, pp. 179–201, The University of Wisconsin Press, Madison, Wisc.

Beermann, W., editor, 1972 *Developmental Studies on Giant Chromosomes*, Springer-Verlag, Berlin.

Bellet, A. J. D., 1969 Relationships among the polyhedrosis and granulosis viruses of insects. *Virology* **37**:117–123.

Berendes, H. D. and H. G. Keyl, 1967 Distribution of DNA in heterochromatin and euchromatin of polytene nuclei of *Drosophila hydei*. *Genetics* **57**:1–13.

Bianchi, A. G., 1972 Bioquímica da secreção de *Rhynchosciara americana*. Ph.D. Dissertation, Universidade de São Paulo, São Paulo.

Bier, K., W. Kunz and D. Ribbert, 1967 Struktur und Funktion der Oöcytenchromosomen und Nukleolen sowie der Extra-DNS während der Oögenese panoistischen und meroistischen Insekten. *Chromosoma (Berl.)* **23**:214–254.

Boveri, T. H., 1887 Über Differenzierung der Zellkerne während der Forschung des Eies von *Ascaris megalocephala*. *Anat. Anz.* **2**:688–693.

Boveri, T. H., 1892 Über die Entstehung des Gegensatzes zwischen den Geschlechtszellen und den Somatischen Zellen bei *Ascaris megalocephala*. *S.-B. Ges. Morphol. Physiol. (München)* **8**:114–125.

Bradshaw, W. S. and J. Papaconstantinou, 1970a Differential incorporation of 5-bromodeoxyuridine into DNA puffs of larval salivary gland chromosomes in *Rhynchosciara*. *Biochem. Biophys. Res. Commun.* **41**:306–312.

Bradshaw, W. S. and J. Papaconstantinou, 1970b Differential synthesis of salivary gland DNA during development of *Rhynchosciara angelae*. *Fed. Proc.* **29**:670a.

Breuer, M. E., 1967 Cromossomos politênicos das glândulas salivares de *Rhynchosciara angelae* Nonato et Pavan 1951. *Rev. Bras. Biol.* **27**:105–108.

Breuer, M. E., 1969 Revision of the genus Rhynchosciara Rübsaamen (Diptera, Sciaridae) in the neotropical region. *Arq. Zool. (São Paulo)* **17**:167–198.

Breuer, M. E. and C. Pavan, 1952 Gens na diferenciação. *Cienc. Cult. (São Paulo)* **4**:141.

Breuer, M. E. and C. Pavan, 1954 Salivary gland chromosomes and differentiation. *Proc. IX Interntl. Congr. Genet. Caryologia Suppl.* **6(1)** (Part II):728.

Breuer, M. E. and C. Pavan, 1955 Behavior of polytene chromosomes of *Rhynchosciara angelae* at different stages of larval development. *Chromosoma (Berl.)* **7**:371–386.

Brown, D. D. and I. B. Dawid, 1968 Specific gene amplification in oöcytes. *Science (Wash., D.C.)* **160**:272–280.

Brown, S. W. and H. S. Chandra, 1973 Inactivation system of the mammalian X chromosome. *Proc. Natl. Acad. Sci. USA* **70**:195–199.

Burnett, R. G. and R. C. King, 1962 Observations on a microsporidian parasite of *Drosophila willistoni* Sturtevant. *J. Invertebr. Pathol.* **4**:104–112.

Casartelli, C., 1970 Estudo do desenvolvimento dos testículos de *Rhynchosciara angelae* e da síntese de acidos nucleicos e proteinas. M. A. Thesis, Universidade de São Paulo, São Paulo.

Cordeiro, M. and R. Meneghini, 1972 The rate of DNA replication in the polytene chromosomes of *Rhynchosciara angelae*, *Cell Differentiation* **1**:167–177.

Crouse, H. V., 1939 An evolution change in chromosome shape in *Sciara*. *Am. Nat.* **73**:476–480.

Crouse, H. V., 1943   Translocations in *Sciara*: Their bearing on chromosome behavior and sex determination. *Mo. Univ. Res. Bull.* **379**:1–79.

Crouse, H. V., 1947   Chromosome evolution in *Sciara*. *J. Hered.* **38**:278–288.

Crouse, H. V., 1960   The controlling element in sex chromosome behavior in *Sciara*. *Genetics* **45**:1429–1443.

Crouse, H. V., 1968   The role of ecdysone in "DNA-puff" formation of *Sciara coprophila*. *Proc. Natl. Acad. Sci. USA* **61**:971–978.

Crouse, H. V. and H. G. Keyl, 1968   Extra replications in the "DNA-puffs" of *Sciara coprophila*. *Chromosoma (Berl.)* **25**:357–364.

Crouse, H. V. and H. Smith-Stocking, 1938   New mutants in *Sciara* and their genetic behavior. *Genetics* **23**:275–282.

Crouse, H. V., A. Brown and B. C. Mumford, 1971   L-chromosome inheritance and the problem of chromosome "imprinting" in *Sciara* (Sciaridae, Diptera). *Chromosoma (Berl.)* **34**:324–339.

da Cunha, A. B. and C. Pavan, 1969   Alguns problemas da diferenciacão celular em Sciarideos. *Cienc. Cult. (São Paulo)* **21**:18–19.

da Cunha, A. B., J. S. Morgante, C. Pavan and M. C. Garrido, 1968   Studies on cytology and differentiation in Sciaridae. I. Chromosome changes induced by a gregarine in *Trichosia sp.* (Diptera, Sciaridae). *Caryologia* **21**:271–282.

da Cunha, A. B., J. S. Morgante, C. Pavan and M. C. Garrido, 1969*a*   Studies on cytology and differentiation in Sciaridae. II. DNA redundancy in salivary gland cells of *Hybosciara fragilis* (Diptera, Sciaridae). *Genetics Suppl.* **61(1)**:335–349.

da Cunha, A. B., J. S. Morgante, C. Pavan and M. C. Garrido, 1969*b*   Studies on cytology and differentiation in Sciaridae. III. Nuclear and cytoplasmic differentiation in the salivary glands of *Bradysia sp.* (University of Texas Publication 6918), *Stud. Genet.* **V**:1–11.

da Cunha, A. B., C. Pavan, J. J. Biesele, R. W. Riess and L. C. G. Simões, 1972   An ultrastructural study of the development of a nuclear polyhedrosis with effects on giant polytene chromosomes. (University of Texas Publication 7213), *Stud. Genet.* **VII**:117–143.

da Cunha, A. B., J. S. Morgante, C. Pavan, M. C. Garrido and J. Marques, 1973   Studies in cytology and differentiation in salivary glands of *Bradysia elegans* (Diptera, Sciaridae). *Caryologia* **26**:83–100.

Dasgupta, B. and H. N. Ray, 1954   Occurrence of intranuclear inclusions in the larvae of *Anopheles subpictus*. *Bull. Calcutta Sch. Trop. Med.* **2**:57–58.

Dasgupta, B. and H. N. Ray, 1957   The intranuclear inclusions in the midgut of the larvae of *Anopheles subpictus*. *Parasitology* **47**:194–195.

Davidheiser, B., 1943   Inheritance of the X chromosome in exceptional males of *Sciara ocellaris* (Diptera). *Genetics* **28**:193–199.

Debaisieux, P. and L. Gastaldi, 1919   Les microsporidies parasites des larves de *Simulium*. *Cellule* **30**:187–213.

de Souza, H. M. L. and C. Pavan, 1972   Change in the X chromosome during ontogeny of *Sciara ocellaris* inducing selective segregation of the mutated chromosome. *Genetics Suppl.* **74** (2, part 2):s61.

Diaz, M. and C. Pavan, 1965   Changes in chromosomes induced by microorganism infection. *Proc. Natl. Acad. Sci. USA* **54**:1321–1327.

Dickson, E., J. B. Boyd and C. D. Laird, 1971   Sequence diversity of polytene chromosome DNA from *Drosophila hydei*. *J. Mol. Biol.* **61**:615–627.

Du Bois, A. M., 1932   Elimination of chromosomes during cleavage in the eggs of *Sciara* (Diptera). *Genetics* **18**:352–355.

Dreyfus, A., E. Nonato, M. E. Breuer and C. Pavan, 1951   Cromosomas politênicos em vários órgãos de *Rhynchosciara angelae* Nonato et Pavan (Diptera). *Rev. Bras. Biol.* **11**:439–450.

Eckhardt, R. A. and J. G. Gall, 1971   Satellite DNA associated with heterochromatin in *Rhynchosciara. Chromosoma (Berl.)* **32**:407–427.

Edström, J. E., 1964   Chromosomal RNA and other nuclear RNA fractions. In *The Role of Chromosomes in Development,* edited by M. Locke, p. 137, Academic Press, New York.

Evans, N. L., 1956   The effect of cold treatment on the deoxyribonucleic acid (DNA) content of cells of selected plants and mammals. *Cytologia (Tokyo)* **21**:417–432.

Ficq, A. and C. Pavan, 1957   Autoradiography of polytene chromosomes of *Rhynchosciara angelae* at different stages of larval development. *Nature (Lond.)* **180**:983–984.

Gabrusewycz-Garcia, N., 1964   Cytological and autoradiograph studies in *Sciara coprophila* salivary gland chromosomes. *Chromosoma (Berl.)* **15**:312–344.

Gall, J. G., 1968   Differential synthesis of the genes for ribosomal RNA during amphibian oögenesis. *Proc. Natl. Acad. Sci. USA* **60**:553–560.

Gall, J. G., 1969   The genes for ribosomal RNA during oögenesis. *Genetics Suppl.* **61(1)**:127–132.

Gerbi, S. A., 1971   Localization and characterization of the ribosomal RNA cistrons in *Sciara coprophila. J. Mol. Biol.* **58**:499–511.

Geyer-Duszyńska, I., 1959   Experimental research on chromosome elimination in Cecidomyidae (Diptera). *J. Exp. Zool.* **141**:391–446.

Gil, R., P. Alonso and J. Perez-Silva, 1972   Ultrastructure of the macronuclear anlage in *Stylonychia mitilus. Exp. Cell Res.* **72**:509–518.

Greig-Holmes, A. P. and M. W. Shaw, 1971   Polymorphism of human constitutive heterochromatin. *Science (Wash., D.C.)* **174**:702–704.

Grossbach, U., 1968   Cell differentiation in the salivary glands of *Camptochironomus tentans* and *C. pallidivitatus. Ann. Zool. Fenn.* **5**:37–40.

Grossbach, U., 1969   Chromosomen-Aktivität und biochemische Zelldifferenzierung in den Speicheldrüsen von *Camptochironomus. Chromosoma (Berl.)* **28**:136–187.

Guaraciaba, H. L. B. and L. F. A. Toledo, 1967   Age determination of *Rhynchosciara angelae* larvae. *Rev. Bras. Biol.* **27**:321–332.

Guaraciaba, H. L. B. and L. F. A. Toledo, 1968   Morphological changes in the salivary chromosomes of *Rhynchosciara angelae. Arq. Inst. Biol. (São Paulo)* **35**:89–98.

Guevara, M., 1971   Estudo citológico da fisiologia e diferenciacão cromossômica durante o desenvolvimento larval de *Rhynchosciara angelae.* Ph.D. Dissertation, Universidade de São Paulo, São Paulo.

Guevara, M. and R. Basile, 1973   DNA and RNA puffs in *Rhynchosciara, Caryologia* **26**:275–295.

Helmsing, P. and H. D. Berendes, 1971   Induced accumulation of non-histone proteins in polytene nuclei of *Drosophila hydei. J. Cell Biol.* **50**:893–896.

Hinton, T., 1942   A comparative study of certain heterochromatic regions in the mitotic and salivary gland chromosomes of *Drosophila melanogaster. Genetics* **27**:119–127.

Jones, K. W., J. O. Bishop, and A. B. da Cunha, 1973   Complex formation between poly-r(U) and various chromosomal loci in *Rhynchosciara. Chromosoma (Berl.)* **43**:375–390.

Jurand, A., L. C. G. Simões and C. Pavan, 1967   Changes in the ultrastructure of salivary gland cytoplasm in *Sciara ocellaris* (Comstock, 1882) due to microsporidian infection. *J. Insect Physiol.* **13**:795–803.

Karlson, F., 1966   Steroid hormones in insects. *Proc. 2nd Interntl. Congr. Hormonal Steroids*: 146–153.

Kellen, W. R., T. B. Clark and J. E. Lindgren, 1963   A possible polyhedrosis in *Culex tarsalis* Coq. (Diptera, Culicidae). *J. Insect Pathol.* **5**:98–103.

Kramer, J. P., 1964   *Nosema kingi* sp. n., a microsporidian from *Drosophila willistoni* Sturtevant, and its infectivity for other muscoids. *J. Insect Pathol.* **6**:491–499.

Kudo, R., 1924   Studies on microsporidia parasitic in mosquitoes. III On *Thelohania legeri* Hesse. *Arch. Protistenkd.* **49**:147–162.

Kunz, W., H.-H. Trepte and K. Bier, 1970   On the function of the germline chromosomes in the oögenesis of *Wachtliella persicariae* (Cecidomyidae). *Chromosoma (Berl.)* **30**:180–192.

Lainson, R., P. C. C. Garnham, R. Kellick-Kendrick and R. G. Bird, 1964   Nosematosis, a microsporidial infection of rodents and other animals, including man. *Br. Med. J.* **2**:470–472.

Lara, F. J. S. and F. M. Hollander, 1967   Changes in RNA metabolism during the development of *Rhynchosciara angelae*. *Natl. Cancer Inst. Monogr.* **27**:235–242.

Lara, F. J. S., H. Tamaki and C. Pavan, 1965   Laboratory culture of *Rhynchosciara angelae*. *Am. Nat.* **99**:189–191.

Lima-de-Faria, A., 1959   Differential uptake of tritiated thymidine into hetero- and euchromatin in *Melanoplus* and *Secale*. *J. Biophys. Biochem. Cytol.* **6**:457–466.

Lima-de-Faria, A., 1962   Metabolic DNA in *Tipula oleracea*. *Chromosoma (Berl.)* **13**:47–59.

Lima-de-Faria, A. and H. Jaworska, 1968   Late DNA synthesis in heterochromatin. *Nature (Lond.)* **217**:138–142.

Lima-de-Faria, A. and M. J. Moses, 1966   Ultrastructural and cytochemistry of metabolic DNA in *Tipula*. *J. Cell Biol.* **30**:177–192.

Lima-de-Faria, A., M. Birnstiel and H. Jawonski, 1969   Amplification of ribosomal cistrons in the heterochromatin of *Acheta*. *Genetics (Suppl.)* **61**(1):145–159.

Lom, J. and J. O. Corliss, 1967   Ultrastructural observations on the development of the microsporidian protozoan *Plistophora hyphessobryconis* Schaperclaus. *J. Protozool.* **14**:141–152.

Malvaldi, G. and M. P. Viola-Magni, 1972   DNA turnover in adrenal medullary cells of different strains of rats and its enhancement after intermittent exposure to cold. *Cell Tissue Kinet.* **5**:103.

Mattingly, E. and S. Ogle, 1969   A new culture method for *Rhynchosciara*. *Ann. Entomol. Soc. Am.* **62**:94–96.

Mattingly, E. and C. Parker, 1968   Sequence of puff formation in *Rhynchosciara* polytene chromosomes. *Chromosoma (Berl.)* **23**:255–270.

Mendelsohn, M. L., B. H. Mayall, E. Bogart, D. H. Moore and B. H. Perry, 1973   DNA content and DNA-based centromeric index of the 24 human chromosomes. *Science (Wash., D.C.)* **179**:1126–1129.

Meneghini, R. and M. Cordeiro, 1972   DNA replication in polytene chromosomes of *Rhynchosciara angelae*. *Cell Diff.* **1**:167–177.

Meneghini, R., H. A. Armelin and F. J. S. Lara, 1968   Change in pattern of inhibition of actinomycin D of uridine-H³ incorporation into salivary gland RNA of *Rhynchosciara* at different larval ages. *Biochem. Biophys. Res. Commun.* **32**:846–851.

Meneghini, R., H. A. Armelin, J. Balsamo and F. J. S. Lara, 1971   Indication of gene amplification in *Rhynchosciara* by RNA–DNA hybridization. *J. Cell. Biol.* **49**:913–916.

Metz, C. W., 1934   Evidence indicating that in *Sciara* the sperm regularly transmits two sister sex chromosomes. *Proc. Natl. Acad. Sci. USA* **20**:31–36.

Metz, C. W., 1938   Chromosome behavior, inheritance, and sex determination in *Sciara*. *Am. Nat.* **72**:485–520.

Metz, C. W. and E. G. Lawrence, 1938   Preliminary observations on *Sciara* hybrids. *J. Hered.* **29**:179–186.

Metz, C. W. and M. L. Schmuck, 1931   Studies on sex determination and the sex chromosome mechanism in *Sciara*. *Genetics* **16**:225–253.

Miller, O. L., 1964   Extrachromosomal nucleolar DNA in amphibian oöcytes. *J. Cell Biol.* **23**:20A.

Miller, O. L., 1966   Structure and composition of peripheral nucleoli of salamander oöcytes. *Natl. Cancer Inst. Monogr.* **23**:53–66.

Morgante, J. S., 1969   Estudo sôbre a biologia, ecologia e sistemática de três espécies brasileiras de Sciaridae (Diptera, Menatocera). M. A. Thesis, Universidade de São Paulo, São Paulo.

Morgante, J. S., 1972   Rhynchosciara angelae: Aspectos da ecologia e da patologia celular induzida por virus de poliedrose nuclear. Ph.D. Dissertation, Universidade de São Paulo, São Paulo.

Morgante, J. S., A. B. da Cunha, C. Pavan, J. J. Bieselle, R. W. Riess, and M. C. Garrido, 1974   Development of a nuclear polyhedrosis in cells of *Rhynchosciara angelae* (Diptera, Sciaridae) and patterns of DNA synthesis in the infected cells. *J. Invertebr. Pathol.* **24**:93–105.

Morgante, J. S. and M. Guevara, 1969   Caracterização dos estadios larvais de *Rhynchosciara angelae* Nonato et Pavan 1951. *Cienc. Cult. (São Paulo)* **21**:288–289.

Morgante, J. S., J. Marques, A. B. da Cunha and I. Romeo, 1970   Métodos para a criação de alguns sciarídeos (Diptera). *Rev. Bras. Entomol.* **14**:33–40.

Moritz, K. B., 1970   DNS-Variation im Leimbahnbegrenztenchromatin und autoradiographische Befunde zu seines Funktion bei *Parascaris equorum*. *Verh. Dtsch. Zool. Ges.* **64**:36–42.

Müller, H. J., D. Raffel, S. M. Gershenson and A. A. Prokofjeva-Belgovskaya, 1937   A further analysis of loci in the so-called "inert region" of the X chromosome of *Drosophila*. *Genetics* **22**:87–93.

Muñoz de Hoyos, P., 1972   Relationship between two species of *Microsporidia* (Sporozoa) and two related species of *Rhynchosciara* (Diptera). M. A. Thesis, The University of Texas, Austin, Texas.

Nagl, W., 1972   Evidence of DNA amplification in the orchid *Cymbidium in vitro*. *Cytobios* **5**:145–154.

Nonato, E. and C. Pavan, 1951   A new species of *Rhynchosciara* Rübsaamen 1894 (Diptera, Mycetophilidae). *Rev. Bras. Biol.* **11**:435–437.

Papaconstantinou, J., W. E. Bradshaw, E. T. Chiu and E. M. Julku, 1972   Synthesis of satellite DNA in *Rhynchosciara hollaenderi*. *Dev. Biol.* **28**:649–661.

Pardue, M. L., S. A. Gerbi, R. A. Eckhardt and J. G. Gall, 1970   Cytological localization of DNA complementary to ribosomal RNA in polytene chromosomes of Diptera. *Chromosoma (Berl.)* **29**:268–290.

Pavan, C., 1946   Two types of heterochromatin in *Drosophila nebulosa*. *Proc. Natl. Acad. Sci. USA* **32**:137–145.

Pavan, C., 1958 Morphological and physiological aspects of chromosomal activities. *Proc. X. Interntl. Congr. Genet.* **1**:321–336.

Pavan, C., 1959 Organization of the chromosome. In *Organization of the Chromosome in Biological Organization. Cellular and Sub-cellular,* edited by C. H. Waddington, pp. 72–89, Pergamon Press, London.

Pavan, C., 1965a Nucleic acid metabolism in polytene chromosomes and the problem of differentiation. *Brookhaven Symp. Biol.* **18**:222–241.

Pavan, C., 1965b Nucleic acid metabolism in polytene chromosomes and the problem of differentiation. *Natl. Cancer Inst. Monogr.* **18**:309–323.

Pavan, C. and R. Basile, 1966a Invertebrate pathology, cytology, and development. *J. Invertebr. Pathol.* **8**:131–132.

Pavan, C. and R. Basile, 1966b Chromosome changes induced by infections in tissues of *Rhynchosciara angelae. Science (Wash., D.C.)* **151**:1556–1558.

Pavan, C. and M. E. Breuer, 1952 Polytene chromosomes in different tissues of *Rhynchosciara. J. Hered.* **23**:150–157.

Pavan, C. and M. E. Breuer, 1955 Differences in nucleic acid content of the loci in polytene chromosomes of *Rhynchosciara angelae* according to tissue and larval stages. In *Symposium on Cell Secretions,* edited by G. Schreiber, pp. 90–99, Belo Horizonte, Brazil.

Pavan, C. and A. B. da Cunha, 1968 Chromosome activities in normal and infected cells of Sciaridae. In *Proceedings of the International Seminar on the Chromosome—Its Structure and Function,* edited by A. K. Sharma and A. Sharma, Supplementary Volume, pp. 183–196, *The Nucleus,* Calcutta.

Pavan, C. and A. B. da Cunha, 1969a Chromosomal activities in *Rhynchosciara* and other Sciaridae. *Annu. Rev. Genet.* **3**:425–450.

Pavan, C. and A. B. da Cunha, 1969b Gene amplification in ontogeny and phylogeny of animals. *Genetics Suppl.* **61**(1):289–304.

Pavan, C. and A. L. P. Perondini, 1967 Heterozygous puffs and bands in *Sciara ocellaris* Comstock 1882. *Exp. Cell Res.* **48**:202–205.

Pavan, C., A. L. P. Perondini and T. Picard, 1969 Changes induced in chromosomes and in development of cells of *Sciara ocellaris* induced by microsporidian infections. *Chromosoma (Berl.)* **28**:328–345.

Pavan, C., A. B. da Cunha and C. Morsoletto, 1971a Virus–chromosome relationships in cells of *Rhynchosciara* (Diptera, Sciaridae). *Caryologia* **24**:371–389.

Pavan, C., J. L. Sanders and R. C. Richmond, 1971b Effects of irradiation on neuroendocrine glands and puffs in *Rhynchosciara. Abstr. 11th Annu. Meet. Am. Soc. Cell Biol.:* 220.

Pavan, C., J. J. Biesele, R. W. Riess and A. V. Wertz, 1971c XIII. Changes in the ultrastructure of *Rhynchosciara* cells infected by microsporidia. (University of Texas Publication 7103), *Stud. Genet.* **VI**:241–271.

Pelc, S. R., 1972 Metabolic DNA in ciliated protozoa, salivary gland chromosomes, and mammalian cells. *Interntl. Rev. Cytol.* **32**:327–358.

Perondini, A. L. P., 1968 Fisiologia dos cromossomos politênicos de *Bradysia tritici* (Coquillet 1895). Ph.D. Dissertation, Universidade de São Paulo, São Paulo.

Perondini, A. L. P. and E. M. Dessen, 1969 Heterozygous puffs in *Sciara ocellaris. Genetics Suppl.* **61**(1):251–260.

Rennie, J., 1923 Polyhedral disease in *Tipula paludosa* (Meig.) *Proc. R. Phil. Soc. Edin. A* **20**:265–267.

Ritossa, F., 1968 Unstable redundancy of genes for ribosomal RNA. *Proc. Natl. Acad. Sci. USA* **60**:509–516.

Ritossa, F. and G. Scala, 1969 Equilibrium variations in redundancy of DNA. *Genetics Suppl.* **61(1)**:305–317.

Roberts, P. A., R. F. Kimball and C. Pavan, 1967 Response of *Rhynchosciara* chromosomes to microsporidian infection. *Exp. Cell Res.* **47**:408–422.

Rübsaamen, H., 1894 Die aussereuropäische Trauermücken des Königl. Museums für Naturalkunde zu Berlin. *Berl. Ent. Zeitschr.* **39**:17–42.

Rudkin, G. T., 1965 Non-replicating DNA in giant chromosomes. *Genetics* **52**:470.

Rudkin, G. T., 1969 Non-replicating DNA in *Drosophila*. *Genetics Suppl.* **61(1)**:227–238.

Rudkin, G. T. and S. L. Corlette, 1957 Disproportionate synthesis of DNA in a polytene chromosome region. *Proc. Natl. Acad. Sci. USA* **43**:964–968.

Sanders, P. F. and C. Pavan, 1972 Heterochromatin in development of normal and infected cells. In *Proceedings of the First Conference on Cell Differentiation* (Nice, France), pp. 287–300, Munksgaard, Copenhagen.

Sauaia, H., E. M. Laicine and M. A. Alves, 1971 Hydroxyurea-induced inhibition of DNA puff development in the salivary chromosomes of *Bradysia hygida*. *Chromosoma (Berl.)* **34**:129–151.

Sharman, G. B., 1970 Reproductive physiology of marsupials. *Science (Wash., D.C.)* **167**:1221–1228.

Sharman, G. B., 1971 Late DNA replication in paternally derived X chromosomes of female kangaroos. *Nature (Lond.)* **230**:231–232.

Siegel, A., D. Lightfood, O. G. Ward and S. Keener, 1973 DNA complementary to ribosomal RNA: Relation between genomic proportion and ploidy. *Science (Wash., D.C.)* **179**:682–683.

Simões, L. C. G., 1967 Síntese de DNA durante o desenvolvimento larval de *Rhynchosciara sp.* Ph.D. Dissertation, Universidade de São Paulo, São Paulo.

Simões, L. C. G., 1970 Studies on DNA synthesis during larval development of *Rhynchosciara sp.* *Rev. Bras. Biol.* **30**:191–199.

Simões, L. C. G. and A. N. Cestari, 1969 Behavior of polytene chromosomes *in vitro*. *Genetics Suppl.* **61(1)**:361–372.

Smith, K. M., 1967 *Insect Virology*, Academic Press, New York.

Smith, K. M. and N. Xeros, 1953 Development of virus in cell nuclei. *Nature (Lond.)* **172**:670–671.

Sprague, V., 1965 *Nosema sp.* (Microsporidia, Nosematidae) in the musculature of the crab *Callinectes sapidus*. *J. Protozool.* **12**:66–70.

Stocker, A. J., C. Pavan and C. Charlton, 1972 Induction of DNA puffs in *Rhynchosciara* by ecdysterone. Abstract, Annual Meetings of the Genetics Society of America, Minneapolis, August, 1972.

Stoltz, D. B., C. Pavan and A. B. da Cunha, 1973 Nuclear polyhedrosis virus: A possible example of *de novo* intranuclear membrane morphogenesis, *J. Gen. Virol.* **19**:145–150.

Summerfelt, R. C., 1964 A new microsporidian parasite from the Golden Shiner, *Notemigonus cripoleucas*. *Trans. Am. Fish. Soc.* **93**:6–10.

Swift, H., 1962 Nucleic acids and cell morphology in Dipteran salivary glands. In *Molecular Control of Gene Activity*, (edited by J. M. Allen, pp. 73–125, McGraw-Hill, New York.

Terra, W. R., 1972   Aspectos bioquímicos da hemolinfa e do casulo coletivo de *Rhynchosciara americana*. Ph.D. Dissertation, Universidade de São Paulo, São Paulo.

Thomson, H. H., 1960   A list and brief description of the microsporidia infecting insects. *J. Insect Pathol.* **2**:346–385.

Tobler, H., K. D. Smith and H. Ursprung, 1972   Molecular aspects of chromatin elimination in *Ascaris lumbricoides*. *Dev. Biol.* **27**:190–203.

Toledo, S. A., S. H. Yang and C. Pavan, 1973   Isoenzymes during the development of *Rhynchosciara hollaenderi*. *Genet. Iber.*, **24**:263–281.

Turpin, R. and J. Lejeune, 1965   *Les Chromosomes Humains,* Gauthier-Villars, Paris.

Viola-Magni, M. P., 1965   Changes in the DNA content of adrenal medulla nuclei of rats intermittently exposed to cold. *J. Cell Biol.* **25**:415–433.

Weiser, J., 1965   *Nosema muris* n. sp., a new microsporidian parasite of the white mouse (*Mus musculus*). *J. Protozool.* **12**:78–83.

Wertz, A. V., 1970   Host–parasite relationships in *Rhynchosciara* infected by *Thelohania sp.* M.A. Thesis, University of Texas, Austin, Texas.

White, M. J. D., 1950   Cytological studies on gall midges (Cecidomyidae), University of Texas Publication 5007, pp. 1–80, Austin, Texas.

White, M. J. D., 1954   *Animal Cytology and Evolution,* Cambridge University Press, London.

Whitten, J. M., 1965   Differential deoxyribonucleic acid replication in the giant food-pad cells of *Sarcophaga bullata*. *Nature (Lond.)* **208**:1019–1021.

Wiedemann, C. R. W., 1821   *Diptera Exotica,* Kiel, Germany.

Wilson, E. B., 1925   *The Cell in Development and Heredity,* Macmillan, New York.

Wobus, U., R. Panitz and E. Serfling, 1970   Tissue specific gene activity and proteins in the Chironomus salivary gland. *Mol. Gen. Genet.* **107**:215–223.

Wobus, U., E. Serfling and R. Panitz, 1971   Salivary gland protein of a *Chironomus thummi* strain with an additional Balbiani-ring. *Exp. Cell Res.* **65**:240–245.

9

Sciara coprophila

NATALIA GABRUSEWYCZ-GARCIA

Introduction

During the last ten years considerable interest has focused on the study of chromosomal puffs, which have been widely interpreted to represent synthetically active sites of the genome [see review by Pelling (1972)]. In most of these studies the larval salivary chromosomes of *Drosophila* and *Chironomus* have been used. Larvae of the Sciarid family are of interest because in all species so far examined, the salivary chromosomes develop prior to metamorphosis special puffs which show a localized increase in DNA content (Rudkin and Corlette, 1957: Crouse and Keyl, 1968; Rasch, 1970a). These extremely large puffs appear to form under hormonal control (Crouse, 1968; Gabrusewycz-Garcia and Margless, 1969). The morphology, cytochemistry, and metabolic characteristics of DNA puffs have been investigated in several laboratories (Poulson and Metz, 1938; Swift, 1962; Gabrusewycz-Garcia, 1964; Pavan and da Cunha, 1969; Sauaia *et al.*, 1971; Goodman and Benjamin, 1973).

Sciarid flies are also of interest to the cytogeneticist because of a peculiar mechanism of sex determination where chromosome elimination plays an important role (see pages 208–217). The two species most widely used for both genetic and developmental studies are *Sciara coprophila* and *Rhynchosciara angelae*. The biology of *Rhynchosciara* is reviewed by Pavan *et al.* in Chapter 8 of this volume. The following brief account of

NATALIA GABRUSEWYCZ-GARCIA—Onondaga Community College and Department of Anatomy, State University of New York, Syracuse, New York.

the life cycle, culture methods, and cytology applies primarily to *Sciara coprophila*, although a number of other *Sciara* species share many of its biologic characteristics and are easily maintained in the laboratory by following essentially the same techniques.

Notes on the Biology of *Sciara*

Although frequently unnoticed by the casual observer, adults of the genus *Sciara* are ubiquitous. They are frequent in suburban yards, greenhouses, mushroom cellars, and around potted plants. I have collected them in cow barns, on the windshield of my car and, on one occasion, eclosing from the garbage disposal in my own kitchen! The larvae are less conspicuous and may be found in moist locations among decomposing vegetation or in the potting soil. They are very sensitive to dessication. In the older literature, *Sciara* larvae are said to cause extensive damage to the softer parts of many plants, especially the young root system. The plants cited range from lettuce, cucumbers, tomatoes, wheat, and corn to geraniums and African violets (Hungerford, 1916).

Taxonomy of Sciaridae

This appears to be a very entangled subject, at least to the uninitiated. Fortunately, a new revision of the genera within the family Sciaridae has recently appeared (Steffan, 1966). According to this new publication, the correct name for *Sciara coprophila* is *Bradysia coprophila*. Unfortunately, there is now a literature of considerable size which uses the former name, and it seems that the cytologists favor *Sciara* as the generic name. The following references on taxonomy may also be consulted: Johannsen (1912) and Shaw (1953). To the cytologist, the publications of Metz and his students are very useful. Based on descriptions and chromosome drawings published by McCarthy (1945), I was able to identify correctly *S. pauciseta* and *S. prolifica*. Good drawings of the chromosomes from salivary gland cells of *S. impatiens* (prior to the appearance of DNA puffs) are also available (Carson, 1944).

Collection of Adults

Probably the easiest places for collection are greenhouses and cow barns. Single gravid females are trapped on the glass panes by covering them with small vials which are either partially filled with agar or contain moist filter paper. Once in the laboratory, oviposition may be induced in the following way. Females are etherized and placed on agar in small Petri dishes. The wings may be pushed into the agar thus immobilizing the fly. Taking a blunt instrument, one then presses the abdomen in such a way as to cause extension of the ovipositor. If the female is "ripe," continued stroking will eventually bring about oviposition, but injury to the fly must be carefully avoided. Another option is to let the female lay eggs of her own accord. Frequently she will use cracks in the agar or the inside of gelled agar bubbles or "hide" her eggs under particles of straw or potting soil. Once hatched, the larvae are maintained according to the procedure described below. When the next generation of adults ecloses, brother–sister matings keep the culture going. In a unisexual species, the hope is to get female and male producers simultaneously in the same collection. Newly collected flies are often heavily infested with mites. These have to be picked off carefully and destroyed if infestation of the cultures is to be avoided. For anti-mite operations, see Spencer (1950). Pavan *et al.* in Chapter 8 in this volume have helpful suggestions for controlling bacterial, mold, and nematode infections.

Laboratory Culture

The smaller species, such as *S. coprophila, S. impatiens,* and *S. pauciseta,* are maintained in the laboratory by following the techniques described below. Glass vials (35 mm in diameter and 100 mm in height) are partially filled (about 3 cm deep) with a 2 percent agar solution. For best results the vials should be poured one day previous to use, left to stand for a couple of hours at room temperature, plugged with cotton, and stored in a tin box in a cool place. Care should be taken not to overcrowd the vials with flies. Around 30 individuals per vial seems the optimum for female larvae, but males are smaller and may tolerate larger groups. Larvae may be fed either on vegetable matter or dry yeast. Newly hatched larvae should be lightly sprinkled with yeast. A light mat of fine straw or potting soil is scattered over the yeast. Eventually all the larvae will crawl under the mat of straw and yeast. Second- and later-instar larvae may be fed on squares of spinach leaves. Fresh leaves are added once or twice a week, depending on larval age, and old, dried out leaves are removed. Larvae of all stages, but especially prepupae, are very sensitive to the water content of the agar. If the agar is soft enough so that the larvae can burrow into it, they should be transferred to a fresh vial. During the second half of the fourth instar, when larvae are getting closer to pupation, there should be plenty of fine straw in the vial. Shortly after the imagoes eclose, matings are set up in fresh vials. Flies may be lightly etherized. With the right amount of moisture, the straw, remnants of yeast, etc., will not fall out when the vial is inverted. No special provisions are made to feed the adults. It appears that they may suck up the yeast in the fluid which collects on the surface of the agar.

The stocks of *S. coprophila* now used by several different laboratories are all derived from collections made by C. W. Metz around 1925 and later maintained by Dr. H. V. Crouse. It is a pleasure to acknowledge the generosity of Dr. Crouse for sharing her stocks with other workers in the field.

Life Cycle of *Sciara coprophila*

The number of eggs laid by a single female is variable and ranges from about 20 to 200. As a rule, large females will produce more eggs than smaller ones. Within limits, the size of the flies is determined by the conditions under which they developed as larvae. When kept at 19–20°C, the eggs hatch within a period of 4–5 days. The newly hatched larvae are about 0.65 mm long. After two days they molt and become second-instar larvae. The second molt occurs 2.5–3 days later, and the third molt is reached after another 2.5 days. The larvae do not develop in perfect synchrony, and the first and last adults may eclose several days apart even under "constant" conditions. Therefore, it may be desirable to choose larvae that are developing at similar rates. This is often done at the third molt. At each molt the old larval cuticle and the black head capsule are discarded, so that newly molted larvae are completely transparent. The new head capsule undergoes gradual darkening which, at room temperature, takes 2.5–3 hours. Molting and postmolt individuals may thus be identified and transferred to separate vials. The fourth larval instar is the longest, and at this stage the normal schedule of development may be profoundly affected by factors such as moisture, availability of food, crowding, and even handling of the larvae.

The best criterion for distinguishing each stage within the fourth instar is the appearance and increase in size of the imaginal eye anlagen or "eyespots" (Gabrusewycz-Garcia, 1964). At 19–20°C, the eyespots are first visible (under a stereomicroscope) on day 6 in female larvae and on day 5 in male larvae. From this point on, the developmental schedule of males and females diverge. The following description applies to females; a description of male development is found in Rieffel and Crouse (1966). If desirable, larvae may also be selected at the time eyespots can first be seen. This stage is referred to as small eyespots (SES). In another 2–3

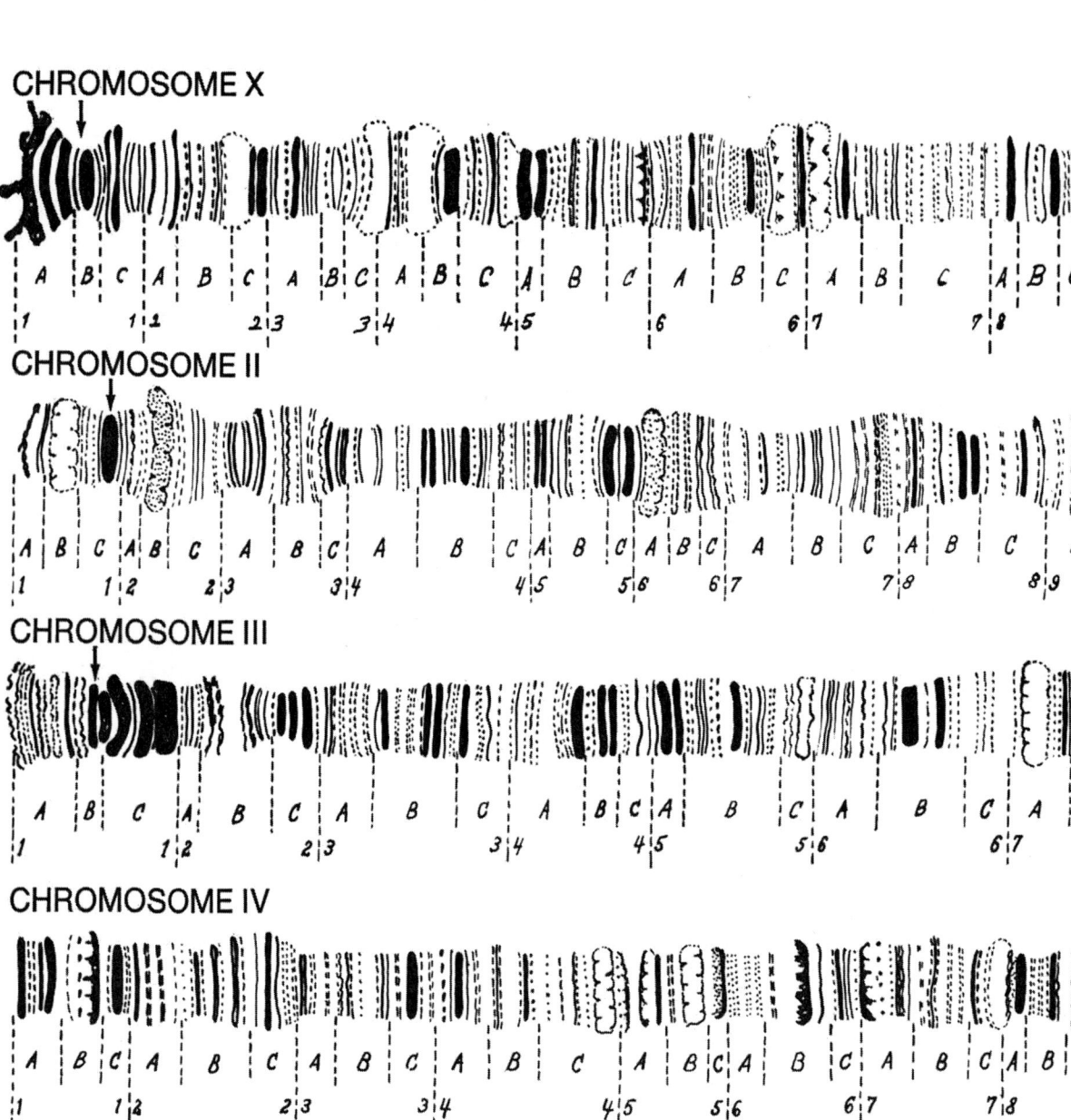

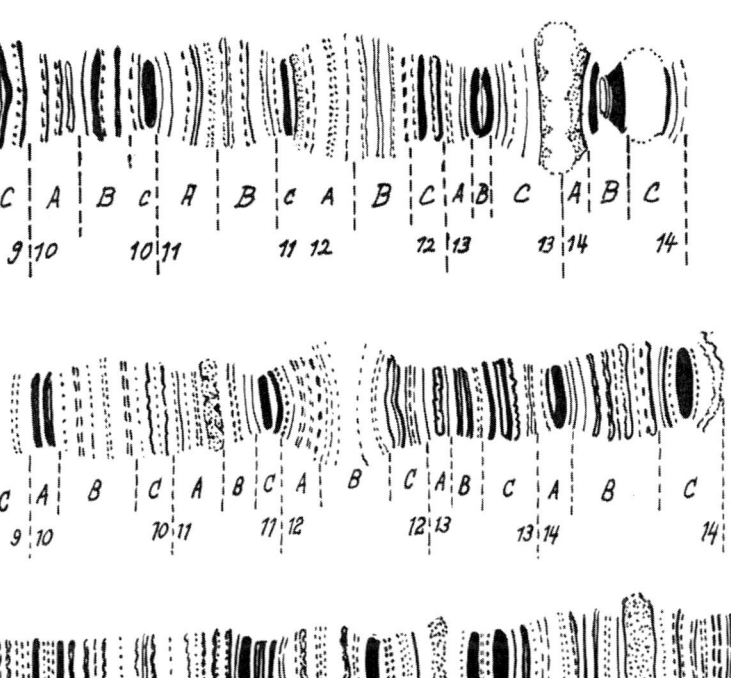

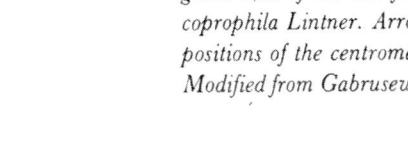

Figure 1. The polytene c[...]
gland cells of the late fo[...]
coprophila Lintner. Arro[...]
positions of the centrome[...]
Modified from Gabrusew[...]

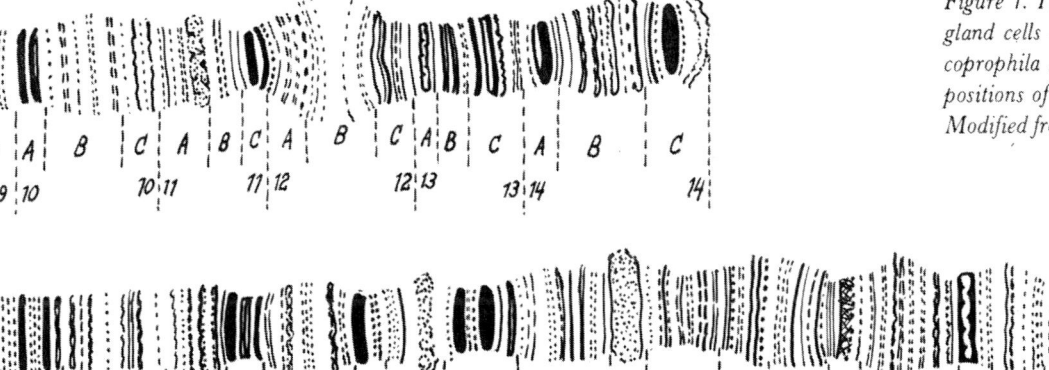

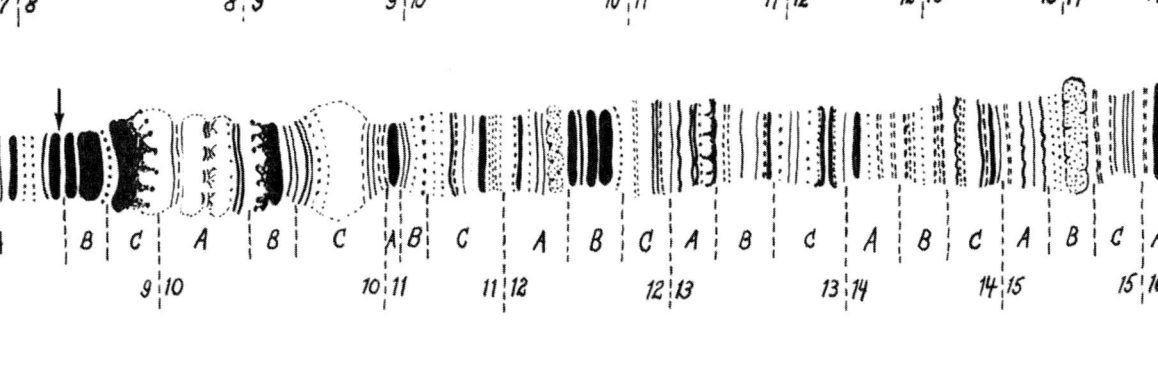

s of the salivary
larva of Sciara
he approximate
fication 1250×.
(1964).

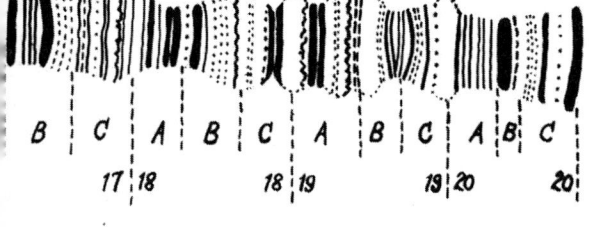

days the larvae grow to the medium-eyespot size (MES), and after one
more day they become large-eyespot (LES) larvae. For more details and
photographs of different stages, see the excellent review by Rasch (1970*a*).
The DNA puffs appear shortly after the eyespots, usually between days 7
and 8 of the fourth instar. In addition to eyespots, other characteristics
may be used to estimate larval age. They are: the amount and pattern of
fat deposition, the mobility of the larvae, the feeding behavior (feeding
stops at LES), and the color of the gastric caeca. The exact onset of the
prepupal stage is difficult to define. I have arbitrarily used the time of
lateral displacement of the eyespots as the transition point between the
LES larva and the prepupa. At the LES stage, larvae start to prepare for
pupation by digging little holes in the agar, most frequently between the
agar and the glass of the vial. They coat the agar side of the hole with
their salivary secretion which, together with extraneous material, forms a
"flimsy coccoon" which serves as the pupal chamber (Hungerford, 1916).
While working on the coccoon, larvae bend their bodies into a *U*-shaped
curve. After completion of the chamber, the larva shortens to about 4 mm,
from its previous length of about 1 cm, and soon it loses its ability to
crawl, even when disturbed. The pupal molt takes place in the pupal
chamber 16–20 hours after eyespot displacement. The chamber seems to
be necessary for normal development since I have noticed that a large proportion of the individuals pulled out of their coccoons fail to molt normally. At the pupal molt, both the larval cuticle and the dark head
capsule are shed. The pupal period lasts for another 5–6 days, and then
eclosion occurs. At 19–20°C the whole life cycle takes place in approximately one month.

The Salivary Gland and Its Secretion

Each larva has a pair of salivary glands, which by the end of fourth
instar are about 1 cm in length (in females). The salivary glands are attached to the fat body and are folded. The secretion enters the mouth of
the larva by means of a common salivary duct. Distally the duct divides to
provide drainage to each member of the gland pair. Between the duct and
the gland proper lies the small anlage of the imaginal salivary gland. The
larval salivary gland is a tubular structure with a single layer of cells arranged around a narrow lumen. After embryogenesis the gland cells do
not divide, but they increase in size by polytenization. The salivary gland
may be subdivided into several segments. The anterior segment (also
referred to as the reservoir) consists of two opposing rows of large cells.
There are usually 15 cells in each row. The fine structure of this portion

of the gland has been studied by Phillips and Swift (1965) and by Phillips (1965), especially with respect to its secretory product. The next portion is generally referred to as the neck and consists of seven pairs of smaller cells. Their nuclei have a lower range of DNA values. Prior to and during the appearance of eyespots, I have observed that the neck cells become filled with large granules (1.3–1.5 μm in diameter) which, at the electron microscope level, are somewhat similar to the electron-lucid granules described by Phillips and Swift (1965) in the cells of the anterior portion of the gland. The posterior portion of the gland is the longest and consists of approximately 120 large cells. The lumen here is not straight, rather it describes a zigzagging line, with the cells distributed in a characteristically alternating pattern. The distal or "tip" portion of the gland consists of about 24 cells which exhibit a low degree of polyteny. At about the time the eyespots appear, the lumen becomes greatly distended with secretion. The anterior and posterior gland portions differ with respect to several DNA puffs and a few RNA puffs (see below).

The salivary secretion is a clear, viscous fluid which, once extruded, forms silklike fibers. It may be produced by larvae of all ages. In certain cultures these fibers are fastened to pieces of straw or bits of food to form a communal net under which the larvae move. It appears that larvae may eat the net when there is shortage of food. Such "netted" cultures always develop rapidly and seem to have a high rate of metabolism as judged by the level of incorporation of labeled precursors into protein and nucleic acids of the larval salivary gland cells. Reference has already been made to the use of the salivary secretion in the construction of the pupal chamber. The secretion also seems to lubricate the larval cuticle (Been and Rasch, 1972) and to serve in digestion (Phillips and Swift, 1965). A recent publication deals with the analysis of protein from both whole salivary glands and from samples of the secretion (Been and Rasch, 1972).

Chromosome Cytology of *Sciara coprophila*

This species has a haploid complement of four chromosomes, three autosomes (II, III, and IV), and one sex chromosome (X). Mitotic figures show that two of the autosomal pairs are rod-shaped (II and III) and one is V-shaped (IV). The sex chromosome is rod-shaped. In addition, the germline nuclei contain 2 to 3 large V-shaped, limited chromosomes (Rieffel and Crouse, 1966). Although in *Sciara* several larval tissues develop polytene nuclei, only those from the salivary gland are large enough for detailed cytological studies. Cytophotometric estimates of DNA content of these and other nuclei of *Sciara* have been made by Rasch (1970*b*, 1971).

The polytene salivary complement consists of four elements with the following length relationships: 1(X) : 1.07 (II), and 1.25 (III) : 1.71 (IV). Chromosome IV, the longest of the group is metacentric and measures, on the average, 264 μm. Salivary chromosome maps were published by Crouse in 1943. Later these were revised and much cytological detail has been added (Gabrusewycz-Garcia, 1964). Figure 1 is a slightly modified drawing of the maps from the latter publication. In the salivary nuclei there is no definitive chromocenter. The only reliable way to determine the position of the centromeres is by cytogenetic techniques. Using reciprocal translocations and a number of mutants, Crouse (1943) was able to identify the approximate map positions of the centromeres. Their locations on the revised maps are as follows: 1A–C (X); 1C (II); 1B (III); 9B (IV). The positions of the centromeres are marked by dense, heterochromatic bands. These, as well as other heavy bands, may often adhere to each other. This phenomenon is referred to as ectopic pairing. Autoradiographic observations show that the majority of such bands replicate their DNA at a specific time period and out of cycle with the remainder of the complement (Gabrusewycz-Garcia, 1964). The nucleolar organizer (NOR) is located on the X chromosome in region 1A, in the so-called proximal heterochromatin (Gabrusewycz-Garcia and Kleinfeld, 1966; Gerbi, 1971). During late developmental stages, the amount of nucleolar material may vary from a small clump at the NOR to numerous masses scattered within the nucleus (micronucleoli). More details on the nucleolar material, including description of fine structure, may be found in a recent publication (Gabrusewycz-Garcia, 1972).

Nine major DNA puffs were described in my 1964 publication. Since then, nine other smaller DNA puffs have been added to this group. Table 1 lists all DNA puffs known to occur in *S. coprophila* to date, as well as their location on the salivary chromosomes. Table 1 also shows the major differences in the puffing pattern between the anterior and the posterior segments of the salivary gland. A list of the more conspicuous RNA puffs (bulbs) will be found in Gabrusewycz-Garcia (1964). However, in *Sciara* the developmental patterns of RNA puffing have not been studied in detail.

Puffing starts in MES larvae, approximately on day 7 of the fourth instar. In most larvae, DNA puffs arise fairly simultaneously in the chromosomes of both the anterior and the posterior portions of the salivary gland. However, it appears that in some larvae DNA puffs in the posterior segment may precede those in the anterior segment by a 24-hour period (Cannon, 1965). During their development, large DNA puffs pass through a sequence of stages, each with its distinct morphology and metabolic characteristics. For convenience, four stages may be recognized.

TABLE 1.   The DNA Puffs of the Chromosomal Complement of the
             Salivary Gland Cells of S. coprophila.[a]

Chromosome	Puff location	Puff size in anterior part of gland	Puff size in posterior part of gland
X	7A	Small	Small
	11B	Small	Small
II	2B	Large	Large
	6A	Large	Large
	9A	Large	Large
	11A	Small or absent	Large
	13A	Small	Small
	14B	Small	Larger
III	2B	Large	Absent
	10A	Large	Large
	11A	Large	Large
	15B	Large	Absent
IV	5C	Small	Small
	8C	Small	Small
	10B	Small	Small
	12A	Small	Absent
	15B	Absent	Large
	19A	Small	Small

[a] Modified from Gabrusewycz-Garcia (1971).

Stage I is characterized by small puffs. The chromosomal diameter at the puff site is slightly enlarged. Small puffs are compact and stain intensely with orcein or Feulgen. In autoradiographs they show a very high rate of ^{3}H-thymidine uptake relative to other chromosomal regions (Gabrusewycz-Garcia, 1964). Stage II is characterized by larger or expanding puffs. A further increase in diameter and an expansion of the DNA puff bands takes place. However, expansion along the chromosomal axis is not as advanced and neighboring bands are not yet obliterated. The puffs are intensely stained with orcein or Feulgen and show a rate of ^{3}H-thymidine uptake comparable to that of stage I. Stage III is characterized by large or expanded puffs, with maximal expansion of the puff both laterally and in the direction of the chromosomal axis. A number of neighboring bands are obliterated and the puff now is approximately spherical in shape. Staining with orcein or Feulgen is faint but a diffuse, metachromatic staining with basic dyes may be detected. ^{3}H-thymidine uptake is decreased relative to previous stages. Stage IV is characterized by regressed or compacted puffs. There is some decrease in puff diameter. Presumably as a result of compaction, staining with orcein and Feulgen increases, while metachromasy tends to disappear. There is further decrease in ^{3}H-thymidine uptake. See Crouse and Keyl (1968) for photomicrographs of stages I–IV.

Observations in this laboratory show that not all DNA puffs are necessarily synchronous with respect to these stages. Table 2 shows the developmental sequence of seven large DNA puffs of the *S. coprophila* complement. It will be seen that two puffs, 9A (II) and 15B (IV) are fairly large already in MES larva, suggesting that they may slightly precede the rest of the group of puffs. During the prepupal stages the same puffs regress somewhat in advance of the others. Puff 19B (IV) is unusual in that it is absent in the late larval stages but is first seen in 2- to 3-hour-old prepupa. This puff is present through most of the later prepupal stage and regresses shortly before the pupal molt.

All *Sciara* species examined so far show DNA puffs during late developmental stages. In addition to *S. coprophila*, the following species have been examined in my laboratory: *S. impatiens, S. pauciseta I,* and *S. pauciseta II,* as well as *S. prolifica.* The number of large DNA puffs is fairly constant (around nine) in the above species, and the total number of discernible DNA puffs is around 20 (Gabrusewycz-Garcia, 1971). This finding suggests that, in the future, it may be possible to trace homologies between DNA puffs in related *Sciara* species.

Mutants

In *S. coprophila* there are two widely used, sex-linked mutants. Wavy (*W*) is a dominant located on the X′ (X-prime) chromosome; it normal allele is found on the X chromosome. Swollen (*sw*) is a recessive

TABLE 2. *Developmental Sequence of Seven Large DNA Puffs of S. coprophila[a]*

Puff location[b]	Medium or large spots	Large spots or young prepupa	Young prepupa	Old prepupa[c]
2B (II)	Puff stage I	II	III	III–IV
9A (II)	II	III	III–IV	IV
2B (III)	I	II	III	III–IV
10A (III)	I	I–II	III	III–IV
11A (III)	I	I–II	III	III–IV
15B (IV)	III	III	III–IV	IV
19B (IV)	Absent	Absent	Absent	Expanded

[a] For description of other stages in larval-pupal transformation, as well as for description of puff stages, see text.
[b] Roman numerals next to the map location indicate the chromosome number.
[c] Old prepupa is considered that stage when locomotion is entirely lost.

localized on the X chromosome, while its dominant, normal allele is found on the X' chromosome. Phenotypic effects are a curly wing in the case of *W* and an irregular, patchy enlargement of the wing veins in the case of *sw*. In predicting the sex of progeny of female flies, either or both mutants are useful since they serve as markers for the X and X' chromosomes. For details of sex determination, see Chapter 8 Pavan *et al.* in this volume. Several translocations between the autosomes and the sex chromosomes are also known (Crouse, 1943).

Acknowledgment

I would like to thank my mother, Mrs. Maria Muzychenko, who, like the Biblical Martha, helped me by taking upon herself more than her share of the domestic chores.

Literature Cited

Been, A. C. and E. M. Rasch, 1972   Cellular and secretory proteins of the salivary glands of *Sciara coprophila* during the larval–pupal transformation. *J. Cell Biol.* **55**:420–432.

Cannon, G. B., 1965   Puff development and DNA synthesis in *Sciara* salivary gland chromosomes in tissue culture. *J. Cell Comp. Physiol.* **65**:163–182.

Carson, H. L., 1944   An analysis of natural chromosome variability in *Sciara impatiens* Johannsen. *J. Morphol.* **75**:11–59.

Crouse, H. V., 1943   Translocations in *Sciara,* their bearing on chromosome behavior and sex determination. *Univ. Mo. Agric. Exp. Stn. Res. Bull.* **379**:1–75.

Crouse, H. V., 1968   The role of ecdysone in DNA puff formation and DNA synthesis in the polytene chromosomes of *Sciara coprophila*. *Proc. Natl. Acad. Sci. USA* **61**:971–978.

Crouse, H. V. and H. G. Keyl, 1968   Extra replications in the "DNA puffs" of *Sciara coprophila*. *Chromosoma (Berl.)* **25**:357–364.

Gabrusewycz-Garcia, N., 1964   Cytological and autoradiographic studies in *Sciara coprophila* salivary gland chromosomes. *Chromosoma (Berl.)* **15**:312–344.

Gabrusewycz-Garcia, N., 1971   Studies in polytene chromosomes of *Sciarids*. I. The salivary chromosomes of *Sciara (Lycoriella) pauciseta* Felt. *Chromosoma (Berl.)* **33**:421–435.

Gabrusewycz-Garcia, N., 1972   Further studies of the nucleolar material in salivary gland nuclei of *Sciara coprophila*. *Chromosoma (Berl.)* **38**:237–254.

Gabrusewycz-Garcia, N. and R. G. Kleinfeld, 1966   A study of the nucleolar material in *Sciara coprophila*. *J. Cell Biol.* **29**:347–359.

Gabrusewycz-Garcia, N. and S. Margless, 1969   Induction of DNA puffs by ecdysterone. *J. Cell Biol.* **43**:41A.

Gerbi, S. A., 1971   Localization and characterization of the ribosomal RNA cistrons in *Sciara coprophila*. *J. Mol. Biol.* **58**:499–511.

Goodman, R. M. and W. B. Benjamin, 1973   Nucleoprotein methylation in salivary gland chromosomes of *Sciara coprophila*. Correlation with DNA synthesis. *Exp. Cell Res.* **77**:63–72.

Hungerford, H. B., 1916   *Sciara* maggots injurious to potted plants. *J. Econ. Entomol.* **9**:538–549.

Johannsen, O., 1912   The fungus gnats of North America. Part IV. *Maine Agric. Exp. Stn. Bull.* **200**:57–146.

McCarthy, M. D., 1945   Chromosome studies on eight species of *Sciara* (Diptera) with special reference to chromosomal changes of evolutionary significance. *Am. Nat.* **79**:104–245.

Pavan, C. and A. B. da Cunha, 1969   Chromosomal activities in *Rhynchosciara* and other *Sciaridae*. *Annu. Rev. Genet.* **3**:425–450.

Pelling, C., 1972   Transcription in giant chromosomal puffs. In *Results and Problems in Cell Differentiation*, Vol. 4, edited by W. Beermann, pp. 87–99, Springer Verlag, Heidelberg.

Phillips, D. M., 1965   An ordered filamentous component in *Sciara* (Diptera) salivary gland nuclei. *J. Cell Biol.* **26**:677–683.

Phillips, D. M. and H. Swift, 1965   Cytoplasmic fine structure of *Sciara* salivary glands. *J. Cell Biol.* **27**:395–409.

Poulson, D. F. and C. W. Metz, 1938   Studies on the structure of nucleolus-forming regions and related structures in the giant salivary gland chromosomes of Diptera. *J. Morphol.* **63**:363–395.

Rasch, E. M., 1970*a*   Two-wavelength cytophotometry of *Sciara* salivary gland chromosomes. In *Introduction to Quantitative Cytochemistry*, Vol. II, edited by G. L. Wied and G. F. Bahr, pp. 335–355, Academic Press, New York.

Rasch, E. M., 1970*b*   DNA cytophotometry of salivary gland nuclei and other tissue systems in Dipteran larvae. In *Introduction to Quantitative Cytochemistry*, Vol. II, edited by G. L. Wied and G. F. Bahr, pp. 357–397, Academic Press, New York.

Rasch, E. M., 1971   Estimated differences in the DNA content of male gametes from two species of *Bradysia* (Sciaridae). Paper 470, *Abstracts of Papers, Eleventh Annual Meeting of the American Society for Cell Biology, New Orleans, Louisiana*, p. 239.

Rieffel, S. M. and H. V. Crouse, 1966   The elimination and differentiation of chromosomes in the germ line of *Sciara*. *Chromosoma (Berl.)* **19**:231–276.

Rudkin, G. T. and S. L. Corlette, 1957   Disproportionate synthesis of DNA in a polytene chromosome region. *Proc. Natl. Acad. Sci. USA* **43**:964–968.

Sauaia, H., E. M. Laicine and M. A. R. Alves, 1971   Hydroxyurea-induced inhibition of DNA puff development in the salivary gland chromosomes of *Bradysia hygida*. *Chromosoma (Berl.)* **34**:129–151.

Shaw, F., 1953   A review of some of the more important contributions to our knowledge of the systematic relationships of the *Sciaridae* (Diptera). *Proc. Hawaii. Entomol. Soc.* **15**:25–32.

Spencer, W. P., 1950   Collection and laboratory culture. In *Biology of Drosophila*, edited by M. Demerec, pp. 535–590, John Wiley & Sons, New York.

Steffan, A., 1966   *A Generic Revision of the Family Sciaridae (Diptera) of America North of Mexico*. Univ. of Calif. Publ. Entomol. 44, University of California, Calif.

Swift, H., 1962   Nucleic acids and cell morphology in Dipteran salivary glands. In *The Molecular Control of Cellular Activity*, edited by J. Allen, pp. 73–125, McGraw-Hill, New York.

10

Chironomus

KLAUS HÄGELE

The Biology of *Chironomus*

Chironomus thummi thummi Kieffer

The gnatlike midge of this species has a length of 6–8 mm and is grayish brown. The male possesses one pair of large, plumed antennae, whereas the female has simpler ones. Unlike gnats, these midges raise their forelegs when at rest. They have no piercing organs and do not feed (Miall and Hammond, 1900).

The egg-masses of *Ch. thummi* contain 400–800 eggs, which are invested in a gelatinous envelope. The moment the egg-mass touches the water, the envelope swells and the eggs float. The female midge moors the egg-mass by gelatinous cords to a fixed object at the surface of the water. Under optimal culturing conditions in water at 18°C, the larvae hatch 2–3 days after oviposition. At the bottom of a water basin, for example, the larvae build tubes in which they grow and pupate. The tubes consist of mud and food particles spun together by the larvae using the secretion products of their salivary glands.

Each of the first, second, and third larval instars has a duration of 2–3 days. The fourth instar begins at days 8 and 9 and lasts until days 15–17. The hemolymph of these larvae is intensely red. The fully grown larva is 12–15 mm long and weighs 10–12 mg. It has a head capsule and

KLAUS HÄGELE—Institute for Genetics, Ruhr-University Bochum, Bochum, West Germany.

12 body segments. The first and last body segments carry on the ventral side one pair of appendages with a circle of hooklets for locomotion. Two pairs of tube-building appendages (tubuli) are present on the lateral side of the eleventh segment. The last (twelfth) segment has on its dorsal side a tuft of bristles and four anal papillae, one pair on the dorsal and the other pair on the ventral side of the anus.

The prepupal stage begins 16 days after hatching from the egg. Pupation has an average duration of 2 days. Immediately before eclosion, the pupa moves to the surface of the water. The males hatch some hours before the females. The adults live about 5 days.

Mating takes place during flight. Swarm formation of a number of male midges is a prerequisite to mating. A single pair of midges will produce no fertilized eggs.

Chironomus (Camptochironomus) tentans Fabricius

This species and *Ch. thummi* differ in the following ways: *Ch. tentans* is larger than *Ch. thummi* and needs 5–6 weeks for its generation cycle. The egg-masses contain 800–1200 eggs. The females drop the egg-masses on the water and do not moor them to a fixed object (Sadler, 1936).

Each of the first three larval instars has a duration of about 8 days. The fourth instar lasts approximately 16 days. However, the time the larvae need for development is quite variable in different stocks. The fully grown larva is 20–25 mm in length. It carries at each lateral side of the tenth segment one additional short appendage. The adult has a length of 10–12 mm.

Swarm formation in *Ch. tentans* is not a prerequisite for mating as it is for *Ch. thummi*. A single pair of midges will mate in a glass tube, for example, and oviposition will also take place if some water is present.

Larval Tissues that Provide Polytene Chromosomes for Cytological Study

All tissues of *Chironomus* possess polyploid nuclei, with the exception of most ganglion cells and all anlage cells. The chromosomes of the cells of the salivary glands and the Malpighian tubules are excellent in both species. In *Ch. tentans,* the cells of the rectum and the anterior portion of the mid-gut also contain chromosomes suitable for study in squash preparations. The oenocytes, hypodermal cells, the cells of the remainder of the digestive tube, the anal papillae, and the fat body do not contain well-banded polytene chromosomes.

Laboratory Culturing Procedures

Chironomus are reared at 18°C during a schedule of 15 hours of illumination and 9 hours of darkness. They are fed a paste made of powdered stinging nettles (4 parts), cellulose (1 part), and water. The following fluid serves as a substitute for pond water: 100 ml salt solution plus 10 liters of double-distilled water. The salt solution contains 0.35 g NaCl, 0.30 g $MgSO_4$, 0.27 g $CaCl_2$, 0.05 g $NaHCO_3$, 0.02 g KH_2PO_4, 0.1 ml of 1 percent aqueous $FeCl_3$, and 100 ml double-distilled water. The mass culturing of stock cultures takes place in a basin of dimensions 110 cm (length) × 45 cm (width) × 20 cm (height) and containing perforations for air hoses. The basin is filled with fluid to a depth of 6 cm, and one tablespoon of food paste is added per 100 larvae. A swarming cage is put on top of the basin. The cage is a frame 110 cm × 45 cm × 50 cm, and its top is covered with a fine mesh gauze. A port is provided through which food can be added to the culture and egg-masses can be collected. In situations where one wishes to produce large larvae for cytological studies, smaller numbers of animals are reared in plastic dishes about 20 cm in diameter. The culturing fluid is maintained at a depth of 5 cm, and about 70 larvae are reared with two tablespoons of food. A glass cap about 23 cm in diameter is used to cover the dish. The cap is perforated to allow passage of a plastic tube from a blower unit. It is essential that the culture fluid in either setup be well aerated.

The Salivary Gland Chromosomes of *Chironomus thummi thummi*

The salivary gland nuclei of this species contain four polytene chromosomes: three long elements (chromosomes I, II, and III) and a short one (chromosome IV). Sex chromosomes are not formed. How sex is determined is not known.

The first detailed chromosome maps were published by Keyl (1957). In his drawings the right arms were drawn to the left, and *vice versa*. In later work these maps have been used as standards, and, therefore, maps shown here are not arranged as is the convention for *Drosophila*.

The average length of the chromosomes follows the sequence I-II-III-IV, chromosome I being the longest (Keyl, 1957; Keyl and Keyl, 1959). A prominent swelling occurs near the middle of each of the long chromosomes (see Figure 1). In the short chromosome (IV) the swelling is terminal. These swollen regions presumably correspond to the centromere regions (Bauer, 1935). They subdivide each of the long chromosomes into a right and a left arm.

TABLE 1.   *Prominent Chromosome Regions in Ch. th. thummi*[a]

Region	Description
CHROMOSOME I	
Centromere region (submedian)	Region D1k-D2; the region is swollen and contains four dark-staining groups of bands
Right arm	Region A4/B1; contains a constriction which is bordered in A4 by three groups of heavy bands and followed proximally by two bands
Left arm	In adult larvae region G1 frequently contains a striking puff which is bordered at the distal side by two dark-staining bands
Inversions	In(I, L-1)-F2i/F3a-F2i/F3a-; In(I, L-2)-F3h/F31-F3h/F31-
CHROMOSOME II	
Centromere region (median)	Region C3c-C4b; this region is slightly swollen, its center contains five closely packed, heavy bands
Right arm	A characteristic constriction is found near the distal end in A2; the center of the constriction contains four bands; these bands are followed distally and proximally by a group of dark-staining bands
Left arm	A characteristic sequence of dark-staining bands in regions E1, E2, and E3
Inversions	In (II, R-1)-B5o/C3c-B5o/C3c-; In (II, R-2)-C2h/C21-C2h/C21-
CHROMOSOME III	
Centromere region (submedian)	Region B2; the centromere swelling contains closely packed, heavy bands and a faintly staining region with three small bands
Right arm	In region A2 band A2i often forms a dark-staining bulb; at the distal side it is followed by three groups of heavy bands
Left arm	The distal section has about half the diameter of the right arm; region C4 contains three doublet bands; these are followed distally by two doublets and by another doublet in D1
Inversion	In (III, L-1)-B4g/C3g-B4g/C3g-; In (III, R-1)-B1h/B1r-B1h/B1r-
CHROMOSOME IV	
Centromere region (terminal)	Region Ee; the terminal swelling with one dark-staining band
	In regions B and C two Balbiani rings (Balbiani, 1881) are formed; region D contains the nucleolus.

[a] See Figure 1.

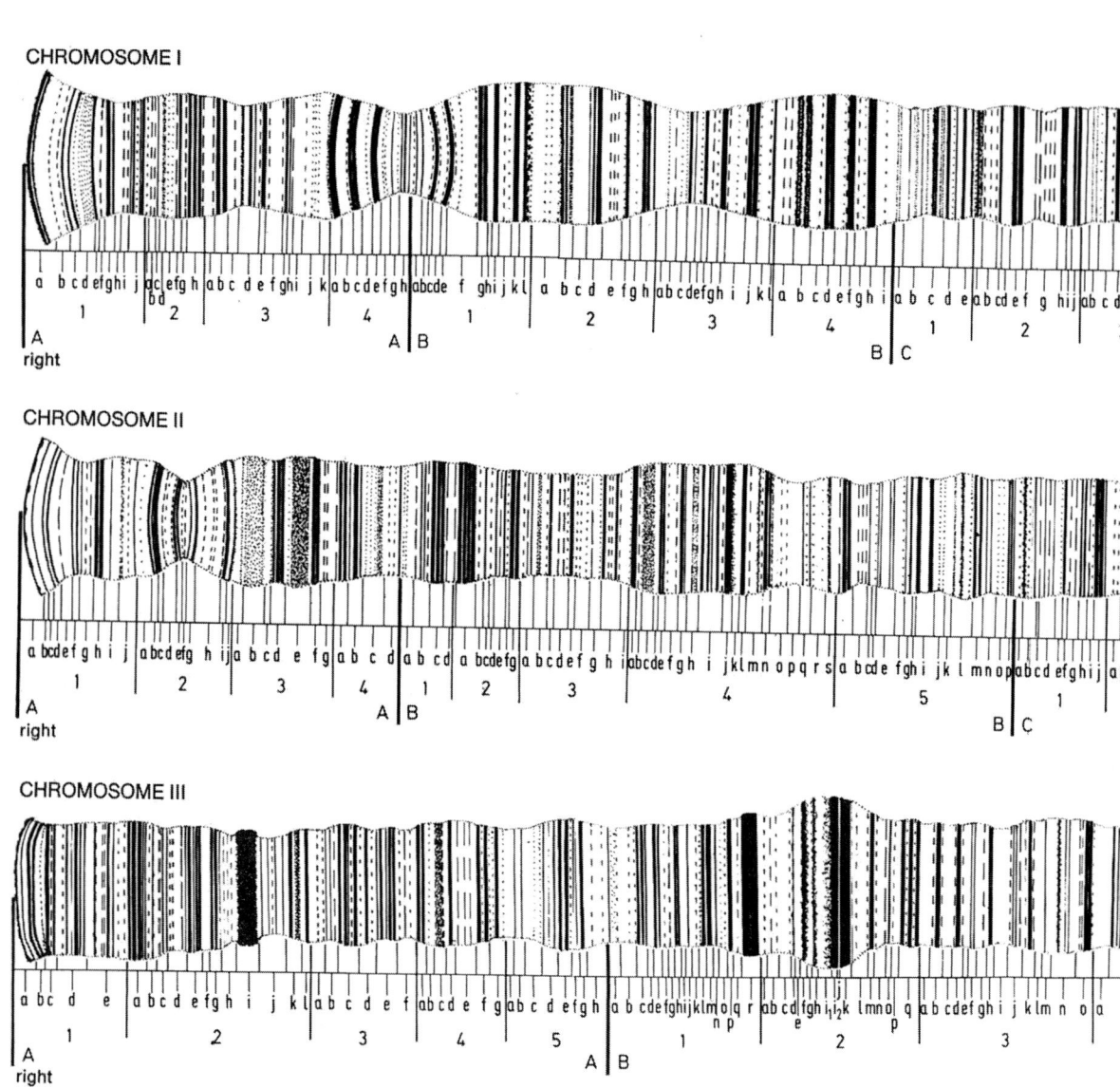

Figure 1. Chromosome maps of the salivary gland chromosomes of Chironomus thummi thummi Kieffer.

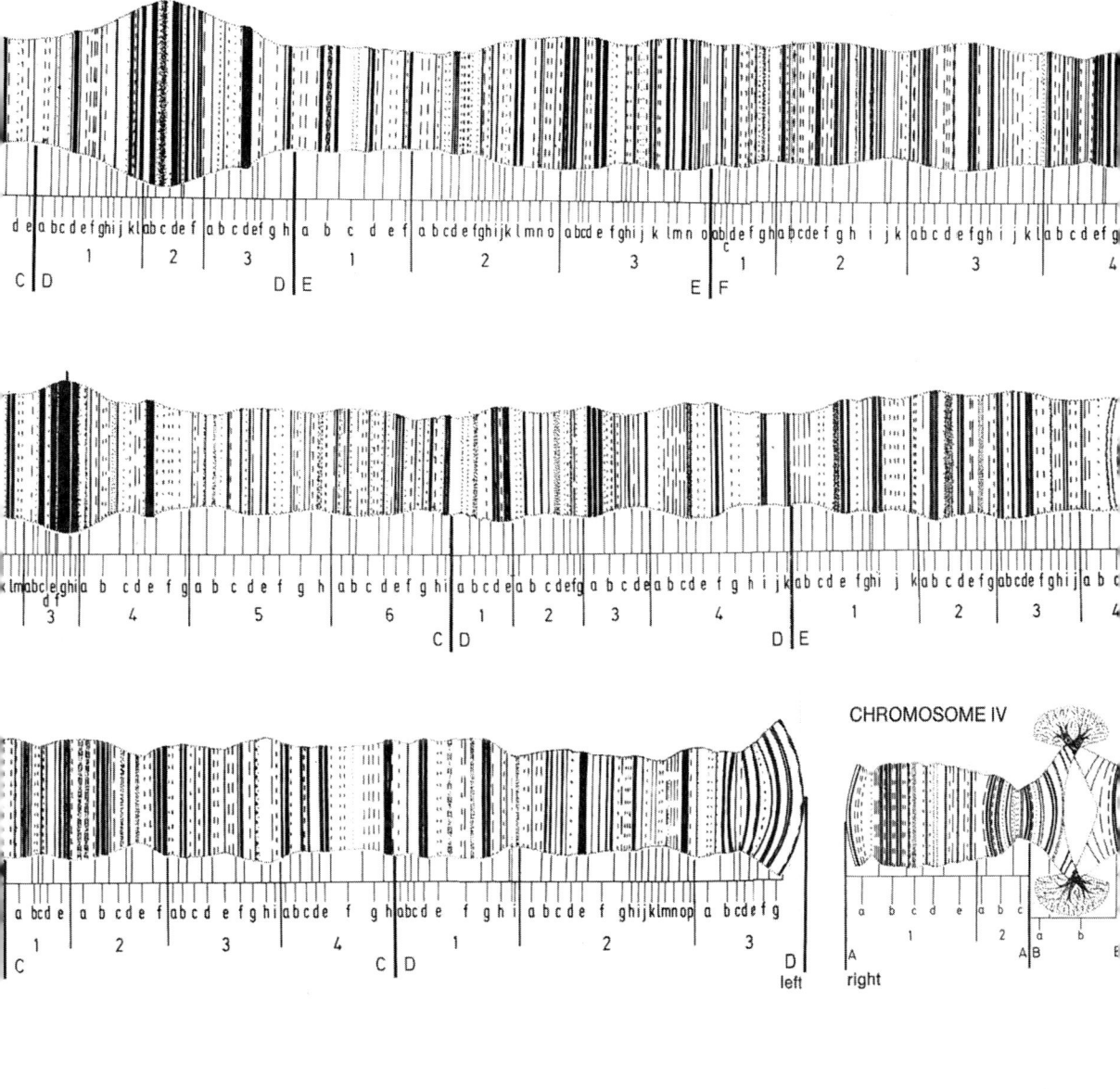

CHROMOSOME IV

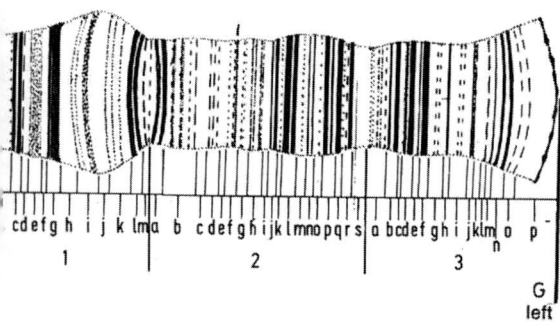

cdefg h i j k lma b cdefghijklmnopqrs a bcdefg h i jklm o p

1   2   3
                                                          n

G
left

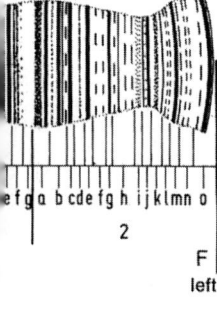

efga bcdefgh ijklmn o

2

F
left

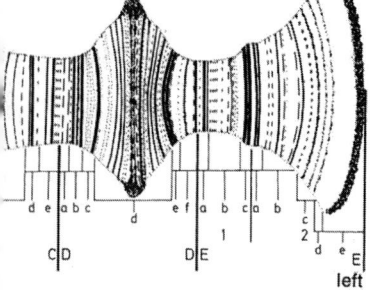

d e a b c   d   e f a b c a b   c
                                    2
           C D   D E   1   d   e   E

left

CHROMOSOME I

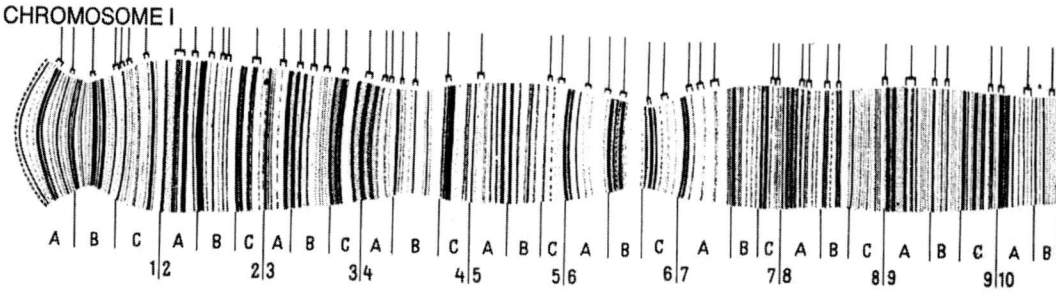

CHROMOSOME II

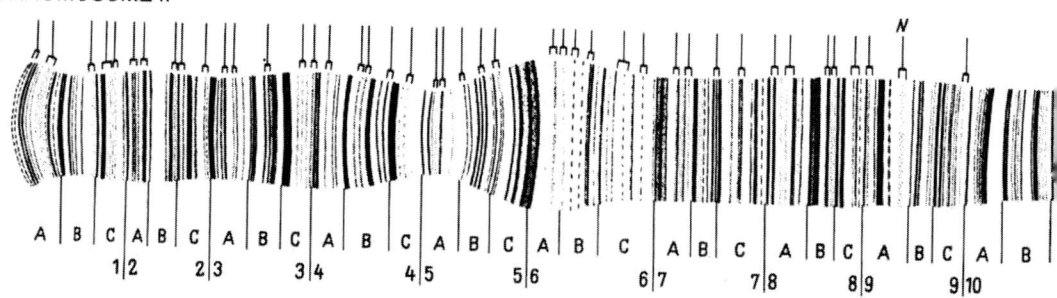

CHROMOSOME III

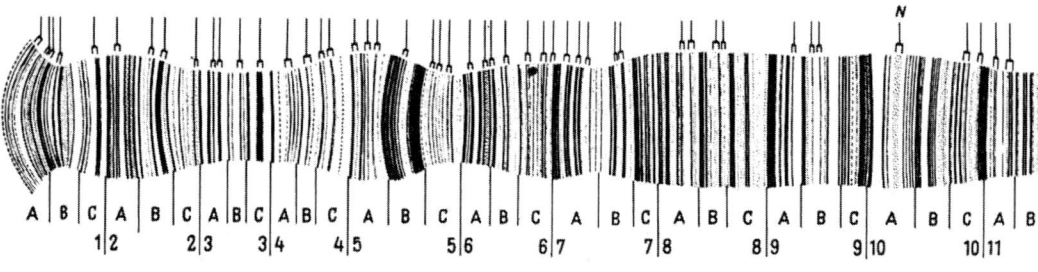

Figure 2. Chromosome maps of the salivary gland chromosomes of Chironomus tentans Fabricius. From I

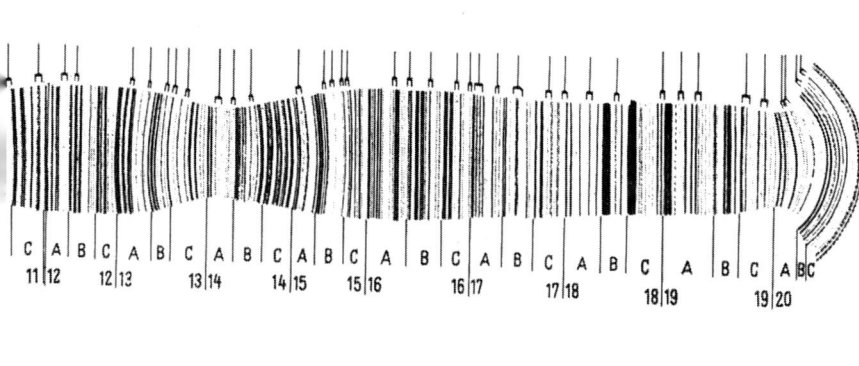

C | A | B | C | A | B | C | A | B | C | A | B | C | A | B | C | A | B | C | A | B | C | A | B | C | A | B C
11|12   12|13   13|14   14|15   15|16   16|17   17|18   18|19   19|20

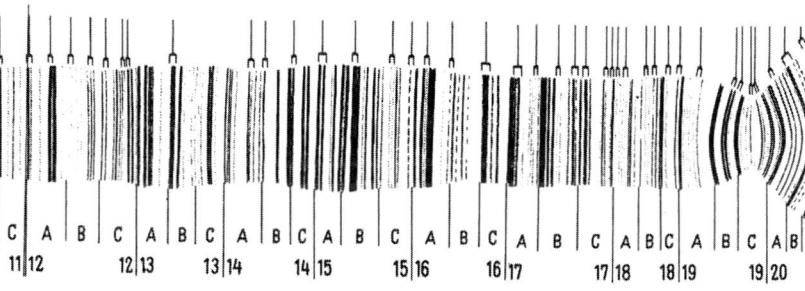

C | A | B | C | A | B | C | A | B | C | A | B | C | A | B | C | A | B | C | A | B | C | A | B C
11|12   12|13   13|14   14|15   15|16   16|17   17|18   18|19   19|20

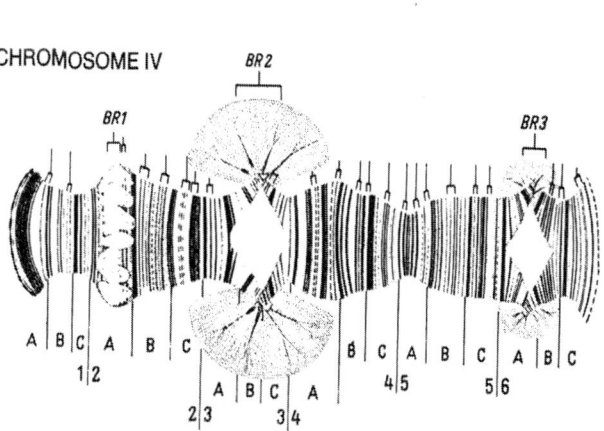

CHROMOSOME IV

BR1   BR2   BR3

B | C | A | B | C | A | B | C | A | B | C | A | B | C
12|13   13|14   14|15   15|16

A | B | C | A | B | C   B | C | A | B | C | A | B | C
    1|2   4|5   5|6

A | B | C | A
  2|3   3|4

n (1952) (revised).

TABLE 2. *Prominent Chromosome Regions in Ch. tentans*[a]

Region	Description
CHROMOSOME I	
Centromere region	Position within region 10–12
Right arm	Region 18B-19A contains a group of three doublet bands; the distal end of the chromosome is fan-shaped; region 17B with an RNA bulb
Left arm	Region 1C-3B near the distal end is swollen
Inversions	In(1L-1) b.p.[b] 4C/5A, 8B; In(1L-2)b.p. 5C, 7B; In(1L-3)b.p. 4A, 4C; In(1L-4)b.p. 4C, 5B; In(1R-1)b.p. 12A, 18C; In(1R-2)b.p. 13C, 18A; the complex inversion In(1-k1)b.p. 11A, 18B/9A, 10B contains the inversion In(1R-2) and is found only in the heterozygous condition in the male (Y_1 chromosome)
CHROMOSOME II	
Centromere region	Position within region 10B-12B
Right arm	In region 19 a constriction is found which is bordered proximally by three dark-staining bands
Left arm	In region 9A a nucleolus is formed
Inversions	In (2L-1)b.p. 1A, 9C, this inversion acts alternately either as X_{2L} or Y_{2L}; In(2L-k1) 1A/4B-8A/1C-1B/4B-1C/8A-, this complex inversion is found in the heterozygous condition only; it represents the Y_{2L} chromosome of the male; In(2L-k1a) 1A/4B-8A/1C-1B/4B-2A/9C-8A/1C-2A/9C-; In(2L-k2)-1B6/6B2-7A1/x/7C-8A/1C-6C/x/7A2-7C/1B7-1C/8A-; In(2R-1)b.p. 12C, 17C/18A
CHROMOSOME III	
Centromere region	Position within region 10B-11B
Right arm	A characteristic banding pattern in region 15A-15B with dark-staining bands
Left arm	In region 5B two dark-staining bands are followed proximally by a group of closely packed, heavy bands; in region 10A a nucleolus is formed
Inversions	In(3L-1)b.p. 2A, 8C; In(3L-2)b.p. 2B, 8A; In(3L-k1)b.p. ?; In(3R-1) b.p. 14A, 14C; In(3R-k1)b.p. 14A, 14C (+?)
CHROMOSOME IV	
Centromere region	Position presumably in region 1A; three Balbiani rings, Br1 in region 2A, Br2 in region 3 and Br3 in region 6A
Inversions	In(4-1)b.p. 1A, 6C

[a] See Figure 2.
[b] Here, b.p. = breakpoint.

Heterochromatic chromosome regions are not present, and a chromocenter is never found in any tissue. The total number of registered bands of the chromosome set is 1474 (Hägele, 1970). This number is distributed over the chromosomes as follows: I = 512, II = 457, III = 340, IV = 165.

Heterozygous inversions have been found in each of the long chromosomes (Hägele, unpublished). For a detailed description of organization and function of polytene chromosomes see, for example, Bauer (1935, 1936a,b), Bauer and Beermann (1952), Beermann (1952, 1955a, 1962, 1964), Beermann and Bahr (1954), Berendes and Beermann (1969), and Clever (1961, 1966).

In the salivary gland anlage of *Ch. th. thummi* mitotic activity ceases after 15 hours of embryonic development (Keyl, 1958). Further development takes place by cell growth and polytenization of the chromosomes. During the four larval instars the chromosomes undergo up to twelve successive replications. Replication includes all parts of the genome throughout polytenization. By ^{3}H-thymidine autoradiography it is demonstrated that polytene bands or groups of bands complete duplication at specifically different times (Keyl and Pelling, 1963). Three types of chromosomal labeling patterns can be distinguished: (1) discontinuous labeling at the beginning of a replication cycle (small bands and interbands labeled, centromere regions unlabeled), (2) continuous labeling at an intermediate phase of replication (chromosomes are completely labeled) and (3) discontinuous labeling at the very end of a replication cycle (only the swollen centromere regions show labeling) (Hägele, 1970).

The pattern of chromosomal RNA puffing changes characteristically during larval development (Kroeger, 1964; Laufer and Holt, 1970). The location of the nucleolus and of the Balbiani rings is constant. These structures contain large quantities of RNA.

In different strains of *Ch. th. thummi* DNA differences occur in particular bands (I D1d; II B5p, C1j; III B1r, B3h, C1c). The DNA values of these bands differ by a factor of 2, 4, or 8. Within heterozygotes, these bands are identifiable by the difference in size of the halves of the bands. It is postulated that the DNA differentiation of these bands has been established during chromosome evolution by mutational events causing a localized increase of DNA content by a series of doublings (Keyl, 1965).

The Salivary Gland Chromosomes of *Chironomus tentans*

The salivary gland nuclei of this species contain three long polytene chromosomes (chromosomes I, II, and III) and a short one (chromosome

IV) (Figure 2). The relative lengths of the four chromosomes are in proportions of 1.0 : 1.0 : 0.8 : 0.3 (Beermann, 1952). The long chromosome that does not have a nucleolus is designated as chromosome I. Chromosome II has a nucleolus and so does chromosome III, which is the shortest of the long chromosomes. Chromosome IV exhibits three Balbiani rings. The number of bands is distributed over the chromosomes as follows: I = 483, II = 393, III = 410, IV = 158 (Pelling, 1964). Chromosomes I, II, and III contain no heterochromatic elements; in chromosome IV, a heterochromatic band occurs terminally. The positions of the centromere regions are not exactly known. However, the mitotic chromosome complement consists of three pairs of mediocentric chromosomes and one short pair of telocentrics (Beermann, 1952).

In *Ch. tentans* a large number of chromosomal rearrangements is found (inversion polymorphism). Inversions occur in both homozygous and heterozygous conditions (Beermann, 1955*a*).

Morphologically distinguishable sex chromosomes are not present. The sex-determining system is a complex one. Chromosome I and chromosome arm II2L are alternately sex chromosomes or autosomes. The inheritance of sex-linked inversions shows heterogamety in the male. Two inversions [In(1k-1), In(2L-k1)] are sex-linked in the male and act without exception as Y chromosomes (Y_1, Y_{2L}). Moreover, gene sequences in chromosome I represent alternately either X chromosomes or autosomes, and most inversions in chromosome arm II2L mark either the X_{2L} or the Y_{2L} chromosome (Beermann, 1955*b*).

Larvae of *Ch. tentans* complete the four larval instars in approximately six weeks. The largest nuclei of fully grown larvae contain 10^{13} times the diploid amount of DNA (Daneholt and Edström, 1967). The nuclei within a gland replicate asynchronously, and the frequency of replicating nuclei varies from larva to larva. The number of DNA-synthesizing nuclei is highest during the intermolt, and declines sharply at each molting period (Darrow and Clever, 1970).

The DNA of *Ch. tentans* is of the A-T-type with an overall G+C content of about 30 percent. In the chromosome complement of fourth-instar larvae up to 277 chromosomal segments (272 puffs, 3 Balbiani rings, and 2 nucleolar organizers) are active in RNA synthesis (Pelling, 1964). Nucleolar and cytoplasmic RNAs are nearly symmetric in their A/U and their G/C ratios. In contrast, the RNA base compositions of the three Balbiani rings is asymmetric (AU-ratios are 2.2, 1.5, and 1.7). The RNA of Balbiani rings contains both high-molecular-weight RNA and low-molecular-weight RNA. The high-molecular-weight RNA presumably represents messenger-type RNA and the low-molecular-weight RNA, transfer RNA (Edström and Daneholt, 1967; Daneholt and Edström,

1969; Pelling, 1970; Berendes and Beermann, 1969). It is assumed that the asymmetric base composition is the consequence of the transcription of one of the DNA strands only (Beermann, 1964). The nuclear sap RNA of *Ch. tentans* contains heterogeneous high-molecular-weight RNA and low-molecular-weight RNA (Lambert *et al.*, 1972). Cytological RNA–DNA hybridization experiments show that a large percentage (55–70 percent) of the nuclear sap RNA is derived from the RNA of Balbiani ring 2 (Br2) (Lambert *et al.*, 1972, 1973*b*). The molecular weight of this Br2-RNA is estimated to be $15–35 \times 10^6$ daltons (Daneholt, 1972). The DNA of Br2 contains repeated sequences (Sachs and Clever, 1972; Lambert *et al.*, 1972) with a gene redundancy of about 200 (Lambert, 1972). Such a single large Balbiani ring is able to synthesize about 15 percent of the total cellular RNA and apparently contains as much RNA as the long chromosome I (Pelling, 1972). The two other long chromosomes (II and III) synthesize rRNA at their nucleolar organizer regions. A sequence similarity of the RNA from the two different nucleoli of chromosomes II and III is indicated (Lambert *et al.*, 1973*a*).

Acknowledgment

I am very much indebted to Dr. C. Pelling, Tübingen, who has placed the chromosome maps of *Chironomus tentans* at my disposal.

Literature Cited

Balbiani, E. G., 1881   Sur la structure du noyau des cellules salivaires chez les larves de *Chironomus. Zool. Anz.* **4**:637–641.

Bauer, H., 1935   Der Aufbau der Chromosomen aus den Speicheldrüsen von *Chironomus thummi* Kieffer (Untersuchungen an den Riesenchromosomen der Dipteren. I.). *Z. Zellforsch.* **23**:280–313.

Bauer, H., 1936*a*   Beiträge zur vergleichenden Morphologie der Speicheldrüsen-Chromosomen (Untersuchungen an den Riesenchromosomen der Dipteren. II.). *Zool. Jb. Abt. Allg. Zool. Physiol.* **56**:239–276.

Bauer, H., 1936*b*   The structure of the salivary gland chromosomes in *Chironomidae. Am. Nat.* **70**:164–170.

Bauer, H. and W. Beermann, 1952   Die Polytänie der Riesenchromosomen. *Chromosoma (Berl.)* **4**:630–648.

Beermann, W., 1952   Chromosomenkonstanz und spezifische Modifikationen der Chromosomenstruktur in der Entwicklung und Organdifferenzierung von *Chironomus tentans. Chromosoma (Berl.)* **5**:139–198.

Beermann, W., 1955*a*   Cytologische Analyse eines *Camptochironomus* Artbastards. I. Kreuzungsergebnisse und die Evolution des Karyotyps. *Chromosoma (Berl.)* **7**:198–259.

Beermann, W., 1955*b* Geschlechtsbestimmung und Evolution der genetischen Y-Chromosomen bei *Chironomus. Biol. Zentralbl.* **74**:525–544.

Beermann, W., 1962 Riesenchromosomen. In *Protoplasmatologia VI, D,* edited by M. Alfert, H. Bauer and C. V. Harding, pp. 1–161, Springer, Vienna.

Beermann, W., 1964 Structure and function of interphase chromosomes. *Gent. Today (Proc. XIth Internatl. Congr. Genet., The Hague)*: 375–384.

Beermann, W. and G. F. Bahr, 1954 The submicroscopic structure of the Balbiani-ring. *Exp. Cell Res.* **6**:195–201.

Berendes, H. D. and W. Beermann, 1969 Biochemical activity of interphase chromosomes (polytene chromosomes). In *Handbook of Molecular Cytology,* edited by A. Lima-de-Faria, pp. 500–519, North-Holland, Amsterdam.

Clever, U., 1961 Genaktivitäten in den Riesenchromosomen von *Chironomus tentans* und ihre Beziehungen zur Entwicklung. I. Genaktivierung durch Ecdyson. *Chromosoma (Berl.)* **12**:607–675.

Clever, U., 1966 Induction and repression of a puff in *Chironomus tentans. Dev. Biol.* **14**:421–438.

Darrow, J. M. and U. Clever, 1970 Chromosome activity and cell function in polytene cells. III. Growth and replication. *Dev. Biol.* **21**:331–348.

Daneholt, B., 1972 Giant RNA transcript in a Balbiani ring. *Nat. New Biol.* **240**:229–232.

Daneholt, B. and J.-E. Edström, 1967 The content of deoxyribonucleic acid in individual polytene chromosomes of *Chironomus tentans. Cytogenet.* **6**:350–356.

Daneholt, B. and J.-E. Edström, 1969 The DNA base composition of individual chromosomes and chromosome segments from *Chironomus tentans. J. Cell Biol.* **41**:620–624.

Edström, J.-E. and B. Daneholt, 1967 Sedimentation properties of the newly synthesized RNA from isolated nuclear components of *Chironomus tentans* salivary gland cells. *J. Mol. Biol.* **28**:331–343.

Hägele, K., 1970 DNS-Replikationsmuster der Speicheldrüsen-Chromosomen von Chironomiden. *Chromosoma (Berl.)* **31**:91–138.

Keyl, H.-G., 1957 Untersuchungen am Karyotypus von *Chironomus thummi.* I. Mitteilung. Karten der Speicheldrüsen-Chromosomen von *Chironomus th. thummi* und die cytologische Differenzierung der Subspezies *Ch. th. thummi* und *Ch. th. piger. Chromosoma (Berl.)* **8**:739–756.

Keyl, H.-G., 1958 Untersuchungen am Karyotypus von *Chironomus thummi.* II. Mitteilung. Strukturveränderungen an den Speicheldrüsen-Chromosomen nach Röntgenbestrahlung von Embryonen und Larven. *Chromosoma (Berl.)* **9**:441–483.

Keyl, H.-G., 1965 A demonstrable local and geometric increase in the chromosomal DNA of *Chironomus. Experientia (Basel)* **21**:191–193.

Keyl, H.-G. and I. Keyl, 1959 Die cytologische Diagnostik der Chironomiden. I. Bestimmungstabelle für die Gattung *Chironomus* auf Grund der Speicheldrüsen-Chromosomen. *Arch. Hydrobiol.* **56**:43–57.

Keyl, H.-G. and C. Pelling, 1963 Differentielle DNS-Replikation in den Speicheldrüsen-Chromosomen von *Chironomus thummi. Chromosoma (Berl.)* **14**:347–359.

Kroeger, H., 1964 Zellphysiologische Mechanismen bei der Regulation von Genaktivitäten in den Riesenchromosomen von *Chironomus thummi. Chromosoma (Berl.)* **15**:36–70.

Lambert, B., 1972 Repeated DNA sequences in a Balbiani ring. *J. Mol. Biol.* **72**:65–75.

Lambert, B., L. Wieslander, B. Daneholt, E. Egyházi and U. Ringborg, 1972 *In situ* demonstration of DNA hybridizing with chromosomal and nuclear sap RNA in *Chironomus tentans. J. Cell Biol. 53:*407–418.

Lambert, B., E. Egyházi, B. Daneholt and U. Ringborg, 1973*a*   Quantitative micro-assay for RNA/DNA hybrids in the study of nucleolar RNA from *Chironomus tentans* salivary gland cells. *Exp. Cell Res.* **76:**369–380.

Lambert, B., B. Daneholt, J.-E. Edström, E. Egyházi and U. Ringborg, 1973*b*   Comparison between chromosomal and nuclear sap RNA from *Chironomus tentans* salivary gland cells by RNA/DNA hybridization. *Exp. Cell Res.* **76:**381–389.

Laufer, H. and T. K. H. Holt, 1970   Juvenile hormone effects on chromosomal puffing and development in *Chironomus thummi. J. Exp. Zool.* **173:**341–351.

Miall, L. C. and A. R. Hammond, 1900   *The Structure and Life History of the Harlequin Fly,* pp. 1–191, Clarendon Press, Oxford.

Pelling, C., 1964   Ribonukleinsäure-Synthese der Riesenchromosomen. Autoradiographische Untersuchungen an *Chironomus tentans. Chromosoma (Berl.)* **15:**71–122.

Pelling, C., 1970   Puff RNA in polytene chromosomes. *Cold Spring Harbor Symp. Quant. Biol.* **35:**521–531.

Pelling, C., 1972   Transcription in giant chromosomal puffs. In *Developmental Studies on Giant Chromosomes,* edited by W. Beermann, pp. 87–99, Springer-Verlag, Berlin.

Sachs, R. I. and U. Clever, 1972   Unique and repetitive DNA sequences in the genome of *Chironomus tentans. Exp. Cell Res.* **74:**587–591.

Sadler, W. O., 1936   Biology of the midge *Chironomus tentans* Fabricius and methods for its propagation. *Cornell Univ. Agric. Exp. Stn. Chem.* **173:**1–24.

11

Glyptotendipes

Ludwig Walter

Culture of *Glyptotendipes barbipes*

It is very difficult to keep *Glyptotendipes barbipes* in mass cultures, because the adults seldom copulate. However, copulation can be artifically stimulated using the procedure of Fischer (1969). Larvae are cultivated in plastic bowls in a well-aerated liquid medium. This is made according to the following formula: 100 liter distilled water, 0.05 g $NaHCO_3$, 3.5 g NaCl, 2.7 g $CaCl_2$, 0.2 g KH_2PO_4, 3.0 g $MgSO_4$, and 1 ml of a 1 percent aqueous $FeCl_3$ solution. A mixture of cellulose and stinging nettle powder serves as the substratum. Stinging nettle powder is prepared by grinding leaves of the stinging nettle (*Urtica dioica*). In Germany it is supplied by Christoph Mix, über Bad Kitzingen, Postfach, 8711 Abtswind, West Germany. The density of larvae should not exceed 1 larva per 4 cm².

Chromosome Morphology

The salivary gland chromosomes of the *G. barbipes* were first studied by Bauer (1936), who described the heavily stained, drum-shaped heterochromatic regions. Later these were interpreted to represent centromere sites because of their correspondence to the position of constrictions on mitotic chromosomes (Basrur, 1957). In the nuclei of the Malpi-

Ludwig Walter—Institute for Genetics, Ruhr-University Bochum, Bochum, West Germany.

ghian tubules these heterochromatic bulbs fuse together into a large chromocenter. The dense-staining chromocenters are always present in the nuclei of cells of the brain, adipose tissue, and intestinal tract, as well as in spermatocytes (Bauer, 1936).

The chromosome number of each of the *Glyptotendipes* subspecies is $2n = 8$. The germ cells of *G. barbipes*, *G. cauliginellus*, and *G. gripekoveni* have 3 pairs of long metacentric chromosomes. The smallest chromosomal pair in all three subspecies is acrocentric. The acrocentric elements are equal in *G. cauliginellus* and *G. gripekoveni*. However, in some cells of *G. barbipes* the acrocentrics are unequal (Dvorak *et al.*, 1970).

The nucleus of the salivary gland cell of *G. barbipes* contains 4 chromosomes, numbered I–IV in a decreasing order of size. The drum-shaped heterochromatic regions in the middle of each of the three long chromosomes and at one end of chromosome IV form prominent landmarks. The lengths of the three smaller salivary gland chromosomes relative to the length of chromosome I, are 0.9, 0.7, and 0.3, and the positioning of the heterochromatic "drums" divides each chromosomes into a longer left arm and a shorter right arm.

Morphological characteristics of the four chromosomes are listed below and illustrated in Figure 1. Chromosome I: the position of the centromere is in section D3, a nucleolus resides in section D2 of the right arm, and a puff occurs in section A3 of the left arm. Chromosome II: the position of the centromere is in section C3, a strong constriction occurs in section F2 of the right arm, and a nucleolus is seen in section C2 of the left arm. Chromosome III: the position of the centromere is in section C1, and a nucleolus resides in section A2 of the left arm. Chromosome IV: the position of the centromere is the terminal section D2, and two Balbiani rings occur in sections A2 and B1 of the left arm.

In chromosome II a heterozygous inversion is found at A2–B2 in about 50 percent of the salivary gland chromosomes analyzed. This inversion has been found in a population from Stratford, England as well as in a German stock (Basrur, 1957). An analysis of the chromosomes of the testis and salivary glands did not reveal any evidence for a sex-linked inversion as found in *Chironomus annularius* (Beermann, 1955; Keyl and Keyl, 1959).

In the Stratford population, Basrur (1957) found three other rearrangements: (1) in the short arm of chromosome I with breakpoints in sections E2 and F2, (2) in chromosome II in the left arm in sections A3–B1, and (3) in chromosome III with rearranged segments in C2–D3.

According to Miseiko *et al.* (1971*b*) certain Russian populations of *G. barbipes* are more extensively polymorphic. In 141 of 150 larvae

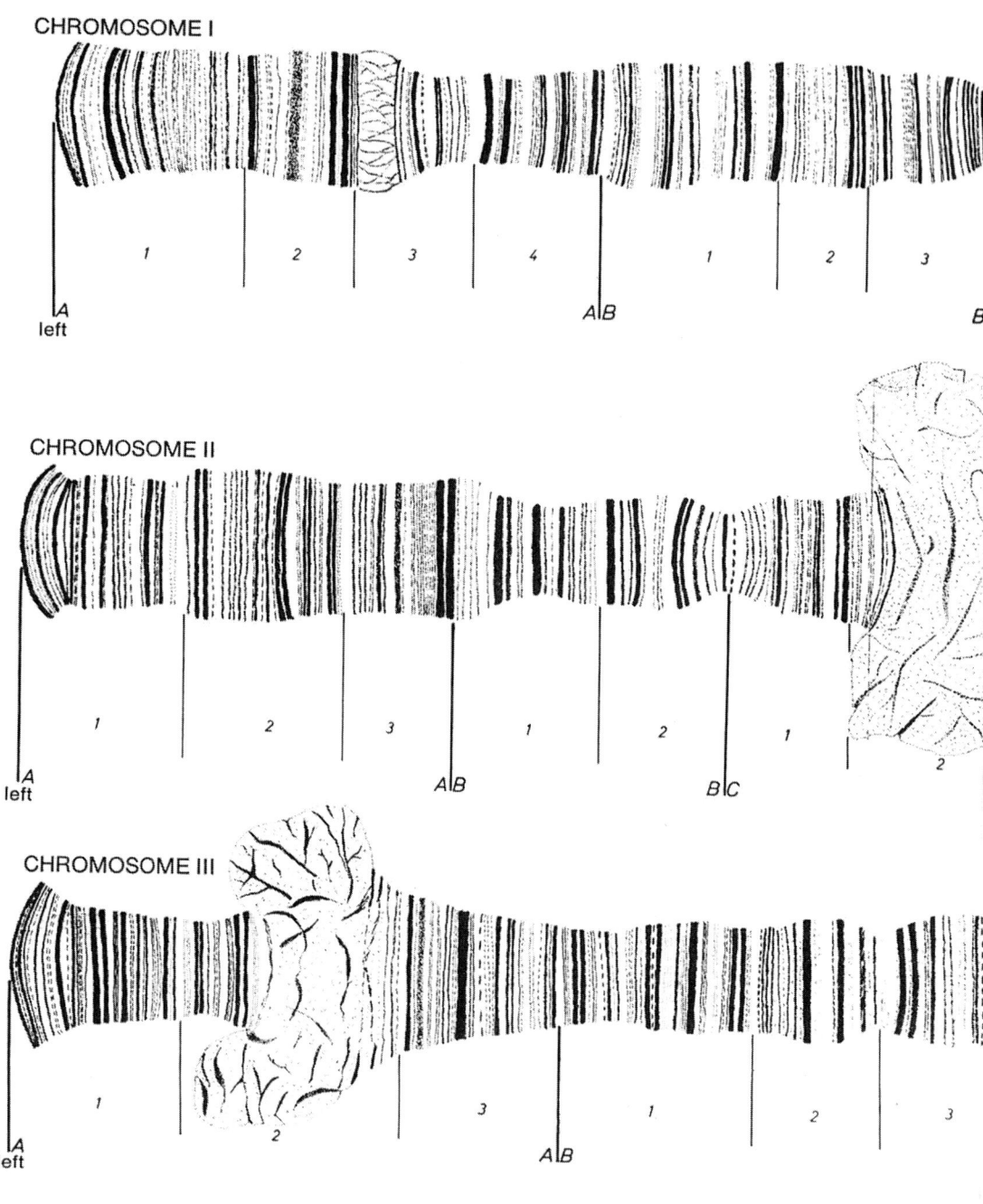

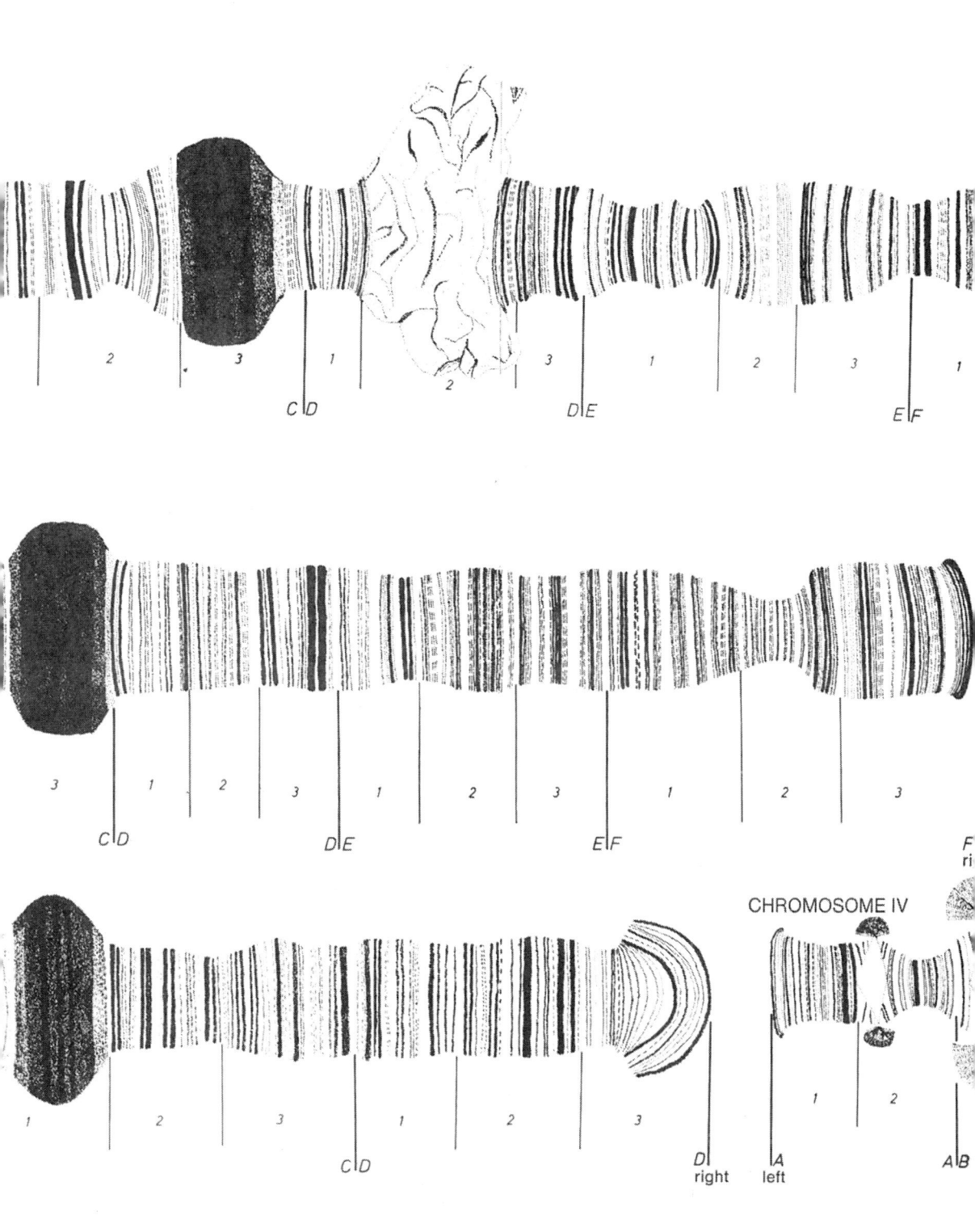

CHROMOSOME IV

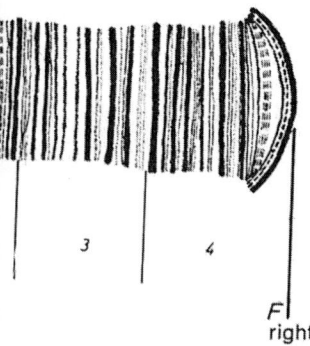

3   4

F
right

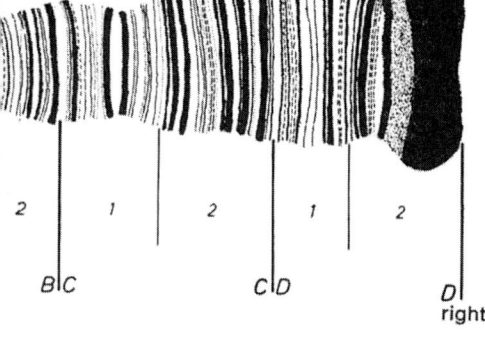

2   1   2   1   2

B *C*   *C* *D*   *D*
right

examined, 5 different kinds of inversions were observed. A morphological comparison between Canadian, German, and Novosibirsk populations suggests an endemic inversion in the latter.

Puffs may be induced by temperature shocks and x rays at the heterochromatic regions of the salivary gland chromosomes of *G. barbipes* (Stich and Naylor, 1957; Keyl, 1962; Walter, 1973). Cytophotometric measurements by Stich and Naylor yielded different values for the DNA content of puffed and unpuffed heterochromatic bulbs. These data suggested that this DNA has a metabolic function. More recent measurements (Keyl, 1962; Walter, 1973) have shown that the DNA undergoes the same number of replications in the heterochromatic and euchromatic regions, and that the puffing of the heterochromatic regions is not accompanied by a decrease in DNA. Furthermore, there is no measurable RNA synthesis at these puffs, although small amounts of the typical puff proteins are produced. In *Glyptotendipes* the relationship between DNA replication and the composition of proteins in the salivary gland chromosomes has been studied with autoradiographic methods using ^{14}C-thymidine, ^{3}H-lysine, and ^{3}H-arginine. In contrast to ^{14}C-thymidine, the radioactive amino acids are steadily incorporated into the chromosomes without any differences in concentration corresponding to the banding pattern. A banded pattern of silver grains could only be obtained after a long-period incorporation of ^{3}H-lysine.

The autoradiographic results, the cytophotometric measurements on DNA content, and the data on protein distribution in single, isolated salivary gland chromosomes all support the conclusion that the precursors of protein are steadily incorporated into the chromosomes. However, these precursors are only recognizably linked with DNA (to form a banding pattern) after a considerable time. This conclusion is compatible with the hypothesis that protein links to DNA long after its replication.

According to Miseiko *et al.* (1971a) about 16 percent of the larvae of *G. barbipes* examined in a Russian population characteristically exhibit supernumerary microchromosomes (B chromosomes). Microchromosomes have not been reported in the subspecies *G. paripes* and *G. glaucus*.

Literature Cited

Basrur, V. R., 1957 Inversion polymorphism in the midge *Glytotendipes barbipes*. *Chromosoma (Berl.)* **8**:597–608.

Bauer, H., 1936 Beiträge zur vergleichenden Morphologie der Speicheldrüsen-Chromosomen. *Zool. Jahrb.* **56**:239–276.

Beermann, W., 1955 Geschlechtsbestimmung und Evolution der genetischen Y-Chromosomen bei *Chironomus*. *Biol. Zentralbl.* **74**:525–544.

Dvorak, J., J. M. van Brink and B. Kiauta, 1970 A note on the germ cell chromosomes of the genus *Glyptotendipes*. *Genen Phaenen* **14**:5–8.

Fischer, G., 1969 Zur Fortpflanzungsbiologie von *Chironomus nuditarsis* Str. *Rev. Suisse Zool.* **76**:23–55.

Keyl, H. G., 1962 DNS-Konstanz im Heterochromatin von *Glyptotendipes*. *Exp. Cell Res.* **30**:245–247.

Keyl, H. G. and I. Keyl, 1959 Die cytologische Diagnostik der Chironomiden. I. Bestimmungstabelle für die Gattung *Chironomus* auf Grund der Speicheldrüsen-Chromosomen. *Arch. Hydrobiol.* **56**:43–57.

Miseiko, G. H., I. I. Kiknadze and B. K. Minsarinova, 1971*a* Supplementary microchromosomes in Chironomidae. *Dokl. Akad. Nauk SSSR* **200**:709–711.

Miseiko, G. N., B. K. Minsarinova and I. I. Kiknadze, 1971*b* The karyotype structure in natural populations of *Glyptotendipes barbipes* (Diptera, Chironomidae). *Tsitologiya* **13**:1501–1505.

Stich, H. F. and J. M. Naylor, 1958 Variation of desoxyribonucleic acid content of specific chromosome regions. *Exp. Cell Res.* **14**:442–445.

Walter, L., 1973 Syntheseprozesse an den Riesenchromosomen von Glyptotendipes. *Chromosoma (Berl.)* **41**:327–360.

PART J
MOSQUITOES AND
FLIES OF GENETIC
INTEREST

12

Anopheline Mosquitoes

Mario Coluzzi and James B. Kitzmiller

Introduction

The world catalog of the *Culicidae* or mosquitoes (Stone *et al.*, 1959) divides them into three subfamilies, *Anophelinae, Toxorhynchitinae,* and *Culicinae.* The subfamily *Anophelinae* has three genera: the neotropical *Chagasia,* the Australasian *Bironella,* and the nearly cosmopolitan *Anopheles.* The first two genera include 4 and 7 known species, respectively, while the genus *Anopheles* contains more than 350 species grouped in six subgenera: *Stethomyia* with 5 species, *Lophopodomyia* with 6, *Kerteszia* with 6, *Nyssorhynchus* with 25, *Anopheles* with about 150, and *Cellia* with about 160 (Reid, 1968). The last four subgenera include all the known vectors of human malaria, as well as important vectors of Bancroftian filariasis and arbovirus.

The development of genetic studies on anopheline mosquitoes has been closely linked to their medical importance. However, many species represent suitable material for purely genetic approaches because they possess a number of favorable characteristics. They are relatively easy to sample in the field and to breed in the laboratory, they have a short generation span and high reproductive potential, and they possess chromosomes that are excellent for cytological study. Moreover, anopheline mosquitoes are among the best-known groups of insects. A large body of information has been accumulated on their systematics, physiology,

Mario Coluzzi—Institute of Parasitology, University of Rome, Rome Italy. James B. Kitzmiller—Florida Medical Entomology Laboratory, Vero Beach, Florida.

ecology and behavior, and numerous sophisticated study techniques are available. The literature is scattered through a number of periodicals, but key references are easily found in various general books on mosquitoes [see Bates (1949), Muirhead-Thompson (1951), Clements (1963), Mattingly (1969), and Gillett (1971)]. A list of references on rearing and experimental techniques is provided by Gerberg (1970).

The genetics of the anophelines began with the discovery of the European sibling species of the *Anopheles maculipennis* complex (Falleroni, 1926). The early studies on this species group included hybridization experiments by various authors [see references in Bates (1949)] and the first observations on salivary gland chromosomes (Frizzi, 1947a). However, in recent years the genetics of anophelines has expanded greatly, particularly in relation to the study of sibling species and to problems involved in chemical and genetical control. The present attempt to summarize the work done in this field will deal particularly with the most recent contributions. The earlier reviews by Kitzmiller (1953, 1963, 1967), Davidson and Mason (1963), and Kitzmiller and Mason (1967) should be consulted for a more complete list of references.

Formal Genetics

Little work has been carried out on the formal genetics of anophelines, whereas many studies have been devoted to insecticide resistance and cytogenetics. The few contributions on formal genetics are scattered among the various malaria vectors, e.g., *A. quadrimaculatus, A. atroparvus, A. albimanus, A. stephensi, A. pharoensis,* and species A and B of the *gambiae* complex. Markers are available in some of these species for all three or for two linkage groups, though few linkage data are as yet published.

Morphological Mutants

A considerable number of morphological variants have been recorded in anophelines. More than 60 variants, occurring in different species, are listed by Kitzmiller and Mason (1967), and 50 variants were recently reported by Aslamkhan *et al.* (1972) from a natural population of *A. stephensi.* Few of these variants, however, were shown to be hereditary. The possible hereditary basis of many others has not been investigated, or the experiments gave data difficult to interpret. Difficulties due to inbreeding depression were also frequently encountered in stock isolation and maintenance.

One of the morphological characters for which the genetic basis has been determined concerns the presence of a broad, light, dorsal stripe which can be recognized in larvae, pupae, and adults. The non-stripe mutation is inherited as an autosomal recessive. This mutant, recorded in several species, was investigated in *A. quadrimaculatus* (French, 1963; French and Kitzmiller, 1963), *A. albimanus* (Keppler, 1965), and *A. pharoensis* (Mason, unpublished). The stripe phenotype also occurs in *A. albitarsis, A. noroestensis, A. triannulatus* and *A. evansae*. Rozeboom (1963) presents evidence for a genetic basis for the *bisignatus* and *trisignatus* forms of *A. albimanus*. The data given suggest that both are recessive mutants with complete penetrance. Other morphological markers have been investigated in *A. gambiae* species A, *A. gambiae* species B, and *A. pharoensis* (Mason, 1964; Mason and Davidson, 1966). Two of these are the sex-linked, nonallelic, eye-color mutants white eye and pink eye. The pattern of inheritance of these genes showed that in these three species there is a *Drosophila*-type of sex linkage, in agreement with the cytological evidence (see the section Cytogenetics). Good autosomal marker genes, collarless and diamond, have also been isolated in *A. gambiae* species A. Linkage studies using the DDT- and dieldrin-resistance genes (see the section Applied Genetical Investigations) showed that the collarless gene segregates independently (Mason, 1964, 1967), while Haridi (1971) produced linkage data between diamond and the two resistance genes. Tests for linkage were also carried out in *A. pharoensis* between the autosomal genes non-stripe, green larva, dieldrin-resistance, and DDT-resistance. These tests showed that whereas the non-stripe gene segregated independently, the other three genes were linked [see Kitzmiller and Mason (1967)]. In *A. stephensi* the black larva gene is partially dominant and lethal in the homozygous state (Mason and Davidson, 1966). The character is linked with DDT- and dieldrin-resistance. In *A. atroparvus* a red eye mutant (*or*) was studied by Laudani *et al.* (1970).

Biochemical Mutants

An increasing number of publications deal with electrophoretically detectable enzyme variants. Bianchi (1968a) working with *A. stephensi,* gave the first description of an esterase gene–enzyme system. Further studies on esterases were carried out by Bianchi and Rinaldi (1970) on ·a laboratory strain of *A. atroparvus* in which four isoallelic molecular variants were demonstrated. Six autosomal loci specifying esterases have been identified in *A. punctipennis* by Narang and Kitzmiller (1971a,b) and designated *A, B, C, D, E,* and *F.* The alleles of the *Est-A* and *Est-B* loci control the synthesis of esterases which hydrolize alpha-naphthyl acetate, while the alleles at the *Est-C* and *Est-D* loci are specific for the beta substrate. Genetic analysis showed the existence of three alleles at locus *C* and as many as 7 alleles at loci *A, B,* and *E.* The occurrence of "null" alleles at both *Est-A* and *Est-B* loci was recorded. Analysis of a natural population from Monticello (Illinois) indicates that *Est-C* homozygotes have a higher frequency and *Est-C* heterozygotes a lower frequency than expected on the basis of a Hardy-Weinberg equilibrium. Electrophoretic variants of the enzyme xanthine dehydrogenase were observed by Bianchi and Chessa (1970) in a laboratory strain of *A. atroparvus,* but only in the adult females. Further studies on dehydrogenase polymorphism were carried out by Narang and Kitzmiller (1972) in *A. punctipennis* from Monticello. The xanthine dehydrogenase-active sites were found to be controlled by 2 independent autosomal loci, *Xdh-1* and *Xdh-2,* with 3 and 2 alleles, respectively. Data obtained on the octanol dehydrogenase variants suggested that these bands are under the control of a single, autosomal locus. However, the interpretation of the dehydrogenase zymograms was difficult because of the interference of tetrazolium oxidase activity.

Phosphoglucomutase electrophoretic variants were studied in *A. stephensi* by Bullini *et al.* (1971a,b) utilizing four laboratory colonies having different geographic origins. The genetical data showed in this species the existence of an autosomal locus *Pgm* with four codominant alleles variably distributed in the four strains examined.

Mutagenesis

Few mutagenesis experiments have been conducted with anophelines. Frizzi and Jolly (1961) irradiated adult males of *A. atroparvus* with doses ranging from 2000 to 6000 r and examined the larvae which survived until the fourth instar for chromosomal mutations. The 6000-r dose gave complete sterility, whereas 3500 r produced the highest rate of chromosomal aberrations. Paracentric inversions were most common, followed by pericentric inversions, a few deficiencies, and one translocation. Frizzi (1963) exposed pupae and adult males to a ^{60}Co source, and he then mated the males hatched from treated pupae with normal females. The treated males were mated with successive groups of females at 5-day intervals. Embryogenesis occurred only in eggs from the second mating. Frizzi infers that the spermatids are more sensitive to the induction of dominant lethals than are the spermatozoa. Inversions and translocations were found among the progeny. French (1963) carried out an extensive series of experiments on the mutagenic effects of x-rays in *A. quadrimaculatus.* Untreated females mated with males given a dose of 2500 r produced only about 30 percent as many viable offspring as did the control females. An elaborate protocol for screening F_1, F_2, and F_3 progeny resulted in the discovery of 42 different phenotypic variants among about 20,000 progeny. However, French found similar variants in controls and in other unirradiated stocks, and he therefore concluded that irradiation, at least under his conditions, does not increase the numbers or kinds of visible mutants in *A. quadrimaculatus.* Further experiments on mutagenesis were recently carried out to induce translocations for use in genetic control (see the section Applied Genetical Investigations).

Cytogenetics

Anopheline mosquitoes are favorable material for cytogenetic studies. The diploid chromosomal number is low ($2n = 6$), and mitotic, meiotic, and polytene preparations may be easily obtained (French *et al.,* 1962). Large-banded polytene chromosomes are present in the larval salivary gland cells (Frizzi, 1947*a*) as well as in the ovarian nurse cells of the adult (Coluzzi, 1968). Polytene chromosomes from the Malpighian tubules, although less well developed, have been also utilized (Mason and Brown, 1963).

The Chromosomal Complement

The first chromosomal observations on anophelines were carried out on the *maculipennis* group of the subgenus *Anopheles* (Frizzi, 1947*a*, 1949, 1953*b*). This pioneer work was followed by a series of studies on this and other groups belonging to the subgenera *Anopheles, Cellia* and *Nyssorhynchus.* Two of the six species of subgenus *Kerteszia* (*A. bellator* and *A. cruzii*) were also investigated by Kitzmiller and his co-workers, but the salivary chromosomes were found unfavorable for cytological study. A list of the species whose polytene chromosomes have been described in detail (with maps and/or photographs) is presented in Table 1 with key references. Such contributions also include, with few exceptions, information on the mitotic karyotype. Recent papers specifically dealing with mitotic karyotypes are those of Avirachan *et al.* (1969), Aslamkhan and Baker (1969), and Narang *et al.* (1972*b*). The last paper deals with both the karyotype and the process of spermatogenesis. Previous karyotype

TABLE 1.   *Polytene Chromosome Studies on the Genus Anopheles*

Species		References
Subgenus *Anopheles*		
Anopheles series		
	algeriensis	Kitzmiller (1966)
	plumbeus	Coluzzi and Cancrini (1971)
maculipennis group[a] (Palearctic spp. complex)	*atroparvus* *labranchiae* *maculipennis* *melanoon* *messeae* *sacharovi*	Frizzi (1947a, 1949, 1953b)
maculipennis group[a] (Nearctic spp.)	*atropos* *aztecus*	Kreutzer *et al.* (1969a) Baker and Kitzmiller (1964b)
	earlei	Kitzmiller and Baker (1965)
	freeborni	Kitzmiller and Baker (1963)
	occidentalis	Baker and Kitzmiller (1965)
	quadrimaculatus	Klassen *et al.* (1965)
punctipennis group	*bradleyi* *crucians* *perplexens* *punctipennis*	Kreutzer *et al.* (1970) Baker and Kitzmiller (1964a), Kreutzer and Kitzmiller (1971b)
pseudopunctipennis group	*hectoris* *franciscanus*	Baker *et al.* (1966) Smithson and McClelland (1972)
	pseudopunctipennis	Baker *et al.* (1965)
Myzhorhynchus series	*barbirostris* *nigerrimus*	Chowdaiah *et al.* (1970) Seetharam and Chowdaiah (1971)

descriptions and studies of spermatogenesis have been summarized by Kitzmiller (1967). Sex chromosomes appear to be present in all species of *Anopheles* so far studied, with XX in females and XY in males.

The polytene chromosome complement typically consists of five synapsed, banded chromosomal arms (Figure 1), all connected in the region of their centromeres, usually without a chromocenter as found in

TABLE 1. Continued

Species		References
Arribalzagia series	*neomaculipalpus*	Kitzmiller *et al.* (1966)
	punctimacula	Kreutzer *et al.* (1969*b*)
	vestitipennis	Chowdaiah *et al.* (1966)
Subgenus *Cellia*		
Pyretophorus series	*gambiae* sp. A	Frizzi and Holstein (1956),
gambiae complex	*gambiae* sp. B	Coluzzi (1966, 1968,
	gambiae sp. C	1970), Coluzzi and
		Sabatini (1967, 1968)
		Green (1972*a*)
	gambiae sp. D	Davidson and Hunt (1972)
	melas	Coluzzi and Sabatini
	merus	(1969)
	subpictus	Narang *et al.* (1973*a*)
Neocellia series	*maculatus*	Narang *et al.* (1973*b*)
	pulcherrimus	Baker *et al.* (1968)
	stephensi	Rishikesh (1959*b*), Sharma *et al.* (1969)
	superpictus	Coluzzi *et al.* (1970)
Neomyzomyia series	*farauti* sp. 1	Bryan and Coluzzi (1971)
	farauti sp. 2	
	tessellatus	Narang *et al.* (1974)
	annulipes (complex)	Green (1972*b*)
Subgenus *Nyssorhynchus*		
	albimanus	Hobbs (1962), Keppler *et al.* (1973)
	aquasalis	Frizzi and Ricciardi (1955)
	darlingi	Kreutzer and Kitzmiller (1972*b*)
	nuneztovari	Kitzmiller *et al.* (1973)
	argyritarsis	Kreutzer (1972)

a For further references, see also Kitzmiller *et al.* (1967).

Drosophila. One of the arms, characteristically the shortest, unpaired and less distinctly banded in the male, often is found isolated in squash preparations and represents the telocentric (probably subtelocentric) X chromosome. In some species (e.g., *A. aquasalis*) a second arm of the X has been described. The four autosomal arms belong to two metacentric chromosomes, but they do not always separate in pairs. Therefore, in

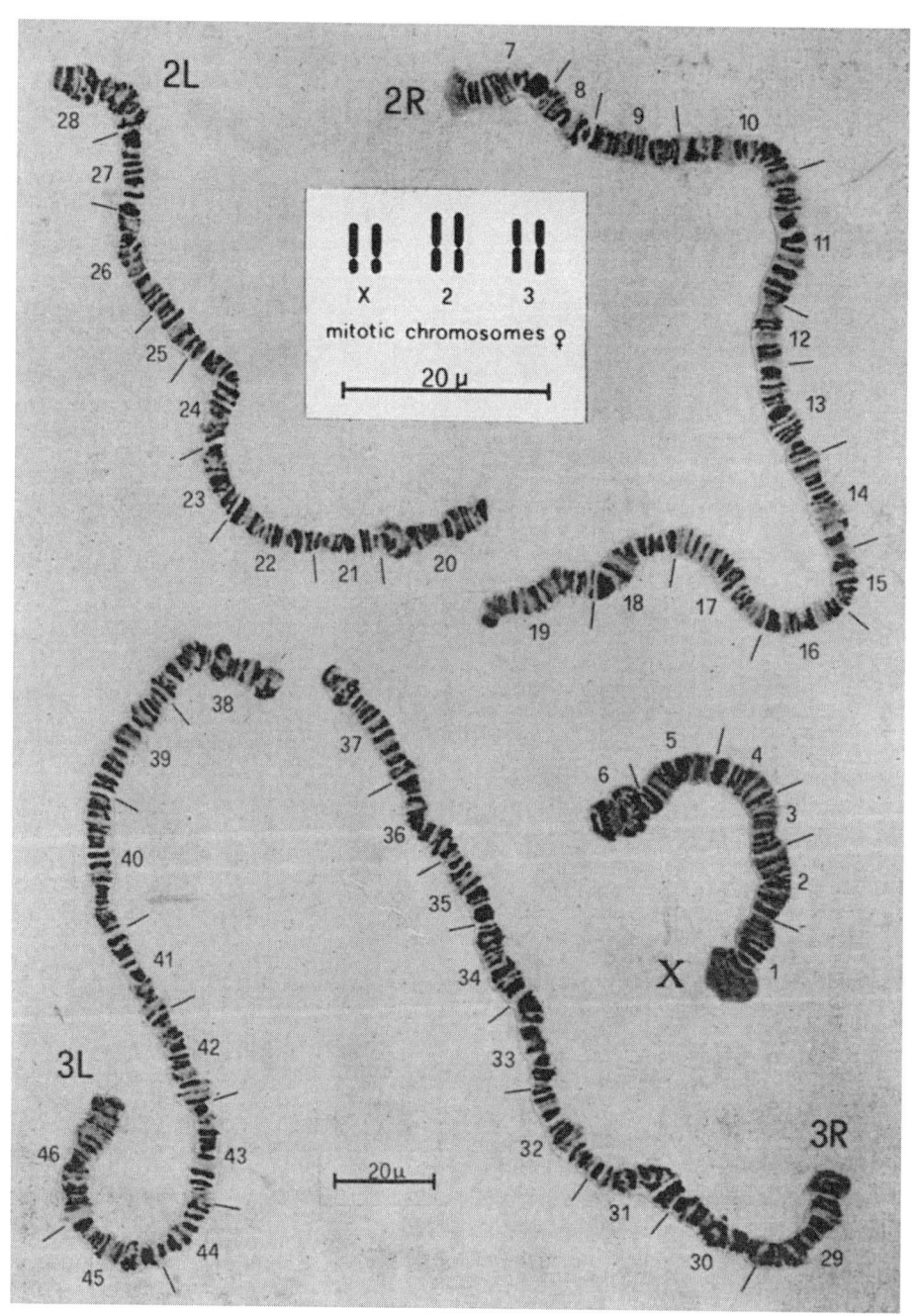

Figure 1. Mitotic karyotype and polytene chromosome complement of A. superpictus. The polytene chromosomes are from ovarian nurse cells. From Coluzzi et al. (1970).

some species it is very difficult to interpret their associations. They have been generally designated as 2L–2R and 3R–3L, following the *Drosophila* nomenclature.

Most of the polytene chromosome studies listed in Table 1 are based on the examination of the salivary gland chromosomes. The only detailed observations on ovarian nurse cells chromosomes were carried out on the *gambiae* complex (Coluzzi, 1968, 1970; Green, 1972a; Davidson and Hunt, 1972) and on *A. superpictus* and *A. stephensi* (Coluzzi *et al.*, 1970). The comparative analysis of the banding pattern in the ovarian and salivary chromosomes of these species showed, as expected, differences in the puffing patterns. The ovarian polytene chromosomes appeared remarkably well developed, reaching the maximum size in connection with yolk synthesis at each gonotrophic cycle. They are easy to manipulate and might represent a good material for developmental studies. Nuclei of all seven nurse cells show polyteny, but the chromosomes are larger in the three nurse cells connected directly to the oocyte. However, not all anophelines show favorable ovarian polytene chromosomes, and no organized polytene arms were detectable in species of the *punctulatus* complex (Bryan and Coluzzi, 1971).

The mitotic complement of anophelines consists of two autosomal pairs and one pair of sex chromosomes; the X–Y dimorphism being obvious in some species, less so in others. Typical somatic pairing has been generally observed. As yet no differences in chromosomal number have been recorded. The two pairs of autosomes are of about equal length, but they generally can be distinguished, one being metacentric or nearly so and the other submetacentric. The position of the centromere in the X chromosome varies in different species so that metacentric, submetacentric, subtelocentric, and telocentric chromosomes have been observed. The evidence from heteropycnosis and from the polytene complement suggests that at least half of the X chromosome is heterochromatic, while the Y chromosome is completely heterochromatic. Two principal types of X chromosomes can be recognized considering the position of the euchromatic zones. In the first type, which can be designated *maculipennis* type (Kitzmiller, 1967), one of the chromosomal arms is euchromatic while the other is completely or mostly heterochromatic. The euchromatic arm is usually the shortest, and its length (1–2 μm) is fairly constant in different species. The length of the heterochromatic arm varies greatly, and determines whether the X is subtelocentric, submetacentric, or metacentric. The *maculipennis* type of X chromosome appears to be widespread in the subgenus *Anopheles*, but it has also been observed in species of the subgenera *Cellia* and *Nyssorhynchus*. The second type of X chromosome can be designated as the *gambiae* type and shows a telocentric or subtelocentric shape. The short arm, presumably heterochromatic, is almost undetectable, since it is no more than 0.5 μm in length. The long arm includes both euchromatic and heterochromatic zones, and it reaches a total length of 2.5–3 μm. The *gambiae* type of X chromosome was recorded in all the species of the *gambiae* complex except *A. melas,* which showed an X chromosome of the *maculipennis* type (Coluzzi and Sabatini, 1967, 1969). An X chromosome of the *gambiae* type appears to be present in *A. subpictus* (Avirachan *et al.,* 1969; Aslamkhan and Baker, 1969), in *A. farauti* (Bryan and Coluzzi, 1971), and in *A. tessellatus* (Narang *et al.,* 1972b). A pericentric inversion can be assumed to explain the origin of the *gambiae* type of X chromosome from the *maculipennis* type, or *vice versa* (Coluzzi and Sabatini, 1969).The Y chromosome is usually quite similar in shape and size to the corresponding X chromosome. However, in many species it can be recognized by having one or both arms shorter than those of the X chromosome.

Information on meiosis in anopheline mosquitoes is found in the papers by Frizzi (1947b, 1953a) on *A. atroparvus* and *A. claviger,* by Rishikesh (1959a) on *A. stephensi,* and by Narang *et al.* (1972b) on *A. tessellatus, A. maculatus, A. annularis, A. culicifacies,* and *A. subpictus.* No leptotene or zygotene stages have been observed. The first visible prophase stage shows very thick and coiled pachytene threads, suggesting that the intimate pairing is retained from the previous pairing of mitotic anaphase and telophase. Subsequent meiotic stages are typical and have been illustrated and described in detail by Narang *et al.* (1972b). During diakinesis the autosomal bivalents show two chiasmata each, but only one chiasma has been recorded in the sex bivalent. Asynchronous separation of homologs was observed in various species, the sex chromosomes moving precociously towards the poles. According to Narang *et al.* (1972b) the sex chromosome as well as the autosomes divide reductionally during anaphase I, while the first division was said to be equational by Rishikesh (1959a).

Chromosomal Polymorphism

Almost all the chromosomal polymorphisms so far recorded in *Anopheles* involve paracentric inversions. One pericentric inversion was observed in the heterozygous state in *A. pulcherrimus* (Baker *et al.,* 1968). A possible polymorphism involving the length of the heterochromatic arm of the X chromosome was noted in *A. punctipennis* (Baker and

Kitzmiller, 1964*a*). No translocation heterozygotes have been observed in natural populations.

Inversion polymorphisms appear to be widespread in *Anopheles*. At least one inversion polymorphism was recorded in about half of the species listed in Table 1, and it must be taken into account that in many cases chromosomally monomorphic material was represented by laboratory colonies. The highest numbers of chromosomal inversions were recorded in *A. punctipennis* (Baker and Kitzmiller, 1964*a*) and in *A. gambiae* species B (Coluzzi and Sabatini, 1967). Eleven chromosomal inversions were observed in a natural population of *A. gambiae* species B recently studied in Nigeria (Coluzzi, unpublished). These inversion polymorphisms are not randomly distributed on the various chromosomes or chromosomal arms. Most of the rearrangements were observed on the longest autosomal arm, which has been designated 3R in subgenus *Anopheles* (Frizzi, 1947*a*) and 2R in subgenus *Cellia* (Frizzi and Holstein, 1956). Inversions were frequently observed also on the X chromosome. No detailed study on the seasonal or geographical change in frequency of chromosomal inversions has been carried out so far on natural populations of *Anopheles,* but such studies are being developed in species of the *gambiae* complex (Coluzzi, unpublished). Laboratory observations were carried out on inversion polymorphisms in *A. stephensi* (Coluzzi *et al.,* 1973). The comparative examination of the carriers of two alternative gene arrangements showed differences involving the time of adult emergence (Coluzzi, 1972) and the egg size (Coluzzi *et al.,* 1972). Inversion polymorphism has been also studied in relation to insecticide resistance (see section Applied Genetical Investigation below).

Evolutionary Genetics

The wide interest in anopheline mosquitoes, and particularly in groups of closely related or sibling species, has provided data of considerable evolutionary interest. These include, together with a large catalog of facts on morphology, ecology, and biogeography that can not be treated here, genetic data mainly from chromosomal and hybridization studies.

Chromosomal and Genic Differences

Polytene chromosome relationships are known for most of the species listed in Table 1. In the *maculipennis* and *gambiae* groups very detailed comparative analyses of the banding patterns in the various siblings were carried out. The homologies and rearrangements were shown both by direct comparison of the chromosomal complements and by the study of the pairing configuration in the hybrids. This has been also done for other pairs of closely related species such as *farauti* species 1 and 2, *crucians* and *bradleyi*, *perplexens* and *punctipennis*, *superpictus* and *stephensi* (see Table 1 for references). Interspecific chromosomal differences were evident in almost every comparison, while homosequential species [*sensu* Carson *et al.* (1967)] appear to be exceptional. A case of homosequential species is represented by *A. atroparvus* and *A. labranchiae*, two almost completely allopatric siblings of the Palearctic *maculipennis* complex [see Frizzi (1949) and Coluzzi (1970)]. The pattern of chromosomal differentiation generally observed appears to involve paracentric inversions. In many cases the two alternative gene arrangements were found to be fixed in the homozygous state in different species, but sometimes the inversion remained polymorphic in one of the siblings. Interspecific overlapping or included inversions were frequently noted, and evidence of nonrandom distribution of the breakpoints was obtained (see the papers listed in Table 1 on the *gambiae* complex and on *A. crucians* and *A. bradleyi*). As noted with inversion polymorphism, the longest autosomal arm and the X chromosome appear to be those more frequently involved in interspecific rearrangements.

Concerning the chromosome relationships between groups and series, clear homologies were observed between species belonging to groups of the same series and also between some species belonging to different series. In the subgenus *Anopheles* the banding patterns of species of *Arribalzagia*, *Myzorhynchus*, and *Anopheles* were easily homologized. The free ends of the autosomal arms appear to be particularly conservative and show very little variation in all the species of the subgenus *Anopheles* so far studied. A comparative analysis of the banding pattern was also successfully carried out in the subgenus *Cellia* between species of *Pyretophorus* and *Neocellia*. In this case, a translocation and a pericentric inversion appear to be involved together with paracentric inversions in the chromosomal change, but most of the banding pattern can be homologized (Narang *et al.*, 1973a). However, when examining the polytene chromosomes of species of *Neomyzomyia* (a primitive series of subgenus *Cellia*), no obvious homologies were observed with *Pyretophorus* and *Neocellia* (Bryan and Coluzzi, 1971).

Comparatively very few investigations were carried out on genic differences between species of anophelines. Bianchi (1968b) showed that two sibling species of the *maculipennis* complex (*atroparvus* and *labranchiae*) are characterized by different alkaline phosphatase allozymes. Different phosphoglucomutase allozymes were recorded between *A. stephensi* and *A. superpictus* and between *A. merus* and the other members of the *gambiae* complex (Bullini and Coluzzi, 1972).

Crossing Experiments

Some interspecific crosses are easily obtained in laboratory cages. The precopulatory isolating mechanisms between the species often break down in this artificial environment. When dealing with species unable to mate in cages, copulation can be forced with special techniques (McDaniel and Horsfall, 1957; Baker, 1964). Crossing studies have been widely utilized to demonstrate the existence of sibling species in various groups, e.g., *maculipennis* (DeBuck *et al.*, 1934; Corradetti, 1934; Bates and Hackett, 1939; Barr, 1954), *gambiae* (Davidson and Jackson, 1962; Paterson *et al.*, 1963; Davidson, 1964; Davidson and Hunt, 1972), *claviger* (Coluzzi, 1963), and *punctulatus* (Bryan and Davidson, 1967; Bryan, 1973). Further hybridization experiments were recently carried out between *A. crucians* and *A. bradleyi* (Kreutzer and Kitzmiller, 1971a), *A. stephensi* and *A. superpictus* (Coluzzi *et al.*, 1971), *A. punctipennis* and *A. perplexens* (Kreutzer and Kitzmiller, 1972a), and *A. maculatus, A. stephensi,* and *A. tessellatus* (Narang *et al.*, 1972a). The results show various degrees of genetic incompatibility, characterized by (1) more or less pronounced hybrid sterility involving only the male or both hybrid sexes (the F_1 sex ratio is often distorted); (2) hybrid inviability, with death soon after emergence, during the preimaginal metamorphosis, or late during embryonic development; (3) lack of fertilization or very early death of the embryo. A fairly good agreement has been observed between phylogenetic distance, as estimated from morphological and chromosomal differences, and the degree of incompatibility as shown by the crossing experiments. Hybrid sterility associated with hybrid vigor was generally observed between sibling species whose homologous polytene chromosomes in the F_1 hybrids appeared mostly paired in spite of paracentric inversions. In the attempt to discover postmating barriers to gene flow, various hybridization experiments were carried out between geographical populations of some widely distributed species such as *A. stephensi, A. punctipennis,* and *A. albimanus* [see Davidson and Kitzmiller (1970)]. The results indicated that geographical isolation *per se* does not affect the cross-fertilizing capacity.

The genetical origin of hybrid sterility has not been studied in detail. The chromosomal rearrangements shown between species are due to paracentric inversions, which should not cause hybrid sterility. Genic sterility appears more likely to be involved.

Mechanisms of Reproductive Isolation

Hybrid sterility appears to develop rapidly during *Anopheles* speciation, but it often involves only the hybrid males. The female hybrids remain in many cases perfectly fertile, and a backcross with either parental species represents, at least in the laboratory, an efficient bridge for gene flow. Such a situation exists for some siblings of the *maculipennis* complex and of the *gambiae* complex, but no evidence of introgression between these species has been obtained in nature. In the case of the *gambiae* complex, species A and B occur sympatrically in large areas of Africa, breeding and presumably swarming in the same places. The wide application of the cytotaxonomic method to these species is providing good and reliable estimates of the extent of natural hybridization. Natural hybrids were first observed cytologically in Tanzania (White, 1970) and later in Nigeria (Shidrawi, 1972; Coluzzi, unpublished). We currently estimate from observations on more than 12,000 chromosomal preparations from wild individuals examined from areas of sympatrism, that the percentage of F_1 hybrids is less than 0.1 percent. This finding clearly indicates that premating ethological barriers have a primary importance in keeping these sibling species reproductively isolated. Indirect evidence of the existence of important differences in mating behavior originates also from various observations showing that pairs of sibling species often differ in their ability to mate in laboratory cages.

Applied Genetical Investigations

The development of chemical and biological control of anophelines and the analysis of vectorial capacity involve some important genetical approaches, which are briefly mentioned here.

Insecticide Resistance

In a recent monograph on insecticide resistance in arthropods (Brown and Pal, 1971), 15 species of *Anopheles* are listed which have developed physiological resistance to DDT and 37 species which have developed resistance to dieldrin. The DDT-resistant species, with two exceptions only, are also resistant to dieldrin. These data originate from field observations carried out all over the world in connection with malaria eradication and control programs [see Brown and Pal (1971) for details on the methods of investigations and for a complete list of references]. Laboratory experiments on the inheritance of resistance to DDT and to dieldrin and on the pattern of cross resistance to related insecticides were carried out on *A. albimanus, A. atroparvus, A. funestus, A. gambiae* species A and B, *A. pharoensis, A. pseudopunctipennis, A. quadrimaculatus, A. sacharovi, A. sergenti, A. stephensi,* and *A. sundaicus.* Such studies, mainly undertaken in the Ross Institute, London, by Davidson and his co-workers, are summarized by Davidson (1958), Davidson and Mason (1963), Brown (1967), and Brown and Pal (1971). Dieldrin resistance, as first shown by Davidson (1956), is inherited as a single, autosomal, partially dominant factor. Almost 100 percent discrimination of phenotypes has been found to be possible since dieldrin resistance is always of a high order. A dominant type of dieldrin resistance was also recorded in *A. albimanus* (Rozeboom and Johnson, 1961) and in *A. gambiae* species A (Davidson and Hamon, 1962). Haridi (1971) has recently shown that the major factors responsible for dominant and partially dominant dieldrin resistance are allelic in *A. gambiae* species A. The study of the frequencies of the various phenotypes for dieldrin resistance has been carried out in natural populations of *A. gambiae* species A and B in various parts of Africa [see Hamon and Garrett-Jones (1963)]. The dieldrin-resistance gene appears to be particularly widespread in West African populations of *gambiae* species A and B, where frequencies of heterozygotes higher than 5 percent were frequently recorded in untreated populations. The frequency of resistant homozygotes reached 45 percent in an untreated village near Kaduna, Nigeria (Service and Davidson, 1964). Single-factor inheritance is also indicated for DDT resistance, but the expression of this factor appears, at least in some species, to be more dependent on the genetic background, and the discrimination of the resistant, susceptible, and heterozygote phenotypes was generally found to be more difficult. Resistance to carbamate or organophosphorus insecticides has recently been observed in *A. albimanus* in Nicaragua and El Salvador (Ariaratnam and Georghiou, 1971; A. Zahar, private communication).

Chromosomal Inversions and Insecticide Selection Pressure

Soon after the discovery of insecticide resistance in malaria vectors a series of investigations developed on possible relationships of this phenomenon with chromosomal inversions (Holstein, 1957; D'Alessandro *et al.,* 1957, 1958; Mosna *et al.,* 1958, 1959). Holstein (1957), working with laboratory colonies of *A. gambiae*, found a greater chromosomal polymorphism in a dieldrin-resistant strain from Sokoto (Nigeria) than in a dieldrin-susceptible strain from Lagos previously studied by Frizzi and Holstein (1956). However, it is now known that two sibling species of the *gambiae* complex were involved in this comparison, the Lagos strain belonging to species A and the Sokoto strain to species B. In various areas the latter species shows a higher chromosomal polymorphism than its sibling (Coluzzi and Sabatini, 1967). D'Alessandro *et al.* (1957, 1958) studied three DDT-tolerant strains of *A. atroparvus* originated by selection from a parent strain polymorphic for an inversion on chromosome 3L. They found that the frequency of the heterozygotes for this inversion was higher in the selected material than in the parental stock. Further selection resulted in a remarkable excess of heterozygotes, and these became more than twice as abundant as the two homozygotes taken together. Similar results were obtained by Mosna *et al.* (1958, 1959), who studied the same inversion system using both DDT and dieldrin. It is not clear from these experiments to what extent the obvious differential survival of the heterokaryotype was specifically dependent on the insecticide selection pressure. Similar increases in the frequency of inversion heterozygotes were also induced by the application of certain rearing procedures, so that the greater survival ability of the heterozygotes could be interpreted as a case of "vigor tolerance" (D'Alessandro *et al.*, 1962). No chromosomal inversion polymorphisms were recorded in a comparative study of insecticide-resistant and susceptible strains of *A. quadrimaculatus* (Mason and Brown, 1963).

Genetical Changes in Behavior and Insecticide Selection Pressure

Behavioral changes were reported in various malaria vectors under insecticide selection pressure, and the term "behavioristic resistance" was introduced to indicate the development of an ability to avoid a dose of toxicant which would prove lethal (Brown, 1958). Although some of these behavioral differences originated by differential survival of two previously unknown sibling species (Mattingly, 1967), evidence of genetic changes in behavior were obtained at least in *A. albimanus* in Panama and in *A. pseudopunctipennis* in Mexico [see Zulueta (1964) for details and references]. Very little is known on the inheritance of the behavioral traits involved with insecticide avoidance. Gerold and Laarman (1964, 1967) selected a strain of *A. atroparvus* for its ability to escape from a tube treated with DDT. A marked response to selection was observed for 8–10 generations, both selecting for escapers and nonescapers. The possibility of selection for anthropophily *versus* zoophily has been demonstrated by Gillies (1964) working with *A. gambiae* species A. Although the heritable component of host selection appears relatively slight compared with environmental effects, a clear difference in behavior between the selected lines was evident in the F_2 and F_3 generations.

Cytotaxonomy

The identification of sympatric sibling species of anophelines has an obvious practical importance in malariology, and the cytotaxonomic approach proved to be very useful (Frizzi, 1953a; Coluzzi, 1970). The chromosomal differentiation accompanying anopheline speciation provides a number of reliable cytotaxonomic characters. Cytotaxonomic identifications were first carried out on the Palearctic sibling species of the *maculipennis* complex [see references in Kitzmiller (1967)], and they are currently done in the *gambiae* complex in various parts of Africa, using both salivary and ovarian polytene chromosomes (Coluzzi, 1968; White, 1970; Service, 1970; Green, 1970; and others). This method is also being used on the morphologically similar and taxonomically difficult members of the subgenus *Nyssorhynchus* (Kitzmiller *et al.*, 1973). The vector population of *A. nuneztovari* in Colombia and Venezuela may be distinguished from the nonvector populations in Brasil by means of an inversion on the X chromosome.

Vector Capacity

Most of the studies on the genetics of vector capacity were carried out using *Aedes aegypti* and *Culex pipiens* as models. Some selection experiments involving the susceptibility of *A. quadrimaculatus* to *Plasmodium* are summarized by MacDonald (1967). More recent experiments were carried out by Corradetti *et al.* (1970), who showed that the host–parasite relationships between *A. stephensi* and *Plasmodium gallinaceum* can be greatly modified selecting both the parasite and the arthropod.

Genetic Control

Various attempts to apply genetic methods to the control of anophelines have been carried out in recent years. The genetic control with sterile males was shown to be theoretically feasible by laboratory observations indicating that secondary insemination does not occur in female anophelines (French and Kitzmiller, 1963). Monogamy is caused by "matrone," a substance produced by the male accessory glands (Craig, 1967), and even sterile hybrid males, provided that they have active accessory glands, can render their mates refractory to insemination (Bryan, 1968, 1972; Davidson, 1969). Release experiments of conspecific sterilized males were made with *A. quadrimaculatus* (Weidhaas *et al.*, 1962; Patterson *et al.*, 1968), while in a field trial against *A. gambiae* species A, the insects released were sterile hybrids obtained by crossing two sibling species of the *gambiae* complex (Davidson *et al.*, 1970). These preliminary attempts were, on the whole, unsuccessful, presumably because of the low competitive ability of the released males [see Davidson and Kitzmiller (1970)].

Translocations have been induced in the laboratory in *A. stephensi* (Aslamkhan and Aaqil, 1970), in *A. albimanus* (Rabbani and Kitzmiller, 1972), and in *A. gambiae* species A and B (Krafsur, 1972*a,b*; Hunt and Krafsur, 1972), but no field attempts to use them in genetic control have been carried out so far.

Literature Cited

Ariaratnam, V. and G. P. Georghiou, 1971   Selection for resistance to carbamate and organophosphorus insecticides in *Anopheles albimanus. Nature (Lond.)* **232**:642–644.

Aslamkhan, M. and M. Aaqil, 1970   A preliminary report on the γ-induced translocations and semisterility in the malaria mosquito, *Anopheles stephensi. Pak. J. Sci. Res.* **22**:183–190.

Aslamkhan, M. and R. H. Baker, 1969   Karyotypes of some *Anopheles, Ficalbia* and *Culex* mosquitoes of Asia. *Pak. J. Zool.* **1**:1–7.

Aslamkhan, M., M. Aaqil and M. Hafeez, 1972   Genetical and morphological variations in a natural population of the malaria mosquito, *Anopheles stephensi* from Karachi, Pakistan. *Biologia* **18**:29–41.

Avirachan, T. T., P. L. Seetharam and B. N. Chowdaiah, 1969   Karyotype studies in oriental anophelines. *Cytologia (Tokyo)* **34**:418–422.

Baker, R. H., 1964   Mating problems as related to the establishment and maintenance of laboratory colonies of mosquitoes. *Bull. WHO* **31**:467–468.

Baker, R. H. and J. B. Kitzmiller, 1964*a*   Salivary gland chromosomes of *Anopheles punctipennis, J. Heredity* **55**:9–17.

Baker, R. H. and J. B. Kitzmiller, 1964*b*   The salivary gland chromosomes of *Anopheles aztecus. Revta. Inst. Salubr. Enferm. Trop.* **24**:43–54.

Baker, R. H. and J. B. Kitzmiller, 1965   The salivary gland chromosomes of *Anopheles occidentalis. Bull. WHO* **32**:575–580.

Baker, R. H., J. B. Kitzmiller and B. N. Chowdaiah, 1965   The salivary gland chromosomes of *Anopheles pseudopunctipennis pseudopunctipennis. Bull. WHO* **33**:837–841.

Baker, R. H., J. B. Kitzmiller and B. N. Chowdaiah, 1966   The salivary gland chromosomes of *Anopheles hectoris. Chromosoma (Berl.)* **19**:126–136.

Baker, R. H., A. S. Nasir and M. Aslamkhan, 1968   The salivary gland chromosomes of *Anopheles pulcherrimus* Theobald. *Parassitologia* **10**:167–177.

Barr, A. R., 1954   Hybridization experiments with some American dark-winged anophelines. *Exp. Parasitol.* **3**:445–457.

Bates, M., 1949   *The Natural History of Mosquitoes,* MacMillan, New York, 379 pp.

Bates, M. and L. W. Hackett, 1939   The distinguishing characteristics of the populations of *Anopheles maculipennis* found in southern Europe. *Vehr. VII Interntl. Kongr. Entomol. (Berl.)* **3**:1555–1569.

Bianchi, U., 1968*a*   Genetica formale di una proteina dotata di attività catalitica esterasica in *Anopheles stephensi. Rend. Accad. Naz. Lincei* **45**:60–62.

Bianchi, U., 1968*b*   Homologous alkaline phosphatases and homologous loci in two sibling species of European anopheline mosquitoes. *Nature (Lond.)* **217**:382–383.

Bianchi, U. and G. Chessa, 1970   Alloenzimi ad attività xantin-deidrogenasica in *Anopheles atroparvus. Boll. Zool.* **37**:477.

Bianchi, U. and A. Rinaldi, 1970   New gene–enzyme system in *Anopheles atroparvus*: occurrence and frequencies of four alleles at the Est6 locus. *Can. J. Genet. Cytol.* **12**:325–330.

Brown, A. W. A., 1958   Laboratory studies on the behaviouristic resistance of *Anopheles albimanus* in Panama. *Bull. WHO.* **19**:1053–1061.

Brown, A. W. A., 1967   Genetics of insecticide resistance in insect vectors. In *Genetics of Insect Vectors of Disease,* edited by J. W. Wright and R. Pal, pp. 505–552, Elsevier, Amsterdam.

Brown, A. W. A. and R. Pal, 1971   *Insecticide Resistance in Arthropods,* WHO Monograph Series No. 38, World Health Organization Geneva, 491 pp.

Bryan, J. H., 1968   Results of consecutive matings of female *Anopheles gambiae* species "B" with fertile and sterile males. *Nature (Lond.)* **218**:489.

Bryan, J. H., 1972   Further studies on consecutive matings in the *Anopheles gambiae* complex. *Nature (Lond.)* **239**:519–520.

Bryan, J. H., 1973   Studies on the *Anopheles punctulatus* complex. II. Hybridization of the member species. *Trans. Roy. Soc. Trop. Med. Hyg.,* **67**:70–84.

Bryan, J. H. and M. Coluzzi, 1971   Cytogenetic observations on *Anopheles farauti* Laveran. *Bull. WHO.* **45**:266–267.

Bryan, J. H. and G. Davidson, 1967   The *Anopheles punctulatus* complex. *Trans. R. Soc. Trop. Med. Hyg.* **61**:455.

Bullini, L. and M. Coluzzi, 1973   Electrophoretic studies on gene–enzyme systems in mosquitoes. *Parassitologia* **15**:221–248.

Bullini, L., G. Cancrini, A. P. Bianchi Bullini and M. Di Deco, 1971*a*   Further studies on the phosphoglucomutase gene in *Anopheles stephensi*: evidence for a fourth allele. (*Diptera, Culicidae*). *Parassitologia* **13**:435–438.

Bullini, L., M. Coluzzi, G. Cancrini and C. Santolamazza, 1971*b*   Multiple phosphoglucomutase alleles in *Anopheles stephensi. Heredity* **26**:475–478.

Carson, H. L., F. E. Clayton and H. D. Stalker, 1967   Karyotypic stability and speciation in Hawaiian *Drosophila. Proc. Natl. Acad. Sci. USA* **57**:1280–1285.

Chowdaiah, B. N., R. H. Baker and J. B. Kitzmiller, 1966   The salivary chromosomes of *Anopheles vestitipennis. Cytologia (Tokyo)* **31**:144–152.

Chowdaiah, B. N., T. T. Avirachan and P. L. Seetharam, 1970   Chromosome studies of oriental anophelines. I. The salivary gland chromosomes of *Anopheles barbirostris*. *Experientia (Basel)* **26**:315–317.

Clements, A. N., 1963   *The Physiology of Mosquitoes*, Pergamon Press, Oxford, 393 pp.

Coluzzi, M., 1963   Le forme di *Anopheles claviger* Meigen indicate con i nomi *missirolii* e *petragnanii* sono due specie riproduttivamente isolate. *Rend. Accad. Naz. Lincei* **32**:1025–1030.

Coluzzi, M., 1966   Osservazioni comparative sul cromosoma X nelle specie A e B del complesso *Anopheles gambiae. Rend. Accad. Naz. Lincei* **40**:671–678.

Coluzzi, M., 1968   Cromosomi politenici delle cellule nutrici ovariche nel complesso *gambiae* del genere *Anopheles. Parassitologia* **10**:179–184.

Coluzzi, M., 1970   Sibling species in *Anopheles* and their importance in malariology. *Misc. Publ. Entomol. Soc. Am.* **7**:63–77.

Coluzzi, M., 1972   Inversion polymorphism and adult emergence in *Anopheles stephensi. Science* (Wash., D.C.) **176**:59–60.

Coluzzi, M. and G. Cancrini, 1971   I cromosomi salivari di *Anopheles plumbeus* Stephens. *Parassitologia* **13**:145–149.

Coluzzi, M. and A. Sabatini, 1967   Cytogenetic observations on species A and B of the *Anopheles gambiae* complex. *Parassitologia* **9**:73–88.

Coluzzi, M. and A. Sabatini, 1968   Cytogenetic observations on species C of the *Anopheles gambiae* complex. *Parassitologia* **10**:155–165.

Coluzzi, M. and A. Sabatini, 1969   Cytogenetic observations on the salt water species, *Anopheles merus* and *Anopheles melas,* of the *gambiae* complex. *Parassitologia* **11**:177–187.

Coluzzi, M., G. Cancrini and M. Di Deco, 1970   The polytene chromosomes of *Anopheles superpictus* and relationships with *Anopheles stephensi. Parassitologia* **12**:101–112.

Coluzzi, M., G. Cancrini and M. Di Deco, 1971   Esperimenti d'incrocio tra *Anopheles stephensi* e *Anopheles superpictus. Parassitologia* **13**:445–448.

Coluzzi, M., G. Cancrini and M. Di Deco, 1972   Polimorfismo cromosomico e lunghezza dell'uovo in *Anopheles stephensi. Parassitologia* **14**:261–266.

Coluzzi, M., M. Di Deco and G. Cancrini, 1973   Chromosomal inversions in *Anopheles stephensi. Parassitologia* **15**:129–136.

Corradetti, A., 1934   Ricerche sugli incroci tra le varietà di *Anopheles maculipennis. Riv. Malariol.* **13**:707–720.

Corradetti, A., G. L. Dojmi Di Delupis, C. Palmieri and G. Piccione, 1970   Modello sperimentale, realizzato con *Plasmodium gallinaceum* e *Anopheles stephensi,* per selezionare popolazioni di plasmodio adatte a vivere in un vettore apparentemente refrattario, e per selezionare popolazioni di vettore suscettibili a un plasmodio apparentemente inadatto a vivere in esso. *Parassitologia* **12**:81–99.

Craig, G., 1967   Mosquitoes: Female monogamy induced by male accessory gland substance. *Science (Wash., D.C.)* **156**:1499–1501.

D'Alessandro, G., G. Frizzi and M. Mariani, 1957   Effect of DDT selection pressure on the frequency of chromosomal structures in *Anopheles atroparvus. Bull. WHO.* **16**:859–864.

D'Alessandro, G., G. Frizzi and M. Mariani, 1958   Ulteriori osservazioni sui rapporti tra ordinamenti cromosomici e resistenza al DDT in *Anopheles atroparvus. Riv. Parassitol.* **19**:67–72.

D'Alessandro, G., M. Mariani and C. Bruno-Smiraglia, 1962   Ricerche sul polimorifsmo cromosomico in *Anopheles atroparvus* ed in *Anopheles labranchiae*. *Riv. Parassitol.* **23**:227–234.

Davidson, G., 1956 Insecticide resistance in *Anopheles gambiae* Giles, a case of simple Mendelian inheritance. *Nature (Lond.)* **178**:863–864.

Davidson, G., 1958 Studies on insecticide resistance in anopheline mosquitos. *Bull. WHO.* **18**:579–621.

Davidson, G., 1964 The five mating types in the *Anopheles gambiae* complex. *Riv. Malariol.* **43**:167–183.

Davidson, G., 1969 The potential use of sterile hybrid males for the eradication of member species of the *Anopheles gambiae* complex. *Bull. WHO.* **40**:221–228.

Davidson, G. and J. Hamon, 1962 A case of dominant dieldrin resistance in *Anopheles gambiae* Giles. *Nature (Lond.)* **196**:1012.

Davidson, G. and R. Hunt, 1973 The crossing and chromosome characteristics of a new, sixth species in the *Anopheles gambiae* complex. *Parassitologia* **15**:121–128.

Davidson, G. and C. E. Jackson, 1962 Incipient speciation in *Anopheles gambiae*, Giles. *Bull. WHO.* **27**:303–305.

Davidson, G. and J. B. Kitzmiller, 1970 Application of new procedures to control anophelines. *Misc. Publ. Entomol. Soc. Am.* **7**:118–129.

Davidson, G. and G. F. Mason, 1963 Genetics of mosquitoes. *Annu. Rev. Entomol.* **8**:177–196.

Davidson, G., J. A. Odetoyinbo, B. Colussa and J. Coz, 1970 A field attempt to assess the mating competitiveness of sterile males produced by crossing two member species of the *Anopheles gambiae* complex. *Bull. WHO.* **42**:55–67.

DeBuck, A., E. Schoute and N. H. Swellengrebel, 1934 Cross-breeding experiments with Dutch and foreign races of *Anopheles maculipennis*. *Riv. Malariol.* **13**:237–263.

Falleroni, D., 1926 Fauna anofelica italiana e suo "Habitat." *Riv. Malariol.* **5**:553–593.

French, W. L., 1963 *Studies on the Genetics and Cytogenetics of* Anopheles quadrimaculatus. Thesis, University of Illinois, Urbana, Ill.

French, W. L. and J. B. Kitzmiller, 1963 Tests for multiple fertilization in *Anopheles quadrimaculatus*. *Proc. N.J. Mosq. Exterm. Assoc.* **50**:374–380.

French, W. L., R. H. Baker and J. B. Kitzmiller, 1962 Preparation of mosquito chromosomes. *Mosq. News* **22**:377–383.

Frizzi, G., 1947a Cromosomi salivari in *Anopheles maculipennis*. *Sci. Genet.* **3**:67–79.

Frizzi, G., 1947b Determinazione del sesso nel genere *Anopheles*. *Sci. Genet.* **3**:80–88.

Frizzi, G., 1949 Genetica di popolazioni in *Anopheles maculipennis*. *Ric. Sci.* **19**:544–552.

Frizzi, G., 1953a Extension of the salivary chromosome method to *Anopheles claviger, quadrimaculatus* and *aquasalis*. *Nature (Lond.)* **171**:1072.

Frizzi, G., 1953b Etude cytogénétique d'*Anopheles maculipennis* en Italie. *Bull. WHO* **9**:335–344.

Frizzi, G., 1963 Effetti delle radiazioni di una sorgente di Co-60 su ninfe ed adulti di *A. maculipennis atroparvus*. *Atti A.G.I.* **8**:242–250.

Frizzi, G. and M. Holstein, 1956 Etude cytogénétique d'*Anopheles gambiae*. *Bull. WHO* **15**:425–435.

Frizzi, G. and M. S. Jolly, 1961 Mutazioni indotte con raggi X in *Anopheles maculipennis*. *Atti A.G.I.* **6**:285–290.

Frizzi, G. and I. Ricciardi, 1955 Introduzione allo studio citogenetico della fauna anofelica del Brasile. *Rev. Bras. Malar. Doenç. Trop.* **7**:399–407.

Gerberg, E. J., 1970   *Manual for Mosquito Rearing and Experimental Techniques,* Am. Mosq. Control Association Bulletin, No. 5.

Gerold, J. L. and J. J. Laarman, 1964   Selection of some strains of *Anopheles atroparvus* with different behavioural responses to contacts with DDT. *Nature (Lond.)* **204**:500–501.

Gerold, J. L. and J. J. Laarman, 1967   Behavioural responses to contact with DDT in *Anopheles atroparvus. Nature (Lond.)* **215**:518–520.

Gillett, J. D., 1971   *Mosquitos,* R. Clay (The Chaucer Press), Bungay, Suffolk, England.

Gillies, M. T., 1964   Selection for host preference in *Anopheles gambiae. Nature (Lond.)* **203**:852–854.

Green, C. A., 1970   Identifications of member species of the *Anopheles gambiae* complex in the Zambesi valley. *Centr. Afr. J. Med.* **16**:207–209.

Green, C. A., 1972a   Cytological maps for the practical identification of females of the three freshwater species of the *Anopheles gambiae* complex. *Ann. Trop. Med. Parasitol.* **66**:143–147.

Green, C. A., 1972b   The *Anopheles annulipes* complex of species. *Proc. 14th Interntl. Congr. Entomol. Canberra (abstracts)*:286.

Hamon, J. and C. Garrett-Jones, 1963   La résistance aux insecticides chez des vecteurs majeurs du paludisme et son importance opérationelle. *Bull. WHO* **28**:1–24.

Haridi, A. M., 1971   DDT and dieldrin resistance in species A and species B of the *Anopheles gambiae* complex. Thesis, University of London, London.

Hobbs, J. H., 1962   Cytogenetics of *Anopheles albimanus* (Diptera, Culicidae). *Ann. Entomol. Soc. Am.* **55**:245–251.

Holstein, M., 1957   Cytogenetics of *Anopheles gambiae. Bull. WHO.* **16**:456–458.

Hunt, R. H. and E. S. Krafsur, 1972   Cytological demonstration of some heterozygous reciprocal translocations in *Anopheles gambiae* species A. *Trans. R. Soc. Trop. Med. Hyg.* **66**:23–24.

Keppler, W. J., 1965   *Genetic, Cytological and Chemical Studies on Anopheles albimanus.* Thesis, Univeristy of Illinois, Urbana, Ill.

Keppler, W. J., J. B. Kitzmiller and M. G. Rabbani, 1973   The salivary gland chromosomes of *Anopheles albimanus. Mosq. News* **33**:42–49.

Kitzmiller, J. B., 1953   Mosquito genetics and cytogenetics. *Rev. Bras. Malar. Doenç. Trop.* **5**:285–359.

Kitzmiller, J. B., 1963   Mosquito cytogenetics. *Bull WHO* **29**:345–355.

Kitzmiller, J. B., 1966   The salivary gland chromosomes of *Anopheles algeriensis. Riv. Malariol.* **45**:51–59.

Kitzmiller, J. B., 1967   Mosquito cytogenetics. In *Genetics of Insect Vectors of Disease,* edited by J. W. Wright and R. Pal, pp. 133–150, Elsevier, Amsterdam.

Kitzmiller, J. B. and R. H. Baker, 1963   The salivary chromosomes of *Anopheles freeborni. Mosq. News* **23**:254–261.

Kitzmiller, J. B. and R. H. Baker, 1965   The salivary chromosomes of *Anopheles earlei. Can. J. Genet. Cytol.* **7**:275–283.

Kitzmiller, J. B. and G. F. Mason, 1967   Formal genetics of anophelines. In *Genetics of Insect Vectors of Disease,* edited by J.W. Wright and R. Pal, pp. 3–15, Elsevier, Amsterdam.

Kitzmiller, J. B., R. H. Baker and B. N. Chowdaiah, 1966   The salivary gland chromosomes of *Anopheles neomaculipalpus. Caryologia* **19**:1–12.

Kitzmiller, J. B., G. Frizzi and R. H. Baker, 1967   Evolution and speciation within the *maculipennis* complex of the genus *Anopheles*. In *Genetics of Insect Vectors of Disease,* edited by J. W. Wright and R. Pal, pp. 151–210, Elsevier, Amsterdam.

Kitzmiller, J. B., R. D. Kreutzer and E. Tallaferro, 1973 Chromosomal differences in populations of *Anopheles nuneztovari. Bull. WHO* **48:**435–455.

Klassen, W., W. L. French, H. Laven and J. B. Kitzmiller, 1965 The salivary chromosomes of *Anopheles quadrimaculatus* Say. *Mosq. News* **25:**328–334.

Krafsur, E. S., 1972*a* Production and isolation of reciprocal translocations in the *Anopheles gambiae* species complex. Thesis, University of London, London.

Krafsur, E. S., 1972*b* Production of reciprocal translocations in *Anopheles gambiae* species A. *Trans. R. Soc. Trop. Med. Hyg.* **66:**22–23.

Kreutzer, R. D., 1972 Chromosomal similarity between *Anopheles argyritarsis* and *Anopheles darlingi. Am. Zool.* **12:**25–26.

Kreutzer, R. D. and J. B. Kitzmiller, 1971*a* Hybridization between *Anopheles crucians* and *Anopheles bradleyi. Evolution* **25:**195–206.

Kreutzer, R. D. and J. B. Kitzmiller, 1971*b* Chromosomal similarity between *Anopheles perplexens* and *Anopheles punctipennis. Mosq. News* **31:**409–415.

Kreutzer, R. D. and J. B. Kitzmiller, 1972*a* Hybridization between two species of mosquitoes *Anopheles punctipennis* Say and *Anopheles perplexans* Ludlow. *J. Hered.* **63:**191–196.

Kreutzer R. D., J. B. Kitzmiller and E. Ferreira, 1972*b* Inversion polymorphism in the salivary gland chromosomes of *Anopheles darlingi* Root. *Mosq. News* **32:**555–565.

Kreutzer, R. D., S. L. Narang and J. B. Kitzmiller, 1969*a* The salivary gland chromosomes of *Anopheles atropos. Mosq. News* **29:**223–230.

Kreutzer, R. D., T. Tadano, S. L. Narang and J. B. Kitzmiller, 1969*b* The salivary gland chromosomes of *Anopheles punctimacula. Rev. Bras. Malar. Doenç. Trop.* **21:**559–570.

Kreutzer, R. D., S. L. Narang and J. B. Kitzmiller, 1970 A comparison of the salivary gland chromosomes of *Anopheles crucians* and *Anopheles bradleyi. Cytologia (Tokyo)* **35:**527–551.

Laudani, U., M. Porcu and A. R. Lecis, 1970 Genetic analysis of a red eye mutant (*or*) of *Anopheles atroparvus. Mosq. News* **30:**648–649.

McDaniel, I. N. and W. R. Horsfall, 1957 Induced copulation of aedine mosquitoes. *Science (Wash., D.C.)* **125:**745.

MacDonald, W. W., 1967 The influence of genetic and other factors on vector susceptibility to parasites. In *Genetics of Insect Vectors of Disease,* edited by J. W. Wright and R. Pal, pp. 567–584, Elsevier, Amsterdam.

Mason, G. F., 1964 *Cytogenetics and Genetics of Strains in the Anopheles gambiae Complex.* Thesis, University of London, London.

Mason, G. F., 1967 Genetic studies on mutations in species A and B of the *Anopheles gambiae* complex. *Genet. Res.* **10:**205–217.

Mason, G. F. and A. W. A. Brown, 1963 Chromosome changes and insecticide-resistance in *Anopheles quadrimaculatus. Bull. WHO.* **28:**77–81.

Mason, G. F. and G. Davidson, 1966 Morphological mutants in anopheline mosquitoes. *Trans. R. Soc. Trop. Med. Hyg.* **60:**20.

Mattingly, P. F., 1967 Genetics of behaviour. In *Genetics of Insect Vectors of Disease,* edited by J. W. Wright and R. Pal, pp. 553–566, Elsevier, Amsterdam.

Mattingly, P. F., 1969 *The Biology of Mosquito-Borne Disease,* Allen and Unwin, London, pp. 184.

Mosna, E., L. Rivosecchi and K. R. S. Ascher, 1958   Studies on insecticide-resistant anophelines. 1. Chromosome arrangements in a dieldrin-selected strain of *Anopheles atroparvus. Bull. WHO.* **19**:297–301.

Mosna, E., C. Palmieri, K. R. S. Ascher, L. Rivosecchi and I. Neri, 1959   Studies on insecticide-resistant anophelines. 2. Chromosome arrangements in laboratory-developed DDT-resistant strains of *Anopheles atroparvus. Bull. WHO.* **20**:63–74.

Muirhead-Thompson, R. C., 1951   *Mosquito Behaviour in Relation to Malaria Transmission and Control in the Tropics,* Edward Arnold, London.

Narang, S. and J. B. Kitzmiller, 1971*a*   Esterase polymorphism in a natural population of *Anopheles punctipennis.* I. Genetic analysis of the esterase A–B system. *J. Hered.* **62**:259–264.

Narang, S. and J. B. Kitzmiller, 1971*b*   Esterase polymorphism in a natural population of *Anopheles punctipennis.* II. Analysis of the Est–C system. *Can. J. Genet. Cytol.* **13**:771–776.

Narang, S. and J. B. Kitzmiller, 1972   Dehydrogenase polymorphism in *Anopheles punctipennis* (Diptera: Culicidae). Genetics of xanthine and octanol dehydrogenases. *Ann. Entomol. Soc. Am.* **65**:798–804.

Narang, N., S. Narang and J. B. Kitzmiller, 1972*a*   Lack of gene flow among three species of anopheline mosquitoes. *Syst. Zool.* **21**:1–6.

Narang, N., S. Narang and J. B. Kitzmiller, 1972*b*   Karyological studies on four species of *Anopheles,* subgenus *Cellia. Caryologia* **25**:259–274.

Narang, N., S. Narang and J. B. Kitzmiller, 1973*a*   The salivary gland chromosomes of *Anopheles subpictus. Parassitologia* **15**:99–120.

Narang, N., S. Narang, J. B. Kitzmiller, G. P. Sharma and O. P. Sharma, 1973*b*   Evolutionary changes in the banding patterns of salivary gland chromosomes in the genus *Anopheles,* subgenus *Cellia. J. Med. Entomol.* **10**:13–22.

Narang, N., S. Narang and J. B. Kitzmiller, 1974   The salivary gland chromosomes of *Anopheles tessellatus. Cytologia (Tokyo)* **39**:1–10.

Paterson, H. E., J. S. Paterson and G. J. VanEeden, 1963   A new member of the *Anopheles gambiae* complex. *Med. Proc.* **9**:414–418.

Patterson, R. S., C. S. Lofgren and M. D. Boston, 1968   The sterile-male technique for control of mosquitoes. A field cage study with *Anopheles quadrimaculatus. Fla. Entomol.* **51**:77–82.

Rabbani, M. G. and J. B. Kitzmiller, 1972   Chromosomal translocations in *Anopheles albimanus* Wiedemann. *Mosq. News* **32**:421–432.

Reid, J., 1968   *Anopheline mosquitoes of Malaya and Borneo,* Studies from the Institute of Medical Research Malaysia No. 31, Kuala Lumpur, 520 pp.

Rishikesh, N., 1959*a*   Chromosome behaviour during spermatogenesis of *Anopheles stephensi sensu stricto. Cytologia (Tokyo)* **24**:447–458.

Rishikesh, N., 1959*b*   Morphology and development of the salivary glands and their chromosomes in the larvae of *Anopheles stephensi sensu stricto. Bull. WHO.* **20**:47–61.

Rozeboom, L. E., 1963   Mutant forms of *Anopheles albimanus* Wiedemann. *Proc. Entomol. Soc. Wash.* **65**:110–114.

Rozeboom, L. E. and R. Johnson, 1961   Inheritance of resistance to dieldrin in *Anopheles albimanus* Wiedemann. *Am. J. Trop. Med. Hyg.* **10**:775–781.

Seetharam, P. L. and B. N. Chowdaiah, 1971   Chromosome studies of oriental anophelines. II. The salivary gland chromosomes of *Anopheles nigerrimus. Parassitologia* **13**:429–434.

Service, M. W., 1970 Identification of the *Anopheles gambiae* complex in Nigeria by larval and adult chromosomes. *Ann. Trop. Med. Parasitol.* **64**:131–136.

Service, M. W. and G. Davidson, 1964 A high incidence of dieldrin-resistance in *Anopheles gambiae* Giles from a unsprayed area in northern Nigeria. *Nature (Lond.)* **203**:209–210.

Sharma, G. P., R. Parshad, S. L. Narang and J. B. Kitzmiller, 1969 The salivary chromosomes of *Anopheles stephensi stephensi. J. Med. Entomol.* **6**:68–71.

Shidrawi, G. R., 1972 The distribution and seasonal prevalence of members of the *Anopheles gambiae* species complex (species A and B) in Garki district, northern Nigeria. WHO/MAL/72.776.

Smithson, T. W. and G. A. H. McClelland, 1972 Salivary gland chromosome map of *Anopheles pseudopunctipennis franciscanus. Mosq. News* **32**:80–87.

Stone, A., K. L. Knight and H. Starcke, 1959 *A Synoptic Catalogue of the Mosquitoes of the World (Diptera: Culicidae)*, Thomas Say Foundation, Vol. 6, Entomol. Society of America Washington, D.C.

Weidhaas, D. E., C. H. Schmidt and E. L. Seabrook, 1962 Field studies on the release of sterile males for the control of *Anopheles quadrimaculatus. Mosq. News* **22**:283–291.

White, G. B., 1971 Chromosomal evidence for natural interspecific hybridization by mosquitoes of the *Anopheles gambiae* complex. *Nature (Lond.)* **231**:184–185.

White, G. B., S. A. Magayuka and P. F. L. Boreham, 1972 Comparative studies on sibling species of the *Anopheles gambiae* Giles complex (Dipt., Culicidae): Bionomics and vectorial activity of species A and species B at Segera, Tanzania. *Bull. Entomol. Res.* **62**:295–317.

Zulueta, J. de, 1964 Ethological changes in malaria vectors. A review of the situation in the light of recent findings. *Riv. Malariol.* **43**:29–36.

13

Aedes

KARAMJIT S. RAI AND W. KEITH HARTBERG

Introduction

Because of their biological and medical importance, more work has been done with mosquitoes than with any other family of invertebrates. Nevertheless, until about 15 years ago, the emphasis of this work had been on systematics, bionomics, physiology, and public health importance of various species. Consequently, several important areas, particularly those dealing with genetic aspects, lagged behind. However, the last 15 years have seen a remarkable expansion of research in mosquito genetics.

Among mosquitoes, the genus *Aedes* constitutes one of the most important genera. It is a large genus containing over 700 species (Stone *et al.*, 1959; Stone, 1961, 1963, 1967, 1970), several species of which transmit important human diseases. Most pest mosquitoes in the United States are of this genus. In California, *Aedes nigromaculis* is resistant to all conventional insecticides. In the midwest, *A. triseriatus* is the principal vector of California encephalitis virus. *A. vexans* and *A. stimulans* are among the commonest pest species. *A. aegypti* is still rampant in southeast United States in spite of the 65-million-dollar campaign of the U. S. Public Health Service to eradicate it during 1964–1969. It has re-invaded several countries which had previously claimed to have eradicated it. These include Brazil, El Salvador, Honduras, Mexico, and Panama. In

KARAMJIT S. RAI—Department of Biology, University of Notre Dame, Notre Dame, Indiana. W. KEITH HARTBERG—Institute of Arthropodology and Parasitology, Department of Biology, Georgia Southern College, Statesboro, Georgia.

several parts of the world, this species transmits several arbovirus diseases, e.g., yellow fever, hemorrhagic fever, and dengue, and is unquestionably one of the most important vectors of human disease. Dengue fever swept several islands in the Caribbean from 1963 through 1966 and continues to be an important public health problem in Asia. Hemorrhagic fever, which appeared for the first time in 1956, is an even more serious problem in southeast Asia. This disease has a significant mortality rate, and its outbreaks have occured in India, Thailand, Burma, Malaysia, Singapore, Laos, Vietnam, and the Philippines (Rudnick, 1967).

A. aegypti is well suited for basic studies on genetics and cytogenetics and for the development and application of genetic methodology for population control. It has a low chromosome number, is easily maintained and manipulated in the laboratory, has a rich source of genetic variability, and has global distribution. As a result of all these attributes, among mosquitoes, the most extensive amount of genetical work has been done with *A. aegypti*. Consequently, today we know far more about its genetic biology than about any other mosquito species. Accordingly, the emphasis of this paper will be on *A. aegypti,* although work with other species of *Aedes* will be mentioned.

It should be emphasized that this paper is not intended as an extensive review on the subject. Rather, as desired by the editor, it is a compendium listing and briefly describing the thrust of the work on genetics, cytogenetics, and genetic control of *Aedes* mosquitoes.

Formal Genetics

Prior to the publication of the monograph on *Mosquito Genetics and Cytogenetics* by Kitzmiller (1953), the study of the genetics of mosquitoes had been essentially nonexistent, or haphazard at best. The publication of this monograph, along with the discovery of the development of insecticide resistance in mosquitoes during the late 1940's and early 1950's, provided the impetus needed to focus the attention of entomologists on the research possibilities and need for genetic studies with mosquitoes. Since Kitzmiller's monograph, several major reviews of the field of mosquito genetics have been published which deal wholly or in part with *Aedes* mosquitoes. These include Rozeboom and Kitzmiller (1958), Mattingly (1957, 1958), McClelland (1962, 1967), Davidson and Mason (1963), and Craig and Hickey (1967).

In general, the methods used for the isolation of mutants and genetic research with *Aedes* mosquitoes have followed those given by Craig and VandeHey (1962). An essential reference for anyone contemplating working with mosquitoes is Gerberg (1970), with its exhaustive list of references on rearing and techniques. Mutant nomenclature and designation in *Aedes* mosquitoes has generally followed the practices which have been used by *Drosophila* workers.

Morphological Mutants

Most of the genetic research with *A. aegypti* and other *Aedes* mosquitoes to date has dealt with the isolation and characterization of morphological mutants. The morphological mutants comprise the basic tools needed for genetic analysis and are the easiest characters to isolate and study. In the most recent review of the genetics of *A. aegypti*, Craig and Hickey (1967) compiled a list of 87 mutants in three linkage groups (1 sex-linked, 2 autosomal) known to occur in this species. Of these, 81 are morphological (51 affect structure and 30 affect color). Of the remaining 6 they list, 2 affect insecticide resistance, 3 affect vectorial capacity, and 1 distorts the sex ratio. If one were to take into consideration the papers published since 1967 dealing with individual mutants and also the unpublished data, the actual count of known mutants in *A. aegypti* probably stands at over 100. Considering problems of reduced penetrance, expressivity, and viability, which make many mutants difficult to work with and maintain, only about half of the mutants are useful genetic markers. Craig and Hickey (1967) should be consulted for the symbols, names, linkage, and description of most mutants in *A. aegypti*, as well as for the extensive bibliography they present. In addition, the following references present more detailed information on some of the mutants as well as information on morphological mutants not presented in Craig and Hickey (1967): McClelland (1966), Bhalla and Craig (1967), Bhalla (1968*a*), Dunn and Craig (1968), Roberts (1973), Hartberg (1975), and Petersen *et al.* (1974).

A. mascarensis is probably the closest relative of *A. aegypti*. Since those variations seen in *A. mascarensis* involve characteristics shared by typical *A. aegypti*, *A. mascarensis* may be a relict of the ancestral population from which *A. aegypti* evolved (McClelland, 1967; Hartberg and McClelland, 1973). To date, 11 morphological variants have been described in *A. mascarensis* in which linkage and/or the mode of inheritance has been determined (McClelland, 1962; Hartberg and Craig, 1973, 1974; Hartberg and McClelland, 1973). In addition, Hartberg and McClelland (1973) suggest that the genetic basis for variation in several morphological traits in field populations of *A. mascarensis* is monofactorial. The variability in *A. mascarensis* is extensive and provides much raw material for genetic analysis.

A. aegypti and *A. mascarensis* can be easily hybridized and fertile off-spring produced (McClelland and Mamet, 1962), thus making it possible to transfer genetic material between the two species. Craig and Hickey (1967) have already transferred one *A. mascarensis* character (silver), to the genetic background of *A. aegypti,* and it has been used as a marker in studies of field populations of *A. aegypti* (Fay and Craig, 1969; Bond *et al.,* 1970). Other characters of *A. mascarensis* could be used in a similar way.

Another *Aedes* mosquito in which several morphological mutants have been isolated is *A. albopictus.* Bat-Miriam and Craig (1966) reported 8 mutants in *A. albopictus,* 7 of which are morphological. In their study a number of other structural abnormalities were observed, but no information was collected on the heritability of the abnormalities. A more extensive analysis of one of the mutants, proboscipedia, is presented by Quinn and Craig (1971). As in *A. aegypti* and *A. mascarensis,* the raw material for genetic analysis is abundant in *A. albopictus.*

Many phenotypic variants have been described in other species of *Aedes,* but no genetic studies have been undertaken to analyze the genetic basis of the variants. It would seem that genetic studies of other species of *Aedes* should be pursued to lay the foundation for the development of a comparative genetics for aedine mosquitoes.

In those closely related species in which fertile hybrids, F$_2$'s, and backcross progeny are produced, it is possible to determine the genetic basis for the differences between them. A few studies of this nature have been undertaken. McClelland (1962) established the mode of inheritance and/or linkage of some of the factors determining morphological dif-ferences between *A. aegypti* and *A. mascarensis.* The genetic basis of the differences in the male genitalia of these two species has been determined by Hartberg and Craig (1973). In all characters studied the differences were controlled by single genes.

Using forced mating, McClelland (1962) was able to cross *A. simpsoni* and *A. woodi* and to obtain fertile hybrids. In the F$_2$ generation and in backcrosses to *A. woodi,* he noted in some progeny that characters of *A. woodi* assorted independently. These findings suggested monofac-torial control. Hartberg (1972) analyzed F$_1$, F$_2$, and backcross progeny obtained from forced matings between *A. simpsoni* and *A. woodi* and pos-tulated from his findings that single factors form the genetic basis of some of the differences between the two species. His findings suggest that (1) the shape of the anterolateral spots on the mesonotum is controlled by a single, semidominant factor, with the *A. simpsoni* character being semi-dominant over the *A. woodi* character, and (2) the phenotype of the submedian lines on the mesonotum is controlled by a single factor, with the *A. woodi* condition dominant. His observations also strongly suggest that the scaling on the lateral lobes of the scutellum is controlled by a single factor, with the *A. woodi* dark-lobed character recessive to the silver-scaled lobes of *A. simpsoni*.

In backcross and F$_2$ progeny obtained from forced matings between *A. hendersoni* and *A. triseriatus,* Truman and Craig (1968) found that several characters, which are used for specific separation of the larvae of these two species, behaved as if they were controlled by single genes. The characters segregated in simple Mendelian ratios.

These types of studies should be pursued as they will contribute to an understanding of the comparative genetics of *Aedes* mosquitoes, as well as to a better understanding of evolution in the genus.

Miscellaneous Genetic Studies

O'Meara and Craig (1969) analyzed the mode of inheritance of auto-geny in several strains of *A. atropalpus* and concluded that autogeny in this mosquito is controlled by a single, dominant, autosomal gene. The expression of autogenous reproduction in *A. atropalpus* has been shown to be influenced by the interaction of both dietary and genetic factors (O'Meara and Krasnick, 1970). Autogeny in *A. detritus* also appears to be controlled by a single, dominant, autosomal gene (Rioux *et al.,* 1973). Thomas and Leng (1972) concluded that autogeny in *A. togoi* is controlled by a polygenic mechanism. Other genetic studies have shown that the regulation of fecundity in autogenous strains of *A. atropalpus* is under polygenic control (O'Meara, 1972), and that the genetic basis of resistance to desiccation in *A. aegypti* and *A. atropalpus* is multifactorial (Machado-Allison and Craig, 1972).

The genetic analysis of behavior in *Aedes* mosquitoes has not received the attention it warrants. There is ample evidence of intraspecific variation in behavior patterns, and investigations into the genetic basis of these would be profitable. Anyone interested in the genetics of behavior in *Aedes* mosquitoes should consult Craig and Hickey (1967) and Mattingly (1967) for key references and background information.

Some of the more recent investigations in the genetics of behavior in *Aedes* are those of Schoenig (1967, 1968, 1969) and Gwadz (1970). Schoenig (1968) presents evidence that oviposition on a solid surface (paper) in *A. aegypti* is largely controlled by a single, sex-linked gene with incomplete dominance. Spontaneous movement of both adult and larval *A. aegypti* appears to be controlled by a semidominant, autosomal gene which is influenced by other genes (Schoenig, 1967, 1969).

Gwadz (1970) analyzed hybrids and backcrosses between an autogenous strain of *A. atropalpus* which showed an early onset of sexual receptivity and an anautogenous strain with a prolonged refractory period to sexual receptivity. His data indicated that early sexual receptivity is under the control of a single, autosomal, semidominant gene.

Biochemical Mutants

The first gene–enzyme system to be described in *A. aegypti* was for an esterase (Trebatoski and Craig, 1969). Trebatoski and Craig obtained results which indicated that one esterase, which existed in two forms distinguishable by starch gel electrophoresis, was controlled by a single pair of codominant alleles at a single gene locus ($Est-6^a$, $Est-6^b$) on linkage group 2. Their data also suggested that a third codominant allele, $Est-6^c$, was also present, but the data were not sufficient for a conclusive statement. Townson (1972) separated esterases of individual *A. aegypti* by electrophoresis on polyacrilamide gels. He found mosquitoes which differed in the mobility of the most intensely staining band, and was able to distinguish four phenotypes based on band mobility: F (fast), S (slow), FS (both bands), and a null phenotype with neither band. On the basis of single-pair matings, Townson postulates that the F and S forms of the enzyme are controlled by two codominant alleles, $Est-\alpha^f$ and $Est-\alpha^s$, with a third allele, $Est-\alpha^x$, producing the null phenotype when homozygous. No linkage data were obtained. The relationship between the esterase phenotypes reported by Townson (1972) and those described by Trebatoski and Craig (1969) remains to be established.

Bullini *et al.* (1970a,b) have described another gene–enzyme system in *A. aegypti,* that for phosphoglucomutase (PGM), using electrophoretic techniques. It has been demonstrated that at least four codominant alleles of an autosomal *Pgm* gene exist in *A. aegypti* (Bullini *et al.,* 1972), and linkage studies have placed *Pgm* on linkage group 2. Coluzzi *et al.* (1971) examined natural populations of *A. zammitii* and *A. mariae*. Each population showed nonpolymorphic double-band PGM patterns, and the populations were easily separated by comparing their PGM electrophoretic patterns. Their data suggest that the PGM patterns in the *A. mariae* and *A. zammitii* populations are the phenotypic expression of a single locus. They have assumed two codominant alleles, Pgm^A and Pgm^B, with the *A. zammitii* and *A. mariae* populations being homozygous

Pgm^A/Pgm^A and Pgm^B/Pgm^B, respectively, while the F_1 hybrids represent the heterozygotes Pgm^A/Pgm^B. In another study, Bullini and Coluzzi (1972) studied populations of *A. aegypti* and *A. mariae* of different geographic origin for the distribution of PGM alleles. They reported 5 different alleles in both *A. aegypti* and *A. mariae* and showed that certain of the alleles are more frequent than others. Their findings suggest that protein polymorphism is most probably caused by some form of balancing selection.

The study by Coluzzi and Bullini (1971) of reproductive isolation of *A. mariae* and *A. zammitii* clearly shows the value of enzyme variants in the study of precopulatory isolating mechanisms. The excellent review of electrophoretic studies of gene–enzyme systems in mosquitoes by Bullini and Coluzzi (1974) gives a thorough review of the literature and greater detail than is possible in this paper and should be consulted by anyone interested in biochemical mutants in mosquitoes. In addition, they clearly point out the possible utilization of electrophoretic data in taxonomic studies and the use of electrophoretic variants as biochemical markers to study such areas as genetic maps, identification of cryptic species, reproductive isolation, competitiveness, reproductive biology, etc.

Patterns of fluorescent compounds from heads of normal and eye-color mutants of *A. aegypti* and *A. mascarensis* were determined by Bhalla (1968*b*) by means of paper chromatography. He was able to demonstrate qualitative and quantitative differences among various mutants within a species as well as among phenotypically similar mutants of the two species.

Vectorial Capacity

Most, if not all, genetic studies dealing with vectorial capacity of *Aedes* mosquitoes have been limited to *A. aegypti*. Roubaud (1937) demonstrated variability in the susceptibility of different strains of *A. aegypti* to *Dirofilaria immitis,* and suggested that susceptibility was an inherited character. Similar experiments were made by Kartman (1953), who was successful in selecting more susceptible and more refractory stocks from his original colony. Zielke (1973) has shown by a series of crosses and backcrosses that susceptibility of *A. aegypti* to *D. immitis* is controlled by a sex-linked, recessive gene. In addition, Zielke (1973) found that the genes determining the susceptibility of *A. aegypti* to infection of *D. immitis* and *Brugia pahangi* are located on the same chromosome but at different loci.

Macdonald (1962) concluded that a sex-linked, recessive gene, which he labeled f^m, controlled the susceptibility of *A. aegypti* to subperiodic *B. malayi.* Later studies (Macdonald, 1963*a,b*; Macdonald and Sheppard, 1965) showed that f^m does not exhibit complete penetrance, has variable expressivity, and is located 3–4 crossover units from the sex locus. The influence of the gene f^m on the susceptibility of *A. aegypti* to seven strains of *Brugia, Wuchereria,* and *Dirofilaria* was studied by Macdonald and Ramachandran (1965). Their studies showed that the gene f^m controlled development of subperiodic *B. malayi,* periodic *B. malayi, B. pahangi,* periodic *W. bancrofti,* and subperiodic *W. bancrofti*; however, *D. immitis* and *D. repens* were not influenced by the gene.

McGreevy *et al.* (1974) selected stocks of *A. aegypti* that were susceptible and refractory to *D. immitis* infection. By crossing these stocks and determining the susceptibility rate of the F_1 and backcross progeny, they established that susceptibility of *A. aegypti* to *D. immitis* infection is controlled by a sex-linked, recessive gene that they have designated *ft* (filarial susceptibility, Malpighian tubules). Their studies indicated that the variation in development of *D. immitis* in the hybrids between different *A. aegypti* stocks probably resulted from the influence of the different genetic backgrounds on the expression of the *ft* allele. The study by McGreevy *et al.* (1974) also shows that the genes *ft* and *fm* (Macdonald, 1962) are distinct. Their findings are similar to those reported by Zielke (1973). The gene reported by Zielke (1973) and the one reported by McGreevy *et al.* (1974) also shows that the genes *ft* and f^m (Macdonald, donald and Ramachandran, 1965; Coluzzi and Gironi, 1971; Zielke, 1973; McGreevy *et al.,* 1974) indicate that the susceptibility of mosquitoes to different filaria is often controlled by different genes.

Trager (1942) was able to increase the level of susceptibility of *A. aegypti* to *Plasmodium lophurae,* a malaria of ducks, through selection for six generations. His studies indicated that the susceptibility was an inherited character, but no conclusions could be drawn about the mode of inheritance of the trait. The genetic aspects of the susceptibility of *A. aegypti* to the chicken malaria, *P. gallinaceum,* were investigated by Ward (1963). He concluded that a single pair of genes or a block of closely linked genes with incomplete dominance was responsible. To explain his results, Ward proposed a model where $S_1 S_1$ gave refractory mosquitoes and $S_1 S_2$ or $S_2 S_2$ were susceptible. His studies gave no linkage information for his proposed gene.

In a study undertaken to establish more complete information on the genetic aspects of susceptibility of *A. aegypti* to *P. gallinacium,* Kilama and Craig (1969) discovered a new genetic factor entirely different from that reported by Ward (1963). Their observations established that the refractory condition is controlled by a simple, autosomal (linkage group 2), recessive factor, designated *pls* (plasmodium susceptibility). Female *A. aegypti* that are homozygous for *pls* cannot develop oocysts of *P. gallinaceum*.

Kilama (1973) undertook a study to determine the distribution of the gene *pls* in populations of *A. aegypti*. He did not find the gene in strains from Asia or the Americas; however, it was present in all 8 strains tested from Africa. The frequency of the *pls* trait in different populations might account for the absence of *P. gallinaceum* in some localities (Kilama and Craig, 1969).

To date, no studies have demonstrated that susceptibility of *Aedes* to viruses is under genetic control. It would be reasonable to assume that genetic factors do play a role in the transmission of arboviruses. Research in this area should prove fruitful.

The fine review article by Macdonald (1967) on the influence of genetic and other factors on vector susceptibility to parasites is an excellent starting point for anyone interested in vectorial capacity of invertebrates.

Genetics of Insecticide Resistance

Coker (1958) and Qutubuddin (1958) provided the initial evidence that established monofactorial inheritance for DDT resistance in *A. aegypti* larvae. Linkage studies have shown that this gene is inherited as an incompletely dominant gene (designated DDT or R^{DDT}) on linkage group 2 (Brown and Abedi, 1962; Klassen and Brown, 1964; Wood, 1967). Other genetic factors can influence this gene (Wood, 1965, 1970). The results obtained by Wood (1967) confirmed that a gene, R^{DDT1}, on linkage group 2 has the major influence on DDT resistance in *A. aegypti* larvae. However, his findings indicate that a different gene, R^{DDT2}, on linkage group 3, controls adult DDT resistance. This conclusion conflicts with other studies which found DDT resistance in both larvae and adults to be associated solely with linkage group 2 (Brown and Abedi, 1962; Klassen and Brown, 1964; Coker, 1966). Pillai and Brown (1965) found that when DDT resistance resulted from selection with the DDT substitute WARF, linkage groups 2 and 3 contributed to DDT resistance. There are no ready explanations for the disparity between the studies.

Larval resistance apparently involves an increase in dehydrochlorination of DDT to harmless DDE by the enzyme DDT-dehydrochlorinase (Chattoraj and Brown, 1960; Abedi *et al.*, 1963; Kimura and Brown,

1964). The basis of adult resistance is not known, but behavorial factors may be involved (Brown and Pal, 1971).

Dieldrin resistance in *A. aegypti* has been shown to be controlled by a single gene on linkage group 2 (Khan and Brown, 1961). Klassen and Brown (1964) showed that *Dl* (dieldrin resistance) is distinct from the gene determining DDT resistance, but closely linked to it. Lockhart *et al.* (1970) should be consulted for the most recent linkage data for *Dl* and *DDT*. *Dl* is an excellent marker gene, in contrast to *DDT*. There is evidence that modifier genes may enhance dieldrin resistance in *A. aegypti*.

Factors affecting malathion resistance have been located on linkage groups 2 and 3 (Pillai and Brown, 1965).

Hazard *et al.* (1964) reported the development of tolerance to apholate (a chemosterilant) in *A. aegypti*. A tolerance to metepa, another chemosterilant, was reported by Klassen and Matsumura (1966). The results of genetic crosses undertaken by Seawright (1972) indicated that apholate resistance in *A. aegypti* was a quantitative trait with a marked paternal influence on the resistance of F_2 and backcross progeny.

For an in-depth review of insecticide resistance and the genetics of resistance the reader should consult Klassen (1966) and Brown and Pal (1971).

Evolutionary Genetics

A considerable amount of information has been collected concerning speciation and evolution in *Aedes* mosquitoes, especially in the subgenus *Stegomyia*. A review of evolutionary genetics is beyond the scope of this paper. Anyone interested in this topic should consult the excellent review *Speciation and Evolution in Aedes* by McClelland (1967).

The mechanisms which reproductively isolate one species from another are among the most important attributes of a species, since they are by definition the species criteria. Several recent studies have dealt with reproductive isolation in aedine mosquitoes. Leahy and Craig (1967) demonstrated at least five reproductive barriers between *A. aegypti* and *A. albopictus*. Hybrid breakdown was demonstrated in crosses involving *A. hendersoni* and *A. triseriatus* (Truman and Craig, 1968).

Hartberg and Craig (1968) demonstrated sexual isolation between *A. aegypti* and *A. mascarensis*. They also found differential mating preference between *A. aegypti formosus* and *A. a. aegypti*. Hybrid breakdown was demonstrated between *A. aegypti* and *A. mascarensis* (Hartberg and Craig, 1970). The hybrid breakdown only appeared when the genetic contribution of *A. aegypti* was above 50 percent and the male-determining chromosome of *A. mascarensis* was present. Two hypothetical genetic mechanisms controlling the observed hybrid breakdown were suggested.

McClelland (1962) presents data which indicates that hybrid breakdown is one of the isolating barriers between *A. woodi* and *A. simpsoni*. In a later study, Hartberg (1972) indicates that other isolating mechanisms separating these two species include behavior, mechanical isolation, and gametic isolation.

Gubler (1970) suggests that both precopulatory and postcopulatory barriers exists between *A. polynesiensis* and *A. albopictus*. Some genetic divergence and reproductive barriers have been shown to exist between strains of *A. polynesiensis* (Tesfa-Yohannes, 1973).

Nijhout and Craig (1971) have shown that the recognition of females by the males of several species of *Aedes* is independent of flight sound or ultrasonic frequencies. Their findings suggest that recognition is effected by contact chemoreception, and that the receptors for the recognition stimulus are contained in the tarsi of the males.

Cytogenetics

Somatic Cytology

The morphology of somatic chromosomes from brain tissues of young fourth-instar larvae in eleven species of *Aedes* has been studied by Rai (1963a, 1966): *A. (Stegomyia) aegypti* Linn., *A. (Stegomyia) albopictus* Skuse, *A. (Stegomyia) mascarensis* MacGregor, *A. (Stegomyia) polynesiensis* Marks, *A. (Stegomyia) simpsoni* Theobald, *A. (Stegomyia) vittatus* Bigot, *A. (Ochlerotatus) sierrensis* Ludlow, *A. (Ochlerotatus) stimulans* Walker, *A. (Finlaya) togoi* Theobald, *A. (Finlaya) atropalpus* Coquillett, and *A. (Aedimorphus) vexans* Meigen. The somatic cytology of some of these same and a few other species of *Aedes* has also been undertaken by Breland (1960), Akstein (1962), Mukherjee *et al.* (1966), Baker and Aslamkhan (1969), and others.

The diploid chromosome number of all species examined is six, and the chromosome complement consists of three homomorphic pairs. These were designated I, II, III in the order of increasing size (Rai, 1963a). Furthermore, they can be often distinguished by the position of the centromeres and the secondary constriction. Intimate somatic pairing of homologous chromosomes occurs in all species.

In *A. aegypti,* one of the chromosome pairs is small and the other two pairs are relatively large. The smallest and the largest pairs are metacentric. The other large pair, which is intermediate in length, is submetacentric, usually with a 4 : 3 arm length ratio. Among the other *Aedes,* the chromosomes of *A. atropalpus* closely resemble those of *A. aegypti.* However, each resting nucleus of *A. atropalpus* shows two conspicuous Feulgen-positive particles at opposite poles. The other species of *Aedes* cannot yet be separated on cytological criteria. All of these possess three pairs of metacentric chromosomes, with two large and one somewhat smaller pair.

On the whole, this work and work done by several other workers with *Culex* and *Anopheles* has disclosed considerable uniformity of karyotypes in aedine mosquitoes and a remarkable variability of these in anophelines. On the basis of this work Rai (1966) proposed that the mechanism of speciation may be different in different genera of mosquitoes and that some of them (e.g., *Anopheles*) may have undergone much more chromosomal repatterning than such genera as *Aedes.* The latter may have depended more on point or genic mutations. There is some genetic corroboration of this idea; many mutants are known in *A. aegypti,* and relatively few in *Anopheles* or *Culex.* Whereas VandeHey (1964) and colleagues have demonstrated a range of 0.7–2.8 mutants per mosquito in different populations of *A. aegypti,* the comparable figures for Culex is 0.2 (VandeHey, private communication), and it may probably be even lower for *Anopheles.*

Furthermore, the work on somatic karyotypes has demonstrated that gross changes in whole chromosomes or chromosome complements have not played any part in mosquito speciation.

Chromosome multiplication, causing extensive polyploidy, followed by several divisions in the absence of chromosomal replication, and resulting in the so-called somatic reduction, has been reported in the larval epidermis of *A. aegypti* (Risler, 1959).

Cell Cultures

In view of the importance of the use of *in vitro* cell cultures as a tool to probe various facets of the genetics, pathogenicity, and physiology of refractoriness and susceptibility of mosquitoes to transmit filarial infections and arboviruses, considerable work has been done on the establishment of mosquito cell lines. Out of approximately 20 such lines, 10 lines (Table I) are in existence in *Aedes* (Singh, 1967 and Schneider, 1972).

The procedure for establishing mosquito cell lines is largely standarized. Most of these lines were originally derived from minced,

TABLE 1. *Cell Lines in Aedes*

Species	Number of Lines
A. aegypti	5–6
A. albopictus	1
A. taeniorhynchus	1
A. vittatus	1
A. w. albus	1

trypsinized, neonate larvae. Although the genetic basis of susceptibility of *A. aegypti* to several filarial infections has been demonstrated (Macdonald and Ramachandran, 1965), the underlying physiological mechanisms remain almost completely unexplored. The field of *in vitro* studies has developed to the point that a fruitful comparision could be made of the ability of cells derived from known susceptible and refractory strains of mosquitoes to promote the development of arthropod stages of filariae *in vitro*. It could well be that refractoriness (inability of the parasite to complete development in the mosquito host) may be a consequence of some nutritional deficiency. The available cell lines could prove invaluable in such studies.

In addition, using radioautography in a cell line of *A. albopictus*, Bianchi *et al.* (1972) have studied chromosome replication and correlated late-replicating regions during the S period on various chromosomes with constitutive heterochromatin. However, in chromosome pairs 2 and 3, distal, late-replicating regions were not associated with the presence of constitutive heterochromatin. According to the authors, these areas possibly correspond to the location of facultative heterochromatin in the genome.

More recently, interphylum, somatic-cell hybridization of an *A. aegypti* and human (HeLa) cell line has been accomplished by using ultraviolet-inactivated Sendai virus to induce fusion (Zepp *et al.*, 1971). Chromosomes characteristic of both the mosquito and human cell lines were observed in the hybrid.

Effect of Radiation on Division Cycle

Cytogenetic effects of different doses of x rays in *A. aegypti* have been studied (Rai, 1963*b*). Early fourth-instar larvae were irradiated with doses ranging from 500 r to 4000 r and were fixed 0–72 hours after irradiation. Mitotic chromosomes were studied from squash preparations of larval brains. Mitotic activity was measured in terms of the total number of dividing cells per brain.

In unirradiated controls, the average number of dividing cells per fourth-instar larval brain was 113, 125, 159, 161, 148, 139, and 79 at 0, 1.5, 6, 12, 18, 36 and 72 hours, respectively, following irradiation (Rai, 1963b). In irradiated larvae, initially, x-irradiation inhibited cell division. Mitotic activity was almost completely suppressed 1.5 hours after irradiation. The duration of the arrested mitotic activity depended on the dose. This inhibition of mitotic activity may be due to either an x-ray-induced delay in the onset of mitosis and/or a reversion of some of the dividing nuclei, especially those at early prophase at the time of irradiation, to a nondividing interphase state following irradiation. After a time (depending on the dose used), this effect was replaced by a great increase in mitotic activity. Twelve hours after irradiation, the larvae exposed to 500 r and 1000 r, for example, showed about twice as many mitotically dividing cells as did the unirradiated controls. The increase in mitotic activity at higher doses was less extreme and took longer to occur.

The increased mitotic activity following irradiation may ensue from a simultaneous release from an inhibition of a population of cells which accumulated in prophase. At doses of 500 r and 1000 r, the increase above the normal mitotic activity after recovery appeared to compensate for the initial fall below normal.

Among the chromosomal aberrations noted were deletions, inversions, exchanges, rings, dicentrics, and anaphase bridges.

F_1 hybrids of crosses between certain strains of *A. aegypti* showed marked resistance to radiation damage (Asman and Rai, 1967). Furthermore, these hybrids showed a higher rate of mitosis when compared with the parental stocks. It is likely that because of this higher rate of cell division, repair of radiation damage was more readily effected in the hybrids.

Meiotic Cytology and Spermatogenesis

In a preliminary report, Akstein (1962) provided information on some stages of meiosis in *A. aegypti*. Mescher and Rai (1966) followed male meiosis in detail in this species. They have shown that visible leptotene and zygotene stages do not occur during male meiosis in this species. This obviously results from the fact that during the earliest stages of meiosis, the chromosomes retain the intimate pairing of the previous mitotic anaphase and telophase.

Ved Brat and Rai (1973a) analyzed chiasma frequencies in 5 different stocks of *A. aegypti* with diverse genetic backgrounds (2 multiple-marker stocks, 2 wild-type strains collected from the field, and 1 hybrid strain obtained by crossing a wild-type and a mutant stock). Abnormalities such as asynapsis and chromosome breakage presumably arising from inbreeding depression were observed in two mutant stocks. The chiasmata frequencies varied from 3.0 to 5.2 chiasmata per cell in different individuals in different stocks. Within different individuals, the chiasmata distribution was random between both the arms of different bivalents, though most chiasmata were distal in position at metaphase I. Statistical analysis of distributions of chiasmata in the two arms of a bivalent in various stocks was undertaken and the data were interpreted to indicate lack of interference in chiasma formation across the centromere, contrary to the conclusions of Callan and Montallenti (1947) in *Culex pipiens*. More than two chiasmata per bivalent were relatively rare, though observed.

Jost (1971) studied some aspects of meiosis in *A. albopictus,* and Smith and Hartberg (1974) presented a more detailed study of meiosis in this species. Bhalla (1971) provided some details about meiosis in diploid and tetraploid forms of *A. aegypti.*

Chromosome Ultrastructure

Roth (1966) provided details on the ultrastructure of the synaptonemal complex in the meiotic prophase in the oocytes of *A. aegypti* and proposed a general model of a prophase I bivalent based on this structure. He has shown that the synaptonemal complex appears during zygonema in the oocytes, is present throughout pachynema, and disappears from the paired homologs at diplonema. Its role in genetic recombination seems well established. Roth (1966) observed that following a blood meal, numerous polycomplexes appear in the post-pachytene oocyte nuclei in *A. aegypti.* There has been considerable debate concerning the origin and function of these polycomplexes (Wolfe, 1972). Roth regarded these as stacks of discarded medial complexes without any function. Based on electron microscopy of serial sections of complete nuclei in oocytes at all developmental stages from early meiotic prophase till egg laying, and on the large quantity of polycomplexes present, Fiil and Moens (1973), on the other hand, proposed that these polycomplexes serve a specific function. They have suggested that a relationship exists, "by origin or by specialization, between the synaptic structures and nuclear envelope."

Polytene Chromosomes

Because of a number of technical difficulties, it has not been possible so far to map polytene chromosomes (Mescher, 1963). These chromosomes are present in salivary glands, certain cells of the alimentary canal, anal papillae of larvae, and Malpighian tubules of larvae and adult females (Gillham, 1957). Even a considerable refinement in techniques, e.g., rearing the larvae at low densities, at a temperature range of 18–28°C, and the addition of small amounts of brewer's yeast and ribonucleic acid, did not materially improve the quality of polytene chromosome preparations (Mescher, 1963). Possibly, because of the large size of the polytene chromosomes (as compared with other diptera), the ends and other parts of chromosomes become entangled with each other and do not spread properly. However, certain strains give much better preparations than others. Additional research on proper pretreatments and fixation procedures is very much needed in order to bypass the above-mentioned difficulties in *A. aegypti* and other aedine species.

Chromosomal Rearrangements

Chromosomal rearrangements have been studied extensively in several insect species. In *D. melanogaster* such work provided the foundations of classical cytogenetics. During the last approximately 10 years, there has been a great deal of interest in such studies with insect vectors of disease and for the application of the knowledge thus gained for genetic control purposes. Among insect vectors, extensive studies have been undertaken on various aspects of the following types of chromosomal rearrangements in *A. aegypti.*

Translocations: Isolation, Identification, and Characterization. In our laboratory at the University of Notre Dame, detailed cytogenetic studies on 75 radiation-induced chromosomal translocations have been completed. Thirty of these translocations were isolated from a wild-type laboratory stock, *ROCK* (Rai et al., 1970; Rai and McDonald, 1972), and 45 were from a freshly collected field stock from Delhi, India (Hallinan, Lorimer, and Rai, unpublished). Another approximately 80 translocations in field stocks from Mombasa, Kenya have been induced and studied by Dr. P. T. McDonald at the Mosquito Biology Unit of the University of Notre Dame and International Centre of Insect Physiology and Ecology in Mombasa (P. T. McDonald, unpublished).

All translocations were isolated following irradiation of young, wild-type males which were crossed with multiple-marker stocks in which each chromosome was marked. F_1's thus obtained were backcrossed with the multiple-marker stock, and cultures showing pseudolinkage were identified and characterized.

The chromosomes involved in all these translocations have been identified, and the radiation-induced breakpoints on each linkage group mapped. Further, all translocations have been characterized with regard to fertility, and some for fecundity, longevity, competitive mating ability, and transmission of the translocation complex to progeny. A detailed analysis of the recombination data in the case of 45 translocations studied from the Delhi stock indicated that the distribution of the radiation-induced breaks on chromosome 3 was nonrandom, whereas it was random for chromosomes 1 and 2. In the case of chromosome 3, breakage occured more frequently in the vicinity of the nucleolus organizing region (Hallinan *et al.*, 1975).

Bhalla (1973) has also studied the cytogenetics of seven sex-linked reciprocal translocations in this species.

Translocations: Double-Translocation Heterozygotes. By intercrossing translocations involving different chromosomes, individuals heterozygous for two different translocations have been synthesized. The differential region in the double-translocation heterozygote between the first two translocations studied showed a sevenfold increase in genetic recombination over the control. Also, recombination in this region was associated with the origin of a "new" chromosome carrying pieces of all three chromosomes (McDonald and Rai, 1970*a*).

Translocations: Chromosome–Linkage Group Correlation. A study of the cytology of T(1;2) and T(1;3), the first two translocations obtained, and the double heterozygote between them allowed correlation of the linkage groups with the individual chromosomes (McDonald and Rai, 1970*b*). The shortest chromosome possesses the sex locus and corresponds to linkage group I, the medium length to linkage group III, and the largest chromosome corresponds to linkage group II. Among approximately 2500 species and subspecies, this was the first chromosome–linkage group correlation in any mosquito species. The linkage group–chromosome correlations have been subsequently confirmed through an analysis of several other translocations and inversions.

Using these rearrangements, McDonald and Rai (1970*b*) and Ved Brat and Rai (1973*b*) have established preliminary cytological maps for *A. aegypti.*

As mentioned earlier, Rai (1963*a*) arbitrarily numbered the chromosomes of *A. aegypti* from I to III in increasing order of their length, with chromosome I being the smallest and III being the largest. However, with the demonstration that linkage group 3 corresponds to Rai's (1963*a*) chromosome II (median length) and linkage group 2 corresponds to the longest chromosome or Rai's (1963*a*) chromosome III, McDonald and Rai (1970*b*) proposed that the chromosomes be numbered as shown in Table 2. The advantage of the new system is that the linkage groups and the chromosomes have the same designations.

Translocations: Homozygotes. The advantages of the use of translocation homozygotes for (1) introduction of desirable genes, such as refractoriness to a particular disease, conditional lethals, etc., into pest populations (and thereby bring about population replacement) and (2) for genetic control have been emphasized by Curtis (1968) and Lorimer *et al.* (1972), respectively. Such homozygotes are also useful in obtaining stocks of multiple translocations, in which the genome is progressively rearranged, resulting in much higher sterility (Whitten, 1970). Because of these features, one important objective of our work with translocations in *A. aegypti* has been to investigate the prospects of obtaining homozygotes for each of the heterozygous translocations induced.

The procedure that we follow for this purpose is to (1) cross females and males heterozygous for each translocation and for certain genetic markers, (2) score the proportion of wild-type to mutant progeny (if homozygotes are viable, a 3 : 1 ratio is expected, otherwise it is a 2 : 1 ratio), (3) select wild-type progeny, and (4) progeny test the same by crossing to an appropriate multiple-marker stock. Those individuals which produce only wild-type progeny in these crosses are expected to be translocation homozygotes. Such individuals are then confirmed through additional crosses, cytology, and fertility studies.

Based on the above studies, 2 of the approximately 30 radiation-induced translocations isolated from the wild-type laboratory stock *ROCK* have yielded viable homozygotes—one for a sex-linked, T(1;3)b, one for an autosomal T(2;3)c translocation. Their fertilities are 19 percent, and 55 percent, respectively, when sib-mated and 45 percent and 46 percent,

TABLE 2.   Chromosome Numbering Systems

	Chromosome length		
System	Shortest	Median	Longest
Old system (Rai, 1963*a*)	I	II	III
New system (McDonald and Rai, 1970*b*)	1	3	2

respectively, when outcrossed (Lorimer *et al.*, 1972). Similarly, approximately 40 of the 45 translocations induced in the Delhi stock were tested for translocation homozygosity. Of these, two, T(2;3)12H and T(1;3)6L have yielded viable homozygotes. Their fertilities are 59 percent and 55 percent, respectively, when sibmated and 82 percent and 88 percent, respectively, when outcrossed with Delhi stock (Hallinan *et al.*, 1975).

Inversions. In view of the importance of inversions as genetic tools, particularly to suppress effective recombination in certain chromosomal segments and for the detection of lethal mutations (Rai, 1967), considerable work has been done with these rearrangements in *A. aegypti* during the last few years. Bhalla (1970) and McGivern and Rai (1972) have studied the cytogenetics of three paracentric inversions in *A. aegypti*. These inversions were originally detected through suppression of recombination in certain marked regions of the linkage groups and confirmed by cytological analysis. McGivern and Rai (1972) showed that heterozygosity for an autosomal paracentric inversion, In(2)a, on linkage group 2 markedly increased recombination in the other two linkage groups, indicating an interchromosomal effect of this inversion on recombination. The increase in recombination was not uniform when measured in three regions on linkage group 1 and two regions of linkage group 3. It was markedly less in the region encompassing the centromere than in the distal regions of the chromosomes.

More recently, McGivern and Rai (1974) studied the cytogenetics of a compound chromosomal rearrangement (translocation and inversion) designated T(1;2)1Mc + In(2)b. This rearrangement was originally detected through suppression of recombination between certain markers in linkage group 1 and 2 and through observation of pseudolinkage between markers on these same linkage groups. The genetic data were confirmed by cytological analysis.

Interestingly, crosses involving normal females and males heterozygous for this compound rearrangement produced nearly twice as many females as males. This distorted sex ratio has been attributed to single genetic exchanges in the inverted region and the subsequent elimination of one of the chromatids carrying the male (M) locus through its involvement in a dicentric bridge. This distortion in sex ratio confirms (1) the genic mode of sex determination and (2) the occurence of crossing over at the four-strand stage in *A. aegypti*.

Duplication-Deficiency Heterozygotes. Crossing over in the interstitial segment of a multiple translocation or non-disjunctional segregation of adjacent chromosomes in a translocation heterozygote gives rise to duplication-deficiency gametes (Figure 1). Usually such gametes are inviable. During cytogenetical studies of a multiple translocation, T(1;2;3), which involves interchanges of both arms of chromosome 2 with chromosomes 1 and 3, evidence has been collected suggesting viability of duplication-deficiency heterozygotes carrying a standard chromosome 3 along with translocated chromosomes 1 and 2. The duplication involves part of chromosome 3 (attached to chromosome 2) and deletion for the same amount of chromosome 2. Cytologically, such heterozygotes show the presence of a homomorphic bivalent for chromosome 3 and an interchange complex of four chromosomes with unequal arms following an interstitial chiasmata (Ved Brat and Rai, 1974).

One duplication-deficiency heterozygote (a male pupae) was found to show a very high frequency of chiasmata in the interstitial region of the long arm of the translocated chromosome 2. Furthermore, the frequency of chiasmata in this interstitial region was found to correspond with the frequency of equational segregation of the two unequal chromatids for one of the arms of a pair at anaphase I. Of the 58 primary spermatocytes scored, 53 (91.4 percent) showed the presence of an interstitial chiasmata. An analysis of 74 anaphase I cells in the same pupa showed that 63 (85.1 percent) had unequal chromatids for one arm (anaphase I, Figure 1).

This is the first report of a duplication-deficiency heterozygote studied in a mosquito species.

Aneuploidy–Polyploidy. On rare occasions, trisomic ($2n = 7$) and triploid individuals ($2n = 9$) have been observed and studied. Both these types were detected while studying the cytology of male pupae, and both originated from crosses where one parent was heterozygous for a reciprocal translocation. In the trisomic, the extra chromosome was present either as a univalent or in a trivalent association at metaphase I (Rai, 1968). In the case of the triploid, the chromosomal associations ranged from three trivalents to three bivalents plus three univalents at metaphase I (Rai, unpublished). Bhalla (1971) has also described the meiotic behavior in tetraploid *A. aegypti*.

Chemosterilization

Extensive studies have been conducted concerning the cytogenetic and developmental basis of chemically induced sterility in *A. aegypti*. It has been demonstrated that rearing the larvae in a 15 ppm solution of a commonly used mutagenic, alkylating chemical, apholate, induces drastic chromosomal aberrations in somatically dividing brain cells, (Rai, 1964*a*), sexual sterility (Rai, 1964*b*), and various cellular and histopathological

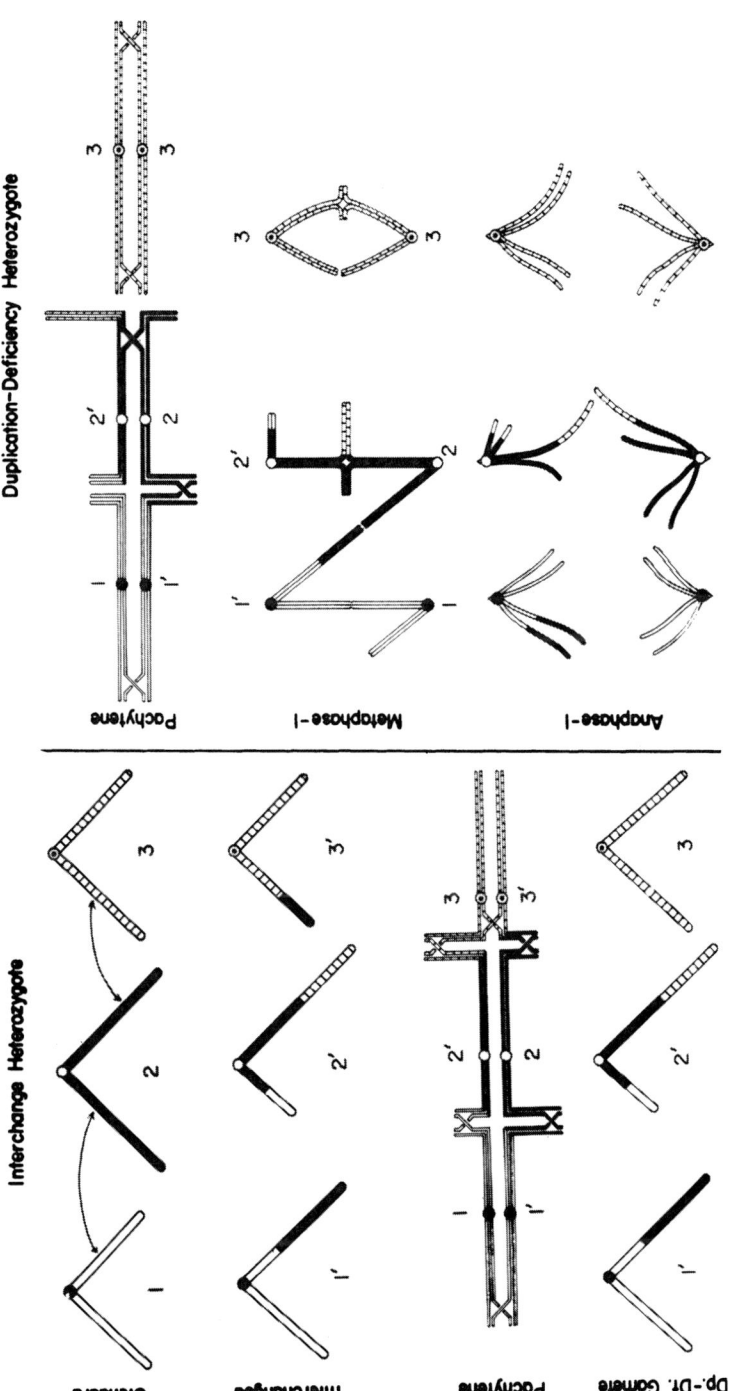

Figure 1. Model explaining the origin of a duplication-deficiency heterozygote owing to the formation of interstial chiasmata in chromosome 3 in the interchange heterozygote. The expected metaphase-I configuration with interstitial chiasma in the long arm of chromosome 2' and the consequent equational segregation at anaphase I in the duplication-deficiency heterozygote are also shown. (From Ved Brat and Rai, 1974.)

abnormalities in nerve fibers and the mid-gut epithelium (Sharma and Rai, 1969). Furthermore, by undertaking ovarian transplants from chemically treated to wild-type abdomens, and *vice versa,* it was shown that chemically induced female infecundity ensues from the effect of apholate on the ovaries themselves rather than through an interference with the production or availability of either neuronal or endocrine secretions (Rai and Sharma, 1971). More recently, Mathew and Rai (1975, unpublished) have investigated chemosterilant-induced ultrastructural changes during oogenesis in *A. aegypti.* Highly condensed (electron-dense) chromatin in pro-nurse cells, oocytes, and follicular epithelial cells; extremely reduced cytoplasm with poor development of polysomes and endoplasmic reticulum; relatively high frequency of autophagic vacuoles with enclosed nuclear material, endoplasmic reticulum, mitochondria and ribosomes; disrupted plasma membranes and nuclear envelopes, and segregation of granular and fibrous components of the nucleolus were observed in chemically treated, poorly developed, and atrophied ovaries. At higher dosages (30 ppm), scanning electron microscopy showed complete absence of ovarioles resulting from total destruction of gonial cells.

Genetic Control

Considerable progress has been made during the last 15 years in developing formal genetics and cytogenetics of *A. aegypti.* Such studies have not only contributed toward making this one of the genetically best-studied species among mosquitoes, but it has also generated many potential mechanisms which could be applied for genetic control of natural populations.

Features Favorable for Genetic Control

Craig (1967) and Rai *et al.* (1974) have reviewed the status of genetic control of *A. aegypti.* Because of several favorable attributes, e.g., the ease of its laboratory culture, a relatively short life cycle, availability of extensive information dealing with its genetic biology, physiology and ecology, and of several potentially useful genetic mechanisms for population manipulation, this species is regarded as a "promising subject for genetic control" (Knipling *et al.,* 1968). In addition, certain features of its ecolgy, such as its breeding often in domestic water containers and its dispersal over relatively small areas, minimizing immigration problems, may make this species particularly suitable for genetic control. Furthermore, preliminary results obtained at the WHO/ICMR* Research Unit on Genetic Control of Mosquitoes in New Delhi, India indicate that the population recovery potential may be relatively low, so that even moderate levels of sterility may be expected to cause significant suppression of adult populations.

Currently Available Mechanisms

Sterile-Male Technique. This technique is based on the induction of sexual sterility in males through the use of radiation or chemical sterilants and on releasing large numbers of such males in natural populations (Knipling, 1959). Morlan *et al.* (1962) field tested this method with *A. aegypti* and released approximately 3,482,850 male pupae sterilized by exposure to 11,000–18,000 r of gamma radiation in two test areas in Pensacola, Florida during 1960–1961. The trials were unsuccessful possibly because the massive doses of radiation used to sterilize pupae reduced their vigor and competitive mating ability. Work in our laboratory has shown that a much smaller dose of 7000 r administered to either pupae or adult males induces almost 100 percent male sterility. More importantly, Hallinan and Rai (1973) have demonstrated that it is possible to avoid the reduced vigor and mating ability and to produce competitive adults if males are irradiated in nitrogen rather than in air. They have shown that male pupae and young adults irradiated to a sterilizing dose of 7000 r or higher in nitrogen were as competitive as normal males in matings with females; whereas males air-irradiated at the same doses were not.

This finding may increase the potential of the sterile male technique for the control of *A. aegypti*. Alternatively, chemosterilized males could be used for sterile-male releases.

Sex-Ratio Distortion. Hickey and Craig (1966) described a genetic factor, distorter, situated at or close to the sex locus on chromosome 1 which distorts sex ratios in favor of males. They suggested that release of such male producing genotype into a natural population could lead to population collapse with time. Such a system could also be used to transport desirable genes into natural populations. As would be mentioned in the next section, another use of this system is in combination with the translocations.

Chromosomal Translocations. In a panel convened by the World Health Organization to discuss "Cytogenetics of Vectors of Disease

* World Health Organization/Indian Council of Medical Research.

of Man " (Anonymous, 1968) Rai (1967) proposed the use of genetic sterility associated with chromosomal translocations for population control of *A. aegypti*. For genetic control, one of the postulated advantages of the use of translocations over the use of sterile males is that following a release of translocations, partial sterility would persist in the wild population for several generations. The extent of this sterility and its persistance would depend upon the number of homozygotes (or heterozygotes) released and most importantly on the fertility, survival, and mating competitiveness of the translocation homozygotes, single heterozygotes, and double heterozygotes of the translocations used.

Computer simulations using the available data with the heterozygous translocations in *A. aegypti* were performed. These indicated the potential role of sex-linked *versus* autosomal translocations for genetic control under various release strategies (McDonald and Rai, 1971). Collaborative arrangements were subsequently developed with the World Health Organization to test the feasibility of the use of the translocation method for population control at its Research Unit on Genetic Control of Mosquitoes in New Delhi, India.

Field Releases.   Following is a brief outline of the results obtained from field releases.

A Heterozygous Translocation and a Genetic Marker.   In order to determine whether an alien genotype can be introduced into and propagated in a wild population, a male-linked, heterozygous translocation and a dominant genetic marker, silver mesonotum, were released in natural populations in two tire dumps in the vicinity of Delhi in August, 1971. In each case, releases were made for approximately three weeks. It was demonstrated that both the genetic marker and the translocation were incorporated and maintained in the wild populations (Rai *et al.*, 1973). There was evidence that the translocation also caused some degree of sterility. Furthermore, the genetic marker was subsequently detected in the next breeding season in 1972 in the tire-dump population. This was the first demonstration of its type among any mosquito species and indicated that, with proper manipulation, it should be possible to use translocations for genetic control.

Double-Translocation Heterozygotes.   As mentioned earlier, four translocations which were viable as homozygotes, two isolated from the *Rock* strain (T_1 and T_2) and two from the Delhi strain (T_3 and T_4) at the University of Notre Dame were colonized at the World Health Organization/ICMR, New Delhi Unit during the summers of 1972 and 1973, respectively. It was expected that such homozygotes could be maintained as true-breeding colonies and crossed to yield highly sterile, double-translocation heterozygotes for field releases. Following appropriate studies on the fitness of the individual homozygotes and the double heterozygotes, limited releases of the T_1 and T_2 double heterozygotes were made in Mahavir Colony in the town of Sonepat located approximately 40 km north of Delhi during a 19-day period in August, 1973. Mahavir Colony consists of 165 houses. The *A. aegypti* population in this colony was relatively low, with maximum daily adult emergence ranging from 270 to 1116 during August, 1973 (WHO/ICMR Delhi Unit Monthly Report, August, 1973). However, after releases of 10,600 males, contamination of the parental stocks by karyotypically standard individuals with normal fertility was observed and the releases were terminated. The results from this limited study, nevertheless, showed that released, double-translocation, heterozygote males mated with wild females and injected a certain amount of sterility (WHO/ICMR Delhi Unit Monthly Report, September, 1973). Another important result of the program was the development and refinement of the necessary quality control tests and monitoring techniques.

Future Plans. A major release experiment has now been planned to begin in February, 1975 with the following objectives:

1. To demonstrate the incorporation of high levels of sterility (and/or sex-ratio distortion) in the target population.
2. To show population suppression as a consequence.
3. To study this area over a sufficient period following releases to obtain information on the dynamics of the population after application of control measures.

The whole town of Sonepat, with a population of approximately 62, 000 people, will be used for these releases. This area is geographically large enough to demonstrate genetic control on an operational basis. Breeding of mosquitoes occurs throughout the year in this town and the natural population is well isolated because of the lack of breeding in surrounding rural areas. Furthermore, although there are differences of densities of *A. aegypti* populations in different parts of Sonepat, the overall population density is relatively low.

Releases of an appropriate double-translocation heterozygote with high sterility either alone or linked with the sex-ratio-distorter gene (Hickey and Craig, 1966) are planned. The combination of the two mechanisms will provide an integrated effect of sex-ratio distortion and translocation-associated sterility. Further, this combination will also enhance the efficiency of mass production. A sex-ratio-distorting stock with the Sonepat genetic background has already been isolated which produces an average sex ratio of 6 : 1 ($\male : \female$). A crossing scheme to link the distorter gene with sex-linked homozygous translocations has resulted in a distorter T_1 line which shows strong sex-ratio distortion ($15\delta : 1\female$). Furthermore, sex-ratio distortion and partial sterility is found in double-translocation heterozygotes produced by crossing distorter T_1 males with T_3 translocation and distortion-sensitive (m^d) homozygous females. The distorter–translocation stocks has been put together by Curtis and co-workers at the WHO/ICMR Delhi Unit (Monthly Report for February, 1974). It appears that this integrated system may provide an effective means of genetic control of *A. aegypti.*

The mean frequency of the distortion-sensitive gene (m^d) estimated from females collected as pupae from various sectors of Sonepat is about 65 percent (WHO/ICMR Delhi Unit Monthly Report for January, 1974).

Besides the work at the WHO/ICMR Unit in Delhi, India, work along more-or-less similar lines is also underway at the University of Notre Dame's Mosquito Biology Unit at the International Center of Insect Physiology and Ecology in Mombasa, Kenya.

Competitive Displacement. Through population replacement, innocuous forms unable to transmit a disease could be substituted for pests that fill similar ecological niches. For example, competition between populations of *A. polynesiensis,* a major vector of filariasis in Polynesia, and *A. albopictus,* results in elimination of the former. This happens in relatively small and large walk-in cages (Rozeboom, 1971). A preliminary field trial based on this principle of competitive exclusion was conducted by Rozeboom and Rosen (private communication) on a small island in the Pacific and was inconclusive. Additional tests are planned.

The use of translocations (Curtis, 1968) and/or compound chromosomes (Foster *et al.,* 1972) to fix desirable genes such as disease refractoriness, conditional lethals, etc., has been proposed. The purpose of such gene fixation is to replace an insect pest with a desired genotype, which in certain cases could be subjected to additional manipulation or insecticidal or climatic control (Klassen *et al.,* 1970).

Cytoplasmic Incompatibility. Members belonging to the *A. scutellaris* species complex are important vectors of filariasis in many islands of Pacific Oceania. Since breeding of their larvae often occurs in inaccessible habitats, including artificial containers, tree holes, and coconut husks, these mosquitoes are particularly difficult to control with insecticides. However, their island distribution may make them good targets for genetic control.

Woodhill (1949, 1950) demonstrated cases of nonreciprocal fertility between various members of the *A. scutellaris* complex. For example, whereas crosses among *A. scutellaris scutellaris* (S) females from New Guinea and *A. scutellaris Katherinensis* (K) males produce normal, viable progeny, the reciprocal cross between K females and S males produce no progeny. Inheritance of this sterility is maternal, being transmitted from mothers to daughters. Smith-White and Woodhill (1954) suggested that this sterility may ensue from some incompatibility factor in the cytoplasm of the eggs of K which kills the sperm of S before karyogamy.

This incompatibility could be used either to bring about genetic control or population replacement of vectors by nonvectors.

Mosquito Data Bank

Considerable emphasis has been placed on the establishment of a computerized Mosquito Data Bank at the University of Notre Dame (MODABUND). More than 26,000 references dealing with all aspects of research on mosquitoes published since 1940 have been computerized. Key words such as *genetics of Aedes* mosquitoes allow quick retrieval of bibliographies. For example, in a recent computer search of references during the decade 1960–1969 with "Chromosome, Karyotype and Cytology" as the key words, taken on behalf of one of us (Rai) the Data Bank provided a print-out of 1066 references listed first by subject and then by author. The details on the mechanics of MODABUND are provided by Crovello (1972).

World Health Organization International Reference Center for *Aedes*

The World Health Organization International Reference Center (W.H.O.I.R.C.) for *Aedes* is located at the Vector Biology Laboratory of the University of Notre Dame. Over 30 species, most of them belonging to the genus *Aedes,* and 150 strains of mosquitoes are maintained at this center. Emphasis of this germ plasm is on *A. aegypti,* and the stocks include various standard strains, geographic strains, inbred lines, single- and multiple-marker genetic stocks with as many as eight genetic markers, and single and multiple chromosome rearrangement stocks, particularly for translocations and inversions. Any of these stocks maintained in the W.H.O.I.R.C. are available on request to interested research workers. During the past seven years, more than 500 requests for such stocks were filled.

Acknowledgments

Some of the work on this manuscript was completed while K. S. Rai was on sabbatical leave (1973–1974) at the Department of Biology, Guru Nanak University, Amritsar, Punjab, India. Much of the research reviewed received support from Atomic Energy Commission Contract AT(11-1)-38 with the Radiation Laboratory at the University of Notre Dame. This is AEC document No. C00-38-966.

Literature Cited

Abedi, Z. H., J. R. Duffy and A. W. A. Brown, 1963   Dehydrochlorination and DDT resistance in *Aedes aegypti. J. Econ. Entomol.* **56**:511–517.

Akstein, E., 1962   The chromosomes of *Aedes aegypti* and of some other species of mosquitoes. *Bull. Res. Counc. Israel* **11**:146–155.

Anonymous, 1968   *Cytogenetics of Vectors of Disease of Man.* World Health Organization Technical Report Series No. 398, World Health Organization, Geneva.

Asman, Sr. M. and K. S. Rai, 1971   Gamma radiation and heterosis in *Aedes aegypti. Bull. Entomol. Soc. Am.* **13**:201.

Baker, R. H. and M. Aslamkhan, 1969   Karyotypes of some Asian mosquitoes of the subfamily culicinae (Diptera: Culicidae). *J. Med. Entomol.* **6**:44–55.

Bat-Miriam, M. and G. B. Craig, Jr., 1966   Mutants in *Aedes albopictus* (Diptera: Culicidae). *Mosq. News* **26**:13–22.

Bhalla, S. C., 1968a   White-eye, a new sex-linked mutant of *Aedes aegypti. Mosq. News* **28**:380–385.

Bhalla, S. C., 1968b   Genetic aspects of pteridines in mosquitoes. *Genetics* **58**:249–258.

Bhalla, S. C., 1970   Paracentric inversions and detection of sex-linked lethals in *Aedes aegypti. Can. J. Genet. Cytol.* **12**:635–650.

Bhalla, S. C., 1971   Meiotic behavior of diploid and tretraploid *Aedes aegypti. Mosq. News* **31**:397–401.

Bhalla, S. C., 1973   Sex-linked translocations, semisterility and linkage alterations in the mosquito *Aedes aegypti. Can. J. Genet. Cytol.* **15**:9–20.

Bhalla, S. C. and G. B. Craig, Jr., 1967   *Bronze,* a female-sterile mutant of *Aedes aegypti. J. Med. Entomol.* **4**:467–476.

Bianchi, N. O., M. S. Bianchi and B. H. Sweet, 1972   Chromosome replication in cells of a continuous line derived from *Aedes albopictus* (Skuse) Larvae. *Experientia* (Basel) **28**:1495–1496.

Bond, H. A., G. B. Craig, Jr. and R. W. Fay, 1970   Field mating and movement of *Aedes aegypti. Mosq. News* **30**:394–402.

Breland, O. P., 1960   Restoration of the name *Aedes hendersoni* Cockerell and its elevation to full specific rank (Diptera: Culicidae). *Ann. Entomol. Soc. Am.* **53**:600–606.

Brown, A. W. A. and Z. H. Abedi, 1962   Genetics of DDT-resistance in several strains of *Aedes aegypti. Can. J. Genet. Cytol.* **4**:319–332.

Brown, A. W. A. and R. Pal, 1971   *Insecticide Resistance in Arthropods.* World Health Organization Monograph Series No. 38, World Health Organization, Geneva.

Bullini, L. and M. Coluzzi, 1972   Natural selection and genetic drift in protein polymorphism. *Nature (Lond.)* **239**:160–161.

Bullini, L. and M. Coluzzi, 1974   Electrophoretic studies on gene–enzyme systems in mosquitoes (Diptera: Culicidae). WHO/VBC/74.483. Mimeographed document, World Health Organization, Geneva.

Bullini, L., M. Coluzzi, A. M. Gironi and M. Morellini, 1970a   Phosphoglucomutase polymorphism in *Aedes aegypti*. *Parassitologia* **12**:27–30.

Bullini, L., A. M. Gironi, A. P. Bianchi Bullini and M. Coluzzi, 1970b   Further observations on phosphoglucomutase polymorphism in *Aedes aegypti*. *Parassitologia* **12**:113–117.

Bullini, L., A. M. Gironi, A. P. Bianchi Bullini and M. Coluzzi, 1972   Phosphoglucomutase gene in *Aedes aegypti*: A fourth allele and preliminary linkage data. *Biochem. Genet.* **7**:41–44.

Callan, H. G. and G. Montalenti, 1947   Chiasma interference in mosquitoes. *J. Genet.* **48**:110–136.

Chattoraj, A. N. and A. W. A. Brown, 1960   Internal DDE production by normal and DDT-resistant larvae of *Aedes aegypti*. *J. Econ. Entomol.* **53**:1049–1051.

Coker, W. Z., 1958   The inheritance of DDT-resistance in *Aedes aegypti*. *Ann. Trop. Med. Parasitol.* **52**:443–455.

Coker, W. Z., 1966   Linkage of the DDT-resistance gene in some strains of *Aedes aegypti* (L.). *Ann. Trop. Med. Parasitol.* **50**:347–356.

Coluzzi, M. and L. Bullini, 1971   Enzyme variants as markers in the study of pre-copulatory isolating mechanisms. *Nature (Lond.)* **231**:455–456.

Coluzzi, M. and A. M. Gironi, 1971   Osservazioni preliminari sulla selezione di ceppi di *Aedes aegypti* sensibli e resistenti all infezione da *Dirofilaria repens*. *Parassitologia* **12**:151–152.

Coluzzi, M., L. Bullini, and A. P. Bianchi Bullini, 1971   Phosphoglucomutase (PGM) allozymes in two forms of the *mariae* complex of the genus *Aedes*. *Biochem. Genet.* **5**:253–255.

Craig, G. B., Jr., 1967   Genetic control of *Aedes aegypti*. *Bull. WHO* **36**:628–632.

Craig, G. B., Jr. and W. A. Hickey, 1967   Genetics of *Aedes aegypti*. In *Genetics of Insect Vectors of Disease*, edited by J. W. Wright and R. Pal, pp. 67–131, Elsevier, Amsterdam.

Craig, G. B., Jr. and R. C. VandeHey, 1962   Genetic variability in *Aedes aegypti* (Diptera: Culicidae). I. Mutations affecting color pattern. *Ann. Entomol. Soc. Am.* **55**:47–58.

Crovello, T. J., 1972   MODABUND—The computerized mosquito data bank at University of Notre Dame. *Mosq. News* **32**:548–554.

Curtis, C., 1968   Possible use of translocations to fix desirable genes in insect pest populations. *Nature (Lond.)* **218**:368–369.

Davidson, G. and G. F. Mason, 1963   Genetics of mosquitoes. *Annu. Rev. Entomol.* **8**:177–196.

Dunn, M. A. and G. B. Craig, Jr., 1968   Small-antenna, a sex-linked mutant of *Aedes aegypti*. *J. Hered.* **59**:131–140.

Fay, R. W. and G. B. Craig, Jr., 1969   Genetically marked *Aedes aegypti* in studies of field populations. *Mosq. News* **29**:121–127.

Fiil, A. and P. B. Moens, 1973   The development, structure and function of modified synaptonemal complexes in mosquito oocytes. *Chromosoma (Berl.)* **41**:37–62.

Foster, G. G., M. J. Whitten, T. Prout and R. Gill, 1972   Chromosome rearrangements for the control of insect pests. *Science (Wash., D.C.)* **176**:875–880.

Gerberg, E. J., 1970   *Manual for Mosquito Rearing and Experimental Techniques,* American Mosquito Control Assoc. Bulletin No. 5, AMCA, Selma, Calif.

Gillham, N. W., 1957   Genetic studies in *Aedes.* I. The distribution of polytene chromosomes in *Aedes aegypti. Am. Nat.* **91**:265–268.

Gubler, D. J., 1970   Induced sterility in *Aedes (Stegomyia) polynesiensis* Marks by cross-insemination with *Aedes (Stegomyia) albopictus* Skuse. *J. Med. Entomol.* **7**:65–70.

Gwadz, R. W., 1970   Monofactorial inheritance of early sexual receptivity in the mosquito, *Aedes atropalpus. Anim. Behav.* **18**:358–361.

Hallinan, E. and K. S. Rai, 1973   Radiation sterilization of *Aedes aegypti* in nitrogen and implications for sterile male technique. *Nature (Lond.)* **244**:368–369.

Hallinan, E., N. Lorimer and K. S. Rai, 1975   A Cytogenetic study of radiation-induced translocations in the Delhi, India strain of *Aedes aegypti,* in preparation.

Hartberg, W. K., 1972   Hybridization between *Aedes simpsoni* and *Aedes woodi* with observations on the genetic basis of morphological differences. *Bull. WHO* **46**:345–352.

Hartberg, W. K., 1975   Palp-extended, a sex-linked and sex-limited mutant of *Aedes aegypti. Mosq. News* **35**:34–41.

Hartberg, W. K. and G. B. Craig, Jr., 1968   Reproductive isolation in *Stegomyia* mosquitoes. I. Sexual isolation between *Aedes aegypti* and *A. mascarensis. Ann. Entomol. Soc. Am.* **61**:865–870.

Hartberg, W. K. and G. B. Craig, Jr., 1970   Reproductive isolation in *Stegomyia* mosquitoes. II. Hybrid breakdown between *Aedes aegypti* and *A. mascarensis. Evolution* **24**:692–703.

Hartberg, W. K. and G. B. Craig, Jr., 1973   Gene-controlled morphological differences in male genitalia of *Aedes aegypti* and *Aedes mascarensis* (Diptera: Culicidae). *Mosq. News* **33**:206–214.

Hartberg, W. K. and G. B. Craig, Jr., 1974   Three new mutants in *Aedes mascarensis:* current-eye, small-antenna and yellow. *J. Med. Entomol.* **11**:447–454.

Hartberg, W. K. and G. A. H. McClelland, 1973   *Aedes mascarensis* MacGregor on Mauritius. II. Genetic variability of field populations (Diptera: Culicidae). *J. Med. Entomol.* **10**:577–582.

Hazard, E. I., C. S. Lofgren, D. B. Woodward, H. R. Ford and B. M. Glancey, 1964   Resistance to the chemical sterilant, apholate, in *Aedes aegypti. Science (Wash., D.C.)* **145**:500–501.

Hickey, W. A. and G. B. Craig, Jr., 1966   Genetic distortion of sex-ratio in a mosquito, *Aedes aegypti. Genetics* **53**:1177–1196.

Jost, E., 1971   Meiosis in the male of *Culex pipiens* and *Aedes albopictus* and fertilization in the *pipiens*-complex. *Can. J. Genet. Cytol.* **13**:237–250.

Kartman, L., 1953   Factors influencing infection of the mosquito with *Dirofilaria immitis* (Leidy, 1856). *Exp. Parasitol.* **2**:27–78.

Khan, N. H. and A. W. A. Brown, 1961   Genetical studies on dieldrin-resistance in *Aedes aegypti* and its cross-resistance to DDT. *Bull. WHO* **24**:519–526.

Kilama, W. L., 1973   Distribution of a gene for susceptibility to *Plasmodium gallinaceum* in populations of *Aedes aegypti* (L.). *J. Parasitol.* **59**:920–924.

Kilama, W. L. and G. B. Craig, Jr., 1969   Monofactorial inheritance of susceptibility to *Plasmodium gallinaceum* in *Aedes aegypti. Ann Trop. Med. Parasitol.* **63**:419–432.

Kimura, T. and A. W. A. Brown, 1964   DDT-dehydrochlorinase in *Aedes aegypti. J. Econ. Entomol.* **57**:710–716.

Kitzmiller, J. B., 1953   Mosquito genetics and cytogenetics. *Rev. Bras. Malariol. Doencas Trop.* **5**:285–359.

Klassen, W., 1966   Genetics of resistance in mosquitoes. *Mosq. News* **26**:309–318.

Klassen, W. and A. W. A. Brown, 1964   Genetics of insecticide resistance and several visible mutants in *Aedes aegypti. Can. J. Genet. Cytol.* **6**:61–73.

Klassen, W. and F. Matsumura, 1966   Resistance to a chemosterilant, Metepa, in *Aedes aegypti* mosquitoes. *Nature (Lond.)* **200**:1155–1156.

Klassen, W., J. F. Creech and R. A. Bull, 1970   *The Potential of Genetic Suppression of Insect Populations by their Adaptations to Climate,* U.S. Dept. Agr. ARS Misc. Publ. No. *1178,* U.S. Department of Agriculture, Washington, D.C.

Knipling, E. F., 1959   Sterile-male method of population control. *Science (Wash., D.C.)* **130**:902–904.

Knipling, E. F., H. Laven, G. B. Craig, Jr., R. Pal, J. B. Kitzmiller, C. N. Smith and A. W. A. Brown, 1968   Genetic control of insects of public health importance. *Bull. WHO* **38**:421–438.

Leahy, Sr. M. G. and G. B. Craig, Jr., 1967   Barriers to hybridization between *Aedes aegypti* and *Aedes albopictus.* (Diptera: Culicidae). *Evolution* **21**:41–58.

Lockhart, W. L., W. Klassen and A. W. A. Brown, 1970   Crossover values between dieldrin-resistance and DDT-resistance and linkage-group-2 genes in *Aedes aegypti. Can. J. Genet. Cytol.* **12**:407–414.

Lorimer, N., E. Hallinan and K. S. Rai, 1972   Translocation homozygotes in the yellow-fever-mosquito, *Aedes aegypti. J. Hered.* **63**:158–166.

McClelland, G. A. H., 1962   A contribution to the genetics of the mosquito *Aedes aegypti* (L.) with particular reference to factors determining colour. Ph.D. Thesis, University of London, London.

McClelland, G. A. H., 1966   Sex-linkage at two loci affecting eye pigment in the mosquito *Aedes aegypti* (Diptera: Culicidae). *Can. J. Genet. Cytol.* **8**:192–198.

McClelland, G. A. H., 1967   Speciation and evolution in *Aedes.* In *Genetics of Insect Vectors of Disease,* edited by J. W. Wright and R. Pal, pp. 277 311, Elsevier, Amsterdam.

McClelland, G. A. H. and R. Mamet, 1962   *Aedes aegypti* (L.) and *Aedes mascarensis* MacGregor in Mauritius: A case of gene survival following species eradication? *Nature (Lond.)* **195**:965.

McDonald, P. T. and K. S. Rai, 1970a   *Aedes aegypti*: Origin of a "new" chromosome from a double translocation heterozygote. *Science (Wash., D.C.)* **168**:1229–1230.

McDonald, P. T. and K. S. Rai, 1970b   Correlation of linkage groups with chromosomes in the mosquito, *Aedes aegypti. Genetics* **66**:475–485.

McDonald, P. T. and K. S. Rai, 1971   Population control potential of heterozygous translocations as determined by computer simulations. *Bull. WHO* **44**:829–845.

Macdonald, W. W., 1962   The genetic basis of susceptibility to infection with semi-periodic *Brugia malayi* in *Aedes aegypti. Ann. Trop. Med. Parasitol.* **56**:373–382.

Macdonald, W. W., 1963a   Further studies on a strain of *Aedes aegypti* susceptible to infection with sub-periodic *Brugia malayi. Ann. Trop. Med. Parasitol.* **57**:452–460.

Macdonald, W. W., 1963b   A preliminary cross-over value between the gene f^m (filarial susceptibility, *Brugia malayi*) and the sex locus in *Aedes aegypti. Ann. Trop. Med. Parasitol.* **57**:461–465.

Macdonald, W. W., 1967   The influence of genetic and other factors on vector susceptibility to parasites. In *Genetics of Insect Vectors of Disease,* edited by J. W. Wright
and R. Pal, pp. 567–584, Elsevier, Amsterdam.

Macdonald, W. W. and C. P. Ramachandran, 1965   The influence of the gene f^m
(filarial susceptibility, *Burgia malayi*) on the susceptibility of *Aedes aegypti* to seven
strains of *Brugia, Wuchereria* and *Dirofilaria. Ann. Trop. Med. Parasitol.* **59:**64–73.

Macdonald, W. W. and P. M. Sheppard, 1965   Cross-over values in the sex chromosomes of the mosquito *Aedes aegypti* and evidence of the presence of inversions.
Ann. Trop. Med. Parasitol. **59:**74–87.

McGivern, J. J. and K. S. Rai, 1972   A radiation-induced paracentric inversion in *Aedes
aegypti* (L.): Cytogenetic and interchromosomal effects. *J. Hered.* **63:**247–255.

McGivern, J. J. and K. S. Rai, 1974   Sex-ratio distortion and directed alternate
segregation of interchange complexes in a mosquito. *J. Hered.* **65:**71–77.

McGreevy, P. B., G. A. H. McClelland and M. M. Lavoipierre, 1974   Inheritance of
susceptibility to *Dirofilaria immitis* infection in *Aedes aegypti. Ann. Trop. Med.
Parasitol.* **68:**97–109.

Machado-Allison, C. E. and G. B. Craig, Jr., 1972   Geographic variation in resistance to
desiccation in *Aedes aegypti* and *A. atropalpus* (Diptera: Culicidae). *Ann. Entomol.
Soc. Am.* **65:**542–547.

Mathew, G. and K. S. Rai, 1975   Chemosterilant(Apholate)-induced ultrastructural
changes during oogenesis in *Aedes aegypti. Cytobios,* in press.

Mattingly, P. F., 1957   Genetical aspects of the *Aedes aegypti* problem. I. Taxonomy
and bionomics. *Ann. Trop. Med. Parasitol.* **51:**392–407.

Mattingly, P. F., 1958   Genetical aspects of the *Aedes aegypti* problem. II. Disease relationships, genetics, and control. *Ann. Trop. Med. Parasitol.* **52:**5–17.

Mattingly, P. 1967   Genetics of behavior. In *Genetics of Insect Vectors of Disease,* edited
by J. W. Wright and R. Pal, pp. 553–566, Elsevier, Amsterdam.

Mescher, Sr. A. L., 1963   A comparative analysis of the morphology and post-embryonic
development of the salivary glands of *Aedes aegypti* (L.) (Diptera: Culicidae). Ph.D.
Thesis, University of Notre Dame, Notre Dame, Ind.

Mescher, Sr. A. L. and K. S. Rai, 1966   Spermatogenesis in *Aedes aegypti. Mosq. News*
26:45–51.

Morlan, H. B., E. M. McCray, Jr. and J. W. Kilpatrick, 1962   Field tests with sexually
sterile males for control of *Aedes aegypti. Mosq. News* **22:**295–300.

Mukherjee, A. B., D. M. Rees and R. K. Vickery, 1966   A comparative study of the karyotypes of four genera and nineteen species of mosquitoes present in Utah. *Mosq.
News* **26:**150–155.

Nijhout, H. F. and G. B. Craig, Jr., 1971   Reproductive isolation in *Stegomyia* mosquitoes. III. Evidence for a sexual pheromone. *Entomol. Exp. Appl.* **14:**399–412.

O'Meara, G. F., 1972   Polygenic regulation of fecundity in autogenous *Aedes atropalpus.
Entomol. Exp. Appl.* **15:**81–89.

O'Meara, G. F. and G. B. Craig, 1969   Monofactorial inheritance of autogeny in *Aedes
atropalpus. Mosq. News* **29:**14–22.

O'Meara, G. F. and G. J. Krasnick, 1970   Dietary and genetic control of the expression
of autogenous reproduction in *Aedes atropalpus* (Coq.) (Diptera: Culicidae). *J. Med.
Entomol.* **7:**328–334.

Petersen, J. L., J. R. Larsen and G. B. Craig, Jr., 1975   Palp-antenna, a homeotic
mutant in *Aedes aegypti.,* manuscript in preparation.

Pillai, M. K. K. and A. W. A. Brown, 1965   Physiological and genetical studies on resistance to DDT substitutes in *Aedes aegypti. J. Econ. Entomol.* **58**:255–266.

Quinn, T. C. and G. B. Craig, Jr., 1971   Phenogenetics of the homeotic mutant proboscipedia in *Aedes albopictus. J. Hered.* **62**:2–12.

Qutubuddin, M., 1958   The inheritance of DDT-resistance in a highly resistant strain of *Aedes aegypti* (L.). *Bull. WHO* **19**:1109–1112.

Rai, K. S., 1963a   A comparative study of mosquito karyotypes. *Ann. Entomol. Soc. Am.* **56**:160–170.

Rai, K. S., 1963b   A cytogenetic study of the effects of x-irradiation in *Aedes aegypti. Caryologia* **17**:595–607.

Rai, K. S., 1964a   Cytogenetic effects of chemosterilants in mosquitoes. I. Apholate-induced aberrations in the somatic chromosomes of *Aedes aegypti. Cytologia (Tokyo)* **29**:346–353.

Rai, K. S., 1964b   Cytogenetic effects of chemosterilants in mosquitoes. II. Mechanism of apholate-induced changes in fecundity and fertility of *Aedes aegypti* (L.). *Biol. Bull.* **127**:119–131.

Rai, K. S., 1966   Further observations on the somatic chromosome cytology of some mosquitoes (Diptera: Culicidae). *Ann. Entomol. Soc. Am.* **59**:242–246.

Rai, K. S., 1967   Techniques for the study of cytogenetics and genetics of vectors. In *Genetics of Insect Vectors of Disease*, edited by J. W. Wright and R. Pal, pp. 673–701, Elsevier, Amsterdam.

Rai, K. S., 1968   Techniques for studying the effects of radiation on meiosis and related processes in mosquitoes with particular reference to *Aedes aegypti*. In *Effects of Radiation on Meiotic Systems*, edited by C. N. Welsh, pp. 185–200, International Atomic Energy Agency Press, Vienna.

Rai, K. S. and P. T. McDonald, 1972   Application of radiation-induced translocations for genetic control of *Aedes aegypti. Proc. W.H.O./ICMR Seminar "Genetics and Our Health," New Delhi, India, Tech. Rep. Series* **20**:77–94.

Rai, K. S. and V. P. Sharma, 1971   Cytogenetic effects of chemosterilants in mosquitoes. III. Development of transplanted ovaries in normal and chemosterilized females in *Aedes aegypti. J. Genet.* **60**:266–271.

Rai, K. S., P. T. McDonald and Sr. M. Asman, 1970   Cytogenetics of two radiation-induced, sex-linked translocations in the yellow-fever mosquito, *Aedes aegypti. Genetics* **66**:635–651.

Rai, K. S., K. K. Grover and N. Suguna, 1973   Genetic manipulation of the mosquito, *Aedes aegypti*. I. Incorporation and maintenance of a genetic marker and a chromosomal translocation in natural populations. *Bull. WHO* **48**:49–56.

Rai, K. S., N. Lorimer and E. Hallinan, 1974   The current status of genetic methods for controlling *Aedes aegypti*. In *The Use of Genetics for Insect Control*, edited by R. Pal and M. Whitten, pp. 119–132, Elsevier North-Holland., Amsterdam.

Rioux, J., H. Croset, A. Gabinaud, B. Papierok and A. Belmonte, 1973   Hérédité monofactorielle de l'autogenise chez *Aedes (Ochlerotatus) detritus* (Haliday, 1833) (Diptera: Culicidae). *C. R. Hebd. Seances Acad. Sci. Ser. D Sci. Nat.* **276**:991–994.

Risler, H., 1959   Polyploidie und somatische Reduktion in der Larvenepidermis von *Aedes aegypti* (Culicidae). *Chromosoma (Berl.)* **10**:184–209.

Roberts, J. R., Jr., 1973   Proboscipedia, a homeotic mutant in *Aedes aegypti* (L.) (Diptera: Culicidae). M. Sci. Thesis, Georgia Southern College, Statesboro, Georgia.

Roth, T. F., 1966 Changes in the synaptinemal complex during meiotic prophase in mosquito oocytes. *Protoplasma* **61**:346–386.

Roubaud, E., 1937 Nouvelles recherches sur l'infection du moustique de la fievre jaune par *Dirofilaria immitis* Leidy. Les races biologiques d'*Aedes aegypti* et l'infection filarienne. *Bull. Soc. Pathol. Exot.* **30**:511–519.

Rozeboom, L. E., 1971 Relative densities of freely breeding populations of *Aedes* (*S.*) *polynesiensis* Marks and *A.* (*S.*) *albopictus* Skuse. *Am. J. Trop. Med. Hyg.* **20**:356–362.

Rozeboom, L. E. and J. B. Kitzmiller, 1958 Hybridization and speciation in mosquitoes. *Annu. Rev. Entomol.* **3**:231–248.

Rudnick, A., 1967 *Aedes aegypti* and haemorrhagic fever. *Bull. WHO* **36**:528–532.

Schneider, I., 1972 Mosquito cell culture. *Proc. "Workshop on Development of Filariae in Mosquitoes," (U.S. Japan Cooperative Medical Science Program, Univ. of Calif., Los Angeles, March 20–21, 1972)*: 52–54.

Schoenig, E., 1967 Strain variation in behavior of *Aedes aegypti* (Diptera: Culicidae). Part I. Strain variation in spontaneous movement. *Philippine Sci. Ser. F* **I(IV)**:55:82.

Schoenig, E., 1968 Strain variation in behavior of *Aedes aegypti* (Diptera: Culicidae). II. Strain variation in oviposition behavior. *Philippine Sci. Ser. F* **V**:29–59.

Schoenig, E., 1969 Strain variation in behavior of *Aedes aegypti* (Diptera: Culicidae). III. Strain variation in the speed of vertical movement of the larvae. *Philippine Sci. Ser. F* **VI**:51–57.

Seawright, J. A., 1972 A genetic study of apholate resistance in *Aedes aegypti*. *J. Econ. Entomol.* **65**:1357–1361.

Sharma, V. P. and K. S. Rai, 1969 Histopathological and developmental effects of the chemosterilant, apholate, on the mosquito *Aedes aegypti*. *Mosq. News* **29**:9–14.

Singh, K. R. P., 1967 Cell Cultures derived from larvae of *Aedes albopictus* (Skuse) and *Aedes aegypti* (L.). *Curr. Sci. (Bangalore)* **36**:506–508.

Smith, R. P. and W. K. Hartberg, 1974 Spermatogenesis in *Aedes albopictus* (Skuse). *Mosq. News* **34**:42–47.

Smith-White, S. and A. R. Woodhill, 1954 The nature and significance of non-reciprocal fertility in *Aedes scutellaris* and other mosquitoes. *Proc. Linn. Soc. N.S.W.* **79**:163–176.

Stone, A., 1961 A synoptic catalog of the mosquitoes of the world, supplement I. *Proc. Entomol. Soc. (Wash., D.C.).* **63**:29–62.

Stone, A., 1963 A synoptic catalog of the mosquitoes of the world, supplement II. *Proc. Entomol. Soc. (Wash., D.C.).* **65**:117–140.

Stone, A., 1967 A synoptic catalog of the mosquitoes of the world, supplement III. *Proc. Entomol. Soc. (Wash., D.C.).* **69**:197–224.

Stone, A., 1970 A synoptic catalog of the mosquitoes of the world, supplement IV. *Proc. Entomol. Soc. (Wash., D.C.).* **72**:137–171.

Stone, A., K. L. Knight and H. Starke, 1959 *A Synoptic Catalog of the Mosquitoes of the World,* Vol. 6, Thomas Say Foundation, Washington, D.C.

Tesfa-Yohannes, T.-M., 1973 Genetic relationships of three strains of *Aedes* (*S.*) *polynesiensis* Marks. *J. Med. Entomol.* **10**:490–492.

Thomas, V. and Y. P. Leng, 1972 The inheritance of autogeny in *Aedes* (*Finlaya*) *togoi* (Theobald) from Malaysia and some aspects of its biology. *S.E. Asian J. Trop. Med. Publ. Hlth.* **3**:163–174.

Townson, H., 1972 Esterase polymorphism in *Aedes aegypti*: The genetics and K_m

values of electrophoretically heterogenous forms. *Ann. Trop. Med. Parasitol.* **66**:255–266.

Trager, W., 1942 A strain of the mosquito *Aedes aegypti* selected for susceptibility to the avian malaria parasite *Plasmodium lophurae. J. Parasitol.* **28**:457–465.

Trebatoski, A. M. and G. B. Craig, Jr., 1969 Genetics of an esterase in *Aedes aegypti. Biochem. Genet.* **3**:383–392.

Truman, J. W. and G. B. Craig, Jr., 1968 Hybridization between *Aedes hendersoni* and *Aedes triseriatus. Ann. Entomol. Soc. Am.* **61**:1020–1025.

VandeHey, R. C., 1964 Genetic variability in *Aedes aegypti* (Diptera: Culicidae) III. Plasticity in laboratory populations. *Ann. Entomol. Soc. Am.* **57**:488–496.

Ved Brat, S. and K. S. Rai, 1973a An analysis of chiasma frequencies in *Aedes aegypti. Nucleus* **16**:184–193.

Ved Brat, S. and K. S. Rai, 1973b Cytological map of chromosome 3 in *Aedes aegypti. Proc. XIII Interntl. Congr. Genet.* **74**:S283–S284.

Ved Brat, S. and K. S. Rai, 1974 Duplication-deficiency heterozygotes in *Aedes aegypti. Heredity* **32**:225–230.

Ward, R. A., 1963 Genetic aspects of the susceptibility of mosquitoes to malarial infection. *Exp. Parasitol.* **13**:328–341.

Whitten, M. J., 1970 Use of chromosome rearrangements for mosquito control. *Interntl. Atomic Energy Agency Symp. "The Sterility Principle for Insect Control or Eradication," Athens*: 399–410.

Wolfe, S. L., 1972 *Biology of the Cell,* pp. 408–412, Wadsworth Publishing Co., Belmont, Calif.

Wood, R. J., 1965 A genetical study on DDT-resistance in the Trinidad strain of *Aedes aegypti* (L.). *Bull. WHO* **32**:563–574.

Wood, R. J., 1967 A comparative genetical study on DDT resistance in adults and larvae of the mosquito *Aedes aegypti* (L.). *Genet. Res.* **10**:219–228.

Wood, R. J., 1970 The influence of the *y* locus on DDT resistance in the mosquito *Aedes aegypti* (L.). *Genet. Res.* **16**:37–47.

Woodhill, A. R., 1949 A note on experimental crossing of *Aedes* (*Stegomyia*) *scutellaris scutellaris* Walker and *Aedes* (*Stegomyia*) *scutellaris katherinesis* Woodhill (Diptera: Culicidae). *Proc. Linn. Soc. N. S. W.* **74**:224–226.

Woodhill, A. R., 1950 Further studies on experimental crossing within the *Aedes scutellaris* group of species. (Diptera: Culicidae). *Proc. Linn. Soc. N. S. W.* **75**:251–253.

Zepp, H. D., J. H. Conover, K. Hirshhorn and H. L. Hodes, 1971 Human–mosquito somatic cell hybrids induced by ultraviolet-inactivated Sendai virus. *Nat. New Biol.* **229**:119–121.

Zielke, E., 1973 Untersuchungen zur Vererbung der Empfanglichkeit gegenuber der Hundefilarie *Dirofilaria immitis* bei *Culex pipiens fatigans* und *Aedes aegypti. Z. Tropenmed. Parasitol.* **24**:36–44.

14

Culex

A. Ralph Barr

Introduction

Culex pipiens is the most widely distributed species of mosquito in the world. It has two well-characterized forms, *quinquefasciatus* (= *fatigans*), which is found throughout the tropics and extends into the temperate regions of the Northern and Southern Hemispheres, and *pipiens,* which is found in temperate areas of the world and perhaps in tropical Africa as well (Mattingly, 1951). Where these two forms come together there is evidence of extensive intergrading in the field (Bekku, 1956; Barr, 1957; McMillan, 1958).

C. *p. quinquefasciatus* is a relatively uniform commensal of man which breeds primarily in natural and artificial containers, usually in moderately polluted water. The adult female requires blood for egg development and commonly feeds on people when they sleep in exposed places at night. This form is said to be the most important vector of periodic Bancroftian filariasis in much of the tropics and may transmit virus diseases as well. The uniformity of populations of this form suggests that it is of relatively recent origin and that it spread through the warm parts of the world rapidly (Barr, 1967). Adult males form swarms during periods of decreased light intensity, but mating usually occurs readily in the laboratory, even when the adults are kept in rather small cages.

The typical subspecies, *pipiens,* is found in cooler areas of the world

A. Ralph Barr—School of Public Health, University of California, Los Angeles, California.

and populations vary rather remarkably from one area to another (Marshall and Staley, 1937). The variation seen in this form suggests a very old, rather sedentary, form which is broken up into smaller populations which vary morphologically and biologically. This nominate subspecies seems to be a rather unexceptional *Culex* which invaded the Palearctic region from the Ethiopian region, since its relatives are largely found there. It is said to breed principally in ground pools in relatively clean water. For the most part, it feeds on birds. Large swarms of males characteristically form at periods of reduced illumination, and there may be difficulty in inducing adults to mate in cages in the laboratory.

This form has at various times in the past invaded highly polluted waters such as cesspools and septic tanks, which are closely associated with man and which frequently have restricted access. In such places there is intense selection for reproduction without feeding on blood (autogeny). (Autogeny is found in low frequency in several species related to *C. pipiens.*) Under these peculiar conditions strains have developed which can reproduce generation after generation in septic tanks, living in a rich organic medium, in almost total darkness, mating in restricted quarters, and reproducing autogenously. Such populations are found all over the range of the subspecies *pipiens* and, although these populations are readily dispersed by human commerce, the variation among strains indicates that this biotype has probably arisen many times. These autogenous strains are frequently called by the vernacular name "molestus," which implies only that they are autogenous. Usually these strains can mate in a very small space and the females do not hibernate as do those of the typical biotype. Even though autogeny is found in many culexes related to *C. pipiens,* there appear to be no authentic records of autogeny in the tropical subspecies, *C. fatigans* [but see Bhatnagar *et al.* (1958)]. This point is easily checked by examining the genitalia of males of autogenous populations (Sundaraman, 1949). McMillan (1958) described an autogenous strain whose males had genitalia clearly intermediate between those of *pipiens* and *quinquefasciatus.* This apparently was a hybrid swarm in a part of the range of *quinquefasciatus* (southern California) which was only a few hundred miles from populations of pure autogenous *pipiens.*

Autogenous strains of *pipiens* are easily transportable by man, and there is ample evidence that this has happened on a massive scale. Drummond (1951) first recorded the autogenous form in Australia and associated its appearance with the entry of American troops. Autogeny has also been observed in *pipiens* strains from both South America and Africa, so it is probable that all typical *pipiens* populations of the

Southern Hemisphere are northern stocks which were transplanted. It appears that truly anautogenous stocks of typical *pipiens* are absent from California, at least from the well-studied areas, and that all autogenous strains are ones (Iltis, 1970) which have been introduced. The situation is even clearer in Japan, where there is a native *pipiens* population which is differentiated into *quinquefasciatus* in the south. Superimposed on this is an autogenous *pipiens* population which is clearly an introduced one since it maintains a high degree of incompatibility with the native populations (Sasa *et al.*, 1966). The distribution of "crossing types" in Europe (Laven, 1967*b*) also argues for the ready transportation of autogenous strains.

In places where both autogenous and anautogenous populations of *Culex pipiens* occur, the autogenous population may be able to exist indefinitely by ecological separation [as is thought to be the case in Britain (Marshall and Staley, 1937)], by behavioral differentiation (Spielman, 1964, 1967, 1971), or even by incompatibility (Sasa *et al.*, 1966). In Egypt there does not seem to be a separation into autogenous and anautogenous populations; all populations seem to have the genes for autogeny in low frequency (Knight and Malek, 1951).

In areas of the world where *pipiens* and *quinquefasciatus* come together they interbreed more or less freely, so that rather widespread intermediate populations are produced. These have been most extensively studied in Japan by Bekku (1956) and in North America by Barr (1957), McMillan (1958), and Iltis (1970). The Asian intermediate form is frequently called *C. p. pallens*, but, as pointed out by Bekku, is clearly intermediate between *pipiens* and *quinquefasciatus*.

In Australia *quinquefasciatus* has been known for many years but the autogenous form of *pipiens* was first recognized in 1942. It is not clear whether or not it was a new introduction at that time. Another form, *australicus*, was described by Dobrotworsky and Drummond (1952) in 1952, and the male genitalia of this form are indistinguishable from those of laboratory hybrids of *pipiens* and *quinquefasciatus*. There is little doubt that *australicus* is of hybrid origin, but it is not clear whether it formed in Australia or was introduced. Typical anautogenous *pipiens* has not been described in Australia. On the other hand, Dobrotworsky's statements that some Australian autogenous strains are sterile (probably incompatible) with one another and that *australicus* is sterile in one direction with both *quinquefasciatus* and autogenous *pipiens* suggest that there have been several introductions of *C. pipiens* forms into Australia from different areas. There is another *pipiens* form in Australia, *globocoxitus*, which must be considered indigenous since the male has peculiar genitalia which have not been observed elsewhere. Irving-Bell (1974) suggests that *australicus* and *globocoxitus* are both indigenous to Australia since they are infected by a hereditary virus rather than *Wolbachia*, which is found in all other members of the complex which have been studied (see page 351). It seems more likely that the absence of *Wolbachia* in these forms is related to the presence of the virus.

In summary, *C. pipiens* is differentiated into *quinquefasciatus* in warmer climates and typical *pipiens* in cooler climates. Where the forms come together, intermediate populations occur. The typical form may be differentiated into more-or-less autogenous and anautogenous biotypes, but this is not the case universally.

Hybridization

The literature on hybridization of forms within the *C. pipiens* complex has been reviewed elsewhere (Rozeboom and Kitzmiller, 1958). When the various forms are hybridized, in many instances, the cross is sterile. In all cases which have been investigated, however, the sterility is caused by cytoplasmic incompatibility. It appears that all of the forms in this complex (*pipiens, quinquefasciatus,* "molestus," "pallens," "australicus," etc.) are closely related genetically; there do not appear to be major, or perhaps even minor, chromosomal differences between them. Maps of the salivary gland chromosomes have been prepared for *quinquefasciatus* (Sharma *et al.,* 1969; Kanda, 1970) and the autogenous form of *pipiens* (Dennhöfer, 1968; Tewfik and Barr, 1974), and no chromosomal differences have been found which could be related to subspecies. Generally speaking, all forms in the *pipiens* complex seem to be genetically compatible with one another, except for crosses in which cytoplasmic incompatibility occurs. The various names applied in the scientific literature to this complex are summarized in Table 1.

Cytoplasmic Incompatibility

Marshall and Staley (1937) first observed crosses of *pipiens* forms in which insemination occurred, but nonviable eggs were laid. These observations were extended by Laven [reviewed in Laven (1967b)], who showed that in such crosses many of the nonhatching eggs evidenced some development, and these were laid by inseminated females. Uninseminated females lay eggs which evidence no development at all [but see Kitzmiller (1959)]. Laven, in a series of "genome-replacement" experiments, showed that the crossing potentiality of an individual was the same as that of its mother and was not influenced by that of its father. Crossing potentiality

TABLE 1. *Names Most Commonly Used in the Culex pipiens Complex*

Name	Form
pipiens Linnaeus, 1758	Temperate form
quinquefasciatus Say, 1823	Tropical form
fatigans Wiedemann, 1828	Synonym of *quinquefasciatus*
australicus Dobrotworsky & Drummond, 1953	Intermediate form in Australia
molestus Forskål, 1775	Autogenous *pipiens*
autogenicus Roubaud, 1935	Synonym of *molestus*
berbericus Roubaud, 1935	Synonym of *molestus*
sternopallidus Roubaud, 1945	Synonym of *molestus*
sternopunctatus Roubaud, 1945	Synonym of *molestus*
pallens Coquillett, 1898	Intermediate form in Asia
dipseticus Dyar and Knab, 1909	Intermediate form in North Amerca
comitatus Dyar and Knab, 1909	Intermediate form in North America
calloti Rioux and Pech, 1959	Synonym of *molestus?*

was therefore demonstrated to be inherited through the cytoplasm of the female and not through the chromosomes. No satisfactory genetic explanation has been offered for this phenomenon [see for example McClelland (1967)]. Hertig (1936) has shown, however, that the gonads of *C. pipiens* are abundantly supplied with a rickettsialike microorganism, *Wolbachia pipientis,* and it has been suggested that these organisms, which occur only in *C. pipiens* (wide sense) and are transmitted only transovarially, are the cause of incompatibility (Yen and Barr, 1973). Removal of the organisms from the male abolishes all incompatibility reactions of the male.

Parthenogenesis

In incompatible crosses an occasional larva is produced (Laven, 1967*b*). These exceptional larvae have been shown to contain no genetic material from the male and so are parthenogenetic. Parthenogenesis is known only in incompatible crosses and is therefore said to be induced [but see Kitzmiller (1959)].

The Rearing of *Culex* in the Laboratory

Rearing of *C. pipiens* has been described in the manuals by Trembley (1955) and Gerberg (1970) and by DeMeillon and Thomas (1966) and Chapman and Barr (1969). Mass rearing was described by Gerberg *et al.* (1969).

C. *pipiens* offers some advantages and some disadvantages over other mosquitoes for genetic studies. Colonies may be maintained autogenously, so that a blood source is not required. The eggs are laid in a raft; a raft therefore, contains eggs laid by a single female, and in most instances the female mates but once (Kitzmiller and Laven, 1958). A raft, therefore, usually represents the progeny of a single pair mating. Adults may usually be kept in very small cages, although some strains do not mate well in such restricted quarters. If natural light cycles are utilized, this difficulty can frequently be overcome. Larvae of C. *pipiens* are usually rather tolerant of polluted water and so are reared more easily in the laboratory than are those of many other mosquitoes.

On the other hand, no stage of C. *pipiens* can be stored for any length of time; unfed adults can be kept for a month or so, but subsequent blood feeding is not certain. Adults of C. *pipiens* frequently feed poorly on blood, even when all precautions are observed; this limits their usefulness in studies which require blood feeding.

Chromosomes

In C. *pipiens,* as in all mosquitoes, the diploid number of chromosomes is six, although most body cells appear to have only three chromosomes because of close pairing of the homologs. In anaphase, 3 pairs of metacentric chromosomes may be seen to pass to each cell. One pair of chromosomes, that associated with sex determination (Jost and Laven, 1971; Dennhöfer, 1972), is markedly shorter than the other two. The two pairs of autosomes differ only slightly in length and probably cannot be distinguished reliably, except in salivary gland preparations. Chromosomes have been studied in cells of the brain, nerves, body wall, Malpighian tubules, imaginal discs, gut, ovary, testis, and in cells in culture.

Polyploidy

Holt (1917) found that the gut cells became polyploid in pupae and afterward disintegrated. Moffett (1936) described occasional tetraploid spermatocytes. Berger (1937) found that the cells of the ileum are polyploid in pupae, but these cells divide rapidly at metamorphosis so that ploidy is reduced (somatic reduction). Rai (1963) saw a few polyploid cells in the brains of larvae.

Giant Chromosomes

Giant polytene chromosomes occur in the salivary gland and Malpighian tubules of larvae. Usually no chromocenter is seen. The salivary gland chromosomes are difficult to examine because they have many cross connections and do not spread easily. However, chromosome maps have been prepared by several investigators [reviewed by Tewfik and Barr (1974)].

A list of *C. pipiens* mutants is given in Table 2.

Chromosomal abnormalities have not been found commonly in *C. pipiens*. None were found by Kitzmiller (1956), Dennhöfer (1968), or Kanda (1970). Kuzoe *et al.* (1966) described chromosome fragments in the testes which may be the result of crossing over within inversions.

Chromosomal abnormalities have been induced by irradiation. Laven (1969) described 7 translocations which involved the sex-determining chromosome. Laven and Jost (1971) claim that after irradiation, translocations are 2 or more times as frequent in *C. pipiens* as in *Drosophila*, perhaps because of the longer chromosomes of the former. Dennhöfer (1972) showed by translocation analysis that the smallest chromosome was the sex-determining one, and that chromosomes 2 and 3 were associated with linkage groups 2 and 3, respectively. She found a radiation-induced pericentric inversion in chromosome 2. A deletion has been found in the sex chromosome in an irradiated stock and a paracentric inversion has been found in a stock of uncertain history (Tewfik and Barr, unpublished). Sweeny (1972) described a factor which causes breakage of the female-determining chromosome during spermatogenesis. This causes a deficiency of female-determining sperm and an excess of males in the progeny.

Sex Determination

There are no heterochromosomes in *C. pipiens* or in other Culicine mosquitoes. Gilchrist and Haldane (1947) showed that sex determination could be explained by assuming that maleness is produced by a dominant (*M*). A male heterozygous for *w* (white-eye) transmits this trait preferentially to his female offspring if he received it from his mother; or to his male offspring if he received it from his father. A female heterozygote, on the other hand, transmits *w* equally to her male and female offspring. In the male *w* showed recombination with *M* in 6.3 percent of the offspring.

TABLE 2.   *Mutants of Culex pipiens*

Symbol	Description	Reference
a^1, a^2, a^3	Autogeny; spontaneous; codominants; chromosome 3; controlled by alleles at D locus on chromosome 1	Aslamkhan and Laven (1970)
Ant	Reduced or clubbed antenna; spontaneous (?); dominant; chromosome 2; full penetrance; slight variation in expression; lethal when homozygous; adult	Laven (1967a), Aslamkhan and Laven (1970)
ani	Interrupted anal vein; spontaneous; inheritance not worked out; seen only in males; variably expressive; adult	VandeHey (1969)
b	Bleached; spontaneous; recessive; chromosome 1; incompletely penetrant; variably expressive; affects all stages	McClelland (unpublished)
ba	Broken antenna; spontaneous; recessive; chromosome 2; incomplete penetrance; variably expressive; sex-influenced expression; partially lethal; pupa, adult	VandeHey (1969), Barr (unpublished)
Bl	Black head capsulse (larva); spontaneous; dominant; chromosome 1; fully penetrant; sex-influenced expression; larva	VandeHey (1967)
c	Intersex; spontaneous; recessive; sex limited; chromosome 1; incompletely penetrant; variably expressive; pupa, adult (female)	Barr (unpublished)
cu_1	Interrupted cu_1 (wing vein); x-ray induced	Kitzmiller (1958)
cus	Cubital scales; x-ray induced; recessive (?); autosomal (?); completely penetrant; sex-influenced expression; associated with *sch*; adult; lost	Kitzmiller (1958)

TABLE 2. Continued

Symbol	Description	Reference
D, d^+	Autogeny control gene (autogeny dominant over anautogeny); spontaneous; dominant; chromosome 1; expression of autogeny conditioned by *a* alleles on chromosome 3; adult	Aslamkhan and Laven (1970)
de	Divided-eye; spontaneous (?); recessive; chromosome 1; incompletely penetrant; variably expressive; larva, pupa, adult	Barr (1969)
di	Sex ratio distorter; spontaneous (?); recessive; chromosome 1; incompletely penetrant (?); variably expressive (?); sex limited (male); adult	Sweeny (1972)
du	Dunkel (dark); recessive; spontaneous (?); chromosome 2; completely penetrant; larva; not allelic with *mel* or *Bl*	Dennhöfer (1973)
Est^4, Est^5	Esterases; spontaneous; codominants; autosomal; complete penetrance; variably expressive (?); adult	Garnett and French (1971)
et	Enlarged tergum; spontaneous; recessive; chromosome 2; incompletely penetrant; variably expressive; pupa	Barr and Narang (1972)
g	Green; spontaneous; probably polyfactorial, one component is *yg*; dominant to *y*; chromosome 2; said to be fully penetrant; variably expressive; larva, pupa	Huff (1929*a*), Laven (1957)
Gd	Gold; spontaneous; dominant, lethal when homozygous; chromosome 2; fully penetrant; variably expressive (?); adult	McClelland and Smithson (1968)
gyn	Gynander (sex mosaic; binucleate egg?); spontaneous; recessive (polyfactorial?); autosomal (?); adult; lost	Laven (1957, 1967*a*)

TABLE 2. Continued

Symbol	Description	Reference
4j	Four-jointed (female maxillary palp); x-ray induced; recessive; autosomal; completely penetrant (?); sex limited (female); variably expressive; associated with *sch*; adult; lost	Kitzmiller (1958)
kfl	Short-wing (kurzflügelig); spontaneous; recessive; chromosome 2; completely penetrant; variably expressive; adult	Laven (1957)
kps	Clubbed palp symmetrical (male); x-ray induced; recessive (semidominant ?); chromosome 3; incompletely penetrant; variably expressive; sex-limited (male); adult	Laven (1955*b*, 1957), Kitzmiller (1958), Dennhöfer (1972), Tadano and Barr (unpublished)
Kpu	Clubbed palp unsymmetrical (male); x-ray induced; dominant; chromosome 1; incompletely penetrant; variably expressive; partially lethal; sex limited (male); adult; lost	Laven (1955*b*, 1957), Kitzmiller (1958)
Kuf	Short-wing (kurzflügelkeit); spontaneous; dominant; autosomal (3?); complete penetrance; adult	Laven (1957)
l¹	Sex-linked lethal; x-ray induced (?); recessive; homozygote dies as embryo; complete penetrance (?); may be a deletion in the sex chromosome	Barr and Tewfik (unpublished)
la	Curved larval antenna; spontaneous; recessive; chromosome 2; complete penetrance; variably expressive; larva, pupa; lethal	Barr and Myers (1966*b*)

TABLE 2. *Continued*

Symbol	Description	Reference
lh	Larval head (pupa does not shed larval head capsule); spontaneous; recessive (?), perhaps polyfactorial; chromosome 1 (?); variably expressive; pupa; lethal	Barr (unpublished)
M	Maleness; spontaneous; dominant; chromosome 1; complete penetrance; no variation in expression; larva, pupa, adult	Gilchrist and Haldane (1947)
m_3	Proximal m_3 wing vein missing; x-ray induced; recessive (?); lost	Kitzmiller (1958)
mar	Maroon-eye; spontaneous; recessive; chromosome 1; complete penetrance; no variation in expression; larva, pupa, adult	Barr (unpublished)
mel	Melanotic; spontaneous; recessive; chromosome 3; complete penetrance; slight variation in expression; lethal; larva, pupa	Kitzmiller (1953), Laven and Chen (1956), Tadano and Barr (unpublished)
mi	Interrupted m_3 and r_2 wing veins; spontaneous (?); probably polyfactorial; incompletely penetrant; variably expressive; adult; lost	Laven (1957, 1967a), Vandehey (1969)
p	Pigmented-paddle; spontaneous; recessive; chromosome 2; complete penetrance; no variation in expression; pupa; partially lethal	Cheng (1972)
Pfl	Scale patch on male palp; x-ray induced; semidominant; chromosome 3 (?) (probably coupled with *kps* and *sch*); incompletely penetrant; variably expressive; sex-limited (male); adult; lost	Laven (1957)

TABLE 2. *Continued*

Symbol	Description	Reference
Pgm^A, Pgm^B, Pgm^C	Phosphoglucomutases; spontaneous; codominants; autosomal; complete penetrance; adult	Bullini *et al.* (1971)
pl	Plum-eye; spontaneous; recessive; chromosome 3; incompletely penetrant; variably expressive; larva, pupa, adult; partially lethal	Barr (unpublished)
r	Red-eye; spontaneous; recessive; chromosome 1; complete penetrance; variably expressive; embryo, larva, pupa, adult	Wild (1963), Spinner (1964), Laven (1967a), Barr (1969)
R_2	Fused r_2 and r_3 wing veins (closed radial cell); x-ray induced; dominant (?); chromosome 1 (?); incomplete penetrance; variably expressive; sex-influenced expression; adult; lost	Kitzmiller (1958)
Rap	Reduced antennae, palpi; X-ray induced; dominant; chromosome 2 (?); complete penetrance; no variation in expression; lethal when homozygous; adult	Laven (1955b, 1957)
ru	Ruby-eye; spontaneous; recessive; chromosome 2; complete penetrance; no variation in expression; larva, pupa, adult	Iltis *et al.* (1965) McClelland and Smithson (1968), Barr and Narang (1972), Dennhöfer (1972)
Sch (sch)	Scale row (schuppenreihe); x-ray induced; semidominant (?); chromosome 3 (?); incompletely penetrant (?); variably expressive; adult; lost	Laven (1957), Kitzmiller (1958)
Spot	Black scales on *r-m*; x-ray induced; semidominant (?); chromosome 1 (?); incomplete penetrance (?); sex-influenced expression; adult; lost	Kitzmiller (1958)

TABLE 2. *Continued*

Symbol	Description	Reference
var	Verschmelzung der Adern in Bereich des Radius, fusion of r_3 and r_{4+5}; x-ray induced; recessive; chromosome 1; complete penetrance; variably expressive; adult	Laven (1955*b*, 1957)
w	White-eye; spontaneous; recessive; chromosome 1; complete penetrance; no variation in expression; epistatic over *r* and *ru*; larva, pupa; adult	Gilchrist and Haldane (1947), Wild (1963), Seal (1966), Laven (1967*a*), Bhalla (1968), Tadano (1969*b*)
y	Yellow fat body; spontaneous; semidominant; chromosome 2; complete penetrance; variably expressive; late larva, pupa	Laven (1957), Umino (1965), Iltis *et al.* (1965), McClelland and Smithson (1968), Barr and Narang (1972)
yg	Yellow-green; modifier, when homozygous turns wild-type fat-body color bright green	Barr (unpublished)
y^l	Yellow fat body (sex-linked); spontaneous; recessive; chromosome 1; complete penetrance; variably expressive; late larva, pupa; partially lethal	Barr (unpublished)
zwi	Intersex (zwitterfaktor); spontaneous; chromosome 3; complete penetrance (?); variably expressive; sex-limited (male); adult	Laven (1955*a*, 1957)

Intersexes

Laven (1955*a*) described zwitter (*zwi*), a recessive, autosomal (linkage group 3), incompletely penetrant, sex-limited factor which feminizes males. Barr (unpublished) has found a recessive, sex-linked, incompletely penetrant, sex-limited factor (*c*) which masculinizes females.

Sex Mosaics

"Gynandromorphs" have been found commonly in *C. pipiens* as well as in other mosquitoes [reviewed by Brust (1966)]. Mosaics may be produced for a variety of sex-linked or autosomal characteristics as well as for sex: white-eye (*w*), maroon-eye (*mar*), and ruby-eye (*ru*). The most likely explanation for these is polyspermy. It is possible to mark male-determining sperm with wild-type eye and female-determining sperm with white-eye and look for black–white-eye mosaics in the offspring of *w* females; most such eye mosaics are also sex mosaics (Barr, unpublished). Laven (1967*a*) also mentions mosaics of the melanotic (*mel*) and short-wing (*Kuf*) autosomal mutants.

Spermatogenesis

Spermatogenesis has been described by Lomen (1914), Taylor (1914), Whiting (1917), and Moffett (1936). Multiplication of spermatogonial cells takes place mostly in young larvae, meiosis in older larvae and pupae. The testis is not divided into well-defined sperm cysts. In meiosis I each of the three tetrads ordinarily has 1 or more chiasmata, which indicates crossing over between the homologs. The sex-determining tetrad frequently divides precociously. The secondary spermatocytes are about two-thirds as large as the primary spermatocytes.

The testes are infected with a symbiote, *Wolbachia pipientis,* which appears to cause a certain amount of pathology (Lomen, 1914; Whiting, 1917; Yen and Barr, 1974). Gonial cells destroyed at this stage are probably not replaceable but represent a loss in reproductive capacity of the male. The testes of aposymbiotic males have not been studied.

Pätau (1941) concluded from an analysis of Moffett's (1936) data that the formation of a chiasma in a tetrad tended to suppress the formation of a second chiasma in that tetrad. Callan and Montalenti (1947) confirmed these findings and pointed out that interference seemed to operate across the centromere. The latter workers produced evidence that the degree of interference varied significantly from one individual to another. This is another way of saying that the frequency of recombination varied from one individual to another. The variation in recombination frequency seen in this species is very large, which makes genetic mapping rather uncertain. This variation has been noted in cytological preparations by Moffett (1936) and Callan and Montalenti (1947), and in genetic data by Gilchrist and Haldane (1947), Iltis *et al.* (1965), McClelland and Smithson (1968), Barr (1969), and Barr and Narang (1972).

Sanders and Barr (1966) found more variation in recombination ratios between males than in progenies sired by a single male.

Oogenesis

The developing ovarian follicle contains an oocyte and 7 nurse cells. When the oocyte is completely developed, it passes, posterior end first, into a lateral and then the common oviduct. According to Nath (1925), meiosis begins before oviposition but is probably not completed until after the egg is laid. The egg is probably fertilized as it passes the opening of the spermathecal duct. At fertilization the egg nucleus lies at the middle of the egg [Taylor (1917), but see Nath (1925)]. The sperm enters the egg and moves, tail and all, down into the egg. It passes through a mass of symbiotes just under the micropyle (Yen and Barr, 1973). The tail of the sperm has 2 rodlike mitochondria, which probably supply the energy required for moving the sperm head through the egg. Polyspermy is not uncommon; Davis (1967) says that each egg usually receives 6–10 sperm, but Jost (1970) says that usually only 1 or 2 sperm enter an egg.

The meiotic divisions probably occur after fertilization of the egg, according to Nath (1925) and Davis (1967). Eggs laid by virgin females invariably show no development at all [but see Kitzmiller (1959)]. According to Nath (1925), fertilization in a cytological sense does not occur until half an hour after oviposition, but segmentation nuclei have been seen an hour after oviposition. Yen and Barr (1973) present evidence which suggests that the symbiotes facilitate meiosis. Aposymbiotic strains are seen to have a greatly reduced reproductive capacity, many eggs in their rafts showing no development even though laid by inseminated females. Aposymbiotic females when mated with normal (symbiotic) males lay eggs which usually show no development at all, their egg rafts being similar to those laid by virgin females. Rarely an egg from such a raft shows some development and very rarely may even produce a larva. These findings suggest that symbiotes in the testis of the male change sperm in such a way that they are no longer capable of inducing meiosis in eggs; it has, however, not been proved that the sperm actually enter the eggs.

Eye-Color Mutants

Wild-type *C. pipiens* have black larval and adult eyes. In adults there is usually a metallic sheen which varies from greenish to violet. The first good mutant described in this species was white-eye (*w*) (Gilchrist and Haldane, 1947). This spontaneous mutant was found in England. Subsequently it has been found in Germany (Wild, 1963), Japan (Tadano, 1969*b*), Louisiana (Seal, 1966), and Brazil (Rai, private communication). It results in a complete lack of pigmentation in the eyes of larvae and adults. It can also be detected in unhatched embryos and in pupae. Red-eye (*r*) was discovered in an irradiated strain from Germany by Wild (1963), but Spinner (1964) found it in an unirradiated subline of the same strain. It affects larval and adult eyes and can be detected in pupae and, with some difficulty, in embryos as well. It varies in expression from scarlet to almost colorless but is typically pale red. Ruby-eye (*ru*) was described as a spontaneous mutant in a strain from Dixon, California (Iltis *et al.*, 1965) and has subsequently been found in Brazil (Bhalla, private communication). It affects larval and adult eyes. In larvae the eyes are a dark brick-red and in the later instars can be easily distinguished from wild-type eyes, which are black. In first instars and embryos the distinction is difficult. Young adults have red or brown eyes, which later darken and may be confused with wild-type eyes. Maroon-eye (*mar*) has not been previously described. It was isolated as a spontaneous mutant from a strain from Lake Charles, Louisiana. It is closely sex-linked and can be distinguished in later-instar larvae and pupae. Plum-eye (*pl*) is another undescribed spontaneous mutant isolated from a strain from Dixon, California. It can be detected in late-instar larvae and pupae. Individuals homozygous for *pl* have reduced viability. In preliminary linkage experiments *pl* shows about 40 percent recombination with *kps* (clubbed palp symmetrical) and is thus a useful marker, since it is in the third linkage group.

All of these eye-color mutants are recessive to wild type. Usually a single, wild-type gene is sufficient to produce full pigmentation of the eyes, but in some strains heterozygous individuals may have lighter eyes and thus resemble maroon-eye homozygotes.

Spinner (1964) found that wild-type eyes contained isoxanthopterin, riboflavin, sepiapterin, and HB-pterine; *r* individuals contained all of these and another material, perhaps erythropterin. Bhalla (1968), on the other hand, found that wild-type *pipiens* contained compound A, flavin mononucleotide, 2 amino-4-hydroxypteridine, sepiapterin, biopterin, and compound B; *r* individuals contained all of these but compound B; *ru* individuals contained all but biopterin and compound B; and *w* individuals contained none of these. The block in pigment synthesis in *w* individuals prevents the formation of all eye pigments, so *w* is epistatic over *r* and *ru*. Dennhöfer (1971*b*) says that *r* is epistatic over *ru*; wild-type and *r* individuals contained both an ommochrome and sepiapterin 1, while *w* individuals contained neither.

Mutations Affecting Cuticular Pigmentation

A pale-skinned mutant, bleached (*b*), has been described by Mc-Clelland (unpublished) in a strain from Dixon, California. It is sex linked and affects all stages: eggs, larvae, pupae, and adults. VandeHey (1967) described *Bl* (pigmented head capsule) a spontaneous mutant in a strain from Germany. It is sex linked, completely dominant in males, partially dominant in females, and is associated with slowed development. Kitzmiller (1953) described the melanotic (*mel*) mutant as a spontaneous mutant with dark pigmentation in the epidermis in a strain from Illinois. It affects larvae and pupae and is lethal; most homozygotes die as fourth-instar larvae. Laven and Chen (1956) found by paper chromatography a reduced amino acid content in melanotic individuals. Tadano (unpublished) showed that this recessive gene was in the third linkage group. McClelland and Smithson (1968) described the Gold (*Gd*) mutant, which lightens adults. This dominant is lethal in early larvae when homozygous; it is in the second linkage group. Dennhöfer (1973) described the dunkel (*du*) mutant, a completely penetrant recessive in linkage group 2. Cheng (1972) described the pigmented-paddle (*p*) mutant from a mongrel laboratory strain. It also darkens the integument and is most readily detected in pupae. It is a completely penetrant recessive, but adults do not fly well, and females oviposit with difficulty. Like *du*, it is in linkage group 2 and rather distant from *ru*. Crosses of *p* and *du* must be done to see if they are allelic.

Mutants Affecting Fat-Body Pigmentation

C. pipiens larvae are normally a dark violet color in the field; in laboratory colonies they are usually violet or bluish green. The yellow fat body (*y*) has been described by Ghelelovitch (1950), Laven (1957), Spielman (1957), Iltis *et al.* (1965), and Umino (1965). It is expressed as an orange body color in late fourth-instar larvae and pupae, is completely penetrant, and recessive. Umino (1965) was not able to identify useful subtypes of yellow. A second type of pale larva (*y'*), which is closely sex linked, has been isolated from a mongrel laboratory strain (Barr, unpublished). It is easily confused with *y* and has reduced viability. Green larvae have been described by Huff (1929*a*), Ghelelovitch (1950), and Laven (1957). Huff (1929*a*) found that green was recessive to brown. Ghelelovitch (1950) found that green was dominant over yellow. Laven (1957) found that green was incompletely dominant over yellow. We have selected for green, blue, and violet and found that none of these colors responded to selection. A green strain from Germany, courtesy of Dr. Laven, yielded a factor (*yg*) which turned *y* homozygotes greenish. This factor when introduced into wild-type strains produced bright green individuals which bred true. It appears that dominance is lacking among these fat-body-pigment genes, and all could be detected in the heterozygous state by proper analytical methods.

Mutations Affecting Adult Characters

Kitzmiller (1958) described a number of antennal variants seen in x-irradiated adults: moniliform-antennae, stunted-antennae, and withered-antennae; the short-antenna mutation was seen only in males, and fused-antennae was thought to be a recessive. The deformed-head phenotype might not have been heritable. Several palpal variants were seen: naked-palp, clubbed-palp, and hooked-palp (which was thought to be a dominant). The clavate-palp and wart-palp mutations were seen only in males and were thought to be recessive. The bent-wing, blister-wing, and curled-wing-tip mutations were thought not to be heritable. The shortened-wing mutation was perhaps a sex mosaic. The curled hind tarsi mutation may not be heritable. The flared-abdominal-sternites mutation also was x-ray induced.

Kitzmiller (1953) described a wings-held-out mutation which was spontaneous and perhaps polyfactorial; it interfered with normal flight. Laven (1957) described a double wing vein fusion (r_{2+3} and m_{2+3}) which was x-ray induced, recessive (?), and sex influenced.

Ghelelovitch (1950) found that dark scales on sternites (punctation) was incompletely dominant over pale scales on sternites and was not sex linked. Since punctation was also inherited independently of *y*, it should be in linkage group 3.

The behavior of characters of the male genitalia in crosses is discussed by Barr and Kartman (1951) and Iltis (1970), among others.

Lethal Mutations

A number of lethals have been described, including *Ant*, *Gd*, *l¹*, *la*, *lh*, *mel*, and *Rap*. In addition, Barr and Myers (1971) described the female-lethal mutation which killed practically all females as embryos; its inheritance was not worked out, and the trait was subsequently lost. The distorter mutation, described by Sweeny (1972), resulted in the elimination of female-determining sperms. A number of traits are partially lethal.

Behavior of Larval Characters in Crosses

The behavior of a number of larval characteristics of taxonomic significance has been studied in crosses: number of teeth on mentum (Callot, 1947), subdorsal hairs (Kitzmiller, 1953), pecten teeth (Buck, 1935), siphonal index (Callot, 1947; Kitzmiller, 1953; Ishii, 1969), siphonal tufts (Callot, 1947; Ishii, 1971 and earlier).

Chromosome 1 (Linkage Group 1)

This is the smallest of the three chromosomes and is involved in sex determination, according to Jost and Laven (1971), Dennhöfer (1972), and Sweeny (1972). Other mutants in linkage group 1 are *b, Bl, c, D, de, di, Kpu, l', lh*(?), *mar, r, R₂*(?), *Spot, var, w,* and *y'*. Only a few of these mutants have been mapped. It would appear that the correct order of loci is *de-r-M-b-w-c*, the estimated interlocal distances being 0.30, 0.01, 0.016, 0.02, and 0.025. Thus, *de* is well removed from the other loci, which are all close together.

McClelland (unpublished) has found that there is about 20 percent recombination between *r* and *b* in females, but only about 2–4 percent in males; in both sexes, however, there is about 2–4 percent recombination between *b* and *w*.

Tewfik (unpublished) has found a deletion in the right arm of chromosome 1 which is close to the centromere and involves about 12 percent of the length of the chromosome. The deletion, although very large, is not lethal in heterozygotes but probably is in homozygotes. It is likely that the deletion is the same as the mutation *l'*. Genetically this factor appears to be very close to the sex locus, so the sex locus seems to be fairly close to the centromere.

Chromosome 2 (Linkage Group 2)

Dennhöfer (1972) found that the middle-length chromosome was associated with *ru*. Other mutants in this linkage group are *Ant, ba, du, et, g*(?), *Gd, kfl, la, p, Rap*(?), and *y*, as well as resistance to DDT *(DDT)*, malathion *(MR)*, fenthion *(FR)*, abate *(RAbT)*, and fenitrothion *(RS)*. The correct order of genes seems to be *MR-FR-ru-y-p-et-Gd-DDT*, the interlocal distances being 0.13, 0.48, 0.20, 0.04, 0.14(?), 0.04(?), and 0.01. The genes for abate resistance and fenitrothion resistance *(RAbT, RS)* are close to *MR*; *la* is close to *y*. Iltis *et al.* (1965) found that recombination between *y* and *ru* was significantly higher (0.07) in females than in males. McClelland and Smithson (1968) also found significantly more recombination between y and ru in females (0.238) than in males (0.172), but recombination between y and Gd did not differ significantly in the two sexes (0.216). Cheng (1972) also found significantly more recombination between y and ru in females (0.279) than in males (0.167). Dorval and Brown (1970), on the other hand, found substantially more recombination between y and ru (0.08) and between fenthion-resistance and y (0.027) in males than in females. Dennhöfer (1972) found a pericentric inversion in an irradiated strain. Tewfik (unpublished) has found a paracentric inversion in the right arm which involves about 18.1 percent of the length of the arm.

Chromosome 3 (Linkage Group 3)

Dennhöfer (1972) found that the longest chromosome was associated with kps. Other mutants in linkage group 3 are a, Kuf, mel, $Pfl(?)$, pl, Sch, and zwi. The locus pl is about 40.2 crossover units from kps (unpublished). Dennhöfer (1971a) found that the factors conferring susceptibility or resistance to infection with *Plasmodium cathemerium* are in this linkage group.

Physiological Genetics

The inheritance of autogeny has been most effectively studied by Spielman (1957) and Aslamkhan and Laven (1970). Spielman found that autogeny could be best explained by 3 factors, inherited on the sex chromosome and one of the autosomes, no dominance being involved. Aslamkhan and Laven (1970), on the other hand, found that autogeny was controlled by two loci, the D locus on the sex chromosome and the a locus on chromosome 3. D, which conferred autogeny, was dominant over d which produced anautogeny when homozygous. Three alleles were described at the a locus, various combinations of which produced autogeny or anautogeny.

The esterases of *C. pipiens* have been studied by Garnett and French (1971). Two major bands, Est^4 and Est^5, appear to be controlled by 2 co-dominant alleles at the same locus, which was on one of the autosomes. Bullini *et al.* (1971) described three bands of phosphoglucomutases which appeared to be controlled by 3 codominant alleles at a single locus; in a wild population in Rome, combinations of the three alleles occurred according to their Hardy-Weinberg expectations.

The Genetics of Insecticide Resistance

Tadano and Brown (1967) showed that DDT resistance was inherited as a dominant on chromosome 2; dieldrin resistance was inherited as a partial dominant on chromosome 3. Suzuki and Umino (1969) found that diazinon resistance was inherited as a partial dominant. Tadano (1969a) found that malathion resistance was inherited as a partial dominant on chromosome 2. Fenthion resistance (1969c) was not allelic with malathion resistance but was also in linkage group 2. Abate resistance (1970) was not allelic with either fenthion or malathion resistance but was also in linkage group 2.

Inheritance of Susceptibility to Parasites

Huff (1929b) found that 11–41 percent of the females of a laboratory strain were susceptible to infection with *Plasmodium cathemerium*. By familial selection he was able to increase the susceptibility of some strains to 50–70 percent and to decrease the susceptibility of other strains to 0 percent. In a later paper (1931) he said that in crosses, susceptibility was inherited as a recessive.

Dennhöfer (1971a) also studied the inheritance of susceptibility to infection with *P. cathemerium*. He produced lines completely susceptible and completely refractory to infection. Susceptibility was inherited as a semidominant in the third linkage group.

Partono and Oemijati (1970), in Indonesia, found that 71.2 percent of a strain of *quinquefasciatus* from the field were susceptible to infection with a strain of periodic *Wuchereria bancrofti*. Three generations of selection for susceptibility or refractoriness did not alter the proportion susceptible appreciably (83.3 percent and 68.9 percent, respectively). Thomas and Ramachandran (1970), on the other hand, did similar studies in Malaysia with an *Anopheles*-transmitted strain. Strains of *quinquefasciatus* from various areas showed susceptibility rates of 7–28 percent. Two strains were selected for susceptibility for 6 generations. In one strain susceptibility rose from 7 percent to 54 percent and in the other it increased from 20 percent to 100 percent.

Zielke (1973) found that 4.8–17.6 percent of the Rangoon strain of *quinquefasciatus* were susceptible to infection with *Dirofilaria immitis*. Selection for susceptibility for 9 generations increased the proportion to 44.8 percent. In a parallel strain selected for resistance, only 2.2 percent were susceptible after 8 generations.

The Genetics of Related Species

Culex tritaeniorhynchus

C. tritaeniorhynchus has 3 pairs of chromosomes (Baker and Aslamkhan, 1969). The smallest pair (1) is associated with sex determination, as has been shown by the study of pericentric inversions (Baker *et al.*, 1971*a*) and translocations (Sakai *et al.*, 1971). The two pairs of autosomes are longer and approximately equal in length. The submetacentric pair carries Rs on its short arm and has been designated chromosome 2 (Sakai *et al.*, 1971; Baker *et al.*, 1971*b*). The metacentric pair (3) presumably carries *st* and *cl*.

There is an almost complete lack of crossing over in females, so recombination values are measured in males (Baker and Rabbani, 1970). Linkage group 1 includes golden (Baker, 1968), $l(1)$ $E1$ (egg lethal), rough, white-eye (Baker, 1969), singed, w^{re}, w^{ch}, w^{D}, $l(1)2$ (lethal), maleness, and delta (Baker and Sakai, 1972). The interlocal distances tentatively assigned are 0.045, 0.056, 0.005, 0.04, 0.020, 0.005, 0.067, 0.033, 0.010, and 0.019 (Baker, 1972). The rose mutation (Baker and Sakai, 1973) is an allele at the w locus and is expressed only in w individuals; it is also codominant with w. Linkage group 2 includes the Red-spotted eye (Rabbani and Baker, 1970), ebony (Sakai *et al.*, 1972), and Alkaline phosphatase (Sakai *et al.*, 1973) loci; the distances between them are 0.355 and 0.020 (Baker, 1972). Linkage group 3 includes the straw body, alcohol dehydrogenase, and curved leg loci, the distances between them being 0.0461 and 0.1290 (Sakai *et al.*, private communication). The esterase locus (Iqbal *et al.*, 1973) is also in this linkage group (Baker, 1972). Heterogeneity of recombination data is sometimes a problem (Baker and Sakai, 1972), as in other mosquitoes. Multiple matings are uncommon (Sakai and Baker, 1972) as in other mosquitoes. Umino and Suzuki (1969) found that dieldrin resistance was inherited as an autosomal semidominant.

Culex tarsalis

M. Asman (private communication) is presently describing the mitotic and meiotic chromosomes of *C. tarsalis*. In a future paper she will describe translocations which have been induced by radiation. Barr and Myers (1966*a*) described 2 spontaneous mutants, yellow fat-body (*y*) and white-eye (*w*) in this species. The *y* mutant is sex linked and shows about 6 percent recombination with sex in males; *w* is autosomal. When *y w* individuals were crossed with *y w Culex pipiens*, three F_1 hybrids reared were yellow but had wild-type eye color. Therefore, *w* is not allelic in the two species; *y* may possibly be allelic, but since the two factors are in different linkage groups, this seems unlikely. Since *y* is a semidominant in each species, individuals heterozygous for each of the *y* genes would probably be rather yellow.

Plapp *et al.* (1961) found that resistance to malathion was dominant over susceptibility. DDT resistance, on the other hand was recessive to susceptibility. Calman and Georghiou (1970) found that malathion resistance was a semidominant trait and was not linked with *w*. It is not clear, however, whether or not malathion resistance is sex linked.

Culex nigripalpus

O'Meara (1970) found that orange and lavender-green fat-body colors are regulated by sex-linked genes.

Strain Retention Centers

Numerous strains of *C. pipiens* are maintained in the laboratories of the writer and of Prof. Hannes Laven, Institüte für Genetik, Johannes-Gutenberg Universität, Mainz, West Germany. Strains of *C. tritaeniorhynchus* are maintained in the laboratory of Dr. R. H. Baker, Pakistan Medical Research Center, Lahore, West Pakistan. Strains of *C. tarsalis* are maintained by Dr. Monica Asman, Division of Entomology, University of California, Berkeley. Strains of *C. nigripalpus* are maintained by Dr. G. F. O'Meara, Entomological Research Center, Vero Beach, Florida. Current information on mosquito genetics is reviewed in the *Information Circular on Insecticide Resistance, Insect Behaviour and Vector Genetics,* which is issued at irregular intervals by the Vector Biology and Control Unit of the World Health Organization, Geneva.

Literature Cited

Aslamkhan, M. and H. Laven, 1970 Inheritance of autogeny in the *Culex pipiens* complex. *Pak. J. Zool.* **2**:121–147.

Baker, R. H., 1968 The genetics of 'golden' (*go*), a new sex-linked colour mutant of the mosquito *Culex tritaeniorhynchus* Giles. *Ann. Trop. Med. Parasitol.* **62**:193–199.

Baker, R. H., 1969 White eye, a female-sterile and sex-linked mutant of *Culex tritaeniorhynchus. Mosq. News* **29**:571–573.

Baker, R. H., 1972 Genetics of *Culex tritaeniorhynchus*: I. Basic research. In

Japan–U.S. Cooperative Medical Science Program, Joint Conference on Parasitic Diseases, pp. 10–13.

Baker, R. H. and M. Aslamkhan, 1969   Karyotypes of some Asian mosquitoes of the subfamily Culicinae (Diptera: Culicidae). *J. Med. Entomol.* **6**:44–52.

Baker, R. H. and M. G. Rabbani, 1970   Complete linkage in females of *Culex tritaeniorhynchus* mosquitoes. *J. Hered.* **61**:59–61.

Baker, R. H. and R. K. Sakai, 1972   The genetics of *delta,* a dominant sex-linked mutant of the mosquito, *Culex tritaeniorhynchus. Can. J. Genet. Cytol.* **14**:353–361.

Baker, R. H. and R. K. Sakai, 1973   Genetics of *Rose,* an allele of the white locus in a mosquito. *J. Hered.* **64**:19–23.

Baker, R. H., R. K. Sakai and A. Mian, 1971*a*   Linkage group–chromosome correlation in *Culex tritaeniorhynchus. Science (Wash., D.C.)* **171**:585–587.

Baker, R. H., R. K. Sakai and A. Mian, 1971*b*   Linkage group–chromosome correlation in a mosquito. Inversions in *Culex tritaeniorhynchus. J. Hered.* **62**:31–36.

Barr, A. R., 1957   The distribution of *Culex p. pipiens* and *C. p. quinquefasciatus* in North America. *Am. J. Trop. Med. Hyg.* **6**:153–165.

Barr, A. R., 1967   Occurrence and distribution of the *Culex pipiens* complex. *Bull. WHO* **37**:293–297.

Barr, A. R., 1969   Divided-eye, a sex-linked mutation in *Culex pipiens* L. *J. Med. Entomol.* **6**:393–397.

Barr, A. R. and L. Kartman, 1951   Biometrical notes on the hybridization of *Culex pipiens* L. and *C. quinquefaciatus* Say. *J. Parasitol.* **37**:419–420.

Barr, A. R. and C. M. Myers, 1966*a*   Two spontaneous mutants of *Culex tarsalis* (Diptera: Culicidae). *Proc. Entomol. Soc. Wash.* **68**:49–52.

Barr, A. R. and C. M. Myers, 1966*b*   Inheritance of a lethal affecting larval antennae in *Culex pipiens* L. (Diptera: Culicidae). *J. Parasitol.* **52**:1163–1166.

Barr, A. R. and C. M. Myers, 1971   Female-lethal, a heritable factor in *Culex pipiens* L. *Mosq. News* **31**:428–434.

Barr, A. R. and S. L. Narang, 1972   The inheritance of enlarged tergum in *Culex pipiens. J. Med. Entomol.* **9**:560–563.

Bekku, H., 1956   Studies on the *Culex pipiens* group of Japan. I. Comparative studies on the morphology of those obtained from various localities in the Far East. *Nagasaki Igakkai Zassi* **31**:956–966.

Berger, C. A., 1937   Additional evidence of repeated chromosome division without mitotic activity. *Am. Nat.* **71**:187–190.

Bhalla, S. C., 1968   Genetic aspects of pteridines in mosquitoes. *Genetics* **58**:249–258.

Bhatnagar, V. N., D. Singh and N. G. S. Raghavan, 1958   A note on autogeny in *C. fatigans* Wied. *Bull. Natl. Soc. India Malariol.* **6**:125–126.

Brust, R. A., 1966   Gynandromorphs and intersexes in mosquitoes (Diptera: Culicidae). *Can. J. Zool.* **44**:911–921.

Buck, A. de, 1935   Beitrag zur Rassenfrage bei *Culex pipiens. Z. Angew. Entomol.* **22**:242–252.

Bullini, L., M. Coluzzi, A. P. Bianchi-Bullini and G. Bleiner, 1971   Phosphoglucomutase polymorphism in *Culex pipiens* (Diptera, Culicidae). *Parassitologia* **13**:439–443.

Callan, H. G. and G. Montalenti, 1947   Chiasma interference in mosquitoes. *J. Genet.* **48**:119–134.

Callot, J., 1947   Etude sur quelques souches de *Culex pipiens (sensu lato)* et sur leurs hybrides. *Ann. Parasitol. Hum. Comp.* **22**:380–393.

Calman, J. R. and G. P. Georghiou, 1970   Linkage relationships between the *white eye* mutant and malathion resistance in *Culex tarsalis* Coquillett. *J. Med. Entomol.* 7:585–588.

Chapman, H. C. and A. R. Barr, 1969   Techniques for successful colonization of many mosquito species. *Mosq. News* **29**:532–535.

Cheng, M. L., 1972   The inheritance of pigmented-paddle in *Culex pipiens*. M.Sc. Thesis, University of California, Los Angeles, Calif.

Davis, C. W. C., 1967   A comparative study of larval embryogenesis in the mosquito *Culex fatigans* Wiedemann (Diptera: Culicidae) and the sheep-fly *Lucilia sericata* Meigen (Diptera: Calliphoridae). I. Description of embryonic development. *Aust. J. Zool.* **15**:547–579.

DeMeillon, B. and V. Thomas, 1966   *Culex pipiens fatigans* Wied. In *Insect Colonization and Mass Production,* edited by C. N. Smith, pp. 101–114, Academic Press, New York.

Dennhöfer, L., 1968   Die speicheldrüsen Chromosomen der Stechmücke *Culex pipiens* I. Der normale Chromosomenbestand. *Chromosoma (Berl.)* **25**:365–376.

Dennhöfer, L., 1972   Die Zuordnung der Koppelungsgruppen zu den Chromosomen bei der Stechmücke *Culex pipiens* L. *Chromosoma (Berl.)* **37**:43–52.

Dennhöfer, L., 1973   Eine neue Larvenfarbmutation bei der Stechmücke *Culex pipiens* L. *Z. Naturforsch. Sect. B* **28**:754–756.

Dennhöfer, U., 1971*a*   Erblichkeit der Übertragungsfähigkeit bzw. Resistenz gegen Vogelmalaria bei der Stechmücke *Culex pipiens* L. *Anz. Schaedlingskd. Pflanzenschutz* **44**:84–91.

Dennhöfer, U., 1971*b*   Augenfarbmutationen bei der Stechmücke *Culex pipiens* L. -ihre chemische und genetische Ursache. *Z. Naturforsch. Sect. B* **26**:599–603.

Dobrotworsky, N. V. and F. H. Drummond, 1952   The *Culex pipiens* group in southeastern Australia. II. *Proc. Linn. Soc. N.S.W.* **78**:131–146.

Dorval, C. and A. W. A. Brown, 1970   Inheritance of resistance to fenthion in *Culex pipiens fatigans* Wied. *Bull. WHO* **43**:727–734.

Drummond, F. H., 1951   The *Culex pipiens* complex in Australia. *Trans. R. Entomol. Soc. Lond.* **102**:369–371

Garnett, P. and W. L. French, 1971   A genetic study of an esterase in *Culex pipiens quinquefasciatus*. *Mosq. News* **31**:379–386.

Gerberg, E. J., 1970   Manual for mosquito rearing and experimental techniques. *Am. Mosq. Control Assoc. Bull.* **5**:1–109.

Gerberg, E. J., T. M. Hopkins and J. W. Gentry, 1969   Mass rearing of *Culex pipiens* L. *Mosq. News* **29**:382–385.

Ghelelovitch, S., 1950   Étude génétique de deux charactères de pigmentation chez *Culex autogenicus* Roubaud. *Bull. Biol. Fr. Belg.* **84**:217–224.

Gilchrist, B. M. and J. B. S. Haldane, 1947   Sex linkage and sex determination in a mosquito, *Culex molestus*. *Hereditas* **33**:175–190.

Hertig, M., 1936   The rickettsia, *Wolbachia pipientis* (gen. et sp. n.) and associated inclusions of the mosquito, *Culex pipiens*. *Parasitology* **28**:453–486.

Holt, C. M., 1917   Multiple complexes in the alimentary tract of *Culex pipiens*. *J. Morphol.* **29**:607–618.

Huff, C. G., 1929*a*   Color inheritance in larvae of *Culex pipiens* Linn. *Biol. Bull. (Woods Hole)* **57**:172–175.

Huff, C. G., 1929*b*   The effects of selection upon susceptibility to bird malaria in *Culex pipiens* Linn. *Ann. Trop. Med. Parasitol.* **23**:427–442.

Huff, C. G., 1931   The inheritance of natural immunity to *Plasmodium cathemerium* in two species of *Culex*. *J. Prev. Med.* **5**:249–259.

Iltis, W. G., 1970   Biosystematics of the *Culex pipiens* complex in Northern California. Ph.D. Thesis, University of California, Davis, Calif.

Iltis, W. G., A. R. Barr, G. A. H. McClelland and C. M. Myers, 1965   The inheritance of yellow-larva and ruby-eye in *Culex pipiens*. *Bull. WHO* **33**:123–128.

Iqbal, M. P., R. K. Sakai and R. H. Baker, 1973   The genetics of an esterase in *Culex tritaeniorhynchus*. *Mosq. News* **33**:72–75.

Irving-Bell, R. J., 1974   Cytoplasmic factors in the gonads of *Culex pipiens* complex mosquitoes. *Life Sci.* **14**:1149–1151.

Ishii, T., 1969   On the *Culex pipiens* group in Japan, Part II, III. Selection experiment for the siphonal index of the fourth instar larvae of *Culex pipiens molestus* Forskål (Diptera, Culicidae). *Jap. J. Sanit. Zool.* **20**:177–185.

Ishii, T., 1971   On the *Culex pipiens* group in Japan, Part II, VII. Siphonal hair types from the type 5-5 population of *Culex pipiens molestus* Forskål (Diptera, Culicidae). *Jap. J. Sanit. Zool.* **22**:14–18.

Jost, E., 1970   Untersuchungen zur Inkompatibilität im *Culex pipiens*-Komplex. *Wilhelm Roux' Arch. Entwicklungsmech. Org.* **166**:173–188.

Jost, E. and H. Laven, 1971   Meiosis in translocation heterozygotes in the mosquito *Culex pipiens* (Diptera, Culicidae). *Chromosoma (Berl.)* **35**:184–205.

Kanda, T., 1970   The salivary gland chromosomes of *Culex pipiens fatigans* Wiedemann. *Jap. J. Exp. Med.* **40**:335–345.

Kitzmiller, J. B., 1953   Mosquito genetics and cytogenetics. *Rev. Bras. Malariol. Doencas Trop.* **5**:285–359.

Kitzmiller, J. B., 1956   Salivary gland chromosomes in the *Culex pipiens-molestus-fatigans* complex. *Proc. Interntl. Congr. Genet. (1954)* **9**:674–677.

Kitzmiller, J. B., 1958   X-ray induced mutation in the mosquito, *Culex fatigans*. *Exp. Parasitol.* **7**:439–462.

Kitzmiller, J. B., 1959   Parthenogenesis in *Culex fatigans*. *Science (Wash., D.C.)* **129**:837–838.

Kitzmiller, J. B. and H. Laven, 1958   Tests for multiple fertilization in *Culex* mosquitoes by the use of genetic markers. *Am. J. Hyg.* **67**:207–213.

Knight, K. L. and A. A. Malek, 1951   A morphological and biological study of *Culex pipiens* in the Cairo area of Egypt (Diptera-Culicidae). *Soc. Fouad. 1er d'Entomol. Bull.* **35**:175–185.

Kuzoe, F. A. S., J. J. B. Gill and W. W. MacDonald, 1966   Evidence of inversions in the chromosomes in the testes of *Aedes aegypti* and *Culex pipiens fatigans*. *Trans. R. Soc. Trop. Med. Hyg.* **60**:21.

Laven, H., 1955a   Erbliche Intersexualität bei *Culex pipiens*. *Naturwissenschaften* **42**:517.

Laven, H., 1955b   Strahleninduzierte Mutationen bei *Culex pipiens* L. *Z. Naturforsch. Sect. B* **10b**:320–322.

Laven, H., 1957   Vererbung durch Kerngene und das Problem der ausserkaryotischen Vererbung bei *Culex pipiens*. I. Kernvererbung. *Z. Indukt. Abstammungs-Vererbungsl.* **88**:443–477.

Laven, H., 1967a   Formal genetics of *Culex pipiens*. In *Genetics of Insect Vectors of Disease*, edited by J. W. Wright and R. Pal, pp. 17–65, Elsevier, Amsterdam.

Laven, H., 1967b   Speciation and evolution in *Culex pipiens*. In *Genetics of Insect Vec-*

tors of Disease, edited by J. W. Wright and R. Pal, pp. 251–275, Elsevier, Amsterdam.

Laven, H., 1969   Eradicating mosquitoes using translocations. *Nature (Lond.)* **221**:958–959.

Laven, H. and P. S. Chen, 1956   Genetische und papierchromatograpische Untersuchungen an einer letalen Mutante von *Culex pipiens. Z. Naturforsch. Sect. B* **11b**:273–276.

Laven, H. and E. Jost, 1971   Inherited semisterility for control of harmful insects. I. Productions of semisterility due to translocation in the mosquito, *Culex pipiens* L., by X-rays. *Experientia (Basel)* **27**:471–473.

Lockhart, W. L., W. Klassen and A. W. A. Brown, 1970   Crossover values between dieldrin-resistance and DDT-resistance and linkage-group-2 genes in *Aedes aegypti. Can. J. Genet. Cytol.* **12**:407–414.

Lomen, F., 1914   Der Hodden von *Culex pipiens* (Spermatogenese, Hodenwandungen und Degenerationen). *Jenaische Z. Naturwissenschaft.* **52**:567–628.

McClelland, G. A. H., 1967   Speciation and evolution in *Aedes.* In *Genetics of Insect Vectors of Disease,* edited by J. W. Wright and R. Pal, pp. 277–311, Elsevier, Amsterdam.

McClelland, G. A. H. and T. W. Smithson, 1968   Linkage of *Gold,* its recessive lethality and sex-related variation in crossing-over in *Culex pipiens* (Diptera: Culicidae). *Can. J. Genet. Cytol.* **10**:374–384.

McMillan, H. L., 1958   Study of a naturally occurring population intermediate between *Culex p. pipiens* and *C. p. quinquefasciatus. Am. J. Trop. Med. Hyg.* **7**:505–511.

Marshall, J. F. and J. Staley, 1937   Some notes regarding the morphological and biological differentiation of *Culex pipiens* and *Culex molestus. Proc. R. Entomol. Soc. Lond., Ser. A Gen. Entomol.* **12**:17–26.

Mattingly, P. F., 1951   The *Culex pipiens* complex. Introduction. *Trans. R. Entomol. Soc. Lond.* **102**:331–342.

Moffett, A. A., 1936   The origin and behaviour of chiasmata. XIII. Diploid and tetraploid *Culex pipiens. Cytologia (Tokyo)* **7**:184–197.

Nath, V., 1925   Egg follicle of *Culex. Quart. J. Microscop. Sci.* **69**:151 175, 2 pl.

O'Meara, G. F., 1970   The inheritance of fat body pigmentation in *Culex nigripalpus. Entomol. Soc. Am., Program 1970 Meet.*: 61.

Partono, F. and S. Oemijati, 1970   Susceptibility of *Culex pipiens fatigans* to *Wuchereria bancrofti* in Djakarta, Indonesia. *Southeast Asian J. Trop. Med. Public Health* **1**:516–518.

Pätau, K., 1941   Cytologischer Nachweis einer positiven Interferenz über das Centromer (Der Paarungskoeffizient. I). *Chromosoma (Berl.)* **2**:36–63.

Plapp, F. W. Jr., D. E. Borgard, D. I. Darrow and G. W. Eddy, 1961   Studies on the inheritance of resistance to DDT and to malathion in the mosquito *Culex tarsalis* Coq. *Mosq. News* **21**:315–319.

Rabbani, M. and R. H. Baker, 1970   Red-spotted eye in the mosquito. An autosomal, conditionally codominant mutant. *J. Hered.* **61**:134–138.

Rai, K. S., 1963   A comparative study of mosquito karyotypes. *Ann. Entomol. Soc. Am.* **56**:160–170.

Rozeboom, L. E. and J. B. Kitzmiller, 1958   Hybridization and speciation in mosquitoes. *Annu. Rev. Entomol.* **3**:231–248.

Sakai, R. K. and R. H. Baker, 1972   A method for detecting and measuring concealed variability in the mosquito, *Culex tritaeniorhynchus. Genetics* **71**:287–296.

Sakai, R. K., R. H. Baker and A. Mian, 1971   Linkage group–chromosome correlation in a mosquito. Translocations in *Culex tritaeniorhynchus*. *J. Hered.* **62**:90–100.

Sakai, R. K., R. H. Baker and M. P. Iqbal, 1972   Genetics of *ebony*, a nonlethal recessive melanotic mutant in a mosquito. *J. Hered.* **63**:275–279.

Sakai, R. K., M. P. Iqbal and R. H. Baker, 1973   Genetics of an alkaline phosphatase in a mosquito, *Culex tritaeniorhynchus*. *Ann. Entomol. Soc. Am.* **66**:913–916.

Sanders, R. D. and A. R. Barr, 1966   Variation in crossing-over between two autosomal loci in males of *Culex pipiens*. *Exp. Parasitol.* **19**:21–24.

Sasa, M., A. Shirasaka and T. Kurihara, 1966   Crossing experiments between *fatigans, pallens* and *molestus* colonies of the mosquito *Culex pipiens s. l.* from Japan and Southern Asia, with special reference to hatchability of hybrid eggs. *Jap. J. Exp. Med.* **36**:187–210.

Seal, C. W., 1966   A white-eyed mutant in *Culex pipiens quinquefasciatus* (Say) (Diptera: Culicidae). *Proc. La. Acad. Sci.* **29**:137–138.

Sharma, G. P., R. Parshad, S. L. Narang and P. Kaur, 1969   Salivary gland chromosomes of *Culex p. fatigans*. *Res. Bull. Panjab Univ. Sci.* **20**:541–546.

Spielman, A., 1957   The inheritance of autogeny in the *Culex pipiens* complex of mosquitoes. *Am. J. Hyg.* **65**:404–425.

Spielman, A., 1964   Studies on autogeny in *Culex pipiens* populations in nature. I. Reproductive isolation between autogenous and anautogenous populations. *Am. J. Hyg.* **80**:175–183.

Spielman, A., 1967   Population structure in the *Culex pipiens* complex of mosquitos. *Bull. WHO* **37**:271–276.

Spielman, A., 1971   Studies on autogeny in natural populations of *Culex pipiens*. Part II. Seasonal abundance of autogenous and anautogenous populations. *J. Med. Entomol.* **8**:555–561.

Spinner, W., 1964   Rote Augen als Mutante bei *Culex pipiens* L. *Experientia (Basel)* **20**:527–528.

Sundararaman, S., 1949   Biometrical studies on intergradation in the genitalia of certain populations of *Culex pipiens* and *Culex quinquefasciatus* in the United States. *Am. J. Hyg.* **50**:307–314.

Suzuki, T. and T. Umino, 1969   Some genetical studies on *Culex pipiens* complex. Part VII. Mode of inheritance of diazinon-resistance in *Culex pipiens molestus* larvae. *Jap. J. Sanit. Zool.* **20**:205–208.

Sweeny, T. L., 1972   Sex ratio caused by meiotic drive in *Culex pipiens* L. Ph.D. Thesis, University of California, Los Angeles, Calif.

Tadano, T., 1969a   Genetical linkage of malathion-resistance in *Culex pipiens* L. *Jap. J. Exp. Med.* **39**:13–16.

Tadano, T., 1969b   The crossover between the sex factor and *w* (white eye) in *Culex pipiens molestus*. *Jap. J. Sanit. Zool.* **20**:69–71.

Tadano, T., 1969c   Genetical relationships between malathion resistance and fenthion resistance in larvae of *Culex pipiens pallens* Coq. *Jap. J. Sanit. Zool.* **20**:158–160.

Tadano, T., 1970   Genetics of cross-resistance to organophosphates, abate, fenitrothion and malathion in larvae of *Culex pipiens pallens* Coquillett. *Jap. J. Exp. Med.* **40**:59–66.

Tadano, T. and A. W. A. Brown, 1967   Genetical linkage relationships of DDT-resistance and dieldrin-resistance in *Culex pipiens fatigans* Wiedemann. *Bull. WHO* **36**:101–111.

Taylor, M., 1914   The chromosome complex of *Culex pipiens. Quart. J. Microscop. Sci.* **60**:377–398 + 3 pl.

Taylor, M., 1917   The chromosome complex of *Culex pipiens.* Part II. Fertilisation. *Quart. J. Microscop. Sci.* **62**:287–301 + 2 pl.

Tewfik, H. R. and A. R. Barr, 1974   The salivary gland chromosomes of *Culex pipiens* L. *Mosq. News* **34**:47–54.

Thomas, V. and C. P. Ramachandran, 1970   Selection of *Culex pipiens fatigans* for vector ability to the rural strain of *Wuchereria bancrofti*—A preliminary report. *Med. J. Malaya* **24**:196–199.

Trembley, H. L., 1955   Mosquito culturing techniques. *Am. Mosq. Control Assoc. Bull. No.* **3**:1–73.

Umino, T., 1965   Some genetical studies on *Culex pipiens* complex. (III). Experimental studies on the fertilization, larval colour phenotypes and autogeny of the hybrids between autogenous and anautogenous colony. *Jap. J. Sanit. Zool.* **16**:282–287.

Umino, T. and T. Suzuki, 1966   Some genetical studies on *Culex pipiens* complex. (V). Studies on the mode of inheritance of malathion-resistance in larvae of *Culex pipiens fatigans. Jap. J. Sanit. Zool.* **17**:191–195.

Umino, T. and T. Suzuki, 1969   Studies on the mode of inheritance of dieldrin-resistance in larvae of *Culex tritaeniorhynchus. Jap. J. Sanit. Zool.* **20**:201–205.

VandeHey, R. C., 1967   Inheritance of pigmented larval head capsules in *Culex pipiens. Mosq. News* **27**:69–73.

VandeHey, R. C., 1969   Incidence of genetic mutations in *Culex pipiens. Mosq. News* **29**:183–189.

Whiting, P. W., 1917   The chromosomes of the common house mosquito, *Culex pipiens. J. Morphol.* **28**:523–577.

Wild, A., 1963   A red eye colour mutation in *Culex pipiens* after X-irradiation. *Nature (Lond.)* **200**:917–918.

Yen, J. H. and A. R. Barr, 1973   The etiological agent of cytoplasmic incompatibility in *Culex pipiens. J. Invertebr. Pathol.* **22**:242–250.

Yen, J. H. and A. R. Barr, 1974   Incompatibility in *Culex pipiens.* In *The Use of Genetics in Insect Control,* edited by R. Pal and M. J. Whitten, pp. 97–118, Elsevier/North-Holland, Amsterdam.

Zielke, E., 1973   Untersuchungen zur Vererbung der Empfänglichkeit gegenüber der Hundefilarie *Dirofilaria immitis* bei *Culex pipiens fatigans* und *Aedes aegypti. Z. Tropenmed. Parasitol.* **24**:36–44.

15

The House Fly, *Musca domestica*

Riccardo Milani

Introduction

The interest in the house fly as a genetical tool arose with the appearance and rapid spreading of resistance to chlorinated insecticides in this species between 1946 and 1947. However, earlier valuable data on the chromosomal complement and genetic variability are available.

The ease of handling, the rapid developmental cycle which is continuous throughout the year, the high fertility, and the genetic variability have facilitated genetical studies on this species, which stands now among the genetically best-known insects. The reader is referred to Hewitt (1914), West (1951), and West and Peters (1972) for further data on this species.

Taxonomical Notes

A member of the family Muscidae (Diptera Cyclorrhapha Schizophora Caliptratae), the genus *Musca* includes, with several other species, the *domestica* complex.

In temperate and hot countries not belonging to the Ethiopian

Riccardo Milani—Istituto di Zoologia, Università di Pavia, Pavia, Italy.

biogeographic realm, this complex contains a cline of intergrading forms, originally described as good species, viz., *domestica, vicina,* and *nebulo* (Saccà, 1967; Spielman and Kitzmiller, 1967; Paterson, 1970).

In the Ethiopian realm two other forms (*calleva* and *curviforceps*) are found with intergrading and/or distinct populations. Distinct sympatric populations that behave as good species do occur. Morphological, geographical, and chromosomal data, as well as studies on hybrids, demonstrate a clear-cut separation of *calleva* and *curviforceps* from the three other forms.

Traits used for taxonomical purposes, like frons width and abdominal color pattern, are modified both by developmental conditions and by the genetic background. Other traits, like chetotaxis and shape of paralobi, may also show great genetic variation among and within populations. Inferential evidence indicates that the load of hidden heterozygosity is high and differs among populations, both qualitatively and quantitatively (Milani, 1967). Genetically marked crossover suppressors have recently been developed which may allow direct measurement of the genetic heterogeneity of some autosomes (McDonald, 1971*a*).

Life Cycle

At temperatures of 22–25°C for the imagoes and 27–30°C for the larval cultures, the life cycle takes 9–12 days. Strains from the warmer countries tend to have the shorter developmental times. The imagoes obtained from eggs laid within a period of few hours will all emerge within a period of 2–3 days.

Matings may begin within the first day of adult life if food and water are available. Starvation effectively prevents mating. Females tend to be monogamous.

Oviposition usually starts between the third and fifth day after emergence. Each female lays a clutch of 100–150 eggs in crevices in the oviposition sites. Each female can lay several clutches, at intervals from one to several days. Under mass-culturing conditions, females congregate to lay eggs in large masses. Hatching occurs about one day after oviposition. The larva passes through its three instars in 4 or 5 days. Larvae feed on juices from fermenting organic materials and then migrate to dryer places for pupation. The pupal period lasts another 4 or 5 days.

Fecundity and the length of the life cycle differ among the various strains and are very sensitive to environmental factors, especially temperature, nutrition, and humidity. Imagoes can be stored at 10–12°C for a couple of months, provided that twice a month they are brought to a higher temperature (20–25°C) for about 30 minutes and are supplied with food.

Rearing Methods

A survey of some of the more important works on various aspects of fly rearing and handling techniques has been published by Sawicki and Holbrook (1961).

I have found the following rearing method to be quite reliable. Eggs are collected on cotton-wool pads that were previously soaked with milk and gently squeezed. Egg masses are transferred onto the larval medium, a mixture of wheat bran (2 parts), fresh milk* (2 parts) and water (1 part), to which the fungicide Nipagine and some drops of yeast suspension are added.

The larval medium is placed in aluminum buckets, filled to a third of their height with about 1 g of medium per larva, and covered with thick muslin. Cultures are kept at 75 percent relative humidity and a temperature of 28°C.

Just before pupation, which occurs 5 days after oviposition, the upper layer of caked food is removed, and the stock cultures are covered with a layer of sand 3–5 cm thick. The pupae are collected on the seventh day by sieving the sand and transferring the pupae in small containers to the adult cages, or to jars, if the imagoes are to be examined. Poorly viable cultures and cultures for genetical work do not receive sand in order to avoid selection against late-pupating larvae.

Adult cages are provided with sugar cubes and with separate cotton-wool squares saturated with fresh milk and with water.

In the United States a standard mixture for the larval pabulum is commercially available [Chemical Specialities Manufacturer's Association (CSMA); Ralston Purina, St. Louis, Mo.]. Difficulties are often encountered when the rearing method is suddenly changed. Ether and CO_2 anesthesia are well tolerated by the house fly. Ethyl ether is specially suitable for immobilizing flies for a fairly long time, as generally required for genetical work. CO_2 can be safely administered in a single exposure, for obtaining a brief immobilization and a quick recovery, or in a continuous flow, when prolonged anesthesia is necessary.

---

* During breeding in various laboratories powdered milk has often been found unsuitable.

Cytology

The Complement

The normal diploid complement is $2n = 12$, and all chromosomes are metacentric or submetacentric. Somatic pairing regularly occurs at mitosis.

The Heterosomes

Two heterosomes are generally present. The condition most frequently described is that females have two heterosomes of equal size (X chromosomes) and males have one X and a distinctly shorter Y chromosome. Both the X and Y chromosomes are isobrachial. Natural and laboratory populations exist in which both sexes have two X chromosomes, sex determination being controlled by autosomal male- or female-determining factors (see pages 384–386). The Y chromosome has been found in females of remote (Milani, 1967; Milani *et al.*, 1967; Kerr, 1970) or recent field origin (Boyes, 1967). Both X and Y chromosomes are polymorphic and are known in at least two and three forms, respectively, possibly more for the Y (Boyes, 1967; Milani, 1967; Milani *et al.*, 1967; Rubini, 1967).

Aneuploids for the heterosomes have normal phenotype and are regularly fertile, both in the hypo- and hyperploid condition. Flies with six X chromosomes or with four Y chromosomes have been obtained by selection (Rubini and Palenzona, 1967; Rubini, private communication). No flies or larvae completely lacking heterosomes have been observed (Boyes, 1967; Milani, 1967; Milani *et al.*, 1967; Kerr, 1970).

The X chromosome seems to be neutral with regard to sex determination. The Y chromosome can be dissociated from the male sex, but it resumes its strict male-limited condition when a suitable genotype is restored (see page 386).

Autosomes

Autosomes show some variation in shape. Autosome 1 is polymorphic. No secondary constrictions, one constriction in one or both members of the pair, and four constrictions in both members have been described for this autosome. Autosome 2 shows, in the preparations of some authors, a quite conspicuous secondary constriction that is not mentioned in other descriptions (Boyes, 1967).

Polytene Chromosomes

Preparations of polytene chromosomes have been obtained from trichogen cells of 4-day-old pupae reared at 27°C (Vecchi and Rubini, 1973). Studies of these chromosomes demonstrate that (1) the arms differ greatly in length, in agreement with the structure of mitotic and meiotic chromosomes; (2) a nucleolar organizer is present; (3) all arms converge in a small centric region; and (4) the longer arms show a tendency to entangle distally. These polytene chromosomes have a clear pattern of bands, constrictions, enlarged segments, and various other peculiarities which provide easily recognizable landmarks (see Figure 1). There are several asynaptic regions, in some of which the banding patterns clearly differ in the two facing elements. Incomplete homologies of this sort may effectively act to suppress crossing over in the regions involved.

Translocations, Inversions, and Compound Chromosomes

I know of no descriptions of naturally occurring inversions and translocations, but these types of chromosomal aberrations have been recovered after x-ray treatments and have been fixed in strains suitable for genetic engineering (McDonald, 1971b; Wagoner *et al.*, 1974). Compound chromosomes have been induced by combining radiation treatments (1500 R) with sophisticated crossing and breeding techniques (Wagoner *et al.*, 1974). Such compound chromosomes have two homologous arms attached to a single centromere.

Some 11 possibly compound flies out of 305,560 examined have been obtained from irradiated males carrying recessive markers. These males have been mated 14 days after treatment to females heterozygous for translocations or inversions and have then been given heat shocks to increase nondisjunction (Wagoner *et al.*, 1974).

Aneuploidy and Polyploidy

Aneuploidy has been described only for sex chromosomes, both of wild and laboratory-bred flies (see page 384). A triploid, of otherwise normal male phenotype (XXY 3A), and a third chromosome trisomic have been recorded (Rubini *et al.*, 1972). The trisomic fly was an intersex.

Mutant Types

The mutant types so far described number about 200. This is an overestimate of known loci because of synonymy and allelism. Most

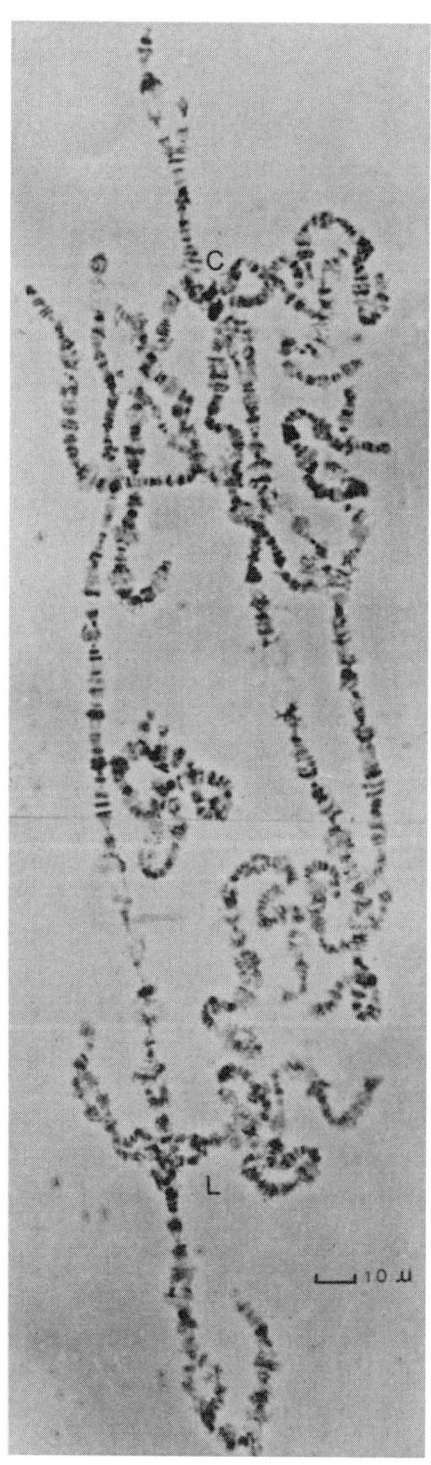

Figure 1. Polytene chromosomes of a tri-chogen cell from a 4-day-old pupa. C = chromocenter.

mutants come from field populations or from old, established laboratory strains and can be defined as spontaneous. Others have been isolated after x-ray treatment. Mutants generally have lower viability than normal flies, but their performance is largely dependent on the genetic background (Milani, 1967). While the commonest mutants have poor phenotypic properties, more than 60 loci have been assigned to linkage groups by using those mutants with high penetrance and expressivity. Dominant mutants are rare and are often lethal when homozygous. A number of inherited syndromes have been found, each showing regularly the same complex combination of highly pathological abnormalities (Milani, 1967). Some of these conditions, although generally appearing as a phenotypic unit, have a polygenic control; the nature of the close association between their component traits is not known.

Inheritance

A large majority of the mutants so-far recorded have variable expressivity and/or incomplete penetrance. These phenotypic properties are specially common among mutants affecting wing venation, wing margins, chetotaxis, or the shape of the compound eyes. Selection for better expressivity and penetrance is often rapidly effective, and the improvement may allow reliable genetical tests. The mutants most suitable as genetic markers are those affecting the color of the body or of the compound eyes, the shape of the wings, enzyme activities and some types of insecticide resistance.

In segregating families, mutants tend to concentrate among late-emerging flies, and their number is generally lower than that expected, with irregular distribution among families. When first recovered by in-breeding from field populations, the average frequencies of mutants are much lower than Mendelian expectation. Laboratory colonization, however, rapidly improves their suitability as genetical tools.

All mutants are autosomal, but autosomal, male-determining factors, limited to some field populations and laboratory strains, cause holandric inheritance of the genes linked to them. The peculiarity of sex determination in the house fly (see below) allows diagynic transmission and crossover recombination of these autosomes.

Meiotic crossing over is limited to female gametogenesis; records of crossing over in the male are very rare and, to my knowledge, limited to loci on chromosome 3.

The correlation between linkage groups and chromosomes has been recently assessed (Wagoner, 1967, 1969a), and, for one chromosome, in-

TABLE 1.   *A Comparison of the Numbering System Used for Autosomal Linkage Groups in Musca*

Wagoner	Hiroyoshi	Milani
1	6	3
2	5	5
3	2	2
4	4	6
5	3	4

dications of the positions of marked loci with respect to the centromere are available (McDonald, 1971*b*). In papers published before 1967 (and sporadically later) the systems for numbering the linkage groups of Milani or Hiroyoshi have been used (see Table 1). The system of Wagoner is used in this account.

Sex Ratio and Sex Determination

Although the sex ratio generally approaches 1♂ : 1♀, gross distortions have been recorded, both for field populations and laboratory strains. By crosses between strains having different methods of sex determination, one can obtain progenies made only by males, only by females, or by both sexes with frequencies traceable to modified Mendelian ratios (e.g., 1 : 3; 7 : 9). Various types of sex determination have been detected in field populations and/or in laboratory strains, and other types have been synthesized in laboratory.

Heterosomal Sex Determination

In most strains of house flies, females have two X chromosomes, and males have one X and one Y. Occasionally, one X can be missing in either sex (♀ XO; ♂ YO) or extra ones can be present; aneuploids for the X are fertile males or females, according to presence or absence of the Y chromosome. This suggests that the Y chromosome is male-determining while the X is neutral.

Cytologically recognizable Y-autosomal translocations recovered after x-ray treatments cause holandric inheritance of the autosomes involved (Wagoner, 1969*a*), in agreement with expectation on the hypothesis of the Y chromosome determining maleness. The XX–XY type of sex determination shall be considered as typical in the following descriptions. Various types of X and Y chromosomes have been described. These differ in the relative length of the arms but show no difference in respect to sex determination (Boyes, 1967; Milani, 1967; Milani *et al.*, 1967; Rubini, 1967).

Autosomal Male-Determining Factors

In an old, established laboratory strain originally started with flies from Florida (and in others derived from it) both females and males are XX; but males are heterozygous for a factor on chromosome 3, which behaves as a dominant male determinant. Males can be coded as $M\,m$, females as $m\,m$. Chromosomal preparations made by conventional methods have so far failed to provide evidence for a detectable translocation of a portion of the Y chromosome to autosome 3. Both reciprocal crosses between flies of these atypical strains and typical ones give hybrid populations having regular $1\male : 1\female$ ratios in the F_1 and following generations, because either M or the Y chromosome are present in the hybrid population's genome.

Crossover frequencies show that this maleness factor, for which the symbol $M(3)$ has been adopted, is near the *pcv* locus (Rubini and Franco, 1969). Therefore, according to the position assigned to this marker (McDonald, 1971*b*), $M(3)$ should be placed toward the centromere. Other, similar, male-determining factors have been recorded recently on other autosomes (Kerr, 1970; Wagoner, 1969*b*).

Recessive genes having a normal allele linked to M cannot become homozygous in the male (apart from very special conditions). This allows the establishing of true-breeding lines with homozygous recessive females and heterozygous normal males (Milani *et al.*, 1967). One of these lines contains a temperature-sensitive lethal factor which kills the female larvae reared at 33°C, but not those reared at 26°C (McDonald, 1971*c*).

Natural populations with two X chromosomes in both sexes and autosomal male-determining factors also have been reported from Japan and Australia (Milani *et al.*, 1967; Wagoner, 1969*b*).

Evidence for Female-Determining Factors

In a strain derived from the one mentioned in the previous paragraph, again both sexes are XX, and most flies of either sex are homozygous $M\,M$. A feminizing factor (F in the following) passes from female to female and is epistatic to *M M*. For the purpose of diagraming crosses, F can be treated as a unit (♀♀ *F f*; ♂♂ *f f*), but all attempts to assign it to a linkage group have failed. However, substitution of X chromosomes has proved that heterosomes are not involved. When *F* is present, intersexes and gynandromophs occur. Selection and crossing experiments suggest that *F* can be broken into subunits of lowered activity (Rubini and Franco, 1968).

When *F* is introduced into an X–Y system, it suppresses the action of the Y chromosome, allowing the appearence of fertile XY females; however, the Y chromosome will resume its association to masculinity, if *F* is removed from the genome. The cross XY ♀ × XY ♂ gives fertile YY flies of both sexes.

Lines in which both sexes have two Y and no X chromosomes and have *F* as the sex-determining mechanism have been repeatedly synthetized and successfully used in crossing experiments (Rubini, 1967).

The presence of different autosomal male factors has been assessed in a strain from Australia for which a factor *F* has been postulated on inferential evidence (Wagoner, 1969*b*).

Maternally Induced Sex Determination

A very unusual sex-determining mechanism has been added to the already complex series of sex mechanisms described for the house fly. A dominant gene, which does not have any recognizable morphological effect on either sex, acts on females only, causing them to lay eggs predetermined to develop as males, independent of the genetic potentialities of the zygote. Therefore, these carrier females have all-male progeny, but one half of their sons are genetically females. These "shunted" males are fully fertile and, when mated to normal females, they generate only female progeny, as expected from the fact that they do not carry any male-determining factors. Thus, the effects of the dominant gene are manifest with a one-generation delay and provide a quite unique male-producing mechanism. The gene gives very good Mendelian segregation ratios. It recombines freely with markers of four autosomes, while showing well-defined linkage relations with the remaining one (autosome 1). Because of its action it has been called "arrhenogenous" (male-generating) and given the symbol *Ag*.

Strains in which *Ag* has been introduced to provide the sole source of males (by excluding from the gene pool all other known male-determining factors) show an excess of females with periodic fluctuations. One such strain has been maintained for more than 70 generations (Rubini *et al.,* 1972; Vanossi Este, 1971; Vanossi Este *et al.,* 1972).

Gynandromophs and Intersexes

Sexually abnormal flies have been observed frequently in field populations, in laboratory strains, and in experimental crosses. Higher relative frequencies have been recorded from field flies captured in the winter (Milani, 1967).

Flies intermediate between the male and female phenotype and recorded as intersexes are common among the progeny of females carrying the *F* factor (or fractions of it). Phenotypic variability may extend up to full expressivity of somatosexual traits of either sex in various parts of the same fly, thus mimicking gynandromorphism.

True gynandromorphism associated with mosaicism has been often recorded; in one case the mosaic involved sexually dimorphic traits and markers of three different chromosomes.

Genetic Control of Biochemical Processes

Studies on the genetical control of biochemical processes have taken advantage of the fairly numerous genes affecting the pigments of the eyes, the color of the cuticle, and sensitivity to insecticides.

Eye Pigments

The eye pigments of the house fly are mainly ommochromes, but pterines are also present. In normal flies the ommochromes show quantitative differences among strains, between sexes, and between flies reared under different light conditions. Males have more ommochromes, as do flies exposed to light (Grigolo and Cima, 1969; Grigolo *et al.,* 1969; Sacchi *et al.,* 1972).

Eye-color mutants are due either to blocks in the tryptophane–ommochrome biosynthetic pathway or to the amount and deposition of available pigments.

The block occurs between tryptophane and kynurenine in *ge* flies and between kynurenine and 3-hydroxykynurenine in *ocra* flies; whereas the mutants *ye* and w^3 have all the ommochrome precursors but fail to synthesize the final pigments. All these mutants have yellow or whitish eyes of various shades (Laudani and Grigolo, 1969); *ge* and *ocra* are nonautonomous in mosaics, and these larvae, when reared in presence of normal ones, may occasionally develop into adults with eyes of various shades of pink (Ward and Hammen, 1957; Milani, 1967).

The mutants having eye colors of various reddish shades (*cm, rb, bu, car, pink*) have ommochromes in smaller amounts than normal (Grigolo and Cima, 1969); the pigments may concentrate in deeper or more superficial cells of the ommatidia, giving a translucent or opaque appearance (Mosconi Bernardini, 1967, and private communication).

Most pterin pigments (drosopterin, xanthopterin, sepiapterin, and others) found in the compound eyes of other brachicerans, are missing in the house fly (Grigolo *et al.*, 1969). Flies homozygous for w^3 accumulate biopterine only, while all other house flies produce isoxanthopterin. The synthesis of this substance has been demonstrated earlier in development than that of 2-amino-4-hydroxpteridine.

Electroretinograms have shown that light sensitivity is greater in flies having lower ommochrome content in the eyes (Pietra *et al.*, 1971). Notwithstanding the high light sensitivity, flies with white or yellowish eyes have very reduced reactions to visual stimuli.

Body Color

The o-diphenoloxidasic activity is greater in *bwb* mutants (brown body) than in normal flies. Electron paramagnetic resonance tests suggest no difference in the melanin component of the cuticle. However, differences are detectable with analysis of *in toto* cuticle and puparia. These findings indicate that other substances are involved, possibly tanned proteins or sclerotines (Cima *et al.*, 1970).

Insecticide Resistance

Most cases of resistance to synthetic organic insecticides have been traced to specific enzymatic activities involving monofactorial inheritance (Brown, 1967; Tsukamoto, 1969).

Among the genes known to impart DDT resistance are a gene on chromosome 2 controlling dechlorinating activity (*Deh*), a gene on chromosome 3 causing very delayed knockdown with decreased nerve sensitivity (*kdr*), and a gene on chromosome 5 causing microsomal oxidation of DDT (*DDT-md*). The reaction controlled by gene *DDT-md* which is responsible for this type of resistance can be inhibited by Sesamex. A description of this synergist is given by O'Brien (1967).

Resistance to dieldrin has been traced to a chromosome-4 gene of unknown action, and to a minor factor on chromosome 2. A gene (*Ox*) for microsomal cyclodiene epoxidase is situated at about 32 units from the *Deh* gene, strikingly close to a diazinon-resistance gene (Khan, 1969).

The resistance to organophosphorous (OP) insecticides is partly due to modified aliesterases, each capable of degrading the P esters to which resistance is displayed. The locus involved (*a*) is on chromosome 2, very near to *Deh*. Enhancing genes have been attributed to chromosomes 3, 4, and 5. A gene for diazinon resistance has crossover rates strikingly coincident with those of the *Ox* gene. The *a* gene has been considered the main cause of carbamate resistance. A chromosome-5 gene, acting also on OP resistance may also contribute to this form of resistance (Bell, 1968; Hoyer and Plapp, 1968). The relationships between low aliesterase activity, OP resistance, and high microsomal oxidase activity still require elucidation (Tsukamoto, 1969). The reader is referred to O'Brien (1967) and Epstein and Legator (1971) for information on the chemistry and metabolism of various insecticides.

Potentialities of Genetic Methods for the Control of House Fly Populations

Some genetic properties of the house fly seem to be potentially useful for control programs.

The "male-sterility" method, when applied to isolated house fly populations, has already given very encouraging results (Saccà, 1969). The cost and the nuisance of released flies in control programs based on this principle would be greatly decreased by the use of femaleless populations obtained either by crossing strains with suitable sex formulae (Milani, 1971) or by exploiting the female-limited, temperature-sensitivity, lethal factor (McDonald, 1971c).

Some of the x-ray-induced translocations have been subjected to laboratory and small field trials as means for reducing fertility. Positive, very promising results have been obtained in the laboratory with two autosomal translocations (Wagoner *et al.,* 1971).

The present status of genetic mechanisms potentially useful for the control of house fly populations has been thoroughly reviewed by Wagoner *et al.* (1974). These authors discuss the theoretical background of the problem, illustrate the technical refinements of the preparatory basic research, examine all published, pertinent information, and add quotations of still unpublished data. The topics covered include: translocations, crossover suppressors, compound chromosomes, meiotic drive, sex-ratio distortion, hybrid sterility, cytoplasmic incompatibility, and conditional lethals. The results of the earliest attempts to reduce fertility in a native house fly population by the introduction into its genetic pool of specific genetic aberrations are also reported. These experiments have provided valuable information on the behavior in the field of laboratory-reared translocation strains and have also met some success at the control level.

A WHO Collaborating Center on *Musca domestica*

The World Health Organization has designated the Institute of Zoology of the University of Pavia as "WHO Collaborating Center for Maintenance and Distribution of Standardized Strains of *Musca domestica*." Among the functions of this Center is the supply of strains of *M. domestica* to the interested workers. The Center has in stock a standardized-insecticide-reference susceptible strain (WHO/IN/*Musca domestica*/1), eight genetically marked strains largely isogenic to the previous one, and a collection of 47 mutant strains. A list of these appears in the newsletter *Vector Genetics* (see page 399). The requests for these strains should be addressed to: Vector Biology and Control, World Health Organization, 1211 Geneva 27, Switzerland.

The coding of the standardized strains conforms to the suggestions which appear in Appendix B (Standardized Strains of Insects of Public Health Importance) of Wright and Pal (1967).

The Mutants of *Musca*

The present list of mutants (Table 2) is limited to mutants described since 1967 and to those mutants described earlier that are referred to in the text. Extensive lists of earlier descriptions have appeared both in a formal publication (Milani, 1967) and in a mimeographed document of limited circulation (*Vector Genetics 1968:* WHO/VBC/68.76). In most cases the description presented is a digest of the original, and efforts have been made to use wording of the original authors. When necessary, the symbols have been adapted to conform with the rules for symbolization recommended by the Committees on Genetic Symbols and Nomenclature (1957; 1968) or to current practice for *Drosophila* mutants.

The data given include the symbol and name; author and date of publication; chromosome; origin of the mutant (spontaneous, induced),

TABLE 2. List of Mutants

Symbol	Name	Description	Chromosome location	Reference
a	aliesterase activity	Spontaneous; controls aliesterase activity and OP resistance	2	Franco and Oppenoorth (1962)
a[C.F.K.G.H]		Five spontaneous ali-esterase alleles, cause different types of OP resistance and low ali-esterase activity	2	Van Asperen (1964)
apt	apterous	Spontaneous; wings and halterers exremely reduced; full penetrance, but variable expressivity	5	Vanossi Este et al. (1967)
bu	brunette	Spontaneous; eye color translucent reddish brown	2	Tsukamoto et al. (1961)
brab	brown body	Spontaneous; basic color of the body brown instead of black; analogous to yellow of Drosophila; very good marker	3	Milani (1956)
car	carnation	Spontaneous; compound eyes pinkish red; good marker	2	Hiroyoshi (1960)
cm	carmine	Spontaneous; compound eyes dark ruby, semitransparent; good marker	2	Hiroyoshi (1960)
cyw	curly wings	From the classic wing strain; wing tips curled on top toward the body about 270 deg.; expressivity variable and penetrance fair	4	Hoyer (1966)
cyw[2]	curly wings[2]	Wings divergent and curled up; full penetrance and uniform expressivity [called conv (convoluted), before its allelism to cyw was demonstrated]	4	Vanossi Este et al. (1967)

TABLE 2. Continued

Symbol	Name	Description	Chromosome location	Reference
Deh	Dehydrochlorinase	Controls the activity of DDT-dehydrochlorinase	2	Khan (1969)
dl	dilution	Spontaneous; body and wing veins yellowish in color and tarsal segments and proboscis nearly uncolored; recessive; full penetrance and uniform expressivity	Not yet localized; independence from autosomes 2, 3, and 4 suggested by preliminary tests	Vanossi Este (1969)
DDT-md	Microsomal detoxication	Microsomes degrade DDT to at least four products of higher polarity; the ensuing DDT resistance can be overcome by Sesamex	5	Oppenoorth and Houx (1968)
$e_3^+, e_5^+, e_6^+,$ e_7^+, e_8^+, e_{10}^+	esterases	Independent esterase-controlling genes, all but e_{10}^+ having nonactive alleles		Velthuis and Van Asperen (1963)
$e_1^+, e_{2,4}^+$	esterase	Esterase-controlling genes; Nonactive alleles not found; possibly allelic	2	Velthuis and Van Asperen (1963)
ge	green	Spontaneous; compound eyes pale yellow-green; excellent marker	3	Zingrone et al. (1959)
kdr	knockdown resistance	Spontaneous; causes extreme delay of knockdown by DDT and resistance to this insecticide; good marker	3	Milani (1956)

In(2)1	Inversion(2)1	x-rays; pericentric inversion greatly reducing genetic recombination		Wagoner *et al.* (1974)
In(3)1	Inversion(3)1	x-rays; paracentric inversion greatly reducing genetic recombination; viable as homozygote	3	McDonald (1971*b*)
In(3)2	Inversion(3)2	x-rays; paracentric inversion greatly reducing genetic recombination	3	McDonald (1971*b*)
In(4)1	Inversion(4)1	x-rays; paracentric inversion greatly reducing genetic recombination; viable as homozygote		Wagoner *et al.* (1974)
In(5)1	Inversion(5)1	x-rays; pericentric inversion greatly reducing genetic recombination		Wagoner *et al.* (1974)
M(3)	Maleness	Spontaneous, male-determining factor, giving about 8 percent recombination with *pcv*	3	Rubini and Franco (1969)
Mk	Masked	The compound eye of *Mk* heterozygotes reduced to a small vertical slit; lethal in the homozygous condition	2	Nickel and Wagoner (1970)
ocra	ocra	Spontaneous; compound eyes yellowish, lighter in color at emergence; nonautonomous; good marker; synonymous with *occhi gialli* (La Face, 1956)	5	Milani (1954)
Ox	Oxidase	Controls the activity of microsomal epoxidase	2	Khan (1969)
pw	pointed wings	Serrated pointed wings		
rb	ruby	Spontaneous; compound eyes bright red, paler than *cm*; see also *rb₁* and *rb₂*	3	Nickel and Wagoner (1970); Hiroyoshi (1960)
rb₁	ruby 1	Spontaneous; recessive gene causing ruby color of the eyes when *rb₂* has simultaneous expression	3	Wagoner (1969*c*)

TABLE 2. Continued

Symbol	Name	Description	Chromosome location	Reference
rb_2	ruby 2	Spontaneous; recessive gene causing ruby color of the eyes if rb_1 has simultaneous expression	4	Wagoner (1969c)
ring	ring	Spontaneous; partial duplication of the fourth longitudinal vein, resulting in a ringlet near the anterior crossvein and/or more distally; sections of L4 occasionally missing in the same region; generally recessive, occasionally partially dominant; complete penetrance; expressivity quite variable	3(?)	Vanossi Este et al. (1967)
Rl	Rolled	Spontaneous; wing rolled up tightly; in homozygous condition body smaller and less polished than normal; heterozygotes somewhat intermediate; very variable	1	Tsukamoto et al (1961)
ro	rough	Spontaneous; irregular arrangement and fusion of facets of compound eyes; good marker	3	Hiroyoshi (1960)
rp	rufipes	Spontaneous; legs, frons, proboscis and hypopigium of a rufous color, body lighter in color than normal; recessive; full penetrance and uniform expressivity	2	Vanossi Este (1969)
Sc	Scalloped	Inner portion of the wings missing in the homozygous state; heterozygote varies	3	Nickel and Wagoner (1970)

from the homozygous phenotype to small chips out of inner edge of the wings; not fully penetrant

spot	spot	Spontaneous; dark spots on the posterior cross vein and on the fourth longitudinal vein, near the wing margin; fully penetrant, espressivity rather variable	1(?)	Vanossi Este et al. (1967)
T(2;4)10-33	Translocation (2;4)	x-rays; associate to *Rl* wings; a marker not fully penetrant		Nickel and Wagoner (1970)
T(2;5)10-53	Translocation (2;5)	x-rays; associate to *ro*		Nickel and Wagoner (1970)
T(3;4;5)11-33	Translocation (3;4;5)	x-rays; associated with a fully penetrant, dominant, cut wing		Nickel and Wagoner (1970)
tin	organotin-R	Spontaneous; incompletely recessive conferring resistance to tributyl tin chloride (TBTC)	3	Hoyer and Plapp (1968)
tsl	temperature-sensitive lethal	Spontaneous; homozygous flies die in the late larval or pupal stage when reared at 33.3°C, viable when reared at 25.6°C	3	McDonald (1971c)
w³	white³	Spontaneous; eye color pale grayish white	3	Tsukamoto et al. (1961)
ye	yellow eyes	Eye color mimic of *ocra* and *ge*		K. A. Lord (private communication)

when known; and a brief description, followed by information on phenotypic and physiologic properties, when available. The linkage groups have been numbered according to the system of Wagoner (1967).

Literature Cited

Bell, J. D., 1968   Genetical investigations on a strain of houseflies resistant to organophosphates and carbamates. *Bull. Entomol. Res.* **58**:191–199.

Boyes, J. W., 1967   The cytology of muscoid flies. In *Genetics of Insect Vectors of Disease,* edited by J. W. Wright and R. Pal, pp. 371–384, Elsevier, Amsterdam.

Brown, A. W. A., 1967   Genetics of insecticide resistance in insect vectors. In *Genetics of Insect Vectors of Disease,* edited by J. W. Wright and R. Pal, pp. 505–552, Elsevier, Amsterdam.

Cima, L., L. Zanotti, A. Grigolo and L. Laterza, 1970   Caratterizzazione delle melanine di *Musca domestica* L. mediante risonanza paramagnetica elettronica. *Riv. Parassitol.* **31**:221–226.

Committee on Genetic Symbolism and Nomenclature, 1957   Report of International Union of Biological Sciences, Series B, No. 30, p. 6. 1970. Report to I.U.B.S. (August 27, 1968) published in *Genet. Agrar.* **22**:395–396.

Drosophila Information Service, Vol. 27–31, available from E. Novitski, Department of Biology, University of Oregon, Eugene, Oregon.

Epstein, S. S. and M. S. Legator, 1971   *The Mutagenicity of Pesticides,* Massachusetts Institute of Technology Press, Cambridge, Mass.

Franco, M. G. and F. J. Oppenoorth, 1962   Genetical experiments on the gene for low aliesterase activity and organophosphate resistance in *Musca domestica* L. *Entomol. Exp. Appl.* **5**:119–123.

Grigolo, A. and L. Cima, 1969   Variazioni quantitative degli omocromi in vari ceppi di *Musca domestica* L. *Riv Parassitol.* **30**:243–248.

Grigolo, A., L. Sacchi and L. Cima, 1969   Le pterine di *Musca domestica* L. *Genet. Agrar.* **22**:382–393.

Hewitt, C. G., 1914   *The Housefly Musca domestica Linn.,* Cambridge University Press, London.

Hiroyoshi, T., 1960   Some new mutants and linkage groups of the house fly. *J. Econ. Entomol.* **53**:985–990.

Hoyer, R. F., 1966   Some new mutants of the house fly, *Musca domestica,* with notations of related phenomena. *J. Econ. Entomol.* **59**:133–137.

Hoyer, R. F. and F. W. Plapp, Jr., 1968   Insecticide resistance in the housefly: Identification of a gene that confers resistance to organotin insecticides and acts as an intensifier of Parathion resistance. *J. Econ. Entomol.* **61**:1269–1276.

Insect Toxicologists' Information Service (Issued annually in 400 copies) edited by F. J. Oppenoorth and N. W. H. Houx, Laboratory for Research on Insecticides, Prinses Marijkeweg 22, Wageningen, Holland.

Kerr, R. W., 1970   Inheritance of DDT resistance in a laboratory colony of the housefly, *Musca domestica. Aust. J. Biol. Sci.* **23**:377–400.

Khan, M. A. Q., 1969   Some biochemical characteristics of the microsomal cyclodiene epoxidase system and its inheritance in the housefly. *J. Econ. Entomol.* **62**:388–392.

La Face, L., 1956 Su una mutazione ad occhi gialli in *Musca domestica. Rend. Ist. Super. Sanità* **19**:1061–1071.

Laudani, U. and A. Grigolo, 1969 Ommochrome precursors and U.V. fluorescent substances in eye colour mutants of *Musca domestica* L. *Monit. Zool. Ital.* **3**:99–104.

McDonald, J. C., 1971*a* A technique for revealing hidden heterozygosity on autosome 3 of the housefly. *J. Hered.* **62**:45–47.

McDonald, J. C., 1971*b* Orientation and position of the linkage map on chromosome 3 of the housefly. *J. Hered.* **62**:246–247.

McDonald, J. C., 1971*c* A male-producing strain of the housefly. *Science (Wash., D.C.)* **172**:3982.

Milani, R., 1954 The genetics of the housefly. Preliminary note, In Atti IX Congresso Internazionale di Genetica, Bellagio, 1953. *Caryologia (Suppl.)*: 791–796.

Milani, R., 1956 Recenti sviluppi delle ricerche genetiche sulla mosca domestica. *Boll. Zool.* **23**:749–764.

Milani, R., 1967 The genetics of *Musca domestica* and other muscoid flies. In *Genetics of Insect Vectors of Disease*, edited by J. W. Wright and R. Pal, pp. 315–369, Elsevier, Amsterdam.

Milani, R., 1971 Genetics of factors affecting fertility and of sex-ratio distortions in the house fly. Sterility principle for insect control or eradication. In *Proceedings of a Symposium, Athens, 14–18 Sept. 1970, Jointly Organized by the IAEA and FAO*, pp. 381–397, International Atomic Energy Agency Proceedings Series, Vienna.

Milani, R., P. G. Rubini and M. G. Franco, 1967 Sex determination in the housefly. *Genet. Agrar.* **21**:385–411.

Mosconi Bernardini, P., 1967 Esame istochimico e fluoromicroscopico dell' occhio normale e mutante di *Musca domestica* L. *Boll. Zool.* **XXXIV**:147.

Nickel, C. A. and D. E. Wagoner, 1970 Some new mutants of the house flies and their linkage groups and map positions. *J. Econ. Entomol.* **63**:1385–1390.

O'Brien, R. D., 1967 *Insecticides: Action and Metabolism*, Academic Press, New York.

Oppenoorth, F. J. and N. W. H. Houx, 1968 DDT resistance in the housefly caused by microsomal degradation. *Entomol. Exp. Appl.* **11**:81–93.

Paterson, H. E., 1970 Population genetic studies in areas of overlap of two subspecies of *Musca domestica* L. *Monogr. Biol.* **14**:244–254.

Pietra, P., L. Cima, A. Grigolo and B. Taglietti, 1971 Influenza dei pigmenti schermanti sui processi visivi di *Musca domestica* L. *Boll. Zool.* **38**:553.

Rubini, P. G., 1967 Ulteriori osservazioni sui determinanti sessuali di *Musca domestica* L. *Genet. Agrar.* **21**:363–384.

Rubini, P. G. and M. G. Franco, 1968 Osservazioni sui determinanti sessuali presenti in un ceppo YY di *Musca domestica* L. *Boll. Zool.* **35**:437.

Rubini, P. G. and M. G. Franco, 1969 Localizzazione genetica del fattore autosomico di mascolinita *M* in *Musca domestica* L. *Boll. Zool.* **36**:414.

Rubini, P. G. and D. Palenzona, 1967 Response to selection for high number of heterosomes in *Musca domestica* L. *Genet. Agrar.* **21**:101–110.

Rubini, P. G., M. G. Franco and S. Vanossi Este, 1972 Polymorphisms for heterochromosomes and autosomal sex-determinants in *Musca domestica* L. In *Atti del IX Congresso Nazionale Italiano di Entomologia, Siena, 1972*, pp. 341–352, Tip. Bertarelli e Piccardi, Florence.

Saccà, G., 1967 Speciation in *Musca*. In *Genetics of Insect Vectors of Disease*, edited by J. W. Wright and R. Pal, pp. 385–399, Elsevier, Amsterdam.

Saccà, G., 1969 Il metodo della sterilita nella lotta contro *Musca domestica* L.: sintesi delle recenti ricerche effettuate dall'Istituto Superiore di Sanità. *Mem. Soc. Entomol. Ital.* **XLVIII:**179–188.

Sacchi, L., A. Grigolo and L. Cima, 1972 Influenza della luce sull'accumulo degli ommocromi in *Musca domestica* L. *Riv. Parassitol.* **33:**231–235.

Sawicki, R. M. and D. V. Holbrook, 1961 The rearing, handling and biology of houseflies (*Musca domestica* L.) for assay of insecticides by the application of measured drops. *Pyrethrum Post* **6:**3–18.

Spielman, D. and J. B. Kitzmiller, 1967 Genetics of populations of medically important arthropods. In *Genetics of Insect Vectors of Disease,* edited by J. W. Wright and R. Pal, pp. 459–480, Elsevier, Amsterdam.

Tsukamoto, M., 1969 Biochemical genetics of insecticide resistance in the housefly. *Residue Rev.* **25:**289–314.

Tsukamoto, M., Y. Baba and S. Hiraga, 1961 Mutations and linkage groups in Japanese strains of the housefly. *Jap. J. Genet.* **36:**168–174.

Van Asperen, K., 1964 Biochemistry and genetics of esterases in houseflies (*Musca domestica*) with special reference to the development of resistance to organophosphorus compounds. *Entomol. Exp. Appl.* **7:**205–214.

Vanossi Este, S., 1969 Osservazioni su due nuovi mutanti del colore del corpo in *Musca domestica* L. *Boll. Zool.* **XXXVI:**377.

Vanossi Este, S., 1971 Nuovi equilibri nella determinazione del sesso in *Musca domestica* L. *Boll. Zool.* **38:**566.

Vanossi Este, S., G. Biscaldi and M. G. Franco, 1967 New mutants isolated from laboratory strains of *Musca domestica* L. *Insect Toxicol. Inf. Serv.* **X:**198–199. (Mimeographed newsletter.)

Vanossi Este, S., P. G. Rubini, M. G. Franco and C. Rovati, 1972 Arrenogenia in *Musca domestica* L. e sua ereditarietà. *Boll. Zool.* **39:**669.

Vecchi, M. L. and P. G. Rubini, 1973 Polytene chromosomes of trichogen-cells in *Musca domestica* L. *Genet. Agrar.* **27:**456–463.

Velthuis, H. H. W. and K. Van Asperen, 1963 Occurrence and inheritance of esterases in *Musca domestica. Entomol. Exp. Appl.* **6:**79–87.

Wagoner, D. E., 1967 Linkage group–karyotype correlation in the housefly determined by cytological analysis of X-ray-induced translocations. *Genetics* **57:**729–739.

Wagoner, D. E., 1969a Linkage group–karyotype correlation in the housefly, *Musca domestica* L., confirmed by cytological analysis of X-ray-induced Y-autosomal translocations. *Genetics* **62:**115–121.

Wagoner, D. E., 1969b Presence of male determining factors found on three autosomes in the housefly *Musca domestica. Nature (Lond.)* **223(5202):**187–188.

Wagoner, D. E., 1969c The ruby eye-color mutants in the housefly, *Musca domestica* L., a case of duplicate genes. *Genetics* **62:**103–113.

Wagoner, D. E., O. A. Johnson and C. A. Nickel, 1971 Fertility reduced in a caged native housefly strain by the introduction of strains bearing heterozygous chromosomal translocations. *Nature (Lond.)* **234:**473–475.

Wagoner, D. E., I. C. McDonald and D. Childress, 1974 The present status of genetic control mechanisms in the house fly, *Musca domestica* L. In *The Use of Genetics in Insect Control,* edited by R. Pal and M. J. Whitten, pp. 183–197, Elsevier/North Holland, Amsterdam.

Ward, C. L. and C. S. Hammen, 1957 New mutations affecting tryptophan-derived eye pigments in three species of insects. *Evolution* **11:**60–64.

West, L. S., 1951 *The Housefly,* Comstock Publ. Co., Ithaca, N. Y.

West, L. S. and O. B. Peters, 1972 *An Annotated Bibliography of Musca domestica Linnaeus,* Dawsons of Pall Mall, Cannon House, Folkestone, Kent, England.

World Health Organization Publications, Vector Biology and Control Section, Division of Environmental Health, Geneva, Switzerland.

Vector Genetics, Mutation and Stock List of Arthropod Vectors, WHO/VBC/68.76.

Information Circulars on Insecticide Resistance, Insect Behavior and Vector Genetics (formerly: *Information Circular on Insecticide Resistance*).

Wright, J. W. and R. Pal, editors, 1967 *Genetics of Insect Vectors of Disease,* Elsevier, Amsterdam.

Zingrone, L. D., W. N. Bruce and G. C. Decker, 1959 A mating study of the female housefly. *J. Econ Entomol.* **52**:236.

16

The Australian Sheep Blowfly, *Lucilia cuprina*

Maxwell J. Whitten, Geoffrey G. Foster,

James T. Arnold, and Christine Konowalow

Introduction

The Australian sheep blowfly, *Lucilia cuprina* (Wiedemann) (Calliphoridae) has been the subject of intensive research in a variety of fields over the past three decades. Its suitability as a laboratory organism has attracted its use as a model species for studies in population dynamics (Nicholson, 1957), biochemistry (Williams and Birt, 1972), physiology and mating behavior (Waterhouse, 1950; Barton Browne *et al.,* 1969). Its importance as a major pest of the sheep industry in Australia has ensured that its ecology has come under close scrutiny (Waterhouse, 1947; Norris, 1959), and attempts for its containment by various biological control agents [for review see Norris (1959)] and insecticides have been examined (Shanahan, 1965; Arnold and Whitten, 1975a,b). The possibility of controlling *L. cuprina* by genetic means is currently being investigated (Foster and Whitten, 1974). With this end in mind, the formal genetics of the

Maxwell J. Whitten, Geoffrey G. Foster, James T. Arnold and Christine Konowalow—Division of Entomology, Commonwealth Scientific and Industrial Research Organization, Canberra City, Australia.

species is being elucidated, along with more detailed studies of its ecology and population dynamics.

Biology of L. cuprina

L. cuprina was recognized as a major myiasis blowfly of sheep in Australia around 1900. *L. cuprina dorsalis,* the form common in Australia, was probably introduced into Australia from South Africa or India during the last century (Waterhouse and Paramonov, 1950). There is indirect evidence to suggest that *L. cuprina* has only recently switched from being a carrion breeder to the parasitic myiasis habit, and that this evolutionary switch is still being perfected. The extent to which the availability of large numbers of susceptible sheep has influenced the shift in life habit is unknown, although the fact that *L. cuprina* is a carrion breeder in areas of northern Australia and New Guinea, where there are no sheep, may afford an opportunity to examine this evolutionary question.

Unlike the screw-worm fly, *Cochliomyia hominivorax* Coq., *L. cuprina* is not restricted to attacking animals with pre-existing lesions, but it can initiate wounds in the skin of living sheep. Typically, females deposit clusters of eggs in the fleece and, if the fleece and skin are sufficiently moist, larvae hatch from the eggs within 12 hours and migrate to the skin surface, which they rasp with their mouthparts until the skin is broken and fluid exudes. Subsequently, more *L. cuprina* and several other blowfly species may oviposit near the wound, which, if untreated, may spread until the animal dies. After passing through two moults, fully fed third-instar larvae (approximately 3 days old) leave the host and pupate under the soil surface. In warm weather (25–30°C) adult flies may emerge within 2 weeks, and females are ready to mate and oviposit after 4 days, if they have fed on sufficient protein to mature their eggs. Thus, in the long Australian summer, at least five or six generations are possible in a season. This, combined with the ability of females to survive several weeks in the field (Norris, 1959; Whitten *et al.*, 1973), contributes to a high incidence of myiasis in a favorable season, with consequent severe economic losses to the sheep industry.

In addition to causing myiasis on sheep, *L. cuprina* is capable of breeding on carrion under field conditions, although competition from native blowflies, particularly the *Calliphora* and *Chrysomya* species, drastically reduces the chances of its larvae developing to the point where they are capable of completing their life cycle successfully (Waterhouse,

1947). However, eggs laid on sheep, particularly the fine wool Merino breed, over areas of the fleece that are contaminated with urine stain, feces, or bacterial fleece rot, can complete larval development before the wound or "strike" attracts secondary and tertiary blowflies.

In the laboratory, larvae are routinely reared on animal protein, normally sheep's liver rendered unfit for human consumption by the presence of hydatid cysts and liver fluke. The presence of such parasites in these livers acts as an admirable bioassay to indicate that the livers are devoid of drenching chemicals, such as carbon tetrachloride, which destroy their suitability as a larval diet. "Healthy" livers are sometimes saturated with chemicals that are lethal to flies and whose effects on man are not fully understood.

At 25°C the eggs take 12-24 hours to hatch, and larval feeding continues for 5-6 days. A brief, third-larval-instar wandering stage is followed by pupal development, which takes 6-7 days in the male and 7-8 days in the female. Development is temporarily arrested if fully grown larvae which have cleared their guts are held below 10°C. Thus, stocks can be held for several months in cold storage.

Adult males survive on a diet of sugar and water, although a protein meal may enhance their sexual drive. They are ready to mate after 2 days and are capable of inseminating as many as 17 females over their full life cycle. Females require a protein meal for ovarian development, although a capacity for autogeny does exist and can be selected for (Nicholson, 1957). Females are unwilling to mate until their ovaries are partly developed, a fact which facilitates the collection of virgin females within the first 24 hours after emergence. Females rarely mate more than once, although it is possible to select for polygamy (Whitten and Taylor, 1970). Under laboratory conditions females become gravid 3-4 days after a protein meal. Egg laying is normally gregarious, but there is no difficulty in obtaining egg masses from individual females. Egg clusters of 200-300 eggs can be collected, on small cubes of liver, from individual females every 3 or 4 days for several weeks. The availability of large numbers of eggs at roughly the same stages of development has proved extremely useful for genetic studies.

Approaches to the Control of *L. cuprina*

The most effective measures for the control of blowfly myiasis, which causes an estimated loss of 20-40 million dollars annually, include the

Mules operation and the application of insecticides (Shanahan, 1965). The Mules operation consists of the surgical removal of folds of skin around the breech in ewes, reducing the soiling in this region and rendering it less attractive for oviposition. Since breech or crotch myiasis constitutes the most common form of fly myiasis, this simple measure reduces the susceptibility of sheep, although other areas of the body can be stricken, particularly in hot, humid seasons, in pastures where the grass is long. In the early postwar period DDT was used extensively for fly control, but in 1955, dieldrin, which proved both cheaper and easier to apply, displaced DDT as the major insecticide. Within two seasons high levels of resistance to dieldrin and other cyclodienes had become widespread in field populations due to the spread of a single gene (*Rdl* in Table 1) on chromosome 5 (Shanahan, 1965). Since the cessation of the use of dieldrin, control has depended on organophosphorus insecticides (OP's), particularly diazinon and, to a lesser extent, on carbamates. Low levels of resistance to the OP's appeared in the late sixties, reducing the period of protection for sheep from some 12 weeks to less than 4. However, in the absence of more effective alternatives, OP insecticides still constitute the major form of control of the sheep blowfly. Although resistance to DDT has not been detected in *L. cuprina,* problems of environmental contamination and residue restrictions by overseas markets prevent the reuse of this insecticide for control of the sheep blowfly.

The absence of cheap and effective alternative insecticides, the decreasing availability of new groups of insecticides which do not exhibit cross resistance with the earlier groups, and the general dissatisfaction by the community and overseas markets with insecticides, has created a need for "clean" methods of pest management.

Early attempts by Froggatt (1918) at the biological control of the sheep blowfly using pupal parasites were unsuccessful. There have been no serious attempts at biological control since that time, primarily because effective parasites or predators are unknown for any blowfly.

Since the classical biological control approach does not appear promising for the control of the sheep blowfly, attention has been devoted to ways of using the sheep blowfly for its own control. Such "autocidal" methods are, of necessity, genetic in nature. The simpler genetic approaches, such as the now-classical sterile-insect release method (*SIRM*) used by E. F. Knipling and colleagues for the control of the screw-worm fly in the southern United States (Bushland, 1971), do not require any formal genetics. However, the more sophisticated approaches which are outlined later in this paper require extensive information on the formal genetics of the insect to be controlled.

Genetics of *L. cuprina*

Some 45 visible mutations, in addition to mutations to insecticide resistance at three loci, are maintained in single- and multiple-marker stocks in the CSIRO Division of Entomology (Table 1). These constitute the residue of a much larger number of mutations that have been screened to include only those which are highly penetrant and whose viabilities are near 100 percent. Most (41) of the visibles are recessive to wild type, while three are expressed in heterozygotes (*Sh* and *Bl* are recessive lethals, and *Tw* has an enhanced phenotype in the homozygote). The mutations conferring insecticide resistance are all expressed as heterozygotes, and the effect is additive in homozygotes (Arnold and Whitten, 1975*a*).

The mutations are mostly of spontaneous origin, pre-existing in laboratory stocks or in strains recently derived from the field, or they were induced with gamma irradiation or ethyl methanesulfonate. It is interesting to note that 15 visible mutations were detected in one field population during the course of experiments designed to test the incorporation of genetic material from laboratory strains into a field population (Whitten *et al.*, 1973).

Linkage Maps

The absence of crossing over in males permits rapid partition of mutants into six linkage groups, which correspond to the pairs of chromosomes in the species. The X chromosome, which is largely heterochromatic, is represented by one marker, black body (*b*). The other mutations occur in the five autosomal linkage groups (Figure 1). Chromosome 4, with 13 markers, is currently the best marked autosome, whereas chromosome 2, with seven markers, is the least well marked. Map distances (Figure 1) are derived from information accumulated over a number of years from numerous crosses, and which will be published elsewhere. The order of mutations indicated in Figure 1 is mostly based on the results of standard three-point test crosses or on crosses involving the mapping of chromosome rearrangements. Exceptions to this rule are noted in the caption to Figure 1. One inconsistency between the present map and a previously published map (Foster and Whitten, 1974) should be noted. Earlier, *Rdl* was placed to the right of linkage group 5 on the basis of one cross which suggested loose linkage to *sk*; the present position of *Rdl* at the left end of chromosome 5 is based on the results of two different five-point crosses and linkage to the new marker, *to²*.

TABLE 1.   Lucilia cuprina Mutation List

Symbol	Name of mutant	Chromosome	Description
ar	arista	3	Aristae lack plumage
b	black body	X	Metallic body color, shiny black instead of green
Bl	Bristle	6	Thoracic bristles, especially scutellar sublateral marginals and posterior sternopleurals, short and pointed; dominant, homozygous lethal[a]
bp[1]	black puparium	2	Puparium black instead of normal brown color
bp[2]	dark puparium	2	Puparium reddish black; allele of bp[1]
bu	bubble	4	Prominent bubbles in one or both wings
bz	bronze	5	Bronze-colored body
cu	curled	5	Wings curled upward and thorax a dark color
cy	curly	4	Wings curled upward
dfw	deformed wings	6	Wings twisted or undulating, sometimes with prominent bubbles
drm	double radial-median crossvein	3	r-m crossvein thicker than normal, as is proximal portion of R_{1+2} vein[a]
f	forked	3	Most thoracic bristles twisted and with molten appearance
gl	golden	4	Golden-colored calypters and parafacial pubescence
gla	glazed	2	Eye has glazed surface and irregularly arrayed facets
gp	grape	4	Eye color dark purple
hk	hooked	4	Thoracic bristles about half normal length and hooked at tips
ho	held-out	6	Wings held at right angle to body and contain extra dotlike veinlets
m_1	M1 veinless	5	All or a portion of M1 vein missing[a]
ms	missing bristles	2	Major thoracic bristles, scutellars especially, missing or very short; sockets present
ol	olive	5	Body a dark metallic green color, instead of normal bright green
pb	purple body	2	Metallic body color a shiny purple
pt	purple thorax	2	Thorax plus first abdominal segment a dull purple color; scutellum the normal green color
Rdl	Dieldrin resistance	5	Very high resistance to dieldrin[b]
Rop-1	Diazinon resistance	4	Resistance to diazinon[b] (see text)
Rop-2	Diazinon resistance	6	Moderate levels of resistance to diazinon[b] (see text)
ra	radials	4	Gaps in radial (R_{1+2}) and Sc wing veins[a]

TABLE 1. *Continued*

Symbol	Name of mutant	Chromosome	Description
re	reduced	4	Eye size reduced, facet pattern irregular
ru	rusty	3	Wing veins, legs a light brown color instead of normal black; normal green coloring of body takes longer to form in newly emerged homozygotes
sa	sabre	2	Wings complete but narrow and tapered, frequently deformed and folded
sb	stubble	2	Most major bristles reduced in size, thickened at bases, and sharply pointed
sbd	stubbloid	3	Bristles short and pointed
sblk	stubblelike	4	Like *sbd*
sby	stubby	5	Like *sbd*
Sh	Short	4	Major bristles short blunt; dominant; usually homozygous lethal
sk	sockets	5	Many major bristles absent; sockets present
st	stumpy	6	Scutellar and other major thoracic bristles shortened and stumplike
sv	singed vibrissae	4	Stigmatal, ventral propleural, posterior sternopleural bristles, and oral vibrissae short and with singed appearance[a]
tg	tangerine	4	Eye color ranging from yellowish to scarlet
thv	thick veins	4	Irregular thickenings in wing veins
ti	tiny bristles	6	Like *sbd*
to^1	topaz^1	5	Eye color yellow
to^2	topaz^2	5	Eye color scarlet; allele of *to*^{1}; *to*^{1}/*to*^{2} has orange eyes
Tw	Twisted	6	Dorsal thoracic and scutellar bristles twisted and truncated; expression in homozygote more extreme than in heterozygote
vg	vestigial	6	Wings missing large pieces or reduced to stumps
w	white	3	Eyes colored white
wy	wavy	3	Wings undulating instead of flat
y	yellow	6	Eyes colored yellow
yw	yellowish	3	Eye color ranging from yellow to orange

[a] For details of bristle and wing-vein nomenclature, consult Colless and McAlpine (1970).
[b] Resistance to diazinon and dieldrin is intermediate in heterozygote.

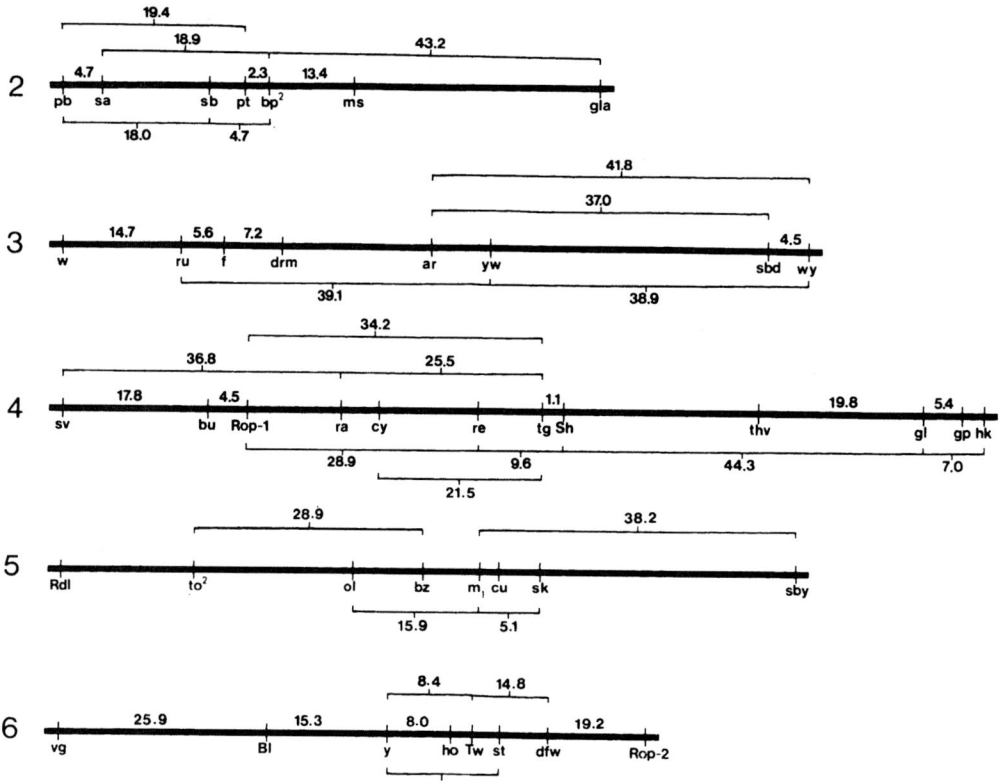

Figure 1. Autosomal linkage maps in Lucilia cuprina. Relative orders of the following marker combinations have not been determined critically: sbd-wy, ra-cy-re, gp-hk, ol-bz, ho-Tw-st. The position of ti (not shown) is assumed to be at the right end of linkage group 6, since it appears to be unlinked to Rop-2 and to In(6)2+3, and is not covered by Dp(6L;Y)19, which includes the terminal half of the left arm of chromosome 6. The position of sblk (not shown) is assumed to be near the middle of linkage group 4, since it is unlinked to sv and gl.

Cytogenetics

The chromosome complement, comprising five autosomal pairs and a heterochromatic sex pair, was first described by Ullerich (1963) and then by Childress (1969). Preparations of brain mitoses using the method of Lewis and Smith Riles (1960) and meiotic squashes, using acetic–alchohol (1 : 3) fixative for 30 seconds and then staining in aceto-orcein, are illustrated in Figure 2.

Using mutant stocks and translocations, Childress established a correspondence between the linkage groups and the five autosomes. Our own investigations have led to a revision of Childress' (1969) linkage group–chromosome correlation (Foster and Whitten, 1975). We have identified linkage group 4 with the largest chromosome in the complement (Figure 2), whereas Childress had concluded that the largest autosome corresponded to linkage group 3. Our decision is based on the availability of a pericentric inversion on chromosome 4 which shifts the centromere of chromosome 4 from a medial position to a subterminal position (Figure 2E). We suggest for adoption our numbering system given in Table 2, so that the chromosome number is identical to the linkage group number.

Note that following the discovery of a mutation on the X chromosome, this chromosome has been designated linkage group 1, and we have redesignated Childress' (1969) linkage group 1 as linkage group 6. Chromosome 4 is the largest in the complement, chromosome 3 is the next largest, while chromosome 2 is discernible by a prominent secondary constriction (Figure 2H). Chromosome 6 is the smallest element and has the highest long arm : short arm ratio.

Good polytene chromosome preparations have been obtained from pupal trichogen cells (Childress, 1969; and Figure 2D), but not from salivary glands or pupal footpads. There is only a very weak chromocentral attraction, and whole chromosomes are often recovered separate from the other chromosomes in squash preparations. Our own observations on translocation preparations have confirmed the linkage group–polytene chromosome correlation of Childress (1969) for linkage groups 2, 3, and 6, but indicate that arms 4L and 4R should be interchanged with arms 5L and 5R, respectively (Foster and Whitten, 1975; and Figure 2D). Allowing for this correction, the labeling of chromosome ends adopted by us corresponds to that of Childress (1969) in her Figure 2 photograph, rather than in her drawing, in which the ends are transposed.

*TABLE 2. Linkage Group
Numbering Systems*

Ullerich	Childress	Present authors
X	X	1
II	2	2
V	4	3
I	3	4
IV	5	5
III	1	6

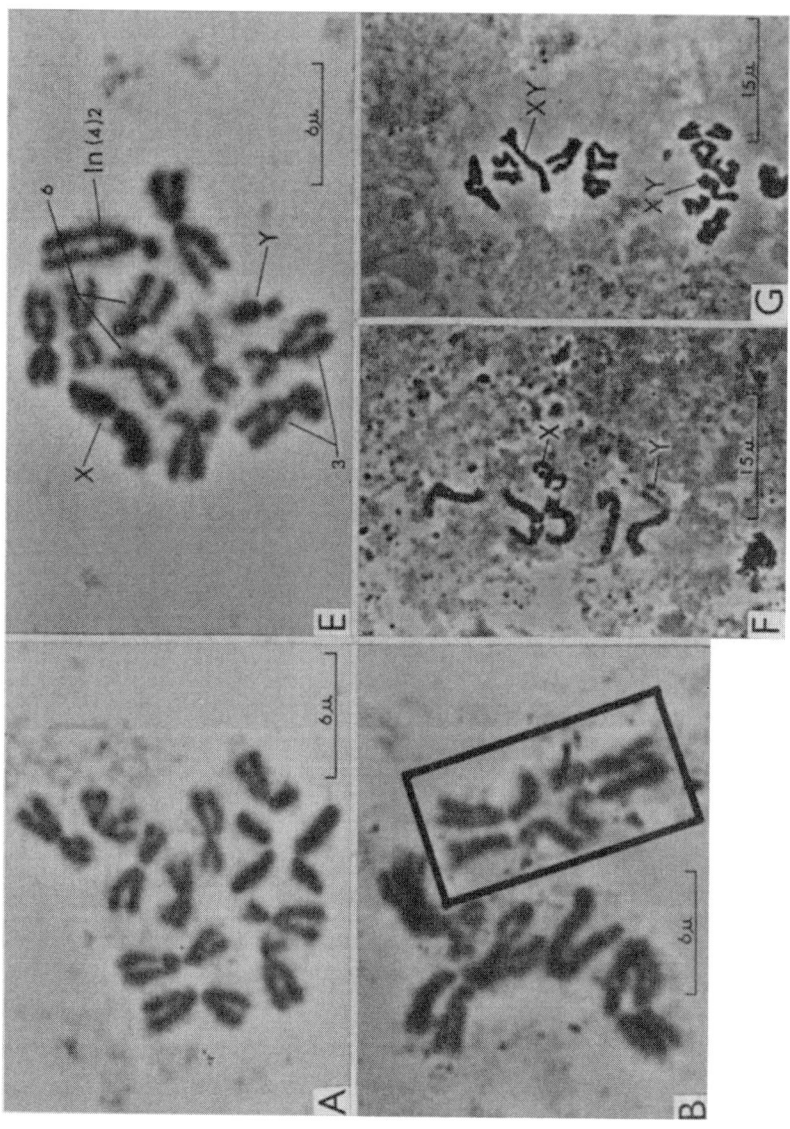

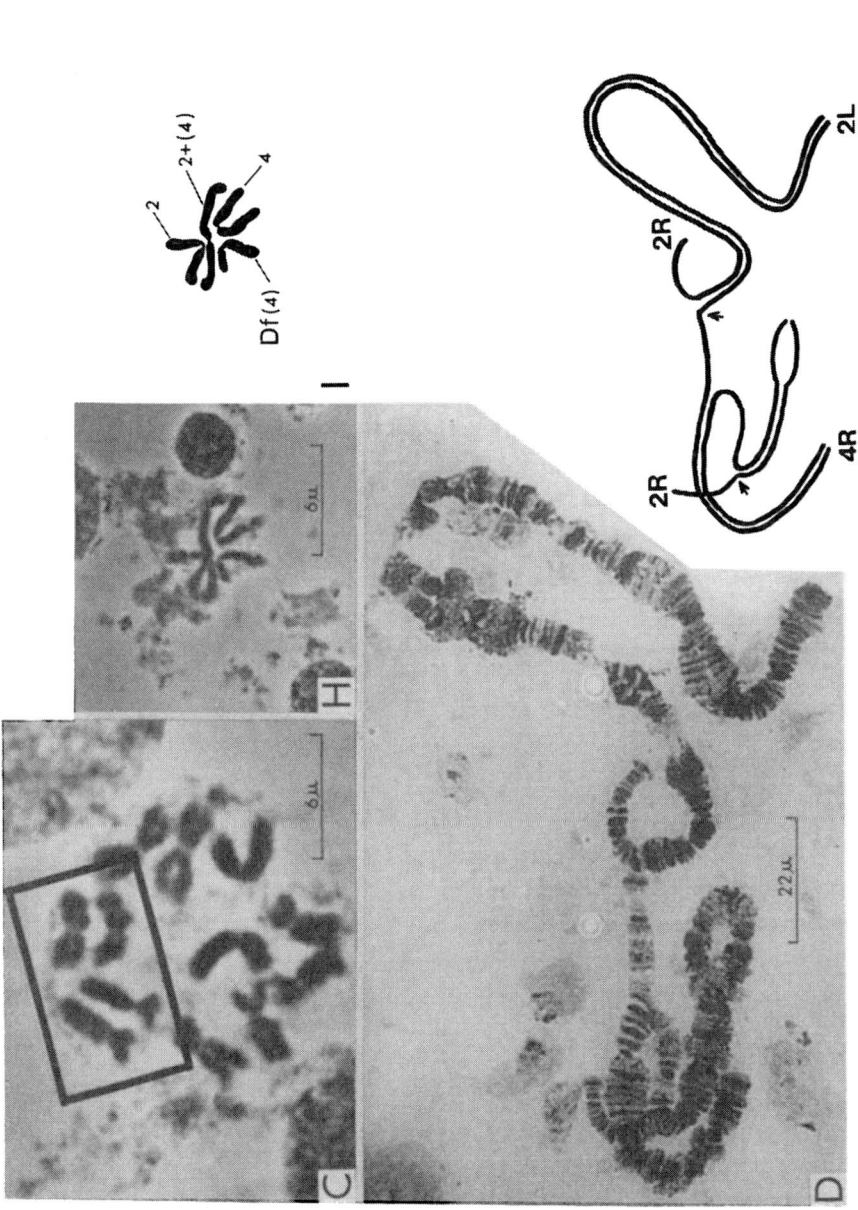

Figure 2. (A, B, C, E, H) Brain squashes of L. cuprina: (A) normal female; (B) heterozygote for translocation T(2;6)A27; (C) female homozygous for T(2;6)A27; (E) male heterozygous for pericentric inversion In(4)2, indicating centromere shift; (H) incomplete mitotic plate showing an insertional translocation of a segment of chromosome 4 into chromosome 2. (I) Line-drawing of fig. 2H. (D) Polytene chromosomes from trichogen cells of T(2;4)A50 strain, showing translocated chromosomes (the left arm of chromosome 4 is missing). (F,G) Prophase and early anaphase from spermatogonial squashes of normal karyotype.

Chromosome Rearrangements

Inversions. Systematic screening procedures involving the detection of reduced crossing over in the female progeny of irradiated males, have led to the recovery of inversions on chromosomes 3, 4, and 6 (Figure 3). In addition, inversions have been recovered on chromosomes 2, 3, 4, and 5 by the routine cytological screening of translocations. One crossover suppressor between *tg* and *gl* on chromosome 4 has been identified as an insertional translocation of a segment of chromosome 4 into chromosome 2 (Figure 2H,I), and another on chromosome 3 is associated with an X;3 translocation. The various chromosome 4 inversions have been combined with the dominant marker, *Sh,* and the recessive marker, *gl,* preparatory to the synthesis of a crossover balancer stock for chromosome 4 (Foster and Whitten, 1974). Similarly, a balancer strain is being developed for chromosome 6.

Translocations. Over 150 translocations have been recovered following ^{60}Co treatment of mature sperm. Of these, 30 were tested for homozygous viability, but only one translocation was viable (Foster and

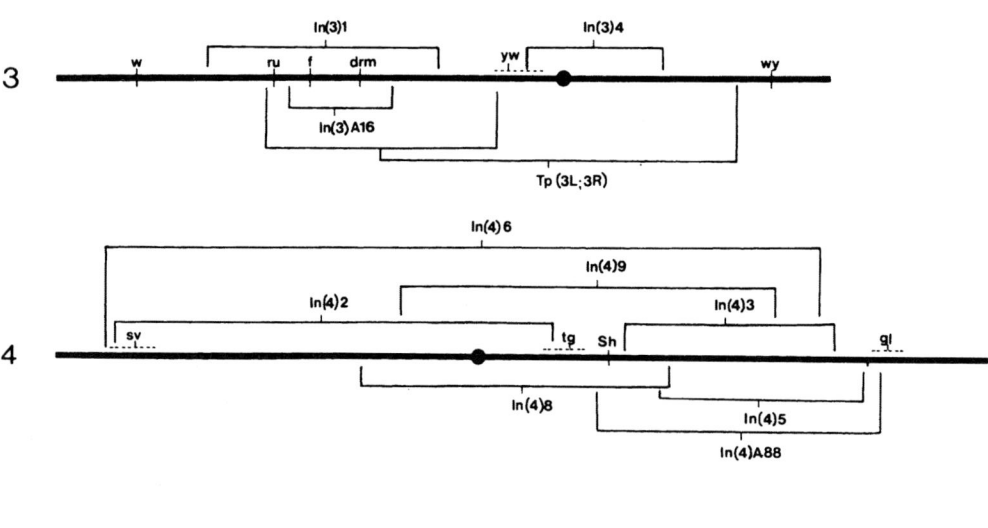

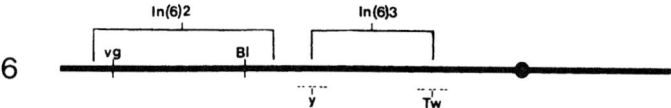

Figure 3. Relative cytological positions of crossover suppressors and mutations on chromosomes 3, 4, and 6.

Whitten, 1974, and see Figure 2). These studies were originally undertaken preliminary to attempts at genetic control through the release of translocation homozygotes (Whitten, 1971). However, the difficulty of obtaining homozygous translocations and the discovery that a type of rearrangement known as a compound autosome should be more ideally suited to the needs of genetic control (Foster *et al.,* 1972; Foster and Whitten, 1974) have led us to suspend the homozygous-translocation approach. Instead, newly synthesized translocations are screened cytologically to provide the intermediate strains necessary for compound-autosome synthesis (Foster *et al.,* 1972).

Duplications. In males carrying Y-autosome translocations, normal alternate segregation results in chromosomally normal females and in males carrying the translocation. Adjacent-I segregations occur frequently, however, and some of the aneuploid products survive as holandrically inherited terminal duplications of autosomal material. Duplications on each of the autosomes have been isolated in this manner and are being used in genetic mapping and in studies of aneuploid viability.

Organophosphorus-Insecticide Resistance

The formal genetics of OP resistance in Australian populations of *L. cuprina* has been examined (Arnold and Whitten, 1975*a*). There is a single locus (*Rop-1*) on chromosome 4 with four allelic states: wild type and three resistance allelles, *Rop-1^A*, *Rop-1^B*, *Rop-1^C*. Another locus on chromosome 6, *Rop-2,* exists in two allelic states: wild type and resistant.

The levels of resistance for larval and adult blowflies conferred by these alleles have been determined (Arnold and Whitten, 1975*c*) and are summarized in Table 3. There appears to be no consistent relationship between the respective levels of larval and adult resistance relative to wild type for the different *Rop-1* alleles. Resistance levels for both the larval and adult stages are additive when *Rop-1* alleles are heterozygous with one another. The relationship between *Rop-2* and the *Rop-1* alleles, however, appears to be multiplicative, consistent with the hypothesis that the two loci determine different resistance mechanisms (Arnold and Whitten, 1975*c*).

A survey of OP resistance levels and gene frequencies in field populations has indicated that variations in levels of population resistance are accountable in terms of change in frequency of the resistance alleles (Arnold and Whitten, 1975*b*). There is evidence to suggest that in the absence of organophosphorus insecticide the resistance alleles are severely deleterious,

TABLE 3.   Relative Larval and
Adult Resistances to Diazinon of
Different Homozygous Rop Mutations
in L. cuprina

Allele	Larval	Adult
Rop^+	1	1
$Rop\text{-}1^A$	45	9.0
$Rop\text{-}1^B$	60	4.8
$Rop\text{-}1^C$	123	7.7
$Rop\text{-}2$	2	4.2

and, consequently, fluctuations in gene frequency may be associated with the usage of these insecticides in the field (Arnold and Whitten, 1975*b*).

The Potential Uses of Genetics in Controlling *L. cuprina*

The formal genetics described above may be put to use in controlling *L. cuprina* in several ways. In the first instance they may provide useful adjuncts to other systems of control, or secondly they may lead to the development of entirely new systems, of which alterations to the genome of the insect are an integral part.

Sex-Killing Systems

As an example of the first point (above), practical sexing systems could be developed as an aid to SIRM. The coupling of the *bp* trait with a (Y;2) translocation has permitted simple sexing of *L. cuprina* at the pupal stage (Whitten, 1969). Similarly, the combination of conditional-lethal mutations which act earlier in the life cycle with sex-linked translocations would permit the development of sex-killing systems which would eliminate the waste inherent in rearing both sexes to maturity and then discarding one. One method which can be used to develop female-killing systems in many insect species involves the coupling of an appropriate insecticide-resistance gene to a sex chromosome with a suitable translocation (Whitten and Foster, 1975). Such a female-killing system has been developed in *L. cuprina* using a *T(Y;5)Rdl* strain and dipping first-instar larvae into a dieldrin solution to kill the susceptible females. Details of this method will be reported elsewhere (Whitten *et al.*, 1975).

The amount of genetics required for the development of sex-killing systems is not extensive and their use would lower the cost of rearing flies for use in a sterile-insect-release program. Thus, the contribution by geneticists to the field of applied entomology could be significant, if appropriate co-operation between these disciplines is nurtured.

Control by Genetic Load and Genetic Manipulation

Genetic systems which permit the release of fertile insects whose descendants manifest sterility can initiate genetic loads considerably higher than those produced by the direct release of sterile insects. For example, if we could release fertile males whose progeny will be sterile, a 9 : 1 ratio of the released fertile males to native males would produce a genetic load of 99-percent in the following generation compared with a 90-percent load produced immediately for a comparable release of fully sterile males. The method usually suggested for generating this type of sterility is the release of strains differing for a number of reciprocal translocations (Curtis and Hill, 1971; Whitten, 1971). Another possibility is that self-perpetuating systems of genetic load can be established by the release of both sexes of several homozygous-translocation strains (Curtis and Hill, 1971; Whitten, 1971) or compound-autosome races (Foster and Whitten, 1974).

The concept of pest control by modifying the genetic composition of natural populations to reduce their effectiveness (e.g., destroy vector capacity) or by introducing conditionally lethal traits has been discussed by many authors (Whitten, 1971; Foster *et al.,* 1972; Waterhouse *et al.,* 1975). To be able to introduce a gene rapidly into a population, some type of transporting mechanism is necessary. The most effective mechanism known to date relies on negative heterosis. If the hybrid between a released strain and the field population is either sterile or lethal, an unsteady state exists and whichever strain is more frequent will rapidly displace its competitor. Theoretically, either homozygous-translocation or compound-autosome races could generate the sort of negative heterosis necessary for population genome replacement (Curtis, 1968; Whitten, 1971; Foster *et al.,* 1972), although compound autosomes offer major advantages over translocations (Foster *et al.,* 1972). Using compound autosomes in *D. melanogaster,* Foster *et al.* (1972) demonstrated the possibility of using negative heterosis for the complete displacement of a population.

These approaches to genetic control of insect pests have not been tested under field conditions since the genetics of few suitable pests is sufficiently well advanced to provide the chromosome rearrangements necessary for adequate testing of the methods. For example, although the concept of compound chromosomes is simple, their actual construction is quite difficult. The general scheme for their synthesis, which is being followed for *L. cuprina,* is described by Foster *et al.* (1972). Much of the formal genetics which has been described above has been developed for this specific purpose. *L. cuprina* is currently unique in that, besides our having a reasonable knowledge of its genetics, considerable ecological information is being accumulated on its population dynamics (Foster *et al.,* 1975), and, also, the species is a major pest. We are now in a position to assess the possibility of synthesizing chromosomally altered strains which are competitive under field conditions.

Concluding Remarks

Apart from the practical implications of strains bearing chromosome rearrangements, their release into natural populations would represent interesting perturbation experiments. Population genetics is particularly depauperate in large-scale field experiments which disturb equilibrium situations. The effects of persisting genetic loads created by such releases will allow investigation of the rarely studied interface between population dynamics and genetics.

There has also accumulated over the years considerable information, largely of a descriptive nature, on inter- and intraspecific variation in chromosome numbers. Based on this type of data for grasshoppers, White (1970) has proposed a theory of stasipatric speciation. Novel chromosome rearrangements which arise spontaneously and become fixed by chance in small subpopulations are presumed to display heterozygous disadvantage in the hybrids because of irregularities during meiosis. White suggests that, under certain circumstances, this incipient speciation may be reinforced by the evolution of behavioral premating isolation, which ultimately leads to the formation of new species. The release of strains which exhibit complete postmating genetic isolation (e.g., compound-chromosome strains) will provide an opportunity to assess the ability of a species to evolve premating isolating mechanisms as an escape from the pressures imposed by the presence of otherwise incompatible strains. If premating isolation does evolve during a particular control program, although creating problems from a control viewpoint, it will illuminate an important aspect of the speciation process.

The work outlined above provides a demonstration that the formal genetics of a species need not simply be a repetition of Mendel's work or a "drosophilization" of *L. cuprina,* but it may be put both to practical uses, hopefully for controlling an important pest species, and to more esoteric uses, such as the analysis of hitherto untreated areas of population genetics and speciation mechanisms.

Acknowledgments

We wish to thank Messrs. A. T. Mills, R. A. Helman, D. Pfitzner, and Mrs. G. Maffi for technical assistance during these genetic studies.

Literature Cited

Arnold, J. T. and M. J. Whitten, 1975*a* The genetic basis of resistance to organophosphorus insecticides in the Australian sheep blowfly, *Lucilia cuprina*. unpublished.

Arnold, J. T. and M. J. Whitten, 1975*b* The population genetics of organophosphorus insecticide resistance in the Australian sheep blowfly, *Lucilia cuprina*. unpublished.

Arnold, J. T. and M. J. Whitten, 1975*c* Measurement of resistance in *Lucilia cuprina* larvae and absence of correlation between organophosphorus-resistance levels in larvae and adults. *Entomol. Exp. et Appl.* (in press).

Barton Browne, L., R. J. Bartell and H. H. Shorey, 1969 Pheromone-mediated behaviour leading to group oviposition in the blowfly *Lucilia cuprina*. *J. Insect Physiol.* **15**:1003–1014.

Bushland, R. C., 1971 Sterility principle for insect control. Historical development and recent innovations. In *Sterility Principle for Insect Control or Eradication*, pp. 3–14, International Atomic Energy Agency, Vienna.

Childress, D. C., 1969 Polytene chromosomes and linkage group-chromosome correlations in the Australian sheep blowfly *Lucilia cuprina* (Diptera: Calliphoridae). *Chromosoma (Berl.)* **26**:208–214.

Colless, D. H. and D. K. McAlpine, 1970 Diptera. In *The Insects of Australia*, pp. 656–740, C.S.I.R.O., Melbourne University Press, Melbourne.

Curtis, C. F., 1968 Possible use of translocations to fix desirable genes in insect pest populations. *Nature (Lond.)* **218**:368–369.

Curtis, C. F. and W. G. Hill, 1971 Theoretical studies on the use of translocations for the control of tsetse flies and other disease vectors. *Theoret. Pop. Biol.* **2**:71–90.

Foster, G. G. and M. J. Whitten, 1974 The development of genetic methods of controlling the Australian sheep blowfly, *Lucilia cuprina*. In *The Use of Genetics in Insect Control*, edited by R. Pal and M. J. Whitten, Elsevier/North-Holland, Amersterdam.

Foster, G. G. and M. J. Whitten, 1975 Revised linkage group–karyotype correlations and polytene chromosome maps of the Australian sheep blowfly *Lucilia cuprina* (Diptera:Calliphoridae). unpublished.

Foster, G. G., R. L. Kitching, W. G. Vogt, and M. J. Whitten, 1975 Sheep blowfly and its control in the pastoral ecosystem of Australia. *Proc. Ecol. Soc. Aust.* **9**:213–229.

Foster, G. G., M. J. Whitten, T. Prout and R. Gill, 1972 Chromosome rearrangements for the control of insect pests. *Science (Wash., D.C.)* **176**:875–880.

Froggatt, J. L., 1918 An economic study of *Nasonia brevicornis*, a hymenopterous parasite of muscid Diptera. *Bull. Entomol. Res.* **9**:257–262.

Lewis, E. B. and L. Smith Riles, 1960   A new method of preparing larval ganglion chromosomes. *Drosophila Inf. Serv.* **34**:118–119.

Nicholson, A. J., 1957   The self-adjustment of populations to change. *Cold Spring Harbor Symp. Quant. Biol.* **22**:153–173.

Norris, K. R., 1959   The ecology of sheep blowflies in Australia. In *Biogeography and Ecology in Australia, Monographiae Biologicae,* Vol. VIII, pp. 514–544,

Shanahan, G. J., 1965   A review of the flystrike problem of sheep in Australia. *J. Aust. Inst. Agric. Sci.* **31**:11–24.

Ullerich, F., 1963   Geschlechtschromosomen und Geschlechtsbestimmung bei einigen Calliphorinen (Calliphoridae, Diptera). *Chromosoma (Berl.)* **14**:45–110.

Waterhouse, D. F., 1947   The relative importance of live sheep and of carrion as breeding grounds for the Australian sheep blowfly *Lucilia cuprina.* Council for Scientific and Industrial Research, Bulletin No. 217 (Melbourne, 1947).

Waterhouse, D. F., 1950   Studies of the physiology and toxicology of blowflies. *Aust. J. Sci. Res. Ser. B* **3**:76–112.

Waterhouse, D. F. and S. J. Paramonov, 1950   The status of the two species of *Lucilia* (Diptera, Calliphoridae) attacking sheep in Australia. *Aust. J. Sci. Res.* **3**:310–336.

Waterhouse, D. F., L. E. LaChance and M. J. Whitten, 1975   Use of autocidal methods. In *Theory and Practice of Biological Control,* edited by C. Huffaker, P. DeBach and P.S. Messenger, Academic Press, New York.

White, M. J. D., 1970   Cytogenetics of speciation. *J. Aust. Entomol. Soc.* **9**:1–6.

Whitten, M. J., 1969   Automated sexing of pupae and its usefulness in control by sterile insects. *J. Econ. Entomol.* **62**:272–273.

Whitten, M. J., 1971   Insect control by genetic manipulation of natural populations. *Science (Wash., D.C.)* **171**:682–684.

Whitten, M. J. and G. G. Foster, 1975   Genetical methods of pest control. *Annu. Rev. Entomol.* **20**:461–475.

Whitten, M. J. and W. C. Taylor, 1970   A role for sterile females in insect control. *J. Econ. Entomol.* **63**:269–272.

Whitten, M. J., G. G. Foster and R. L. Kitching, 1973   The incorporation of laboratory-reared genetic material into a field population of the Australian sheep blowfly, *Lucilia cuprina. Can. Entomol.* **105**:893–901.

Whitten, M. J., G. G. Foster and J. T. Arnold, 1975   The use of insecticide resistance to eliminate females during mass rearing for autocidal control of insect pests. unpublished.

Williams, K. L. and L. M. Birt, 1972   A study of the quantitative significance of protein synthesis during the metamorphosis of the sheep blowfly, *Lucilia cuprina. Insect Biochem.* **2**:305–320.

PART K
THE GENUS
DROSOPHILA

17

The Phylogeny, Ecology, and Geography of *Drosophila*

Lynn H. Throckmorton

Introduction

The genus *Drosophila* is large, diverse, and widely distributed. Its members are found from sea level to high mountains and from the tropics to the edges of the tundra. Plains, deserts, swamps, and savannas all play host to them, but woodlands and forests are their habitat of choice and their centers of greatest abundance. Within the ecosystem, the species of *Drosophila* are important in saprophytic food chains because their immature stages are dependent upon organisms causing fermentation or decay. Efficient exploitation of this food niche accounts for much of the success of the genus and for many of its patterns of geographic distribution.

In spite of its size and diversity, the genus *Drosophila* cannot be treated apart from the other members of the family Drosophilidae. Too often, genera, subgenera, and species groups arise from a single common ancestor, and to treat some and exclude others would make biogeographic

Lynn H. Throckmorton—Department of Biology, University of Chicago, Chicago, Illinois.

analysis impossible. It would also obscure fruitful and challenging opportunities for research that contemporary biology can profit from. The evolutionary patterns among *Drosophila* and its close relatives show only the most recent working out of a success story that began with the founding of the family. Hence, if one is to fully understand the complex ways adaptive change, opportunity, time, and accident are interwoven in the history of *Drosophila,* this deep perspective is needed. Some mention must be made of other genera of drosophilids, but limitations of space prevent a detailed treatment of such a large group. This discussion of phylogeny, ecology, and geography can only be a summary, but it should be sufficient to illustrate the knowledge accumulated to date, to introduce the resources provided by *Drosophila* and its relatives, and to expose gaps in our understanding that can be filled by careful work in many areas.

A Guide to the Literature on *Drosophila*

The monograph, *Evolution in the Genus Drosophila,* by Patterson and Stone (1952), is still the most valuable single reference to the genus *Drosophila.* I use the distributions of *Drosophila* species mostly as they are given there, with some revisions where more recent work has altered the general pattern. I also depend on this work to provide the reader with an adequate bibliography of the earlier (prior to 1950) literature, so I will touch on that only lightly. Among the most significant of the older works are those of Sturtevant (1921, 1942). The University of Texas Publications, *Studies in the Genetics of Drosophila,* edited by Patterson (1940–1957), and *Studies in Genetics,* edited by M. R. Wheeler (1962–1972), are indispensible for many major papers on the taxonomy, biology, and distribution of drosophilids. The work of Wheeler (1952, 1954) is likewise indispensible, particularly for taxonomy and distribution, but also for genetics and ecology of *Drosophila.* His major catalogs (Wheeler, 1959, 1965, 1970; Wheeler and Hamilton, 1972) provide access to the earlier and more specialized literature of drosophilid taxonomy, which, for that reason, I omit from this listing. The studies of Okada (1956, 1962, 1966*b*, 1968*a*) are invaluable references to the oriental and Asian faunas and are important also for information they provide on the ecology, immature stages, and internal anatomy of many drosophilids other than *Drosophila.* Momma (1957) and Takada (1958, 1960) list species of Hokkaido, and Takada and Lee (1958) list species of Korea. Wheeler and Takada (1964) and Wheeler and Kambysellis (1966) treat faunas of the islands of the Pacific, and Mather (1955, 1956*a*, 1960) and Bock (in preparation) treat that of Australia. Hardy (1965, 1966, 1969) and Hardy and Kaneshiro (1968, 1969, 1972) describe the spectacular Hawaiian drosophilid fauna, while Carson *et al.* (1970) summarize the evolutionary biology of these forms. Burla (1951, 1954, 1956) has published much valuable work on the European and African species and on the neotropical *Hirtodrosophila* and *Zygothrica*. Lachaise (1974*a,b*), Lachaise and Tsacas (1974) and Tsacas and Lachaise (1974) provide extremely valuable work, particularly on the ecology of African species. Basden (1956), Basden and Harnden (1956), and Wheeler and Throckmorton (1960) treat arctic and subarctic faunas, and Hackman (1955, 1957) treats with north European forms. Dobzhansky and his co-workers have dealt extensively with Neotropical and Nearctic forms, and this literature is accessible through citations in Patterson and Stone (1952) and Dobzhansky (1970). Brncic (1970) summarizes the biology of Chilean species. Dobzhansky (1965) and Carson (1965) discuss cosmopolitan forms.

Phylogenetic relationships among Drosophilidae, aside from those implicit in taxonomic treatments, have been studied mostly within major groups, and the more important of this work has involved chromosome studies. Foremost among these is the work of Wasserman (1963) on species of the *repleta* group, of Patterson, Stone, and co-workers on species of the *virilis* group [reported by Stone, *et al.* (1960)], and of Dobzhansky and his co-workers on species of the *obscurà* group [summarized by Dobzhansky (1970)]. Miller and his associates deal with chromosomes of species of the *affinis* subgroup (Miller and Stone, 1962; Miller and Voelker, 1968, 1969*a,b*; Miller and Sanger, 1968), Stalker (1966) with the *melanica* group, Heed and Russell (1971) with the *cardini* group, Kastritsis (1966, 1969) with the *tripunctata* and *guarani* groups, Mather (1956*b,c*, 1960) with the subgenus *Scaptodrosophila* (= *Pholadoris*), Carson and Stalker [see Carson *et al.* (1970) for references], Carson (1970, 1971), Clayton *et al.* (1972), and Yoon *et al.* (1972*a,b,c*) with Hawaiian drosophilids, Ward and Heed (1970) with the subgenus *Sordophila* and its relatives, and Brncic *et al.* (1971) with species of the *mesophragmatica* group. Stalker (1972) has published on intergroup chromosome phylogeny, Kastritsis *et al.* (1970) have commented on relationships between the *guarani* and *tripunctata* groups, and Yoon *et al.* (1972*a*) have shown intergeneric chromosome homologies.

Special studies of relationships between major groups have been made mostly by Sturtevant (1942), Patterson and Stone (1952), Nater (1953), Okada (1956, 1963*a,b*, 1966*a*, 1967, 1968*b*, 1971), and Throckmorton (1962*a,b*, 1966, 1968). Bächli (1971) has made a computer study of phenetic distances within and between the genera *Leucophenga* and *Paraleucophenga*, but he has not yet followed this with a covariation analysis to discover the phylogenetic relationships therein.

Biogeographic studies of *Drosophila* and its relatives are rare, at least at the level of the group as a whole. The most comprehensive treatment is that of Patterson and Stone (1952), but this is more a report of distribution than of biogeography. Okada (1970) has published a faunal analysis of drosophilids in the area around New Guinea.

Fossil drosophilids are known from only two sources. Wheeler (1963) describes specimens of *Neotanygastrella* from Mexican amber of Oligocene–Miocene age. Hennig (1965) describes the genus *Electrophortica* from Baltic amber which is generally taken to be of Eocene origin.

Explanation of Tables and Figures

Table 1 is a taxonomic listing of the groups treated herein, together with their distributions and culturability. I have departed somewhat from the traditional procedure of indicating distribution by zoogeographic regions. Instead, I indicate the land masses across which the species are found. The primary purpose of biogeography is to interrelate history, ecology, and distribution of organisms, aiming toward a more complete understanding of existing ecosystems and of ecological and evolutionary theory. Movements from continent to continent are a critical feature of history. Accordingly, I am most concerned with the five continental areas of the globe, excluding Antarctica and Greenland for obvious reasons. Further aspects of distribution can be read from Figure 6. I have not been overly concerned with islands, either those of the Pacific or of the Caribbean. Their faunas mostly show relationships with those of adjacent continents, or of interconnecting island chains. The fauna of the Hawaiian Islands is rather a special case, and I will comment on it later. New Zealand has no endemic drosophilid fauna (Hennig, 1960).

With regard to distribution, I am concerned with general patterns rather than finer details of pattern (altitude, seasonality, etc.). These are very incompletely known and will be of concern later, when the overall picture is completed. In consequence, I list the distributions only by continent or by some well-known descriptive term (Holarctic, Pantropical, etc.). I include Malaysia, New Guinea, the Philippines, and so on as part of Eurasia (EA in Table 1). I have considered it necessary to exclude the widespread cosmopolitan or domestic species when listing distributions. Thus, the *melanogaster* group is listed as being found in Africa, Eurasia, Australia, and the Pacific islands (Micronesia, etc., excluding the East In-

TABLE 1. *Taxonomic Listings of Groups, Distribution, Culture, and Figure where Phylogenetic Position is Shown*

Group	Culture[a]	Distribution[b]	Figure
FAMILY: DROSOPHILIDAE			
Subfamily: Steganinae			
Amiota		WW	1, 5
Amiota	0		
Phortica	0		
Electrophortica	—	Baltic amber	1
Gitona	0	AF, EA, NW	1
Leucophenga	0	WW	1
Oxyphortica	0	EA	1
Paraleucophenga	0	AF, EA	1
Pararhinoleucophenga	0	EA	1
Protostegana	0	WW	1
Rhinoleucophenga	0	NW	1
Stegana		WW	1, 5
Stegana	0		
Steganina	0		
Subfamily: Drosophilinae			
Chaetodrosophilella	+, B	EA, PI	4, 6
Chymomyza	+–0, B	WW	2, 6
Dettopsomyia	+–0, B	WW	3
Drosophila			
Dorsilopha	+, B	EA	4, 6
Drosophila			
annulimana	+–?, B	NW	3, 6
bizonata	+–?, C	EA	—
bromeliae	±–?, B	NW	3, 6
canalinea	+–?, B	NW	3, 6
carbonaria	0	NA	3, 6
cardini	+, B	NW	4, 6
carsoni	+, B	NA	3, 6
castanea	+, B	NW	3, 6
dreyfusi	+, B	NW	3, 6
funebris	+, B, C	HO	2, 6
guaramunu	+, B	NW	4, 6
guarani	+, B	NW	4, 6
histrio	±, B	EA	—
immigrans	+–0, B, C	EA, AU, PI, AF	4, 6
macroptera	±, B	NA	4, 6
melanderi	±, S	HO	4

[a] Abbreviations for culture are as follows: B =banana medium, C =corn meal medium, S =special techniques; +=readily cultured, ± =difficult, 0 =not successfully cultured to date, ? =probably culturable.

[b] Abbreviations for distributions are as follows: AF=Africa, Ea=Eurasia, AU=Australia, PI=Pacific Islands, HI =Hawaiian Islands, NA =North America, SA =South America, WW =World-wide, PT = Pantropical, HO =Holarctic, NW =New World.

TABLE 1.   Continued

Group	Culture[a]	Distribution[b]	Figure
melanica	+, B, C	HO	3, 6
mesophragmatica	+–?, B	NW	3, 6
nannoptera	+, B	NA	3, 6
pallidipennis	+, B	NW	4, 6
peruviana	±, B	SA	3, 6
pinicola	±, S	NA	4, 6
polychaeta	+, B	EA, PI, NW	3, 6
quinaria	+–?, B	HO	4, 6
repleta			
fasciola	+–±, B	NW	3, 6
hydei	+, B	NW	3, 6
melanopalpa	+, B	NW	3, 6
mercatorum	+, B	NW	3, 6
mulleri	+, B	NW	3, 6
robusta	+, B, C	HO	3, 6
rubrifrons	+, B	NA	4, 6
sternopleuralis	±, B, C	EA	—
sticta	+, B	SA	4, 6
testacea	±, B	HO	4, 6
tripunctata	+–?, B	NW	4, 6
virilis	+, B	HO	3, 6
Engiscaptomyza	?, S	HI	4
Hirtodrosophila			
denticeps	0	EA	4, 6
duncani	+, B	NA	4, 6
hirticornis	±–0, S	EA, NW	4, 6
quadrivittata	±–0, S	EA	4, 6
Other species	±–0, S	WW	4
Phloridosa	0	NW	3, 6
Scaptodrosophila			
bryani	+, B, S	AF, EA, AU, PI	2, 6
coracina	+, B, S	EA, AU, PI	2, 6
subtilis	+, B, S	EA	2, 6
victoria	+, B, S	HO	2, 6
Other species	?, S	AF, EA, AU, PI	2
Siphlodora	0	NW	4, 6
Sophophora			
melanogaster	+, C, B	AF, EA, AU, PI	2, 6
obscura	+, C, B	HO	2, 6
populi	0	NA	6
saltans	+, C, B	NW	2, 6
willistoni	+–0, C, B	NW	2, 6
Sordophila	+, B, S	NA	3, 6
Hawaiian drosophiloids	+–0, S	HI	4, 6
Hypselothyrea	0	AF, EA	2, 6

TABLE 1. *Continued*

Group	Culture[a]	Distribution[b]	Figure
Liodrosophila	±–0	EA, AU, PI	2, 6
Microdrosophila	±–0, S	AF, EA, AU, PI, NW	1
Mycodrosophila	+–0, S	WW	4, 6
Neotanygastrella	0–?, S	AF, EA, PI, NW Miocene amber	4, 6
Nesiodrosophila	0–?, S	EA, PI	4, 6
Paramycodrosophila	0–?, S	EA, AU, PI, NW	6
Samoaia	±, B, S	PI	4, 6
Scaptomyza	+–?, S	WW	4, 6
Titanochaeta	0	HI	4, 6
Zaprionus	+–?	AF, EA, PI	4, 6
Zapriothrica	0	NW	—
Zygothrica	0–?, S	NW, PI	4, 6
Not placed in subfamily			
Lissocephala	0	PT	1, 5

dies, Hawaii, and New Zealand), even though some cosmopolitan species are found in the New World and Hawaii. When groups are indicated as being present in an area, this should not be taken as implying that they completely occupy that area, although they may do so. Hence, by worldwide I mean only that the group is represented by presumably noncosmopolitan species in Africa, Eurasia, North America, and South America. It may or may not also be present in Australia, for that fauna is poorly known, and it may be present in some islands I take no special note of, as those of the Caribbean, for example.

Culturability is shown in Table 1 by symbols (+, ±, etc.). They indicate the ease of culture, but only in a very general way, since members of a given group are not always cultured with comparable ease. The culture medium is indicated (B = banana, C = corn meal, S = special), and in some cases the probable range of culturability within the group is also shown (+–±, etc.). Recipes, general culture methods, and a key to the United States species of *Drosophila* are given by Strickberger (1962). Special methods are quite varied and depend somewhat on the investigator. The methods of Wheeler and Clayton (1965) and Speith (1972) are useful for many forms that are otherwise impossible to maintain in the laboratory.

Finally, a word needs to be said about terminology. I shall be referring to radiations, and in the figures these are represented by several, or even many, lineages arising at one level in the dendrogram. In part, or in places, this will be an evolutionarily realistic picture of diversification. Certainly there is no reason to suppose that populations do not at times fragment, effectively founding several or many independent lineages simultaneously. In other cases radiations will reflect lack of evidence as to the sequence of events by which diversification proceeded at a given time. For these, relevant character states are discovered in so many of their possible combinations that no hierarchical pattern is discernible. In some of these instances future work may discover patterns of character covariation where none are now seen. In others, true radiation, rapid diversification within a new adaptive zone, habitat, or geographical area, will remain the parsimonious inference. The radiations referred to here must be regarded as conservative indications of covariation patterns in the data. Future work may show certain branches from a radiation to be more closely related than is presently indicated; it is unlikely that they will be shown to be less closely related. Finally, neither vertical nor horizontal dimensions in the figures have significance. These were determined at the whim of the illustrator. Only sequence of diversification is to be read from the dendrograms.

Phylogeny, Ecology, and Biogeography

Origin and Early Radiations of the Family Drosophilidae

The family Drosophilidae stems from a cluster of families of Acalypterae, the Drosophiloidea (Hennig, 1958). Of these (Curtonotidae, Drosophilidae, Diastatidae, Camillidae, Ephydridae), the Diastatidae are most closely related to the Drosophilidae (Figure 5). Members of the two major families of this radiation, the ephydrids and the drosophilids, have larval stages depending for food on organisms or organic matter in a liquid or semiliquid medium. The larval stages of many ephydrids are aquatic, but some are found in foul muds, manures, or carrion, while others mine the stems of aquatic or terrestrial plants. The diastatids are saprophagous in leafmold (Hennig, 1965), as are a considerable number of species of somewhat more distantly related families (Oldroyd, 1964). Okada (1962) has suggested that larval feeding on sap of bleeding trees was the primitive drosophilid condition, but I suspect the group was not quite so specialized in the earliest times. The drosophilids of the primitive radiations (Figure 1) are quite varied in their habits. Some species of

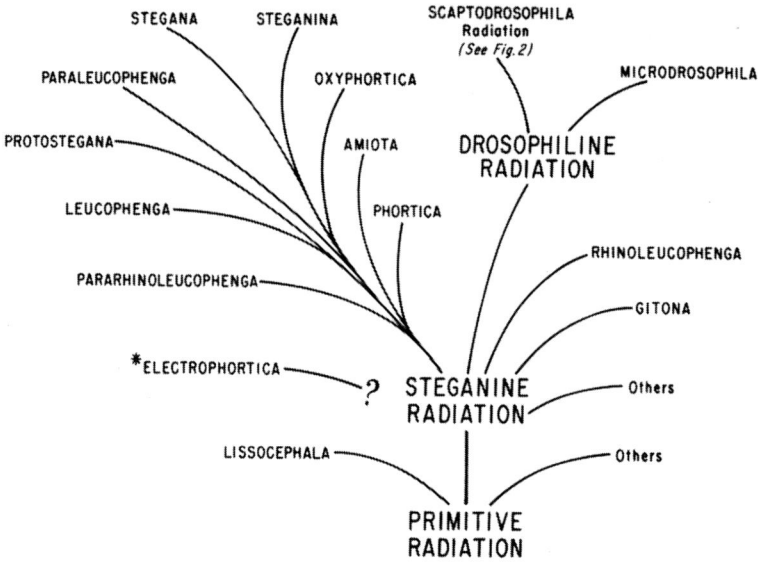

Figure 1. The early radiations of the family Drosophilidae showing the origin of the genus Drosophila from among the early drosophiline genera with the appearance of the subgenus Scaptodrosophila (upper right). The genus Electrophortica (*) is described from Baltic amber of Eocene age.

Amiota are sap feeders and some are fungivorous. Species of *Leucophenga* are fungivorous, larvae of *Stegana* are reported under bark [Morge (1956) cited by Okada (1968a)] and in flowers (Buruga and Olembo, 1971), species of *Gitona* are reported in broken plant parts, flowers, fruits, rotting cactus, and as parasites of mealybugs, a species of *Rhinoleucophenga* is parasitic on coccids, and so on. Many drosophiline species are reported in rotting leaves and decaying or fermenting fruit, as well as in fungus, sap, flowers, and pollen (Wheeler, 1952; Heed, 1957; Cole, 1969; Okada, 1956, 1962, 1968a; Pipkin, 1964). To me, this adds up to a pattern of opportunism and versatility centering around the saprophagous leafmold habit of some primitive acalypterates. It is not uncommon for drosophilids to exhibit considerable breadth in their choice of breeding site. Thus, for example, Basden (1954) reports *D. subobscura* as breeding naturally in the saps of elm, willow, and sycamore, in iris root, in toadstools, and in fermenting fruit and oak galls; this very nearly embraces all the basic food types exploited by the family, excepting only flowers and the parasitic modes of existence. It is not improbable that the earliest drosophilid was an opportunist of this sort, capable of exploiting many alternative resources but perhaps preferring one of these over the others. On present evidence it seems simplest to visualize the diversification of the Drosophiloidea as being founded on the food resources of rotting leafmold, with two major lineages diverging and specializing from this. On the one hand the ephydrids exploited the wetter, more foul muds and related organic decay, with some eventual specialization on algae. On the other hand the drosophilids evolved more toward decaying leaves, fermenting vegetables and fruits, saps, and fungi, with specialization mostly on yeasts. At one time or another both have adjusted to mining tissues of plants.

The most primitive genus of drosophilids is *Lissocephala* (Figures 1 and 5). It is pantropical in distribution and provides sound evidence for the tropical origin of the Drosophilidae. The food habits of these species are not well known, but I have swept them from compost. Wheeler and Kambysellis (1966) report sweeping them from garbage, Buruga and Olembo (1971) report them on fruit, and Carson (Carson and Wheeler, 1973) discovered larvae of one of these species developing on land crabs on Christmas Island.

The major genera of the steganine radiation (*Amiota, Leucophenga, Stegana*) also have their main distributions in the tropics, and this lends support to the conclusion that the family originated there. The genus *Amiota* is world-wide in distribution, and so is *Stegana* (Table 1), with *Stegana* being proportionately less well represented in the temperate fauna than *Amiota*. *Gitona* is found in Africa, Europe, and North America, but the assignment of some of the North American species to specific genera is uncertain (McAlpine, 1968), and these may represent a group endemic to North America (Wheeler and Takada, 1971). Some of the remaining genera are also restricted to certain regions, as *Rhinoleucophenga* to the Americas, *Pararhinoleucophenga* to Taiwan, and *Oxyphortica* to New Guinea, Taiwan, and Southeast Asia.

The major steganine genera, and the minor genera associated with them (to the left in Figure 1), form a coherent lineage, sharing much, both of internal and external anatomy. Of these, *Amiota* combines more of both drosophiline and steganine attributes, and among the Steganinae it is the most generalized group. In collecting, it has been my experience that *Amiota* tends to be of the shaded forest, *Leucophenga* is more often of the brighter and less humid forest edges, savannas, and brushy meadows, and *Stegana* is of stream sides, mossy banks and logs, and humid ravines. *Oxyphortica* resembles *Leucophenga* in being found in drier and more-open places, particularly in the upper reaches of valleys or the drier valley edges. Hence, in spite of some close resemblance and overlap in food choice among the members of this kindred, resources seem generally to be partitioned along habitat boundaries, and direct competition between individuals of these genera must be limited.

Most of these species can be collected by sweeping brush and vegetation in appropriate habitats, with special attention to tree trunks, fallen logs, and mossy banks. Fungus is important also, as are slime fluxes and bleeding trees, and an aspirator is often the most convenient way to collect from these. *Leucophenga* occasionally comes to fermenting baits, or local fungus can be gathered and used as bait. Males of *Amiota* have a habit of buzzing around the head of a person walking through the woods, and then they can be netted. Basden (1954) reports obtaining good numbers of both males and females of a species of *Amiota* using fermenting apple bait placed high up in oak and chestnut trees. He also reports collection of *Stegana* near fungus, and on several occasions I have collected female *Stegana* directly off mushrooms.

Hennig (1965) describes a fossil genus, *Electrophortica,* from Baltic amber. He notes that in some keys for the family it would be in the genus *Amiota,* but it might equally well belong to the stem group for all recent species, or it could be the ancestral species itself. Baltic amber may be from Eocene times, and the presence of a drosophilid then and there is fully consistent with the conclusion one reaches from steganine distributions. These indicate dispersion at a time when tropical corridors connected Asia and North America, and the middle of the Oligocene period is very nearly the latest time when that might have been true. This fossil seems to have existed before then, and probably much before then. Depending on the reliability of dates for Baltic amber, the family Drosophilidae may be 50 million years old, or older.

The Early Drosophiline Radiations

The genus *Microdrosophila* is treated taxonomically by Okada (1968b). It has a world-wide distribution through the tropics, and there are several representatives in the temperate zone. The greater number of known species is from Southeast Asia and the adjacent islands. Okada (1968a) reports eggs, larvae, and pupae from rotting sweet potatoes and rotting bamboo leaves, and adults can be collected by sweeping brush, garbage, and rotting fruit. Some of the species can be cultured on standard *Drosophila* medium, but culture is generally difficult.

The primary distribution of the *Scaptodrosophila* radiation (Figures 2 and 6), exclusive of the *subtilis* and *victoria* groups, is in the tropics. It is probably represented in the New World by the genus *Zapriothrica,* individuals of which have been collected from flowers of *Datura* (Wheeler, 1956). As the subgenus *Scaptodrosophila,* members of this radiation are distributed through the Old World tropics from Africa to Australia and the

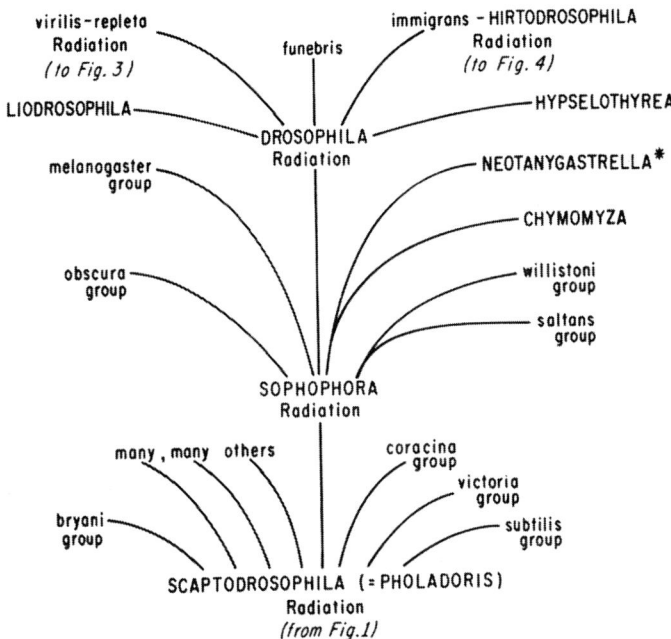

Figure 2. The early radiations of Drosophila and derived genera (continued from Figure 1).

Pacific, and this defines the place of origin of the genus. Although there has been a sizeable expansion of *Scaptodrosophila* into Australia [44 of 46 recognized species are regarded as endemic (I. R. Bock, private communication)], no evidence indicates that the group originated there. Much evidence points to its origin in tropical Asia (Throckmorton, unpublished).

Species of *Scaptodrosophila* are collected from tree sap, palm sap, fungus, fruit, and flowers. Okada (1968a) reared *D. throckmortoni* Okada 1973 (=*D. rufifrons* Okada 1956) from slime flux on oak and *D. coracina* from fallen leaves. Hence, the feeding diversity encountered among the steganine genera is still encountered here, but with a shift in emphasis toward more feeding on fermenting fruit. Burla (1954), Lachaise (1974a,b), and Lachaise and Tsacas (1974) describe the ecology of African species, Mather (1955, 1956a) and I. R. Bock (in preparation) discuss the Australian species, and Wheeler and Takada (1964) and Wheeler and Kambysellis (1966) list Pacific island species.

In contrast to the other species of this radiation, the *victoria* and *subtilis* groups have primary distributions in the north temperate zone. The *subtilis* group is from China and Japan, while the *victoria* group has a disjunct distribution, with species in Europe, the Middle East, and North America. The distributions of these two groups do not bear directly on the problem of the origin of the genus *Drosophila*. Anatomically they are clearly derivative within *Scaptodrosophila*. The *victoria* group breeds on bleeding cottonwoods, and its disjunct distribution almost certainly originated at the disruption of the temperate deciduous forest in late Miocene times. Judging by present distributions, the *Scaptodrosophila* radiation occurred prior to the middle of the Oligocene period, so the *victoria* group would have arisen later than that but well prior to mid-Miocene, presumably by invasion of the temperate deciduous forest at the northern border of the Old World tropics.

Many of these species can be collected fairly easily from the standard, fermenting fruit baits, or by sweeping or aspirating from bleeding trees, fungus, or fallen fruit. Some of these species show less diurnal periodicity than is usual for *Drosophila,* tending to come to baits in the hotter parts of the afternoon and preferring fresher baits than do the better-known species (*D. melanogaster,* etc.). Some flies do well on various "instant" *Drosophila* media, and I have been able to bring otherwise recalcitrant species into culture through exposing them to a light regimen of long days and short nights. The *victoria* group in North America is reviewed most recently by Pipkin (1961). At present, the known species are concentrated in the Southwest, but one or more species do exist in the United States east of the Rockies (Wheeler, 1949; L. Throckmorton, unpublished).

The Sophophoran Radiation

This radiation (Figures 2 and 6) is comprised of the *saltans–willistoni* lineage in the New World tropics, the *melanogaster* lineage in the Old World tropics, and the *obscura* group distributed throughout the Holarctic temperate zone. It also includes isolated species such as *D. populi,* and the two genera, *Chymomyza* (world-wide) and *Neotanygastrella* (pantropical).

Although I have not myself seen *Neotanygastrella,* I include it here because two fossil specimens, tentatively assigned to this genus, are described by Wheeler (1963) from Mexican amber of Oligocene or early Miocene age. Frota-Pessoa and Wheeler (1951) and Burla (1954) regard *Chymomyza* and *Neotanygastrella* as being very close, so I include them in one lineage in the figure. I note that Burla's figure (1954, his p. 52) shows internal details that place *Neotanygastrella* closer to *D. populi* than to *Chymomyza,* so *D. populi* may be very near the stem from which these two genera arose. *D. populi* was collected over fallen cottonwood in Alaska (Wheeler and Throckmorton, 1960), and I have collected two closely related species from Taiwan. Hence, *D. populi* seems to be a northern relict of a subtropical group that was once distributed through that region. *Neotanygastrella* and *Chymomyza* are both attracted to cut tree trunks, *Chymomyza* is attracted to peeled bark of aspen, alder, fir, pine, and birch (Wheeler, 1952; Basden, 1954). *C. amoena* breeds in acorns and *C. aldrichi* larvae have been found under aspen bark [Spieth, reported by Wheeler (1952)]. Wheeler (1963) suggests an Afro-Asian origin for the *Chymomyza* complex, with the African species representing the ancestral type that gave rise to both *Chymomyza* and *Neotanygastrella*. This suggestion is compatible with other available evidence. These genera relate through forms such as *D. populi* to Afro-Asian *Scaptodrosophila* similar to *D. bryani* or *D. latifasciaeformis,* which themselves represent the primitive group out of which the sophophoran radiation emerged. Here, as for the previous radiation, the New World lineages are derivative relative to the Old World forms, and none of the higher lineages show any indication of having been derived from them. The Old World forms, on the other hand, intergrade in many features, both with members of lower and higher radiations. Hence, parsimoniously, the sophophoran radiation can be regarded as originating in the Old World tropics. From distribution, the time for this would again be very much before mid-Oligocene times. The fossils indicate the same thing, since the sophophoran radiation must have occurred well before the Oligocene–Miocene times from which the fossils are recorded.

The *melanogaster* group, of 76 named species, is reviewed by Bock and Wheeler (1972). Aside from four widespread species, its distribution is within the tropical and subtropical regions of the Old World. In south Asia it extends from India and Nepal east to Korea, Japan, and the other islands offshore (Taiwan, Philippines, New Guinea, etc.), thence east and south to the islands of the Pacific, and then along the northern edge of Australia. Members of the group are also widespread in Africa.

There are four species of nearly cosmopolitan distribution. *D. kikkawai* is from Asia, the Pacific islands and South America; *D. ananassae* is found in Africa, Asia, Australia, the Pacific islands, and the New World; and *D. simulans* and *D. melanogaster* are both world-wide, being excluded only from the polar regions. As noted by Bock and Wheeler, however, *D. melanogaster* is more common in colder regions, while *D. simulans* is more common in the warmer areas. From patterns of distribution it can be concluded that the *melanogaster* subgroup, including both *D. melanogaster* and *D. simulans,* arose in Africa (but see Bock and Wheeler for a less parsimonious alternative, and see Tsacas and Lachaise, 1974, for their views), and they probably coevolved with man throughout their period of coexistence with him. The *melanogaster* group itself almost surely arose in south Asia, and it has diversified and dispersed from there. While the group, or at least a *protomelanogaster* group, must have existed prior to mid-Oligocene times, its major radiation has quite obviously occurred since the New and Old World tropics became isolated from each other. A secondary radiation of the group has occurred in Africa, possibly starting in the late Oligocene times. Although the *melanogaster* group is represented in Australia, present evidence suggests no great amount of evolution there (I. R. Bock, private communication). In view of the history of the Australian continent, this may not be surprising. From the time when the *melanogaster* group originated in south Asia, Australia has been connected to that region only through island chains. They may not have been efficient corridors for *Drosophila* migration until quite recently, and even now, possibilities for movement across them are not great. That regardless, the subgenus *Scaptodrosophila* did achieve a greater radiation in Australia, presumably because it originated earlier and arrived there sooner.

The ecology of species in this group has not been greatly studied. The majority can be collected at fermenting fruit baits or swept over fallen fruit. Carson (1965) lists a great variety of breeding sites for widespread species of this group, including more than twenty different kinds of fruit, living flowers, potatoes, slime fluxes, mushrooms, rotting plant tissues, stale beer, and human feces. At least one endemic species of the Philippines, *D. elegans,* is collected from flowers, as was discovered by C. Kanapi (unpublished). Most of the members of this group can be cultured in the laboratory on standard media, though many of them are considerably more difficult to care for than is *D. melanogaster.*

The *saltans* and *willistoni* groups are products of a single sophophoran lineage. They are distinct from all other sophophoran groups but very close to each other, and they are derivative within the subgenus. A review of the *saltans* group by Magalhaes (1962) includes a map of distributions and a key to the species. Two species have been described since then (Mourão and Bicudo, 1967), for a total of 21 species in five subgroups. These show an orderly progression from the more primitive *cordata* and *elliptica* subgroups, through the *sturtevanti* and *parasaltans* subgroups, to the *saltans* subgroup, which is unequivocally the most derivative cluster of species. Members of the primitive subgroups are distributed from Mexico to Brazil. Most of the *saltans* subgroup species are in South America. They show a distribution pattern typical of groups that evolved on the South American continent and then spread northward after the building of the present Isthmus of Panama in the late Pliocene period, perhaps 4.5 million years ago. The evidence from distribution thus suggests origin of the *saltans* group in tropical North America, colonization of South America at least once prior to the building of the present Isthmus of Panama, diversification in South America to produce at least the *parasaltans* and *saltans* subgroups, and finally diffusion of the *saltans* subgroup northward into Central America, Mexico, and the Caribbean. Except for Pipkin's observations (1965), the ecology of these species is not well known. Some do not come readily to bait, but *D. saltans* is reported as being bred from pineapple (Magalhaes, 1962), *D. sturtevanti* from citrus (Heed, 1957) and from fallen fruits and blossoms, and *D. prosaltans* from fallen fruits and blossoms (Pipkin, 1965). The larvae skip, which is a habit often associated with sap-feeding forms, but in this case it may only indicate the retention of one of the characters of *Scaptodrosophila* ancestors.

The *willistoni* group (25 species) divides into three major clusters. One of these, morphologically the most primitive form, is comprised of *D. willistoni* and its siblings, a second contains only *D. fumipennis,* and the third contains all the remaining species, including the *alagitans–bocainensis* complex of Wheeler and Magalhaes (1962). The distribution of these clusters presents almost a reverse image of that of the *saltans* group. Here it is the primitive group that is found predominantly in South America (Spassky *et al.,* 1971). The derivative group extends from Mexico south to Argentina (Wheeler and Magalhaes, 1962). *D. fumipennis* is reported from Costa Rica south to Brazil (Wheeler, 1970). In light of these distributions, a fragile case might be made for the hypothesis that the *saltans* group originated in tropical North America while the *willistoni* group originated in South America, perhaps evolving there in isolation after an early crossing of the water gap then existing between the two continents. Subsequent crossings in both directions could complete existing patterns, and not all of these need to have been prior to the formation of the Isthmus of Panama. The most recent evolutionary event would have been the blossoming of sibling clusters in each lineage. Those of both the *saltans* and the *willistoni* groups seem to have originated in South America, but the diversification of the *willistoni* siblings seems to have been nearly complete at the time when these species moved northward into Central America, whereas the *saltans* cluster was still actively evolving at that time. Several of the *willistoni* siblings are found together in most Central American localities (Spassky *et al.,* 1971), as if an entire fauna had moved northward, but in the *saltans* cluster the pattern is more one of individual populations spreading northward, with some speciation in the process. Thus, the species *D. saltans,* with a distribution from Costa Rica to Mexico, is largely parapatric with *D. prosaltans,* as if this were one of the most recent speciation events in that cluster, and there is apparently much less sympatry among the *saltans* siblings than among the *willistoni* siblings. The diversification of the semispecies of *D. paulistorum* (Spassky *et al.,* 1971; Dobzhansky, 1972) is apparently still continuing. One can speculate that at least part of this diversification was induced by Pleistocene events, but population shifts seem not to have been great, and genetic differentiation seems to have been comparatively minor (Ayala *et al.*, 1974).

Only slightly more is known of the ecology of the *willistoni* group than is known for the species of the *saltans* group. These species can be collected from the standard fruit baits or by sweeping over fallen fruits. *D. sucinea, D. nebulosa, D. fumipennis,* and the *willistoni* siblings have been reared from fruits and flowers (Pipkin, 1965) and some have been swept from acorns (Heed, 1957; Pipkin *et al.*, 1966). *D. willistoni* and its closest relatives are cultured readily, but attempts to culture many of the remaining species have been unsuccessful. *D. capricorni* has been reared from flowers, and flower feeders are all difficult to rear in the laboratory.

The 23 species of the *obscura* group are distributed throughout the North Temperate Zone. Ten species are recorded from Eurasia, being distributed from North Africa, Spain, the British Isles, and Scandinavia through the Middle East to Japan and Korea. Thirteen species are from the New World, with a distribution extending from Alaska, Manitoba, and Quebec south to Florida, Mexico, Guatemala, and central South America. Although phylogenetic relationships are known for several species clusters within the group, no overall phylogeny is available. Dobzhansky and Epling (1944) and Heed *et al.* (1969) describe the relationships and distribution of *D. pseudoobscura* and its relatives in western North America. Miller (1958) outlines the distribution of the remainder of the North American species, and Sulerud and Miller (1966) give a key to these species.

The *obscura* group is most closely related to the *melanogaster* group and to the subgenus *Scaptodrosophila* of the Old World tropics. Although several species have distributions bordering or extending into the tropics, there is no indication that any of these represents ancestral links to tropical species. The available evidence suggests that the group originated from a *protomelanogaster* lineage of the Old World tropics. Following adaptation to temperate habitats, diversification occurred in the Palearctic and the group spread to North America through the temperate deciduous forest prior to mid-Miocene times. Within the Palearctic, the members of this group present no clear pattern of diversification. Somewhat more of a pattern is discernible in North America, where two relatively distinct subgroups are present. The *obscura* subgroup (5 species) is western, with a distribution from British Columbia south through the Rocky Mountains to Mexico, Guatemala, and Colombia. The *affinis* subgroup has both a western (4 species) and an eastern (4 species) branch, with one species (*D. athabasca*) having both eastern and western–northern forms. The western branch extends from Oregon south through the Rocky Mountains to

Colombia, Venezuela, Bolivia, and Haiti. The eastern cluster extends from southern Canada south to Florida and west through the Great Plains almost to the eastern face of the Rockies. In the west, *D. athabasca* extends from New Mexico north to Alaska, then east to northern Manitoba (Throckmorton, unpublished) and Quebec, and then south to Tennessee and Nebraska (Miller, private communication).

Tentatively, the New World evolution of the *obscura* group appears as follows: Either before arrival in the New World or shortly thereafter, two main types existed. Presumably both of these were western, but eventually one or more of the *affinis* subgroup types extended the distribution to the east. Ecological separation of the North American continent by grasslands of the Great Plains dates from the Miocene era, and it may have been this partial barrier that isolated the eastern and western branches of the *affinis* subgroup and that restricted the *obscura* subgroup to the West. Much of the area occupied by *D. athabasca* was covered by ice during the Pleistocene so that part of the range must have been occupied quite recently. The eastern and western–northern forms of *D. athabasca* overlap in a zone extending from Minnesota to Maine (Miller, private communication), and significant barriers to gene exchange between them have been demonstrated (Miller, 1958; Miller and Westphal, 1967; Miller and Voelker, 1968, 1969a,b). Most of the distribution of these species to the Neotropics has been at higher altitudes, and the present pattern undoubtedly represents the end result of chance colonizations, of island hopping from mountain top to mountain top over several millions of years, with just three successes (*D. azteca, D. tolteca,* and *D. pseudoobscura*) out of unnumbered trials. One colonization, that of Colombia by *D. pseudoobscura*, is thought to have occurred within the last few decades (Prakash, 1972).

Dobzhansky and Epling (1944, their pages 147–183) discuss paleoecology and the evolution of the *obscura* subgroup in company with the development of the western paleoflora. There is little reason to doubt that many of its chromosome inversions have persisted since Miocene times, or earlier.

As usual, the ecology of these species is by no means well known. The most important natural breeding site seems to be in sap of trees such as oak, sycamore, willow, and elm. *D. pseudoobscura* has also been reared from cactus (Heed, private communication), *D. pseudoobscura, D. persimilis,* and *D. affinis* from the sap of wild grape vines (Patterson and Stone, 1952), and *D. pseudoobscura* from slime flux on fir (Carson, 1965). Both *D. athabasca* and *D. algonquin* have been reared from fungi, but this is probably not an important natural breeding site for these species (Carson and Stalker, 1951; Miller and Sanger, 1968). *D. affinis* has been reared from ripe blackberries (Miller and Weeks, 1964). *D. subobscura* has also been reared from toadstools, fermenting fruits, and so on, and probably many of these species are similarly general in their tastes. Most of the *obscura* subgroup species can be collected readily at baits and cultured fairly easily. The *affinis* subgroup species are also easy to collect, but some of them are troublesome to keep in culture for any length of time. They tend to be sensitive to propionic acid as a mold inhibitor, and they are often easier to maintain if some alternative chemical is used for the suppression of molds.

The Drosophila Radiation

This radiation is comprised primarily of major subradiations (Figures 2 and 6). In addition, several groups are clearly related at this point to the higher Drosophilinae, yet they show none of the special features of any of the well-defined lineages. *Liodrosophila* and *Hypselothyrea* are distinctive, small flies. *Liodrosophila* is the more diverse of the two, and it is distributed from South Asia to the Pacific islands. *Hypselothyrea* is from Africa and south Asia. The groups themselves are compact, but they differ as much from each other as from the other groups associated with this radiation. They can be regarded as independent lineages arising from early species of the *Drosophila* radiation. As lineages they probably existed by Oligocene times, but since they are not represented in the New World, a major part of their diversification may have occurred during the Miocene times or later, which would be consistent with their distinctiveness as groups as well as with their present distribution. Individuals of both groups are most readily collected by sweeping low shrubs, thick leafy vegetation, and tall grass in shaded areas under trees. Okada (1956) reports collecting *Liodrosophila* from tree sap, and some species of *Liodrosophila* can be cultured on standard *Drosophila* culture medium.

The *funebris* group is also associated with this radiation. In contrast to the two previous groups, its species share derivative features with species of both major subradiations. Hence, it cannot be assigned definitely to either one. Of the six species in this group, two are Oriental, three are Nearctic, and one, *D. funebris,* is cosmopolitan. The group's primary distribution is within the temperate zone, and its relationships are with species of the Old World tropics. As a member of the temperate deciduous forest fauna, it most probably dispersed to the New World prior to mid-Miocene times. Within the Nearctic region, *D. macrospina* is represented by a cluster of subspecies. The form *D. macrospina macrospina* is distributed from Texas and Arizona north to Montana, east to New York, and thence south to Florida. *D. m. limpiensis* is reported from Texas, Arizona, and Mexico, while *D. m. ohioensis* is reported from Ohio, Michigan, and New York. The two species *D. subfunebris* and *D. trispina* are distributed to California and Washington, and California and Arizona, respectively. This distribution pattern is a very common one for *Drosophila* species of the temperate deciduous forest. It will be commented upon during discussion of the next cluster of species. The Nearctic form, *D. m. limpiensis,* is reported as breeding in bracket fungus on willow (Patterson and Stone, 1952), and *D. maculinotata* of Japan is reported from bleeding trees (Okada, 1968*a*). The cosmopolitan *D. funebris* is reported from fungi, walnut husks, fruit, potatoes, and onions (Carson, 1965).

The *virilis–repleta* Radiation

This radiation (Figures 3 and 6), while complex in appearance, is basically simple. The primary radiation occurred in the Old World tropics, and I have seen representatives of it from Taiwan and Luzon. Eventually it extended from the Old to the New World tropics, and since that time there have been two centers of evolution for it. Out of this radiation in the Old World tropics came at least one temperate lineage, and the *repleta* group developed out of the Neotropical branch. The *repleta* lineage has also shown considerable diversification into the temperate zone and has produced several cosmopolitan species.

The early tropical radiation is represented by a heterogeneous assemblage of groups. The two species of the *tumiditarsus* group are both Oriental. The *polychaeta* group is represented in both the New and Old Worlds. *D. polychaeta* itself is distributed from the United States through Central America to Brazil, as well as to several Pacific islands, with the last probably being the result of human transport. The ranges of other New World species are within that of *D. polychaeta. D. daruma* of Japan is a member of this group (Okada, private communication), and the species of this group seem mostly to be associated with fallen fruit. The *annulimana* group is wholly Neotropical, being distributed to Mexico and Brazil. One of these species, *D. gibberosa,* has been reared from fruit. The genus *Dettopsomyia* is world-wide in distribution. *D. nigrovittata* has been reported from California, but it is primarily from the Old World tropics. *D. formosa* is the only Neotropical representative. Outside of Central America it is also found on several islands of the Pacific and In-

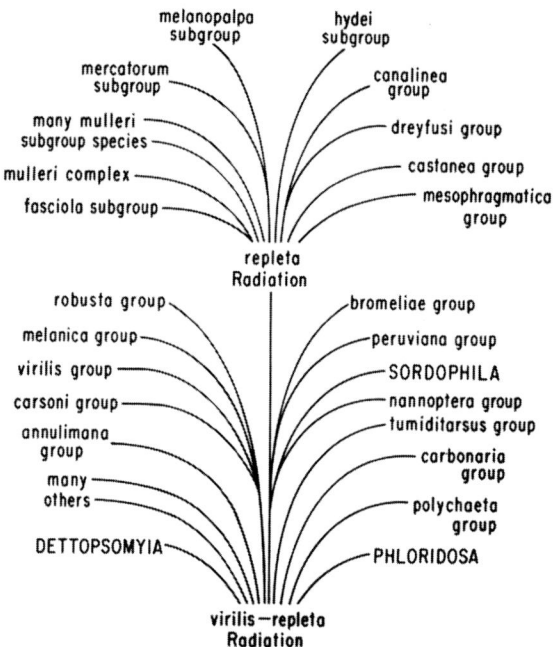

Figure 3. The virilis–repleta radiation continued from the upper left of Figure 2.

dian Oceans. It breeds in rotting banana stems and presumably was distributed through much of this region by man. The subgenus *Phloridosa* is a small cluster of flower feeders whose larvae utilize the pollen of *Datura, Hibiscus,* and so on. It is distributed from the southern United States south to Chile and Argentina, but it is mostly Neotropical. The *carbonaria* group contains only *D. carbonaria,* a species that breeds in bleeding mesquite, and its distribution is from the southern United States into Mexico (Patterson and Stone, 1952).

Several major temperate-forest groups emerged from the Old World limb of this radiation. Three of these now have a Holarctic distribution and one is Nearctic only. They seem to represent a single lineage that adapted to the temperate zone, diversified there, and eventually spread through the temperate deciduous forest to the New World. The *virilis, melanica,* and *robusta* groups are well represented in the literature of *Drosophila,* and each of these presents disjunct distribution patterns typical of groups associated with the temperate deciduous forests of the Holarctic region. The *robusta* group is comprised of eight species in the Orient and two species, *D. robusta* and *D. colorata,* in the Nearctic region. *D. robusta* breeds in the slime flux of elm (Carson and Stalker,

1951) and *D. sordidula* breeds in the sap of oak trees (Okada, 1968*a*). It is probable that other members of the group have similar habits. These species can be collected with standard baits, although many of them are quite rare, and most of them can be cultured on standard media.

Stalker (1966) treats the distribution and chromosome phylogeny of six North American members of the *melanica* group. Aside from these, there is one European species (Burla and Gloor, 1952) and one Oriental species (Okada and Kurokawa, 1957). Another species, *D. melanissima* of North America, may be a member of this group. In Eurasia the group's distribution is widely disjunct, although this may in part represent our lack of information regarding the *Drosophila* of central Asia. Disregarding *D. melanissima,* there are four eastern forms in North America and three species have east–west disjunct patterns. *D. melanura* shows a spotty distribution across the northern United States, *D. melanica* is scattered across the center of the continent, and *D. micromelanica* shows a comparable pattern across the south. *D. melanura* and *D. micromelanica,* together with an eastern form, *D. nigromelanica,* are phylogenetically the oldest representatives of the *melanica* group in North America (Stalker, 1966), and this disjunct pattern probably results from the fragmenting of the North American forests in Oligicene–Miocene times with the rise of the Rocky Mountains and the cooling and drying of the climate of western North America at that time. *D. melanica, D. paramelanica,* and *D. euronotus* exhibit a south–north–south pattern of speciation that might reflect Pleistocene changes (Stalker, 1966). Most of these species are readily cultured and can be collected with standard fermenting banana baits. Carson and Stalker (1951) report rearing *D. paramelanica* from slime fluxes on red oak, black locust, and elm. In Nebraska I have collected *D. paramelanica* in numbers from a bleed on willow where they congregated, but I did not attempt to rear them from it. *D. micromelanica* has been reared from a slime flux on oak (Heed, private communication).

The *virilis* group is discussed at length by Patterson and Stone (1952), and more recently by Stone *et al.* (1960). The group is presently comprised of twelve species; four European, one Oriental, six North American, and one cosmopolitan form, *D. virilis.* The group is divided cytologically into phylads (Stone *et al.,* 1960), and information from proteins shows the group to be comprised of two phylads that are completely consistent with the evidence from the chromosomes (Throckmorton and J. L. Hubby, unpublished). Both phylads are represented in the Nearctic and Palearctic regions. The group appears to have originated in Asia as a species of the temperate deciduous forest associated predominantly with riparian communities. This is the present habitat of most members of the *virilis* phylad, and *D. americana* has been bred from under the bark of willow (Blight and Romano, 1953). Members of the *montana* phylad are associated mostly with riparian communities of the boreal and montane forests. One of these species, *D. lacicola,* has been bred from the rotting phloem of aspen (Spieth, 1951), and this is probably the most important breeding site for the American members of this phylad. However, Wheeler (private communication) has reared *D. flavomontana,* a North American species of the intermontane west, from slime flux on the narrow-leaved cottonwood, and *D. montana* breeds in red alder (Moorhead, 1954). Basden (1954) reports rearing *D. littoralis,* a European member of the *montana* phylad, from the stumps of recently felled sycamore in Scotland.

In North America the group shows an east–west pattern similar to that noted earlier for the *victoria, obscura, funebris,* and *melanica* groups. Each phylad has eastern and western species, and again the pattern would reflect the disjunction of the North American forest in Oligocene–Miocene times. The present distributions of *D. montana, D. borealis,* and *D. lacicola* are partly or wholly in areas formerly covered by ice during the Pleistocene, and for one of these, *D. montana,* studies of proteins have shown that populations in areas formerly occupied by ice exhibit a distinct genotype. This genotype is distributed from high altitudes in the Colorado Rockies to the coastal plain in western Alaska, and it seems to represent a single "ecogenotype" that expanded from some Pleistocene refugium to occupy this broad area (Throckmorton and J.L. Hubby, unpublished). In Eurasia an east-west disjunct pattern is also seen, with *D. ezoana* in Japan and Korea, and *D. littoralis, D. lummei, D. lakovaarai* and *D. ovivororum* in Europe and Scandinavia. *D. virilis* is cosmopolitan but it was probably endemic in Asia (Patterson and Stone, 1952).

The *carsoni* group is comprised of only one species. It is represented by eastern (South Dakota to Maine) and western (New Mexico and Wyoming) populations in North America. These differ slightly morphologically, and breeding tests might disclose more than one species to be involved here. This is a rare species and nothing is known of its biology. It can be bred in the laboratory and collected on the usual baits.

Taken together, the *carsoni, virilis, melanica,* and *robusta* groups show remarkable parallels in distribution and ecology. They seem to be predominantly sap feeders, with some known from under bark near cuts or breaks and others from slime flux. Their distribution is that of the temperate deciduous forest, and there is no reason to assume other than that they achieved this distribution when the forest itself was continuous. The disjunction between Palearctic and Nearctic branches is attributed to the Miocene events that severed the Beringian connection, and the east–west disjunction within both the Palearctic and Nearctic can be attributed also to mountain-building episodes of these early periods. Since these groups are derived from a radiation that itself occurred early enough so some of its members could reach the New World through tropical or subtropical corridors, the influence of Miocene events on intragroup distribution patterns is not at all improbable, which is not to say that parts of the patterns may not have been generated during the Pleistocene, as was noted earlier regarding late speciation events in the *melanica* group. The profound disjunctions exhibited by the groups in Eurasia, if real, may also partly reflect the severe effects of Pleistocene conditions on temperate faunas there. While it is conceivable that a series of evolutionary accidents produced all the parallels mentioned, parsimony does not permit us to take seriously such a compounding of coincidence. There can be little question that common environmental changes, effecting a common substrate, the deciduous-forest community, evoked the parallel responses exhibited by the four groups just discussed, by the *victoria, obscura,* and *funebris* groups mentioned earlier, and by the *quinaria, testacea,* and *melanderi* groups, which are yet to be discussed in connection with a higher radiation in the genus.

The remainder of the *virilis–repleta* radiation is centered in the tropics of the New World. It is comprised of the large *repleta* lineage and a smaller cluster of groups closely related to it. These latter groups are rather diverse on casual inspection, and their habits also are quite varied, but several share unique features with the *repleta* lineage and these were probably derived from a single original group in the New World. Ward and Heed (1970) have demonstrated that *D. acanthoptera* (of the monotypic subgenus *Sordophila*), *D. pachea,* and an unnamed species make up a cytological lineage that includes *D. nannoptera.* Through their courtesy I have been able to examine all these species. Morphologically, the first three comprise a tight cluster. They are very similar to each other and share several derivative features. *D. nannoptera* obviously shares a common ancestor with these, but it has no more in common with them than it does with the *bromeliae* group or *D. peruviana.* Hence, *D. nannoptera* can be regarded as the primitive representative of the lineage leading to *D. acanthoptera* and its relatives. *D. acanthoptera, D. nannoptera,* and the unnamed species are from dry habitats in southern Mexico, and *D. pachea* is found in the Sonoran desert of northern Mexico and Baja California. They all breed in cactus and all are fairly easy to rear in the laboratory. *D. pachea,* however, breeds only on senita cactus and requires medium that is supplemented with that cactus or with a specific sterol from it (Kircher and Heed, 1970). The *bromeliae* group is small, and I have seen only two species from it. They are collected from flowers and are distributed from Mexico through Colombia to Brazil.

They do not breed well in the laboratory, but with constant attention they can be maintained. Internally they have much in common with *D. nannoptera* and with *D. peruviana*. This latter species represents a cluster of small yellow forms of which I have seen several undescribed species. Together with the *bromeliae* group, these form a link between *D. nannoptera* and the *repleta* lineage. *D. peruviana* is from Peru and Brazil, and the undescribed species are also from South America. Pipkin *et al.* (1966) report breeding *peruviana*-like forms from flowers, and many of the flower-feeding species described by Pipkin (1964) appear to be derived from this radiation. The *flavopilosa* group of flower feeders (Wheeler *et al.*, 1962) is derived either from this radiation or from the *repleta* radiation. I have made no direct observation of these species.

The *repleta* radiation (Figure 3) includes the *castanea, canalinea, dreyfusi,* and *mesophragmatica* groups, as well as the large *repleta* group. With the exception of the *mesophragmatica* group, all of these have been shown to be related cytologically. Wasserman (1963) summarizes his work with this cluster of species, and morphological details permit the remainder of the pattern to be filled in. *D. castanea,* the sole member of its group, is distributed from Colombia and Venezuela to Mexico. It shares derivative morphological features with both the *mesophragmatica* and *peruviana* groups. The *mesophragmatica* group of eight species is reviewed by Brncic *et al.* (1971), who give the distribution and a cytological phylogeny. These are predominantly Andean species, but *D. gaucha* is also found in southern Brazil, Uruguay, and Argentina. They are collected with standard, fermenting-fruit baits and most can be cultured. The *canalinea* and *dreyfusi* groups are both distributed from Brazil to Central America, with *D. canalinea* ranging northward into Mexico. Pipkin (1965) classes these species among those preferring small, dry fruits and fallen blossoms as feeding and breeding sites.

The *repleta* group of about eighty species is comprised of five subgroups, and these are related to each other and to the *canalinea, dreyfusi,* and *castanea* groups through the *repleta* standard gene arrangement (Wasserman, 1963). The *canalinea* and *dreyfusi* groups share a common branch off the standard gene arrangement, the *mulleri* and *fasciola* subgroups share a second branch, the *hydei* subgroup makes up a single independent branch and so also does the *castanea* group, and the *melanopalpa* and *mercatorum* subgroups share a fifth branch. *D. peninsularis,* morphologically a member of the *mulleri* subgroup, is also a member of this last branch. Members of the *hydei* subgroup are found from the southern United States through Mexico and Central America to Colombia, Venezuela, and Peru. *D. hydei* is a cosmopolitan species. The *melanopalpa* subgroup extends from Oregon and Idaho in western North America southward through Mexico and Central America to Peru and Brazil. *D. repleta* of this subgroup is cosmopolitan. The *mercatorum* subgroup is distributed from the United States through Mexico, Central America, and Colombia to Brazil, Chile, Peru, and Bolivia. *D. mercatorum* itself is also distributed to Hawaii (Carson, 1965). The *fasciola* subgroup is distributed from Arizona and Mexico to the West Indies, and to Central and South America. The *mulleri* subgroup, the largest of all, is distributed from central California, Nebraska, Tennessee, and Florida south to Argentina and Chile. *D. buzzatii* is also distributed to the Mediterranean region and Australia.

The *repleta* radiation, and the *nannoptera, bromeliae,* and *peruviana* groups, appear to have originated in or near present-day Mexico. On anatomical grounds, the *nannoptera* line was the earliest to branch off as a separate lineage, and these species are presently restricted to the deserts and arid lands of Mexico. Parsimony requires that this be regarded as the general area of origin for these groups, and other evidence indicates the same thing. The anatomically more-primitive species of the *hydei* subgroup (*D. bifurca, D. nigrohydei*) are northern species (Texas, Arizona, Mexico), and so is *D. fulvalineata,* the most primitive of the *fasciola*-subgroup species. The biology and distribution of these forms suggests that diversification occurred largely in association with the developing American deserts. It probably began in tropical or subtropical forests of North America and spread through chance colonization to secondary centers of radiation in South America. The *canalinea, dreyfusi, mesophragmatica, peruviana,* and *castanea* groups are forest forms and center in South America. The first four of these probably originated there, and the *castanea* and *bromeliae* groups could have originated either in North or South America. All the subgroups of the *repleta* group seem to have originated in North America, with the possible exception of that of *D. mercatorum.* Wasserman (1962a) suggests that this subgroup originated in Brazil.

The species of the *repleta* group are mostly desert forms associated with cactus (Patterson and Stone, 1952; Wasserman, 1963; Fellows and Heed, 1972), but the *fasciola* subgroup is found in wetter areas of rain and cloud forest and on banana and coffee plantations of Central and South America. *D. californica* breeds in bleeding trees (Patterson and Stone, 1952), and *D. hydei, D. repleta, D. melanopalpa,* and *D. fasciola* have been reared from fallen fruits and flowers (Pipkin, 1965). Since the morphologically and cytologically primitive member of the *fasciola* subgroup, *D. fulvalineata,* is a desert species, Wasserman (1962b) suggests that the group originated as a desert form, then returned to the ancestral forest habitat. A more parsimonious alternative, consistent with the cytological, morphological, ecological, and distributional evidence, would suggest that the *fasciola* subgroup represents the primitive type out of which the *repleta* radiation evolved. The group that first invaded the desert would have included initially both forest and desert forms, and these could easily have shared the more-primitive gene arrangements presently distributed among these lineages.

This lineage, from the *nannoptera* cluster to the *repletas,* engaged in considerable ecological experimentation (forest, flowers, cactus), with at least two radiations into the desert and major expansions into both high altitudes and temperate zones. As already indicated, the lineage almost surely arrived in the New World as a member of the tropical or sub-tropical forest fauna, presumably by mid-Oligocene times. Its diversification partly involved colonization of South America across the Caribbean water gap (*mesophragmatica,* etc.) and partly involved ecological experimentation and adaptation to diverse food types (flowers, rotting cactus) and climates (desert, temperate) or altitudinal regions. It is reasonable to infer that much of this latter development reflects responses to environmental stress attending the development of the New World mountains and deserts during Oligocene and Miocene times. And it would equally reflect exploitation of novel opportunities presented to these species with the expansion of new ecological communities in arid regions and the flourishing of unusual plant types such as cactus. These species are readily collected and cultured, and they are among the most promising research materials available in the genus *Drosophila* today.

The *immigrans–Hirtodrosophila* radiation

When grasped in its entirety, this last major radiation is seen to have a basic structure very similar to that of the *virilis–repleta* radiation. It originated and diversified first in the Old World tropics, spread from there, and sent two separate lineages (*tripunctata* and *Hirtodrosophila*) to the New World tropics. Then, from both of these centers the temperate zone was entered, with the major impetus for this coming from the Old World. A similar dominance of the Old World was seen in the *virilis–repleta* radiation, and the reason seems simple. In the Old World, and particularly in east Asia, the tropical and temperate forests intergrade on a wide front. This provides abundant and continuing opportunity for tropical faunas to spread into and master temperate environments. In the New World the situation is different. As climatic and altitudinal zonation became more pronounced in Oligocene and Miocene times, the tropics were more and more isolated from temperate North America by deserts that developed across what is now northern Mexico. The progenitors of the *tripunctata* radiation depended for their living on fungus and on flowers and fruits fermenting slowly on the humid forest floor. The expanding deserts crowded them southward. The species of the *virilis–repleta* radiation, on the other hand, responded to the growing deserts by adjusting to them, a circumstance encouraged by their utilization of oozing saps and rotting parts of still-living plants (rot pockets of cactus, for example). Hence, they continued to occupy a large part of arid southwestern North America, but since they had specialized so much toward cactus, they did not have efficient entry into the temperate deciduous forest. Those forms, of the *melanica, robusta,* and *virilis* groups, for example, came eventually from Asia, as did comparable forms of the *quinaria, melanderi,* and *testacea* groups from this radiation.

The *immigrans, denticeps,* and *pinicola* groups make up a complex that forms the core of the higher Drosophilinae. The *melanderi* group and the subgenus *Siphlodora* are very close to these, so close in fact that it is difficult to make sharp distinctions among them for characters of phylogenetic significance at this level. On many other characters they are easily distinguished, and the extremes of this radiation are sharply separate from each other. Figure 4 exaggerates the closeness of some of these groups, particularly those near *Hirtodrosophila,* and at the same time it underemphasizes the similarities of *immigrans, denticeps,* and so on.

According to Wilson *et al.* (1969) the *immigrans* group contains about 70 "nominal" species, which they assign to five subgroups plus a sixth that contains species of uncertain relationships. This group is part of a larger cluster of about 100 species, the taxonomy of which remains confused. Various generic and subgeneric names have been applied to some of the more conspicuous phenotypes, but the entire cluster is, in reality, a close-knit lineage little justifying the nomenclatural industry expended on it. Except for one cosmopolitan species (*D. immigrans*), the *immigrans* group is distributed in Africa, the Seychelles, south Asia north to Japan, Australia, and the Pacific islands. In Southeast Asia it intergrades broadly with related lineages, both of its own radiation and of earlier radiations, so it must be regarded as originating there. The genus *Zaprionus* predominates in Africa, where there are 25 species, and several more species of dubious relationship are found elsewhere. The seven species of *Samoaia* are endemic to Samoa (Wheeler and Kambysellis, 1966). The genus *Chaetodrosophilella* is small and is found in Southeast

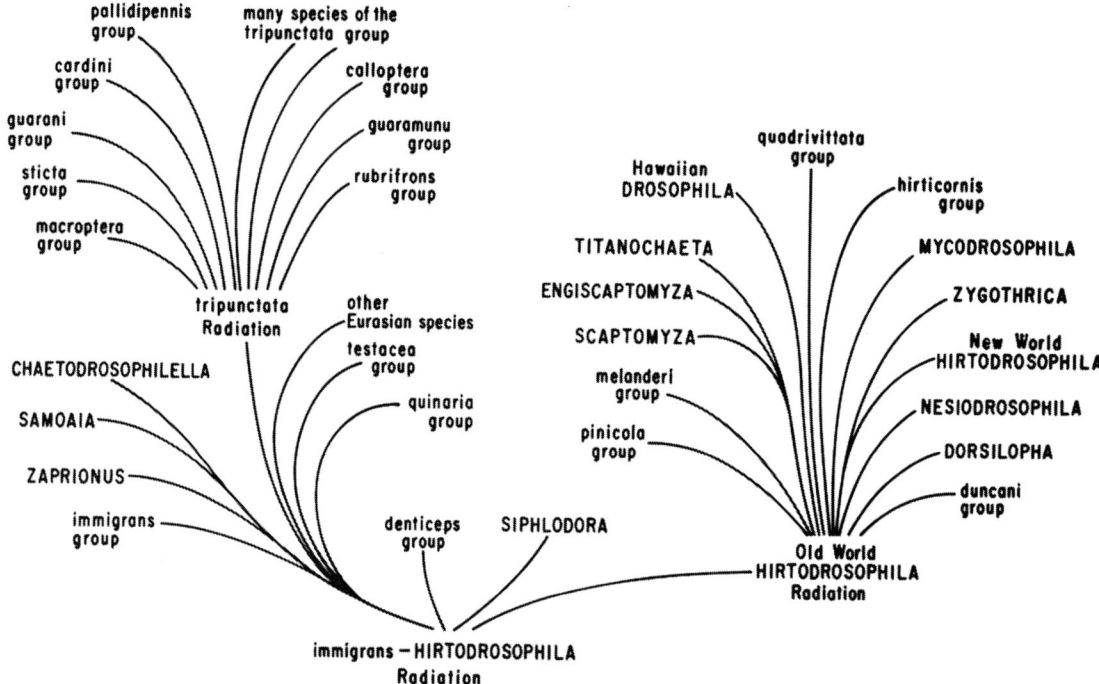

Figure 4. The immigrans–Hirtodrosophila radiation continued from the upper right of Figure 2.

Asia and the Pacific islands. Where the ecology of the species is known, species of the *immigrans* cluster are associated with fungus, fallen fruit, flowers, tree sap, slime flux, or rotting vegetables and leaves. Many of them cannot be cultured, even though they come to fruit baits and are swept over fallen fruit. Together with species of the *melanogaster* group they make up the greater part of the drosophilid fauna in parts of the Old World tropics (Bock and Wheeler, 1972).

The *tripunctata* radiation centers in the New World tropics, and individuals from it make up a large part of collections from South and Central America. The *tripunctata* group itself is comprised of nearly 60 species, and it seems to be related to the other groups of this cluster, very much as the genus *Drosophila* is related to the higher Drosophilinae. That is to say, it is the group out of which, at different times and at different levels, other groups arose. On cytological grounds Kastritsis *et al.* (1970) drew attention to a relationship of this sort among the *tripunctata, guaramunu,* and *guarani* groups, and distribution and morphology point to a similar relationship for the remaining ones. This evolutionary pattern is also observed among groups of the *repleta* radiation, and it is seen also among those of the *Hirtodrosophila* radiation. The major treatments of the *tripunctata* group are by Frota-Pessoa (1954), Heed and Wheeler (1957), Pipkin and Heed (1964), and Kastritsis (1966). It is distributed from the eastern United States to Mexico, Central America, the West Indies, and South America, with perhaps its highest concentration of species being in Brazil, where it ranks second only to the *willistoni* group in population densities (Frota-Pessoa, 1954). The species of this group have diverse feeding habits. Some are fungivorous, some are sap-feeding, and some are ground-feeding forms associated with fallen flowers, small fruits, and decaying pulpy vegetation (Heed, 1957; Heed and Wheeler, 1957; Patterson and Stone, 1952; Pipkin, 1965). The group originated in the New World tropics, but whether in North or South America remains uncertain. The one United States species, *D. tripunctata*, is derived from the south, and it represents the single, successful colonization of the eastern deciduous forest by this group. Taken together, the Caribbean and the deserts of northern Mexico have been very effective barriers to a northward dispersion of the *tripunctata* radiation.

The *cardini* group is summarized by Heed and Russell (1971). They divide the group into continental and island clusters, each of eight species. The continental subgroup is distributed from Georgia, Texas, Mexico, and the West Indies south to Chile and Brazil. The island subgroup is from the West Indies, except for *D. acutilabella*, which also extends northward into Florida. Heed (1957) reports some of these species from fallen fruits and fungus, and Pipkin (1965) classifies some of them as utilizing fleshy fruits for feeding and breeding sites. The *rubrifrons* and *macroptera* groups are both North American, with the first being distributed from New Mexico and Arizona south into Mexico and the second from Colorado and Texas south to Guatemala. The two groups together comprise no more than a dozen species. Heed (private communication) has reared both *D. macroptera* and *D. rubrifrons* from fungus. The *calloptera*, *guarani*, *guaramunu*, *pallidipennis*, and *sticta* groups are also small, with fewer than two dozen species all told. Species of the *calloptera* group are most distinctive, with dark, patterned bodies and patterned wings. *D. sticta* is not greatly different from species of the *tripunctata* group. Both of these groups are part of the ground-feeding fauna associated with fallen flowers and fruits (Pipkin, 1965). The *calloptera* and *pallidipennis* groups are distributed from Mexico through Central America to Peru and Brazil, the *sticta* group is from Colombia and Central America, and the *guarani* and *guaramunu* groups are found from Mexico to Brazil.

When species of this radiation are better known it is probable that a pattern of distribution and evolution similar to that for the *saltans* group will be evident. The ancestors of the radiation were members of the tropical fauna that arrived in the New World prior to mid-Oligocene times. Mountain building and desert formation fragmented former continuous distributions, leaving the species of the *rubrifrons* and *macroptera* groups scattered and isolated from Mexico north to the Colorado Rockies. The remaining groups all have a conspicuously southern distribution. They may well have originated in South America and spread northward with the building of the Isthmus of Panama in Pliocene times. Species of the *cardini* group can be cultured with relative ease. They have skipping larvae, whatever that signifies, and so also do several other species of this radiation. Some members of the other groups can be cultured readily but many cannot. When problems of culturing these species are solved they will provide outstanding materials for studying evolutionary ecology.

The temperate limb of this radiation evolved out of some Eurasian species having features in common with the *immigrans, denticeps, pinicola,* and *melanderi* groups. As representatives of this evolutionary level I have seen *D. sternopleuralis, D. bizonata, D. histrio,* and *D. confusa,* all from Japan. Some of these have more in common with the *quinaria* section, some more with *Hirtodrosophila,* and they can hardly be regarded as an evolutionary unit. Regardless of that, they serve my present purpose very well, for they provide a strong link to the *quinaria* group and support the conclusion that it originated in the Old World.

The *quinaria* group is comprised of 25 species, 4 from Europe (Burla, 1954; Basden, 1954), 5 from the Orient (Okada, 1956), and 16 from North America (Patterson and Stone, 1952; Wheeler, 1960). This distribution is exactly that noted previously for the species of the temperate forest, and the resemblance is further enhanced by the distribution of the North American species. Nine of these are western, with an overall range from Alaska to Mexico. Only one of these, *D. subquinaria,* extends very much north of southern Canada and, like *D. athabasca* of the *obscura* group and *D. montana* of the *virilis* group, it achieved this distribution through expansion northward with the retreat of the continental glaciations of the Pleistocene.

There are two groups of predominantly eastern forms. One of these is an evolutionary lineage comprised of *D. palustris, D. subpalustris,* and *D. guttifera* (possibly also *D. deflecta,* which I have not seen). These are distributed from Nebraska, Manitoba, and Ontario south to Texas and Florida. *D. quinaria* ranges from Manitoba and Quebec south to Missouri and Virginia. Its nearest relatives are among the western forms. Likewise *D. recens* and *D. falleni* represent northeastern extensions of the western types, with the first ranging from North Dakota and Ontario east to Quebec and Maine, and the second ranging from British Columbia and Quebec south to Colorado, Texas, and Alabama. Most of the species breed in fungus or in rotting vegetation (Patterson and Stone, 1952; Basden, 1954; Okada, 1956, 1968a). *D. palustris* and its relatives breed in decaying water plants such as *Sagittaria* (Patterson and Stone, 1952). *D. transversa* has been reared from meat and mushroom baits placed into vole burrows (Hackman, 1963).

The *testacea* group is small. *D. putrida* is from eastern North America, where it ranges from Ontario south to Texas and Florida. In North America *D. testacea* ranges from Alaska south to Washington and California and east to Quebec and the southern Appalachians. It is also found in Europe and Japan. *D. putrida* is reported from fungi, and Okada (1968a) has reared *D. testacea* from fallen leaves.

The *melanderi* group is derived from the *Hirtodrosophila* radiation, but since it is part of the temperate fauna it is convenient to deal with it now. One species of the group, *D. mankinoi*, is Oriental and three are North American. Two of the latter are from the eastern United States and one, *D. melanderi*, is western, ranging from Alaska and Oregon east to Montana and Minnesota. Spieth recently reared *D. melanderi* from fungi, and through his courtesy I was able to examine some of these individuals. The group is very near the *pinicola* group and to *Hirtodrosophila*, particularly species of the American southwest such as *D. orbospiracula*. *D. pinicola* and *D. flavopinicola* of the *pinicola* group were also recently provided me by Spieth. The *pinicola* group is known only from western North America, where it ranges from southern California to British Columbia. These species are fungivorous (Spieth, private communication). Again, these groups exhibit the disjunct patterns of the temperate forest species, and they reinforce the conclusion presented earlier that the temperate forest fauna originated, in all its varied lineages, prior to mid-Miocene times.

Before turning to the remainder of the *Hirtodrosophila* radiation, two smaller groups should be discussed. The subgenus *Siphlodora* is comprised of three species, one of which (*D. sigmoides*) is distributed through southeastern North America from Illinois and New York south to Texas and Alabama. The other two are distributed from Mexico and the West Indies south to Brazil. *D. sigmoides* has been reared from inflorescences of *Tripsacum* (Butler and Mettler, 1963). *D. sigmoides* combines characteristics of both the *tripunctata* and the *Hirtodrosophila* radiations. The subgenus is closest to the *denticeps* group, which is placed by Okada in the subgenus *Hirtodrosophila*. *D. denticeps* itself is a leaf miner (Okada

1968*a*), and it is quite possible that some species of the subgenus *Siphlodora* are also. The *denticeps* group of four species is reviewed by Okada (1971). This group is distributed from Nepal to Taiwan and Japan. I have seen one species from Japan and at least two from Taiwan, including one undescribed form. The group is at least as close to the *immigrans* cluster, *D. histrio,* and *D. confusa,* as it is to the more typical *Hirtodrosophila.* Thus, the subgenus *Siphlodora,* together with the *pinicola* and *melanderi* groups already mentioned, provides the link to the remainder of this radiation.

The subgenus *Hirtodrosophila* is treated most recently by Burla (1956) and Okada (1967). It is divided into eight species groups and, as usual, some of the more conspicuous phenotypes have been segregated out as subgenera or genera (Figure 4). In his review of the Old World *Hirtodrosophila,* Okada notes 27 Palearctic, 11 Oriental, 7 Australian, and 4 Ethiopian forms, for a total of 42 species. Within the Palearctic some species have invaded the Far North, and Hackman (1969) has described one species, *D. subarctica,* from northern Finland. There is an overlap of three species between the Palearctic and Oriental regions and of three species between the Oriental and Australian regions. There are, in addition, a great number of undescribed species. In one visit to Taiwan I obtained data on a minimum of 36 species of *Hirtodrosophila* and this was by no means all that were there. In the New World there are 27 Neotropical species, with three of these extending into Florida or Texas. Of the ten Nearctic species, three are southwestern (Texas, New Mexico, Arizona, Mexico) and four are distinctly northern. Taken together, these latter range from Nebraska and Ontario east to Rhode Island, then south to Alabama and Texas. *D. duncani,* of the eastern United States, is morphologically the most primitive species in the subgenus. The *Hirtodrosophila* are fungivorous, except for *D. denticeps,* which is a leaf-mining species.

The genus *Zygothrica* is from the New World tropics, with some species endemic to Samoa (Wheeler and Kambysellis, 1966). On the basis of external morphology, *Zygothrica* is very close to *Hirtodrosophila* (Burla, 1956), and internal morphology shows it to be derived from the New World types. The adults are numerous over fungi. Dr. Alan Young sent me a collection he had made over one fungus in Costa Rica, and out of it I sorted 31 species. Wheeler (1970) lists only 59 species of *Zygothrica* from the entire New World, so it appears that there is a large job of discription remaining here also. Pipkin *et al.* (1966) report rearing *Zygothrica* from flowers, so for some species the larval feeding site may be quite different from that of the adults.

The subgenus *Dorsilopha*, with its single species, *D. busckii*, is world-wide in distribution, but species very close to it exist in Southeast Asia, and its origin is almost certainly there. It breeds in a great variety of rotting vegetables as well as in fungus (Heed, 1968). The genus *Nesiodrosophila* is from Southeast Asia, the Pacific islands, and Africa (Wheeler and Takada, 1964; Okada, 1970). There is no report of its biology. *Paramycodrosophila* is from South Asia, the Pacific islands, and the New World, where five species are distributed from the southern United States to the West Indies and Central America. These three groups, plus the typical *Hirtodrosophila* (excluding the *denticeps* and *confusa* groups) comprise a tight cluster that is most probably a phylogenetic unit.

The genus *Mycodrosophila* is world-wide in distribution, though its species are predominantly tropical (only two of the ten New World species have distributions entirely north of Mexico). Its species are fungivorous. The genus *Scaptomyza* is also world-wide in distribution, from Africa to arctic Norway in the Old World, and from Argentina and Chile to Alaska in the New World (Basden, 1956; Hackman, 1959; Wheeler and Takada, 1966). Its species are predominantly miners of fresh leaves, though they occasionally breed in fruit, and Hawaiian *Scaptomyza* have been reared from flowers, fungus, slime flux, leaves, stems, and fruit (Heed, 1968).

The endemic Hawaiian drosophilids are a large, complex, and fascinating group. The biology of these species is reviewed by Carson *et al.* (1970). They are comprised of two major lineages, the so-called drosophiloids (*ca.* 340 species) and the scaptomyzoids (*ca.* 140 species). Hardy estimates a total endemic drosophilid fauna of nearly 700 species, of which one-third would be scaptomyzoids. There are five endemic drosophiloid genera in addition to *Drosophila* (*Antopocerus, Ateledrosophila, Celidosoma, Grimshawomyia, Nudidrosophila*), and the genus *Drosophila* has one endemic subgenus, *Engiscaptomyza*. There is one endemic genus of scaptomyzoids in addition to *Scaptomyza* (*Titanochaeta*) and six endemic subgenera of *Scaptomyza* (*Alloscaptomyza, Bunostoma, Exalloscaptomyza, Rosenwaldia, Tantalia, Trogloscaptomyza*). Some species of *Bunostoma* are found also in the Marquesas, Samoa, and Australia, and *Rosenwaldia* has been reported from the Marquesas. One species of *Trogloscaptomyza* is reported from Tristan da Cunha (Hackman, 1959). Heed (1968) summarizes their ecology as follows: Among drosophiloids, species of the genus *Antopocerus*, and the bristle-tarsi, fork-tarsi, and spoon-tarsi groups, mine fermenting leaves exclusively; those of the light-tip-scutellum group are fungivorous; and some species of the picture-wing, modified-labellum, and ciliated-tarsi groups are polyphagous on leaves, stems, and flowers. Most drosophiloids are from higher altitudes in areas of low light intensity and high humidity. Among species of scaptomyzoids, those of the subgenus *Exalloscaptomyza* breed in flowers and those of *Titanochaeta* breed on spider eggs. Species of *Trogloscaptomyza* are polyphagous and overlap ecologically with the polyphagous drosophiloids, although they tend to utilize substrates in fresher condition. To some extent the scaptomyzoids choose the drier and more exposed habitats of higher light intensity, but they broadly overlap drosophiloids within habitats also. The major evolutionary pattern is one of dispersion from the oldest island (Kauai) to the younger ones (Oahu, Molokai-Maui-Lanai, Hawaii) and of pronounced, single-island endemism. The Maui complex has the greatest number of drosophiloids (160), followed by Hawaii (98), Oahu (84), and Kauai (44). A minimum of 22 interisland founder events was postulated by Carson *et al.* (1970) to account for the distributional and cytological patterns seen among about 100 picture-winged species studied up to that time. The major factors responsible for these patterns seem to be the low variety of usable foods, the dissection and isolation of habitats through volcanic and meterological activity, and the infrequent successful colonization of adjacent islands.

It has been suggested that the Hawaiian drosophilids originated in East Asia (Throckmorton, 1966). Investigations since that time have tended to confirm this (Throckmorton, unpublished; Okada, 1967, 1971). They arise from among the cluster of species groups and genera already discussed, and this cluster is distributed in Asia from the northern subtropics to the cold temperate region. Some representatives of these lineages are also found in the New World (the *melanderi* and *pinicola* groups and *Siphlodora*). These latter are specialized in one way or another, however, giving small probability that they were themselves ancestral to the Hawaiian drosophilids. The highest concentration of related types is in the northern subtropics of East Asia, and it is most probable that the Hawaiian lineages derive from there by some more-or-less direct route. Populations with the requisite genotypes were in existence in that region by Miocene times at the latest, so they were easily available to colonize the Hawaiian chain during the Pliocene times when the present high islands developed, or they could have colonized earlier islands of the central Pacific before the existing Hawaiian Islands emerged.

The problem of the origin of the drosophiloid and scaptomyzoid lineages of Hawaii remains unresolved. It is possible that two introductions to Hawaii were involved, and there is no reason to postulate more than that. However, the Hawaiian drosophiloid and scaptomyzoid lineages intergrade conspicuously for internal morphology (Throckmorton,

1966), behavior (Spieth, 1966), genitalia (Takada, 1966; Kaneshiro, 1969), and external morphology [Hardy, in Carson *et al.* (1970)]. All of this is presumptive evidence for the origin of *Scaptomyza* in Hawaii and its subsequent dispersal from there to achieve its present world-wide distribution. The parsimonious inference from the evidence, in its present state, still favors the origin of all Hawaiian drosophilids from a single introduction. This would have come from subtropical Southeast Asia and from among such related species groups as those including *D. histrio, D. confusa, D. denticeps,* and so on.

Insofar as culture is concerned, the species of the *Hirtodrosophila* radiation are a heterogeneous lot. Forms such as *D. busckii, D. duncani,* and so on can be cultured readily on standard media. So can several species of *Mycodrosophila* and *Scaptomyza.* Many others (the Hawaiian drosophiloids, *D. pinicola, D. melanderi,* etc.) can be cultured with special media or special techniques (Wheeler and Clayton, 1965; Spieth, private communication).

Generalizations and Hypotheses

The family Drosophilidae is one of two major lineages that emerged from a small radiation of acalypterate diptera saprophagous in leafmold. The other major lineage, the ephydrids, specialized toward wetter substrates and aquatic habitats. The Drosophilidae apparently gained their own ascendency through specializing on organisms causing fermentation. This gave them access to a great variety of substrates in a variety of habitats, and presumably to a variety of fermenters, bacteria as well as yeasts. The history of the family is a history of the mastering of this niche complex as it has been accomplished through the last fifty million years or so and over the major continents of the globe.

Originally, the Drosophilidae were probably associated with slowly fermenting leaves and other fleshy plant parts on the humid forest floor and probably also with sap and broken and damaged parts of living plants themselves. It is unlikely that they "saw" a sharp boundary among these, especially if they were oriented more toward fermentation *per se* than toward some specific plant product. This was a relatively austere existence since breaks and other damage may have been infrequent and small, or highly periodic in occurrence (after storms, etc.), and the saps and tissues exploited were not rich in carbohydrates. This provided a step, however, toward exploitation of fleshy fungi, and that transfer was made several times in the history of the family. The first major entrance into such an association was made among the Steganinae by the founders of the *Leu-*

cophenga lineages, and many other and later groups accomplished such a transfer also. The major evolutionary line continued, however, in the fermentation mode, and by the time of the origin of the Drosophilinae, some lines had the capacity to move into richer fermentation sites such as fruits. The first considerable exploitation of these was by the *Scaptodrosophila*. The utilization of fleshy fruits contributed to small expansions of *Scaptodrosophila* and to much larger radiations of sophophorans and the *immigrans* complex. That is, the later radiations have most conspicuously exploited fruits. The utilization of the fleshy fungi promoted the flourishing *Hirtodrosophila* line, together with the genera, subgenera, etc., associated with it. Both of these together enabled the flies to invade the temperate zone in force, as it were, since they could use enriched saps and plant tissues of deciduous forest trees, and the fleshy fungi themselves reach into the arctic and so provide avenues of advance out of the tropics that can be utilized by many species.

Only two major patterns, components of a larger and more inclusive pattern, were generated during the evolution of the Drosophilinae. The sophophoran radiation developed these in almost diagrammatic clarity and can be recalled by way of example. The first pattern is that of the primary tropical disjunction. For sophophorans this involves the *melanogaster* group (*ca.* 80 species) in the Old World tropics and the *saltans–willistoni* lineage (*ca.* 50 species) in the New World. A more limited secondary pattern of only certain subgroups of the *melanogaster* group and of the related *fima* group is seen in Africa, and only individual species of Asian subgroups are found in Australia. The second major pattern is seen in the New and Old World disjunctions among the temperate-forest species and in their secondary east–west disjunctions within Eurasia and North America. For the *obscura* group (*ca.* 22 species) this is seen in the distribution of approximately 5 species to Europe, 2 to East Asia, 10 to the western United States, and 5 to the eastern United States.

The complete pattern closely matches Cenozoic continental and vegetational histories. The older tropical disjunctions involve species groups, subgenera, and genera. The more recent temperate disjunctions involve species subgroups and species. The partial African disjuncts involve species groups, subgroups, and species, which is consistent with the late establishment of contacts with Africa during Oligocene times and the development of the present connection during the Pliocene. Even now, the drosophilid faunas of Asia and Africa are partially isolated by the deserts of the Middle East. The minor radiation into Australia is compatible with its relatively recent approach to Southeast Asia and to the continued presence of a water gap there. The somewhat blurred patterns in the New

World seem to reflect secondary radiations into South America across the Caribbean water gap, evolution in isolation for a time, and a subsequent partial merging of North and South American faunas with the establishment of the Isthmus of Panama in late Pliocene times.

This overall pattern is repeated five times in more or less detail, but always sufficiently to be identified. Simplifying somewhat for the sake of brevity, the five occurrences appear as follows. The first is the *Scaptodrosophila* radiation, with *Scaptodrosophila* in the Old World tropics, *Zapriothrica* in the New, and the *victoria* group of *Scaptodrosophila* showing the temperate disjunct patterns. The second is the sophophoran radiation with the *melanogaster* group in the Old World tropics, the *saltans–willistoni* lineage in the New, and the *obscura* group showing the temperate disjunctions. The third is the *virilis–repleta* radiation, with a nondescript cluster of species, species groups, genera, and subgenera in the Old World tropics, the *repleta* radiation in the New, and the *virilis, melanica,* and *robusta* groups showing the temperate-forest patterns. The fourth is the *immigrans* radiation, with the *immigrans* cluster in the Old World, the *tripunctata* radiation in the New, and the *quinaria* group disjunct through the temperate forests. The fifth and last is the *Hirtodrosophila* radiation, with the Old World tropical *Hirtodrosophila* and related groups, the New World tropical *Hirtodrosophila* and *Zygothrica*, and the *melanderi, pinicola,* and related groups involved in the temperate disjunct patterns.

At some time representatives of each of these radiations spread through the tropics between the New and Old Worlds, and these movements may have been quite widely separated in time; at least there is no reason to suppose that they were synchronous. There is some evidence for a partial restriction of the passage through Beringia, particularly for members of the earliest drosophiline radiations. Both the *Scaptodrosophila* and the sophophoran radiations are represented in the New World by lineages attributable to a single founder each (realizing that the present data are incomplete and appearances may be misleading). The higher radiations all give evidence of greater heterogeneity among the New World founders. As a single example, at least five lineages appear to have been represented among the founders of the radiation of the *virilis–repleta* cluster in the New World tropics. Of all the groups involved, *Scaptodrosophila* and *Sophophora* show the tightest affinity to the tropics. Only one species of each was involved in founding the temperate lineages, but several or many species from each of the higher radiations accomplished this adjustment to temperate habitats. It may be that Beringia never offered more than a warm, temperate avenue to the New World during the time of evolution of *Drosophila* and related genera. Hence, the genus *Drosophila* might have arisen as late as the late Eocene, but not a great deal later. Alternately, *Drosophila* can have originated much earlier, but *Scaptodrosophila* and *Sophophora* may have been minor elements of early faunas and relatively fewer existed to explore the Beringian passage. The limits of the continental shelf in the region of Beringia do not permit this passage to have ever been broad, and optimum conditions for *Drosophila* may have been either infrequent or short-lived. Intermittent closings of the land bridge by a water gap may not have been trivial so far as tropical drosophilids were concerned, and a filtering effect might be inevitable, even granting optimal conditions for tropical species.

The development of temperate faunas may have taken place during a relatively shorter interval and in a more nearly coordinated fashion. The time at which this began cannot be fixed at present. It does seem that the temperate deciduous forest itself came into being rather rapidly during the mid-Tertiary times, and only shortly before it was fragmented by mountain-building episodes (Graham, 1972). If that is true, it seems plausible to suppose that the temperate drosophilid fauna expanded with it. Evidence from the *Drosophila* groups themselves suggests this. The *victoria*, *obscura*, *virilis–melanica–robusta*, and *quinaria* clusters are distinctive and clearly distinct from their tropical relatives. Each group is quite homogeneous and seems to be derived from a founder that had diverged to a characteristic type before diversifying to the cluster of species seen today (in contradistinction to the pattern seen for the *repleta*, *tripunctata* and *Hirtodrosophila* radiations). Each of these founders could have developed in response to some local climatic, altitudinal, or biotic conditions within, or at the northern borders of, the tropical forest. Then they could have marked time, preadapted as it were to temperate forests that did not exist or, if they did exist, that were too limited in distribution to permit much diversification within them. There is a rough parallel between the distinctness and homogeneity of a group and the relative age of the radiation from which it was derived. Thus, the *victoria* group, from the earliest radiation, is sharply distinct from other *Scaptodrosophila* and is very homogeneous. The *obscura* group, from the second radiation, is moderately distinct from other sophophorans and is moderately homogeneous. From later radiations, the *virilis–melanica–robusta* cluster and the *quinaria* group are each distinct, but both overlap close relatives in certain important features and both are considerably more heterogeneous internally than are the *victoria* and *obscura* groups. Thus, the *victoria* founder may have arisen early and existed for a long time as an isolated specialist. The *obscura* founder may have arisen later, existed a shorter

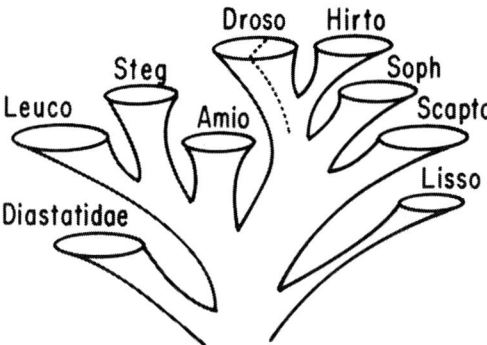

Figure 5. The basic skeleton of the family Drosophilidae as it most probably existed by the middle of the Oligocene age. Abbreviations are as follows: Leuco = Leucophenga, Steg = Stegana, Amio = Amiota, Droso = subgenus Drosophila, Hirto = subgenus Hirto-drosphila, Soph = subgenus Sophophora, Scapto = subgenus Scaptodrosophila, Lisso = Lissocephala.

time before expanding with the temperate forest, etc. Hence, in spite of different times of origin, the five major temperate radiations may have begun diversification nearly at the same time, and the patterns we now see would have developed in consequence.

The parallels and consistencies, both internal and external, from successive radiations are too compelling to be dismissed as accidental or convergent. They reflect in great detail the disjunctions of tropical and temperate floras and of continental relationships during the Cenozoic era; these seem to have influenced each radiation in the same manner and to the same degree, as if the effects were being felt simultaneously by the members of all radiations. Nearly 600 drosophiline species are involved in the tropical disjunctions (*ca.* 60 African, 190 Eurasian, 340 Neotropical) and almost 150 species contribute to the temperate disjunctions (*ca.* 40 European, 35 East Asian, 30 western North American, 20 eastern North American). It is difficult to avoid the conclusion, or to argue otherwise, that the five successive radiations of Drosophilinae occurred before the end of the Eocene age. The individual branches would not have existed then as the fully diversified groups we see today, but at least the basic skeleton of the family, as it is shown in Figures 5 and 6, would have been elaborated. Subsequent to this, the tropical disjunctions occurred in the early Oligocene times, the temperate faunas developed and spread up to the

Figure 6. A flow diagram of the phylogeny and distribution of the higher Drosophilidae. Solid lines indicate major occupations of a zone. Dashed lines indicate only minor incursions.

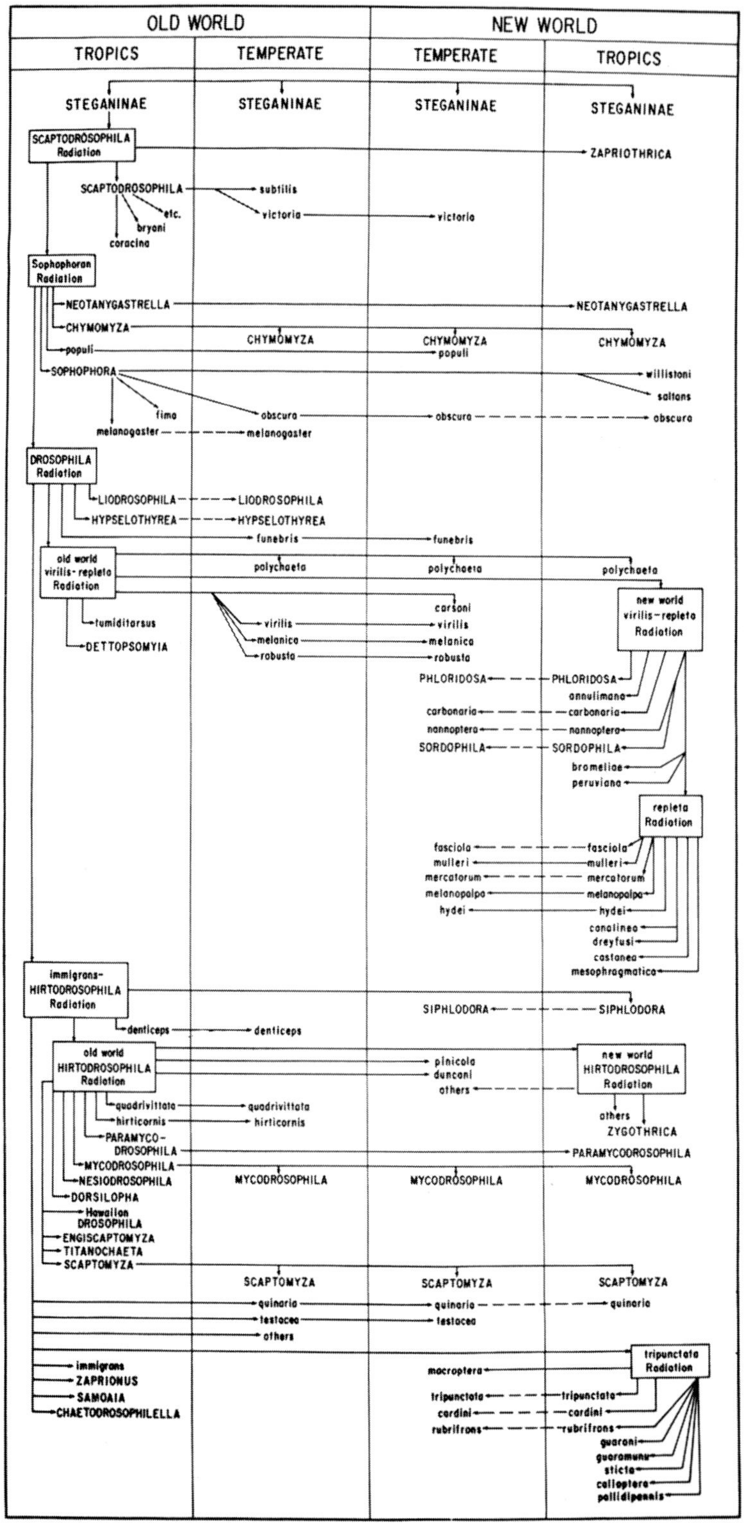
OLD WORLD
NEW WORLD
TROPICS
TEMPERATE
TEMPERATE
TROPICS
STEGANINAE
STEGANINAE
STEGANINAE
STEGANINAE
SCAPTODROSOPHILA Radiation
ZAPRIOTHRICA
SCAPTODROSOPHILA
subtilis
victoria
victoria
etc.
bryani
coracina
Sophophoran Radiation
NEOTANYGASTRELLA
NEOTANYGASTRELLA
CHYMOMYZA
CHYMOMYZA
CHYMOMYZA
CHYMOMYZA
populi
populi
SOPHOPHORA
willistoni
saltans
fima
obscura
obscura
obscura
melanogaster
melanogaster
DROSOPHILA Radiation
LIODROSOPHILA
LIODROSOPHILA
HYPSELOTHYREA
HYPSELOTHYREA
funebris
funebris
old world virilis-repleta Radiation
polychaeta
polychaeta
polychaeta
carsoni
new world virilis-repleta Radiation
tumiditarsus
virilis
virilis
melanica
melanica
robusta
robusta
DETTOPSOMYIA
PHLORIDOSA
PHLORIDOSA
annulimana
carbonaria
carbonaria
nannoptera
nannoptera
SORDOPHILA
SORDOPHILA
bromeliae
peruviana
repleta Radiation
fasciola
fasciola
mulleri
mulleri
mercatorum
mercatorum
melanopalpa
melanopalpa
hydei
hydei
canalinea
dreyfusi
castanea
mesophragmatica
immigrans-HIRTODROSOPHILA Radiation
SIPHLODORA
SIPHLODORA
denticeps
denticeps
old world HIRTODROSOPHILA Radiation
pinicola
duncani
others
new world HIRTODROSOPHILA Radiation
quadrivittata
quadrivittata
hirticornis
hirticornis
others
ZYGOTHRICA
PARAMYCO-DROSOPHILA
PARAMYCODROSOPHILA
MYCODROSOPHILA
MYCODROSOPHILA
MYCODROSOPHILA
MYCODROSOPHILA
NESIODROSOPHILA
DORSILOPHA
Hawaiian DROSOPHILA
ENGISCAPTOMYZA
TITANOCHAETA
SCAPTOMYZA
SCAPTOMYZA
SCAPTOMYZA
SCAPTOMYZA
quinaria
quinaria
quinaria
testacea
testacea
others
tripunctata Radiation
immigrans
macroptera
ZAPRIONUS
SAMOAIA
tripunctata
tripunctata
CHAETODROSOPHILELLA
cardini
cardini
rubrifrons
rubrifrons
guarani
guaramunu
sticta
calloptera
pallidipennis

time of the temperate-forest disjunction in mid-Miocene age, and the final details of present-day patterns were added by speciation events within local regions during the Pliocene and Pleistocene ages, and on into recent times.

Acknowledgments

This work was supported in part by National Institute of Health grant GM 11216 and National Science Foundation grants GH 152 and GH 270.

I am endebted to H. L. Carson, A. E. Emerson, D. E. Hardy, W. B. Heed, D. D. Miller, T. Okada, H. T. Spieth, H. Stalker, H. Takada, K. Wakanama, R. Wenzel, and M. R. Wheeler for reading and commenting on the manuscript, their many helpful comments, and much useful discussion. I am particularly thankful to I. Bock for sharing with me the unpublished results of his studies on the Australian drosophilids.

Literature Cited

Ayala, F. J., M. T. Tracey, D. Hedgecock, and R. C. Richmond, 1974   Genetic differentiation during the speciation process in *Drosophila. Evolution* **28**(4):576–592.

Bächli, G., 1971   *Leucophenga und Paraleucophenga* (Diptera Brachycera) *Fam. Drosophilidae,* Exploration du Parc National de l'Upemba, Mission G. G. de Witte (1946–1949), fasc. 71.

Basden, E. B., 1954   The distribution and biology of Drosophilidae (Diptera) in Scotland, including a new species of *Drosophila. Trans. R. Soc. Edinb.* **72**:603–654.

Basden, E. B., 1956   Drosophilidae (Diptera) within the Arctic Circle. I. General survey. *Trans. R. Entomol. Soc. Lond.* **108**:1–20.

Basden, E. B. and D. G. Harnden, 1956   Drosophilidae (diptera) within the Arctic Circle. II. The Edinburgh University Expedition to subarctic Norway, 1953. *Trans. R. Entomol. Soc. Lond.* **108**:147–162.

Blight, W. C. and A. Romano, 1953   Notes on the breeding site of *Drosophila americana* near St. Louis, Missouri. *Am. Nat.* **87**:111–112.

Bock, I. R. and M. R. Wheeler, 1972   The *Drosophila melanogaster* species group. *Stud. Genet. VII Univ. Texas Publ.* **7213**:1–102.

Brncic, D., 1970   Studies on the evolutionary biology of Chilean species of *Drosophila.* In *Essays in Evolution and Genetics in Honor of Theodosius Dobzhansky,* edited by M. K. Hecht and W. C. Steere, Appleton-Century-Crofts, New York.

Brncic, D., P. S. Nair and M. R. Wheeler, 1971   Cytotaxonomic relationships within the *mesophragmatica* species group of *Drosophila. Stud. Genet. VI Univ. Texas Publ.* **7103**:1–16.

Burla, H., 1951   Systematik, Verbreitung und Oekologic der Drosophila-Arten der Schweiz. *Rev. Suisse Zool.* **58**:23–175.

Burla, H., 1954 Zur Kenntnis der Drosophiliden der Elfenbeinküste (Französisch West-Afrika). *Rev. Suisse Zool.* **61**:1–218.

Burla, H., 1956 Die Drosophilidengattung *Zygothrica* und Ihre Beziehung zur Drosophila-Untergattung *Hirtodrosophila. Mitt. Zool. Mus. Berl.* **32**:189–321.

Burla, H. and H. Gloor, 1952 Zur Systematic der *Drosophila*-Arten Süd-West Europas. *Z. Indukt. Abstammungs.-Vererbungsl.* **84**:164–168.

Buruga, J. H. and R. J. Olembo, 1971 Plant food preferences of some sympatric drosophilids of tropical Africa. *Biotropica* **3**:151–158.

Butler, D. R. and L. E. Mettler, 1963 Ecological and cytological notes on *Drosophila sigmoides. Drosophila Inf. Serv.* **38**:70.

Carson, H. L., 1965 Chromosomal morphism in geographically widespread species of *Drosophila.* In *The Genetics of Colonizing Species,* edited by H. G. Baker and G. Ledyard Stebbins, pp. 503–531, Academic Press, New York.

Carson, H. L., 1970 Chromosome tracers of the origin of species. *Science (Wash., D.C.)* **168**:1414–1418.

Carson, H. L., 1971 Polytene chromosome relationships in Hawaiian species of *Drosophila.* V. Additions to the chromosomal phylogeny of the picture-winged species. *Stud. Genet. VI Univ. Texas Publ.* **7103**:183–192.

Carson, H. L. and H. D. Stalker, 1951 Natural breeding sites for some wild species of *Drosophila* in the eastern United States. *Ecology* **32**:317–330.

Carson, H. L., D. E. Hardy, H. T. Spieth and W. S. Stone, 1970 The evolutionary biology of the Hawaiian Drosophilidae. In *Essays in Evolution and Genetics in Honor of Theodosius Dobzhansky,* edited by M. K. Hecht and W. C. Steere, Appleton-Century-Crofts, New York.

Carson, H. L. and M. R. Wheeler, 1973 A new crab fly from Christmas Island, Indian Ocean (Diptera: Drosophilidae). *Pacific Insects* **15**(2):199–208.

Clayton, F. E., H. L. Carson and J. E. Sato, 1972 Polytene chromosome relationships in Hawaiian species of *Drosophila.* VI. Supplementary data on metaphases and gene sequences. *Stud. Genet. VII Univ. Texas Publ.* **7213**:163–178.

Cole, F. R., 1969 *The Flies of Western North America,* University of California Press, Berkeley, Calif.

Dobzhansky, T., 1965 "Wild" and "Domestic" species of *Drosophila.* In *The Genetics of Colonizing Species,* edited by H. G. Baker and G. Ledyard Stebbins, pp. 533–546, Academic Press, New York.

Dobzhansky, T., 1970 *Genetics of the Evolutionary Process,* Columbia University Press, New York.

Dobzhansky, T., 1972 Species of *Drosophila, Science (Wash., D.C.)* **177**:664–669.

Dobzhansky, T., and C. Epling, 1944 *Contributions to the Genetics, Taxonomy and Ecology of Drosophila pseudoobscura and Its Relatives.* Carnegie Institution of Washington Publication 554, Carnegie Institution, Washington, D.C.

Fellows, D. P. and W. B. Heed, 1972 Factors affecting host plant selection in desert-adapted cactiphilic *Drosophila. Ecology* **53**:850–858.

Frota-Pessoa, O., 1954 Revision of the tripunctata group of *Drosophila* with description of fifteen new species (Drosophilidae, Diptera). *Arq. Mus. Parana.* **10**:253–304.

Frota-Pessoa, O. and M. R. Wheeler, 1951 A revision of the genus *"Neotanygastrella"* Duda (Diptera, Drosophilidae). *Rev. Bras. Biol.* **11**:145–151.

Graham, A., 1972 Outline of the origin and historical recognition of floristic affinities between Asia and eastern North America. In *Floristics and Paleofloristics of Asia and Eastern North America,* edited by A. Graham, Elsevier, Amsterdam.

Hackman, W., 1955   Die Drosophila-Arten Finnlands. *Not. Entomol.* **34**:130–139.

Hackman, W., 1957   Beiträge zur Kenntnis der Drosophiliden des Lenningradgebietes. *Not. Entomol.* **49**:69–72.

Hackman, W., 1959   On the genus *Scaptomyza* Hardy (Diptera, Drosophilidae) with descriptions of new species from various parts of the world. *Acta Zool. Fenn.* **97**:1–71.

Hackman, W., 1963   Studies on the dipterous fauna in burrows of voles (*Microtus, Clethrionomys*) in Finland. *Acta Zool. Fenn.* **102**:1–64.

Hackman, W., 1969   A new *Drosophila* species from northern Fennoscandia (Diptera). *Not. Entomol.* **49**:69–72.

Hardy, D. E., 1965   Diptera: Cyclorrhapha II, Series Schizophora, Section Acalypterae I. Family Drosophilidae. In *Insects of Hawaii*, Vol. 12, University of Hawaii Press, Honolulu, Hawaii.

Hardy, D. E., 1966   Descriptions and notes on Hawaiian Drosophilidae (Diptera). *Stud. Genet. III Univ. Texas Publ.* **6615**:195–244.

Hardy, D. E., 1969   Notes on Hawaiian "idiomyia" (*Drosophila*). *Stud. Genet. V Univ. Texas Publ.* **6918**:71–78.

Hardy, D. E. and K. Y. Kaneshiro, 1968   New picture-winged *Drosophila* from Hawaii. *Stud. Genet. IV Univ. Texas Publ.* **6818**:171–262.

Hardy, D. E. and K. Y. Kaneshiro, 1969   Descriptions of new Hawaiian *Drosophila*. *Stud. Genet. V Univ. Texas Publ.* **6918**:39–54.

Hardy, D. E. and K. Y. Kaneshiro, 1972   New picture-winged *Drosophila* from Hawaii, Part III (Drosophilidae, Diptera). *Stud. Genet. VII Univ. Texas Publ.* **7213**:155–162.

Heed, W. B., 1957   Ecological and distributional notes on the Drosophilidae (Diptera) of El Salvador. *Stud. Genet. Drosophila IX Univ. of Texas Publ.* **5721**:62–78.

Heed, W. B., 1968   Ecology of the Hawaiian Drosophilidae. *Stud. Genet. IV Univ. Texas Publ.* **6818**:387–420.

Heed, W. B. and J. S. Russell, 1971   Phylogeny and population structure in island and continental species of the *cardini* group of *Drosophila* studied by inversion analysis. *Stud. Genet. VI Univ. Texas Publ.* **7103**:91–130.

Heed, W. B. and M. R. Wheeler, 1957   Thirteen new species in the genus *Drosophila* from the neotropical region. *Stud. Genet. Drosophila IX Univ. Texas Publ.* **5721**:17–38.

Heed, W. B., D. W. Crumpacker and L. Ehrman, 1969   *Drosophila lowei*, a new member of the *obscura* species group. *Ann. Entomol. Soc. Am.* **62**:388–393.

Hennig, W., 1958   Die Familien der Diptera Schizophora und ihre phylogenetischen Verwandtschaftsbeziehungen. *Beitr. Entomol.* **8**:505–688.

Hennig, W., 1960   Die Dipteren-Fauna von Neuseeland als systematisches und tiergeographisches Problem. *Beitr. Entomol.* **10**:221–329.

Hennig, W., 1965   Die Acalyptratae des Baltischen Bernsteins. *Stuttg. Beitr. Naturkd.* Nr. 145.

Kaneshiro, K. Y., 1969   The *Drosophila crassifemur* group of species in a new subgenus. *Stud. Genet. V Univ. Texas Publ.* **6918**:79–84.

Kastritsis, C. D., 1966   Cytological studies on some species of the *tripunctata* group of *Drosophila*. *Stud. Genet. III Univ. Texas Publ.* **6615**:413–474.

Kastritsis, C. D., 1969   The chromosomes of some species of the *guarani* group of *Drosophila*. *J. Hered.* **60**:51–57.

Kastritsis, C. D., G. Pasteur and J. Quick, 1970   Relations of the polytene chromosomes of *Drosophila mediostriata* and *D. griseolineata*. *Can. J. Genet. Cytol.* **12**:952–959.

Kircher, H. W. and W. B. Heed, 1970   Phytochemistry and host plant specificity in *Drosophila*. In *Recent Advances in Phytochemistry*, Vol. 3, edited by C. Steelink and V. C. Runeckles, pp. 191–209, Appleton-Century-Crofts, New York.

Lachaise, D., 1974a   Les Drosophilidae des Savanes Préforestières de la Région Tropicale de Lamto (Cote-D'Ivoire). I. Isolement écologique des espèces affines et sympatriques; rythmes d'activité saisonnière et circadienne; rôle des feux de brousse. *Ann. Univ. Abidjan, série E (Écologie)*, Tome VII, fasc. 1, pp. 7–152.

Lachaise, D., 1974b   Les Drosophilides des Savanes Préforestières de la Région Tropicale de Lamto (Cote-D'Ivoire). V. Les Régimes Alimentaires. *Ann. Soc. ent. Fr. (N.S.)* **10**(1):3–50.

Lachaise, D. and L. Tsacas, 1974   Les Drosophilidae des Savanes Préforestières de la Région Tropicale de Lamto (Cote-D'Ivoire). II. Le peuplement des fruits de *Pandanus candelabrum* (Pandanacées). *Ann. Univ. Abidjan, série E (Écologie)*, Tome VII, fasc. 1, pp. 153–192.

McAlpine, J. F., 1968   An annotated key to Drosophilid genera with bare or micropubescent aristae and a revision of *Paracacoxenus* (Diptera: Drosophilidae). *Can. Entomol.* **100**:514–532.

Magalhaes, L. E., 1962   Notes on the taxonomy, morphology, and distribution of the saltans group of *Drosophila*, with descriptions of four new species. *Stud. Genet. II Univ. Texas Publ.* **6205**:135–154.

Mather, W. B., 1955   The genus *Drosophila* (Diptera) in eastern Queensland. I. Taxonomy. *Aust. J. Zool.* **3**:545–582.

Mather, W. B., 1956a   The genus *Drosophila* (Diptera) in eastern Queensland. II. Seasonal changes in a natural population 1952-1953. *Aust. J. Zool.* **4**:65–75.

Mather, W. B., 1956b   The genus *Drosophila* (Diptera) in eastern Queensland. III. Cytological evolution. *Aust. J. Zool.* **4**:76–89.

Mather, W. B., 1956c   The genus *Drosophila* (Diptera) in eastern Queensland. IV. The hybridization relationships of four species of the *Pholadoris* subgenus. *Aust. J. Zool.* **4**:90–97.

Mather, W. .B., 1960   Additions to the *Drosophila* fauna of Australia. *Univ. Queensl. Pap. Dept. Entomol.* **1**:229–239.

Miller, D. D., 1958   Geographical distributions of the American *Drosophila affinis* subgroup species. *Am. Midl. Nat.* **60**:52–70.

Miller, D. D. and W. G. Sanger, 1968   Salivary gland chromosome variation in the *Drosophila affinis* subgroup. II. Comparison of C-chromosome patterns in *D. athabasca* and five related species. *J. Hered.* **59**:323–327.

Miller, D. D. and L. E. Stone, 1962   A reinvestigation of karyotypes in *Drosophila affinis* and related species. *J. Hered.* **53**:12–24.

Miller, D. D. and R. A. Voelker, 1968   Salivary gland chromosome variation in the *Drosophila affinis* subgroup. I. The C chromosome of "western" and "eastern" *Drosophila athabasca*. *J. Hered.* **59**:86–98.

Miller, D. D. and R. A. Voelker, 1969a   Salivary gland chromosome variation in the *Drosophila affinis* subgroup. III. The long arm of the X chromosome in "western" and "eastern" *Drosophila athabasca*. *J. Hered.* **60**:231–238.

Miller, D. D. and R. A. Voelker, 1969b   Salivary gland chromosome variation in the *Drosophila affinis* subgroup. IV. The short arm of the X chromosome in "western" and "eastern" *Drosophila athabasca*. *J. Hered.* **60**:307–311.

Miller, D. D. and L. Weeks, 1964 *Drosophila* collection near the Blue Ridge of southwestern North Carolina. *Am. Midl. Nat.* **72**:93–114.

Miller, D. D. and N. J. Westphal, 1967 Further evidence on sexual isolation within *Drosophila athabasca. Evolution* **21**:479–492.

Momma, E., 1957 *Drosophila* survey of Hokkaido. V. Distribution and habitats of Drosophilid flies. *J. Fac. Sci. Hokkaido Univ. Ser. VI Zool.* **13**:93–98.

Moorehead, P. S., 1954 Chromosomal variation in giant forms of *Drosophila montana. Stud. Genet. Drosophila VIII Univ. Texas Publ.* **5422**:106–129.

Morge, G., 1956 Uber Morphologie und Lebensweise der bisher unbekannten Larven von *Palloptera* and *Stegana coleoptrata* Scopoli (Diptera). *Beitr. Entomol.* **6**:124–137.

Mourão, C. A. and H. E. M. di Campos Bicudo, 1967 Duas novas espécies de *Drosophila* do grupo "Saltans" (Drosophilidae, Diptera). *Pap. Avulsos Zool. Sao Paulo* **20**:123–134.

Nater, H., 1953 Vergleichend-Morphologische Untersuchung des Aussern Geschlechtsapparates innerhalb der Gattung *Drosophila. Zool. Jahrb. Bd. 81. Abt. Syst.*: 437–486.

Okada, T., 1956 *Systematic Study of Drosophilidae and Allied Families of Japan,* Gihodo Co., Tokyo.

Okada, T., 1962 Bleeding sap preference of the Drosophilid flies. *Jap. J. Appl. Entomol. Zool.* **6**:216–229.

Okada, T., 1963*a* Caenogenetic differentiation of mouth hooks in Drosophilid larvae. *Evolution* **17**:84–98.

Okada, T., 1963*b* Cladogenetic differentiation of Drosophilidae in relation to material compensation. *Mushi* **37**:79–100.

Okada, T., 1966*a* Caenogenesis versus palaeogenesis in view of the character continuities. *Proc. Jap. Soc. Syst. Zool.* **2**:21–27.

Okada, T., 1966*b* *Diptera from Nepal. Cryptochaetidae, Diastatidae and Drosophilidae. Bull. Br. Mus. (Nat. Hist.) Entomol. Suppl. 6.*

Okada, T., 1967 A revision of the subgenus *Hirtodrosophila* of the old world, with descriptions of some new species and subspecies (Diptera, Drosophilidae, *Drosophila*). *Mushi* **41**:1–36.

Okada, T., 1968*a* *Systematic Study of the Early Stages of Drosophilidae,* Bunka Zugeisha Co., Tokyo.

Okada, T., 1968*b* Taxonomic treatment of the correlative characters in the genus *Microdrosophila* (Diptera, Drosophilidae). *Proc. Jap. Soc. Syst. Zool.* **4**:1–7.

Okada, T., 1970 A faunal analysis of the drosophilids at genus level centering around New Guinea. *Kontyu* **38**:187–194.

Okada, T., 1971 Systematic and biogeographical analysis of the *denticeps* group, with description of two new species (Diptera, Drosophilidae). *Bull. Biogeogr. Soc. Jap.* **26**:29–38.

Okada, T. and H. Kurokawa, 1957 New or little known species of Drosophilidae of Japan (Diptera). *Kontyu* **25**:2–12.

Oldroyd, H., 1964 *The Natural History of Flies,* Widenfeld and Nicolson, London.

Patterson, J. T., editor, 1940–1957 *Stud. Genet. Drosophila I–IX Univ. Texas Publ.* 4032, 4228, 4313, 4445, 4750, 4920, 5204, 5422, 5721.

Patterson, J. T. and W. S. Stone, 1952 *Evolution in the Genus Drosophila,* Macmillan, New York.

Pipkin, S. B., 1961 Taxonomic relationships within the *Drosophila victoria* species group, Subgenus *Pholadoris* (Diptera: Drosophilidae). *Proc. Entomol. Soc. Wash.* **63**:145–161.

Pipkin, S. B., 1964 New flower breeding species of *Drosophila* (Diptera: Drosophilidae). *Proc. Entomol. Soc. Wash.* **66**:217–245.

Pipkin, S. B., 1965 The influence of adult and larval food habits on population size of Neotropical ground-feeding *Drosophila*. *Am. Midl. Nat.* **74**:1–27.

Pipkin, S. B. and W. B. Heed, 1964 Nine new members of the *Drosophila tripunctata* species group (Diptera: Drosophilidae). *Pac. Insects* **6**:256–273.

Pipkin, S. B., R. L. Rodríguez and J. León, 1966 Plant host specificity among flower-feeding neotropical *Drosophila* (Diptera: Drosophilidae). *Am. Nat.* **100**:135–156.

Prakash, S., 1972 Origin of reproductive isolation in the absence of apparent genic differentiation in a geographic isolate of *Drosophila pseudoobscura*. *Genetics* **72**:143–155.

Spassky, B., R. C. Richmond, S. Perez-Salas, O. Pavlovsky, C. A. Mourão, A. S. Hunter, H. Hoenigsberg, T. Dobzhansky and F. J. Ayala, 1971 Geography of the sibling species related to *Drosophila willistoni*, and of the semispecies of the *Drosophila paulistorum* complex. *Evolution* **25**:129–143.

Spieth, H. T., 1951 The breeding site of *Drosophila lacicola* Patterson. *Science (Wash., D.C.)* **113**:232.

Spieth, H. T., 1966 Courtship behavior of endemic Hawaiian *Drosophila*. *Stud. Genet. III Univ. Texas Publ.* **6615**:245–313.

Spieth, H. T., 1972 Rearing techniques for the Hawaiian species *Drosophila grimshawi* and *Drosophila crucigera*. *Drosophila Inf. Serv.* **48**:155–157.

Stalker, H. D., 1966 The phylogenetic relationships of the species in the *Drosophila melanica* group. *Genetics* **53**:327–342.

Stalker, H. D., 1972 Intergroup phylogenies in *Drosophila* as determined by comparisons of salivary banding patterns. *Genetics* **70**:457–474.

Stone, W. S., W. C. Guest and F. D. Wilson, 1960 The evolutionary implications of the cytological polymorphism and phylogeny of the virilis group of *Drosophila*. *Proc. Natl. Acad. Sci. USA* **46**:350–361.

Strickberger, M. W., 1962 *Experiments in Genetics with Drosophila,* John Wiley & Sons, New York.

Sturtevant, A. H., 1921 *The North American Species of Drosophila,* Carnegie Institution of Washington Publication 301, Carnegie Institution, Washington, D.C.

Sturtevant, A. H., 1942 The classification of the genus *Drosophila*, with descriptions of nine new species. *Univ. Texas Publ.* **4213**:5–51.

Sulerud, R. L. and D. D. Miller, 1966 A study of key characteristics for distinguishing several *Drosophila affinis* subgroup species, with a description of a new related species. *Am. Midl. Nat.* **75**:446–474.

Takada, H., 1958 *Drosophila* survey of Hokkaido. X. Drosophilidae from several localities of Hokkaido. *J. Fac. Sci. Hokkaido Univ. Ser. VI Zool.* **14**:120–127.

Takada, H., 1960 *Drosophila* survey of Hokkaido. XII. Some remarkable or rare species of *Drosophila* from the southern-most area in the Hidaka Mountain range. *Annot. Zool. Jap.* **33**:188–195.

Takada, H., 1966 Male genitalia of some Hawaiian Drosophilidae. *Stud. Genet. III Univ. Texas Publ.* **6615**:315–334.

Takada, H. and J. J. Lee, 1958 A preliminary survey of the Drosophilidae from Kongju and its adjacent localities, South Korea. *Annot. Zool. Jap.* **31**:113–116.

Throckmorton, L. H., 1962*a* The problem of phylogeny in the genus *Drosophila*. *Stud. Genet. II Univ. Texas Publ.* **6205**:207–343.

Throckmorton, L. H., 1962*b* The use of biochemical characteristics for the study of problems of taxonomy and evolution in the genus *Drosophila*. *Stud. Genet. II. Univ. Texas Publ.* **6205**:415–487.

Throckmorton, L. H., 1966 The relationships of the endemic Hawaiian Drosophilidae. *Stud. Genet. III Univ. Texas Publ.* **6615**:335–396.

Throckmorton, L. H., 1968 Concordance and discordance of taxonomic characters in *Drosophila* classification. *Syst. Zool.* **17**:355–387.

Tsacas, L. and D. Lachaise, 1974 Quatre Nouvelles Espèces de la Cote-D'Ivoire du Genre *Drosophila*, Groupe *melanogaster*, et Discussion de l'Origine du Sous-Groupe *melanogaster* (Diptera: *Drosophilidae*). *Ann. Univ. Abidjan, série E (Écologie)*, Tome VII, fasc. 1, pp. 193–211.

Ward, B. L. and W. B. Heed, 1970 Chromosome phylogeny of *Drosophila pachea* and related species. *J. Hered.* **61**:248–258.

Wasserman, M., 1962*a* Cytological studies of the *repleta* group of the genus *Drosophila*. III. The *mercatorum* group. *Stud. Genet. II Univ. Texas Publ.* **6205**:63–71.

Wasserman, M., 1962*b* Cytological studies of the *repleta* group of the genus *Drosophila*. VI. The *fasciola* subgroup. *Stud. Genet. II Univ. Texas Publ.* **6205**:119–134.

Wasserman, M., 1963 Cytology and phylogeny of *Drosophila*. *Am. Nat.* **97**:333–352.

Wheeler, M. R. 1949 The subgenus *Pholadoris* (*Drosophila*) with descriptions of two newspecies. *Stud. Genet. Drosophila VI Univ. Texas Publ.* **4920**:143–156.

Wheeler, M. R., 1952 The Drosophilidae of the nearctic region exclusive of the genus *Drosophila*. *Stud. Genet. Drosophila VII Univ. Texas Publ.* **5204**:162–218.

Wheeler, M. R., 1954 Taxonomic studies on American Drosophilidae. *Stud. Genet. Drosophila VIII. Univ. Texas Publ.* **5422**:47–64.

Wheeler, M. R., 1956 *Zapriothrica*, a new genus based upon *Sigaloessa dispar* Shiner, 1868 (Diptera, Drosophilidae). *Entomol. Soc. Wash.* **58**:113–115.

Wheeler, M. R., editor, 1959 A nomenclatural study of the genus *Drosophila*. In *Biol. Contrib. Univ. Texas Publ.* **5914**:181–205.

Wheeler, M. R., 1960 New species of the quinaria group of *Drosophila* (Diptera, Drosophilidae). *Southwest. Nat.* **5**:160–164.

Wheeler, M. R., editor, 1962–1972 *Stud. Genet. II–VII Univ. Texas Publ.* 6205, 6615, 6818, 6918, 7103, 7213.

Wheeler, M. R., 1963 A note on some fossil Drosophilidae (Diptera) from the amber of Chiapas, Mexico. *J. Paleontol.* **37**:123–124.

Wheeler, M. R., 1965 Family Drosophilidae. In *A Catalogue of the Diptera of America North of Mexico*, Agriculture Handbook 276, pp. 760–772, Agricultural Research Service, United States Department of Agriculture, Washington, D.C.

Wheeler, M. R., 1970 Family Drosophilidae. In *A Catalogue of the Diptera of the Americas South of the United States*, Vol. 79, pp. 1–65, Museu de Zoologia, Universidade de São Paulo, São Paulo.

Wheeler, M. R. and F. E. Clayton, 1965 A new *Drosophila* culture technique. *Drosophila Inf. Serv.* **40**:98.

Wheeler, M. R. and N. Hamilton, 1972 Catalogue of *Drosophila* species names, 1959–1971. *Stud. Genet. VII Univ. Texas Publ.* **7213**:257–268.

Wheeler, M. R. and M. P. Kambysellis, 1966 Notes on the Drosophilidae (Diptera) of Samoa. *Stud. Genet. III Univ. Texas Publ.* **6615**:533–563.

Wheeler, M. R. and L. E. Magalhaes, 1962   The *alagitans–bocainensis* complex of the *willistoni* group of *Drosophila. Stud. Genet. II Univ. Texas Publ.* **6205**:155–173.

Wheeler, M. R. and H. Takada, 1964   Diptera: Drosophilidae. In *Insects of Micronesia* Vol. 14, pp. 163–242, Bernice P. Bishop Museum, Honolulu, Hawaii.

Wheeler, M. R. and H. Takada, 1966   The Nearctic and Neotropical species of *Scaptomyza* Hardy (Diptera; Drosophilidae). *Stud. Genet. III Univ. Texas Publ.* **6615**:37–78.

Wheeler, M. R. and H. Takada, 1971   Male genitalia of some representative genera of American Drosophilidae. *Stud. Genet. VI. Univ. Texas Publ.* **7103**:225–240.

Wheeler, M. R. and L. H. Throckmorton, 1960   Notes on Alaskan Drosophilidae (Diptera), with the description of a new species. *Bull. Brooklyn Entomol. Soc.* **55**:134–143.

Wheeler, M. R., H. Takada and D. Brncic, 1962   The *flavopilosa* species group of *Drosophila. Stud. Genet. II Univ. Texas Publ.* **6205**:395–413.

Wilson, F. D., M. R. Wheeler, M. Harget and M. Kambysellis, 1969   Cytogenetic relations in the *Drosophila nasuta* subgroup of the *immigrans* group of species. *Stud. Genet. V Univ. Texas Publ.* **6918**:207–270.

Yoon, J. S., K. Resch and M. R. Wheeler, 1972*a*   Intergeneric chromosomal homology in the family Drosophilidae. *Genetics* **71**:477–480.

Yoon, J. S., K. Resch and M. R. Wheeler, 1972*b*   Cytogenetic relationships in Hawaiian species of *Drosophila*. I. The *Drosophila hystricosa* subgroup of the "modified mouthparts" species group. *Stud. Genet. VII Univ. Texas Publ.* **7213**:179–200.

Yoon, J. S., K. Resch and M. R. Wheeler, 1972*c*   Cytogenetic relationships in Hawaiian species of *Drosophila*. II. The *Drosophila mimica* subgroup of the "modified mouthparts" species group. *Stud. Genet. VII Univ. Texas Publ.* **7213**:201–212.

18

A Catalog of *Drosophila* Metaphase Chromosome Configurations

Frances E. Clayton and

Marshall R. Wheeler

Introduction

Metaphase chromosome configurations have been described for 513 species and subspecies of *Drosophila,* representing about 40 percent of the total number of species described for the world. In the following catalog list (Table 1), species and species groups are arranged within subgenera alphabetically, generally organized according to the pattern of Throckmorton (Chapter 17 in this volume).

Most of the variations from the primitive condition, 5 pairs of rods and one pair of dots, can be attributed to translocations, pericentric inversions, and varying degrees of heterochromatic additions (either with or without other chromosomal rearrangements; see discussion in Patterson and Stone (1952), Chapter 4). The catalog gives only minimal data on metaphases, the distribution in different species, species groups, and

Frances E. Clayton—Department of Zoology, University of Arkansas, Fayetteville, Arkansas. Marshall R. Wheeler—Department of Zoology, University of Texas at Austin, Austin, Texas.

higher categories, and acknowledges the first publication reporting the information. Other, later reports are included when they provide added significant details or describe a metaphase condition at variance with that first recorded.

Metaphase variations do occur within some species; other reports of variation may be due to errors of analysis of the chromosome preparations, or may result from misidentification of the species being studied. Where feasible, we have shown the geographic origins of the strains when significant variation has been reported. When a report was based upon a misidentification we have indicated (under Remarks) the species name used by the author at the time of his study, but we have listed the species by its currently approved name.

Abbreviations for the metaphases, shown as the haploid complement, are as follows: R and r represent large and small rod-shaped chromosomes; V and v are large and small V-shaped elements; J is J-shaped; and D, Dr, and Dv represent the dot chromosome, a rodlike dot, and a V-shaped dot, respectively.

Literature Cited

Angus, D., 1964   *D. tetrachaeta*: A new species of *Drosophila* from New Guinea. *Univ. Queensl. Pap. Dep. Zool.* **2**:155–159.

Angus, D., 1967   Cytological evolution in the *quadrilineata* species group. *Drosophila Inf. Serv.* **42**:112.

Baimai, V., 1969   Karyotype variation in *Drosophila birchii*. *Chromosoma (Berl.)* **27**:381–394.

Baimai, V., 1970   *Drosophila pseudomayri*, a new species from New Guinea (Diptera: Drosophilidae). *Pacific Insects* **12**:21–23.

Blumel, J., 1949   Additional tests within the *quinaria* species-group of *Drosophila. Univ. Texas Publ.* **4920**:31–38.

Bock, I. R., 1966   *D. argentostriata*: A new species of *Drosophila* from New Guinea. *Univ. Queensl. Pap. Dep. Zool.* **2**:271–276.

Bock, I. R. and V. Baimai, 1967   *D. silvistriata*: a new species of *Drosophila* from New Guinea. *Univ. Queensl. Pap. Dep. Zool.* **3**:19–25.

Bock, I. R. and M. R. Wheeler, 1972   The *Drosophila melanogaster* species group. *Stud. Genet. VII Univ. Texas Publ.* **7213**:1–102.

Brncic, D., 1957   Las especies chilenas de Drosophilidae. *Col. Monografías Biol., Univ. Chile, Santiago (Chile)* **8**:1–136.

Brncic, D. and S. Koref-Santibañez, 1957   The *mesophragmatica* group of species of *Drosophila. Evolution* **11**:300–311.

Burla, H., 1948   Die Gattung *Drosophila* in der Schweiz. *Rev. Suisse Zool.* **55**:272–279.

Burla, H., 1950a   *Drosophila grischuna* species nova, eine neue Art aus der Schweiz. *Arch. J. Klaus-Stift. Vererbungsforsch. Sozialanthropol. Rassenhyg.* **25**:619–623.

(Literature Cited continued on p. 508)

TABLE 1.　*Catalog of Drosophila Metaphase Chromosome Configurations*

Species	Metaphase	Reference	Remarks
Subgenus Dorsilopha			
busckii Coquillett 1901	2 V, 1 R, 1 D	Metz (1916a)	—
	2 V, 1 R	Wharton (1943)	Y may appear J-shaped
Subgenus Drosophila			
annulimana species group			
annulimana Duda 1927	1 V, 3 v, 1 R	Dobzhansky and Pavan (1943)	XO ♂; X is rod- or J-shaped
araicas Pavan and Nacrur 1950	1 V, 3 v, 1 D	Pavan and Nacrur (1950)	—
arapuan da Cunha and Pavan 1947	2 V, 1 R, 1 D	Pavan and da Cunha (1947)	Y is J-shaped
ararama Pavan and da Cunha 1947	4 R, 1 J	Pavan and da Cunha (1947)	—
arassari da Cunha and Frota-Pessoa 1947	5 R, 1 D	Pavan and da Cunha (1947)	—
arauna Pavan and Nacrur 1950	1 V, 3 v, 1 R, 1 Dr	Pavan and Nacrur (1950)	—
gibberosa Patterson and Mainland 1943	5 R	Wharton (1943)	X is long rod with proximal constriction; Y is J-shaped
talamancana Wheeler 1968	1 V, 4 R	Wheeler (1968)	X is rod-shaped; Y is J- or V- shaped
bizonata species group			
bizonata Kikkawa and Peng 1938	3 V, 1 D	Kikkawa and Peng (1938)	—
heterobristalis Tan et al. 1949	2 V, 1 R, 1 D	Tan et al. (1949)	—
meitanensis Tan et al. 1949	2 V, 1 J, 1 D	Tan et al. (1949)	X and Y are J-shaped
bromeliae species group			
bromeliae Sturtevant 1921	2 V, 1 R, 1 D	Metz (1916b)	Y is J-shaped
bromelioides Pavan and da Cunha 1947	1 R, 3 V	Pavan and da Cunha (1947)	—
	4 V	Clayton and Wasserman (1957)	Species identity uncertain

TABLE 1.   Catalog of Drosophila Metaphase Chromosome Configurations

Species	Metaphase	Reference	Remarks
		bromeliae species group (Continued)	
florae Sturtevant 1916	2 V, 1 R, 1 D	Metz (1916*a*)	—
		calloptera species group	
atrata Burla and Pavan 1953	5 R, 1 D	Dobzhansky and Pavan (1943)	Reported as *calloptera*
		Clayton and Ward (1954)	—
calloptera Schiner 1868	3 R, 1 V, 1 D	Metz (1916*a,b*)	—
	4 R, 1 J	Clayton and Ward (1954)	—
ornatipennis Williston 1896	3 R, 1 V, 1 D	Metz (1916*a,b*)	Reported as *calloptera*
	3 R, 1 V, 3 D	Clayton and Wasserman (1957)	—
		canalinea species group	
canalinea Patterson and Mainland 1944	1 R, 1 V, 1 v, 1 D	Patterson and Mainland (1944)	—
canalinoides Wheeler 1957	6 R	Clayton and Wasserman (1957)	—
paracanalinea Wheeler 1957	1 V, 1 J, 1 R, 1 D	Clayton and Wasserman (1957)	J has satellite
		carbonaria species group	
carbonaria Patterson and Wheeler 1942	2 R, 2 J, 1 v, 1 D	Ward (1949)	—
		cardini species group	
acutilabella Stalker 1953	2 V, 1 R, 1 D	Stalker (1953)	—
antillea Heed 1962	2 V, 1 R, 1 D	Heed and Krishnamurthy (1959)	Reported as stock SL

Species	Configuration	Reference	Notes
arawakana Heed 1962	2 V, 1 R, 1 D	Heed and Krishnamurthy (1959)	Reported as stock GU
a. kittensis Heed 1962	2 V, 1 R, 1 D	Heed and Krishnamurthy (1959)	Reported as stock SK
bedicheki Heed and Russell 1971	1 R, 2 V, 1 D	Heed and Russell (1971)	—
belladunni Heed and Krishnamurthy 1959	2 V, 2 R	Heed and Krishnamurthy (1959)	—
cardini Sturtevant 1916	5 R, 1 D	Metz (1916*b*)	Species identity uncertain
	2 V, 1 R, 1 D	Wharton (1943)	
	6 R	Ward (1949), Clayton and Wasserman (1957), Heed and Russell (1971)	—
cardinoides Dobzhansky and Pavan 1943	2 V, 1 R, 1 D	Dobzhansky and Pavan (1943)	—
caribiana Heed 1962	2 V, 1 R, 1 D	Heed and Krishnamurthy (1959)	Reported as stock MA
dunni Townsend and Wheeler 1955	2 V, 1 R, 1 r	Townsend and Wheeler (1955)	—
d. thomasensis Heed 1962	2 J, 1 V, 1 r	Heed and Krishnamurthy (1959)	Reported as stock ST
neocardini Streisinger 1946	2 V, 1 R, 1 D	Streisinger (1946) Ward (1949)	Y is a small V
neomorpha Heed and Wheeler 1957	2 V, 1 R, 1 D	Heed and Wheeler (1957)	Y is rod, shorter than X
nigrodunni Heed and Wheeler 1957	2 V, 1 R, 1 D	Heed and Wheeler (1957)	—
parthenogenetica Stalker 1953	2 V, 1 R, 1 D	Stalker (1953)	Y is short rod
polymorpha Dobzhansky and Pavan 1943	2 V, 1 R, 1 D	Dobzhansky and Pavan (1943)	—
procardinoides Frydenberg 1956	2 V, 1 R, 1 D	Frydenberg (1956)	—
similis Williston 1896	2 V, 1 R, 1 D	Metz (1916*b*) Heed and Krishnamurthy (1959)	Species identity uncertain

TABLE 1. Continued

Species	Metaphase	Reference	Remarks
cardini species group (Continued)			
s. grenadensis Heed 1962	2 V, 1 R, 1 D	Heed and Krishnamurthy (1959)	Reported as stock GR
carsoni species group			
carsoni Wheeler 1957	2 R, 2 J, 1 V, 1 D	Clayton and Wasserman (1957)	—
dreyfusi species group			
briegeri Pavan and Breuer 1954	3 V, 1 D	Pavan and Breuer (1954)	—
camargoi Dobzhansky and Pavan 1950	2 V, 1 J, 1 R	Pavan (1950)	Stock from Brazil
	3 V, 1 J	Clayton and Wasserman (1957)	Stock from Honduras
dreyfusi Dobzhansky and Pavan 1943	2 V, 1 J	Dobzhansky and Pavan (1943)	X and Y are J-shaped
wingei Cordeiro 1964	3 V	Cordeiro (1964)	Largest V has satellite
flavopilosa species group			
flavopilosa Frey 1919	3 R, 2 V, 1 J	Wheeler et al. (1962)	—
funebris species group			
funebris (Fabricius) 1787	5 R, 1 D	Metz (1914)	—
macrospina Stalker and Spencer 1939	5 R, 1 D	Wharton (1943)	—
m. limpiensis Mainland 1941	5 R, 1 D	Patterson and Wheeler (1942)	—
subfunebris Stalker and Spencer 1939	5 R, 1 D	Wharton (1943)	Y has proximal constriction
trispina Wheeler 1949	5 R, 2 D	Ward (1949)	—

Species	Reference	Configuration	Notes
tenuicauda Okada 1956	Kang *et al.* (1964)	4 R, 1 V, 1 D	—
grandis species group			
guaramunu species group			
griseolineata Duda 1927	Dobzhansky and Pavan (1943)	5 R, 1 D	—
guaraja King 1947	King (1947)	1 V, 3 R, 1 D	Y is rod with large satellite; X is short rod
guaramunu Dobzhansky and Pavan 1943	Dobzhansky and Pavan (1943)	5 R, 1 D	—
neoguaramunu Frydenberg 1956	Clayton and Wasserman (1957)	4 R, 1 V	Species identity uncertain
	Frydenberg (1956)	3 V	X is V-shaped; Y is rod
guarani species group			
guarani Dobzhansky and Pavan 1943	Dobzhansky and Pavan (1943)	5 R, 1 V	X and Y are V-shaped
guaru Dobzhansky and Pavan 1943	Dobzhansky and Pavan (1943)	4 R, 1 V, 1 D	Y is J-shaped
subbadia Patterson and Mainland 1943	Wharton (1943)	3 R, 2 V	X is V-shaped; Y is J-shaped
	King (1947)	5 R, 1 V	
histrio species group			
histrio Meigen 1830	Frolova (1926)	5 R, 1 D	—
sternopleuralis Okada and Kurokawa 1957	Okada and Kurokawa (1957)	4 R	—
immigrans species group			
albomicans Duda 1924	Wilson *et al.* (1969)	1 R, 1 V, 1 J	Y is small V; reported as *komaii*
	Kikkawa and Peng (1938)	3 R, 1 V	
argentostriata Bock 1966	Bock (1966)	5 R, 1 D	—
curviceps Okada and Kurokawa 1957	Okada and Kurokawa (1957)	2 R, 1 V, 1 J	—

TABLE 1. *Continued*

Species	Metaphase	Reference	Remarks
immigrans species group (Continued)			
hexastriata Tan et al. 1949	2 R, 1 V, 1 D	Tan et al. (1949)	—
hypocausta Osten-Sacken 1882	2 R, 1 V, 1 D	Pipkin (1956)	—
immigrans Sturtevant 1921	1 V, 1 J, 2 R	Emmens (1937), Wharton (1943)	
	1 V, 3 R	Metz and Moses (1923), Ward (1949), Clayton and Wasserman (1957), Mather (1962)	Y is small V
kepulauana Wheeler 1969	2 R, 1 V, 1 D	Wilson et al. (1969)	X is rod; Y is rod- or J-shaped
kohkoa Wheeler 1969	2 R, 1 V, 1 D	Wilson et al. (1969)	X is rod; Y is rod-, V-, or J-shaped
nasuta Lamb 1914	2 R, 1 V, 1 D	Wakahama and Kitagawa (1972)	X is rod; Y is J-shaped
nixifrons Tan et al. 1949	3 R, 1 V, 1 D	Tan et al. (1949)	—
pallidifrons Wheeler 1969	1 V, 2 R, 1 D	Wilson et al. (1969)	X and Y are rods
pararubida Mather 1961	2 R, 1 V, 1 D	Mather (1961)	—
	1 R, 2 V, 1 D	Mather (1962)	—
pulaua Wheeler 1969	2 R, 1 V, 1 D	Wilson et al. (1969)	X and Y are rods
rubida Mather 1960	1 V, 2 R, 1 D	Mather (1960)	—
	2 R, 2 V	Mather (1962)	—
silvistriata Bock & Baimai 1967	1 V, 3 R, 1 D	Bock and Baimai (1967)	X is long rod; Y is short rod
sulfurigaster Duda 1923	2 R, 1 V, 1 D	Mather (1962)	Reported as setifemur
		Wilson et al. (1969)	X is rod; Y is V- or J-shaped
s. albostrigata Wheeler 1969	1 V, 2 R, 1 D	Wilson et al. (1969)	X is rod; Y is rod-, J-, or V-shaped
s. bilimbata Bezzi 1928	1 V, 2 R, 1 D	Patterson and Wheeler (1942)	Reported as spinofemora
		Wilson et al. (1969)	—

macroptera species group

Species	Reference	Configuration	Notes
macroptera Patterson and Wheeler 1942	Patterson and Wheeler (1942)	5 R, 1 D	—
submacroptera Patterson and Mainland 1943	Wharton (1943)	1 V, 2 v, 1 R, 1 D	X and Y are rods (stock from Guerrero, Mexico)
	Clayton and Wasserman (1957)	2 V, 1 J, 1 D	Stocks from Hidalgo, Puebla, and Vera Cruz, Mexico

melanica species group

Species	Reference	Configuration	Notes
afer Tan *et al.* (1949)	Tan *et al.* (1949)	2 V, 1 R, 1 J, 1 D	—
euronotus Patterson and Ward 1952	Patterson and Ward (1952)	1 V, 1 v, 2 R, 1 D	—
melanica Sturtevant 1916	Metz (1916a)	1 V, 1 v, 2 R, 1 D	Y is J-shaped; X is V-shaped
	Ward (1949)		X is large V; Y is J-shaped
melanura Miller 1944	Miller (1944)	1 V, 1 v, 2 R, 1 Dv	X is large V; Y is V-shaped
	Ward (1949)	1 V, 1 v, 2 R, 1 Dr	—
micromelanica Patterson 1941	Patterson (1941a)	5 R, 1 D	—
	Patterson and Wheeler (1942), Wharton (1943)	1 V, 1 v, 2 R, 1 D	—
	Ward (1949), Clayton and Ward (1954), Stalker (1965)	4 R, 1 v, 1 D	—
nigromelanica Patterson and Wheeler 1942	Ward (1949), Stalker (1965)	4 R, 1 v, 1 Dr	X is large V
	Patterson and Wheeler (1942)	1 V, 1 v, 2 R, 1 D	
	Wharton (1943)	1 V, 1 v, 2 R, 1 Dv	—
	Stalker (1964)	1 V, 1 v, 2 R, 1 Dr	—
	Ward (1949)	1 V, 1 v, 3 R	X is large V; Y is V-shaped
paramelanica Patterson 1942	Griffen (1942), Wharton (1943)	2 V, 2 R, 1 D	—
	Ward (1949)	2 V, 3 R	—
pengi Okada and Kurokawa 1957	Kikkawa and Peng (1938)	1 V, 1 v, 2 R, 1 D	Reported as *melanissima*
	Okada and Kurokawa (1957)		—

TABLE 1. Continued

Species	Metaphase	Reference	Remarks
mesophragmatica species group			
altiplanica Brncic and Koref-Santibañez 1957	1 V, 3 R, 1 D	Brncic and Koref-Santibañez(1957)	One pair of rods bent in middle giving appearance of small V's; dots elongated
brncici Hunter and Hunter 1964	1 V, 3 R, 1 D	Hunter and Hunter (1964)	Dots usually appear as small rods
gasici Brncic 1957	1 V, 3 R, 1 Dr	Brncic (1957)	—
gaucha Jaeger and Salzano 1953	3 R, 1 V, 1 D	Jaeger and Salzano (1953)	Y has subterminal constriction
mesophragmatica Duda 1927	1 V, 3 R, 1 D	Pavan and da Cunha (1947)	—
	1 V, 3 R, 1 r	Brncic and Koref-Santibañez (1957)	—
orkui Brncic and Koref-Santibañez 1957	1 V, 4 R	Brncic and Koref-Santibañez (1957)	One rod is half length others
pavani Brncic 1957	3 R, 1 V, 1 D	Brncic and Koref-Santibañez (1957)	Y has subterminal constriction
viracochi Brncic and Koref-Santibañez 1957	3 R, 1 V, 1 D	Brncic and Koref-Santibañez (1957)	
nannoptera species group			
acanthoptera Wheeler 1949	2 R, 1 V, 2 v	Ward (1949)	X is large V; Y is J-shaped
nannoptera Wheeler 1949	3 V, 1 J, 1 v	Ward (1949)	X is large V; Y is rod
pachea Patterson and Wheeler 1942	2 R, 1 V, 2 J	Ward and Heed (1970)	Y is J-shaped
		Ward and Heed (1970)	Y is short rod; X is large V
pallidipennis species group			
pallidipennis Dobzhansky and Pavan 1943	4 R, 1 V, 1 D	Dobzhansky and Pavan (1943)	X and Y are V-shaped
p. centralis Patterson and Mainland 1944	4 R, 1 V, 1 D	Clayton and Wasserman (1957)	

pinicola species group

Species	Metaphase configuration	Reference	Notes
flavopinicola Wheeler 1954	5 R, 1 D	Clayton and Ward (1954)	—
pinicola Sturtevant 1942	2 V, 1 R	Sturtevant (1942)	—

polychaeta species group

Species	Metaphase configuration	Reference	Notes
polychaeta Patterson and Wheeler 1942	2 R, 2 J, 1 V, 1 D	Patterson and Wheeler (1942)	X and Y are rods

quinaria species group

Species	Metaphase configuration	Reference	Notes
angularis Okada 1956	5 R, 1 D	Tokumitsu et al. (1967)	—
brachynephros Okada 1956	5 R, 1 D	Wharton (1943)	Reported as *transversa*
falleni Wheeler 1960	5 R, 1 D	Wharton (1943)	—
guttifera Walker 1849	5 R, 1 D	Clayton and Ward (1954)	—
innubila Spencer 1943	5 R, 1 D	Spencer (1942)	—
magnaquinaria Wheeler 1954	6 R	Tan et al. (1949)	—
munda Spencer 1942	2 V, 1 R, 1 D	Momma (1954)	—
mutandis Tan et al. 1949	5 R, 1 D	Tokumutsu et al. (1967)	—
nigromaculata Kikkawa and Peng 1938	5 R, 1 D	Spencer (1942)	—
occidentalis Spencer 1942	5 R, 1 D	Wharton (1943)	—
palustris Spencer 1942	5 R, 1 D	Frolova (1926)	—
phalerata Meigen 1830	5 R, 1 D	Metz (1914)	—
quinaria Loew 1865	1 V, 1 J, 1 D	Spencer (1942)	X is rod; Y is J-shaped
suboccidentalis Spencer 1942	5 R, 1 D	Spencer (1942)	—
subpalustris Spencer 1942	5 R, 1 D	Spencer (1942)	—
subquinaria Spencer 1942	5 R, 1 D	Clayton and Ward (1954)	Y is small, V-shaped
suffusca Spencer 1943	1 V, 1 v, 1 R, 1 D	Wharton (1943)	Y is J-shaped
tenebrosa Spencer 1943	3 R, 1 J, 1 D	Blumel (1949)	—
transversa Fallén 1823	3 R, 1 V, 1 D	Frolova (1926), Kim (1965)	—
unispina Okada 1956	5 R, 1 D	Kang et al. (1964)	—

TABLE 1. Continued

Species	Metaphase	Reference	Remarks
repleta species group			
fasciola subgroup			
coroica Wasserman 1962	5 R, 1 D	Wasserman (1960)	Reported as species L
fasciola Williston 1896	5 R, 1 D	Wasserman (1962*c*)	X is rod- or J-shaped
fascioloides Dobzhansky and Pavan 1943	3 V, 1 D	Dobzhansky and Pavan (1943)	—
		Wasserman (1962*c*)	Reported 3 types of X and Y shapes
fulvalineata Patterson and Wheeler 1942	5 R, 1 V	Patterson and Wheeler (1942), Wharton (1943)	X is rod; Y is short rod
		Clayton and Wasserman (1957)	Stock from New Mexico
	1 V, 1 v, 3 R	Clayton and Wasserman (1957)	X is large V, Y is J-shaped; stock from Arizona
moju Pavan 1950	5 R, 1 Dr	Wasserman (1962*c*)	—
mojuoides Wasserman 1962	5 R, 1 D	Wasserman (1960)	Reported as species M
paraguttata Thompson 1957	5 R, 1 D	Clayton and Wasserman (1957)	—
pictilis Wasserman 1962	6 R	Wasserman (1960)	Reported as species J; Y is short rod
pictura Wasserman 1962	4 R, 1 V, 1 J	Wasserman (1960)	Reported as species K; X is J-shaped; Y is short rod
hydei subgroup			
bifurca Patterson and Wheeler 1942	5 R, 1 D	Patterson and Wheeler (1942), Wharton (1943), Ward (1949)	Y is rod
			Y is small, V-shaped

eohydei Wasserman 1962	5 R, 1 D	Wasserman (1962a)	Y is short rod
hydei Sturtevant 1921	4 R, 1 V, 1 D	Kikkawa (1935), Wharton (1943)	X is V; Y is J-shaped
		Kikkawa and Peng (1938), Wasserman (1960)	Y is rod
hydeoides Patterson and Wheeler 1942	6 R	Patterson and Wheeler (1942)	Y is very short rod
neohydei Wasserman 1962	5 R, 1 D	Wasserman (1962a)	X is J-shaped; Y is rod
nigrohydei Patterson and Wheeler 1942	6 R	Patterson and Wheeler (1942)	Y is very short rod
novemaristata Dobzhansky and Pavan 1943	6 R	Dobzhansky and Pavan (1943)	Microchromosome is large dot or short rod
melanopalpa subgroup			
brunneipalpa Dobzhansky and Pavan 1943	5 R, 1 D	Dobzhansky and Pavan (1943)	Y is dotlike
californica Sturtevant 1923	3 V, 1 R	Patterson and Wheeler (1942)	Reported as *fuliginea*
canapalpa Patterson and Mainland 1944	5 R, 1 V	Patterson and Mainland (1944)	—
fulvimacula Patterson and Mainland 1944 *f. flavorepleta* Patterson and Pavan 1952	5 R, 1 D	Clayton and Ward (1954)	—
fulvimaculoides Wasserman and Wilson 1957	5 R, 1 D	Clayton and Wasserman (1957)	Y is J-shaped
limensis Pavan and Patterson 1947	6 R	Pavan and da Cunha (1947)	Y is very short rod
melanopalpa Patterson and Wheeler 1942	4 R, 1 V, 1 J	Patterson and Wheeler (1942)	X is J-shaped; Y is short rod
neorepleta Patterson and Wheeler 1942	4 R, 2 J	Wharton (1943)	

TABLE 1. Continued

Species	Metaphase	Reference	Remarks
repleta species group (Continued)			
repleta Wollaston 1858	5 R, 1 D	Metz (1914), Wharton (1943), Clayton and Wasserman (1957)	—
	4 R, 1 V, 1 D	Metz (1916b)	—
mercatorum subgroup			
carcinophila Wheeler 1960	1 V, 3 R, 1 D	Carson (1967)	XO ♂
mercatorum Patterson and Wheeler 1942	1 V, 3 R, 1 Dv	Patterson and Wheeler (1942), Wharton (1943) Ward (1949), Clayton and Wasserman (1957)	X is rod; Y is short rod
m. pararepleta Dobzhansky and Pavan 1943	1 V, 3 R, 1 D	Dobzhansky and Pavan (1943)	Y is short rod
paranaensis de Barros 1950	1 V, 3 R, 1 D	de Barros (1950), Dreyfus and de Barros (1949)	—
	1 V, 1 v, 3 R	Clayton and Wasserman (1957), Clayton and Ward (1954)	—
mulleri subgroup			
aldrichi Patterson and Crow 1940	5 R, 1 D	Patterson and Crow (1940)	Y is short rod, ⅓ length of X
anceps Patterson and Mainland 1944	6 R	Patterson and Mainland (1944)	—
airzonensis Patterson and Wheeler 1942	} 5 R, 1 D		
buzzatii Patterson and Wheeler 1942		Patterson and Wheeler (1942)	Y is short rod, ⅓ length of X

Species	Configuration	Reference	Notes
eremophila Wasserman 1962	5 R, 1 Dv	Wasserman (1960)	Reported as species F
hamatofila Patterson and Wheeler 1942	5 R, 1 D	Patterson and Wheeler (1942)	Y is small, V-shaped
hexastigma Patterson and Mainland 1944	5 R, 1 D	Patterson and Mainland (1944)	Y is J-shaped
longicornis Patterson and Wheeler 1942	5 R, 1 D	Patterson and Wheeler (1942)	Y is short rod
martensis Wasserman and Wilson 1957	5 R, 1 D	Clayton and Wasserman (1957)	Y is small, V-shaped
meridiana Patterson and Wheeler 1942	5 R, 1 V	Patterson and Wheeler (1942)	Y is short rod
m. rioensis Patterson 1943	1 V, 3 R, 1 D	Wharton (1943)	Y is short rod
meridionalis Wasserman 1962	1 V, 3 R, 1 D	Wasserman (1962b)	Y is short rod; X is rod
mojavensis Patterson and Crow 1940	5 R, 1 D	Patterson and Crow (1940)	Y is short rod
mulleri Sturtevant 1921	5 R, 1 D	Patterson and Crow (1940), Wharton (1943)	—
nigricruria Patterson and Mainland 1943	1 V, 4 R, 1 D	Metz (1916b), Wharton (1943)	Reported as *repleta*, variety b
pachuca Wasserman 1962	5 R, 1 D	Wasserman (1962b)	—
peninsularis Patterson and Wheeler 1942	5 R, 1 D	Patterson and Wheeler (1942)	Y is J-shaped
promeridiana Wasserman 1962	1 V, 3 R, 1 D	Wasserman (1962b)	Y is small, V-shaped
propachuca Wasserman 1962	5 R, 1 D	Wasserman (1962b)	Y is short rod; X is rod
racemova Patterson and Mainland 1944	5 R, 1 D	Patterson and Mainland (1944)	Y is J-shaped
ritae Patterson and Wheeler 1942	5 R, 1 D	Patterson and Wheeler (1942)	—
stalkeri Wheeler 1954	5 R, 1 D	Clayton and Ward (1954)	X and Y are longest rods
tira Wasserman 1962	5 R, 1 D	Wasserman (1962b)	Y is J-shaped

TABLE 1. Continued

Species	Metaphase	Reference	Remarks
		***repleta* species group (Continued)**	
wheeleri Patterson and Alexander 1952	5 R, 1 D	Patterson and Alexander (1952)	Y is short rod
		subgroup uncertain	
aureata Wheeler 1957	5 R, 1 D	Clayton and Wasserman (1957)	Y is J-shaped
betari Dobzhansky and Pavan 1943	1 V, 3 R, 1 D	Dobzhansky and Pavan (1943)	Y is dotlike but larger than autosomal dot
brevicarinata Patterson and Wheeler 1942	5 R, 1 D	Wharton (1943)	—
castanea Patterson and Mainland 1944	2 V, 1 R, 1 D	Clayton and Wasserman (1957)	X is V-shaped; Y is J-shaped
inca Dobzhansky and Pavan 1943	5 R, 1 J	Dobzhansky and Pavan (1943)	—
leonis Patterson and Wheeler 1942	6 R	Wharton (1943)	—
lineareptela Patterson and Wheeler 1942 / *nigrospiracula* Patterson and Wheeler 1942	5 R, 1 D	Patterson and Wheeler (1942)	—
onca Dobzhansky 1943	1 V, 1 J, 1 R, 1 D	Dobzhansky and Pavan (1943)	X is rod; Y is J-shaped
ramsdeni Sturtevant 1916	5 R, 1 D	Metz (1916b)	—
		***robusta* species group**	
cheda Tan et al. 1949	1 V, 1 v, 1 R, 1 D	Tan et al. (1949)	—
colorata Walker 1849	2 R, 2 V, 1 v, 1 J	Wharton (1943)	X is V-shaped; Y is rod

Species	Configuration	Reference	Remarks
lacertosa Okada 1956	1 V, 4 J, 1 d	Momma (1956)	Determined from oogonial metaphase
moriwakii Okada and Kurokawa 1957	1 V, 2 v, 2 R, 1 D	Okada and Kurokawa (1957)	—
pseudosordidula Kaneko et al. 1964	1 V, 1 J, 3 R, 1 r	Tokumitsu et al. (1967)	—
pullata Tan et al. 1949	1 V, 3 R, 1 D	Kaneko et al. (1964)	—
robusta Sturtevant 1916	4 V, 1 D	Tan et al. (1949)	—
	2 V, 1 R, 1 D	Metz (1916a)	—
	3 V, 1 D	Carson and Stalker (1947)	X is largest V; Y is V-shaped
sordidula Kikkawa and Peng 1938	2 V, 2 R, 1 D	Kikkawa and Peng (1938)	—
rubrifrons species group			
parachrogaster Patterson and Mainland 1943	4 R, 1 V, 1 D	Wharton (1943)	—
rubrifrons Patterson and Wheeler 1942	1 J, 4 R, 1 r	Clayton and Ward (1954)	—
sticta species group			
sticta Wheeler 1957	5 R, 1 D	Clayton and Wasserman (1957)	Three forms observed; rods identical but one pair of dots, rods identical but one dot with one short rod, or rods identical but two dots with one short rod
testacea species group			
putrida Sturtevant 1916	2 V, 1 R, 1 D	Wharton (1943)	Stock from Texas
	2 V, 1 R, 2 D	Wharton (1943)	Stock from Florida
testacea von Roser 1840	1 V, 2 R, 1 D	Wharton (1943)	X is rod
tripunctata species group			
albirostris Sturtevant 1921	5 R, 1 D	Clayton and Wasserman (1957)	Y is rod shorter than X
bandeirantorum Dobzhansky and Pavan 1943	4 R, 1 V, 1 D	Dobzhansky and Pavan (1943)	—

TABLE 1. Continued

Species	Metaphase	Reference	Remarks
tripunctata species group (Continued)			
bipunctata Patterson and Mainland 1943	5 R, 1 D	Clayton and Wasserman (1957)	Y is rod shorter than X
blumelae Pipkin and Heed 1964	5 R, 1 D	Pipkin and Heed (1964)	Y is J-shaped
converga Heed and Wheeler 1957	5 R, 1 D	Heed and Wheeler (1957)	—
crocina Patterson and Mainland 1944	5 R, 1 D	Patterson and Mainland (1944)	—
facialba Heed and Wheeler 1957	3 R, 1 V, 1 D	Heed and Wheeler (1957)	Stock from El Salvador
fairchildi Pipkin and Heed 1964	5 R, 1 D	Pipkin and Heed (1964)	—
	5 R	Clayton and Ward (1954)	
fragilis Wheeler 1949	3 R, 1 V, 3 D	Clayton and Wasserman (1957)	Stock from El Salvador
	3 R, 1 J, 1 D		
greerae Pipkin and Heed 1964	5 R, 1 D	Pipkin and Heed (1964)	X is rod, Y is shorter rod
johnstonae Pipkin and Heed 1964	5 R, 1 D	Pipkin and Heed (1964)	Y is J-shaped
mediodiffusa Heed and Wheeler 1957	5 R, 1 D	Heed and Wheeler (1957)	X is double-length rod; Y is short rod
medionotata Frota-Pessoa 1954	5 R, 1 D	Clayton and Wasserman (1957)	Species identity uncertain
mediopictoides Heed and Wheeler 1957	4 R, 1 r, 1 V	Heed and Wheeler (1957)	—
mediopunctata Dobzhansky and Pavan 1943	5 R, 1 D	Dobzhansky and Pavan (1943)	Stock from Brazil
mediosignata Dobzhansky and Pavan 1943	1 V, 1 J, 2 R, 1 D	Clayton and Wasserman (1957)	Stock from El Salvador
	5 R, 1 D	Dobzhansky and Pavan (1943)	—

Species	Metaphase configuration	Reference	Remarks
mediostriata Duda 1925	5 R, 1 D	Dobzhansky and Pavan (1943)	—
metzii Sturtevant 1921	5 R, 1 D	Clayton and Wasserman (1957)	—
paramediostriata Townsend and Wheeler 1955	5 R, 1 D	Townsend and Wheeler (1955)	—
pellewae Pipkin and Heed 1964	5 R, 1 D	Pipkin and Heed (1964)	Y is J-shaped
prosimilis Duda 1927	5 R, 1 D	Dobzhansky and Pavan (1943)	—
roehrae Pipkin and Heed 1964	5 R, 1 D	Pipkin and Heed (1964)	—
setula Heed and Wheeler 1957	4 R, 1 V, 1 D	Clayton and Wasserman (1957)	Stock from Colombia
spinatermina Heed and Wheeler 1957	3 R, 1 V, 1 D	Clayton and Wasserman (1957)	Stock from Panama Canal Zone
trapeza Heed and Wheeler 1957	3 R, 1 V, 1 D	Heed and Wheeler (1957)	—
tranquilla Spencer 1943	5 R, 1 D	Clayton and Wasserman (1957)	—
triangula Wheeler 1949	1 V, 2 R	Wharton (1943)	—
	1 V, 2 R, 1 D	Clayton and Ward (1954)	Stock from Chihuahua, Mexico
trifiloides Wheeler 1957	4 R, 1 J, 1 D	Clayton and Ward (1954)	Stock from Puebla, Mexico
	5 R	Clayton and Wasserman (1957)	—
tripunctata Loew 1862	3 R, 1 V	Metz (1914), Metz (1916b)	—
	5 R, 1 D	Metz and Moses (1923), Wharton (1943)	—
tristriata Heed and Wheeler 1957	5 R, 1 D	Clayton and Wasserman (1957)	One rod is double-length
unipunctata Patterson and Mainland 1943	2 R, 1 V, 1 J, 1 D	Wharton (1943)	—

TABLE 1. Continued

Species	Metaphase	Reference	Remarks
tumiditarsus species group			
tumiditarsus Tan et al. 1949	2 V, 1 J, 1 D	Hsiang (1949)	X is V-shaped; Y is shorter J-shaped
virilis species group			
americana Spencer 1938	2 V, 1 R, 1 D	Hughes (1939), Wharton (1943)	—
borealis Patterson 1952	4 R, 1 v, 1 D	Patterson (1952)	—
ezoana Takada and Okada 1958	4 R, 1 v, 1 D	Stone et al. (1960)	Y is small V
flavomontana Patterson 1952	4 R, 1 v, 1 D	Patterson (1952)	—
lacicola Patterson 1944	4 R, 1 v, 1 D	Patterson (1944)	—
littoralis Meigen 1830	2 R, 1 V, 1 J, 1 D	Clayton and Ward (1954)	X is rod; Y is J-shaped
montana Stone et al. 1942	4 R, 1 v, 1 D	Stone et al. (1942)	—
novamexicana Patterson 1941	5 R, 1 D	Patterson (1941b)	—
texana Patterson 1940	1 V, 3 R, 1 D	Patterson (1941a)	—
virilis Sturtevant 1916	5 R, 1 D	Metz (1914)	Reported as species B
Subgenus Engiscaptomyza			
amplilobus Hardy 1966	1 V, 3 R, 1 D	Clayton (1966)	Reported as crassifemur
crassifemur Grimshaw 1901	1 V, 3 R, 1 D	Clayton (1968)	—
nasalis Grimshaw 1901	2 V, 2 R, 1 D	Clayton (1966)	—
reducta Hardy 1965	1 V, 3 R, 1 D	Clayton (1968)	Reported as crassifemur
Subgenus Hirtodrosophila			
alboralis Momma and Takada 1954	5 R, 1 D	Momma (1954)	Y is shorter than X
confusa Staeger 1844	5 R, 1 D	Burla (1950a)	Reported as grischuna
		Okada and Kurokawa (1957)	Reported as histrioides
	1 V, 3 R, 1 D	Kang et al. (1964)	Reported as histrioides

Species	Configuration	Reference	Notes
duncani Sturtevant 1918	2 V, 2 v, 1 Dv	Wharton (1943)	Microsome considered small V; X is V-shaped; Y is rod
grisea Patterson and Wheeler 1942	5 R, 1 D	Clayton and Ward (1954)	
longala Patterson and Wheeler 1942	5 R, 1 D	Patterson and Stone (1952)	XO ♂
orbospiracula Patterson and Wheeler 1942	5 R, 1 D	Patterson and Wheeler (1942)	
pictiventris Duda 1925	1 V, 1 J, 1 R, 1 D	Clayton and Ward (1954)	
thoracis Williston 1896	5 R, 1 D	Clayton and Ward (1954)	
trivittata Strobl 1893	1 V, 1 v, 2 R, 1 D	Kikkawa and Peng (1938)	—

Subgenus *Scaptodrosophila* (= *Pholadoris*)

Species	Configuration	Reference	Notes
brooksae Pipkin 1961	2 V, 1 v, 1 R	Pipkin (1961)	X is rod; Y is rod with constriction
bryani Malloch 1934	2 V, 1 R		—
cancellata Mather 1955	3 R, 1 r, 1 V	Mather (1956)	
coracina Kikkawa and Peng 1938	2 V, 1 R, 1 D	Kikkawa and Peng (1938)	Y is J-shaped
		Kang *et al.* (1964)	Y is rod
enigma Malloch 1927	4 R, 2 V	Mather (1956)	—
fumida Mather 1960	2 V, 2 R	Mather (1960)	Y is rod, half length of X
latifasciaeformis Duda 1940	1 V, 2 v	Dobzhansky and Pavan (1943)	Reported as *mirim*
lativittata Malloch 1923	6 R	Mather (1956)	One rod is twice the length of the others
lebanonensis Wheeler 1949	2 V, 1 v, 1 R	Ward (1949)	—
l. casteeli Pipkin 1961	2 V, 1 v, 1 R	Pipkin (1961)	—
novamaculosa Mather 1956	6 R	Mather (1956)	—
novopaca Mather 1956	6 R	Mather (1956)	One rod is twice the length of the others
pattersoni Pipkin 1956	1 V, 2 v, 1 R	Pipkin (1956)	Reported as *nitens*; X and Y are small, V-shaped
rufifrons Loew 1873	2 V, 2 v	Buzzati-Traverso (1943)	

TABLE 1. Continued

Species	Metaphase	Reference	Remarks
Subgenus Scaptodrosophila (= Pholadoris) (Continued)			
stonei Pipkin 1956	1 V, 1 J, 1 v, 1 R	Pipkin (1956)	X is rod or J; Y is small, V-shaped; in some, large V's are J-shaped
subtilis Kikkawa and Peng 1938	2 R, 1 V, 2 J	Kikkawa and Peng (1938)	—
victoria Sturtevant 1942	1 V, 1 v, 1 J, 1 R	Wharton (1943)	Species identity uncertain, stock from Mexico
	1 V, 1 v, 2 J	Sturtevant (1942)	Stock from California
Subgenus Siphlodora			
sigmoides Loew 1872	5 R, 1 D	Butler and Mettler (1963)	—
Subgenus Sophophora			
melanogaster sp. group			
		ananassae subgroup	
ananassae Doleschall 1858	4 V	Metz (1916b)	Reported as *caribbea*
		Kikkawa and Peng (1938)	X is large V; Y is J-shaped
atripex Bock and Wheeler 1972	4 V	Kaneshiro and Wheeler (1970)	Reported as "species 2"; Y is J-shaped
bipectinata Duda 1923	4 V	Kikkawa and Peng (1938)	X is medium V; Y is V-shaped
malerkotliana Parshad and Paika 1964	4 V	Kaneshiro and Wheeler (1970)	X and Y are V-shaped; reported as "species 10 and 11"
m. pallens Bock and Wheeler 1972	4 V	Kaneshiro and Wheeler (1970)	Reported as "species 10 and 11;" Y is J-shaped
nesoetes Bock and Wheeler 1972	3 V, 1 R	Kaneshiro and Wheeler (1970)	Reported as "species 3;" X is V-shaped; Y is J-shaped

Species	Configuration	Reference	Notes
pallidosa Bock and Wheeler 1972	3 V, 1 v	Futch (1966)	Reported as "light" *ananassae*; Y is J-shaped
parabipectinata Bock 1971	3 V, 1 v	Kaneshiro and Wheeler (1970)	Reported as "species 7"
phaeopleura Bock and Wheeler 1972	4 V	Kaneshiro and Wheeler (1970)	Reported as "species 5;" Y is J-shaped
pseudoananassae Bock 1971	4 V	Kaneshiro and Wheeler (1970)	Reported as "species 8"
p. nigrens Bock and Wheeler 1972	3 V, 2 v	Kaneshiro and Wheeler (1970)	Reported as "species 9;" X is V-shaped; Y is rod
	5 V	Kaneshiro and Wheeler (1970)	X is V-shaped; Y is rod
varians Bock and Wheeler 1972	4 V	Kaneshiro and Wheeler (1970)	Reported as "species 4;" Y is J-shaped
denticulata subgroup			
denticulata Bock and Wheeler 1972	2 V, 1 R	Bock and Wheeler (1972)	X is rod-shaped; Y is slightly longer rod with spherical expansion at end
elegans subgroup			
elegans Bock and Wheeler 1972	5 R	Bock and Wheeler (1972)	Y is short, J-shaped
eugracilis subgroup			
eugracilis Bock and Wheeler 1972	2 V, 1 R	Bock and Wheeler (1972)	X is short rod; Y is thick heterochromatic rod
ficusphila subgroup			
ficusphila Kikkawa and Peng 1938	2 V, 1 R, 1 D	Kikkawa and Peng (1938)	Y is J-shaped
melanogaster subgroup			
melanogaster Meigen 1830	2 V, 1 R, 1 D	Stevens (1912)	Reported as *ampelophila*
		Metz (1914)	Y is J-shaped
		Patau (1935)	—
simulans Sturtevant 1919	2 V, 1 R, 1 D	Kikkawa and Peng (1938)	X is rod; Y is small rod or J

TABLE 1. Continued

Species	Metaphase	Reference	Remarks
melanogaster sp. group (Continued)			
montium subgroup			
auraria Peng 1937	2 V, 1 R, 1 D	Kikkawa and Peng (1938)	Y is short rod
baimaii Bock and Wheeler 1972	2 V, 1 R		
barbarae Bock and Wheeler 1972	2 V, 1 R	Bock and Wheeler (1972)	X is rod; Y is short
biauraria Bock and Wheeler 1972	2 V, 1 R		
bicornuta Bock and Wheeler 1972	2 V, 1 R, 1 D		
birchii Dobzhansky and Mather 1961	2 V, 1 D, + 1	Baimai (1969)	Pair of sex chromosomes of various types
kanapiae Bock and Wheeler 1972	2 V, 1 R	Bock and Wheeler (1972)	X is rod; Y is small, densely heterochromatic
khaoyana Bock and Wheeler 1972	2 V, 1 R	Bock and Wheeler (1972)	X is rod; Y is short
kikkawai Burla 1954	2 V, 2 R	Ward (1949)	X is rod; Y is rod or small V; reported as *montium*
		Baimai (1969)	Reported extensive variation in metaphases; reported as *montium*.
lini Bock and Wheeler 1972	2 V, 1 R, 2 r	Bock and Wheeler (1972)	X is rod; Y is short
mayri Mather and Dobzhansky 1962	2 V, 1 R, 1 D	Mather and Dobzhansky (1962)	—
montium de Meijere 1916	2 V, 2 R	Kikkawa (1936)	Y is V-shaped; X is rod; species identity uncertain
orosa Bock and Wheeler 1972	2 V, 1 R	Bock and Wheeler (1972)	X is rod; Y is short
parvula Bock and Wheeler 1972	2 V, 1 R	Bock and Wheeler (1972)	X is rod; Y is small, densely heterochromatic
pennae Bock and Wheeler 1972	2 V, 1 R	Bock and Wheeler (1972)	X is long rod; Y is short
pseudomayri Baimai 1970	3 V, 1 D	Baimai (1970)	X is V-shaped; Y is J-shaped

Species	Configuration	Reference	Description
quadraria Bock and Wheeler 1972	2 V, 1 R	Bock and Wheeler (1972)	X is rod; Y is short
rhopaloa Bock and Wheeler 1972	2 V, 1 R, 1 D	Bock and Wheeler (1972)	—
rufa Kikkawa and Peng 1938	2 V, 1 R, 1 D	Kikkawa and Peng (1938)	
serrata Malloch 1927	2 V, 1 R, 1 D	Mather (1956)	
triauraria Bock and Wheeler 1972	2 V, 1 R	Bock and Wheeler (1972)	X is rod; Y is short
vulcana Bock and Wheeler 1972	2 V, 1 R, 1 D	Bock and Wheeler (1972)	X is rod; Y is short, J-shaped
suzukii subgroup			
lucipennis Lin 1972	2 V, 1 R	Bock and Wheeler (1972)	X is rod; Y is small rod
mimetica Bock and Wheeler 1972	2 V, 1 R, 1 D	Bock and Wheeler (1972)	
pulchrella Tan et al. 1949	2 V, 1 R, 1 D	Tan et al. (1949)	Y is J-shaped
suzukii (Matsumura) 1931	2 V, 1 R, 1 D	Kikkawa and Peng (1938)	
takahashii subgroup			
lutea Kikkawa and Peng 1938	2 V, 1 R, 1 D	Kikkawa and Peng (1938)	Y is short rod
paralutea Bock and Wheeler 1972	2 V, 1 R	Bock and Wheeler (1972)	X is rod; Y is short
prostipennis Lin 1972	2 V, 1 R	Bock and Wheeler (1972)	X is rod; Y is short, heterochromatic
pseudotakahashii Mather 1957	2 V, 1 R, 1 D	Mather (1956)	Reported as *takahashii*
takahashii Sturtevant 1927	2 V, 1 R, 1 D	Kikkawa and Peng (1938, Ward (1949)	X is rod; Y is short rod
	2 V, 1 J	Sturtevant (1942)	Dot attached to X; X is J-shaped; Y is short rod
trilutea Bock and Wheeler 1972	2 V, 1 R	Bock and Wheeler (1972)	X is rod; Y is short, heterochromatic
obscura species group			
affinis subgroup			
affinis Sturtevant 1916	3 R, 1 V, 1 D	Metz (1916*a*)	—
	1 R, 2 V, 1 J, 1 D	Kikkawa and Peng (1938)	—
	1 R, 1 V, 2 J, 1 D	Miller and Stone (1962)	X is V-shaped; Y is J-shaped

TABLE 1. Continued

Species	Metaphase	Reference	Remarks
obscura species group (Continued)			
algonquin Sturtevant and Dobzhansky 1936	1 R, 1 V, 2 J, 1 D	Sturtevant and Dobzhansky (1936)	—
		Miller and Stone (1962)	Pericentric inversion in V to form J in some
athabasca Sturtevant and Dobzhansky 1936	3 J, 1 V, 1 D	Sturtevant and Dobzhansky (1936)	—
	2 V, 1 J, 1 R, 1 D	Kikkawa and Peng (1938)	
	1 R, 1 V, 2 J, 1 D	Miller and Stone (1962)	Rod has subterminal centromere; X is V-shaped
azteca Sturtevant and Dobzhansky 1936	3 J, 1 V, 1 D	Sturtevant and Dobzhansky (1936)	—
	2 V, 1 J, 1 R, 1 D	Kikkawa and Peng (1938)	—
	1 R, 1 V, 2 J, 1 D	Miller and Stone (1962)	—
helvetica Burla 1948	1 V, 2 J, 1 R, 1 D	Burla (1948), Miller and Stone (1962)	Like *algonquin* except Y is rod instead of J-shaped
narragansett Sturtevant and Dobzhansky 1936	1 V, 2 J, 1 R, 1 D	Sturtevant (1940), Miller and Stone (1962)	—
tolteca Patterson and Mainland 1944	2 V, 1 J, 1 R, 1 D	Ward (1949)	—
obscura subgroup			
ambigua Pomini 1940	2 V, 2 J, 1 D	Buzzati-Traverso (1941)	X is large V; Y is rod
bifasciata Pomini 1940	2 V, 2 J, 1 D	Buzzati-Traverso (1941)	X is large V; Y is rod; dots are large
imaii Moriwaki *et al.* 1967	4 V, 1 D	Moriwaki *et al.* (1967)	X is V-shaped, Y is rod

Species	Configuration	Reference	Notes
lowei Heed et al. 1969	2 R, 2 V, 1 D	Heed et al. (1969)	X is large V; Y is J-shaped
miranda Dobzhansky 1935	3 R, 1 V, 1 D	Dobzhansky (1935)	In ♂♂ only 9 chromosomes; Y is J-shaped; X_1 is V and unpaired X_2 is rod
obscura Fallén 1823	2 V, 2 J, 1 D	Frolova and Astaurov (1929)	X is V; Y is rod
obscuroides Pomini 1940	1 V, 1 J, 2 R, 1 D	Buzzati-Traverso (1941)	Listed as synonym of *obscura*, but metaphases differ
persimilis Dobzhansky and Epling 1944	3 R, 1 V, 1 D	Dobzhansky (1935)	X is V-shaped; Y is variable
pseudoobscura Frovola 1929	3 R, 1 V, 1 D	Metz (1916a, b)	Reported as *obscura*; X is V, Y is rod
subobscura Collin 1936	5 R, 1 D	Dobzhansky (1935) Emmens (1937)	X is V; Y is variable
tristis Fallén 1823	3 V, 1 J, 1 D	Buzzati-Traverso (1941)	X is V-shaped; Y is J-shaped
saltans species group			
cordata subgroup			
cordata Sturtevant 1942	2 V, 1 R	Sturtevant (1942)	—
elliptica subgroup			
elliptica Sturtevant 1942	4 R, 1 v, 1 j	Sturtevant (1942)	—
	2 V, 1 R	Clayton and Ward (1954), Clayton and Wasserman (1957)	—
emarginata Sturtevant 1942	2 V, 1 R	Sturtevant (1942)	—
neoelliptica Pavan and Magalhaes 1950	2 V, 1 R	Pavan (1950)	—
neosaltans Pavan and Magalhaes 1950			
saltans subgroup			
austrosaltans Spassky 1957	2 V, 1 R	Spassky (1957)	—

TABLE 1. Continued

Species	Metaphase	Reference	Remarks
saltans species group (Continued)			
lusaltans Magalhaes 1962	2 V, 1 R	Magalhães (1962)	—
nigrosaltans Magalhaes 1962	2 V, 1 R	Magalhães (1962)	—
prosaltans Duda 1927	2 V, 1 R	Wharton (1943)	X and Y are V-shaped
		Dobzhansky and Pavan (1943)	Rod X and rod Y; also X and Y are on one arm of V in some
saltans Sturtevant 1916	2 V, 1 R, 1 D	Metz (1916b)	—
	2 V, 1 R	Sturtevant (1942), Wharton (1943)	Reported as sellata
septentriosaltans Magalhães and Buck 1962	2 V, 1 R	Magalhães (1962)	—
sturtevanti subgroup			
rectangularis Sturtevant 1942	2 V, 1 R	Sturtevant (1942)	—
sturtevanti Duda 1927	2 V, 1 R	Sturtevant (1942)	—
		Dobzhansky and Pavan (1943)	X is V-shaped
willistoni species group			
bocainensis Pavan and da Cunha 1947	2 V, 1 R	Pavan and da Cunha (1947)	—
		Clayton and Wasserman (1957)	X is V-shaped; Y is J-shaped
bocainoides Carson 1954	2 V, 1 R	Carson (1954)	—
capricorni Dobzhansky and Pavan 1943	2 V, 1 R	Dobzhansky and Pavan (1943)	—
equinoxialis Dobzhansky 1946	2 V, 1 R	Burla et al. (1949)	—
fumipennis Duda 1925	2 V, 1 R	Dobzhansky and Pavan (1943)	—

Species	Configuration	Reference	Remarks
insularis Dobzhansky 1957	2 V, 1 R	Dobzhansky et al. (1957)	—
mangabeirai Malogolowkin 1951	2 V, 1 R	Carson et al. (1957)	—
nebulosa Sturtevant 1916	2 V, 1 R, 1 D	Metz (1916a), Wharton (1943)	—
parabocainensis Carson 1954	2 V, 1 R	Pavan (1946), Ward (1949), Clayton and Ward (1954)	—
paulistorum Dobzhansky and Pavan 1949	2 V, 1 R	Carson (1954), Dobzhansky and Pavan (1943)	—
pavlovskiana Kastritsis and Dobzhansky 1967	2 V, 1 R	Kastritsis and Dobzhansky (1967)	—
sucinea Patterson and Mainland 1944	2 V, 1 R	Patterson and Mainland (1944)	—
tropicalis Burla and da Cunha 1949	2 V, 1 R	Burla et al. (1949)	—
t. cubana Townsend 1954	2 V, 1 R	Townsend (1954)	—
willistoni Sturtevant 1916	2 V, 1 R, 1 D	Metz (1916b), Wharton (1943), Dobzhansky and Pavan (1943)	—
Subgenus *Spinodrosophila*			
nigrosparsa Strobl 1898	5 R, 1 V	Burla (1950b)	X and Y are V-shaped
Species of uncertain classification			
alexandrei Cordeiro 1951	3 R, 1 V	Cordeiro (1951)	—
andina Dobzhansky and Pavan 1943	1 V, 4 R	Dobzhansky and Pavan (1943)	—
aracea Heed and Wheeler 1957	1 V, 1 J, 1 R	Clayton and Wasserman (1957)	—
caponei Pavan and da Cunha 1947	3 V, 1 D	Pavan and da Cunha (1947)	—
endobranchia Carson and Wheeler 1968	2 V, 1 R, 1 D	Carson and Wheeler (1968)	—

TABLE 1. Continued

Species	Metaphase	Reference	Remarks
Species of uncertain classification (Continued)			
fumosa Pavan and da Cunha 1947	1 R, 2 V, 1 D	Pavan and da Cunha (1947)	—
limbinervis Duda 1925	5 R, 1 D	Clayton and Wasserman (1957)	—
mcclintockae Pipkin 1964	3 R, 1 V, 1 D	Pipkin (1964)	Y is rod
nigrilineata Angus 1967	5 R, 1 D	Angus (1967)	—
pagliolii Cordeiro 1963	1 V, 3 R, 1 D	Cordeiro (1963)	—
pseudotetrachaeta Angus 1967	5 R, 1 D	Angus (1967)	—
tetrachaeta Angus 1964	5 R, 1 D	Angus (1964)	—
Endemic Hawaiian Drosophiloids "picture-winged" group			
adiastola subgroup			
adiastola Hardy 1965	5 R, 1 D	Clayton (1966)	—
cilifera Hardy and Kaneshiro 1968	5 R, 1 D	Clayton (1968)	—
clavisetae (Hardy) 1966	5 R, 1 D	Carson *et al.* (1967)	—
hamifera Hardy and Kaneshiro 1968	5 R, 1 D	Clayton (1971)	—
neogrimshawi Hardy and Kaneshiro 1968	5 R, 1 D	Clayton (1968)	—
ochrobasis Hardy and Kaneshiro 1968			
ornata Hardy and Kaneshiro 1969	5 R, 1 D	Clayton (1969)	—
paenehamifera Hardy and Kaneshiro 1969			
peniculipedis Hardy 1965			

Species	Configuration	Reference	Notes
setosimentum Hardy and Kaneshiro 1968	5 R, 1 D	Clayton (1968)	—
spectabilis Hardy 1965	5 R, 1 D	Clayton (1966)	—
touchardiae Hardy and Kaneshiro 1972	5 R, 1 D	Clayton *et al.* (1972)	—
truncipenna Hardy 1965	5 R, 1 D	Clayton (1969)	One rod is extremely large
varipennis (Grimshaw) 1901	5 R, 1 D	Clayton (1971)	—
paucipuncta subgroup			
basisetae Hardy and Kaneshiro 1968	5 R, 1 D	Clayton (1968)	—
ocellata Hardy and Kaneshiro 1969	5 R, 1 D	Clayton (1969)	—
paucicilia Hardy and Kaneshiro 1972	5 R, 1 D	Clayton *et al.* (1972)	—
paucipuncta Grimshaw 1901 *prolaticilia* Hardy 1965	} 5 R, 1 D	Carson *et al.* (1967)	—
prostopalpis Hardy and Kaneshiro 1968	4 R, 1 V, 1 D	Clayton (1971)	—
punalua Bryan 1934	5 R, 1 D	Clayton (1966)	—
uniseriata Hardy and Kaneshiro 1968	6 R	Clayton (1968)	—
vesciseta subgroup			
alsophila Hardy and Kaneshiro 1971		Clayton (1971)	
assita Hardy and Kaneshiro 1969	5 R, 1 D	Clayton (1971)	—
hexachaetae Hardy 1965	5 R, 1 D	Clayton (1968)	—
montgomeryi Hardy and Kaneshiro 1972	6 R	Clayton *et al.* (1972)	—
vesciseta Hardy and Kaneshiro 1968 *virgulata* Hardy and Kaneshiro 1968	} 5 R, 1 D	Clayton (1968)	—

TABLE 1. Continued

Species	Metaphase	Reference	Remarks
Endemic Hawaiian Drosophiloids			
"picture-winged" group (*Continued*)			
distinguenda subgroup			
distinguenda Hardy 1965	5 R, 1 D	Clayton (1969)	—
divaricata Hardy and Kaneshiro 1971	5 R, 1 D	Clayton (1971)	—
inedita Hardy 1965	5 R, 1 D	Clayton (1969)	Dots are extremely large
odontophallus subgroup			
liophallus Hardy and Kaneshiro 1968	5 R, 1 D	Clayton (1968)	—
macrothrix Hardy and Kaneshiro 1968	5 R, 1 D	Clayton (1971)	—
odontophallus Hardy and Kaneshiro 1968	5 R, 1 D	Clayton (1968)	—
psilophallus Hardy and Kaneshiro 1971	6 R	Clayton (1971)	—
spaniothrix Hardy and Kaneshiro 1968	5 R, 1 D		
tarphytrichia Hardy 1965	5 R, 1 D	Clayton et al. (1972)	—
pilimana subgroup			
aglaia Hardy 1965	5 R, 1 D	Clayton et al. (1972)	—
discreta Hardy and Kaneshiro 1968	5 R, 1 D	Clayton (1968)	—
fasciculisetae Hardy 1965	5 R, 1 D	Carson et al. (1967)	—
glabriapex Hardy and Kaneshiro 1968	5 R, 1 D	Clayton (1968)	—
lineosetae Hardy and Kaneshiro 1968	5 R, 1 D	Clayton (1969)	—

Species	Configuration	Reference	Notes
pilimana Grimshaw 1901	5 R, 1 D	Clayton (1966)	—
grimshawi subgroup			
balioptera Hardy 1965	5 R, 1 D	Clayton (1968)	—
bostrycha Hardy 1965			
conspicua Grimshaw 1901	5 R, 1 D	Carson *et al.* (1967)	—
crucigera Grimshaw 1902	5 R, 1 D	Clayton (1966)	—
disjuncta Hardy 1965	5 R, 1 D	Carson *et al.* (1967)	—
grimshawi Oldenberg 1914	5 R, 1 D	Clayton (1966)	—
pullipes Hardy and Kaneshiro 1972	5 R, 1 D	Clayton *et al.* (1972)	—
attigua Hardy and Kaneshiro 1969	5 R, 1 D	Clayton (1969)	—
primaeva subgroup			
primaeva Hardy and Kaneshiro 1968	5 R, 1 D	Clayton (1968)	—
planitibia subgroup			
cyrtoloma Hardy 1969	5 V, 1 J	Clayton (1968)	Reported as *"perkinsi?"*
hanaulae Hardy 1969	5 R, 1 D	Clayton (1969)	—
hemipeza (Hardy) 1965	5 R, 1 D	Carson *et al.* (1967)	—
heteroneura (Perkins) 1910	5 R, 1 D	Clayton (1968)	—
ingens Hardy and Kaneshiro 1971	5 R, 1 D	Clayton (1969)	Reported as *melanocephala*
melanocephala (Hardy) 1966	5 R, 1 V	Clayton (1969)	Reported as *"melanocephala?"*
neoperkinsi Hardy and Kaneshiro 1968	5 R, 1 D	Clayton (1969)	—
neopicta Hardy and Kaneshiro 1968	5 R, 1 D	Clayton (1968)	—
nigribasis Hardy 1969	5 R, 1 D	Clayton (1968)	Reported as *brunneipennis*
oahuensis (Grimshaw) 1901	5 R, 1 D	Clayton (1968)	—
obscuripes (Grimshaw) 1901	5 R, 1 D	Clayton (1968)	—
picticornis Grimshaw 1901	5 R, 1 D	Clayton (1966)	—
planitibia (Hardy) 1966	5 R, 1 D	Carson *et al.* (1967)	—

TABLE 1. Continued

Species	Metaphase	Reference	Remarks
Endemic Hawaiian Drosophiloids **"picture-winged" group (Continued)**			
setosifrons Hardy and Kaneshiro 1968	5 R, 1 D	Clayton (1969)	—
silvestris (Perkins) 1910	5 R, 1 D	Carson et al. (1967)	Reported as nigrifacies
substenoptera Hardy 1969	5 R, 1 D	Clayton et al. (1972)	—
orphnopeza subgroup			
atrimentum Hardy and Kaneshiro 1971	5 R, 1 D	Clayton (1971)	—
ciliaticrus Hardy 1965	5 R, 1 D	Clayton (1968)	—
claytonae Hardy and Kaneshiro 1969	5 R, 1 D	Clayton (1969)	—
engyochracea Hardy 1965	5 R, 1 D	Clayton (1966)	—
limitata Hardy and Kaneshiro 1968	6 R	Clayton (1968)	—
murphyi Hardy and Kaneshiro 1969	5 R, 1 D	Clayton (1969)	—
obatai Hardy and Kaneshiro 1972	5 R, 1 D	Clayton et al. (1972)	—
ochracea Grimshaw 1901	5 R, 1 D	Carson et al. (1967)	—
orphnopeza Hardy and Kaneshiro 1968	5 R, 1 D	Clayton (1968)	—
orthofascia Hardy and Kaneshiro 1968	5 R, 1 D	Clayton (1968)	—
reynoldsiae Hardy and Kaneshiro 1972	5 R, 1 D	Clayton et al. (1972)	—
sejuncta Hardy and Kaneshiro 1968	5 R, 1 D	Clayton (1969)	—
sobrina Hardy and Kaneshiro 1971	5 R, 1 D	Clayton et al. (1972)	—

sodomae Hardy and Kaneshiro 1968	5 R, 1 D	Clayton (1971)
sproati Hardy and Kaneshiro 1968	5 R, 1 D	Clayton (1968)
villosipedis Hardy 1965	5 R, 1 D	Clayton (1966)
hawaiiensis subgroup		
flexipes Hardy and Kaneshiro 1968	5 R, 1 D	Clayton (1971)
formella Hardy and Kaneshiro 1972	5 R, 1 D	Clayton *et al.* (1972)
gradata Hardy and Kaneshiro 1968	5 R, 1 D	Clayton (1968)
gymnobasis Hardy and Kaneshiro 1971	5 R, 1 D	Clayton (1971)
hawaiiensis Grimshaw 1901	5 R, 1 D	Carson *et al.* (1967)
heedi Hardy and Kaneshiro 1971	6 R	Clayton *et al.* (1972)
hirtipalpus Hardy and Kaneshiro 1968	5 R, 1 D	Clayton (1968)
musaphila Hardy 1965	5 R, 1 D	Clayton (1969)
recticilia Hardy and Kaneshiro 1968	5 R, 1 D	Clayton (1968)
silvarentis Hardy and Kaneshiro 1968	5 R, 1 D	Clayton (1968)
turbata Hardy and Kaneshiro 1969	5 R, 1 D	Clayton (1971)
"Modified mouthparts" group		
anoplastoma Hardy and Kaneshiro 1968	5 R, 1 D	Clayton (1968)
asketostoma Hardy 1965	6 R	Clayton (1966)
biseriata Hardy 1965	1 V, 3 R, 1 D	Clayton *et al.* (1972)
chaetopeza Hardy 1965	5 R, 1 D	Clayton (1966)
comatifemora Hardy 1965	5 R, 1 D	Clayton (1968)
deltaneuron Bryan 1938	2 V, 1 R, 1 D	Clayton *et al.* (1972)

TABLE 1. Continued

Species	Metaphase	Reference	Remarks
Endemic Hawaiian Drosophiloids			
"Modified mouthparts" group *(Continued)*			
diminuens Hardy 1965	5 R, 1 D	Clayton (1968)	—
eurypeza Hardy 1965	5 R, 1 D	Clayton (1966)	—
flavibasis Hardy 1965	5 R, 1 D	Clayton (1966)	—
fuscoamoeba Bryan 1934	5 R, 1 D	Clayton (1968)	
hystricosa Hardy and Kaneshiro 1969	1 V, 3 R, 1 D		Reported as "n. sp. near *caccabata*"
infuscata Grimshaw 1901	5 R, 1 D	Clayton (1966)	—
ischnotrix Hardy 1965	1 R, 2 V, 1 D	Clayton et al. (1972)	—
kambysellisi Hardy and Kaneshiro 1969	6 R		
kauluai Bryan 1934	5 R, 1 D	Clayton (1966)	—
mimica Hardy 1965	6 R	Clayton (1966)	—
mitchelli Hardy 1965	5 R, 1 D	Clayton (1968)	—
polliciforma Hardy 1965		Clayton et al. (1972)	—
ptychochaetae Hardy 1965		Clayton (1966)	—
quadrisetae Hardy 1965		Clayton (1968)	—
"bristle foot" group			
atroscutellata Hardy 1966	5 R, 1 D	Clayton (1966)	Reported as "dark scutellum" species
basimacula Hardy 1965			—
"spoon foot" group			
disticha Hardy 1965	5 R, 1 D	Clayton (1969)	—
percnosoma Hardy 1965	5 R, 1 D	Clayton (1968)	—

Species	Configuration	Reference	Notes
"ciliated tarsus" group			
imparisetae Hardy 1965	5 R, 1 D	Clayton et al. (1972)	—
"split tarsus" group			
freycinetiae Hardy 1965	5 R, 1 D	Clayton (1966)	—
pectinitarsus Hardy 1965	5 R, 1 D	Clayton (1966)	—
"fungus feeding" group			
goureaui Hardy 1972	5 R, 1 D	Clayton (1966)	Reported as *mycetophila*
melanosoma Grimshaw 1901	5 R, 1 D	Clayton (1966)	—
nigra Grimshaw 1901	5 R, 1 D	Clayton (1968)	—
Unassigned species			
parva Grimshaw 1901	1 R, 2 V, 1 D	Clayton (1966)	—
quasianomalipes Hardy 1965	5 R, 1 D	Clayton (1969)	—

Burla, H., 1950*b* Die Chromosomensätze der in der Schweiz vorkommenden *Drosophila*-Arten *D. helvetica, D. kuntzei, D. limbata, D. testacea, D. littoralis* und *D. nigrosparsa. Arch. J. Klaus-Stift. Vererbungsforsch. Sozialanthropol. Rassenhyg.* **25**:496–504.

Burla, H., A. B. da Cunha, A. R. Cordeiro, T. Dobzhansky, C. Malogolowkin, and C. Pavan, 1949 The *willistoni* group of sibling species of *Drosophila. Evolution* **3**:300–314.

Butler, D. R. and L. E. Mettler, 1963 Ecological and cytological notes on *Drosophila sigmoides. Drosophila Inf. Serv.* **38**:70.

Buzzati-Traverso, A., 1941 Genetica di popolazioni in *Drosophila*. II. Cromosomi di 4 specie del "gruppo *obscura*", e la incrociabilita di varie razze geografiche. *Sci. Genet.* **2**:1–18.

Buzzati-Traverso, A., 1943 Morfologia, citologia e biologia di duo nuovo specie di *Drosophila* (Diptera Acalyptera: *Drosophila nitens* n. sp., *Drosophila tigrina* n. sp.). *Reale Istit. Lombardo Sci. Lett. Estrat. Rend. Cl. Sci.* **77**:1–13.

Carson, H. L., 1954 Interfertile sibling species in the *willistoni* group of *Drosophila. Evolution* **8**:148–165.

Carson, H. L., 1967 The association between *Drosophila carcinophila* Wheeler and its host, the land crab *Gecarcinus ruricola* (L.). *Am. Midl. Nat.* **78**:324–343.

Carson, H. L. and H. D. Stalker, 1947 Gene arrangements in natural populations of *Drosophila robusta* Sturtevant. *Evolution* **1**:113–133.

Carson, H. L. and M. R. Wheeler, 1968 *Drosophila endobranchia*, a new Drosophilid associated with land crabs in the West Indies. *Ann. Entomol. Soc. Am.* **61**:675–678.

Carson, H. L., M. R. Wheeler and W. B. Heed, 1957 A parthenogenetic strain of *Drosophila mangabeirai. Univ. Texas Publ.* **5714**:115–122.

Carson, H. L., F. E. Clayton and H. D. Stalker, 1967 Karyotype stability and speciation in Hawaiian *Drosophila. Proc. Natl. Acad. Sci. USA* **57**:1280–1285.

Clayton, F. E., 1966 Preliminary report on the karyotypes of Hawaiian Drosophilidae. *Stud. Genet. III Univ. Texas Publ.* **6615**:397–404.

Clayton, F. E., 1968 Metaphase configurations in species of Hawaiian Drosophilidae. *Stud. Genet. IV Univ. Texas Publ.* **6818**:263–278.

Clayton, F. E., 1969 Variations in the metaphase chromosomes of Hawaiian Drosophilidae. *Stud. Genet. V Univ. Texas Publ.* **6918**:95–110.

Clayton, F. E., 1971 Additional karyotypes of Hawaiian Drosophilidae. *Stud. Genet. VI Univ. Texas Publ.* **7103**:171–181.

Clayton, F. E. and C. L. Ward, 1954 Chromosomal studies of several species of Drosophilidae. *Univ. Texas Publ.* **5422**:98–105.

Clayton, F. E. and M. Wasserman, 1957 Chromosomal studies of several species of *Drosophila. Univ. Texas Publ.* **5721**:125–131.

Clayton, F. E., H. L. Carson and J. E. Sato, 1972 Polytene chromosome relationships in Hawaiian species of *Drosophila*. VI. Supplementary data on metaphases and gene sequences. *Stud. Genet. VII Univ. Texas Publ.* **7213**:163–178.

Cordeiro, A. R., 1951 *Drosophila alexandrei,* una nova especie brasileira. *Publ. Faculdade Fil. Univ. Rio Grande Sul* **3**:1–11.

Cordeiro, A. R., 1963 "*Drosophila pagliolii*" a new species showing unusual chromatographic pattern of fluorescent substances. *Rev. Bras. Biol.* **23**:401–407.

Cordeiro, A. R., 1964 "*Drosophila wingei*" a new Brazilian species of the "*dreyfusi*" group. *Rev. Bras. Biol.* **24**:1–4.

de Barros, R., 1950 A new species of the genus *Drosophila* with discussion about speciation in the *mercatorum* subgroup. *Rev. Bras. Biol.* **10**:265–278.

Dobzhansky, T., 1935 *Drosophila miranda,* a new species. *Genetics* **20**:377–391.

Dobzhansky, T. and C. Pavan, 1943 Chromosome complements of some South American species of *Drosophila. Proc. Natl. Acad. Sci. USA* **29**:368–375.

Dobzhansky, T., L. Ehrman and O. Pavlovsky, 1957 *Drosophila insularis,* a new sibling species of the *willistoni* group. *Univ. Texas Publ.* **5714**:39–47.

Dreyfus, A. and R. de Barros, 1949 Sex ratio chez certains hybrides interspecifiques de *Drosophila* et son interpretation par l'analyse des chromosomes salivaires. *Ric. Sci.* **19 (Suppl.)**:94–104.

Emmens, C. W., 1937 The morphology of the nucleus in the salivary glands of four species of *Drosophila* (*D. melanogaster, D. immigrans, D. funebris,* and *D. subobscura*). *Z. Zellforsch.* **26**:1–20.

Frolova, S. L., 1926 Normale und polyploide Chromosomengarnituren bei einigen *Drosophila*-Arten. *Z. Zellforsch.* **3**:682–694.

Frolova, S. L. and B. L. Astaurov, 1929 Die Chromosomengarnitur als systematisches Merkmal. Eine verleichende untersuchung der russischen und amerikanischen *Drosophila obscura* Fall. *Z. Zellforsch.* **10**:201–213.

Frydenberg, O., 1956 Two new species of *Drosophila* from Peru (Drosophilidae, Diptera). *Rev. Bras. Entomol.* **6**:57–64.

Futch, D. G., 1966 A study of speciation in South Pacific populations of *Drosophila ananassae. Stud. Genet. III Univ. Texas Publ.* **6615**:79–120.

Griffen, A. B., 1942 Relationships of the *melanica* species group. *Univ. Texas Publ.* **4228**:67–73.

Heed, W. B. and N. B. Krishnamurthy, 1959 Genetic studies on the *cardini* group of *Drosophila* in the West Indies. *Univ. Texas Publ.* **5914**:155–179.

Heed, W. B. and J. S. Russell, 1971 Phylogeny and population structure in island and continental species of the *cardini* group of *Drosophila* studied by inversion analysis. *Stud. Genet. IV Univ. Texas Publ.* **7103**:91–130.

Heed, W. B. and M. R. Wheeler, 1957 Thirteen new species in the genus *Drosophila* from the neotropical region. *Univ. Texas Publ.* **5721**:17–38.

Heed, W. B., D. W. Crumpacker and L. Ehrman, 1969 *Drosophila lowei,* a new American member of the *obscura* species group. *Ann. Entomol. Soc. Am.* **62**:388–393.

Hsiang, W., 1949 The distribution of heterochromatin in *Drosophila tumiditarsus. Cytologia (Tokyo)* **15**:149–152.

Hughes, R. D., 1939 An analysis of the chromosomes of two subspecies, *Drosophila virilis virilis* and *Drosophila virilis americana. Genetics* **24**:811–834.

Hunter, A. S. and R. A. Hunter, 1964 The *mesophragmatic* species group of *Drosophila* in Colombia. *Ann. Entomol. Soc. Am.* **57**:732–736.

Jaeger, C. P. and F. M. Salzano, 1953 *Drosophila gaucha,* a new species from Brazil. *Rev. Bras. Biol.* **13**:205–208.

Kaneko, A., T. Tokumitsu and H. Takada, 1964 *Drosophila* survey of Hokkaido. XX. Description of a new species, *Drosophila pseudosordidula* sp. nov. (Diptera, Drosophilidae). *J. Fac. Sci. Hokkaido Univ. Ser. VI Zool.* **15**:374–394.

Kaneshiro, K. and M. R. Wheeler, 1970 Preliminary report on the species of the *ananassae* subgroup. *Drosophila Inf. Serv.* **45**:143.

Kang, Y. S., Y. J. Kim and K. W. Bahng, 1964 Chromosome studies on several wild species of Drosophilidae. *Korean J. Zool.* **7**:83–88.

Kastritsis, C. D. and T. Dobzhansky, 1967 *Drosophila pavlovskiana,* a race or a species? *Am. Midl. Nat.* **78**:244–247.

Kikkawa, H., 1935   An inference as to the constitution of X-chromosome in *Drosophila*. *Proc. Imp. Acad. Jap.* **11**:62–65.

Kikkawa, H., 1936   Two races of *Drosophila montium* (a preliminary note). *Jap. J. Genet.* **12**:137–142.

Kikkawa, H. and F. T. Peng, 1938   *Drosophila* species of Japan and adjacent localities. *Jap. J. Zool.* **7**:507–552.

Kim, K. W., 1965   Chromosomal studies of Korean *Drosophila* species. *Drosophila Inf. Serv.* **40**:69.

King, J. C., 1947   A comparative analysis of the chromosomes of the *guarani* group of *Drosophila. Evolution* **1**:48–62.

Magalhães, L. E., 1962   Notes on the taxonomy, morphology, and distribution of the *saltans* group of *Drosophila,* with description of four new species. *Stud. Genet. II Univ. Texas Publ.* **6205**:135–154.

Mather, W. B., 1956   The genus *Drosophila* (Diptera) in eastern Queensland. III. Cytological evolution. *Aust. J. Zool.* **4**:76–89.

Mather, W. B., 1960   Additions to the *Drosophila* fauna of Australia. *Univ. Queensl. Pap. Dep. Zool.* **1**:229–239.

Mather, W. B., 1961   *D. pararubida,* a new species of *Drosophila* from New Guinea. *Univ. Queensl. Pap. Dep. Zool.* **1**:251–255.

Mather, W. B., 1962   Patterns of chromosomal evolution in the *immigrans* group of *Drosophila. Evolution* **16**:20–26.

Mather, W. B. and T. Dobzhansky, 1962   Two new species of *Drosophila* from New Guinea. *Pacific Insects* **4**:245–249.

Metz, C. W., 1914   Chromosome studies in the Diptera. I. A preliminary survey of five different types of chromosome groups in the genus *Drosophila. J. Exp. Zool.* **17**:45–49.

Metz, C. W., 1916*a*   Chromosome studies in the Diptera. II. The paired association of chromosomes in the Diptera, and its significance. *J. Exp. Zool.* **21**:213–279.

Metz, C. W., 1916*b*   Chromosome studies in the Diptera. III. Additional types of chromosome groups in the Drosophilidae. *Am. Nat.* **50**:587–599.

Metz, C. W. and M. S. Moses, 1923   Chromosomes of *Drosophila.* Chromosome relationships and genetic behavior in the genus *Drosophila*: I. A comparison of the chromosomes of different species of *Drosophila. J. Hered.* **14**:195–204.

Miller, D. D., 1944   *Drosophila melanura,* a new species of the *melanica* group. *J. N. Y. Entomol. Soc.* **52**:85–97.

Miller, D. D. and L. E. Stone, 1962   A reinvestigation of karyotype in *Drosophila affinis* and related species. *J. Hered.* **53**:12–24.

Momma, E., 1954   *Drosophila* survey of Hokkaido. II. Chromosomes of seven wild species. *J. Fac. Sci. Hokkaido Univ. Ser. VI Zool.* **12**:200–208.

Momma, E., 1956   *Drosophila* survey of Hokkaido. IV. On a new member of "*robusta* group" common in woodlands. *Annot. Zool. Jap.* **29**:171–173.

Moriwaki, D., O. Kitagawa and T. Okada, 1967   *Drosophila imaii,* a new sibling species related to *Drosophila bifasciata. Evolution* **21**:109–116.

Okada, T. and H. Kurokawa, 1957   New or little known species of Drosophilidae of Japan (Diptera). *Kontyu* **25**:2–12.

Patau, K., 1935   Chromosomenmorphologie bei *Drosophila melanogaster* und *Drosophila simulans* und ihre genetische Bedeutung. *Naturwissenschaften* **23**:537–543.

Patterson, J. T., 1941a Sterility in crosses of geographical races of *Drosophila micromelanica. Proc. Natl. Acad. Sci. USA* **27**:392–394.

Patterson, J. T., 1941b The *virilis* group of *Drosophila* in Texas. *Am. Nat.* **75**:523–539.

Patterson, J. T., 1944 A new member of the *virilis* group. *Univ. Texas Publ.* **4445**:102–103.

Patterson, J. T., 1952 Revision of the *montana* complex of the *virilis* species group. *Univ. Texas Publ.* **5204**:20–34.

Patterson, J. T. and M. L. Alexander, 1952 *Drosophila wheeleri,* a new member of the *mulleri* subgroup. *Univ. Texas Publ.* **5204**:129–136.

Patterson, J. T. and J. F. Crow, 1940 Hybridization in the *mulleri* subgroup of *Drosophila. Univ. Texas Publ.* **4032**:251–256.

Patterson, J. T. and G. B. Mainland, 1944 The Drosophilidae of Mexico. *Univ. Texas Publ.* **4445**:1–101.

Patterson, J. T. and W. S. Stone, 1952 *Evolution in the Genus Drosophila,* Macmillan, New York.

Patterson, J. T. and C. L. Ward, 1952 *Drosophila euronotus,* a new member of the *melanica* species group. *Univ. Texas Publ.* **5204**:158–161.

Patterson, J. T. and M. R. Wheeler, 1942 Description of new species of the subgenera *Hirtodrosophila* and *Drosophila. Univ. Texas Publ.* **4213**:69–109.

Pavan, C., 1946 Chromosomal variation in *Drosophila nebulosa. Genetics* **31**:546–557.

Pavan, C., 1950 Especies brasileiras de *Drosophila.* II. *Bol. Fac. Filos. Cienc. Letr. Univ. São Paulo No. 111 Biol. Ger.* **8**:3–37.

Pavan, C. and M. E. Breuer, 1954 Two new species of "*Drosophila*" of the "*dreyfusi* group" (Diptera). *Rev. Bras. Biol.* **14**:459–463.

Pavan, C. and A. B. da Cunha, 1947 Especies brasileiras de *Drosophila. Bol. Fac. Filos. Cienc. Letr. Univ. São Paulo, No. 86 Biol. Ger.* **7**:20–64.

Pavan, C. and J. Nacrur, 1950 Duas novas especies de *Drosophila* (Diptera) do grupo *annulimana. Dusenia* **I(5)**:263–274.

Pipkin, S. B., 1956 Two new species of the *Drosophila* subgenus *Pholadoris* and a redescription of *Drosophila hypocausta* Osten-Sacken. *Proc. Entomol. Soc. Wash.* **58**:251–258.

Pipkin, S. B., 1961 Taxonomic relationships within the *Drosophila victoria* species group, subgenus *Pholadoris. Proc. Entomol. Soc. Wash.* **63**:145–161.

Pipkin, S. B., 1964 New flower breeding species of *Drosophila* (Diptera: Drosophilidae). *Proc. Entomol. Soc. Wash.* **66**:217–245.

Pipkin, S. B. and W. B. Heed, 1964 Nine new members of the *Drosophila tripunctata* species group (Diptera: Drosophilidae). *Pacific Insects* **6**:256–273.

Spassky, B., 1957 Morphological differences between sibling species of *Drosophila. Univ. Texas Publ.* **5714**:48–61.

Spencer, W. P., 1942 New species in the *quinaria* group of the subgenus *Drosophila. Univ. Texas Publ.* **4213**:55–66.

Stalker, H. D., 1953 Taxonomy and hybridization in the *cardini* group *Drosophila. Ann. Entomol. Soc. Am.* **46**:343–358.

Stalker, H. D., 1964 The salivary gland chromosomes of *Drosophila nigromelanica. Genetics* **49**:883–893.

Stevens, N. M., 1912 The chromosomes in *Drosophila ampelophila. Proc. VII Interntl. Zool. Congr. Boston:* 380–381.

Stone, W. S., A. B. Griffen and J. T. Patterson, 1942 *Drosophila montana,* a new species of the *virilis* group. *Genetics* **27**:172.

Stone, W. S., W. C. Guest and F. D. Wilson, 1960 The evolutionary implications of the cytological polymorphism and phylogeny of the *virilis* group of *Drosophila*. *Proc. Natl. Acad. Sci. USA* **46**:350–361.

Streisinger, G., 1946 The *cardini* species group of the genus *Drosophila*. *J. N. Y. Entomol. Soc.* **54**:105–113.

Sturtevant, A. H., 1940 Genetic data on *Drosophila affinis* with a discussion of the relationships in the genus *Sophophora*. *Genetics* **25**:337–353.

Sturtevant, A. H., 1942 The classification of the genus *Drosophila*, with descriptions of nine new species. *Univ. Texas Publ.* **4213**:5–51.

Sturtevant, A. H. and T. Dobzhansky, 1936 Observations on the species related to *Drosophila affinis*, with descriptions of seven new forms. *Am. Nat.* **70**:574–584.

Tan, C. C., T. C. Hsu and T. C. Sheng, 1949 Known *Drosophila* species in China with descriptions of twelve new species. *Univ. Texas Publ.* **4920**:196–206.

Tokumitsu, T., T. Shima and A. Kaneko, 1967 *Drosophila* survey of Hokkaido. XXIII. A karyotype study in seven species of the *quinaria* and *robusta* groups. *Jap. J. Genet.* **42**:279–282.

Townsend, J. I. and M. R. Wheeler, 1955 Notes on Puerto Rican Drosophilidae, including descriptions of two new species of *Drosophila*. *J. Agric. Univ. Puerto Rico* **39**:57–64.

Wakahama, K. and O. Kitagawa, 1972 Evolutionary and genetical studies of the *Drosophila nasuta* subgroup. II. Karyotypes of *Drosophila nasuta* collected from the Seychelles Islands. *Jap. J. Genet.* **47**:129–131.

Ward, B. L. and W. B. Heed, 1970 Chromosome phylogeny of *Drosophila pachea* and related species. *J. Hered.* **61**:248–258.

Ward, C. L., 1949 Karyotype variation in *Drosophila*. *Univ. Texas Publ.* **4920**:70–79.

Wasserman, M., 1960 Cytological and phylogenetic relationships in the *repleta* group of the genus *Drosophila*. *Proc. Natl. Acad. Sci. USA* **46**:842–859.

Wasserman, M., 1962a Cytological studies of the *repleta* group of the genus *Drosophila*. IV. The *hydei* subgroup. *Stud. Genet. II Univ. Texas Publ.* **6205**:73–84.

Wasserman, M., 1962b Cytological studies of the *repleta* group of the genus *Drosophila*. V. The *mulleri* subgroup. *Stud. Genet. II Univ. Texas Publ.* **6205**:85–117.

Wasserman, M., 1962c Cytological studies of the *repleta* group of the genus *Drosophila*. VI. The *fasciola* subgroup. *Stud. Genet. II Univ. Texas Publ.* **6205**:119–134.

Wharton, L. T., 1943 An analysis of the metaphase and salivary chromosome morphology within the genus *Drosophila*. *Univ. Texas Publ.* **4313**:282–319.

Wheeler, M. R., 1968 Some remarkable new species of neotropical Drosophilidae. *Stud. Genet. IV Univ. Texas Publ.* **6818**:431–442.

Wheeler, M. R., H. Takada and D. Brncic, 1962 The *flavopilosa* species group of *Drosophila*. *Stud. Genet. II Univ. Texas Publ.* **6205**:395–414.

Wilson, F. D., M. R. Wheeler, M. Harget and M. Kambysellis, 1969 Cytogenetic relations in the *Drosophila nasuta* subgroup of the *immigrans* group of species. *Stud. Genet. V Univ. Texas Publ.* **6918**:207–253.

19

Drosophila ananassae

DAIGORO MORIWAKI AND YOSHIKO N. TOBARI

Introduction

Drosophila ananassae was first described by Doleschall in 1858 from Ambon (= *Amboina*), a small island off the southwestern tip of Ceram, Indonesia. Doleschall's description was extremely brief and vague, and several synonyms of this species were subsequently published [see Bock and Wheeler (1972)]. Recently, two species complexes, the *ananassae* complex and the *bipectinata* complex, were recognized within the *ananassae* subgroup (Kaneshiro and Wheeler, 1970; Bock and Wheeler, 1972). The six species, *ananassae, pallidosa, phaeopleura, nesoetes, atripex,* and *varians* were described in the *ananassae* species complex (Bock and Wheeler, 1972).

D. *ananassae* has been recorded from all six geographical regions, although it is conspicuously absent from some areas and is largely tropical in its distribution (Patterson and Stone, 1952; Bock and Wheeler, 1972). This species is frequently found in domestic habitats (Sturtevant, 1942).

The culture methods devised for D. *melanogaster* have been found to be generally satisfactory for D. *ananassae*. The development time required from egg to adult is about 8 days at 25°C, either on medium composed of corn meal–molasses–agar sprayed with live yeast or on 20 percent boiled yeast–sugar–agar medium (Moriwaki *et al.*, 1956a).

DAIGORO MORIWAKI AND YOSHIKO N. TOBARI—Department of Biology, Faculty of Science, Tokyo Metropolitan University, Tokyo, Japan.

Karyotype

Mitotic chromosomes of *D. ananassae* were first studied by Metz (1916) in flies classified as "*D. caribbea* Sturtevant" collected in Panama and Cuba. He described the female complement (oogonial) as consisting of four pairs of V-shaped chromosomes, one of which is shorter than the other three. His figures and diagrams of spermatogonial chromosomes show a V-shaped X chromosome and rod-shaped Y chromosome. However, Kaufmann (1935, 1936*a, b*) reported that ganglion cells of the larvae of both the Alabama and the Japanese stocks possess an unequal-armed, J-shaped Y chromosome. Kikkawa (1936*a*, 1938) likewise found a J-shaped Y chromosome in spermatogonial cells of his material. Kaufmann (1937*b*) examined the chromosomes of the neurocytes in detail. He showed that three pairs of V-shaped autosomes and a pair of V-shaped X chromosomes in the female and a J-shaped Y chromosome in the male could be distinguished by size and characteristic constrictions, that the fourth chromosomes and the Y chromosome appear totally heteropycnotic in resting and early prophase stages of mitotic cells, and that short, heteropycnotic regions lie adjacent to the spindle-attachment regions of the X chromosomes and the two pairs of large autosomes.

Kaufmann (1937*b*) reported a unique situation of association of the nucleolus with the fourth chromosomes in mitotic prophase of female larvae, as well as with the Y chromosome in the male. He was tempted to postulate that a translocation of the nucleolus-forming region from the X to the fourth chromosome during the processes of speciation.

Hinton (1968) reported that meiotic chromosomes in primary spermatocytes are first visible as fine, dispersed strands not readily equated with standard descriptions of leptonema-zygonema. Heterochromatic blocks, presumed to represent the Y and fourth chromosomes, are intimately associated with the nucleolar surface at this time. The two large autosomes form pachytene bivalents, and these then pass through diplonema, diakinesis, and first meiotic metaphase. Hinton stated that in many cases the arms of the homolog were not held together by chiasmata, and, in fact, that positive identification of chiasmata could not be made. However, more recently, he has found that some of the large autosomal arms are associated by chiasmata (Hinton, private communication). The X, Y, and fourth chromosomes are usually observed as a tangled multivalent. The remainder of the meiotic sequence does not differ significantly from that described for *D. melanogaster* by Cooper (1950).

Polytene Chromosomes

As in *D. melanogaster* the homologous chromosomes of the larval salivary glands undergo somatic pairing and polytenization. Kikkawa (1935*a*) first indicated that the number of arms radiating from chromocenters in salivary gland nuclei of *D. ananassae* was six, rather than the eight to be expected from the conjugation of the paracentric heterochromatin of four pairs of V-shaped chromosomes. The six strands represent the arms of the two longer autosomes and the X chromosome. The fourth chromosome is reduced to a small heterochromatic mass forming part of the chromocenter (Kikkawa, 1936*b*, 1938; Kaufmann, 1936*b*, 1937*a, b*). Kikkawa (1936*b*, 1938) and Kaufmann (1937*b*) have described the few euchromatic bands which represent the fourth chromosome.

R.L. Seecof (Stone *et al.*, 1957) has prepared a salivary gland chromosome map showing the banding pattern over the entire length of the six major arms using a structurally homozygous stock derived from a stock collected on the Pacific island of Majuro. The gene arrangement represented in this stock was referred to by Futch (1966) as the standard for the species. Moriwaki and Ito (1969) have constructed a photomap of *ananassae* to compare the puffing pattern of the structural homozygotes with that of the heterozygotes.

Chromosomal Polymorphisms

Four paracentric inversions (2L, 3L, 2R, and 3R basal) were first described by Kaufmann (1936*b*) from Alabama and Japanese populations. Kikkawa (1937*a*, 1938) discovered a 3–4 reciprocal translocation and four paracentric inversions corresponding to those described by Kaufmann, plus a small inversion in 2L. Dobzhansky and Dreyfus (1943) reported the same four paracentric inversions, a new 3R median inversion, and a 2L–3L translocation. Among them, the three paracentric inversions (2L, 3L, and 3R basal) have been found in most of the wild populations of various regions of the world (Kikkawa, 1938; Dobzhansky and Dreyfus, 1943; Shirai and Moriwaki, 1952; Futch, 1966). In addition to the three cosmopolitan inversions, 18 paracentric inversions with more restricted distribution than the cosmopolitan ones were described by Futch (1966). Freire-Maia (1955) reported 19 paracentric inversions discovered in flies collected from northern Brazil and Argentina during the period 1951–1955.

In *D. ananassae* populations chromosomal variants have been frequently reported that do not exist in other species of *Drosophila*. Dobzhansky and Dreyfus (1943) found an autosomal translocation and short terminal deficiencies in a Brazilian population. Kikkawa (1938) also described extra chromatin bands at the distal end of the chromosome. These bands presumably represent terminal duplications.

Freire-Maia (1955, 1961) reported a new translocation (2R–3R), five pericentric inversions, two heterobrachial shifts, and one deficiency, along with a great number of different extra bands. Futch (1966) observed three pericentric inversions and one translocation from South Pacific populations. Moriwaki and Tanaka (unpublished) found a translocation (2L–3L) and terminal deficiencies (or duplications) in a Hawaiian population. Freire-Maia (1961) has suggested that some special mechanism has developed in *D. ananassae* which enables it to retain gene arrangements in its natural populations that are ordinarily disadvantageous in other species. Alternatively, the many chromosomal variants found in natural populations can be considered to reflect a high mutability in this species.

Extensive studies of balanced chromosomal polymorphisms in artificial populations of *D. ananassae* have been done by Moriwaki and his colleagues. Moriwaki *et al.* (1952, 1953, 1954, 1955, 1956*b*) reported that two 2L chromosome arrangements (which they designated *In2LA* and *In2LB*) reached equilibrium frequencies, ranging from 48 percent to 60 percent for the A arrangement, depending upon the localities from where they were sampled and their initial frequencies. An analysis of the fitness component characters was carried out by Moriwaki *et al.* (1956*a*) and by Ebitani (1971), and they demonstrated the superiority of heterozygotes. A maternal effect on the rate of development of heterozygotes was shown by Moriwaki and Tobari (1963). Still another balanced polymorphic system has been found involving inversions in 3L (Tobari, 1962) and 3R (Moriwaki and Ito, unpublished). In the polymorphic populations, a joint effect of heterosis and frequency dependent selection has been recorded (Tobari, 1964; Tobari and Kojima, 1967, 1968; Kojima and Tobari, 1969). Some interaction between chromosomes 2 and 3 on fitness has been found by Tobari and Kojima (unpublished).

Isozyme Polymorphisms

Johnson *et al.* (1966) examined the electrophoretic variation in several enzymes of Samoan strains of *D. pallidosa* and *D. ananassae*. In both species about 40–50 percent of the loci were variable for two or more alleles. However, the two species have attained different polymorphic balances of one esterase (EST-C). Out of the four enzyme systems studied (ACPH, EST-C, ADH, ODH), the EST-C is also the only system that showed some degree of significant divergence between Samoan and Fijian dark *D. ananassae* populations (Stone *et al.*, 1968). In the ADH and ODH systems, the frequency of the minority allleles is no more than that expected from the theory of mutation-selection balance at the gene locus where minority alleles are recessive in determining fitness. Johnson *et al.* (1969) reported that several systems, EST-C, ACPH, LAP, and APH, were polymorphic, with significant differences in allele frequency distributions among regions and between two forms of *ananassae*. Johnson (1971) summarized the data of isozyme variations in several South Pacific island populations of *ananassae*. Four loci (*Est-C, Acph, Aph,* and *Lap*) showed moderate to high levels of polymorphism, and the allelic frequencies in geographically distant localities tended to be more different than those from localities situated near one another. Three loci (*Adh, Odh,* and *Mdh*) showed low levels of variability and no appreciable differences among localities.

Gillespie and Kojima (1968) reported (1) that the degree of genetic variability of seven enzymes known to be active in energy metabolism (group I) exhibited much less variation than the enzymes which are of unknown physiological function and have broad substrate specificities and (2) that genetic variants in group I enzymes are probably maintained by mutation-selection balance.

Spontaneous Crossing Over in Males

D. ananassae is the only species of *Drosophila* characterized with a considerable frequency of spontaneous crossing over in the male. About 95 percent of the chromosomes from the natural populations of Southeast Asia were accompanied by male crossing over (Moriwaki and Tobari, 1973).

Spontaneous occurrence of male crossing over in this species was first observed by Moriwaki (1937*a*) and Kikkawa (1937*b*) independently. These and all subsequent studies of this phenomenon revealed considerable variation of recombination frequencies among strains and among families for either second- or third-chromosome markers. Although male recombination frequencies may decline with age (Ray-Chaudhuri and Kale, 1966), Kale (1969) found no evidence that would implicate premeiotic origin of crossing over as a source of variability. Kikkawa (1938) and Moriwaki (1938*b*, 1940) located a dominant gene or genes in the third and second chromosomes, respectively, that enhanced crossing over in males. Recently, Hinton's analysis (1970) revealed that the spontaneous occurrence of crossing over in males was controlled by a dominant enhancer which was located in the right arm of chromosome 3 and a dominant suppressor which was mapped in the left arm of chromosome 2, although presence of additional modifiers were suggested. Mukherjee (1961) and Kale (1968) reported some responses to selection for male recombination frequencies. Moriwaki *et al.* (1970) showed that the variation among families was decreased and recombination frequencies were random with respect to families when inbreeding was preceded, indicating probable control of polygenic systems. They found significant differences in recombination frequencies between reciprocal heterozygous males and suggested an effect of the Y chromosome on male crossing over.

Meiotic origin of male crossing over was suggested by Kale (1969) and Moriwaki *et al.* (1970). However, little cytological analysis has been done. Only Hinton (private communication) described the presence of pachytene pairing. At the submicroscopic level, Grell *et al.* (1972) reported that male crossing over in *ananassae* was not accompanied by a detectable synaptonemal complex. Moriwaki and M. Tsujita (1974) examined by electron microscopy the pro-spermatocytes of a strain with a high recombination value in males. They have observed imperfectly developed synaptonemal complexes and incomplete synapsis of homologs and suggest that male crossing over takes place to some extent between these imperfectly synapsed homologs.

Catalog of Mutants

Mutants Discovered before World War II

As it has been ascertained by Kikkawa (1935*b*) that *D. ananassae* is synonymous with *D. caribbea,* the first mutant described in this species was an autosomal recessive, curved, found by Sturtevant (1921). In 1931 Moriwaki began genetic analyses utilizing the mutants he obtained, and shortly thereafter Kikkawa started independent studies. Between 1931 and 1939, over 100 mutants were discovered (see Table 1).

In Table 2 all the mutants are classified into linkage groups. Each mutant is described in turn by its abbreviation, its full name (placed in parentheses), its discoverer, date of discovery, and main character affected. More detailed descriptions can be found in certain issues of the *Drosophila Information Service* (**2, 3, 4, 5, 7, 8, 11**), or in Kikkawa (1938) or Moriwaki (1934, 1935*a, b, c,* 1936, 1937*b,* 1938*a,* 1939, 1940).

TABLE 1.   *Classification of Mutants of D. ananassae Discovered during 1921 to 1939*

Main character affected	1 K	1 M	2 K	2 M	3 K	3 M	4 K	4 M	A S	A M	U M	Total S	Total K	Total M
Wings (W)	7	8	5	10	7	7			1	2	1	1	19	28 = 48
Eyes (E)	4	2	1	3	1			1					6	6 = 12
Legs (Lg)		2		2		1								5 = 5
Bristles (Bs)	6	8	8	7	3	5	1	3					18	23 = 41
Body (Bd)	1	1	1								1		2	2 = 4
Lethal (Lt)		3		1	1								1	4 = 5
Recombination (R)				1	1								1	1 = 2
Total	18	24	15	24	13	13	1	4	1	2	2	1	47	69 = 117

(Columns grouped under *Linkage group*[a]: 1, 2, 3, 4, A, U; Total = S + K + M)

[a] S = Sturtevant, K = Kikkawa, M = Moriwaki. A = autosomal, U = undetermined.

Mutants Discovered after World War II

All the wild and mutant stocks, which had been kept in Japanese laboratories before the War, were lost during or soon after the War. Since 1940, using wild flies collected in various parts of the world, Moriwaki and his colleagues have once again been engaged in discovering mutants. Newly obtained mutants were named independently of the former mutants, when it was uncertain whether or not they were reoccurrences of previously described ones. Some were renamed later according to the identification of the locus, based upon the assumption of allelism, or after referring to Hinton (unpublished).* A catalog of these mutants is given in Table 3. They are listed alphabetically by symbol. The linkage group follows the name.

Linkage and Mapping

Linkage maps of *ananassae* were first constructed by Kikkawa (1938) and Moriwaki (1938a, 1940), analyzing linkage relations between mutants, almost all of which were lost during the World War II years. Using newly obtained mutants, the reconstruction of the maps of the four linkage groups has been carried out. The latest ones, except the fourth

* See Acknowledgment.

TABLE 2. *Catalog of Mutants of D. ananassae Discovered during 1921 to 1939*[a]

X-Chromosome

ab (abnormal) K35f20 Bd
ac (achaete) M36b13 Bs
br (broad) K35d9 W
cb (club) M37k11 W
cl (clumploid) M35d5 W
ch-b (chilblained-b) M39e22 Lg
ck (crooked) M33f26 Lg
ct (cut) K33kl W
ct^2 (cut²) K35k29 W
ct^3 (cut³) M36k24 W
ct^4 (cut⁴) M37e4 W
dp (dwarp) K35i28 W
dp^2 (dwarp²) M38d28 W
dy (dusky) K36k17 W
ex-b (extended-b) M36j13 W
f (forked) K34i16 Bs
f^2 (forked²) K35e22 Bs
g (garnet) K34g4 E
g^2 (garnet²) K34129 E
Gf (Golf) M37e21 Bs
Ir (Interrupted) M32j28 W
l-1 (lethal-1) M34d Lt-H : 1(1)M1
l-3 (lethal-3) M ? Lt-H : 1(1)M3
l-4 (lethal-4) M37a Lt-H : 1(1)M4
M-1a (Minute-1a) K3617 Bs
m (miniature) K33j15 W
N (Notch) K34d21 W
ph (purplish) M35d23 E
sc (scute) M35g 7 Bs
sc^2 (scute²) M36j26 Bs
sc^3 (scute³) M37e20 Bs
sc^4 (scute⁴) M37k30 Bs
sc^5 (scute⁵) M37118 Bs
sc^6 (scute⁶) M38e26 Bs
sm (small bristle) K37a11 Bs
sn (singed) K34j10 Bs
sn^2 (singed²) K35k11 Bs
v (vermilion) K34k10 E
vs (vesiculated) M37a22 W
w (white) M33j19 E
w^a (apricot) K35h19 E
y (yellow) M36125 Bd

Chromosome 2

Bd (Beaded) M37d8 W
bn-b (broken-b) M37a17 W
c-2a (curved-2a) K34c10 W
c-2b (curved-2b) K36112 W
c-2c (curved-2c) M38c10 W
cd (cardinal) K34b24 E
cnt (contracted) M36i16 W
ch (chilblained) M37e21 Lg
cp (crippled) M36131 Lg
D (Dichaete) M36125 Bs
En-2 (Enhancer-2) M361 R-H : En(2)
e (ebony) K36i8 Bd
et^2 (extra²) M37j18 W
ex (extended) M36a22 W
hk (hooked) M37a8 Bs
l-2 (lethal-2) M34e Lt-H : 1(2)M1
la (lance) K34j11 W
M-2a (Minute-2a) K34f25 Bs
M-2b (Minute-2b) K35h8 Bs
M-2c (Minute-2c) K35i30 Bs
M-2d (Minute-2d) M37j27 Bs
ms (missing) M35k13 Bs
ms-b (missing-b) M36h24 Bs
Off (Off) M36b22 Bs
ob (obliterated) K35c4 W
Pt (Plexate) M33k15 W
Pt^2 (Plexate²) K34i10 W
Pu (Puffed) M37g5 E
Pu^2 (Puffed²) M37130 E
pk (prickly) K36k9 Bs
rf (roof) M36i28 W
ro (rough) M37b23 E
rt (retracted) M33126 W
sb (stubble) K35b19 Bs
sd (spread) K36a11 W
sk (ski) M33f26 W
sl (slender) K34h1 Bs
ss (spineless) K35f10 Bs
tb (tiny bristle) K34h15 Bs

Chromosome 3

arc (arc) M3713 W

[a] The date of discovery is given according to the by-laws of the *Drosophila* Information Service (*DIS*), for example, 35f20 means the mutation was discovered in 1935 on June 20. The symbols describing the discoverers and the phenotype are the same as those shown in Table 1 (i.e., H = Hinton, K = Kikkawa, M = Moriwaki, W = wings, E = eyes, etc.).

TABLE 2. Continued

Bb (Barb) K35a14 Bs	*rp* (rippled) M37b27 W
ba (balloon) M33g8 W	*sk-3* (ski-3) M3516 W
bn (broken) K35e31 W	*wp* (warped) M36k28 W
c-3a (curved-3a) K35i27 W	*wy* (wavy) M37a7 W
ck-b (crooked-b) M37a6 Lg	
D-3 (Dichaete-3) M36l18 Bs	**Chromosome 4**
En (Enhancer) K36k R-H : En(3)	*bb* (bobbed) M34k28 Bs
er (erect) M37b23 Bs	*bb²* (bobbed²) K35k11 Bs
et (extra) K35k14 W	*M-4a* (Minute-4a) M36f11 Bs
gp (gap) K35h22 W	*mo* (mottled) M36k24 E
l-3a (lethal-3a) K36h Lt-H : 1(3)a	*Sv* (Shaven) M37b1 Bs
ll (lanceolate) K35b23 W	
M-3a (Minute-3a) K34j24 Bs	**Autosomal**
M-3b (Minute-3b) K34k19 Bs	*c* (curved) Sturtevant 21? W
M-3c (Minute-3c) M3516 Bs	*cr* (crumpled) M32i30 W
M-3d (Minute-3d) M36d22 Bs	*ic* (incomplete) M32b16 W
M-3e (Minute-3e) M37f19 Bs	
Pi (Pinched) K37d4 W	**Undetermined**
Pm (Plum) K35h22 E	*abr* (abrupt) M38c1 W
px (plexus) K34e8 W	*Eg* (Engrailed) M36l25 Bd
rm (rumpled) M37c11 W	

chromosome, though still tentative and rough, are presented in Figures 1–4. Ray-Chaudhuri *et al.* (1959) and Hinton (1970, and unpublished) have also reported some of the linkage relations.

In Figure 1, our current map of the X chromosome is compared with the classical one (Moriwaki, 1938a) and Hinton's (unpublished). According to Hinton, *ct, y,* and *rb* are located in XL, while *f* and *w* are located in XR.

Since the second chromosome often carries a subterminal inversion, *In2L* (or *2LA* according to Futch's designation),* recombination frequencies between markers were determined for both sequences. The maps in Figure 2 are drawn for the entire chromosome containing the standard sequence (*In2LA* or +), while Figure 3 presents the maps for only the in-

---

* Futch (1966) named three paracentric inversions *2LA, 3LA* and *3RA,* and concluded that they were found wherever the species flourishes. Unfortunately, inversions in this species have been named independently and differently by various authors. The subterminal inversion *2LA* (Futch, 1966) corresponds to *CIIL* (Kikkawa, 1938) and *In2L* (Shirai and Moriwaki, 1952). Similarly, the terminal inversion *3LA* is the same as *CIIIL* and *In3L*; the basal inversion *3RA* is identical with *CIIIR* and *In3R*. Hinton (1970, and unpublished) used the symbols as *In(2L)A, In(3L)A,* and *In(3R)A,* naming the "standard" sequence as +. Kikkawa (1938) called A (corresponding to the "standard") and B the reciprocal sequences, respectively, and we followed him.

TABLE 3. *Catalog of Mutants of D. ananassae Discovered after World War II (Mostly at Moriwaki's Laboratory)*[a]

Symbol	Name	Chromosome	Discoverer and Discovery Date[b]	Description
amb	amber	1	C. Kato 71c17 (*DIS* **48**)	Pale yellow body; bristles thin and slightly shortened
app	approximate	3	Moriwaki 67j23 (*DIS* **45**)	Posterior crossvein shifts obliquely toward anterior crossvein
Arc	Arc	2	Moriwaki 66i23 (*DIS* **43**)	Wings bent downward; crossveins absent or traces present; dominant; homozygote viable, almost sterile
b	black	2	Reported by Ray-Chaudhuri (*DIS* **32**)	Hinton (unpublished) changed the symbol to e^2
b[65]	black[65]	2	Moriwaki 65h20 (*DIS* **43**)	Black body color; allelic to *b* [= e^{65} (Hinton, unpublished)]
ba-b	balloon-b	2	Moriwaki 65h20 (*DIS* **43**, *ba*[65])	Wings warped with blisters; different from *ba* (Moriwaki 33g8 chromosome 3)
bb[67]	bobbed[67]	4	Moriwaki 67j23 (*DIS* **45**)	Only in ♀ bristles shortened and often abdomen etched; male shows neither characteristic; normal allele exists in Y chromosome too
bb[2]	bobbed[2]	4	Moriwaki 67k21 (*DIS* **46**)	Bristles shortened; allelic to *bb*[67]
Bd[3]	Beaded[3]	3	Moriwaki 68e16 (*DIS* **45**, *Bd*)	Wings reduced by marginal excisions; dominant; homozygous lethal; viability and fertility of heterozygotes low
bn-b[67]	broken-b[67]	2	Moriwaki 67k21 (*DIS* **45**, *bn*[67])	Posterior crossvein missing or broken; the later-emerging flies are often "normal" in phenotype, especially true of males

bri	bright	3	Reported by Hinton (1970)	Eye color bright red; ocelli colorless
bs	blistered	3	Moriwaki 71g28 (*DIS* **48**)	Wings blistered
bw	brown	2	Reported by Ray-Chaudhuri (*DIS* **32**, *or*); (*DIS* **43**, *bw*^{R})	Brownish wine eye color [= *ca* (Hinton, unpublished)]
bw^{71}	brown^{71}	2	Moriwaki 71d9 (*DIS* **48**)	Allelic to *bw* [= *ca*^{71} (Hinton, unpublished)]
bw^{71e}	brown^{71e}	2	Moriwaki 71e25 (*DIS* **48**)	Allelic to *bw* [= *ca*^{71e} (Hinton, unpublished)]
cd	cardinal	2	Sent from California Institute of Technology, 1950; may be the same as *cd* (Kikkawa, *DIS* **2**); (*DIS* **43**)	Eye color yellowish vermilion; ocelli white
ct^6	cut^6	1	Moriwaki 71g12 (*DIS* **48**, *ct*)	Wings cut, incised at tips
Dl	Delta	2	Moriwaki 69h1 (*DIS* **46**)	End of L2 vein and costa are fused together; dominant; homozygous lethal; when combined with one *px* gene, the manifestation is exaggerated by extra veins; in extreme case, combined with homozygous *px*, additional balloonlike expression appears
Dl^{71}	Delta^{71}	2	Moriwaki 71a22 (*DIS* **48**, *Pt*)	The end of L2 vein fused with costa as delta; extra veins often seen in submarginal cells; the manifestation is variable, depending on the genetic background; dominant; homozygote not necessarily lethal; allelic to *Dl*
ecv	extra crossvein	1	Moriwaki 72d14 (*DIS*50)	L2 and L3 partly fuse with thickness of a crossvein. Less viable, though *amb* seems to improve the viability

[a] Some mutants remain to be analyzed more precisely. Any changes will be reported in future issues of the *Drosophila Information Service*.
[b] See footnote to Table 2.

TABLE 3. *Continued*

Symbol	Name	Chromosome	Discoverer and Discovery Date[b]	Description
ext	extended	2	Moriwaki 69125 (*DIS* **46**)	Wings extending at 75 deg. from body axis, usually showing shortened L3 vein; occasionally only one of those characteristics is expressed, *Dl ext* often manifesting only extended wings
ext^k	kidney	2	Moriwaki 70d30 (*DIS* **48**)	Eye size reduced by indentation of front margin; penetrance low, expressed when combined with *Dl*; allelic to *ext*
eyg	eye gone	2	Fuyama 72d (*DIS* **50**)	Eyes and head much smaller than normal; percent emergence low
f^49	forked[49]	1	Moriwaki 49129 (*DIS* **43**)	Moderate forked phenotype; allelic to *f*
f^72	forked[72]	1	Moriwaki 72c23 (*DIS* **50**)	Allelic to *f*
f	forked	1	Sent from California Institute of Technology, 1950; may be the same as *f* (Kikkawa, *DIS* **2**); (*DIS* **43**)	
gr	grey	2	Moriwaki 65h20 (*DIS* **43**)	Less dark than *b*; sometimes gives intermediate type F₁ with *b*
Ir-a	Interrupted-autosomal	2	Moriwaki 69h1 (*DIS* **48**)	Posterior crossveins missing or broken; expression variable, overlapping the wild type even when homozygous; semidominant
j	jaunty	2	Reported by Ray-Chaudhuri (*DIS* **32**, *cy²*); (*DIS* **43**)	Sharply coiling wings

Symbol	Name	Origin	Chr	Description
kk	kinky	Moriwaki 67a11 (*DIS* **43**)	1	Bristles slightly bent or forked; gives wild type F$_1$ with *f*
kk^c	curly bristles	Moriwaki 70f7 (*DIS* **46**)	1	Bristles curled upward; allelic to *kk*
L	Lobe	T. Oishi 71d28 (*DIS* **50**)	2	Dominant, less viable; homozygous lethal; heterozygous *L* eyes smaller; expression ranges from *Bar*-like to kidney-shaped, depending on genetic backgrounds, sometimes overlaps wild type
l(1)M2	lethal 2 of Moriwaki	Moriwaki 67e (*DIS* **43**, *l-1*)	1	
l(1)M5	lethal 5 of Moriwaki	Moriwaki 72d (*DIS* **50**)	1	Semilethal (*ca.* 70 percent); seemingly located near the end of either arm of XL or XR
M(3)65	Minute(3)65	Moriwaki 65j21 (*DIS* **43**, *M*^{65})	3	Minute bristles; dominant; homozygous lethal
M(3)b67	Minute(3)b67	Moriwaki 67d22 (*DIS* **45**, *M-b*)	3	Minute bristles; dominant; homozygous lethal
M(3)c68	Minute(3)c68	Moriwaki 68a11 (*DIS* **45**, *M-c*)	3	Minute bristles; dominant; homozygous lethal
M(3)d70	Minute(3)d70	Moriwaki 70f (*DIS* **46**, *M-d*)	3	Minute bristles; dominant; homozygous lethal; may be allelic to *M(3)b67*
ma	maroon	Reported by Ray-Chaudhuri (*DIS* **32**, *cd*); (*DIS* **43**)	2	Reddish brown eye color
mot	mottled	Moriwaki 69118 (*DIS* **46**)	3	Eyes mottled, dark-spotted, and rough; expression variable
Ms	Missing	Moriwaki 69112 (*DIS* **48**)	3	Bristles missing, in extreme cases nearly all are absent; semidominant (penetrance about 40 percent); heterozygote, when expressed, anterior scutellars are missing

TABLE 3. *Continued*

Symbol	Name	Chromosome	Discoverer and Discovery Date[b]	Description
od	outstretched	1	S. Ito 67b	Wings very divergent, often at right angles to body, and slightly depressed; mostly expressed in males
od[u]	uplift	1	C. Kato 70j7 (*DIS* **48**)	Wings uplifted at right angles to body; allelic to od
pea	peach	2	Tobari 69a (*DIS* **46**, *pe*)	Eye color translucent yellowish pink; ocelli colored
px	plexus	3	Reported by Ray-Chaudhuri (*DIS* **32**). (*DIS* **43**)	Venation plexus
px[66]	plexus[66]	3	Moriwaki 66h23 (*DIS* **43**, *px*[2])	Venation plexus; semidominant; more pronounced in some minutes; allelic to px
Rf	Roof	3	Moriwaki 66h3 (*DIS* **43**)	Roof-shaped wing; dominant emerge as normal, [Rf] appears almost after 12 hours (Y. Oguma and M. Mitamura, unpublished), the same as Rf of D. *melanogaster*
ri	radius interruptus	3	Moriwaki 70i13 (*DIS* **46**)	Vein L2 interrupted
ri[71]	radius interruptus[71]	3	Moriwaki 71e9 (*DIS* **48**)	Allelic to ri; expression often incomplete in females
ru	roughoid	3	Moriwaki 49112 (*DIS* **43**)	Slight smudge of blackened facets in lower parts of eye; expression varied by modifying genes (A. Ono, unpublished); *ru*[2] (*DIS* **43**) seems identical with ru

rus	russet	2	Moriwaki 72j25 (*DIS* **50**)	Reddish brown eye color; female sterile
scar	scarred	1	C. Kato 71c17 (*DIS* **48**)	Eye surface scarred and wrinkled; postscutellars mostly erect; often wings spread, especially in males
se[T]	sepia[T]	2	Sent from Austin, Texas, 1950, as "brown eye color" (*DIS* **43**)	Eye color sepia; ocelli remain wild type in color
sm[66]	small bristle[66]	3	Moriwaki 66e12 (*DIS* **43**)	Bristles small, not as extreme as *M*
sn[65]	singed[65]	1	Moriwaki 65i27 (*DIS* **43**)	Bristles twisted and gnarled
Snp	Snipped	3	Moriwaki 69b5 (*DIS* **46**)	Tips of wings snipped; dominant, with low penetrance; homozygous sterile, with low viability and *vg*-like expression
Tr	Trident	3	Moriwaki 72c15 (*DIS* **50**)	Posterior crossvein branched with trident shape; extra veins in marginal and submarginal cells; dominant; homozygous lethal; expression variable according to combined mutant genes; for example, combined with homozygous *ri*, tip of L3 thickened as delta
ty	tiny	1	Moriwaki 68111 (*DIS* **46**)	Bristles thin and short, like minute
w[65]	white[65]	1	N. Ebitani 65e14 (*DIS* **43**)	Inseparable from *w*
w[m]	white-mottled	1	C. Kato 71c8 (*DIS* **48**)	Eyes show one or a few red spots on white background; penetrance incomplete, especially in males; allelic to *w*
y[51]	yellow[51]	1	Moriwaki 51b19 (*DIS* **43**)	Yellow body, wings, and bristles
y[66]	yellow[66]	1	Tobari 66h (*DIS* **43**)	Allelic to *y*

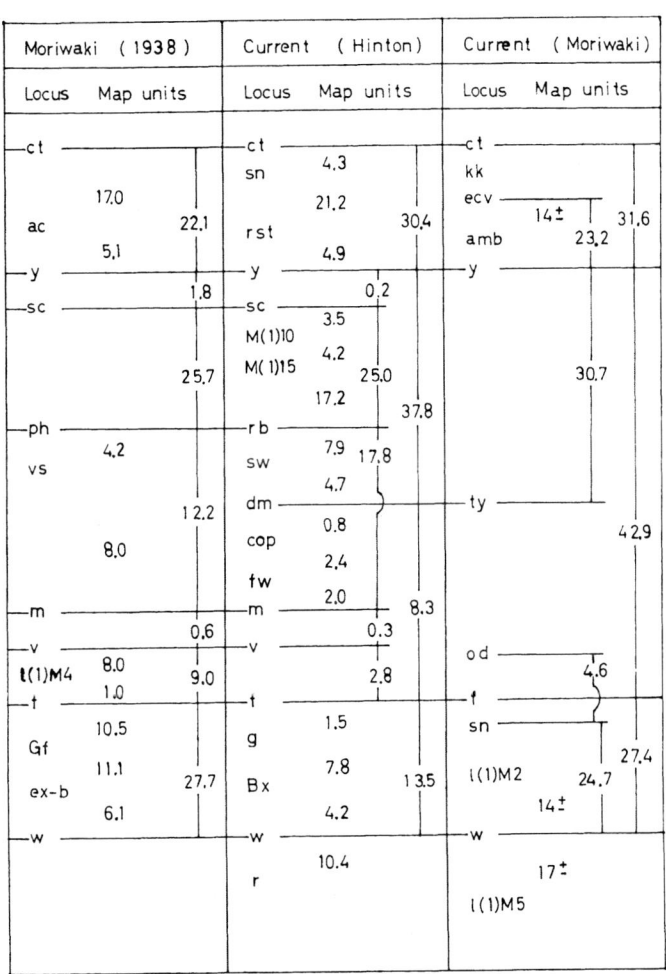

Figure 1. Maps of the X chromosome.

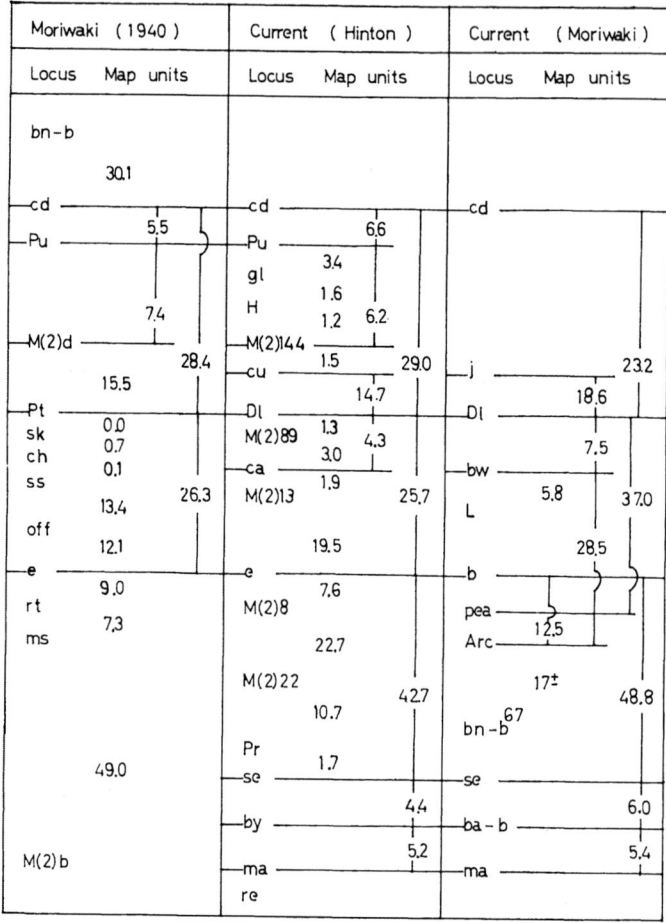

Figure 2. Maps of the second chromosome.

verted sequences for comparison. Concerning the differing results for the two sequences, Hinton (unpublished) states, ''The reversal of the *cd-cu-Dl* sequence with respect to *e* proves that breakpoints of *In(2L)A* lie to the left of *cd* and to the left of *e* . . . it seems probable from consideration of map distances that most of the markers to the right of *e* lie in 2R.'' This conclusion agrees with our results.

Current maps of the third chromosome constructed by Hinton and our laboratory are compared in Figure 4. The original maps (Kikkawa, 1938; Moriwaki, 1938*a*) are not used for the comparison because they contain scarcely any mutants in common with the current maps. The terminal inversion, *In3L,* possibly includes *bri,* which seems to be located on

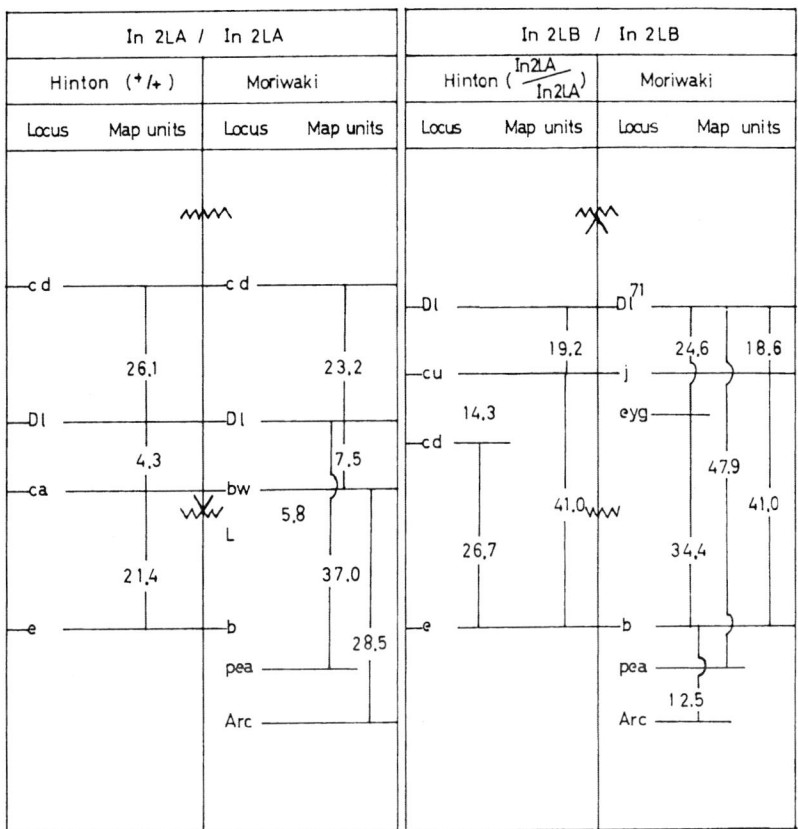

Figure 3. Maps of the In2LA and In2LB sequences in the second chromosome.

the right half of the *In3LA* (or "standard") sequence. The markers, *M(3)65, M(3)b67,* and *Rf,* are believed to lie to the right of the inversion, *In3L,* on the left arm, although the position of centromere remains unknown. Hinton (1970) reported that heterozygosity for *In(3R)A* reduced recombination in the *stw–px* region, and in our laboratory a similar result was obtained in the *M(3)b67–px* region with respect to the basal inversion, *In3R.*

Acknowledgment

Dr. Claude Hinton completed a manuscript on "The Cytogenetics of *Drosophila ananassae*" for inclusion in Vol. 1 of *The Genetics and*

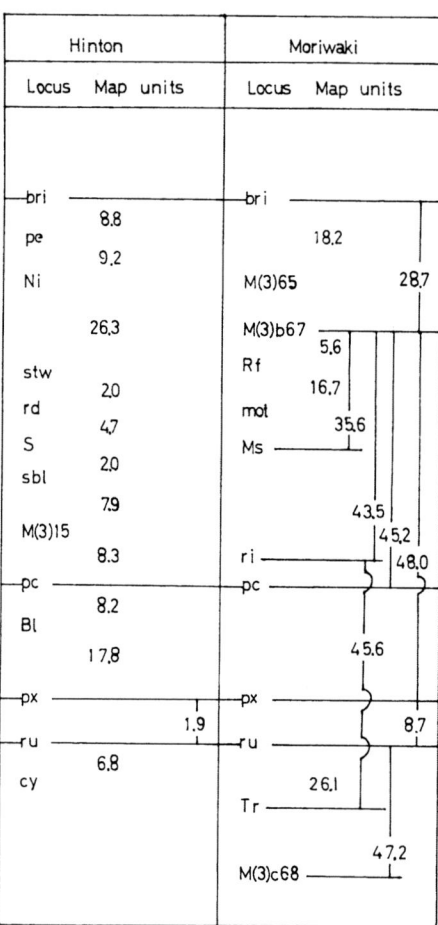

Figure 4. Current maps of the third chromosome.

Biology of Drosophila being edited by Drs. M. Ashburner and E. Novitski. Dr. Hinton kindly provided us with a copy of his manuscript. We referred to this, and many data obtained from it are cited here, each with a note, showing the source as Hinton (unpublished). We wish to express our hearty thanks to Dr. Hinton for his generosity.

Literature Cited

Bock, I. R. and M. R. Wheeler, 1972   The *Drosophila melanogaster* species group. *Univ. Texas Publ.* **7213**:1–102.

Cooper, K. W., 1950   Normal spermatogenesis in Drosophila. In *Biology of Drosophila,* edited by M. Demerec, pp. 1–60, John Wiley & Sons, New York.

Dobzhansky, T. and A. Dreyfus, 1943   Chromosomal aberrations in Brazilian *Drosophila ananassae. Proc. Natl. Acad. Sci. USA* **29**:301–305.

Doleschall, C. L., 1858   Derde bijdrage tot de kennis der dipteren fauna van Nederlandsch Indïe. *Natrk. Tijdschr. Nederland. Indïe (1858–1859)* 17 (ser. 4, 3): 73–128.

Ebitani, N., 1971   Body weight at different developmental stages of inversion homozygotes in *Drosophila ananassae. Jap. J. Genet.* **46**:309–319.

Freire-Maia, N., 1955   Chromosome mutations in natural populations of *D. ananassae. Drosophila Inf. Serv.* **29**:116–117.

Freire-Maia, N., 1961   Peculiar gene arrangements in Brazilian natural populations of *Drosophila ananassae. Evolution* **15**:486–495.

Futch, D. G., 1966   A study of speciation in South Pacific populations of *Drosophila ananassae. Univ. Texas Publ.* **6615**:79–120.

Gillespie, J. H. and K. Kojima, 1968   The degree of polymorphisms in enzymes involved in energy production compared to that in non-specific enzymes in two *Drosophila ananassae* populations. *Proc. Natl. Acad. Sci. USA* **61**:582–585.

Grell, R. F., H. Bank and G. Gassner, 1972   Meiotic exchange without the synaptinemal complex. *Nat. New Biol.* **240**:155–156.

Hinton, C. W., 1968   Meiosis in *Drosophila ananassae* males. *Drosophila Inf. Serv.* **43**:154.

Hinton, C. W., 1970   Identification of two loci controlling crossing over in males of *Drosophila ananassae. Genetics* **66**:663–676.

Johnson, F. M., 1971   Isozyme polymorphism in *Drosophila ananassae:* Genetic diversity among isolated populations in the South Pacific. *Genetics* **68**:77–95.

Johnson, F. M., C. G. Kanapi, R. H. Richardson, M. R. Wheeler and W. S. Stone, 1966   An analysis of polymorphisms among isozyme loci in dark and light *Drosophila ananassae* strains from American and Western Samoa. *Proc. Natl. Acad. Sci. USA* **56**:119–125.

Johnson, F. M., K. Kojima and M. R. Wheeler, 1969   Isozyme variation in *Drosophila* island populations. II. An analysis of *Drosophila ananassae* populations in the Samoan, Fijian and Philippine Islands. *Univ. Texas Publ.* **6918**:187–205.

Kale, P. G., 1968   Spontaneous crossing over in the males of *D. ananassae:* Two-way selection for recombination values. *Jap. J. Genet.* **43**:27–31.

Kale, P. G., 1969   The meiotic origin of spontaneous crossovers in *Drosophila ananassae* males. *Genetics* **62**:123–133.

Kaneshiro, K. and M. R. Wheeler, 1970 Preliminary report on the species of the *ananassae* subgroup. *Drosophila Inf. Serv.* **45**:143.

Kaufmann, B. P., 1935 *Drosophila ananassae (D. caribbea). Drosophila Inf. Serv.* **4**:61.

Kaufmann, B. P., 1936*a* The chromosomes of *Drosophila ananassae. Science (Wash., D.C.)* **83**:39.

Kaufmann, B. P., 1936*b* A terminal inversion in *Drosophila ananassae. Proc. Natl. Acad. Sci. USA* **22**:591–594.

Kaufmann, B. P., 1937*a* Chromosome studies on *Drosophila ananassae. Genetics* **22**:197–198.

Kaufmann, B. P., 1937*b* Morphology of the chromosomes of *Drosophila ananassae. Cytologia (Tokyo)* **Fujii Jubilee Vol.**:1043–1055.

Kikkawa, H., 1935*a* An inference as to the constitution of X-chromosome in *Drosophila. Proc. Imp. Acad. Jap.* **11**:62–65.

Kikkawa, H., 1935*b* *D. ananassae. Drosophila Inf. Serv.* **3**:46.

Kikkawa, H., 1936*a* Chromosomes of *D. ananassae. Drosophila Inf. Serv.* **5**:25.

Kikkawa, H., 1936*b* Chromosomes of *Drosophila ananassae* (a preliminary note). *Jap. J. Genet.* **12**:65–66 (in Japanese).

Kikkawa, H., 1937*a* A terminal inversion found in *Drosophila ananassae* (a preliminary note). *Jap. J. Genet.* **13**:237–239 (in Japanese).

Kikkawa, H., 1937*b* Spontaneous crossing-over in the male of *Drosophila ananassae. Zool. Mag. Tokyo*) **49**:159–160.

Kikkawa, H., 1938 Studies on the genetics and cytology of *Drosophila ananassae. Genetica (The Hague)* **20**:458–516.

Kojima, K. and Y. N. Tobari, 1969 Selective modes associated with karyotypes in *Drosophila ananassae*. II. Heterosis and frequency-dependent selection. *Genetics* **63**:639–651.

Metz, C. W., 1916 Chromosome studies in the Diptera. III. Additional types of chromosome groups in the Drosophilidae. *Am. Nat.* **50**:587–599.

Moriwaki, D., 1934 Mutant characters in a species of *Drosophila. Jap. J. Genet.* **9**:164–168.

Moriwaki, D., 1935*a* Some mutant characters in *Drosophila ananassae. Genetica (The Hague)* **17**:32–46.

Moriwaki, D., 1935*b* *Crumploid*, a sex-linked character of *Drosophila ananassae. Jap. J. Genet.* **11**:302–307.

Moriwaki, D., 1935*c* *Bobbed* mutation in *Drosophila ananassae. Proc. Imp. Acad. Jap.* **11**:340–341.

Moriwaki, D., 1936 The genetics of *Drosophila ananassae. Zool. Mag.* **48**:693–703.

Moriwaki, D., 1937*a* A high ratio of crossing-over in *Drosophila ananassae. Z. Indukt. Abstammungs.-Vererbungsl.* **74**:17–23.

Moriwaki, D., 1937*b* Abnormal inheritance in relation to the "bobbed" character of *Drosophila ananassae. Cytologia (Tokyo)* **Fujii Jubilee Vol.**:228–233.

Moriwaki, D., 1938*a* The genetics of some mutant characters in *Drosophila ananassae. Jap. J. Genet.* **14**:1–23.

Moriwaki, D., 1938*b* Enhanced crossing over in the second chromosome of *Drosophila ananassae* (preliminary note). *Jap. J. Genet.* **14**:283–284.

Moriwaki, D., 1939 Genetical studies in *D. ananassae* (review). *Bot. Zool. (Tokyo)* **7**:280–286 (in Japanese).

Moriwaki, D., 1940 Enhanced crossing over in the second chromosome of *D. ananassae. Jap. J. Genet.* **16**:37–48.

Moriwaki, D. and S. Ito, 1969   Studies on puffing in the salivary gland chromosomes of *Drosophila ananassae. Jap. J. Genet.* **44**:129–138.

Moriwaki, D. and Y. N. Tobari, 1963   Maternal effects and heterosis in *D. ananassae. Genetics* **48**:171–176.

Moriwaki, D. and Y. N. Tobari, 1973   Spontaneous male crossing-over of frequent occurrence in *Drosophila ananassae* from Southeast Asian populations. *Jap. J. Genet.* **48**:167–173.

Moriwaki, D. and M. Tsujita, 1974   Synaptonemal complex and male crossing-over in *Drosophila ananassae. Cytologia (Tokyo)* **39**:829–838.

Moriwaki, D., M. Shirai and Y. H. Yoshida, 1952   Frequency change of different gene arrangements of *D. ananassae* in artificial populations. *Jap. J. Genet.* **27**:220 (in Japanese).

Moriwaki, D., M. Shirai and Y. H. Yoshida, 1953   Frequency change of different gene arrangements of *D. ananassae* in artificial populations (a continuation). *Jap. J. Genet.* **28**:176 (in Japanese).

Moriwaki, D., M. Shirai, Y. H. Yoshida and M. Tsusue, 1954   Frequency change of different gene arrangements of *Drosophila ananassae in artificial populations. III. Jap. J. Genet.* **29**:165–166 (in Japanese).

Moriwaki, D., M. Shirai and Y. H. Yoshida, 1955   Balanced polymorphism attained in some experimental populations of *D. ananassae. Drosophila Inf. Serv.* **29**:143–144.

Moriwaki, D., M. Ohnishi and Y. Nakajima, 1956a   Analysis of heterosis in populations of *D. ananassae. Proc. Interntl. Genet. Symp. 1956 Cytologia Suppl. Vol.* 370–379.

Moriwaki, D., M. Shirai, Y. H. Yoshida and M. Tsusue, 1956b   Frequency changes of two inversion arrangements in artificial populations of *D. ananassae.* In *Shudan Idengaku,* edited by T. Komai and K. Sakai, pp. 95–97, Baifukan, Tokyo.

Moriwaki, D., Y. N. Tobari and Y. Oguma, 1970   Spontaneous crossing over in the male of *Drosophila ananassae. Jap. J. Genet.* **45**:411–420.

Mukherjee, A. S., 1961   Effect of selection on crossing over in the males of *D. ananassae. Am. Nat.* **95**:57–59.

Patterson, J. T. and W. S. Stone, 1952   *Evolution in the Genus Drosophila,* Macmillan, New York.

Ray-Chaudhuri, S. P. and P. G. Kale, 1966   Crossing over in the males of *Drosophila ananassae. J. Cytol. Genet. (Banaras Hindu Univ., India)* **1**:22–29.

Ray-Chaudhuri, S. P., S. Sarkar, A. S. Mukherjee and J. Bose, 1959   Mutation in *Drosophila ananassae* and their linkage map. *Proc. 1st All India Congr. Zool. Pt. 2, Addendum*:i–xi.

Shirai, M. and D. Moriwaki, 1952   Variations of gene sequences in various strains of *D. ananassae. Drosophila Inf. Serv.* **26**:120–121.

Stone, W. S., M. R. Wheeler, W. P. Spencer, F. D. Wilson, J. T. Neuenschwander, T. G. Gregg, R. L. Seecof and C. L. Ward, 1957   Genetic studies of irradiated natural populations of *Drosophila. Univ. Texas Publ.* **5721**:260–316.

Stone, W. S., M. R. Wheeler, F. M. Johnson and K. Kojima, 1968   Genetic variation in natural island populations of members of the *Drosophila nasuta* and *Drosophila ananassae* subgroups. *Proc. Natl. Acad. Sci. USA* **59**:102–109.

Sturtevant, A. H., 1921   *North American Species of Drosophila,* Carnegie Institution of Washington Publication 301, Carnegie Institution, Washington, D.C.

Sturtevant, A. H., 1942   The classification of the genus *Drosophila,* with descriptions of nine new species. *Univ. Texas Publ.* **4213**:5–51.

Tobari, Y. N., 1962   Heterosis relating to a terminal inversion in artificial population of *D. ananassae. Jap. J. Genet.* **37**:302–309.

Tobari, Y. N., 1964   Relation between adaptive values and composition of the population in *D. ananassae. Evolution* **18**:343–348.

Tobari, Y. N. and K. Kojima, 1967   Selective modes associated with inversion karyotypes in *D. ananassae.* I. Frequency-dependent selection. *Genetics* **57**:179–188.

Tobari, Y. N. and K. Kojima, 1968   The selective mode associated with two chromosome polymorphisms in *D. ananassae. Proc. 12th Interntl. Congr. Genet. Tokyo* **1**:227.

20

Drosophila pseudoobscura and Its American Relatives, *Drosophila persimilis* and *Drosophila miranda*

THEODOSIUS DOBZHANSKY AND

JEFFREY R. POWELL

Introduction

Drosophila obscura Fallén was described in 1823 from a locality in southern Sweden. Sturtevant (1921) attributed to this species specimens not only from European localities but also from Oregon and California. Frolova and Astaurov (1929) found that American flies differed from the European ones in their genitalia, chromosomal complements, and inability to cross; the American species was given the name *D. pseudoobscura* Frol. In the same year, Lancefield (1929) discovered that *D. pseudoobscura* consists of two reproductively partially isolated forms, which he designated "races or physiological species," A and B. Although at that

THEODOSIUS DOBZHANSKY—Department of Genetics, University of California, Davis California. JEFFREY R. POWELL—Department of Biology, Yale University, New Haven, Connecticut.

time these forms were believed quite indistinguishable morphologically, Dobzhansky and Epling (1944) recognized them as an instance of sibling species and named "race B" *D. persimilis*. Still earlier, Dobzhansky (1935a) found *D. miranda* in the Pacific Northwest (Washington), a species morphologically barely distinguishable, but reproductively isolated, from *D. pseudoobscura* and *D. persimilis*. In addition, *D. miranda* possesses an extraordinary chromosomal complement (see below). A fourth American species, *D. lowei,* has been described by Heed *et al.* (1969). Meanwhile, eight species, none identical with American ones, were found in Eurasia. These eight, covered only in part in the present review, are *D. alpina* Burla, *D. ambigua* Pomini, *D. bifasciata* Pomini, *D. imaii* Moriwaki and Okada, *D. obscura* Fallén, *D. subobscura* Collin, *D. subsilvestris* Hardy and Kaneshiro, and *D. tristis* Fallén (Buzzati-Traverso and Scossiroli, 1955; Lakovaara *et al.,* 1972).

Morphology, Geography, and Reproductive Isolation

D. pseudoobscura and *D. persimilis* are classical examples of sibling species. The females are quite indistinguishable by externally visible traits; Rizki (1951) did, however, discern a slight but diagnostic difference in the male genitalia, by means of which an experienced and keen-eyed observer can recognize the two species. *D. pseudoobscura* lives in the region from British Columbia to Mexico and Guatemala, and from the Pacific to Rocky Mountains and Texas, in quasicontinuous distribution (Dobzhansky and Epling, 1944). Dr. A. Hunter has discovered a colony in the Andes near Bogotá, Colombia, separated from the main body of the species by a gap of some 1500 miles (Dobzhansky *et al.,* 1963a). The distribution area of *D. persimilis* is included in that of *D. pseudoobscura*; it extends from British Columbia to southern California, and from the Pacific to the Sierra Nevada–Cascades, and to some adjacent mountain ranges eastward (Dobzhansky, 1974). In the zone of the geographic overlap, *D. pseudoobscura* is more frequent in warmer and drier locations and at lower elevations, while *D. persimilis* is abundant under opposite circumstances. Where both species occur together, *D. pseudoobscura* tends to be more frequent in mid-summer, and *D. persimilis* during spring and autumn. In a given locality the abundance of the two species often changes greatly from year to year; the environmental reasons for these changes are not at all obvious. That the two species share at least some breeding sites was proven by Carson (1951). However, they show average differences in diurnal activity: *D. persimilis* comes to baits relatively more often on cool mornings than on warm evenings (Dobzhansky, 1951).

By 1929 Lancefield (1929) had already observed that matings within a species occur more often than between the species *D. pseudoobscura* and *D. persimilis*; this has been confirmed many times since (see below, the discussion of the genetics of behavior). Nevertheless, hybrids between these species are obtainable in laboratory cultures without difficulty, while only a single hybrid female was found in nature among more than 15,000 flies from localities where the two species coexist (Dobzhansky, 1973). This appears to be due to much stronger sexual (ethological) isolation in nature than in laboratory cultures (Dobzhansky, 1951). The reasons for this difference in the intensity of sexual isolation are unknown. Anderson and Ehrman (1969) found no evidence of mating preference or aversion between strains of *D. pseudoobscura* from remote geographic regions, where this species occurs sympatrically with *D. persimilis* or where it lives alone. Whether or not the sexual isolation varies in strength between different strains of these two species is unknown. However that may be, interspecific insemination is followed by production of somatically vigorous hybrid progenies; the F_1 hybrid females are fertile, while the males are completely sterile. Backcrosses of the hybrid females to males of either parental species yield progenies in which both females and males are somatically weak, but some of which are nevertheless fertile (Dobzhansky, 1936; Lamy, 1943). Among the three isolating mechanisms—sexual isolation, hybrid sterility, and hybrid breakdown—it is the first that is most effective in nature. The three of them together doubtless preclude most or all gene flow from the gene pool of one species to that of the other.

D. miranda lives together with *D. persimilis* and *D. pseudoobscura* in Washington, Oregon, in the Coast Ranges, and in the Sierra Nevada of California. Prof. W. W. Anderson (unpublished) found it abundant in a locality in mountains of Idaho. *D. miranda* is larger on the average and more heavily pigmented (especially darker legs and abdominal sternites) than the other species. The discrimination of the species by these traits is not, however, wholly reliable. In laboratory tests, the sexual isolation is stronger between *D. miranda* and either *D. persimilis* or *D. pseudoobscura* than between the latter two species. Moreover, it is greater between sympatric than allopatric strains (Dobzhansky and Koller, 1938). Premating isolating mechanisms are reinforced by natural selection where the species concerned are exposed to the challenge of hybridization and production of sterile or poorly viable progeny. The crosses of *D. miranda* females to *D. psuedoobscura* or *D. persimilis* males give hybrid daughters intermediate in appearance between the parental species and sons that are phenotypically abnormal. The reciprocal crosses yield mostly females and very few males. All hybrids are completely sterile (Dobzhansky, 1937*a*, 1951).

D. lowei is, as far as known, restricted to the mountains of Arizona and Colorado. This species is hard to maintain in laboratory cultures, partly because it undergoes a seasonal diapause during which the females have underdeveloped ovaries and no sperm in their seminal receptacles. Hybrids with *D. psuedoobscura,* a sympatric species, have nevertheless been obtained in the laboratory and possibly in nature as well. The hybrids are sterile (Heed *et al.,* 1969). *D. frolovae* Wheeler, described from Michoacan, Mexico, is inadequately known, but it is seemingly related to the other species mentioned above.

Hybridization experiments conducted in laboratory cultures between the American and the European species of the *obscura* group have been reviewed by Buzzati-Traverso and Scossiroli (1955). In most combinations, either no progeny or at least no adult progeny is obtained. Exceptions are *D. persimilis* × *D. ambigua* and *D. pseudoobscura* × *D. ambigua,* which produce sterile hybrids. The sibling species *D. bifasciata* and *D. imaii,* partly sympatric in Japan, yield fertile female but sterile male hybrids (Moriwaki *et al.,* 1967).

Chromosomes

The first description of the metaphase chromosomes of *D. pseudoobscura* was given by Metz (1916). In his paper the species is misnamed *D. obscura.* A variety of chromosome complements in the *obscura* species group have been brought to light since then [see review in Buzzati-Traverso and Scossiroli (1955)]; the different types are listed in Table 1.

D. miranda shows an extraordinary situation. The female has a metaphase complement like that in *D. persimilis* or *D. pseudoobscura.* The male has V-shaped X and Y chromosomes and an unpaired rod obviously corresponding to one of the autosomes (the third) of its relatives. The chromosome number is consequently odd (9) instead of even (10). It has been shown that *D. miranda* has a "neo-X," the female being $X_1X_1X_2X_2$, and the male X_1X_2Y (Dobzhansky, 1935*b,* 1937). In the salivary gland nuclei of male larvae three pale strands are visible. They correspond to the two limbs of the X_1 and to the X_2; in other species only two strands are pale. MacKnight (1939) found largely heterochromatic sections included in the chromocenter in *D. miranda* males. These are evidently the remains of a chromosome homologous to the X_2 of *D. miranda* and to the third autosome of *D. pseudoobscura* and *D. persimilis.*

A considerable number of chromosome fusions, separations, and inversions have taken place in the phylogeny of the *obscura* species group. It is quite probable that some pericentric inversions have also occurred, breaking and modifying the so-called "elements" of the chromosome set (Sturtevant and Novitski, 1941). The evidence is, however, incomplete, especially for the Old World species.

Linkage and Cytological Maps in *D. pseudoobscura*

A fair number of mutants have been obtained and their linkage relations studied, in only one New World species, namely *D. pseudoobscura* (and in only one Old World species, *D. subobscura*). Lancefield (1922), Crew and Lamy (1935, 1936), and Tan (1936) published linkage maps, the most adequate of which was that for the X chromosome. The length of that map (some 180 Morgan units) suggested that the X of *D. pseudoobscura* must contain materials homologous to the X and to a part of one of the autosomes in *D. melanogaster*. This matter was elaborated further by Donald (1936) and by Sturtevant and Tan (1937). The homologies of the chromosome limbs ("elements") in *D. pseudoobscura* and *D. melanogaster* were found to be thus:

pseudoobscura	XL	XR	II	III	IV	V
melanogaster	X	IIIL	IIIR	IIR	IIL	IV

The map lengths in Morgan units and the numbers of the loci mapped (given in parentheses) were as follows: X chromosome, 181 (29); second, 101 (11); third, 68 (11); fourth, 69 (7); and fifth, 0 (1). Most of the mutants of *D. pseudoobscura* were homologized with those known in *D. melanogaster* on the basis of phenotypic resemblance. Assuming these homologies to be reliable, one reaches the conclusion that, although the

TABLE 1.   *Chromosome Complements*

Species	Autosomes	X chromosome	Y chromosome
D. subobscura	4 Rods, 1 dot	Rod	Rod
D. pseudoobscura	3 Rods, 1 dot	V	Variable
D. persimilis	3 Rods, 1 dot	V	Variable
D. lowei	2 Rods, 1 V, 1 dot	V	Hook shaped
D. bifasciata	3 V's, 1 dot	V	Rod
D. imaii	3 V's, 1 dot	V	Rod
D. ambigua	3 V's, 1 dot	V	Rod
D. tristis	3 V's, 1 dot	V	Hook shaped
D. obscura	2 V's, 2 rods, 1 dot	V	Rod
D. alpina	1 V, no dots	V	V (?)

chromosomal elements remained intact despite fusions or separations, the gene arrangements within the elements were pretty radically scrambled by paracentric inversions.

Tan (1935, 1937) proceeded to identify the genetically established linkage groups with cytologically visible chromosomes, especially the giant chromosomes in the larval salivary gland cells. For this purpose he used the sibling species *D. pseudoobscura* and *D. persimilis* (then designated race A and race B, respectively). Four of the five chromosomal strands in these species differ in inverted blocks of genes, which can easily be seen under the microscope in the salivary gland cells in hybrids. Translocations and some deficiencies were also obtained at that time. Tan established correlations between these cytologically visible features and the mutant markers, and published very rough cytological maps, showing the approximate locations of some gene loci in terms of the disc patterns of the salivary gland chromosomes. Hardly any further progress has occurred in this field since then.

Genetic Burden

With rare exceptions, individuals of a species of *Drosophila* collected in nature are uniform in appearance. There is variation is size, but this is largely a result of abundance or scarcity of food during larval development and the temperature at which the larvae had grown. Observations and experiments on chromosomal variation have, however, shown that despite outward uniformity, a great deal of genetic diversity is present. But even this is only the top of the iceberg. Natural populations carry what at the time of its discovery seemed an astounding amount of recessive genetic variants concealed in heterozygous state.

The pioneer work in this field was done in *D. melanogaster,* beginning with Chetverikov (1927), and in *D. pseudoobscura* by Sturtevant (1937). Comparative study of populations of *D. pseudoobscura* in various localities for lethals and viability modifiers in the third chromosome was started by Dobzhansky and Queal (1938) and Dobzhansky (1939a). The study of the other autosomes (second and fourth chromosomes) had to wait for construction of analyzer chromosomes with inversions and mutant markers (Dobzhansky *et al.,* 1942). Analyzer chromosomes in *D. persimilis* were prepared and utilized by Dobzhansky and Spassky (1953) and Dobzhansky *et al.* (1954).

In every species and every chromosome studied in this respect, the viability of homozygotes for wild chromosomes shows a bimodal distribution. One mode is represented by complete lethals and the other by "quasinormal" chromosomes. Semilethals are relatively rare. "Normal" viability (or fecundity, development rate, etc.) is defined as the average viability in a given environment of individuals having the two homologous chromosomes of each pair taken at random from a given population. With the aid of a statistical technique devised by Wallace and Madden (1953), it is possible to separate the quasinormal chromosomes into subvital, normal, and supervital ones. The lethals, semilethals, and subvitals constitute the genetic burden (or load); the supervitals are the genetic elite of the population (Dobzhansky and Spassky, 1963). Table 2 gives a summary of the frequencies of different classes of chromosomes in *D. pseudoobscura* and *D. persimilis* according to Dobzhansky and Spassky (1953) as corrected by Sankaranarayanan (1965). The frequencies of subvital, normal, supervital, and sterility-inducing chromosomes are shown, of course, among chromosomes that are not lethal or semilethal.

It can easily be seen that very few individuals in nature carry chromosomes which would all give normal viability and fertility if they should become homozygous. Deleterious effects of inbreeding are a consequence of this fact. Although the prevalence of genetic burdens varies somewhat in populations of a species as well as in different species, genetic burdens are probably universal in sexually reproducing and normally outbreeding organisms. Table 2 shows the incidence of chromosomes that, when homozygous, induce viability modifications or complete sterility of one or the other sex. Other kinds of modifications have also been found—morphological mutants, prolonged or speeded up development, and quantitative variations of fertility and fecundity. These last categories have been carefully studied, especially by Marinkovic (1967a,b).

TABLE 2. *Effects of Homozygous Autosomes from Natural Populations of Drosophila pseudoobscura (in Percentages)*

	D. pseudoobscura			D. persimilis		
	Second	*Third*	*Fourth*	*Second*	*Third*	*Fourth*
Lethal and semilethal	33.0	25.0	25.9	25.5	22.7	28.1
Subvital	93.5	78.3	69.9	66.9	79.8	98.4
Normal	6.4	21.7	30.0	32.8	17.5	1.2
Supervital	0.10	0.02	0.04	0.3	2.7	0.4
Female sterile	10.6	13.6	4.3	18.3	14.3	18.3
Male sterile	8.3	10.5	11.8	13.2	15.7	8.4

Release of Genetic Variability by Recombination

The data in Table 2 describe the incidence in populations of lethal, subvital, etc., *chromosomes,* not genes. A chromosome that is lethal in double dose may have a single lethal, it may have two or more gene variants at different loci which are lethal when combined but not when they are separate, or, finally, it may have several subvitals which are lethal in the aggregate.

Dobzhansky (1946) isolated three second chromosomes from a population of *D. pseudoobscura.* One of them (A) was nearly normally viable in double dose at 16°C, semilethal at 21°C, and lethal at 25°C. Two chromosomes (B and C) were normal or supervital at all three temperatures. By appropriate intercrosses, 100 chromosomes were obtained, some of which were combinations of parts of A and B, 29 were combinations of A and C, and 33 were combinations of B and C. Testing these recombination products for their effects in double dose revealed a remarkable variety of situations. Some recombinants were lethal or semilethal at temperatures at which none of the ancestral chromosomes were. These are "synthetic" lethals or semilethals. Others evinced retardations of the development, morphological abnormalities, etc.

Spassky *et al.* (1958), Spiess (1959), Dobzhansky *et al.* (1959), and Levene (1959) studied the release of genetic variability by recombination in *D. pseudoobscura, D. persimilis,* and *D. prosaltans.* The common method adopted in these studies was to isolate 10 quasinormally viable chromosomes from each of two natural populations of each species. Strains with these chromosomes were intercrossed in all combinations— 90 within and 100 between populations. Females carrying each pair of wild chromosomes were bred to males with appropriate mutant markers. Ten sons were taken from each female (900 from intrapopulational and 1000 from interpopulational crosses). The second chromosomes of these sons were analyzed for their viability in homozygous condition.

A great amount of genetic variability is released by recombination of the genes that were carried in the original chromosomes. The viability of the recombinants in homozygous condition ranges from normal, through subvital and semilethal, to lethal. It must be stressed that synthetic lethals and semilethals arise by recombination of chromosomes normally viable when homozygous (although some authors repeatedly misquote these results, alleging that lethals and semilethals come only from pairs of subvital chromosomes). Most important is the fact that the genetic variability released by recombination constitutes a sizeable fraction of the total variability present in natural populations. Estimates of the viability variance in the second chromosomes of *D. pseudoobscura* and *D. persimilis* are given in Table 3. Quasinormal chromosomes are by no means identical "typical" chromosomes of the species. They store an immense amount of genetic diversity.

If lethals can be "synthesized," it should also be possible to "desynthesize" them. Dobzhansky and Spassky (1960) took a sample of 12 synthetic-lethal second chromosomes obtained in the experiment described above and attempted to locate these lethals on the genetic map of the chromosome by recombination with various mutant markers. Only two of the twelve lethals proved to be so localizable; these were presumably single-locus lethals which arose by mutation rather than by recombination. The remaining ten were suppressed by crossing over. Quite similar results with lethal "suppressors" were later obtained in *D. willistoni* by other investigators (see the review of the *willistoni* species group in the present volume).

Heterozygosis and Homeostasis

The viability of the carriers of many genotypes is very sensitive to all sorts of environmental variations, e.g., temperature, larval crowding, kind of food, etc. Moreover, homozygotes for chromosomes carried in wild populations are far more sensitive to environmental changes than are heterozygotes (Dobzhansky and Spassky, 1944); yet chromosomes which give normally viable and even supervital homozygotes still exist (Table 2). Are they as good as heterozygotes? Dobzhansky *et al.* (1955) and Dobzhansky and Levene (1955) attempted to elucidate this problem. From a sample of 128 second chromosomes of a wild population of *D. pseudoobscura,* 19 chromosomes were selected; 10 gave normal or

TABLE 3. *Viability Variance in Second Chromosomes*[a]

Species	Present in nature	Released by recombination
Drosophila pseudoobscura		
All Chromosomes	140	60
Quasinormal	65	48
Drosophila persimilis		
All Chromosomes	110	26
Quasinormal	60	16

[a] Dobzhansky *et al.* (1959).

supervital homozygotes and 9 gave subvital homozygotes under standard test conditions. By means of suitable intercrosses, 10 kinds of heterozygotes were obtained which had both chromosomes normal or supervital, 9 which had one normal and the other subvital, and 8 which had two subvital chromosomes. The 19 homozygotes and 27 heterozygotes were then tested for viability at different temperatures, from 4°C to 27°C, and on culture media inoculated with different species of yeasts. Not a single homozygous chromosome selected for normality or supervitality at standard conditions conserved this status in all the environments in which it was placed. The nine chromosomes subvital at standard conditions sometimes improved and sometimes deteriorated further in changed environments. All heterozygotes were viable in all environments, although some of them were better or worse than others in some environments. What seemed important and significant was that heterozygotes with two normal, two subvital, or one normal and one subvital chromosomes were, on the average, equally viable. The viabilities in homozygous and heterozygous conditions were not correlated. The chromosomes chosen because of their normal to supervital records in homozygotes were "environmentally narrow specialists;" the developmental pattern of heterozygotes was homeostatically buffered.

It should, of course, be kept in mind that the above studies concentrated attention on only some components of genetic burdens or loads, chiefly egg-to-adult viability and fertility *vs.* sterility. However, Darwinian fitness is determined by other factors as well—fecundity, longevity, speed of development, etc. Sved and Ayala (1970) in *D. pseudoobscura* and Mourão *et al.* (1972) in *D. willistoni* cast the dragnet more widely. Having selected chromosomes from wild populations which yielded normal or only mildly subvital homozygotes, they made them compete with heterozygotes carrying the same chromosomes and also chromosomes with certain mutant marker genes. The fitness of the homozygotes turned out to be distinctly below normal.

Geographic Differences in Genetic Burdens

Autosomal recessive lethals are valuable materials for studies on the genetic population structure since their incidence in populations can be simply and unambiguously scored. If the lethals are completely recessive, the mutation rates that produce them uniform, and the genetically effective population size (N_e) large enough to be treated as infinite, then all populations of a species should have the same aggregate frequencies of lethals and the same frequencies of lethals at particular loci. Already

Dobzhansky and Wright (1941) and Wright *et al.* (1942) showed that these expectations are not realized in *D. pseudoobscura*. Percentages of third chromosomes that are lethal in double dose range from 13.9 on Mount San Jacinto and 17.0 in the Death Valley region of California, to 30.0 in Mexico and Guatemala (confirming these estimates with new data would be most desirable). More importantly, 2.13 ± 0.32 percent of the lethals encountered within territories of roughly 10,000 square meters are allelic, compared to 0.88 ± 0.20 percent in localities some 15 miles apart, and 0.41 ± 0.08 percent in localities some hundreds of miles apart. This was originally ascribed to random genetic drift in populations of limited effective size, isolated by distance or by barriers to migration.

About 1 percent of third chromosomes per generation acquire new lethals by mutation in *D. pseudoobscura* and 1.78 percent in *D. persimilis* at similar temperatures in laboratory experiments (Dobzhansky *et al.,* 1954). Wright [in Dobzhansky and Wright (1941)] pointed out that this mutation frequency is about four times greater than necessary to account for the observed frequencies of lethal chromosomes in nature. The discrepancy indicates either that some of the lethals are incompletely recessive and are selected against in heterozygotes or that matings of close relatives are frequent, or that both factors operate to depress the frequencies of lethals. This issue is closely related to the problem discussed in the following section.

Mutational and Balanced Loads

The universal presence in natural populations of deleterious genetic variants may be accounted for by either one of the following two causes, or a combination of both. First, the mutation pressure continuously supplies such variants, and some of them persist for several generations until eliminated by normalizing natural selection; this is the mutational genetic burden (or load). Second, variants deleterious in homozygous condition may be heterotic when heterozygous, or those disadvantageous in one environment may be advantageous in other environments; this is the balanced or segregational genetic load. Much work has been done in *D. melanogaster* and *D. pseudoobscura* attempting to distinguish the mutational and balanced components of genetic burdens.

There is no doubt that a majority of newly arisen mutants are deleterious, both when homozygous and heterozygous. For x-ray-induced mutants this has been shown in *D. pseudoobscura* by Mourad (1962, 1964), and ample evidence is available in *D. melanogaster*. It should, however, be kept in mind that the mutants found in natural populations are not an unbiased sample of mutants that arise owing to the mutation pressure. While some mutants in nature arose in the generation sampled or a few generations earlier, others may have persisted for many generations and thus passed a scrutiny of natural selection. As pointed out above, the mutation rate, at least that observed in laboratory experiments, is much higher than would be expected if the lethal mutants were fully recessive and if no inbreeding occurred in natural habitats. Spassky *et al.* (1960) and Dobzhansky *et al.* (1960) studied the viabilities of homozygotes and heterozygotes for 156 second and 153 third chromosomes at different temperatures. The viability effects of some chromosomes are sensitive to temperature, and other chromosomes are independent of temperature; environmental sensitivity is generally greater in chromosomes with deficient viability (subvitals) than in normal ones. No correlation was found between the viabilities of homozygotes and heterozygotes for the same chromosome, except that some chromosomes which were supervital when homozygous also produced exceptionally viable heterozygotes. This was confirmed by Dobzhansky and Spassky (1963), and also by Wallace and Dobzhansky (1962), using the statistical technique of "ordered homozygotes." Wills (1966) found no deleterious effects of lethals when they were heterozygous, but he found some deleterious effects of subvitals. Interestingly enough, the lightest genetic burden was found in the isolated marginal population of *D. pseudoobscura* from Bogotá, Colombia (Dobzhansky *et al.*, 1963a), while the most flourishing central populations carry the heaviest genetic burdens.

All the experiments referred to above tested the viability effects of chromosomes from natural populations, not only in laboratory environments but also on the genetic backgrounds of laboratory tester stocks. Dobzhansky and Spassky (1968) and Anderson (1969) endeavored to remedy this last defect. By means of a series of crosses, wild second chromosomes, lethal and quasinormal when homozygous, were tested on the genetic backgrounds of *D. pseudoobscura* populations from which they came and also on foreign genetic backgrounds. The same chromosomes were tested also on a mixed Mexican–Guatemalan genetic background. The viability of heterozygotes for lethal chromosomes was equal, or even superior, to that of quasinormal chromosomes on their "native" genetic background; on foreign backgrounds, the lethal chromosomes were equal or inferior to the quasinormal ones.

Morton *et al.* (1956) suggested a statistic which, they believed, could discriminate between mutational and balanced genetic loads. It is based on the loss of viability (or fitness) from genetic causes in outbred populations (A) relative to that which would occur at complete homozygosis (B). The value *B* cannot be observed directly, and it is inferred by extrapolation from viability losses at various low degrees of inbreeding. Dobzhansky *et al.* (1963*b*) compared viabilities (or mortalities) of the progenies of *D. pseudoobscura* collected in nature—individuals not known to be related, brother–sister matings, and half-sib matings. The *B* : *A* ratios of 4.5–5.8 were obtained. Such ratios are ambiguous in the sense that they could occur with various proportions of mutational and balanced loads. The estimation of *B* values is based on the assumption of lack of epistatic (synergistic) interactions of the components of the genetic loads. This assumption was tested by Spassky *et al.* (1965) and found not to be valid for *D. pseudoobscura*. The viability losses were compared in homozygotes for wild second, wild third, and simultaneously for second and third chromosomes. The loss of viability in double homozygotes was greater than expected on the assumption of no epistatic interactions. The problem of relative importance of the mutational and balanced burdens in *D. pseudoobscura* remains open.

Adaptive Changes in Laboratory Cultures

The presence in populations of genetic variance concerned with viability, and also the occurrence of mutations changing the fitnesses of their carriers, invites attempts to create in the laboratory models of adaptive evolution that may also occur in nature. Dobzhansky and Spassky (1947) selected 3 second and 4 fourth chromosomes of *D. pseudoobscura* which were subvital to semilethal in homozygotes. Two strains homozygous for each chromosome and two having these chromosomes balanced in heterozygous condition were prepared. The homozygous strains were bred in deliberately overpopulated cultures, and the heterozygous ones without crowding. One homozygous and one heterozygous culture with each chromosome received 1000 r units of x-rays in every generation, the others were not irradiated. After 50 generations of this regimen, all chromosomes were tested for viability. In five out of the seven the viability improved, sometimes up to normal, in both the irradiated and the unirradiated line; one chromosome showed no improvement with or without radiation, and the last improved in the irradiated but not in the unirradiated line. Strikingly different were the results in lines with balanced chromosomes. In 7 out of 14 lines the chromosomes became lethal, in 1 they become semilethal, and in 6 there was no change or there was only a slight improvement. In the homozygous lines there has clearly been natural selection for genetic variants compensating for the original subvitality;

where the chromosomes were kept balanced in heterozygous condition there was no impediment for further accumulation of genes harmful when homozygous. It was possible to demonstrate that the genetic improvements were sometimes due to the occurrence of new mutations in the chromosomes concerned and sometimes to selection of genetic variants present in the strains.

In 1958, Vetukhiv started six originally identical populations of *D. pseudoobscura* in population cages, two maintained at 16°C, two at 25°C, and two at 27°C. After his untimely death, the populations were maintained and studied by Ehrman (1964), Mourad (1965), Anderson (1966, 1973), and Kitagawa (1967). The populations became genetically different in body size: those bred at the lowest temperature being the largest and those at the highest temperature the smallest. The size differences were of the same order as those obtained by artificial selection directed specifically at body size by Druger (1962) and found in natural populations of different geographic origin by Anderson (1968). The populations became also different in longevity and showed traces of sexual isolation, but these differences were not correlated with temperature. Most remarkably, the outcrosses between the populations tended to produce heterosis in F_1 and hybrid breakdown in F_2 generation.

Allozyme Variation

Populations of *D. pseudoobscura* were among the first of any species to be extensively surveyed for enzyme variation. Hubby and Lewontin (1966) and Lewontin and Hubby (1966) showed how the technique of gel electrophoresis can be used to obtain quantitative estimates of genetic variation in populations. The term *allozyme* was introduced later (Prakash *et al.*, 1969) to describe "the variant proteins produced by allelic forms of the same locus, to avoid the now common confusion with 'isozymes' which are the various polymers produced from monomers specified by different loci." The papers of Lewontin and Hubby should be consulted for the theory underlying the use of this technique as well as the drawbacks and biases inherent to it.

Table 4 gives the amounts of genic variation found in various species of the *obscura* group. In this table, a locus is considered polymorphic if the frequency of the most common allele is 0.95 or less in one half or more of the populations studied. The data summarized in this table are from Prakash *et al.* (1969), Prakash (1969), and Lakovaara and Saura (1971*a,b*). This amount of variation is somewhat less than found in the neotropical group of species related to *D. willistoni* (see Chapter 21 in this volume).

How is this variability distributed among populations? Prakash *et al.* (1969) studied four populations of *D. pseudoobscura*. These populations included one they considered a central population (Strawberry Canyon), two marginal populations (Mesa Verde and Austin), and one isolated population (Bogotá). In general, the three North American populations showed very little genic differentiation. At almost all of the 24 loci studied the same alleles were found in approximately the same frequencies in all populations. What genic differentiation does occur is primarily at loci associated with inversion polymorphisms (see below). The isolated population, Bogotá, is most distinctive, having about one-third less variation. The Bogotá population is fixed, or nearly so, for the most common allele at several loci which are polymorphic in the other populations. However, at three loci the Bogotá population has a high frequency of, or is fixed for, an allele relatively rare in the other three populations. The reduction in variation is due perhaps to a "founder effect," although the founders may not have come from the center of the distribution of the species. The third-chromosome gene-arrangement frequencies indicate that the Guatemala population may well be the origin of the founders of the Bogotá population (Dobzhansky *et al.*, 1963a). Some reproductive isolation exists between the Bogotá and North American populations (Prakash, 1972).

Saura *et al.* (1973) studied 20 enzyme loci in several populations of *D. subobscura*. These included populations from much of the distribution of the species, including some marginal populations from southern Finland. Most loci show very little differentiation among the populations; six loci, however, do show local differences. One locus, *Est-8,* shows considerable differentiation: allele 1.15 varies from a frequency of 0.04 in

TABLE 4. *Amounts of Genic Variation in Species of the obscura Group Detected by Gel Electrophoresis*

Species	Number loci studied	Percent loci polymorphic	Percent heterozygosity per individual
D. pseudoobscura	24	33	12.3
D. persimilis	24	25[a]	10.5
D. subobscura	31	26	7.6
D. obscura	30	33	11.0

[a] Exact frequencies of alleles were not given for this species; this figure is an estimate.

a sample from Finland to 0.94 in a population from eastern Alps. The overall amount of variation is not different in various parts of the distribution area.

Lakovaara and Saura (1971*a*) studied 33 loci in 57 populations of *D. obscura*. Two loci, *Aph-4* and *Est-7* (loci coding for akaline phosphatase and esterase, respectively), exhibited significant north–south clines in the frequencies of their most common alleles. Two highly polymorphic esterase loci, *Est-5* and *Est-6,* showed considerable geographic differentiation. The remainder of the loci showed no significant differentiation among the populations.

Studies of protein variation have also been used to elucidate genic differentiation among various gene arrangements of the third chromosome of *D. pseudoobscura* (Prakash and Lewontin, 1968, 1971). Because recombination is suppressed in inversion heterozygotes over most of the third chromosome, very little mixing of genes between gene arrangements occurs. Evidence of selection of gene arrangements indicates considerable genic differentiation of chromosomes with different gene arrangements (see below). Protein markers can be used to identify specific gene differences among gene arrangements. Three loci on the third chromosome have been shown to be differentiated among the gene arrangements. An allele at a larval protein locus, *Pt-10*$^{1.04}$, is in very high frequency or is fixed in gene arrangements of the standard phylad (ST, AR, and PP). *Pt-10*$^{1.06}$ is characteristic of the Santa Cruz phylad. *D. persimilis* is characterized by allele 1.04, which could be predicted as the species is derived from the ST phylad. Alleles at the α-amylase locus are somewhat less differentiated. The SC phylad is essentially *Amy-1*$^{0.84}$, the ST phylad is *Amy-1*$^{1.00}$, and *D. persimilis* has allele 1.00 plus several alleles not present in *D. pseudoobscura*. Alleles at *Pt-12* show a different pattern of differentiation. The ST phylad in *D. pseudoobscura* and WT in *D. persimilis* are characterized by a high frequency of one allele, while all other gene arrangements in both species have a high frequency of another allele.

The sex-ratio (SR) condition in *D. pseudoobscura* is characterized by an X chromosome with three inversions in the right arm relative to the standard arrangement (ST) (see details below). Alleles at two sex-linked loci have been shown to be differentiated between the two X chromosome gene arrangements (Prakash and Merritt, 1972). Allele 1.04 at the esterase-5 locus is at a frequency of 0.8–0.9 in SR and only about 0.01 in ST. A null allele at the adult acid phosphatase-6 locus is fixed in SR and is found only with a frequency of about 0.6 in ST.

Besides these allozyme–gene arrangement interactions, Zouros and Krimbas (1973) have clearly demonstrated interactions between two enzyme loci in *D. subobscura*. Alleles at *Xdh* (xanthine dehydrogenase locus) and *AO* (acetaldehyde oxidase locus) are nonrandomly associated and exhibit similar significant linkage disequilibria in two widely separated populations. These two loci are 9 centiMorgans apart on the same chromosome. The associations were shown to be independent of chromosome inversion polymorphisms.

Dobzhansky and Ayala (1973) have simultaneously followed seasonal changes in gene arrangements and in allozyme frequencies in two populations of *D. pseudoobscura* and *D. persimilis*. As expected, gene arrangements of the third chromosome of *D. pseudoobscura* showed clear-cut seasonal changes. *D. persimilis* also showed significant changes in third chromosome gene-arrangement frequencies at one locality. Allele frequencies at two enzyme loci, *Pgm-1* (phosphoglucomutase) and *Me-2* (malic enzyme), showed much smaller but significant seasonal changes. Data on those loci known to be associated with the gene arrangements were not presented in this report.

It should be noted that all of these studies on allozyme variation in the various species of the *obscura* group indicate that some form of selection is acting at protein loci. The results are incompatible with the theory that most protein variation is selectively "neutral." Furthermore, it is clear that the population dynamics of and selective pressures on chromosomal polymorphisms and protein polymorphisms must differ in some important aspects [see Powell *et al.* (1972) for a brief discussion of these differences]. Because many species of the *obscura* group exhibit widespread inversion and allozyme polymorphisms, this group affords favorable material for comparative studies.

Allozymes have also been used to study the genetic relationships among various species of the *obscura* group. While differentiation within species tends to be slight, interspecific differences are generally considerable and many of them diagnostic. Lakovaara *et al.* (1972) studied seven European and four American members of the *obscura* group. These species were compared with respect to electrophoretically detectable differences at 27 enzyme loci. In comparing pairs of species it was shown that the major allele is different at 15–85 percent of the loci studied. Because of the limitations of the technique, these are minimal estimates of the total genetic differences. The phylogenetic relationships of these 11 species, as determined by allozyme studies, are in good agreement with the phylogeny based on chromosome and morphological studies [see Lakovaara *et al.* (1972) for references and discussion].

Because of the relatively large allozymic differences among species, electrophoresis can be useful for identification of sibling species (Ayala and Powell, 1972). Among the three North American siblings, *D. pseudoobscura, D. persimilis,* and *D. miranda,* 15–28 percent of the loci studied allow correct diagnosis of species with an accuracy of 99 percent or better; 4–17 percent of the loci allow correct diagnosis of species with an accuracy of 99.9 percent or greater.

Intraspecific Chromosomal Polymorphisms

Every *obscura* group species studied in this respect displays chromosomal polymorphisms of various sorts. Six kinds of Y chromosomes have been encountered in natural populations of *D. pseudoobscura* and three kinds in *D. persimilis* (Dobzhansky, 1935b, 1937b). As seen in metaphase plates in dividing spermatogonial cells, these kinds differ in size and in the locations of their centromeres; in the salivary gland cells the Y chromosome is not conveniently studiable. The commonest type of Y in *D. pseudoobscura* is hook-shaped, with the ratios of the two limbs divided by the centromere either about 1:4 (type IV) or 1:3 (type V). However, in southern Arizona, parts of New Mexico, Colorado, Mexico, and Guatemala some or all males have V-shaped Y chromosomes, seemingly of three different sizes (types I, VI, and VII). *D. persimilis* has a V-shaped metacentric or submetacentric Y (types I, II, and III). In the Northwest (Washington, British Columbia) Y chromosomes seem to be smaller (type II), and in the Sierra Nevada of California they are more unequal-armed (type III). A caveat must be entered at this point—the discrimination of some of the types may not be reliable, although the existence of polymorphism is beyond reasonable doubt.

Only two translocation heterozygotes have ever been encountered in nature, each in a single individual of *D. pseudoobscura.* By far the commonest polymorphisms are paracentric inversions (i.e., not including the centromeres). Moreover, in *D. pseudoobscura, D. persimilis, D. miranda,* and apparently in *D. lowei,* inversion polymorphisms are concentrated mainly in one of the autosomes, designated the third chromosome (III). This is the same chromosome which in *D. miranda* has become transformed into the neo-X (see above). In contrast to the variant Y chromosomes, the variant gene arrangements can be diagnosed quite reliably and accurately. To date, 22 gene arrangements in the third chromosome have been found in *D. pseudoobscura,* and 11 in *D. persimilis* (Dobzhansky, 1970; page 132). Only occasional inversions, found in single individuals or in single localities, have been encountered in the second and fourth chromosomes (Dobzhansky and Epling, 1944). The inversions associated with the "sex-ratio" conditions in the X chromosomes are a separate story and will be dealt with below.

Sturtevant and Dobzhansky (1936*a*) and Dobzhansky and Sturtevant (1938) have distinguished three situations which arise when two or more inversions occur in the same chromosome. The inversion may be independent, one may be included into the other, or they may be overlapping. This last kind is most interesting since it permits inferences of phylogenetic relationships and prediction of yet-undiscovered gene arrangements. It happens that the inversions in the third chromosomes of *D. pseudoobscura* and *D. persimilis* are mostly of the overlapping kind. A phylogeny of the gene arrangements in these species was devised by Dobzhansky and Sturtevant (1938) and improved by Dobzhansky and Epling (1944) and Dobzhansky (1970). As shown in Figure 1, only one gene arrangement, the Standard, occurs in both species, and only one, the hypothetical, has not actually been observed. The phylogenetic "tree" in Figure 1 does not, strictly speaking, define which of the gene arrangements is the ancestral one. However, it is most probable that one of four arrangements is the ancestor: Standard, Hypothetical, Santa Cruz, or Tree Line. In Figure 1 these arrangements are connected by double arrows, the remainder by single arrows. Most of the gene arrangements in the peripheral part of the "tree" are narrowly endemic or have been seen but once; the common ones tend to be found at or near the trunk of the "tree."

Inversion polymorphisms have also been found in the third chromosomes of *D. miranda* (Dobzhansky, unpublished) and of *D. lowei* (Heed *et al.,* 1969). Excellent photographic records of inversion configurations in *D. pseudoobscura* has been published by Kastritis and Crumpacker (1966, 1967).

"Sex-Ratio" Chromosomes

Gershenson (1928), in one of the European species of the *obscura* group, and Sturtevant and Dobzhansky (1936*b*), in *D. pseudoobscura* and *D. persimilis,* observed that some males collected in nature give progenies consisting mostly or only of daughters. These unisexual progenies depend only on the fathers, regardless of what females they are mated with. Sex-ratio (SR) males of *D. pseudoobscura* always have three independent inversions in the right limb of the X chromosome (XR). None of these inversions are found in normal males. The XR of SR *D. persimilis* males differs in a single inversion from normal males. Curiously enough, the XR

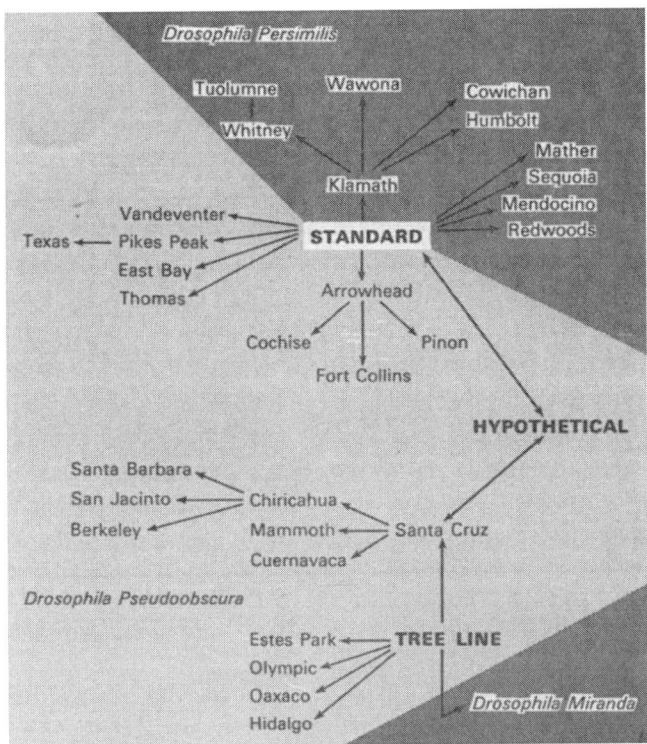

Figure 1. The phylogenetic relationships of the gene arrangements in the third chromosome of D. psuedoobscura and its relatives.

of *D. persimilis* SR is identical in gene arrangement with normal *D. pseudoobscura,* while the XR's of the normal males of the two species always differ in a single inversion. Of course, SR chromosomes occur in females as well as in males, but in the former they have no effect on the proportion of the sexes in the progeny (Sturtevant and Dobzhansky, 1936*b*; Dobzhansky, 1939*b*; Dobzhansky and Epling, 1944).

The mode of action of the SR chromosomes is not entirely clear. Sturtevant and Dobzhansky (1936*b*) believed that in SR males the X chromosome divides twice, the Y chromosome is eliminated, and all sperms carry X chromosomes. Novitski *et al.* (1965) and Polikansky and Ellison (1970) claim that the spermatids receiving a Y but no X chromosome fail to develop into spermatozoa, and the sperm bundles in SR males contain only half as many sperm as in normal males. The X chromosome of the SR kind somehow incapacitates the spermatids that fail to include it.

The frequency of SR is geographically variable. In *D. pseudoobscura* it shows a gradient from the Pacific Northwest, where it is absent or rare, to the southwestern United States and northern Mexico, where it reaches frequencies of 10–20 percent (Dobzhansky and Epling, 1944). What maintains the SR in natural populations is an interesting problem. Since SR males transmit their X chromosomes to their entire progeny while normal males transmit it to only half of their progeny, the SR chromosomes have an inherent selective advantage. If not controlled by some other factor, they should reach frequencies of 100 percent, whereupon the population must either become parthenogenetic or die out. Wallace (1948) studied experimental laboratory populations which were made to contain certain percentages of SR chromosomes. He found that at 25°C the Darwinian fitness of SR males is below that of normal ones, homozygous SR/SR females have a fitness close to zero, while heterozygous females are superior to homozygous normals. At $16 \pm 0.5°$C the SR males are superior to normals, and heterozygous females superior to both homozygotes.

Geography of Autosomal Inversions

Already Dobzhansky and Sturtevant (1938) saw that the populations of *D. pseudoobscura* and *D. persimilis* contain different variant gene arrangements in their third chromosomes in different localities. Dobzhansky and Epling (1944) mapped the distribution areas of both species for their chromosomal polymorphs. A given fly population can be described in terms of relative frequencies of gene arrangements in its gene pool, rather like human populations in terms of blood group alleles in their gene pools. Neighboring populations have generally rather similar chromosome frequencies, while remote populations can be very different. Plotting the frequencies in localities along a geographic transect often reveals gradients (clines), an example of which is shown in Figure 2. A gradient can be steeper in some places than in others. For example, standard chromosomes (ST) wane and arrowhead (AR) wax in frequencies moderately between the Pacific Coast ranges and the Sierra Nevada–Cascades, but east of the mountains the former rapidly dwindle and the later become predominant. Localities only a dozen or so miles apart can be very different in the chromosomal composition of their populations [for example, the three localities on Mount San Jacinto in California (Dobzhansky, 1947), also see Koller (1939)]. Sometimes the chromosomal changes strikingly parallel changes in some environmental factor, as for example the elevation above sea level in the Sierra Nevada (Dobzhansky, 1948a). In *D. persimilis,* the populations of the Sierra Nevada are chromosomally

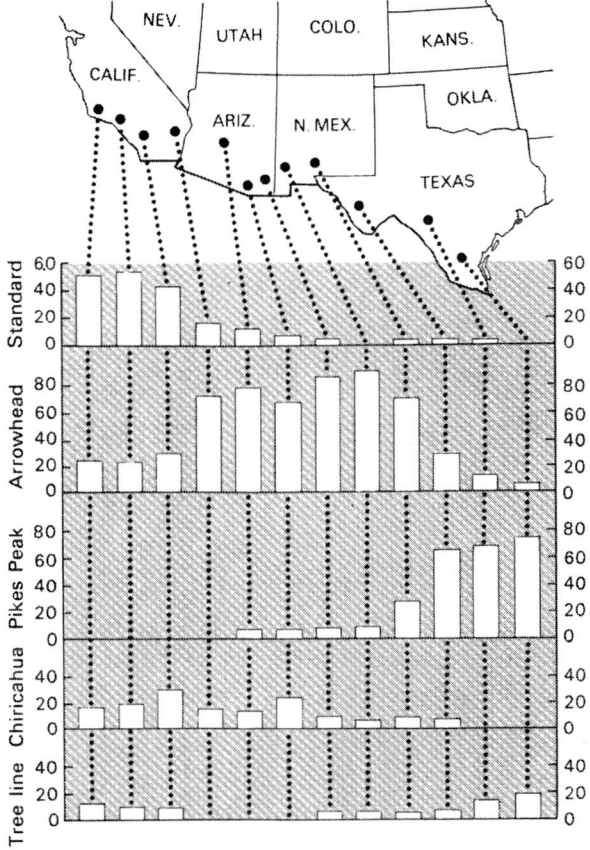

Figure 2. An example of geographic gradient of frequencies of third chromosomes with certain gene arrangements in D. psuedoobscura.

rather different from those of the Coast Ranges of California; these mountains are separated only by the hot valley where the species is rare or absent.

Powell *et al.* (1972) obtained quantitative estimates of the value of knowing the chromosomal composition of an individual for diagnosis of its geographic origin. This value is often considerable. Thus, an individual of *D. pseudoobscura* from southern Mexico will only very rarely have the gene arrangements in its two third chromosomes identical with those of a fly from California, Texas, or Colorado. One can say that this species contains the following geographic races differing in chromosome frequencies: (1) Pacific Coast, (2) Intermountain Plateau, (3) Rocky Mountains and Texas, (4) North Mexico, and (5) South Mexico and Guatemala. Race (2) is nearly monomorphic for the AR gene arrangement while other races are highly polymorphic. Very often a majority of wild individuals are inversion heterozygotes.

Inversion Polymorphism and Natural Selection

The carriers of all gene arrangements in a given species appear to be identical in external appearance. This led early students to assume that chromosomal inversions are adaptively neutral traits, and that differences between populations in inversion polymorphisms arise through random genetic drift. Such assumptions became untenable with the discovery that the relative frequencies of certain inversions in *D. pseudoobscura* undergo cyclic seasonal changes in some localities (Dobzhansky, 1943, 1947*a,b*, 1971). For example, at the Piñon Flats locality, on Mount San Jacinto, California, the frequency of ST chromosomes declines, and that of CH (Chiricahua) increases between March and June, while the opposite change occurs during summer. At Mather, California, some 300 miles north of San Jacinto, ST chromosomes grow and AR diminish in frequency during the summer season; the changes are reversed apparently during winter. At Berkeley, California, ST chromosomes are most frequent during the summer and CH in winter (Strickberger and Wills, 1966).

Although the annual numbers of generations of *D. pseudoobscura* in the above localities are not known for certain, it is clear that the selection intensities needed to produce frequency changes of genetic variants as large and rapid as those observed must be quite considerable. Fortunately, these changes can be reproduced and the selection intensities measured in experimental populations kept in laboratory population cages (Wright and Dobzhansky, 1946; Pavlovsky and Dobzhansky, 1966; Anderson *et al.*, 1968). The cardinal fact that emerges from these experiments is that in any given locality the Darwinian fitness of heterokaryotypes (inversion heterozygotes) tends to be higher than of homokaryotypes (inversion homozygotes). In other words, the heterokaryotypes are heterotic. The carriers of the chromosomes that are common in the population of a given locality are usually more fit than the carriers of rare chromosomes. Despite large and not precisely estimated statistical errors, this can be seen in the example of fitness estimates of chromosomal types from the Mather locality given in Table 5. The estimates are obtained in experiments carried at 25°C, on a laboratory culture medium seeded with baker's yeast. Dobzhansky (1948*b*), Dobzhansky and Spassky (1954), and Levine and Beardmore (1959) showed that the fitness differences observed

TABLE 5.   *Fitness Estimates of Chromosomal Types from
Mather, California*[a]

Homokaryotypes		Heterokaryotypes			
AR/AR	0.58	ST/AR	1.00	AR/PP	0.33
PP/PP	0.45	ST/CH	0.76	PP/TL	0.27
ST/ST	0.35	ST/PP	0.61	CH/PP	0.26
TL/TL	0.35	ST/TL	0.51	AR/CH	0.26
CH/CH	0.26	AR/TL	0.45	CH/TL	0.19

[a] Anderson *et al.* (1968).

in *D. pseudoobscura* at 25°C virtually disappear at 15°C, while in *D. persimilis* the fitness differences are greater at low than at high temperature (Spiess, 1950). The relative fitnesses of the carriers of different chromosomes was modified by da Cunha (1951) by using culture media with different species of yeasts, and Levine (1955) and Levene *et al.* (1958) showed them to be sensitive to the genetic environments (chromosomes other than the third). Birch (1955) found the relative fitnesses quite different when larvae are exposed to crowding than when they are uncrowded. This fact may help to explain the reversals of the direction of selection in some natural populations at different seasons.

Differential Adaptedness of Karyotypes

Heterotic balanced polymorphisms can be maintained indefinitely if the fitness of a heterozygote (or a heterokaryotype) exceeds that of both homozygotes. In principle, this explains the persistence of chromosomal polymorphisms in natural as well as in experimental populations. The situation becomes more complex with three or more alleles or gene arrangements. The maintenance of polymorphisms in nature probably is due to combination of many causes, in addition to heterosis. The environment is always more-or-less heterogeneous in space and time. Genetic variants that coexist in a population may have different environmental optima. The frequency of a chromosomal type will then be a function of how frequent or rare is the environment, or environments, to which that chromosomal type is best adapted.

Rosenbaum-Moos (1955) found in *D. pseudoobscura* that the heterokaryotype ST/CH was superior in longevity to both homokaryotypes, ST/ST and CH/CH. In preadult viability, total fecundity per lifetime, and total fecundity per surviving female, both ST/CH and

ST/ST were superior to CH/CH. In a series of admirable studies, Spiess and his co-workers have brought to light behavioral differences which influence the adaptive values of karyotypes of *D. pseudoobscura* and, particularly, *D. persimilis* (Spiess, 1970; Spiess and Spiess, 1967; Spiess and Langer, 1961, 1964; Spiess *et al.,* 1966, 1971; also, Parsons and Kaul, 1966). Table 6 gives percentages of individuals of three different karyotypes in *D. persimilis* who mated in 60 minutes after they were placed together. Clearly, the carriers of WT chromosomes have a mating advantage over the carriers of KL chromosomes. In the locality where these chromosomes came from, WT is the frequent and KL the rare kind. In Table 7, the advantages of certain heterokaryotypes over homokaryotypes of *D. pseudoobscura* are expressed in terms of Spiess's so-called index of male mating speed. Another factor, also affecting behavior, may play a role in the maintenance of the chromosomal polymorphism in nature. This is the mating advantage of rare kinds of males over males that are common in the same population (see following).

Coadaptation of Gene Arrangements

Why do the chromosomes differing in inversions of blocks of genes make their carriers differ in adaptive values? Two not mutually exclusive hypotheses come under consideration. First, a change in the gene arrangement in a chromosome may induce position effects, some of which may be adaptive. Second, inversions may tie together gene complexes that are coadapted to produce heterosis with other chromosomes present in the same population. Some evidence in favor of the first hypothesis can be found in the work of Sperlich (1966). Evidence in favor of the second hypothesis first came from the observations that the chromosomes with the same gene arrangement but coming from different geographic localities may or may not produce heterosis in heterokaryotypes (Dobzhansky, 1948*b*, 1950).

TABLE 6. *Karyotype Mating Percentages in D. persimilis*

| | Females | | |
Males	WT/WT	WT/KL	KL/KL
WT/WT	84	75	30
WT/RL	74	57	16
KL/RL	63	26	18

TABLE 7. *Spiess's Index of Male*
Mating Speed

Hetero	Homo	Difference
AR/ST	AR/AR	+17.3
AR/TL	AR/AR	+17.6
AR/CH	AR/AR	+ 1.3
AR/PP	AR/AR	+ 2.9
ST/TL	ST/ST	+24.2
ST/CH	ST/ST	+ 5.1
ST/PP	ST/ST	+10.6

To analyze the situation further, Dobzhansky and Pavlovsky (1953, 1957) studied experimental populations of *D. pseudoobscura* in laboratory population cages; in some of these populations the third chromosomes with ST and CH gene arrangements were derived from the same locality in California, and in others ST chromosomes came from California, CH from Mexico, and PP from Texas. Replicate populations in which the chromosomes were of the same geographic origin gave repeatable results. The changes in the chromosomal frequencies were similar within the limits of sampling errors, and so were the equilibrium frequencies that were eventually attained. Surprisingly, with chromosomes of diverse geographic origins replicate experimental populations gave significantly diverse results. In some populations stable equilibria were achieved, but in others one of the competing chromosomal types was eliminated.

How is such "indeterminacy" to be explained? The following four assumptions make the situation comprehensible: (1) Geographic populations of a species may differ in numerous genes. (2) Chromosomes with the same gene arrangement but of different geographic origin may carry different gene complexes (supergenes). (3) Within each natural population the supergenes are coadapted to produce heterotic heterokaryotypes, but the supergenes in geographically remote populations may or may not be coadapted. (4) The fitness of a hetero- or a homokaryotype is a function of the genotype as a whole, i.e., of the chromosome involved in the inversion and of other chromosomes as well.

Evidence in support of assumption 1 has been obtained in *D. pseudoobscura* by Brncic (1954), Vetukhiv (1954, 1956, 1957), and Anderson (1968). They intercrossed populations of different geographic origin. Though morphologically indistinguishable, the F_1 hybrids between the population often exhibit heterosis (superior viability, fecundity, longevity). Not only does this heterosis disappear in the F_2 generation, but the fitness may fall below that of the parental races. It should be noted that MacFarquhar and Robertson (1963) found no evidence of such heterosis or hybrid breakdown in *D. subobscura*.

Dobzhansky and Pavlovsky (1957) reasoned that if the assumptions 2–4 are valid, the repeatability or indeterminacy of the outcomes of selection in populations of mixed geographic origin must depend on whether the populations are descended from many or from small numbers of founders. California populations with AR and Texas populations with PP chromosomes were intercrossed, and F_2 hybrids obtained. The F_2 progeny served as the source of founders for 20 experimental populations in the population cages; ten of them were started with 4000 founders, and ten others with only 20 founders each. Some 18 months later, the populations started with few founders exhibited a significantly greater diversity of chromosome frequencies than those started with many founders. The diversity is the outcome of interaction of deterministic factors (natural selection) and stochastic ones (random genetic drift). Further checks were imposed on the validity of the above interpretation. Dobzhansky and Spassky (1962) compared the results of natural selection in "bichromosomal" and "multichromosomal" populations; the former descended from a single individual of Californian origin with AR and a single Texan with PP chromosomes, the latter had 10 Californian and 10 Texan strains in their ancestry. The divergence among replicate "multichromosomal" populations was greater than among "bichromosomal" ones. Finally, Solima Simmons (1966) compared replicate populations of two sorts— some started with hybrids between two "multichromosomal" populations, and others with flies from just one such population. The replicates of hybrid origin showed considerable diversity of selection outcomes, while no significant diversity was found among the replicates stemming from a single population.

Direct evidence that the coadaptation of the supergenes can be changed in experiments by selection is afforded by the work of Strickberger (1963, 1965). Strains of *D. pseudoobscura* are kept in laboratories usually in culture bottles; experimental populations are kept in population cages. The bottle and cage environments are not identical. Suppose, then, that we start a monomorphic population with AR, and another with CH chromosomes, using as founders flies bred for many generations in bottles. After the lapse of some generations in cages, one can build polymorphic experimental populations in cages of at least four kinds: AR from cages, CH from bottles; AR from bottles, CH from cages; AR and CH from cages; and AR and CH from bottles. Strickberger found that the chromosomes from cages confer on their carriers greater fitness for life in cage environments compared to those from bottles. He also found that these new cages with different combinations of cage and bottle chromosomes do not converge to common equilibria even after three years of life in presumably similar environments. This comes close to a demonstration of irreversibility of evolution. Mourad (1962, 1964) was able to modify the coadaptation as well as the homozygous fitness of AR and CH chromosomes by x-ray treatments. When only one kind of chromosome was treated, it rapidly lost ground in competition. But if radiation exposure was stopped, the treated chromosomes recovered after several generations, sometimes up to very nearly their normal fitness.

Adaptedness of Chromosomally Polymorphic and Monomorphic Populations

Are polymorphic populations in any way better off than monomorphic ones? This problem has been approached experimentally with gene arrangements of *D. pseudoobscura* by Beardmore *et al.* (1960), Dobzhansky *et al.* (1964a), Battaglia and Smith (1961), and Ohba (1967). Population cages were set up polymorphic for AR and CH, and monomorphic for AR and for CH gene arrangements. The average weight and size of the flies were similar in all populations. However, polymorphic populations yielded greater numbers of individuals and a greater biomass than the monomorphic ones per unit of food consumed. Egg to adult viability, longevity, and fecundity of females of different ages were studied in polymorphic and monomorphic populations, and the data were used to compute the r_m (innate capacity for increase). The r_m values of polymorphic populations exceeded those of monomorphic ones kept in similar environments. The superiority of the polymorphic populations depended mainly on greater fecundity of the females rather than on greater viability or longevity. Ohba (1967) raised polymorphic and monomorphic populations under optimal conditions, in contrast with the crowded and stressful environments in earlier experiments. Under optimal conditions polymorphic populations were no longer superior to monomorphic ones.

Polymorphic populations obviously include some heterokaryotypic and homokaryotypic individuals, the latter being the same as in the monomorphic ones. It is an open question whether the superiority of polymorphic populations depends exclusively on the presence of the heterokaryotypes, or also on some kind of mutual stimulation of individuals of different karyotypes present in the same culture medium. That the latter is not a far-fetched possibility has been shown by Levene *et al.* (1954, 1958), and Pavlovsky and Dobzhansky (1966). The homo- and heterokaryotypes formed by ST, AR, and CH chromosomes of *D. pseudoobscura* were studied in different combinations. The relative fitness of karyotypes A and B may depend on whether certain other karyotypes, such as C and D, are present or absent in the same medium. In other words, the fitness of karyotypes is at least in some instances interdependent.

Cyclic and Directional Changes in Chromosome Frequencies

Reference has already been made to the seasonal cyclic changes in relative frequencies of chromosomes with different gene arrangements which occur in some populations of *D. pseudoobscura*. They are caused by selectional responses of the populations to seasonal changes in the environment. Some chromosomes have evidently higher fitness in environments prevailing at some seasons, and other chromosomes at other seasons. The selectional forces involved in seasonal changes are probably similar to those responsible for changes in space, e.g., genetic differences between populations that live at different elevations in mountains. However, it should not be assumed that if changes are seasonally cyclic, the population must have exactly the same composition during a given month of different years. This can hardly be expected because of climatic and other variations from year to year. In fact, seasonally cyclic and year-to-year directional changes in *D. pseudoobscura* were described simultaneously (Dobzhansky, 1947*a,b*).

Since approximately 1940, populations of *D. pseudoobscura* and *D. persimilis* have repeatedly been sampled, and their chromosomal constitution examined, in some 35 localities in western United States and British Columbia (Dobzhansky, 1952, 1956, 1958, 1963, 1971; Dobzhansky *et al.* 1964*b*, 1966; Epling and Lower, 1957). Two populations, those of Piñon Flats on Mount San Jacinto, and of Mather in the Sierra Nevada of California, were sampled more often than the rest, but unfortunately no population was sampled annually. The main features of the situation may be summarized as follows: Year-to-year changes, superimposed where data are available on rather smaller seasonal ones, have been taking place in the Pacific Coast states (California, Oregon, single localities in Washington and British Columbia, and a single locality in Arizona). Little if any changes have been recorded in the territory between the Rocky Mountains and the Sierra Nevada–Cascades. There has also been some instability in the Front Range of the Rockies in Colorado, in New Mexico, and in Texas.

Where changes do occur, they occur in the same direction in all or most localities in extensive territories, rather than in different localities independently. Most spectacular was the behavior of PP gene arrangement in *D. pseudoobscura* in California and other Pacific Coast states. Among approximately 20,000 third chromosomes examined from various localities in California until the mid-1940's, only 4 PP chromosomes were found (this gene arrangement is common in the Rocky Mountains and in Texas). From the late 1940's to late 1950's, the average PP frequency in California was between 6 and 8 percent, and the frequencies of this chromosomes rose also in the Pacific Northwest. Since then, PP declined again, but not to its former status of rarity.

Percentages (rounded to the nearest integer) of the five commonest gene arrangements in *D. pseudoobscura* at Mather, California are shown in Table 8. Between 1945 and 1950, ST chromosomes dwindled and AR grew in frequencies. The opposite trend prevailed from 1950 to 1961; the trend was reversed again between 1961 and 1972. CH chromosomes were waning while PP waxed in frequencies, and *vice versa*. TL chromosomes were gaining ground from mid-1960's to the 1970's. It looks as if certain pairs of gene arrangements acted as "antagonists." Insofar as data are available, similar changes took place throughout California and the Northwest.

The causation of the year-to-year changes is an unsolved problem. For some time it seemed that the changes in the Mather population were correlated with drought and high-precipitation years. This correlation

TABLE 8.   *Percentage Frequencies of Different Kinds of Third Chromosomes of D. pseudoobscura at Mather, California*

Year	ST	AR	CH	PP	TL	Chromosomes
1945	36	36	17	—	10	308
1946	31	37	17	0.3	11	336
1947	30	39	20	0.7	8	425
1950	20	50	17	3	8	812
1951	29	43	11	5	10	856
1954	27	36	13	12	11	1312
1957	45	33	4	10	6	316
1959	40	36	11	4	7	298
1961	64	14	3	6	11	350
1962	54	27	2	9	7	450
1963	54	22	6	7	9	446
1965	36	25	11	6	18	534
1969	38	45	3	2	12	312
1971	34	33	11	3	17	390
1972	22	37	17	6	15	576

proved spurious. Furthermore, no correlation was found with relative abundance of the three commonest species, *D. pseudoobscura, D. persimilis,* and *D. azteca* (Dobzhansky, 1952, 1963). The possibility that contaminations with traces of insecticides were responsible seemed reasonable. Anderson *et al.* (1968) set up population cages polymorphic for four of five gene arrangements commonly found in *D. pseudoobscura* at Mather. In every generation the adult flies from the cages were treated with weak doses of DDT or dieldrin; no meaningful differences between the treated and control populations were observed. Cory *et al.* (1971) finds a correlation between the genetic changes in the populations and the degree of contamination in different localities in California, and believes that preadult stages, rather than the adults, should be exposed to insecticides.

Another possibility is that year-to-year changes are not induced by environmental factors, but are due rather to the emergence, by recombination or mutation, of new supergenes in chromosomes with certain gene arrangements. Suppose, for example, that there appear ST chromosomes which produce less heterotic heterozygotes with AR, but heterozygotes of superior fitness with PP chromosomes present in a certain locality. The "new" ST chromosomes may also give more fit homokaryotypes than the "old" ones. The chromosome pool will be reconstructed, ST and PP chromosomes rising and AR declining in frequencies. Unfortunately, this hypothesis is not easily testable experimentally. Pavlovsky and Dobzhansky (1966) obtained different fitness estimates with chromosomes collected at Mather in 1959 than were obtained in 1945 and 1946. It is, however, difficult to exclude the possibility that the difference could be caused by unperceived differences in the laboratory environments rather than in the chromosomes. Simultaneous testing would be no more conclusive since chromosomes kept for many generations in laboratory cultures change genetically (Strickberger, 1963). The fact that chromosomal changes occur more-or-less contemporaneously over extensive territories, such as the state of California, seemed to argue against the hypothesis of spread of "new" chromosomes since the active dispersal of *D. pseudoobscura* is much too slow for this. Passive transport by wind and other agencies may, however, achieve such spread more readily (Dobzhansky, 1974).

Genetics of Responses to Light and to Gravity

When disturbed, most species of *Drosophila* evince an escape reaction—they move upward and toward light. In this sense, they are positively phototactic and negatively geotactic. Surprisingly, Pittendrigh

(1958) and Lewontin (1959) found that in a Y-shaped tube, one branch of which is shaded and the other light, *D. persimilis* chooses mostly light (positive phototaxis) and *D. pseudoobscura* prefers the dark alternative (negative phototaxis). Pittendrigh suggested a rather intricate explanation to reconcile this behavior with the observation that in nature *D. persimilis* inhabits relatively cool and moist, and *D. pseudoobscura* warmer and drier habitats. Spassky and Dobzhansky (1967) tested 14 laboratory strains of *D. pseudoobscura* and 10 of *D. persimilis* in mazes of the type devised by J. Hirsch and N. M. Hadler. These mazes require the flies to make 15 choices of light or dark, or of upward or downward passages. *D. persimilis* was on the average photopositive and geoneutral, and *D. pseudoobscura* both photo- and geoneutral. Rockwell and Seiger (1973), working with a still different apparatus, found interstrain differences in phototaxis, but no clear difference between the species.

The reactions of *D. pseudoobscura* to light and to gravity can be changed by selection. Dobzhansky and Spassky (1967*a*) and Dobzhansky *et al.* (1969, 1972), using Hirsch–Hadler mazes, obtained sharply photopositive and -negative, and geopositive and -negative populations by selection in a series of generations, starting with populations originally neutral on the average. Realized heritability in the first 10 generations of selection for phototaxis is quite low (0.103 and 0.067), and even lower for geotaxis (0.051 and 0.021). Richmond's (1969) estimates from parent–offspring correlation in one generation are somewhat higher (0.16 for phototaxis and 0.11 for geotaxis). The success of selection in the face of heritabilities that low is due to the high efficiency of the mazes, which permit rigorous selection among fairly large numbers of individuals.

Some interesting phenomena can be observed because of the low heritability, which makes the phenotype of an individual relatively uninformative about its genotype. Pairs of populations were arranged which exchanged migrants in every generation. The populations were selected for different behaviors with respect to light or to gravity; the migrants were also selected in various ways. As an example of the kind of results obtained, consider a population that is being selected for photopositivity, and is in fact becoming more and more photopositive in a sequence of generations; this population sends phenotypically photonegative migrants to another population. With a trait of high heritability, one would expect the receiving population to be influenced toward the negative side. The opposite is observed. The phenotypically photonegative migrants transfer the genes for an average photopositivity of the population of their origin.

The positive or negative populations obtained by selection from originally neutral ones are unstable. When the selection is discontinued, there is a gradual drift back toward neutrality. This is genetic homeostasis. The artificial selection displaces the population average away from the state established in the species by natural selection. When the artificial selection is discontinued, the natural one operates to bring the population back to close to the original state. Levene [in Dobzhansky *et al.* (1972)] computed the "homeostatic drive," which is a measure of this natural selection.

Dobzhansky and Spassky (1967*b*) made two pairs of populations, in which one member was selected for positive or for negative geotaxis and its partner was selected for the ability to develop in culture media with high concentrations of table salt. The members of the pair of populations exchanged migrants in every generation. The populations changed in their responses to gravity as well as in their salt tolerance. The results of selection for the two traits were, however, not independent; but sometimes they reinforced and in other cases they interfered with each other.

Frequency Dependent Sexual Selection

Mating advantages of minority-type males were independently discovered by Petit (1951) in *D. melanogaster* and by Ehrman (Ehrman *et al.*, 1965; Ehrman, 1966) in *D. pseudoobscura*. In essence, the mating success of males of a given genotype or karyotype is augmented when this kind of males is rare, and is decreased when it is frequent in a given environment in relation to some other kind of male. An example of this phenomenon is shown in Table 9. When males of Californian and Texan origins are equally common (12 : 12), the matings occur randomly. When

TABLE 9.   *Numbers of Matings of D. pseudoobscura of Californian (C) and of Texan (T) Origins in Mating Chambers with Different Proportions of the Two Kinds of Flies*[a]

Pairs per chamber		Males mated		Females mated		Chi-square males
		C	T	C	T	
12 C : 12 T	Observed	55	49	50	54	0.39
	Expected	52	52	52	52	
20 C : 5 T	Observed	70	39	84	25	16.96
	Expected	87.2	21.8	87.2	21.8	
5 C : 20 T	Observed	39	65	30	74	19.91
	Expected	20.8	83.2	20.8	83.2	
23 C : 2 T	Observed	77	24	93	8	34.75
	Expected	92.9	8.1	92.9	8.1	
2 C : 23 T	Observed	30	70	12	88	65.76
	Expected	8.0	92.0	8.0	92.0	

[a] After Petet and Ehrman (1969).

either kind of males becomes rare in relation to the other (5:20 or 2:23 ratios), the number of matings per male is statistically significantly greater than for the common kind of males. No such mating advantage accrues to the less-frequent kind of females, or at least such advantages are much less pronounced than in the male sex.

Rare-male mating advantages have been found not only in *D. pseudoobscura* and *D. melanogaster,* but also in *D. persimilis* (Spiess, 1968, 1970; Spiess and Spiess, 1969) and among sibling species of *willistoni* group (Ehrman and Petit, 1968; Petit and Ehrman, 1969). However, they have not been found in *D. immigrans.* Mating advantages of rarity have been ascertained for strains selected for modified geotaxis and phototaxis (Ehrman *et al.,* 1965), for chromosomal variants (Ehrman, 1966, 1968, 1969; Ehrman and Spiess, 1969; Spiess, 1968; Spiess and Spiess, 1969), strains of different geographic origins (Ehrman, 1966; Spiess, 1968, 1970), mutant strains (Petit, 1951; Ehrman, 1970a; Petit and Ehrman, 1969), and even for flies of the same strain raised at different temperatures (Ehrman, 1966; Spiess and Spiess, 1969). However, no mating advantage is conferred upon rare males when they are confronted with females of different species in semispecies; in other words, ethological isolation is not overcome by making foreign males less numerous than conspecific males (Ehrman, 1966, 1970b).

The phenomenon of rare-male mating advantage was so unexpected and incredible that efforts had to be concentrated simply to make its reality beyond doubt. This having been achieved, steps must be taken to clarify its genetic and physiological causation and consequences. Ehrman (1969, 1972) has begun to explore this field. An air current is made to pass through a chamber with many individuals of a certain kind of flies, and to enter a mating observation chamber in which males of this kind are rare compared to other kinds of males. The mating advantage of the rare males is cancelled by this operation. Ehrman has concluded that olfactory cues are involved in the discrimination of "rare" and "common" males [see also Spiess (1970)]. Some similar, and also some inconsistent, results have been obtained by squashing the bodies of certain strains of flies, and "streaking" them on the bottom of a mating observation chamber; the rare-male mating advantage is sometimes cancelled by the presence of such "streaks" (Ehrman, 1972). If rare-male mating advantages exist in natural as well as in laboratory environments, they might play important roles in the maintenance of genetic polymorphisms. Ehrman (1970a) has devised model experiments and found that gene frequencies can be modified owing to mating advantages of rare types of males. Gene frequencies of a given mutant gene which is initially rare increase until males with this gene no longer possess a mating advantage.

Genetics of Ethological Isolation and Other Behavioral Traits

It has been pointed out above (pages 538–539) that ethological (sexual) isolation is the principal reproductive isolating mechanism maintaining the separation of the gene pools of the sibling species of *obscura* group. Experiments of Dobzhansky and Epling (1944), Mayr and Dobzhansky (1945), Mayr (1946), Levene and Dobzhansky (1945), and Dobzhansky (1951) have shown that sexual isolation between *D. pseudoobscura* and *D. persimilis* can be increased or decreased by some environmental agents (temperature, natural *vs.* laboratory environments) but is fairly independent of others (development in the same culture medium, removal of wings). Tan (1946) has carried out experiments marking the X chromosome and the three large autosomes of the above two species by appropriate mutant genes. By backcrossing the hybrid females to males of the parental species, one obtains in the progenies individuals with different combinations of the species chromosomes (see a more detailed account of this technique below). Tan's results indicated that the genes that distinguish the mating behaviors of *D. pseudoobscura* and *D. persimilis* are located mainly in the X and the second chromosomes, although participation of the other autosomes is not excluded.

Koopman (1950) has utilized Mayr's finding (Mayr and Dobzhansky, 1945) that the degree of ethological isolation between *D. pseudoobscura* and *D. persimilis* is diminished at a low temperature (16°C). Koopman placed females and males of *D. pseudoobscura* homozygous for the recessive gene glass and *D. persimilis* homozygous for the recessive gene orange in population cages at that temperature. It is obvious that matings within the species should yield progenies showing the effects of glass and orange, respectively; interspecific matings should yield wild-type offspring. In every generation the wild-type flies were discarded, and glass and orange flies served as parents of the following generation. This procedure amounts to selection for genetic constitutions that favor homogamic (intraspecific) and militate against heterogamic (interspecific) matings. The selection was quite effective, and Koopman obtained populations of the two species which showed isolation both at high (25°C) and at low (16°C) temperatures.

Kessler (1966, 1968, 1969) was able to dispense with the low temperature as a factor aiding the selection. He placed females of *D. pseudoobscura* together with males of *D. persimilis*, or *vice versa*, and selected the individuals which mated soonest and also individuals that failed to mate during the periods of observation (5 hours). Thus he was able to select both for increased and for decreased sexual isolation. The selections were quite effective, and populations of both species showing enhanced as well as diminished isolation were obtained. In other experiments of Kessler and of Parsons and Kaul (1966) selection was made both for increased and for decreased mating speed within the species. This selection was also effective, but Kessler showed that the modified ethological isolation between the species cannot be accounted for simply by the mating-speed factor. There exist genetic factors which modify the sexual behavior of one species with respect to another.

In both *D. pseudoobscura* and in *D. melanogaster,* del Solar (1968) found that females do not oviposite uniformly in all available places, but rather concentrate their eggs in certain places, leaving other seemingly equally favorable sites with few or no eggs. This aggregation tendency is variable from strain to strain, and it can be increased or decreased by selection. The sensory cue used in aggregation seems to be the presence of one or more eggs deposited by another female or females. One can "direct" the flies to a given site by placing one or several eggs on that site.

Hybrid Sterility and Hybrid Breakdown

Notwithstanding the ethological isolation and the fact that they rarely or never hybridize in nature, *D. pseudoobscura, D. persimilis,* and *D. miranda* can be crossed in laboratory cultures in all combinations. The crosses with *D. miranda* give completely sterile hybrids of both sexes; those of *D. pseudoobscura* with *D. persimilis* yield, in the F_1 generation, vigorous and fertile hybrid females but completely sterile hybrid males. The sons of *pseudoobscura* mothers have testes of normal size, while the sons of *persimilis* mothers have small or diminutive testes. The spermatogenesis in the hybrid males is grossly disturbed, but disturbed in different ways in normal-sized and small testes (Dobzhansky, 1934). In neither case do the disturbances stem from failures of the meiotic pairing; this pairing varies all the way from normal bivalent formation to no bivalents at all, depending on the strains of the parental species used. The proximate cause of the sterility is malfunctioning of the spindle mechanism at the first meiotic division. The spindle elongates abnormally in the progeny of *pseudoobscura* mothers; in that of *persimilis* mothers the division is abortive, often with multipolar spindles.

It proved possible to ascertain that the differences between the sterility situations in the hybrid sons of *pseudoobscura* and of *persimilis* mothers are due to maternal effects, i.e., to predetermination of the egg cytoplasm by the chromosomal complex present in the oocyte before meiosis and fertilization (Dobzhansky, 1933b, 1935c; Dobzhansky and

Sturtevant, 1935). The evidence can be summarized as follows: (1) The difference between the progenies of *pseudoobscura* and *persimilis* mothers is manifest in the F_1 hybrid sons, but not in the backcross hybrid progenies. (2) Males of *pseudoobscura* and *persimilis* lacking a Y chromosome (XO males) are sterile, but show no spermatogenesis disturbances like those in hybrid males. (3) Lack of the Y chromosome does not affect the spermatogenesis in F_1 hybrid males—XO hybrid sons of *persimilis* mothers have small testes even if they carry a *pseudoobscura* X chromosome, but hybrid XO sons of *persimilis* mothers have small testes even if they carry a *pseudoobscura* X chromosome. To put it differently, F_1 hybrid males have small testes if they carry a *persimilis* X chromosome in *pseudoobscura* cytoplasm, or if they have hybrid autosomes in *persimilis* cytoplasm. F_1 hybrid males have large testes if they carry a *pseudoobscura* X chromosome in *pseudoobscura* cytoplasm.

Occasional failures of the mitotic mechanism in spermatogonia occur in pure species, and more frequently in hybrid males. The resulting tetraploid spermatocytes offer an opportunity to analyze the cause of the hybrid sterility. It is well known that in many allotetraploid hybrids, especially among plants, meiosis is normal and the fertility is restored, even if the diploid hybrid is sterile with disturbed meiosis. Not so in *pseudoobscura* × *persimilis* hybrids. The chromosome pairing in the tetraploid spermatocytes is neither more nor less irregular than in the diploid ones in the same testes, and the spermatids formed are equally subject to degenerative changes (Dobzhansky, 1933*a*). Chromosomal sterility, due to different gene arrangements in the chromosomes of different species, is relieved in allotetraploids. Genic sterility, due to physiological incompatibility of the genotypes of the species crossed, is not removed in the allopolyploids. The sterility of *pseudoobscura* × *persimilis* hybrids is evidently genic rather than chromosomal.

Since F_1 hybrid females from crosses of *D. pseudoobscura* with *D. persimilis* are fertile, one can obtain backcross progenies with all possible combinations of the chromosomes of the parental species. To identify the chromosomal constitution of individuals, the X chromosomes and the three large autosomes of the species crossed were marked by suitable mutant genes (Dobzhansky, 1936). Ignoring the recombination within chromosomes, a total of 32 chromosome combinations can be distinguished. The size of the testes in a hybrid male can be used as a rough indication of the normality or abnormality of the spermatogenesis. At least some of the males with testes 500 μm or more in length are fertile, all other males are sterile. It is evident that the genes affecting testis size (and hence fertility or sterility) are present in every chromosome. The smallest

testes occur in males having the X chromosome of one species and the autosomes of the other; males which have one foreign third or fourth chromosome are sometimes fertile; however, a foreign second, or a combination of third and fourth chromosomes result in sterility.

The somatic vigor of F_1 hybrids contrasts sharply with a poor viability of the backcross hybrids of *pseudoobscura* × *persimilis*. These latter,
regardless of whether they are fertile or sterile, are somatically frail, and
in crosses between some strains they are altogether inviable (Dobzhansky,
1936; Weisbrot, 1963). This loss of vigor, or hybrid breakdown, was
shown to be due to a form of maternal effect—the eggs deposited by
hybrid females give rise to poorly viable offspring, independent of the
chromosomal constitution which is found in the eggs after fertilization.
Thus, backcross hybrids, both females and males, which carry chromosomes of only one of the parental species are as deficient in viability as
are individuals with chromosome mixtures of *D. pseudoobscura* and *D.
persimilis*. Hybrid breakdown may be an important isolating mechanism
in nature in those very rare cases (Dobzhansky, 1973) when F_1 hybrids
are produced despite the ethological isolation.

Dobzhansky and Beadle (1936) have shown that the sterility of the
pseudoobscura × *persimilis* hybrid males is autonomous in development,
and not dependent on interactions between the gonads and the hybrid
body. Larval gonads can be implanted into other larvae; the transplanted
gonads become attached to the sexual ducts. A hybrid testis can be implanted into larvae of the parental species, and *vice versa*. A testis of
either parental species implanted into a hybrid larva develops normal
sperm and makes a hybrid male fertile. A hybrid testis implanted into
normal males has disturbed spermatogenesis, but it does not interfere with
the spermatogenesis in the testes of the host. No experiments of this sort
have been made on hybrids of *D. miranda* with *D. pseudoobscura* or *D.
persimilis*.

Gene Arrangements in the Chromosomes of Different Species

Comparative studies of the gene arrangements in the giant salivary
gland chromosomes of hybrids of *D. pseudoobscura* with *D. persimilis*
were made by Tan (1935) and Dobzhansky and Epling (1944). The two
species always differ in a moderately long inversion on the left limb of
the X chromosome (SL) and in the second chromosome. They usually differ also in one or more inversions in the right limb of the X (XR) and in
the third chromosomes, but these differences are not constant. The

inversion polymorphisms in these chromosomes have already been discussed above, and it is sufficient to repeat here that one gene arrangement (standard) is common to both species and that the sex-ratio XR of *D. persimilis* is identical in gene arrangement with the normal XR of *D. pseudoobscura*. Only the fourth and the small fifth chromosomes show no differences in the gene arrangements between the species.

D. miranda has diverged in the gene arrangements in its chromosomes from *D. pseudoobscura* and *D. persimilis* much more than the last two named species from each other (Dobzhansky and Tan, 1936). In most *miranda* × *pseudoobscura* and *miranda* × *persimilis* hybrid larvae the salivary gland chromosomes are completely unpaired or paired in only some sections. The homologies have been traced by systematically recording the sections that have been seen paired in at least a single instance. By doing so, one finds chromosome sections of four kinds: (1) identical gene arrangements in both species, (2) paracentric inversions, (3) translocations, and (4) sections which have never been seen paired with their homologs. Ignoring this last group, one must assume at least 49 chromosome breaks to derive the gene arrangements of *D. miranda* from those of either *D. persimilis* or *D. pseudoobscura*.

Some of the chromosomes have been reconstructed relatively less than others. Thus, the XR chromosomes differ only in a single inversion and two short sections that have never been seen paired. The third chromosomes (which became neo-X's in *D. miranda*) are radically altered. Dobzhansky and Tan (1936) believed that the gene arrangement of *D. miranda* is most like that of the Hypothetical gene sequence in the third chromosome of *D. pseudoobscura* (see Figure 1), but Wallace (private communication) proved that it is closer to the Tree-Line gene arrangement in that species. The sections that seem to lie in the different chromosomes in the two species are mostly very short, including only a few salivary chromosome discs. Their interpretation as resulting from translocations is not wholly reliable; most of them have been seen paired only once, and this may possibly be due to nonhomologous (ectopic) pairing. However, even if one discounts these apparent translocations, it remains true that evolution of *D. miranda* from its common ancestor with *D. pseudoobscura* and *D. persimilis* has involved numerous changes in the gene arrangements. The metamorphosis of the third chromosome of the latter two species into the neo-X and neo-Y chromosomes of *D. miranda* must have required radical alteration of the genetic system, and yet these species can still produce hybrids, albeit sterile ones. Here is good evidence that the process of speciation is at least in some instances brought about by what Mayr (1963) has referred to as "genetic revolution."

Dispersion and Gene Flow

Of the several factors which cause changes in gene frequencies in populations, gene flow (migration) is probably the least well studied. With *Drosophila,* technical difficulties have been a major cause of this paucity of data. Nevertheless, some information on dispersion and gene flow is available for *D. pseudoobscura* and some of its American relatives.

Dobzhansky and Wright (1943, 1947) conducted experiments in two localities in California, Mount San Jacinto in 1941 and 1942 and Mather in 1945 and 1946. Laboratory-reared flies, homozygous for the autosomal recessive mutant orange eye, were released at a central point. Trapping was done at fixed intervals from the release point on subsequent days. The rate of dispersion of the released flies is easily calculated and usually expressed as the variance of the distribution of released flies. Four such experiments were conducted at San Jacinto and one at Mather (in 1945). Table 10 gives the standard deviation [(variance)$^{1/2}$] for the various days after release. In the San Jacinto experiments, the temperature during the first experiment was considerably lower than during the other three. The rate of dispersion is likewise much less. For the three experiments at San Jacinto during which the temperature was similar to the temperature during the Mather experiments, the results from the two localities are very similar.

During the summer of 1973, Dobzhansky and Powell (1974) repeated the release experiment at Mather using a different technique (Crumpacker and Williams, 1973). Flies collected in the wild were dusted with micronized flourescent dusts and released almost immediately at the same central point that was used in the 1945. Traps were placed at various distances from the release point, and recaptured flies were examined with ultraviolet light. The last column in Table 10 shows the average results of nine of these experiments. Because fewer flies were released, recapturing after two days yielded very few marked flies. The greater dispersion seen in these experiments may be due to several factors: higher temperature during the experiments, using flies captured in the wild instead of laboratory-reared ones, or using "wild-type" flies instead of mutants. In these experiments, *D. persimilis, D. miranda* and *D. azteca* flies were also marked and recaptured. There was no great difference in dispersion rates among the four species studied. There did however, seem to be indications that males were dispersing further on the average than females. Crumpacker and Williams (1973) conducted experiments similar to the 1973 Mather experiment on *D. pseudoobscura* in a Colorado locality. Their results are fairly close to those obtained in

TABLE 10.   Standard Deviations (in Meters) of Distributions of
Released D. pseudoobscura at Different Times after Release

Days after release	San Jacinto		Mather	
	Exp. I	Exp. II, III, IV	1945	1973
1	39	62	64	147
2	57	94	85	167
3	74	123	119	—
4	72	141	124	—
5	64	142	153	—
6	84	165	169	—
Temperature[a]	61°F	72°F	71°F	79°F

[a] Temperature is mean of the temperature at the time of recapture.

Mather in 1973, although the number of recaptured flies in their experiments is not great.

As described so far, these experiments only indicate the distances adults travel during a certain period of time. Is there any evidence that gene flow follows a similar pattern? For the 1945 Mather experiments (Dobzhansky and Wright, 1947), follow-up experiments were conducted the following summer (1946). Orange heterozygotes (progeny of released orange flies and wild flies) were detected. The highest concentration was still near the release point, but the standard deviation was now about 700 m. These dispersion rates of the four *obscura*-group species studied, *D. pseudoobscura, D. persimilis, D. miranda,* and *D. azteca,* are greater than has been detected in any other species of *Drosophila* studied so far [e.g., see Wallace (1968, 1970)].

Literature Cited

Anderson, W. W., 1966   Genetic divergence in M. Vetukhiv's experimental populations of *Drosophila pseudoobscura.* II. Divergence in body size. *Genet. Res.* 7:255–266.

Anderson, W. W., 1968   Further evidence for coadaptations in crosses between geographic populations of *Drosophila pseudoobscura. Genet. Res.* 12:317–330.

Anderson, W. W., 1969   Genetics of natural populations. XLI. The selection coefficients of heterozygotes for lethal chromosomes in Drosophila on different genetic backgrounds. *Genetics* 62:827–836.

Anderson, W. W., 1973   Genetic divergence in body size among experimental populations of *Drosophila pseudoobscura* kept at different temperatures. *Evolution* 27:278–284.

Anderson, W. W. and L. Ehrman, 1969 Mating choice in crosses between geographic populations of *Drosophila pseudoobscura*. *Am. Midl. Nat.* **81**:47–53.

Anderson, W. W., C. Oshima, P. Watanabe, T. Dobzhansky and O. Pavlovsky, 1968 Genetics of natural populations. XXXIX. A test of the possible influence of two insecticides on the chromosomal polymorphism in *Drosophila pseudoobscura*. *Genetics* **58**:423–434.

Ayala, F. J. and J. R. Powell, 1972 Allozymes as diagnostic characters of sibling species of *Drosophila*. *Proc. Natl. Acad. Sci. USA* **69**:1094–1096.

Battaglia, B. and H. Smith, 1961 The Darwinian fitness of polymorphic and monomorphic populations of *Drosophila pseudoobscura* at 16°C. *Heredity* **16**:475–484.

Beardmore, J. A., T. Dobzhansky and O. Pavlovsky, 1960 An attempt to compare the fitness of polymorphic and monomorphic experimental populations of *Drosophila pseudoobscura*. *Heredity* **14**:19–33.

Birch, C. L., 1955 Selection in *Drosophila pseudoobscura* in relation to crowding. *Evolution* **9**:389–399.

Brncic, D., 1954 Heterosis and the integration of the genotype in geographic populations of *Drosophila pseudoobscura*. *Genetics* **39**:77–88.

Buzzati-Traverso, A. A. and R. E. Scossiroli, 1955 The obscura group of the genus *Drosophila*. *Adv. Genet.* **7**:47–92.

Carson, H. L., 1951 Breeding sites of *Drosophila persimilis* and *Drosophila pseudoobscura* in the transition zone of the Sierra Nevada. *Evolution* **5**:91–96.

Chetverikov, S. S., 1927 Uber die genetische Beschaffenheit wilder Populationen. *Verh. V Interntl. Kongr. Vererbungsl.* **2**:1499–1500.

Cory, L., P. Fjeld and W. Serat, 1971 Environmental DDT and the genetics of natural populations. *Nature (Lond.)* **229**:128–130.

Crew, F. A. E. and R. Lamy, 1935 Linkage groups in *Drosophila pseudoobscura*. *J. Genet.* **30**:15–29.

Crew, F. A. E. and R. Lamy, 1936 The *plexus* chromosome of *Drosophila pseudoobscura* race A. *J. Genet.* **32**:5–15.

Crumpacker, D. W. and J. Williams, 1973 Density, dispersion, and population structure in *Drosophila pseudoobscura*. *Ecological Monographs* **43**:499–538.

da Cunha, A. B., 1951 Modification of the adaptive values of chromosomal types in *Drosophila pseudoobscura* by nutritional variables. *Evolution* **5**:395–404.

del Solar, E., 1968 Selection for and against gregariousness in the choice of oviposition sites by *Drosophila pseudoobscura*. *Genetics* **58**:275–282.

Dobzhansky, T., 1933a On the sterility of the interracial hybrids in *Drosophila pseudoobscura*. *Proc. Natl. Acad. Sci. USA* **19**:397–403.

Dobzhansky, T., 1933b Role of the autosomes in the *Drosophila pseudoobscura* hybrids. *Proc. Natl. Acad. Sci. USA* **19**:950–953.

Dobzhansky, T., 1934 Studies on hybrid sterility. I. Spermatogenesis in pure and hybrid *Drosophila pseudoobscura*. *Z. Zellforsch. Mikrosk. Anat.* **21**:169–223.

Dobzhansky, T., 1935a *Drosophila miranda*, a new species. *Genetics* **20**:377–391.

Dobzhansky, T., 1935b The Y chromosome of *Drosophila pseudoobscura*. *Genetics* **20**:366–376.

Dobzhansky, T., 1935c Maternal effect as a cause of the difference between reciprocal crosses in *Drosophila pseudoobscura*. *Proc. Natl. Acad. Sci. USA* **21**:443–446.

Dobzhansky, T., 1936 Studies on hybrid sterility. II. Localization of sterility factors in *Drosophila pseudoobscura* hybrids. *Genetics* **21**:113–135.

Dobzhansky, T., 1937a Further data on *Drosophila miranda* and its hybrids with *Drosophila pseudoobscura. J. Genet.* **34**:135–151.

Dobzhansky, T., 1937b Further data on the variation of the Y-chromosome in *Drosophila pseudoobscura. Genetics* **22**:340–346.

Dobzhansky, T., 1939a Genetics of natural populations. IV. Mexican and Guatemalan populations of *Drosophila pseudoobscura. Genetics* **24**:390–412.

Dobzhansky, T., 1939b Fatti e problemi della condizione "rapportosessi" (sex-ratio) in *Drosophila. Sci. Genet.* **1**:67–75.

Dobzhansky, T., 1943 Genetics of natural populations. IX. Temporal changes in the composition of populations of *Drosophila pseudoobscura. Genetics* **78**:162–186.

Dobzhansky, T., 1946 Genetics of natural populations. XIII. Recombination and variability in populations of *Drosophila pseudoobscura. Genetics* **31**:269–290.

Dobzhansky, T., 1947a Adaptive changes produced by natural selection in wild populations of *Drosophila. Evolution* **1**:1–16.

Dobzhansky, T., 1947b A directional change in the genetic constitution of a natural population of *Drosophila pseudoobscura. Heredity* **1**:53–64.

Dobzhansky, T., 1948a Genetics of natural populations. XVI. Altitudinal and seasonal changes produced by natural selection in certain populations of *Drosophila pseudoobscura* and *Drosophila persimilis. Genetics* **33**:158–176.

Dobzhansky, T., 1948b Genetics of natural populations. XVIII. Experiments on chromosomes of *Drosophila pseudoobscura* from different geographic regions. *Genetics* **33**:588–602.

Dobzhansky, T., 1950 Genetics of natural populations. XIX. Origin of heterosis through natural selection in populations of *Drosophila pseudoobscura. Genetics* **35**:288–302.

Dobzhansky, T., 1951 Reproductive isolation between *Drosophila pseudoobscura* and *Drosophila persimilis* under natural and under laboratory conditions. *Proc. Natl. Acad. Sci. USA* **37**:792–796.

Dobzhansky, T., 1952 Genetics of natural populations. XX. Changes induced by drought in *Drosophila pseudoobscura* and *Drosophila persimilis. Evolution* **6**:234–243.

Dobzhansky, T., 1956 Genetics of natural populations. XXV. Genetic changes in populations of *Drosophila pseudoobscura* and *Drosophila persimilis* in some localities in California. *Evolution* **10**:82–92.

Dobzhansky, T., 1958 Genetics of natural populations. XXVII. The genetic changes in populations of *Drosophila pseudoobscura* in the American Southwest. *Evolution* **12**:385–401.

Dobzhansky, T., 1963 Genetics of natural populations. XXXII. A progress report on genetic changes in populations of *Drosophila pseudoobscura* and *Drosophila persimilis* in a locality in California. *Evolution* **17**:333–339.

Dobzhansky, T., 1970 *Genetics of the Evolutionary Process,* Columbia University Press, New York.

Dobzhansky, T., 1971 Evolutionary oscillations in *Drosophila pseudoobscura.* In *Ecological Genetics and Evolution,* edited by R. Creed, pp. 109–133, Blackwell, Oxford.

Dobzhansky, T., 1973 Is there gene exchange between *Drosophila pseudoobscura* and *Drosophila persimilis* in their natural habitats? *Am. Nat.* **107**:312–314.

Dobzhansky, T., 1974 Active dispersal and passive transport in *Drosophila. Evolution,* **27**:565–575.

Dobzhansky, T. and F. J. Ayala, 1973 Temporal frequency changes of enzyme and chromosomal polymorphisms in natural populations of *Drosophila*. Proc. Natl. Acad. Sci. USA **70**:680–683.

Dobzhansky, T. and G. W. Beadle, 1936   Studies on hybrid sterility. IV. Transplanted testes in *Drosophila pseudoobscura*. *Genetics* **21**:832–840.

Dobzhansky, T. and C. Epling, 1944   Contributions to the genetics, taxonomy and ecology of *Drosophila pseudoobscura* and its relatives. Carnegie Institution of Washington Publication 554, Carnegie Institution, Washington, D.C.

Dobzhansky, T. and P. C. Koller, 1938   An experimental study of sexual isolation in *Drosophila. Biol. Zentralbl.* **52**:589–607.

Dobzhansky, T. and H. Levene, 1955   Genetics of natural populations. XXIV. Developmental homeostasis in natural populations of *Drosophila pseudoobscura. Genetics* **40**:797–808.

Dobzhansky, T. and O. Pavlovsky, 1953   Indeterminate outcome of certain experiments on *Drosophila* populations. *Evolution* **7**:198–210.

Dobzhansky, T. and O. Pavlovsky, 1957   An experimental study of interaction between genetic drift and natural selection. *Evolution* **11**:311–319.

Dobzhansky, T. and J. R. Powell, 1974   Rates of dispersal of *Drosophila pseudoobscura* and its relatives. *Proc. Royal Soc. London*, B. **187**:281–298.

Dobzhansky, T. and M. Queal, 1938   Genetics of natural populations. II. Genic variation in populations of *Drosophila pseudoobscura* inhabiting isolated mountain ranges. *Genetics* **23**:463–483.

Dobzhansky, T. and B. Spassky, 1944   Genetics of natural populations. XI. Manifestation of genetic variants in *Drosophila pseudoobscura* in different environments. *Genetics* **29**:270–290.

Dobzhansky, T. and B. Spassky, 1947   Evolutionary changes in laboratory cultures of *Drosophila pseudoobscura. Evolution* **1**:191–216.

Dobzhansky, T. and B. Spassky, 1953   Genetics of natural populations. XXI. Concealed variability in two sympatric species of *Drosophila. Genetics* **38**:471–484.

Dobzhansky, T. and B. Spassky, 1960   Release of genetic variability by recombination. V. Breakup of synthetic lethals by crossing over in *Drosophila pseudoobscura. Zool. Jahrb.* **88**:57–66.

Dobzhansky, T. and B. Spassky, 1963   Genetics of natural populations. XXXIV. Adaptive norm, genetic load and genetic elite in *Drosophila pseudoobscura. Genetics* **48**:1467–1485.

Dobzhansky, T. and B. Spassky, 1967a   Effects of selection and migration on geotactic and phototactic behaviour of *Drosophila*. I. *Proc. R. Soc. Lond. Ser. B Biol. Sci.* **168**:27–47.

Dobzhansky, T. and B. Spassky, 1967b   An experiment on migration and simultaneous selection for several traits in *Drosophila pseudoobscura. Genetics* **55**:723–724.

Dobzhansky, T. and B. Spassky, 1968   Genetics of natural populations. XL. Heterotic and deleterious effects of recessive lethals in populations of *Drosophila pseudoobscura. Genetics* **59**:411–425.

Dobzhansky, T. and N. Spassky, 1954   Environmental modification of heterosis in *Drosophila pseudoobscura. Proc. Natl. Acad. Sci. USA* **40**:407–415.

Dobzhansky, T. and N. P. Spassky, 1962   Genetic drift and natural selection in experimental populations of *Drosophila pseudoobscura. Proc. Natl. Acad. Sci. USA* **48**:148–156.

Dobzhansky, T. and A. H. Sturtevant, 1935   Further data on maternal effects in *Drosophila pseudoobscura* hybrids. *Proc. Natl. Acad. Sci. USA* **21**:566–570.

Dobzhansky; T. and A. H. Sturtevant, 1938 Inversions in the chromosomes of *Drosophila pseudoobscura. Genetics* 23:28–64.

Dobzhansky, T. and C. C. Tan, 1936 Studies on hybrid sterility. III. A comparison of the gene arrangement in two species, *Drosophila pseudoobscura* and *Drosophila miranda. Z. Indukt. Abstammungs- Vererbungsl.* 72:88–114.

Dobzhansky, T. and S. Wright, 1941 Genetics of natural populations. V. Relation between mutation rate and accumulation of lethals in populations of *Drosophila pseudoobscura. Genetics* 26:23–51.

Dobzhansky, T. and S. Wright, 1943 Genetics of natural populations. X. Dispersion rates in *Drosophila pseudoobscura. Genetics* 28:304–340.

Dobzhansky, T. and S. Wright, 1947 Genetics of natural populations. XV. Rate of diffusion of a mutant gene through a population of *Drosophila pseudoobscura. Genetics* 32:303–324.

Dobzhansky, T., H. M. Holz and B. Spassky, 1942 Genetics of natural populations. VIII. The allelism of lethals in the third chromosome of *Drosophila pseudoobscura. Genetics* 27:464–490.

Dobzhansky, T., B. Spassky and N. Spassky, 1954 Rates of spontaneous mutation in the second chromosomes of the sibling species, *Drosophila pseudoobscura* and *Drosophila persimilis. Genetics* 39:899–907.

Dobzhansky, T., O. Pavlovsky, B. Spassky and N. Spassky, 1955 Genetics of natural populations. XXIII. Biological role of deleterious recessives in populations of *Drosophila pseudoobscura. Genetics* 40:781–796.

Dobzhansky, T., H. Levene, B. Spassky and N. Spassky, 1959 Release of genetic variability through recombination. III. *Drosophila prosaltans. Genetics* 44:76–92.

Dobzhansky, T., C. Krimbas and M. G. Krimbas, 1960 Genetics of natural populations. XXX. Is the genetic load in *Drosophila pseudoobscura* mutational or balanced? *Genetics* 45:741–753.

Dobzhansky, T., A. S. Hunter, O. Pavlovsky, B. Spassky and B. Wallace, 1963a Genetics of natural populations. XXXI. Genetics of an isolated marginal population of *Drosophila pseudoobscura. Genetics* 48:91–103.

Dobzhansky, T., B. Spassky and T. Tidwell, 1963b Genetics of natural population. XXXII. Inbreeding and the mutational and balanced genetic loads in natural populations of *Drosophila pseudoobscura. Genetics* 48:361–373.

Dobzhansky, T., R. C. Lewontin and O. Pavlovsky, 1964a The capacity for increase in chromosomally polymorphic and monomorphic populations of *Drosophila pseudoobscura. Heredity* 19:597–614.

Dobzhansky, T., W. W. Anderson, O. Pavlovsky, B. Spassky and C. J. Wills, 1964b Genetics of natural populations. XXXV. A progress report on genetic changes in populations of *Drosophila pseudoobscura* in the American Southwest. *Evolution* 18:164–176.

Dobzhansky, T., W. W. Anderson and O. Pavlovsky, 1966 Genetics of natural populations. XXXVIII. Continuity and change in populations of *Drosophila pseudoobscura* in the Western United States. *Evolution* 20:418–427.

Dobzhansky, T., B. Spassky and J. Sved, 1969 Effects of selection and migration on geotactic and phototactic behavior of *Drosophila.* II. *Proc. R. Soc. Lond. Ser. B Biol. Sci.* 173:191–207.

Dobzhansky, T., H. Levene and B. Spassky, 1972 Effects of selection and migration on geotactic and phototactic behaviour of *Drosophila.* III. *Proc. R. Soc. Lond. Ser. B Biol. Sci.* 180:21–41.

Donald, H. P., 1936   The genetical constitution of *Drosophila pseudoobscura,* race A. *J. Genet.* **33**:103–122.

Druger, M., 1962   Selection and body size in *Drosophila pseudoobscura* at different temperatures. *Genetics* **47**:209–222.

Ehrman, L., 1964   Genetic divergence in M. Vetukhiv's experimental populations of *Drosophila pseudoobscura.* I. Rudiments of sexual isolation. *Genet. Res.* **5**:150–157.

Ehrman, L., 1966   Mating success and genotype frequency in *Drosophila. Anim. Behav.* **14**:332–339.

Ehrman, L., 1968   Frequency dependence of mating success in *Drosophila pseudoobscura. Genet. Res.* **11**:135–140.

Ehrman, L., 1969   The sensory basis of mate selection in *Drosophila. Evolution* **23**:59–64.

Ehrman, L., 1970*a*   The mating advantage of rare males in *Drosophila. Proc. Natl. Acad. Sci. USA* **65**:345–348.

Ehrman, L., 1970*b*   Sexual isolation versus mating advantage of rare *Drosophila* males. *Behav. Genet.* **1**:111–118.

Ehrman, L., 1972   A factor influencing the rare male mating advantage in *Drosophila. Behav. Genet.* **2**:69–78.

Ehrman, L. and C. Petit, 1968   Genotype frequency and mating success in the *willistoni* species group of *Drosophila. Evolution* **22**:649–658.

Ehrman, L. and E. B. Spiess, 1969   Rare type mating advantage in *Drosophila. Am. Nat.* **103**:675–680.

Ehrman, L., B. Spassky, O. Pavlovsky and T. Dobzhansky, 1965   Sexual selection, geotaxis, and chromosomal polymorphism in experimental populations of *Drosophila pseudoobscura. Evolution* **19**:337–346.

Epling, C. and W. R. Lower, 1957   Changes in an inversion system during a hundred generations. *Evolution* **11**:248–258.

Fallén, C. F., 1823   Diptera Sveciae. In *Geomyzides.* Literis Berlingianis, Lund, Sweden.

Frolova, S. L. and B. L. Astaurov, 1929   Die Chromosomengarnitur als systematisches Merkmal. *Z. Zellforsch. Mikrosk. Anat.* **10**:201–213.

Gershenson, S., 1928   A new sex ratio abnormality in *Drosophila obscura. Genetics* **13**:488–507.

Heed, W. B., D. W. Crumpacker and L. Ehrman, 1969   *Drosophila lowei,* a new American member of the *obscura* species group. *Ann. Entomol. Soc. Am.* **62**:388–393.

Hubby, J. L. and R. C. Lewontin, 1966   A molecular approach to the study of genic heterozygosity in natural populations. I. The member of alleles at different loci in *Drosophila pseudoobscura. Genetics* **54**:577–594.

Kastritsis, C. D. and D. W. Crumpacker, 1966   Gene arrangements in the third chromosome of *Drosophila pseudoobscura.* I. Configurations with tester chromosomes. *J. Heredity* **57**:151–158.

Kastritsis, C. D. and D. W. Crumpacker, 1967   Gene arrangements in the third chromosome of *Drosophila pseudoobscura.* II. All possible configurations. *J. Hered.* **58**:113–129.

Kessler, S., 1966   Selection for and against ethological isolation between *Drosophila pseudoobscura* and *Drosophila persimilis. Evolution* **20**:634–645.

Kessler, S., 1968   The genetics of *Drosophila* mating behaviour. I. Organization of mating speed in *Drosophila pseudoobscura. Anim. Behav.* **16**:485–491.

Kessler, S., 1969 The genetics of Drosophila mating behavior. II. The genetic archetecture of mating speed in *Drosophila pseudoobscura*. *Genetics* **62**:421–433.

Kitagawa, O., 1967 Genetic divergence in M. Vetukhiv's experimental populations of *Drosophila pseudoobscura*. IV. Relative viability. *Genet. Res.* **10**:303–312.

Koller, P. C., 1939 Genetics of natural populations. III. Gene arrangements in populations of *D. pseudoobscura* from contiguous localities. *Genetics* **24**:22–33.

Koopman, K. F., 1950 Natural selection for reproductive isolation between *Drosophila pseudoobscura* and *Drosophila persimilis*. *Evolution* **4**:135–148.

Lakovaara, S. and A. Saura, 1971*a* Genetic variation in natural populations of *Drosophila obscura*. *Genetics* **69**:377–384.

Lakovaara, S. and A. Saura, 1971*b* Genic variation in marginal populations of *Drosophila subobscura*. *Hereditas* **69**:77–82.

Lakovaara, S., A. Saura and C. T. Falk, 1972 Genetic distance and evolutionary relationships in the *Drosophila obscura* group. *Evolution* **26**:177–184.

Lamy, R., 1943 Hidden divergence in laboratory strains of *Drosophila pseudoobscura*. *Proc. R. Soc. Edinb. Sect. B Biol.* **62**:9–19.

Lancefield, D. E., 1922 Linkage relations of the sex-linked characters in *Drosophila obscura*. *Genetics* **7**:335–384.

Lancefield, D. E., 1929 A genetic study of crosses of two races of physiological species of *Drosophila obscura*. *Z. Indukt. Abstammungs- Vererbungsl.* **52**:282–317.

Levene, H., 1959 Release of genetic variability through recombination. III. Statistical theory. *Genetics* **44**:93–104.

Levene, H. and T. Dobzhansky, 1945 Experiments on sexual isolation in *Drosophila*. V. The effect of varying proportions of *Drosophila pseudoobscura* and *Drosophila persimilis* on the frequency of insemination in mixed populations. *Proc. Natl. Acad. Sci. USA* **31**:274–281.

Levene, H., O. Pavlovsky and T. Dobzhansky, 1954 Interaction of the adaptive values in polymorphic experimental populations of *Drosophila pseudoobscura*. *Evolution* **8**:325–349.

Levene, H., O. Pavlovsky and T. Dobzhansky, 1958 Dependence of the adaptive values of certain genotypes in *Drosophila pseudoobscura* on the composition of the gene pool. *Evolution* **12**:18–23.

Levine, L, 1955 Genotype background and heterosis in *Drosophila pseudoobscura*. *Genetics* **40**:823–849.

Levine, L. and J. A. Beardmore, 1959 A study of an experimental *Drosophila* population in equilibrium. *Am. Nat.* **93**:35–40.

Lewontin, R. C., 1959 On the anomalous response of *Drosophila pseudoobscura* to light. *Am. Nat.* **93**:321–328.

Lewontin, R. C. and J. L. Hubby, 1966 A molecular approach to the study of genic heterozygosity in natural populations. II. Amount of variation and degree of heterozygosity in natural populations of *Drosophila pseudoobscura*. *Genetics* **54**:595–609.

MacFarquhar, A. M. and F. W. Robertson, 1963 The lack of evidence for coadaptation in crosses between geographical races of *Drosophila subobscura*. *Genet. Res.* **4**:104–131.

MacKnight, R. H., 1939 The sex-determining mechanism of *Drosophila miranda*. *Genetics* **24**:180–201.

Marinkovic, D., 1967*a* Genetic loads affecting fecundity in natural populations of *Drosophila pseudoobscura*. *Genetics* **56**:61–71.

Marinkovic, D., 1967b Genetic loads affecting fertility in natural populations of *Drosophila psuedoobscura*. *Genetics* **57**:701–709.

Mayr, E., 1946 Experiments on sexual isolation in Drosophila. VI. Isolation between *Drosophila pseudoobscura* and *Drosophila persimilis* and their hybrids. *Proc. Natl. Acad. Sci. USA* **32**:57–59.

Mayr, E., 1963 *Animal Species and Evolution,* Harvard University Press, Cambridge, Mass.

Mayr, E. and T. Dobzhansky, 1945 Experiments on sexual isolation in *Drosophila*. IV. Modification of the degree of isolation between *Drosophila pseudoobscura* and *Drosophila persimilis* and of sexual preferences in *Drosophila prosaltans*. *Proc. Natl. Acad. Sci. USA* **31**:75–82.

Metz, C. W., 1916 Chromosome studies in the Diptera. II. The paired association of chromosomes in the Diptera and its significance. *J. Exp. Zool.* **21**:213–279.

Moriwaki, D., O. Kitagawa and T. Okada, 1967 *Drosophila imaii,* a new sibling species related to *Drosophila bifasciata. Evolution* **21**:109–116.

Morton, N. E., J. F. Crow and H. J. Muller, 1956 An estimate of the mutational damage in man from data on consanguinous marriages. *Proc. Natl. Acad. Sci. USA* **42**:855–863.

Mourad, A. K. M., 1962 Effects of irradiation in genetically coadapted systems. *Genetics* **47**:1647–1662.

Mourad, A. K. M., 1964 Lethal and semilethal chromosomes in irradiated experimental populations of *Drosophila pseudoobscura. Genetics* **50**:1279–1287.

Mourad, A. K. M., 1965 Genetic divergence in M. Vetukhiv's experimental populations of *Drosophila pseudoobscura*. II. Longevity. *Genet. Res.* **6**:139–146.

Mourão, C. A., F. J. Ayala and W. W. Anderson, 1972 Darwinian fitness and adaptedness in experimental populations of *Drosophila willistoni. Genetica (The Hague)* **43**:552–574.

Novitski, E., W. Y. Peacock and J. Engel, 1965 Cytological basis of "sex ratio" in *Drosophila pseudoobscura. Science (Wash., D.C.)* **148**:516–517.

Ohba, S., 1967 Chromosomal polymorphism and capacity for increase under near optimal conditions. *Heredity* **22**:169–189.

Parsons, P. A. and D. Kaul, 1966 Mating speed and duration of copulation in *Drosophila pseudoobscura. Heredity* **21**:219–225.

Pavlovsky, O. and T. Dobzhansky, 1966 Genetics of natural populations. XXXVII. The coadapted system of chromosomal variants in a population of *Drosophila pseudoobscura. Genetics* **53**:843–854.

Petit, C., 1951 Le rôle de l'isolement sexuel dans l'évolution des populations de *Drosophila melanogaster. Bull. Biol. Fr. Belg.* **85**:392–418.

Petit, C. and L. Ehrman, 1969 Sexual selection in *Drosophila. Evol. Biol.* **3**:177–223.

Pittendrigh, C., 1958 Adaptation, natural selection and behavior. In *Behavior and Evolution,* edited by A. Roe and G. G. Simpson, Yale University Press, New Haven, Conn.

Policansky, D. and J. Ellison, 1970 "Sex ratio" in *Drosophila pseudoobscura*. Spermiogenic failure. *Science (Wash., D.C.)* **169**:888–889.

Powell, J. R., H. Levene and T. Dobzhansky, 1972 Chromosomal polymorphism in *Drosophila pseudoobscura* used for diagnosis of geographic origin. *Evolution* **26**:553–559.

Prakash, S., 1969 Genic variation in a natural population of *Drosophila persimilis. Proc. Natl. Acad. Sci. USA* **62**:778–784.

Prakash, S., 1972   Origin of reproductive isolation in the abscence of apparent genic differentiation in a geographic isolate of *Drosophila pseudoobscura*. *Genetics* **72**:143–155.

Prakash, S. and R. C. Lewontin, 1968   A molecular approach to the study of genic heterozygosity in natural populations. III. Direct evidence of coadaptation in gene arrangements of *Drosophila*. *Proc. Natl. Acad. Sci. USA* **59**:398–405.

Prakash, S. and R. C. Lewontin, 1971   A molecular approach to the study of genic heterozygosity in natural populations. V. Further direct evidence of coadaptation in inversions of *Drosophila*. *Genetics* **69**:405–408.

Prakash, S. and R. B. Merritt, 1972   Direct evidence of genic differentiation between sex ratio and standard gene arrangements of X chromosome in *Drosophila pseudoobscura*. *Genetics* **72**:169–175.

Prakash, S., R. C. Lewontin and J. L. Hubby, 1969   A molecular approach to the study of genic heterozygosity in natural populations. IV. Patterns of genic variation in central marginal and isolated populations of *Drosophila pseudoobscura*. *Genetics* **61**:841–858.

Richmond, R. C., 1969   Heritability of phototactic and geotactic responses in *Drosophila pseudoobscura*. *Am. Nat.* **103**:315–223.

Rizki, M. T. M., 1951   Morphological differences between two sibling species, *Drosophila pseudoobscura* and *Drosophila persimilis*. *Proc. Natl. Acad. Sci.* **37**:156–159.

Rockwell, R. F. and M. B. Seiger, 1973   A comparative study of photoresponse in *Drosophila pseudoobscura* and *Drosophila persimilis*. *Behav. Genet.* **3**:163–174.

Rosenbaum-Moos, J., 1955   Comparative physiology of some chromosomal types in *Drosophila pseudoobscura*. *Evolution* **9**:141–151.

Sankaranarayanan, K., 1965   Further data on the genetic loads in irradiated experimental populations of *Drosophila melanogaster*. *Genetics* **52**:153–164.

Saura, A., S. Lakovaara, J. Lokki and P. Lankinen, 1973   Genic variation in central and marginal populations of *Drosophila subobscura*. *Hereditas:* **75**:33–46.

Solima Simmons, A., 1966   Experiments on random genetic drift and natural selection in *Drosophila pseudoobscura*. *Evolution* **20**:100–103.

Spassky, B. and T. Dobzhansky, 1967   Responses of various strains of *Drosophila pseudoobscura* and *Drosophila persimilis* to light and to gravity. *Am. Nat.* **101**:59–63.

Spassky, B., N. Spassky, H. Levene and T. Dobzhansky, 1958   Release of genetic variability through recombination. I. *Drosophila pseudoobscura*. *Genetics* **43**:844–867.

Spassky, B., N. Spassky, O. Pavlovsky, M. G. Krimbas, C. Krimbas and T. Dobzhansky, 1960   Genetics of natural populations. XXIX. The magnitude of the genetic load in populations of *Drosophila pseudoobscura*. *Genetics* **45**:723–740.

Spassky, B., T. Dobzhansky and W. W. Anderson, 1965   Genetics of natural populations. XXXVI. Epistatics interactions of the components of the genetic load in *Drosophila pseudoobscura*. *Genetics* **52**:653–664.

Sperlich, D., 1966   Equilibria for inversions induced by X-rays in isogenic strains of *Drosophila pseudoobscura*. *Genetics* **53**:835–842.

Spiess, E. B., 1950   Experimental populations of *Drosophila persimilis* from an altitudinal transect of the Sierra Nevada. *Evolution* **4**:14–33.

Spiess, E. B., 1959   Release of genetic variability through recombination. II. *Drosophila persimilis*. *Genetics* **44**:43–58.

Spiess, E. B., 1968 Low frequency advantage in mating of *Drosophila pseudoobscura* karyotypes. *Am. Nat.* **102**:363–379.

Spiess, E. B., 1970 Mating propensity and its genetic basis in Drosophila. In *Essays in Evolution and Genetics,* edited by M. K. Hecht and W. C. Steere, Appleton-Century-Crofts, New York.

Spiess, E. B. and B. Langer, 1961 Chromosomal adaptive polymorphisms in *Drosophila persimilis.* III. Mating propensity of homocokaryotypes. *Evolution* **15**:535–544.

Spiess, E. B. and B. Langer, 1964· Mating speed control by gene arrangement carriers in *Drosophila persimilis. Evolution* **18**:430–444.

Spiess, E. B. and L. D. Spiess, 1967 Mating propensity, chromosomal polymorphism, and dependent conditions in *Drosophila persimilis. Evolution* **21**:672–678.

Spiess, E. B., B. Langer and L. D. Spiess, 1966 Mating control by gene arrangements in *Drosophila pseudoobscura. Genetics* **54**:1139–1149.

Spiess, E. B., R. N. Sherwin and T. Yacker, 1971 Mating propensity of gene arrangement carriers from a Redwoods population of *Drosophila persimilis. Evolution* **25**:461–470.

Spiess, L. D. and E. B. Spiess, 1969 Minority advantage in interpopulational matings of *Drosophila persimilis. Am. Nat.* **103**:155–172.

Strickberger, M. W., 1963 Evolution of fitness in experimental populations of *Drosophila pseudoobscura. Evolution* **17**:40–55.

Strickberger, M. W., 1965 Experimental control over the evolution of fitness in laboratory populations of *Drosophila pseudoobscura. Genetics* **51**:795–800.

Strickberger, M. W. and C. J. Wills, 1966 Monthly frequency changes of *Drosophila pseudoobscura* third chromosome gene arrangements in a California locality. *Evolution* **20**:592–602.

Sturtevant, A. H., 1921 *The North American Species of Drosophila,* Carnegie Institution of Washington Publication 301, Carnegie Institution, Washington, D.C.

Sturtevant, A. H., 1937 Autosomal lethals in wild populations of *Drosophila pseudoobscura. Biol. Bull.* **73**:542–551.

Sturtevant, A. H. and T. Dobzhansky, 1936a Inversions in the third chromosomes of wild races of *Drosophila pseudoobscura,* and their use in the study of the history of the species. *Proc. Natl. Acad. Sci. USA* **22**:448–450.

Sturtevant, A. H. and T. Dobzhansky, 1936b Geographical distribution and cytology of "sex-ratio" in *Drosophila pseudoobscura* and related species. *Genetics* **21**:473–490.

Sturtevant, A. H. and E. Novitski, 1941 The homologies of the chromosome elements in the genus *Drosophila. Genetics* **58**:113–124.

Sturtevant, A. H. and C. C. Tan, 1937 The comparative genetics of *Drosophila pseudoobscura* and *D. melanogaster. J. Genet.* **34**:415–432.

Sved, J. A. and F. J. Ayala, 1970 A population cage test for heterosis in *Drosophila pseudoobscura. Genetics* **66**:97–113.

Tan, C. C., 1935 Salivary gland chromosomes in the two races of *Drosophila pseudoobscura. Genetics* **20**:392–402.

Tan, C. C., 1936 Genetic maps of the autosomes in *Drosophila pseudoobscura. Genetics* **21**:796–807.

Tan, C. C., 1937 The cytological maps of the autosomes in *Drosophila pseudoobscura. Z. Zellforsch. Mikrosk. Anat.* **26**:439–461.

Tan, C. C., 1946 Genetics of sexual isolation between *Drosophila pseudoobscura* and *Drosophila persimilis. Genetics* **31**:558–573.

Vetukhiv, M., 1954   Integration of the genotype in local populations of three species of *Drosophila*. *Evolution* **8**:241–251.

Vetukhiv, M., 1956   Fecundity of hybrids between geographic populations of *Drosophila pseudoobscura*. *Evolution* **10**:139–146.

Vetukhiv, M., 1957   Longevity of hybrids between geographic populations of *Drosophila pseudoobscura*. *Evolution* **11**:348–360.

Wallace, B., 1948   Studies on "sex-ratio" in *Drosophila pseudoobscura*. *Evolution* **2**:189–217.

Wallace, B., 1968   *Topics in Population Genetics*, W. W. Norton & Company, Inc., New York.

Wallace, B., 1970   Observations on the microdispersion of *Drosophila melanogaster*. In *Essays in Evolution and Genetics*, edited by M. Hecht and W. Steere, pp. 381–399, Appleton-Century-Crofts, New York.

Wallace, B. and T. Dobzhansky, 1962   Experimental proof of balanced genetic loads in *Drosophila*. *Genetics* **47**:1027–1042.

Wallace, B. and C. Madden, 1953   The frequencies of sub- and supervitals in experimental populations of *Drosophila melanogaster*. *Genetics* **38**:456–470.

Weisbrot, D. R., 1963   Studies on differences in the genetic architecture of related species of *Drosophila*. *Genetics* **48**:1121–1139.

Wills, C., 1966   The mutational load in two natural populations of *Drosophila pseudoobscura*. *Genetics* **53**:281–294.

Wright, S. and T. Dobzhansky, 1946   Genetics of natural populations. XII. Experimental reproduction of some of the changes caused by natural selection in certain populations of *Drosophila pseudoobscura*. *Genetics* **31**:125–150.

Wright, S., T. Dobzhansky and W. Hovanitz, 1942   Genetics of natural populations. VII. The allelism of lethals in the third chromosomes of *Drosophila pseudoobscura*. *Genetics* **27**:363–394.

Zouros, E. and C. B. Krimbas, 1973   Evidence for linkage disequilibrium maintained by selection in two natural populations of *Drosophila subobscura*. *Genetics* **73**:659–674.

21

The *willistoni* Group of Sibling Species of *Drosophila*

THEODOSIUS DOBZHANSKY AND

JEFFREY R. POWELL

Introduction

The history of the discovery of the cluster of sibling species related to *Drosophila willistoni* is fairly long and somewhat tortuous. A species living on the Isle of St. Vincent in the Caribbean was named *Drosophila pallida* by Williston in 1896. Because this name was preoccupied, Sturtevant changed it in 1916 to *Drosophila willistoni* [see Sturtevant (1921)]. In 1943, Dobzhansky and Pavan found two species fitting the descriptions of *D. willistoni* on the coast of São Paulo, Brazil. One of these was more common and slightly smaller in size than the other. In the laboratory they failed to mate and produce hybrids, and they were easily distinguishable by the disc patterns of the chromosomes of larval salivary gland cells. The common species was taken to be *D. willistoni*, and the rarer one was described as *D. paulista* Dobzhansky and Pavan. This proved to be an er-

THEODOSIUS DOBZHANSKY—Department of Genetics, University of California, Davis, California. JEFFREY R. POWELL—Department of Biology, Yale University, New Haven, Connecticut.

ror; *D. paulista* was in fact *D. willistoni*. The smaller but more common form was then named *D. paulistorum* Dobzhansky and Pavan [in Burla *et al.* (1949)]. Soon three more morphologically very similar but re-productively isolated species were added: *D. equinoxialis* Dobzhansky (1946) from the Amazon Valley, *D. tropicalis* Burla and da Cunha from central Brazil [in Burla *et al.* (1949)], and *D. insularis* Dobzhansky from the islands of the Lesser Antilles (Dobzhansky *et al.*, 1957; and Figure 1).

D. *paulistorum* did not seem a particularly interesting species until it was found to be a cluster of six "semispecies" or "incipient species" (Dobzhansky and Spassky, 1959). These are identical morphologically, exhibit a strong sexual (ethological) isolation, produce fertile female but sterile male hybrids when crossed, and possess distinct though somewhat overlapping geographic-distribution areas (Figure 2). One of the six semispecies (Guianan) was later found to differ enough to be regarded a separate species, *D. pavlovskiana* Kastritis and Dobzhansky (1967). An additional semispecies (Interior) was added by Pérez-Salas *et al.* (1970). Species other than *paulistorum* are less complexly subdivided. Townsend (1954) found, however, that *D. tropicalis* consists of at least two subspecies (*tropicalis* and *cubana*), which yield sterile male but fertile fe-male hybrids when crossed. A similar situation has recently been dis-covered in *D. willistoni* (subspecies *quechua* in western Peru), and in *D. equinoxialis* (subspecies *caribbensis* in Costa Rica, Hispaniola and Puerto Rico) (Ayala, 1973; Ayala *et al.*, 1974).

Morphological Differences

Sibling species are not easily distinguishable by external characteris-tics, but they are not necessarily morphologically identical. Burla *et al.* (1949) recorded average differences in body size, shape of the palpi, spermathecae, and hypandria between *D. willistoni, D. paulistorum, D. equinoxialis,* and *D. tropicalis.* However, it was Spassky (1957) who found slight but diagnostic differences in the male genitalia, which permit-ted identification of single male individuals. Although the females are not themselves distinguishable, they can be classified by inspection of their male progenies. The species can also be recognized by their chromosomes, enzymes, and their behavior in crosses (see below).

Pasteur (1970) has made a biometrical comparison of four semi-species of *D. paulistorum.* He found statistically significant differences in wing and tibia lengths, wing-to-tibia ratios, sexual dimorphism in wing size, numbers of teeth on claspers in males, and length of development. None of these differences are diagnostic. Moreover, similar though smaller differences are found between strains of the same semispecies. The semi-species can be diagnosed only by hybridization experiments, and some-times by the gene arrangements in their chromosomes as seen in prepara-tions of larval salivary glands (see below).

Chromosomes and Chromosomal Maps

As early as 1916, Metz correctly described the chromosome com-plement of *D. willistoni* as consisting of two pairs of metacentric and one pair of acrocentric chromosomes. The dotlike microchromosomes found in many species of *Drosophila* are absent. One of the metacentrics is the X chromosome; the Y chromosome is indistinguishable from the X at metaphase. The same chromosome complement has been found not only in all *willistoni*-like siblings and in all other members of the *willistoni* species group (i.e., *D. nebulosa, D. fumipennis, D. capricorni, D. suc-cinea*), but also in the *saltans* species group of the subgenus *Sophophora*, to which the *willistoni* and *saltans* groups belong.

The uniformity of the metaphase chromosomes contrasts with a mul-tiformity of the disc patterns in the polytene chromosomes of the larval salivary glands. The species are almost always easily recognizable in salivary gland preparations; there has evidently been a great deal of gene rearrangement within the chromosomes during the evolutionary process, while the chromosomes as a whole have remained intact. Composite "maps" of the giant chromosomes in the larval salivary glands of *D. willi-stoni* have been published by Dobzhansky (1950), and of *D. paulistorum* by Kastritsis (1966). There are, like in most though not all *Drosophila* species, five long chromosome "limbs" radiating from a common chromocenter. These limbs can readily be recognized by the disc patterns, most conveniently in their distal (free) ends. It happens that the end parts of the two limbs of the second chromosome of *D. willistoni* appear rather similar, but the right limb (IIR) has a dark-staining area (a "repeat") in a submedial position, which is lacking in the left limb (IIL).

It is fairly easy to identify the corresponding, homologous, limbs in different species. At the same time, the disc patterns in these homologous limbs are characteristically different, and the differences can be used to recognize the species. Compare the *D. willistoni* and *D. paulistorum* maps referred to above. Burla *et al.* (1949) have published drawings that show the diagnostic features of the third chromosomes (III) and of the right limbs of the X chromosomes (XR) in *D. willistoni, D. paulistorum, D. equinoxialis,* and *D. tropicalis.* Drawings and photographs of the diag-nostic features of the chromosomes of *D. pavlovskiana* can be found in

Dobzhansky and Pavlovsky (1962) and in Kastritsis and Dobzhansky (1967). *D. insularis* is chromosomally closest to *D. tropicalis*, but nevertheless distinguishable (Dobzhansky *et al.*, 1957). All in all, it is clear that the gene orders underwent many alterations in the descent of the sibling species of the *willistoni* group. The homologous chromosome limbs in the siblings are, nevertheless, identifiable without much difficulty. The recognition of the homologous chromosome limbs becomes less easy if the sibling species are compared with the less closely related members of the *willistoni* group, e.g., *D. nebulosa,* and very tenuous indeed in other members of the subgenus *Sophophora,* e.g., *D. melanogaster, D. ananassae,* or *D. prosaltans.*

Reproductive Isolation of the Sibling Species

The distribution areas of the sibling species overlap broadly (Figure 1). *D. willistoni* has the widest distribution, including the areas of all other siblings. *D. paulistorum* reaches southward farther, but less far northward, than do *D. equinoxialis* and *D. tropicalis.* Over very extensive areas of South and Central America these four species are sympatric and can be collected on the same bait. *D. insularis* is known only from some of the islands of Lesser Antilles (where it is sympatric with *D. willistoni*), and *D. pavlovskiana* from only two localities in Guyana (where it is sym-

TABLE 1.   *Insemination Frequencies for Reciprocal Crosses between Various Sibling Species of the* willistoni *Group*

Females		Males	Percent inseminated
willistoni	×	*paulistorum*	51.3
willistoni	×	*equinoxialis*	3.8
willistoni	×	*tropicalis*	0
paulistorum	×	*willistoni*	5.7
paulistorum	×	*equinoxialis*	0
paulistorum	×	*tropicalis*	27.8
equinoxialis	×	*willistoni*	1.5
equinoxialis	×	*paulistorum*	12.7
equinoxialis	×	*tropicalis*	0
tropicalis	×	*willistoni*	0
tropicalis	×	*paulistorum*	65.0
tropicalis	×	*equinoxialis*	0

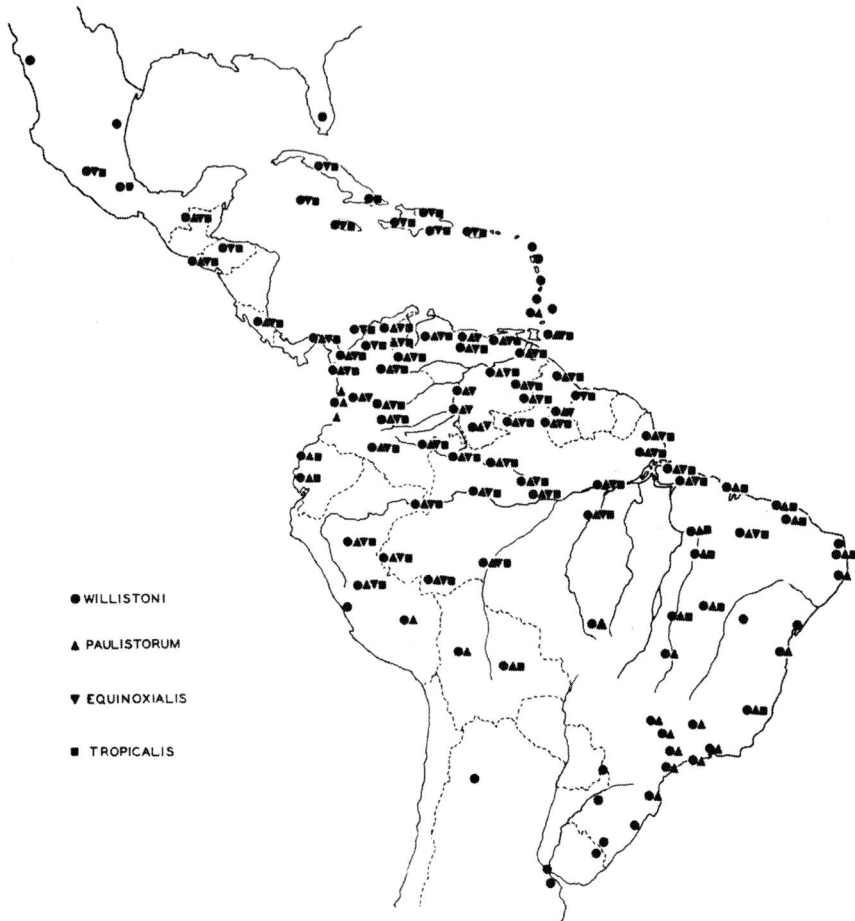

● WILLISTONI

▲ PAULISTORUM

▼ EQUINOXIALIS

■ TROPICALIS

Figure 1. The geographic distribution of the four common sibling species of D. willistoni group.

patric with four other siblings). The question presents itself: What isolating mechanisms preserve the integrity of these sympatric siblings?

Dobzhansky and Pavan (1943) have already noted the failure of laboratory crosses of *D. willistoni* and *D. paulistorum* to produce hybrids, and Dobzhansky (1946) failed to obtain hybrids of *D. equinoxialis* with *D. willistoni*. Burla *et al.* (1949) studied the ethological (sexual) isolation of the *willistoni* group by dissecting the females and examining their sperm receptacles, in experiments in which a choice of mates was available as well as in no-choice experiments. Table 1 provides an extract from their data. The sexual isolation is evidently incomplete, at least in laboratory experiments where females and males are confined together for days or weeks in a bottle or a vial. However, the insemination has never been observed to result in production of hybrid progeny. The situation is different with *D. insularis* (Dobzhansky *et al.*, 1957). Both with availability and absence of mate choice, a small percentage of *insularis* females are inseminated by males of the other four species, and *vice versa*. Furthermore, the crosses *insularis* ♂ × *tropicalis* ♀ and *insularis* ♀ × *willistoni* ♂ produce viable but completely sterile hybrids. The crosses *insularis* ♀ × *equinoxialis* ♂ and *insularis* ♀ × *paulistorum* ♂ result in hybrids that die mostly in preadult stages. Thus, the reproductive isolation between the five siblings is complete. Even if cross-insemination were to occur in nature, the inviability or sterility of the hybrids would prevent gene exchange. Winge and Cordeiro (1963) claimed, however, that certain particular strains of *D. willistoni* and *D. paulistorum* from southern Brazil not only produce viable hybrid progenies, but also that some of the hybrids are fertile. A careful repetition of these experiments by Ehrman (unpublished) failed to substantiate these claims. Working with the same strains, she selected females that had been seen *in copula* with species-foreign males. The eggs deposited by such females yielded no larvae.

The sixth sibling, *D. pavlovskiana,* was believed to be only a "Guianan" semispecies of *D. paulistorum* until Kastritsis and Dobzhansky (1967) found that in the hybrids the chromosomes almost entirely fail to pair in salivary gland cells. Notwithstanding a strong ethological isolation, their crosses produce viable hybrids that are fertile as females but sterile as males. The same phenomenon is observed in the progenies of the crosses of *D. insularis* to *D. tropicalis* and *D. equinoxialis* mentioned above (Dobzhansky, 1957*b*).

Reproductive Isolation of the Semispecies of *Drosophila paulistorum*

As a general rule, no sexual isolation is observed when strains of the same species but of different geographic origin are given opportunity to mate (Dobzhansky and Mayr, 1944). This is true even with respect to the subspecies of *D. tropicalis, D. equinoxialis,* and *D. willistoni* (Ayala and Tracey, 1974; Ayala *et al.*, 1974); but not so with *D. paulistorum.* Dobzhansky and Spassky (1959) found that when strains of this species, allopatric as well as sympatric, are tested for their ability to hybridize, three kinds of situations can be observed: (1) Crosses between strains succeed as easily as intrastrain crosses, and the hybrids are fertile. (2) No mating between strains occurs, and no hybrids are produced. (3) Some interstrain matings do occur, fully viable hybrids are produced, and the hybrid females are fertile but male hybrids completely sterile.

A series of studies unraveled a complex situation (Malogolowkin, 1963; Malogolowkin-Cohen *et al.*, 1965; Carmody *et al.*, 1963; Dobzhansky *et al.*, 1964, 1969; Pérez-Salas *et al.*, 1970; Spassky *et al.*, 1971). *D. paulistorum* is a superspecies composed of six semispecies (or incipient species): Centroamerican, Amazonian, Orinocan, Interior, Andean-Brazilian, and Transitional. The semispecies are not distinguishable morphologically (Pasteur, 1970). They can be diagnosed most easily and reliably by outcrossing unknown strains to a series of six "testers" that represent the six semispecies. With rare exceptions to be considered below, the results of the tests are quite unambiguous—fertile hybrids are produced with one and only one tester, that of the semispecies to which the strain put to the test belongs. Strains of different semispecies show varying degrees of aversion to mating—some mate fairly easily while others are refractory. Repeated trials may be necessary, but sooner or later hybrids between any two strains are probably obtainable. The F_1 hybrid males are completely sterile.

The geographic areas of the semispecies are shown in Figure 2. Although every semispecies inhabits a territory different from the others, in many places two or even three semispecies are sympatric. An interesting exception are Orinocan and Interior semispecies, which are nowhere sympatric. This is reflected in a low degree of sexual isolation. Various coefficients to measure sexual isolation have been proposed; a coefficient of 0 means absence of isolation, and $+1$ means complete isolation. The isolation between Orinocan and Interior semispecies gives coefficients often below 0.5, while that between Amazonian and other semispecies is usually above 0.9. The Amazonian semispecies is often sympatric with one or more of the others. Ehrman (1965) found that the degree of sexual isolation between strains of the same pair of semispecies varies in a very significant fashion: it is higher between sympatric than between allopatric strains. This is the opposite of what would be expected if the semispecies had engaged in hybridization and gene exchange to any significant extent.

The Transitional semispecies is a special case (Dobzhansky *et al.*, 1969). It is most closely related to the Centroamerican, but while some crosses of Transitional × Centroamerican give fertile F_1 hybrid males, the male progenies of other crosses are sterile. The fertility is observed more often when Transitional is the female than when it is the male parent. Furthermore, intercrosses of some Transitional strains with each other also yield sterile male progenies. All tested intercrosses between Centroamerican strains gave fertile male hybrids. There is a similar com-

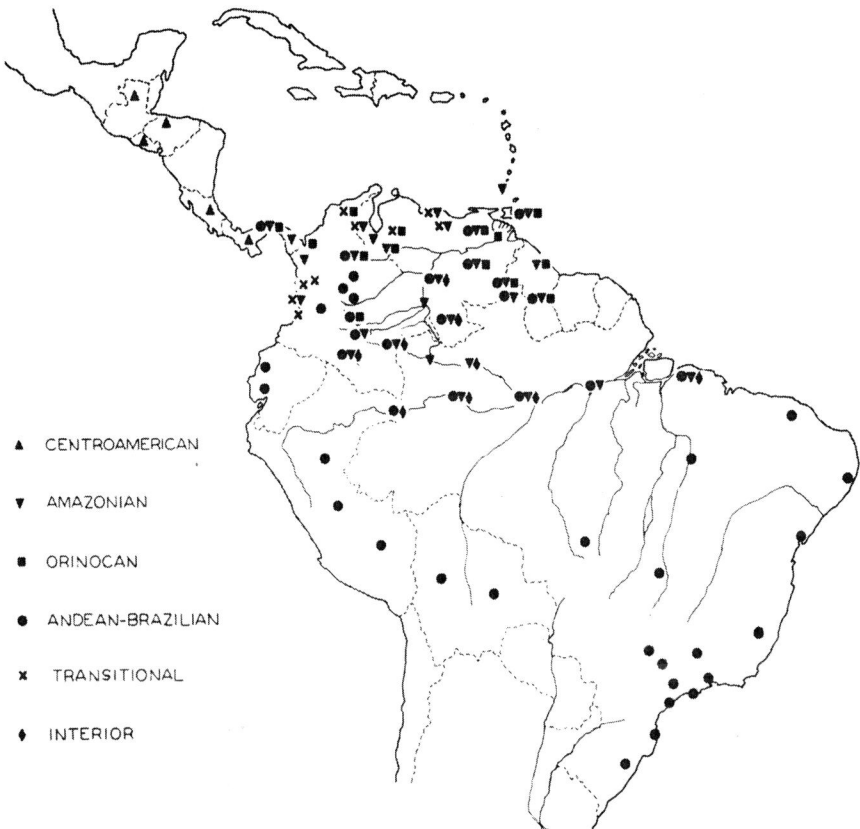

CENTROAMERICAN

AMAZONIAN

ORINOCAN

ANDEAN-BRAZILIAN

TRANSITIONAL

INTERIOR

Figure 2. The geographic distribution of the semispecies of D. paulistorum.

plexity in tests of sexual isolation between Transitional and Centroamerican strains. While some pairs of strains mate almost at random, others give isolation coefficients of up to 0.84. Sterility and sexual isolation are only imperfectly correlated. It can be seen in Figure 2 that the distribution area of the Transitional semispecies is less extensive than that of any of the others, and yet Transitional is the most diversified form of all. The differences between the semispecies in the gene arrangements will be discussed below.

Koref-Santibañez (1972*a,b*) made a painstaking study of the courtship rituals of the semispecies. They are qualitatively alike in the sense that the same stimuli and responses are used by all; yet every semispecies is characteristically different from the others in the relative frequencies of the different movements and activities. Males of every semispecies court females of all others, but semispecies-foreign females reject their advances much more often than they do those of males of their own semispecies.

Genetic Analysis of Isolating Mechanisms between Semispecies

The fertility of female hybrids between the semispecies of *D. paulistorum* makes possible genetic analysis of the semispecific differentials. Having obtained mutant genes to serve as chromosome markers, Ehrman (1960) analyzed the sterility of the hybrid males and (Ehrman, 1961) the sexual isolation. The latter proved to be genetically less unusual than the former. The sexual acceptability of an individual is a function of the proportions of the genetic materials of different semispecies which this individual contains. Usually, though not always, the F_1 hybrids are about equally acceptable to both parental semispecies, but less acceptable than nonhybrid individuals. In the backcross progenies there is range of acceptabilities, from that like an F_1 hybrid to that of the recurrent species parent. Sexual isolation depends upon genes or gene complexes in different chromosomes; it is a polygenic character.

The causes of the sterility of the hybrid males are still imperfectly understood. Ehrman (1960) found that hybrid females backcrossed to males of the parental semispecies give progenies in which all males are completely sterile, although some of these males must contain chromosomes of a single semispecies exclusively. Using backcross females with some chromosome markers, Ehrman concluded that the presence of a single, semispecies-foreign chromosome in the mother causes sterility of all her male progeny. The sterility of a male thus depends not only on his own genetic constitution but also on that of his mother. This suggests some kind of determination of the egg by the maternal chromosomes present in it before meiosis.

As Ehrman herself realized, this cannot be the whole story. The sterility of the F_1 hybrid males is clearly due to their own chromosomal composition and not solely to a predetermination by maternal genes. Crosses between Transitional and Centroamerican strains often give sterile F_1 males, while at least a part of the backcross males are fertile (Ehrman, 1962; Dobzhansky *et al.*, 1969; Pérez-Salas *et al.*, 1970). A strain of Transitional semispecies (Santa Marta) gives sterile male hybrids with an Andean-Brazilian strain (Mesitas) when Santa Marta is used as a female parent, but fertile ones when it is employed as a male parent (Ehrman, 1963). This sterility appears to be due to interaction between the Y chromosome of the Santa Marta strain with the cytoplasm of the Mesitas strain.

Santa Marta and Mesitas strains were used for experiments on "infectious sterility," although similar phenomena were later discovered with other strains (Ehrman and Williamson, 1965, 1969; Ehrman, 1967; Williamson and Ehrman, 1967). Mesitas females were injected, as young adults, with homogenates of Santa Marta males, or of Santa Marta ♀ × Mesitas ♂ F_1 hybrid males. The injected females were then crossed to Mesitas males. The progeny obtained are evidently genetically pure Mesitas, not hybrid at all. Nevertheless, Mesitas sons developing from eggs deposited several days after the injection of the mothers with hybrid male homogenate were sterile, and their sterility resembled cytologically that of the really hybrid males. The injection evidently transferred some factor which has caused the sterility of a part of the progeny of the injected mothers. No sterility arises in the daughters of the injected mothers, or among their nonhybrid progeny.

A quest for identification of the "factor" responsible for the infectious sterility has been pursued by Kernaghan and Ehrman (Kernaghan and Ehrman, 1970a,b; Ehrman and Kernaghan, 1972). Possibly implicated are intracellular inclusions resembling mycoplasma which are present in the testes of nonhybrid fertile males and more abundantly in the sterile males. They have also been seen in the ovaries and in other tissues of *D. melanogaster* by Koch and King (1966), who referred to them as "A-bodies." The working hypothesis is that different populations and semi-species of *D. paulistorum* carry different varieties of mycoplasma, and that each variety of the fly is genetically coadapted to its particular mycoplasma. The coadaptation breaks down as a result of hybridization, and the sterility is a consequence. For the time being, this intriguing and fruitful working hypothesis still needs verification or refutation.

Mutants and Linkage Maps

Lancefield and Metz (1922) and Ferry *et al.* (1923) described 34 mutants in the X, 11 in the second, and 8 in the third chromosomes of *D. willistoni.* A linkage map 84 Morgan units long of the X chromosome was constructed. The authors correctly inferred that the X chromosome of *D. willistoni* contains a part homologous to the X of *D. melanogaster,* and also a part homologous to one of the autosomes in the latter species. In 1941, Sturtevant and Novitski homologized the chromosomes of several species of *Drosophila* in terms of what they called "elements." The elements are five large blocks and one small block of genes, within which but

TABLE 2.   *Chromosome-Limb*
Homologies[a]

D. willistoni	D. melanogaster
XR + XL	X ; IIIL
IIR + IIL	IIR + IIL
III	IIIR
?	IV

[a] After Sturtevant and Novitski.

not between which the gene loci are often rearranged in the course of evolution. Although the mutants described by Lancefield and Metz were by then no longer in existence, Sturtevant and Novitski proposed homologies of the chromosome limbs in *D. willistoni* and *D. melanogaster* as given in Table 2. The smallest element, the fourth microchromosome of *D. melanogaster*, is either lost or translocated to one of the other elements in *D. willistoni*. The constancy and indivisibility of the elements is evidently far from absolute.

New mutants and linkage maps were obtained for *D. willistoni* in the 1940's by Spassky and Dobzhansky (1950) in connection with the studies on the concealed genetic variability, or "genetic loads" (see below). A total of 21 mutants in the X, 22 in the second, and 11 in the third chromosomes were described. The linkage maps are reproduced in Figure 3. The names of the mutants indicate phenotypic similarities with the classical mutants of *D. melanogaster*, and also with the mutants in *D. willistoni* described by Lancefield and Metz (1922). No rigorous proof of the similarities being due to gene homologies can be given, although this is highly probable in many cases. Perhaps the strongest evidence comes from genetic studies of allozymes of different species (see below, and also Lakovaara and Saura, 1972). Mutants like white (w), yellow (y), scute (sc), forked (f) or singed (sn), sepia (se), aristopedia (ss^a), and tardigrade (td) exist in many species of *Drosophila* and are almost certainly homologous. Other similar mutants, within as well as between species, may be mimics. It may be noted that the linkage maps of the X chromosome in *D. willistoni* prepared by Lancefield and Metz and by Dobzhansky and Spassky look rather different. Thus, the genes y and sc are approximately at the midpoint of the map of the former but close to the end of the map of the latter authors. Such differences are not unexpected because of the abundance of chromosomal inversions in natural populations, and also because the initial material of Lancefield and Metz was derived from Puerto Rico, while that of Dobzhansky and Spassky came from Brazil. Several mutants have been

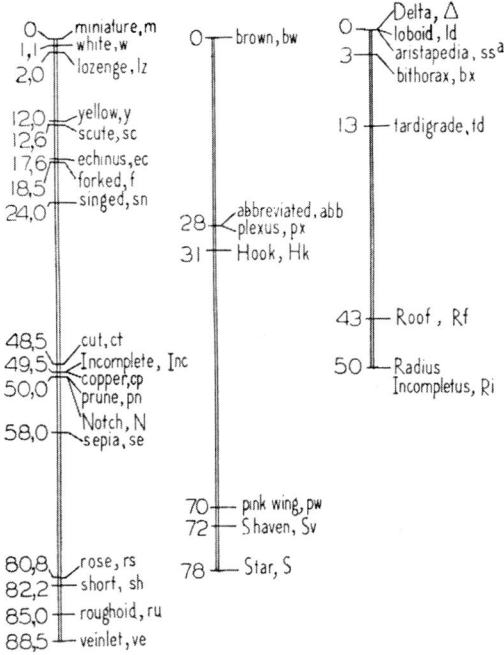

Figure 3. Linkage maps of D. willistoni chromosomes. (Left) X chromosome, (middle) second chromosome, (right) third chromosome. Reproduced from Spassky and Dobzhansky, 1950, Heredity 4:201–215, by permission of Oliver and Boyd, Ltd.

picked up also in *D. paulistorum* and other sibling species, and sketchy linkage maps have been constructed (Malogolowkin and Ehrman, 1960).

Viability and Fertility Variants in Natural Populations

The mutants obtained by Spassky and Dobzhansky (1950) were utilized as chromosome markers to construct "analyzers" of the genetic variability concealed in the second and third chromosomes in natural populations. The analysis can be carried out using either one of the procedures diagramed in Figure 4. The essence of the experimental designs is obtaining in the F_3 generations a class of individuals, $+_1/+_1$, carrying in double dose a chromosome which was present singly in the wild ancestor, $+_1/+_2$. Since the dominant markers, D, are usually lethal in homozygotes, the D/D class is eliminated, and the theoretically expected ratio in F_3 is 33.3 percent of $+_1/+_1$ and 66.7 percent of $+_1/D$. If the $+_1$ chromosome carries a recessive lethal, only flies with the dominant marker appear in the culture. Semilethal and subvital chromosomes give $+_1/+_1$ frequencies below 33.3 percent but above zero; the rare supervitals give frequencies above 33.3 percent. Since the dominant markers, D, may reduce the viability of their carriers, a control experiment is arranged in which flies carrying D appear together with a "wild-type" class, $+_1/+_2$, that has two + chromosomes derived from *different* progenitors from the same natural population. The viability, fertility, development rate, etc., of $+_1/+_2$ individuals is "normal" by definition. The data from the control experiment then permit the expression of the viabilities of the $+_1/+_1$, $+_2/+_2$, etc., flies in terms of percentages of the normal viability. [For a more detailed explanation of this experimental design, see Dobzhansky (1970) pages 75–77, or Pavan *et al.* (1951).]

Pavan *et al.* (1951) submitted 2004 second and 1166 third chromosomes to analysis by the above-described method. The chromosomes came from samples taken in 9 localities in different parts of Brazil. Chromosomes lethal, semilethal, subvital, and quasinormal in double dose were encountered in every sample. Percent frequencies of chromosomes with different viabilities (expressed in percentages of the "normal" viability) are shown in Table 3. It can be seen that, like in all *Drosophila* species studied in this respect, the distribution of the viabilities is bimodal. Chromosomes that are lethal or nearly so in homozygous condition (0–5 percent of the "normal" viability) form one mode, and mildly subvital

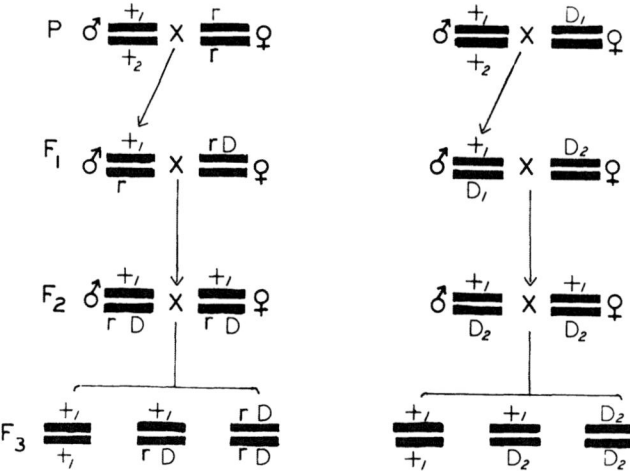

Figure 4. Crosses used to reveal the concealed variability consisting of recessive autosomal genes and gene complexes. Here $+_1$ and $+_2$ are the chromosomes analyzed, r is a recessive, and D_1D_1 and D_2 are dominant marker genes.

TABLE 3. *Viability of Second and Third Chromosomes of D. willistoni in Double Dose*

Chromo-some	Percent normal viability									
	0–5	5–20	20–35	35–50	50–65	65–80	80–95	95–110	110–125	>125
Second	28.6	4.2	3.4	4.5	5.4	12.6	24.7	12.8	3.5	0.3
Third	19.7	5.7	3.2	3.5	5.1	9.4	31.6	20.2	1.6	—

chromosomes (80–95 percent of the "normal" viability) make up the other mode. Semilethals (5–50 percent), strong subvitals (50–80 percent), quasinormals (95–110 percent), and supervitals are relatively rare.

Better estimates of the incidence of subvital second chromosomes have been obtained by Krimbas (1959), using a statistical technique developed by Wallace and Madden (1953). In a sample of 177 second chromosomes coming from localities as far apart as southern Brazil and the West Indies, Krimbas found 65 chromosomes that were lethal or semilethal in double dose; among the remaining 112 chromosomes, 72 percent were subvital, 28 percent quasinormal, and none were supervital. [The much larger sample of Pavan *et al.* (1951) is unfortunately not suitable for analysis.] Krimbas compared the burden of genetic variants reducing the viability in *D. willistoni* with that in *D. prosaltans,* and found the burden heavier in the former than in the latter species. He attributed the difference to the reproductive biologies of these species. *D. willistoni* is a very common, ecologically versatile form, able to live in a great variety of environments. Although the geographic area of *D. prosaltans* is largely the same as that of *D. willistoni,* it is a relatively rare and specialized species. Dobzhansky *et al.* (1952) found that the mutation rates in the second and third chromosomes of *D. willistoni* appear to be higher than in the homologous chromosomes of *D. prosaltans.* The evidence is, however, not conclusive, because differences in mutation rates seem to occur also among strains of the same species.

The genetic technique diagramed in Figure 4 is suitable for detection of all kinds of recessive genetic variants concealed in heterozygous condition in wild flies. Suppose that the chromosome $+_1$ carries a gene, or genes, causing some morphological alteration, or a physiological or a behavioral change in homozygotes. These changes can be detected in the $+_1/+_1$ class in the third generation. Pavan *et al.* (1951) found about 16 percent of the surviving homozygotes for either the second or the third chromosomes in their materials to have clear-cut, visible, mutant traits. About 30 percent of the second chromosomes, and 28 percent of the third chromosomes, caused complete sterility either of the homozygous females or of the males, but rarely of both sexes. Roughly one-third of the viable homozygotes for the second, as well as for the third, chromosomes had their development rates appreciably retarded compared to that of the heterozygotes. Homozygotes with accelerated development were much fewer, but some clear instances were encountered.

It is quite obvious that flies not carrying any concealed recessive variants in any of their chromosomes are encountered rarely or not at all. Most of these variants are to some extent deleterious to their carriers if permitted to become homozygous. They are components of the genetic "burden" or "load," but this is not the whole story of their biological role.

Release of Genetic Variability by Recombination

It should be stressed that the above data on the incidence of recessive lethal, semilethals, sterilities, and other variants pertain to chromosomes rather than to single gene loci. Indeed, the technique shown in Figure 4 generates a class of individuals, $+_1/+_1$, carrying in double dose a chromosome which was present singly in the wild progenitor, $+_1/+_2$. What is observed is, then, a net effect of homozygosis for all loci contained in a certain chromosome. The question that arises is this: Suppose we have two chromosomes with identical effects in double dose (both subvital, or quasinormal, or lethal), can we conclude that these chromosomes are identical in their genes? This question is particularly interesting when asked about "normal" chromosomes. Are all normal chromosomes alike, as certain geneticists naively assume?

Natural populations of several species were tested according to a common plan (*D. melanogaster, D. pseudoobscura, D. persimilis, D. prosaltans,* and *D. willistoni*) (see Chapter 20 on the *Drosophila obscura* group in this volume for more details about this work). The study on *D. willistoni* was carried out by Krimbas (1961). He selected 10 second chromosomes from the same population; 8 of them had normal viability in double dose, and two were subvital. The strains with these chromosomes were intercrossed in all combinations (45 combinations). Females that carried pairs of the chromosomes were allowed to produce offspring, and 10 second chromosomes from each combination (450 chromosomes total) were submitted to tests for viability in homozygotes. If the 10 selected chromosomes were really alike, the products of their meiotic recombinations should also be identical, except for newly arisen mutants. But this is not what the experiments showed. The homozygous viability of the recombination chromosomes ranged all the way from complete lethality to normality and even supervitality. As many as 21 among the 450 recombination chromosomes, or 4.7 $\pm$ 1.0 percent, were lethal. It is particularly important that these synthetic lethals appeared among recombinants of pairs of chromosomes, each of which gave homozygotes of normal viability. If one excludes the two subvital chromosomes, the remaining eight produced 3.9 $\pm$ 1.0 percent synthetic lethals among the recombinations. Thus, contrary to the assertions of some authors who find synthetic lethals uncomfortable for their theories, these lethals are not simply sums of additive effects of pairs of subvital or semilethal chromosomes; they are due to epistatic interactions of the genes brought together by the recombination of seemingly identical "wild-type" chromosomes.

Synthetic lethals are only the extreme products of the recombination process. Krimbas (1961) compared the variance among second chromosomes extracted from flies collected in nature with that among chromosomes obtained by recombination in his experiments. He found that the recombination releases 34.5 percent of the total natural variance, and almost 100 percent of the variance among "natural" quasinormal chromosomes. In another study (Krimbas, 1960), he observed a synthetic sterility in addition to synthetic lethality—some recombination products of chromosomes which make their carriers fertile cause sterility in double dose. Magalhaes *et al.* (1965a,b) and da Cunha *et al.* (1966) produced an elegant confirmation of the work of Krimbas. They observed that some second chromosomes of *D. willistoni* carry recessive "suppressors," which enable homozygotes for certain second chromosome lethals to survive. But it is evident that the removal of a "suppressor" from a nonlethal chromosome transforms this chromosome into a synthetic lethal! Lethal chromosomes can be synthesized as well as desynthesized by recombination.

Relationship of Concealed and Overt Variability in Natural Populations

Most of the recessive genetic variants detected as described above are concealed in heterozygous condition. Like many hereditary diseases in man, they become homozygous and appear on the phenotypic surface owing to occasional inbreeding, or to accidental mating of heterozygous carriers. But the concealment is imperfect because the recessivity is often incomplete. "Normal" or "wild-type" flies in natural populations are genotypically and phenotypically no more alike than "normal" individuals in human populations. Cordeiro and Dobzhansky (1954) tested the viability of many combinations of 5 second chromosomes that were lethal in double dose and 23 chromosomes that gave quasinormal homozygotes. All chromosomes came from populations of *D. willistoni* in southern Brazil. Significant heterogeneity of viabilities was observed among the carriers of different pairs of these chromosomes. The viabilities were measured, of course, by observing the ratios of individuals carrying known combinations of the chromosomes tested, and of individuals with chromosomes marked by suitable mutant genes. The same lethal chromosome may give unlike viabilities in combination with different quasinormal chromosomes, and different lethal chromosomes produce unequally viable heterozygotes with a given quasinormal chromosome. The same is true of quasinormal chromosomes—diverse viabilities are engendered by different pairs. Similar results have recently been described by Kenyon (1972) in *D. melanogaster,* without reference to the findings in *D. willistoni.*

Malogolowkin-Cohen *et al.* (1964) contributed a study bearing on the hotly debated problem of whether the genetic variants deleterious in homozygotes are maintained in natural populations only by mutation pressure or also by balancing natural selection. They used samples of *D. willistoni* from Venezuela, Guyana, and Trinidad. The viability of crossbred and inbred progenies was compared. Two levels of inbreeding, $F = 0.125$ and $F = 0.250$, were arranged. The viability decreased with increased inbreeding, but the estimates of the so-called B/A ratios were appreciably different for different inbreeding levels. This shows that the viability effects of the components of the genetic loads are not additive; epistatic interactions are important, especially at higher inbreeding levels. The relative importance of the mutational and balanced components of the genetic load remains an open question for *D. willistoni.* Equally ambiguous results were obtained by de Toledo *et al.* (1966), comparing the frequencies of recessive lethal chromosomes extracted from wild-collected males and females.

Pavan and Knapp (1954) showed that the genetically effective populations of *D. willistoni,* a very common species in many parts of Brazil, may be treated as indistinguishable from theoretical infinite ones. Intercrosses of strains with chromosomes that are lethal in double dose were made, and the rates of allelism of these lethals determined. For lethals derived from remote localities, the rate is 0.00157, and for those found in the same locality the rate is 0.00169 (not significantly higher). The only exceptions were the populations of small islands in the bay of Angra dos Reis, where the allelism rate was higher, 0.00514. It should also be noted that the magnitude of the genetic burden is apparently quite uniform throughout the area of the species, with a possible exception of some geographically marginal populations (Townsend, 1952).

Chromosomal Polymorphism in *Drosophila willistoni*

Already the first exploratory study of population samples disclosed the ubiquity of heterozygous inversions in the four widespread sibling species—*D. willistoni, D. paulistorum, D. equinoxialis,* and *D. tropicalis* (Burla *et al.,* 1949; Dobzhansky *et al.,* 1950). The more narrowly endemic *D. insularis* and *D. pavlovskiana* are also polymorphic for inversions. Species of the *willistoni* group are unfortunately not favorable for cytological studies of their salivary gland chromosomes; while heterokaryotypes (heterozygous inversions) are scored easily, homokaryotypes are hard to distinguish. Therefore, almost all data are presented in terms of frequencies of heterozygotes for various inversions.

Ayala *et al.* (1971), da Cunha *et al.* (1950, 1959), da Cunha and Dobzhansky (1954), and Dobzhansky (1957*a*) studied population samples of *D. willistoni* from some 85 localities spread over the immense geographic range of this species, from Florida to Argentina. The 50 different inversions recorded are distributed as follows in the five chromosomal limbs seen in the polytene chromosomes:

XL	XR	IIL	IIR	III
11	7	8	6	18

The third chromosome has most inversions, and it happens to be cytologically the longest one. Some of the inversions are narrowly endemic, while others are widespread. Thus, the subterminal inversion *J* in the third chromosome and *E* in the right limb of the second chromosomes are found from Florida to Argentina, and almost everywhere in between. This is quite remarkable, considering that the inversions are almost certainly monophyletic in origin. In other words, there was a time when the inversions *J* and *E* existed each in a single individual; they are now in doubtless many billions of individuals living over millions of square kilometers. Burla *et al.* (1950) found the active dispersal of *D. willistoni* to be slow (slower than in, for example, *D. pseudoobscura*), and the population density of *D. willistoni* and *D. paulistorum* combined to be 10–28 individuals per 100 square meters in a fairly favorable locality in southern Brazil. To achieve a species-wide distribution, a monophyletic genetic variant must be promoted by natural selection, and either be subject to long-distance passive transport by air currents or require long stretches of time, or both.

Populations of different parts of the species area can be characterized by the relative frequencies of the different inversions in their chromosomal pool. Owing to the almost species-wide distribution of the commonest inversions, the chromosomal races in *D. willistoni* are on the whole less sharply distinct than in *D. pseudoobscura,* among others (Powell *et al.,* 1972). The chromosomal races of *D. willistoni* differ in the proportions of individuals that are inversion heterozygotes, and especially in the numbers of heterozygous inversions per individual. The central part of the species area has populations with many heterozygous inversions, up to 9 per average female individual in central Brazil. The average numbers of heterozygous inversions dwindle toward the distribution margins, the West Indies, southern Brazil and Argentina, northeastern Brazil, and coastal Ecuador, where the averages decline to one or fewer than one inversion per individual.

Why should central populations be chromosomally more polymorphic than marginal ones? Dobzhansky, da Cunha, and their colleagues (see references above) argued that, by and large, a species occupies and exploits more diverse environments and resources where it has lived long and is thoroughly "at home" than where it approaches its geographic and ecological limits of tolerance. Genetic polymorphism makes a population able to get hold of a variety of resources and means of existence. A rough quasi-quantitative fit of environmental diversity ratings and of extents of the inversion polymorphisms has been obtained by da Cunha *et al.* (1959). Carson (1959) stresses rather the fact that inversion heterozygosis reduces Mendelian recombination. Geographically, central and chromosomally highly polymorphic populations have, then, more adaptedness than adaptability; the situation is reversed in marginal populations. This way of looking at the problem is clearly not incompatible, but rather complementary, to that of da Cunha *et al.* (1959).

Experimental Demonstration of Coadaptation in Inversion Heterozygotes

Chromosomal inversions do not by themselves enhance the Darwinian fitness of their carriers. They do, however, bind together complexes of genes that interact favorably with other gene complexes present in the same population. These supergenes, locked in the inversions, augment the adaptive values of the inversion heterozygotes in a given population. But the supergenes in one population need not be coadapted with those carried in the inversions in another population. Hybridization and recombination may, then, result in a breakdown of coadaptation.

Dobzhansky and Pavlovsky (1958) have verified the interpretation just presented by experiments on *D. willistoni, D. paulistorum* (Andean-Brazilian semispecies), and *D. tropicalis.* In each of these species populations were found in which approximately half, or more than half, of the individuals were heterozygous for certain inversions. This indicated that in each case the two homokaryotypes were approximately equal in adaptive value, and also that the heterokaryotype was superior to both homokaryotypes. Samples of such populations were kept for a series of generations in laboratory population cages, and the high frequencies of the heterokaryotypes persisted. The relative fitness of the homo- and heterokaryotypes were not greatly different in the natural and in the experimental environments.

Next, pairs of populations of the same species from different localities, but polymorphic for the same inversion, were intercrossed. Population cages were started with hybrids as founders. The problem at issue was whether the chromosomes from different populations would be coadapted as well as those from within a population. The results showed that they were not coadapted. The frequency of heterokaryotypes fell, and one of the homokaryotypes began to considerably outnumber the other. The coadapted supergenes were disrupted by recombination.

Genetic Variation of Behavior

The species differences in the mating rituals have already been mentioned above. Petit and Ehrman (Petit and Ehrman, 1968; Ehrman and Petit, 1968) have shown that in at least three species, *D. willistoni, D. equinoxialis,* and *D. tropicalis,* there exist mating advantages of less-frequent types of males. When females are exposed to two kinds of males of different geographic origin, but of the same species, both kinds of males are equally successful in mating if they are equally frequent. Not so if one kind of male outnumbers the other. The less-frequent males secure on the average more mates per individual than do more-frequent males. The biological role of this mating advantage is a matter of speculation; it may serve to maintain or enhance the genetic polymorphism in populations.

A genetic polymorphism of behavior in a population of *D. willistoni* kept in a laboratory population cage was found by de Souza *et al.* (1968, 1970). Some larvae pupate in the food medium, while others pupate outside the food. The preference for outside pupation seems to be a dominant trait, and pupation in the food a recessive one. Either kind of habit may be advantageous or disadvantageous under certain conditions. Natural selection in different laboratory environments leads to rapid increases of the frequencies of the favored genotypes. It is possible, but not proven, that the sibling species may differ in their circadian rhythms and food preferences (Pavan *et al.,* 1950; da Cunha *et al.,* 1957).

The "Sex-Ratio" Condition

Genetic conditions have been discovered in several species of *Drosophila* which result in production of unisexual progenies, consisting of females only. These conditions are of two sharply distinct kinds: chromosomal and cytoplasmic. The former, not found in species of the *willistoni* group, are due to a gene or a gene complex in the X chromosome, which makes males carrying it produce only or almost only X-bearing sperm. Such males, crossed to any female, give only daughters in the progeny (see Chapter 20). Cytoplasmic sex-ratio is transmitted through females only, and causes a female to produce progeny consisting mostly or only of daughters, regardless of what kind of male it mates with.

Cytoplasmic sex-ratio was studied in the progenies of some wild-collected females of *D. willistoni* and *D. paulistorum* by Malogolowkin (1958) and in *D. equinoxialis* by the same author (Malogolowkin, 1959). How frequent such females are in natural populations is inadequately known, but they are certainly a minority, and most wild-collected flies produce progenies with approximately equal proportions of daughters and sons. Malogolowkin *et al.* (1959) and Malogolowkin and Carvalho (1961) found that the agent responsible for the sex-ratio condition can be transferred artificially from carriers to normal strains by injection of the hemolymph or of the ooplasm from the sex-ratio females to normal females. It can be so transferred not only within but also between species, e.g., from *D. willistoni* to *D. equinoxialis* or to *D. nebulosa*. It cannot be transferred by injection of males, it is transmitted in the egg cytoplasm. However, the agent is not independent of chromosomal genes—crossing sex-ratio females to males of certain strains results in alleviation or "cure" of the condition. A "cure" may also be obtained by heat treatment of the eggs deposited by sex-ratio females.

Poulson and his colleagues (Poulson and Sakaguchi, 1961; Sakaguchi and Poulson, 1961, 1963; Counce and Poulson, 1962; Oishi and Poulson, 1970) discovered that the hemolymph of sex-ratio females is swarming with spirochetes, possibly a species of *Treponema*. These spirochetes are less abundantly present also on fat bodies, thoracic muscles, and ovaries of sex-ratio females, but never in normal females. They are also present in the occasionally surviving sons of sex-ratio mothers. The male zygotes in the progenies of sex-ratio females die owing to gross disturbances in embryogenesis. There is no reasonable doubt that the *Treponema* is the cause of death of the male zygotes, and consequently of the sex-ratio condition. However, the mechanism of its action needs further elucidation, especially after the discovery of a DNA virus associated with the *Treponema*. Oishi and Poulson (1970) rightly say that "The analysis of such three-level systems—virus, spirochete, fly—is of considerable interest not only from the point of view of genetics, but also in terms of their ecological and evolutionary implications."

Allozyme Polymorphisms in the *Drosophila willistoni* Group

Extensive data are available on allozyme (genetically determined enzyme variants) polymorphisms in several of the species of *D. willistoni* group. These studies have centered on four questions: (1) How much genetic variation exists in natural populations? (2) What is the pattern of genetic variation? (3) How much genetic differentiation exists among subspecies, semispecies, and sibling species? (4) What mechanisms might be operating to maintain allozyme polymorphisms?

Table 4 gives a summary of the amounts of genetic variability found in various species and semispecies of the *D. willistoni* group. In this table, if the frequency of the most common allele at a locus is less than or equal to 0.95, then the locus is considered polymorphic. Data on *D. willistoni*, *D. equinoxialis*, and *D. tropicalis* are in Ayala and Powell (1972a) and data for the semispecies of *D. paulistorum* are in Richmond (1972a). It should be borne in mind that the estimates in Table 4 are based on the kind of variation detected by starch gel electrophoresis, and thus are underestimates. The original references should be consulted for the theory behind these estimates and possible errors involved in the technique.

Many species of plants and animals have been studied for allozyme

TABLE 4. *Amounts of Genetic Variation Detected by Electrophoretic Studies of Allozymes*

Species	Semispecies	Number of loci studied	Percent loci polymorphic	Percent average heterozygosity per individuals
D. willistoni		28	58	17.3 ± 3.0
D. equinoxialis		27	71	21.8 ± 3.0
D. tropicalis		25	60	19.2 ± 3.1
D. paulistorum	Centroamerican	13	46	8.0 ± 4.0
	Transitional	15	53	16.0 ± 4.0
	Andean-Brazilian	16	56	18.0 ± 5.0
	Orinocan	11	55	30.0 ± 8.0
	Interior	15	40	15.0 ± 5.0
	Amazonian	14	50	18.0 ± 5.0

polymorphisms. The species and semispecies of the *D. willistoni* group are among the most polymorphic species yet studied. The *D. willistoni* group is, therefore, one of the most polymorphic groups known for both chromosome inversions (see above) and for single-gene polymorphisms detected by electrophoresis.

What is the geographic pattern of frequencies of various allozymes in the *D. willistoni* group? Two generalizations have been formulated to describe the pattern of variation. First, and most remarkable, is that at any given locus, the same allele is (with few and minor exceptions) the most common allele in all populations studied. Since many populations throughout the range of each species have been sampled, it seems safe to conclude that this generalization holds throughout the distributions of the species. The second generalization is that allele frequencies are not identical in all populations of a species. Statistically significant clines in allele frequencies occur at some loci (Ayala *et al.*, 1972*a*; Richmond, 1972*a*). Similar patterns of variation have been noted for other species of *Drosophila* (see Chapter 20 on *obscura* group in this volume). Recent and more extensive data on allozyme polymorphism in the *willistoni* group may be found in Ayala *et al.* (1974*a,b,c*).

There is little or no evidence that allozyme variation decreases as one approaches the geographic margin of a species' distribution. Furthermore, there is only an insignificant decrease in enzyme variability in isolated populations. Ayala *et al.* (1971) studied six Caribbean island populations of *D. willistoni* and four Colombian mainland populations. The average heterozygosity per individual from the islands was 16.9 ± 0.6 percent, and the average from the mainland populations was 18.4 ± 0.8 percent. Again, with few exceptions, the most-frequent alleles on the mainland were the most-frequent ones on the islands; nevertheless, allele frequencies were not identical. These data are in sharp contrast to inversion-polymorphism data mentioned above. Marginal and isolated populations tend to be less chromosomally variable. The six Caribbean populations studied by Ayala *et al.* (1971) had an average mean number of heterozygous autosomal inversions per individual of $0.79 \pm .12$, while Colombian population had 5.27 ± 0.42.

Gillespie and Kojima (1968) have suggested that enzymes involved in glucose metabolism (group I enzymes) should be less variable than other enzymes (group II). The data on the four species listed in Table 4 support this conclusion (Ayala and Powell, 1972*a*; Richmond, 1972*a*).

Besides making it possible to measure amounts and patterns of variability, electrophoretic studies allow comparison of degrees of genetic divergence between taxa. Since the *D. willistoni* group has subspecies, semispecies, sibling species, and morphologically distinct species, this is a good group for comparative studies of different levels of evolutionary divergence. In order to make such comparisons, a quantitative measure of genetic divergence is useful. The genetic distance measure (D) employed here is that of Nei (1972). Table 5 gives a summary of various comparisons. These data are from Ayala and Tracey (1973) and Ayala *et al.* (1974*a,b,c*). An interpretation of the meaning of this measure is that, for example, between populations of different subspecies, an average of 23 electrophoretically detectable allelic substitutions have occurred per 100 loci.

Several conclusions can be drawn from Table 5. First, relatively little genetic divergence has occurred among populations of a given species, semispecies, or subspecies ($\bar{D} = 0.019$). About 7 times more differentiation exists among semispecies and 8 times more among subspecies [also see Richmond (1972*b*)]. On the species level, the average divergence is considerable, even for siblings. More than half of the loci studied, on the average, have diverged between any two of the siblings of the *D. willistoni* group [also see Ayala *et al.* (1970)]. The morphologically distinct member of the group, *D. nebulosa,* is even more distinct. Because of this great amount of divergence between siblings, allozyme variation has proved to be a useful technique for identifying the various siblings of this group. Between any two siblings, an average of 25 percent of the 28 loci studied allow correct diagnosis of species with a probability of 99 percent or greater (Ayala and Powell, 1972*b*). Only 8 percent of the loci on the average allow diagnosis between subspecies with the same degree of accuracy, and no loci have as yet been found diagnostic for the semispecies of *D. paulistorum.*

Because of the large amount of allozyme data on the *D. willistoni* group, much has been learned about the selection values and mechanisms of maintenance of electrophoretically detectable enzyme variants. The

TABLE 5. *Amounts of Genetic Differentiation within and between Various Taxa of the D. willistoni Group*[a]

Comparison	Average genetic distance ($\bar{D}$)
Between populations within a species, semispecies, or subspecies	0.031
Between semispecies of *D. paulistorum*	0.226
Between subspecies of *D. willistoni* and *D. equinoxialis*	0.230
Between sibling species	0.581
Between *D. nebulosa* and siblings of *D. willistoni*	1.056

[a] From Ayala *et al.*, 1974.

most important inference is that the geographic pattern of genetic variation indicates that some form of balancing selection is maintaining these
polymorphisms [for details see Ayala *et al.* (1971, 1972*a,b*) and Richmond (1972*a*)].

Richmond and Powell (1970) found an excess of heterozygotes over
Hardy-Weinberg expectations at the tetrazolium oxidase locus in a
natural population of *D. paulistorum*. This indicated that heterosis may
act to maintain this polymorphism. Powell (1974*b*) supported this interpretation by finding that the excess of heterozygotes persists in laboratory populations. Furthermore, it has been shown that the alleles at this
locus are not associated with inversions. This rules out the possibility that
the heterozygote excess is due to a heterotic inversion system rather than
the locus which is being observed or its immediate neighbors.

That diversifying selection may be acting to maintain allozyme variation in *D. willistoni* was shown by Powell (1971). In experimental populations maintained in various environments, the rate of loss of enzyme
variation was slower in diversified environments than in homogeneous environments. An attempt was also made to measure directly the selective
value of enzyme variants (Powell, 1974*a*). Laboratory populations were
begun with varying frequencies of allozymes at three different loci. Frequency changes were followed for about 2 years. Allele frequencies at two
of the three loci came to the same stable equilibria in all populations.
Allele frequencies at the third locus did not change over this period of
time. Further studies revealed that alleles at the two loci which showed
frequency changes were nonrandomly associated with gene arrangements
of the chromosomes in which they were located [see Lakovaara and Saura
(1972) for the chromosomal location of several enzyme loci in *D. willistoni*]. Thus, it is impossible to unambiguously conclude that the stable
equilibria reached were due to selection at the enzyme loci rather than to
the inversions.

Chromosomal Differentiation of the Semispecies of *Drosophila paulistorum*

Before the existence of the semispecies within the superspecies *D.
paulistorum* had been discovered (Dobzhansky and Spassky, 1959), an exploratory study had shown that natural populations of this species are
chromosomally polymorphic (Dobzhansky *et al.*, 1950). Later work
[Dobzhansky and Pavlovsky (1962), and especially Kastritsis (1966,
1967)] disclosed that, taking the superspecies as a whole, there are a
minimum of 63 inversions, making *D. paulistorum* chromosomally the

most polymorphic *Drosophila* known. The numbers of the inversions per chromosome limb are as follows:

XR	XL	IIL	IIR	III
5	9	7	10	32

The third chromosome is the most variable one. The problem that attracted most attention was whether every semispecies has its own set of chromosomal polymorphs, or polymorphisms are shared by more than one semispecies. The interest of this problem was enhanced by Carson's (1959) hypothesis that new strains arise mostly from peripheral populations of parent species, and that peripheral populations are usually monomorphic. A summary of the Kastritsis (1967) data is presented in Table 6.

Many polymorphisms (P) are evidently shared by two or more semispecies. Although some inversions are found in some semispecies and not in others, none are really diagnostic—they do not permit conclusive identification of the semispecies by the chromosomes of a single larva. Inversion XR–II comes closest to being diagnostic since it is monomorphic (M) in the Amazonian semispecies while the corresponding standard gene arrangement is fixed (S) in Andean, Orinocan, Interior, and Transitional; yet the XR–II inversion has been found heterozygous in one Centroamerican strain. The semispecies have diverged chromosomally much less than the species have. An alternative, but far less probable, explanation of the semispecies being at a much lower level of chromosomal divergence is introgressive hybridization. In other words, one may speculate that the semispecies differences are breaking down rather than increasing. But if so, the shared polymorphisms would be expected where two or more semispecies are sympatric. There is no indication of such a constraint. This is not to imply that there is no gene exchange whatsoever between the semispecies in nature. If this were so they would be full species. In reality, at least some of them have closely approached but not quite achieved the species status.

Origin of an Incipient Semispecies in the Laboratory

The Transitional semispecies has attracted attention because some (though not all) strains give fertile hybrids with the Centroamerican semispecies, and a few strains do so with the Andean semispecies. Even more remarkable is that the intercrosses of some Transitional strains with each other give sterile F_1 hybrid males, but the fertility is restored in the first backcross progenies (Dobzhansky *et al.*, 1969). Although the

TABLE 6.   Chromosomal Polymorphisms among the Semispecies of D. paulistorum[c]

	Semispecies[b]					
Chromosome[a]	Transi-tional	Andean	Centro-american	Amazonian	Orinocan	Interior
XL–II	P	P	P	S	P	P
XL–III	S	P	P	P	P	?
XR–I	P	S	P	S	M	S
XR–II	S	S	P	M	S	S
XR–III	S	P	S	S	S	?
IIL–I	P	P	M	P	P	P
IIR–I	P	S	P	P	P	P
IIR–II	P	S	P	S	P	P
IIR–III	P	S	P	S	S	?
III–V	P	P	P	S	S	P
III–VI	P	P	S	S	S	P
III–VII	P	P	P	S	S	?
III–VIII	P	S	P	S	S	P
III–IX	P	P	S	S	P	P
III–X	P	S	P	S	P	?
III–XI	P	S	P	S	S	?
III–XII	S	P	P	S	S	?
III–XIII	S	P	P	S	S	?
III–XIV	S	P	P	S	S	?
III–XV	S	S	P	P	S	?
III–XXVIII	S	S	S	S	S	P
III–XXIX	S	S	S	S	S	P

[a] Roman numerals refer to different areas of the chromosome.
[b] S =monomorphic for a "standard" gene arrangement, P =polymorphic, and M =monomorphic for a gene arrangement other than standard.
[c] After Kastritsis, 1967.

geographic area of the Transitional semispecies is smaller than those of the other semispecies [see Figure 2 and Spassky et al. (1971)], some cladogenetic processes are taking place within it. The following observations may perhaps throw some light on the nature of these processes.

Orinocan and Interior are related more closely than any other pair of semispecies. They are nowhere sympatric, although their geographic areas closely approach each other (Figure 2). They mate more easily than other semispecies—the average sexual isolation coefficient between them is as low as 0.47 (Pérez-Salas et al., 1970). At least some of the males in back-cross progenies are fertile. A single female captured in March, 1958, in the Llanos of Colombia gave progeny which crossed easily and produced fertile male hybrids with several strains of Orinocan semispecies. The

Llanos strain was accordingly classified as Orinocan. It was not tested with Interior since that semispecies was first discovered in 1963. The Llanos locality, at the foot of the Andes, is geographically marginal or intermediate, since the Orinocan semispecies lives to the North and East, and Interior semispecies to the South and Southeast. In 1963 (but before Interior strains were obtained in the laboratory) the Llanos strain produced sterile hybrids with the Orinocan, and has continued to do so ever since. Later it was found to give fertile hybrids with Interior strains (Dobzhansky and Pavlovsky, 1966, 1967, 1971).

The nature of the change which came to pass in the Llanos strain is unknown. It was certainly not a conversion of an Orinocan into an Interior strain. As pointed out above, the Orinocan and Interior semispecies show a pronounced, though relatively fragile, sexual isolation and a complete sterility of F_1 hybrid males. The Llanos strain, tested after 1963, shows hybrid sterility with the Orinocan semispecies, fertility with the Interior semispecies, and little sexual isolation from either [with the exception of one Interior strain; Pérez-Salas *et al.* (1970)]. Whatever cause made Llanos strain produce sterile male hybrids with the Orinocan, it certainly did not simultaneously induce a sexual isolation between them. Williamson and Ehrman (1967, 1968) found that homogenates of Llanos, of Llanos × Orinocan, or of Llanos × Interior F_1 hybrid males induce sterility in the male progeny of injected Llanos, Orinocan, or Interior females. This led to the hypothesis that the transformation of Llanos may have been caused by acquisition or loss of a symbiotic microorganism, such as a mycoplasma. The hypothesis stands in need of further testing.

Dobzhansky and Pavlovsky (1971) have superimposed a partial sexual isolation on the hybrid sterility between the Llanos and Orinocan strains. This has been done by means of artificial selection favoring the choice of genetically similar mating partners. Recessive mutant genes have been found both in the Llanos strain and in an Orinocan strain. Females of each strain are exposed to mixtures of males of both strains. Matings within a strain produce mutants; and matings between the strains produce wild-type offspring. The latter are discarded in every generation, and the former are used as parents of the next generation. After some 40–50 generations of such selection, the strains no longer breed at random. Isolation coefficients have been obtained which are even slightly higher than between strains of Orinocan and Interior semispecies descended from progenitors collected in the wild. Interestingly enough, the increasing sexual isolation of the Llanos from the Orinocan semispecies has not been accompanied by stronger isolation from the Interior semispecies. The isolating genes are evidently semispecies-specific.

Literature Cited

Ayala, F. J., 1973 Two new subspecies of the *Drosophila willistoni* group. *Pan-Pacific Entom.* **49**:273–279.

Ayala, F. J. and J. R. Powell, 1972*a* Enzyme variability in the *Drosophila willistoni* group. VI. Levels of polymorphism and the physiological function of enzymes. *Biochem. Genet.* **7**:331–345.

Ayala, F. J. and J. R. Powell, 1972*b* Allozymes as diagnostic characters of sibling species of *Drosophila*. *Proc. Natl. Acad. Sci. USA* **69**:1094–1096.

Ayala, F. J. and M. L. Tracey, 1973 Genetic differentiation and reproductive isolation between two subspecies of *Drosophila willistoni*. *J. Hered.* **64**:120–124.

Ayala, F. J., C. A. Mourão, S. Pérez-Salas, R. Richmond and T. Dobzhansky, 1970 Enzyme variability in the *Drosophila willistoni* group. I. Genetic differentiation among sibling species. *Proc. Natl. Acad. Sci. USA* **67**:225–232.

Ayala, F. J., J. R. Powell and T. Dobzhansky, 1971 Polymorphism in continental and island populations of *Drosophila willistoni*. *Proc. Natl. Acad. Sci.* **68**:2480–2483.

Ayala, F. J., J. R. Powell and M. L. Tracey, 1972*a* Enzyme variability in the *Drosophila willistoni* group. V. Genic variation in natural populations of *Drosophila equinoxialis*. *Genet. Res.* **20**:19–42.

Ayala, F. J., J. R. Powell, M. L. Tracey, C. A. Mourão and S. Pérez-Salas, 1972*b* Enzyme variability in the *Drosophila willistoni* group. IV. Genic variation in natural populations of *Drosophila willistoni*. *Genetics* **70**:113–139.

Ayala, F. J., M. L. Tracey, L. G. Barr and J. G. Ehrenfeld, 1974*a* Genetic and reproductive differentiation of *Drosophila equinoxialis caribbensis*. *Evolution* **28**:24–41.

Ayala, F. J., M. L. Tracey, L. G. Barr, J. F. McDonald and S. Pérez-Salas, 1974*b* Genetic variation in natural populations of five *Drosophila* species and the hypothesis of selective neutrality of protein polymorphisms. *Genetics* **77**:343–384.

Ayala, F. J., M. L. Tracey, D. Hedgecock and R. C. Richmond, 1974*c* Genetic differentiation during the speciation process in *Drosophila Evolution* **28**:576–592.

Burla, H., A. B. da Cunha, A. R. Cordeiro, T. Dobzhansky, C. Malogolowkin and C. Pavan, 1949 The *willistoni* group of sibling species of *Drosophila*. *Evolution* **3**:300–314.

Burla, H., A. B. da Cunha, A. G. L. Cavalcanti, T. Dobzhansky and C. Pavan, 1950 Population density and dispersal rates in Brazilian *Drosophila willistoni*. *Ecology* **31**:393–404.

Carmody, G., A. Diaz-Collazo, T. Dobzhansky, L. Ehrman, I. S. Jaffrey, S. Kimball, S. Obrebski, S. Silagi, T. Tidwell and R. Ullrich, 1963 Mating preferences and sexual isolation within and between the incipient species of *Drosophila paulistorum*. *Am. Midl. Nat.* **68**:67–82.

Carson, H. L., 1959 Genetic conditions which promote or retard the formation of species. *Cold Spring Harbor Symp. Quant. Biol.* **24**:87–105.

Cordeiro, A. R. and T. Dobzhansky, 1954 Combining ability of certain chromosomes in *Drosophila willistoni* and in validation of the "wild type" concept. *Am. Nat.* **88**:75–86.

Counce, S. J. and D. F. Poulson, 1962 Developmental effects of the sex-ratio agent in embryos of *Drosophila willistoni*. *J. Exp. Zool.* **151**:17–31.

da Cunha, A. B. and T. Dobzhansky, 1954 A further study of chromosomal polymorphism in *Drosophila willistoni* in its relation to the environment. *Evolution* **8**:119–134.

da Cunha, A. B., H. Burla and T. Dobzhansky, 1950   Adaptive chromosomal polymorphism in *Drosophila willistoni. Evolution* **4**:212–235.

da Cunha, A. B., A. M. T. Shehata and W. de Oliveiza, 1957   A study of the diets and nutritional preferences of tropical species of *Drosophila. Ecology* **38**:98–106.

da Cunha, A. B., T. Dobzhansky, O. Pavlovsky and B. Spassky, 1959   Genetics of natural populations. XXVIII. Supplementary data on the chromosomal polymorphism in *Drosophila willistoni* in its relation to the environment. *Evolution* **13**:389–404.

da Cunha, A. B., L. E. Magalhaes, J. S. de Toledo, S. A. Toledo and H. M. L. de Souza, 1966   On the origin of new lethal chromosomes and its rate in laboratory populations of *Drosophila willistoni. Mutat. Res.* **3**:458–460.

de Souza, H. L., A. B. da Cunha and E. P. dos Santos, 1968   Adaptive polymorphisms of behavior developed in laboratory populations of *Drosophila willistoni. Am. Nat.* **102**:583–586.

de Souza, H. M. L., A. B. da Cunha and E. P. dos Santos, 1970   Adaptive polymorphisms of behavior evolved in laboratory populations of *Drosophila willistoni. Am. Nat.* **104**:175–189.

de Toledo, J. S., L. E. Magalhaes and A. B. da Cunha, 1966   An effect of change of environment on the frequencies of lethal chromosomes in *Drosophila willistoni. Am. Nat.* **100**:693–696.

Dobzhansky, T., 1946   Complete reproductive isolation between two morphologically similar species of *Drosophila. Ecology* **27**:205–211.

Dobzhansky, T., 1950   The chromosomes of *Drosophila willistoni. J. Hered.* **61**:156–158.

Dobzhansky, T., 1957*a*   Genetics of natural populations. XXVI. Chromosomal variability in island and continental populations of *Drosophila willistoni* from Central America and West Indies. *Evolution* **11**:280–293.

Dobzhansky, T., 1957*b*   The X-chromosome in the larval salivary glands of hybrids *Drosophila insularis* and *Drosophila tropicalis. Chromosoma (Berl.)* **8**:691–698.

Dobzhansky, T., 1970   *Gentics of the Evolutionary Process,* Columbia University Press, New York.

Dobzhansky, T. and E. Mayr, 1944   Experiments on sexual isolation in *Drosophila.* I. Geographic strains of *Drosophila willistoni. Proc. Natl. Acad. Sci. USA* **30**:238–244.

Dobzhansky, T. and C. Pavan, 1943   Studies on Brazilian species of *Drosophila. Biol. Facul. Fil Cien. Letr. Univ. São Paulo* **36**:7–72.

Dobzhansky, T. and O. Pavlovsky, 1958   Interracial hybridization and breakdown of coadapted give complexes in *Drosophila paulistorum* and *Drosophila willistoni. Proc. Natl. Acad. Sci. USA* **44**:622–629.

Dobzhansky, T. and O. Pavlovsky, 1962   A comparative study of the chromosomes in the incipient species of the *Drosophila paulistorum* complex. *Chromosoma (Berl.)* **13**:196–218.

Dobzhansky, T. and O. Pavlovsky, 1966   Spontaneous origin of an incipient species in *Drosophila paulistorum* complex. *Proc. Natl. Acad. Sci. USA* **55**:727–733.

Dobzhansky, T. and O. Pavlovsky, 1967   Experiments on incipient species of *Drosophila paulistorum. Genetics* **55**:141–156.

Dobzhansky, T. and O. Pavlovsky, 1971   Experimentally created incipient species of *Drosophila. Nature (Lond.)* **230**:289–292.

Dobzhansky, T. and B. Spassky, 1959   *Drosophila paulistorum* a cluster of species in *statu nascendi. Proc. Natl. Acad. Sci. USA* **45**:419–428.

Dobzhansky, T., H. Burla and A. B. da Cunha, 1950   A comparative study of chromosomal polymorphism in sibling species cf the *willistoni* group of *Drosophila. Am. Nat.* **84**:229–246.

Dobzhansky, T., B. Spassky and N. Spassky, 1952   A comparative study of mutation rates in two ecologically diverse species of *Drosophila. Genetics* **37**:650–664.

Dobzhansky, T., L. Ehrman and O. Pavlovsky, 1957   *Drosophila insularis,* a new sibling species of the *willistoni* group. *Univ. Texas Publ.* **5721**:39–47.

Dobzhansky, T., L. Ehrman, O. Pavlovsky and B. Spassky, 1964   The superspecies *Drosophila paulistorum. Proc. Natl. Acad. Sci. USA* **51**:3–9.

Dobzhansky, T., L. Ehrman and O. Pavlovsky, 1969   Transitional populations of *Drosophila paulistorum. Evolution* **23**:482–492.

Ehrman, L., 1960   The genetics of hybrid sterility in *Drosophila paulistorum. Evolution* **14**:212–223.

Ehrman, L., 1961   The genetics of sexual isolation in *Drosophila paulistorum. Evolution* **16**:1025–1038.

Ehrman, L., 1962   The transitional races of *Drosophila paulistorum*: A study of hybrid sterility. *Proc. Natl. Acad. Sci. USA* **48**:157–159.

Ehrman, L., 1963   Apparent cytoplasmic sterility in *Drosophila paulistorum. Proc. Natl. Acad. Sci. USA* **49**:155–157.

Ehrman, L., 1965   Direct observation of sexual isolation between allopatric and between sympatric strains of the different *Drosophila paulistorum* races. *Evolution* **19**:459–464.

Ehrman, L., 1967   A study of infectious hybrid sterility in *Drosophila paulistorum. Proc. Natl. Acad. Sci. USA* **58**:195–198.

Ehrman, L. and R. P. Kernaghan, 1972   Infectious heredity in *Drosophila paulistorum.* In *Ciba Symposium: Pathogenic Mycoplasmas,* pp. 227–250. Associated Scientific Publishers, Amsterdam.

Ehrman, L., and C. Petit, 1968   Genotype frequency and mating success in the *willistoni* species group of *Drosophila. Evolution* **22**:649–658.

Ehrman, L. and D. L. Williamson, 1965   Transmission by injection of hybrid sterility to nonhybrid males in *Drosophila paulistorum. Proc. Natl. Acad. Sci. USA* **54**:481–483.

Ehrman, L. and D. L. Williamson, 1969   On the etiology of the sterility of hybrids between certain strains of *Drosophila paulistorum. Genetics* **62**:193–199.

Ferry, R. M., R. C. Lancefield and C. W. Metz, 1923   Additional mutant characters in *Drosophila willistoni. J. Hered.* **14**:372–384.

Gillespie, J. H. and K. Kojima, 1968   The degree of polymorphism in enzymes involved in energy production compared to that in nonspecific enzymes in two *Drosophila ananassae* populations. *Proc. Natl. Acad. Sci. USA* **61**:582–585.

Kastritsis, C. D., 1966   A comparative chromosome study in the incipient species of the *Drosophila paulistorum* complex. *Chromosoma (Berl.)* **19**:208–222.

Kastritsis, C. D., 1967   A comparative study of the chromosomal polymorphs in the incipient species of the *Drosophila paulistorum* complex. *Chromosoma (Berl.)* **23**:180–202.

Kastritisis, C. D. and T. Dobzhansky, 1967   *Drosophila pavlovskiana,* a race or a species? *Am. Midl. Nat.* **78**:244–247.

Kenyon, A., 1972 Heterozygous effects on viability of *Drosophila* supergenes that are lethal when homozygous. *Genetica (The Hague)* **43**:536–551.

Kernaghan, R. P. and L. Ehrman, 1970a Antimycoplasmal antibiotics and hybrid sterility in *Drosophila paulistorum*. *Science (Wash., D.C.)* **169**:63–64.

Kernaghan, R. P. and L. Ehrman, 1970b An electron-microscopic study of the etiology of hybrid sterility in *Drosophila paulistorum*. *Chromosoma (Berl.)* **29**:291–304.

Koch, E. A. and R. C. King, 1966 The origin and differentiation of the egg chambers of *Drosophila melanogaster*. *J. Morphol.* **119**:283–304.

Koref-Santibañez, S., 1972a Courtship behavior in the semispecies of the superspecies *Drosophila paulistorum*. *Evolution* **26**:108–115.

Koref-Santibañez, S., 1972b Courtship interaction in the semispecies of *Drosophila paulistorum*. *Evolution* **26**:326–333.

Krimbas, C. B., 1959 Comparison of the concealed variability in *Drosophila prosaltans*. *Genetics* **44**:1359–1369.

Krimbas, C. B., 1960 Synthetic sterility in *Drosophila willistoni*. *Proc. Natl. Acad. Sci. USA* **46**:832–833.

Krimbas, C. B., 1961 Release of genetic variability through recombination. VI. *Drosophila willistoni*. *Genetics* **46**:1323–1334.

Lakovaara, S. and A. Saura, 1972 Chromosomal location of enzyme loci in *Drosophila willistoni*. *Experientia (Basel)* **28**:355–356.

Lancefield, R. C. and C. W. Metz, 1922 The sex-linked group of mutant characters in *Drosophila willistoni*. *Am. Nat.* **56**:211–241.

Magalhaes, L. E., A. B. da Cunha, J. S. de Toledo, S. A. Toledo, H. L. de Souza, H. J. Traga, V. Setzor, and C. Pavan, 1965a On lethals and the suppressors in experimental populations of *Drosophila willistoni*. *Am. Nat.* **56**:211–241.

Magalhaes, L. E., J. S. de Toledo and A. B. da Cunha, 1965b The nature of lethals in *Drosophila willistoni*. *Genetics* **43**:274–286.

Malogolowkin, C., 1958 Maternally inherited "sex-ratio" conditions in *Drosophila paulistorum*. *Genetics* **43**:274–286.

Malogolowkin, C., 1959 Temperature effects on maternally inherited "sex-ratio" conditions in *Drosophila willistoni* and *Drosophila equinoxialis*. *Am. Nat.* **93**:365–368.

Malogolowkin, C., 1963 The interrelationships of the incipient species within the *Drosophila paulistorum* complex. *Evolution* **17**:187–193.

Malogolowkin, C. and G. G. Carvalho, 1961 Direct and indirect transfer of the "sex-ratio" conditions in different species of *Drosophila*. *Genetics* **46**:1009–1012.

Malogolowkin, C. and L. Ehrman, 1960 Mutant genes and linkage relationships in *Drosophila paulistorum*. *Evolution* **14**:266–270.

Malogolowkin, C., D. F. Poulson and E. Y. Wright, 1959 Experimental transfer of maternally inherited abnormal sex-ratio in *Drosophila willistoni*. *Genetics* **44**:59–74.

Malogolowkin-Cohen, C., H. Levene, N. Dobzhansky and A. Solima Simmons, 1964 Inbreeding and the mutational and balanced loads in natural populations of *Drosophila willistoni*. *Genetics* **50**:1299–1311.

Malogolowkin-Cohen, C., A. Solima-Simmons and H. Levene, 1965 A study of sexual isolation between certain strains of *Drosophila paulistorum*. *Evolution* **19**:95–103.

Metz, C. W., 1916 Chromosome studies on the Diptera. III. *Am. Nat.* **50**:587–599.

Nei, M., 1972 Genetic distance between populations. *Am. Nat.* **106**:283–292.

Oishi, K. and D. F. Poulson, 1970 A virus associated with SR-spirochetes of *Drosophila nebulosa*. *Proc. Natl. Acad. Sci. USA* **67**:1565–1572.

Pasteur, G., 1970 A biometrical study of the semispecies of the *Drosophila paulistorum* complex. *Evolution* **24**:156–168.

Pavan, C. and E. N. Knapp, 1954 The genetic population structure of Brazilian *Drosophila willistoni. Evolution* **8**:303–313.

Pavan, C., T. Dobzhansky and H. Burla, 1950 Diurnal behavior of some neotropical sprain of Drosophila. *Ecology* **31**:36–43.

Pavan, C., A. R. Cordeiro, N. Dobzhansky, T. Dobzhansky, C. Malogolowkin. B. Spassky and M. Wedel, 1951 Concealed genetic variability in Brazilian populations of *Drosophila willistoni. Genetics* **36**:13–30.

Pérez-Salas, S., R. C. Richmond, O. Pavlovsky, C. D. Kastritsis, L. Ehrman and T. Dobzhansky, 1970 The interior semispecies of *Drosophila paulistorum. Evolution* **24**:519–527.

Petit, C. and L. Ehrman, 1968 Le role de la sélection sexuelle dans l'évolution des populations. L'avantage des types rares dans le groupe *willistoni* (Genre *Drosophila* sousgenre Sophophora). *Bull. Biol. Fr. Belg.* **102**:433–446.

Poulson, D. F. and B. Sakaguchi, 1961 Nature of "sex-ratio" agent in *Drosophila. Science (Wash., D.C.)* **133**:1489–1490.

Powell, J. R., 1971 Genetic polymorphisms in varied environments. Science **174**:1035–1036.

Powell, J. R., 1973 Apparent selection of enzyme alleles in laboratory populations of *Drosophila. Genetics* **75**:557–570.

Powell, J. R., 1974 Heterosis at an enzyme locus of *Drosophila*: Evidence from experimental populations. *Heredity* **32**:105–108.

Powell, J. R., H. Levene and T. Dobzhansky, 1972 Chromosomal polymorphism in *Drosophila pseudoobscura* used for diagnosis of geographic origin. *Evolution* **26**:553–559.

Richmond, R. C., 1972*a* Enzyme variability in the *Drosophila willistoni* group. III. Amounts of variability in the superspecies, *D. paulistorum. Genetics* **70**:87–112.

Richmond, R. C., 1972*b* Genetic similarities and evolutionary relationships among the semispecies of *Drosophila paulistorum. Evolution* **26**:536–544.

Richmond, R. C. and J. R. Powell, 1970 Evidence of heterosis associated with an enzyme locus in a natural population of *Drosophila. Proc. Natl. Acad. Sci. USA* **67**:1264–1267.

Sakaguchi, B. and D. F. Poulson, 1961 Distribution of "sex-ratio" agent in tissues of *Drosophila willistoni. Genetics* **46**:1665–1676.

Sakaguchi, B. and D. F. Poulson, 1963 Interspecific transfer of the "sex-ratio" condition from *Drosophila willistoni* to *D. melanogaster. Genetics* **48**:841–861.

Spassky, B., 1957 Morphological differences between sibling species of Drosophila. Stud. *Drosophila Genet. Univ. Texas Publ.* **5721**:48–61.

Spassky, B. and T. Dobzhansky, 1950 Comparative genetics of *Drosophila willistoni. Heredity* **4**:201–215.

Spassky, B., R. C. Richmond, S. Pérez-Salas, O. Pavlovsky, C. A. Mourão, A. S. Hunter, H. Hoenigsberg, T. Dobzhansky and F. J. Ayala, 1971 Geography of the sibling species related to *Drosophila willistoni,* and of the semispecies of the *Drosophila paulistorum* complex. *Evolution* **25**:129–143.

Sturtevant, A. H., 1921 The North American species of *Drosophila. Carnegie Institution of Washington Publication,* Carnegie Institution, Washington, D.C.

Sturtevant, A. H. and E. Novitski, 1941 The homologies of the chromosome elements in the genus *Drosophila. Genetics* **58**:113–124.

Townsend, J. I., 1952 Genetics of marginal populations of *Drosophila willistoni*. *Evolution* **6**:428–442.

Townsend, J. I., 1954 Cryptic subspeciation in *Drosophila* belonging to the subgenus *Sophophora*. *Am. Nat.* **88**:339–351.

Wallace, B. and C. Madden, 1953 The frequencies of sub- and supervitals in experimental populations of *Drosophila melanogaster*. *Genetics* **38**:456–470.

Williamson, D. L. and L. Ehrman, 1967 Induction of hybrid sterility in nonhybrid males of *Drosophila paulistorum*. *Genetics* **55**:131–140.

Williamson, D. L. and L. Ehrman, 1968 Infectious hybrid sterility and the "New Llanos" strain of *Drosophila paulistorum*. *Nature (Lond.)* **219**:1266–1267.

Williston, S. W., 1896 On the Diptera of St. Vincent. *Trans. R. Entomol. Soc. Lond.*: 253–446.

Winge, H. and A. R. Cordeiro, 1963 Experimental hybrids between *Drosophila willistoni* Sturtevant and *Drosophila paulistorum* Dobzhansky and Pavan from southern marginal populations. *Heredity* **18**:215–222.

PART L
DROSOPHILA MELANOGASTER

22

Drosophila melanogaster: An Introduction

Robert C. King

Introduction

From the standpoint of genetics, the fruit fly, *Drosophila melanogaster,* is the best known of all multicellular organisms. A catalog of some of the advantages of this insect for laboratory study follows: (1) The adult is small, anatomically complex, readily handled, and it breeds prolifically in the laboratory. (2) Conditions for culturing *Drosophila* are simple, cheap, and readily controlled. Flies can be raised by the hundreds in half-pint milk bottles or by the tens of thousands in population cages. (3) The life cycle is short (9 days). (4) The haploid number of chromosomes is small (four). (5) The polytene chromosomes of the salivary gland cells of the mature larva are gigantic and show a characteristic banding pattern. The homologous chromosomes pair in most somatic tissues, including the salivary gland. This behavior facilitates the identification of chromosomal rearrangements, the mapping of deficiencies, and, as a result, the cytological localization of genes. (6) Homologous chromosomes do not undergo crossing over in the germ cells of the male (Morgan, 1912a), and this peculiarity greatly simplifies the genetic procedures employed. (7) The insect can serve as host to a variety of viruses (see Chapter 31 by

Robert C. King—Department of Biological Sciences, Northwestern University, Evanston, Illinois.

L'Héritier in this volume), and hence the genetics of host–parasite interactions can be studied. (8) A synthetic, minimal medium has been developed upon which the flies can be reared aseptically (Sang, 1956). (9) Media are also available for cell culture, and these are described by Schneider in Chapter 32 of this volume. (10) An encyclopedic body of information for this species is readily accessible through indexed bibliographies (Muller, 1939; Herskowitz, 1952, 1958, 1963, 1969, 1974), and thus a foundation is available from which unexplored areas of research can be attacked. About 25,000 articles dealing with *Drosophila* have been published between 1910 and 1974, and the literature doubles every 12 years! (11) Thousands of mutations and chromosomal aberrations have been discovered, and much of this information is available in the compendium published by Lindsley and Grell (1968). (12) Massive collections of hereditary variations exist, and stocks of various mutants can be readily obtained by any worker in the field. The major collections are housed at *Drosophila* stock centers maintained by Professor I. I. Oster at the Biology Department, Bowling Green State University, Bowling Green, Ohio 43402, and by Professor E. B. Lewis at the Division of Biology, California Institute of Technology, Pasadena, California 91109. (13) A bulletin (*Drosophila Information Service*) is published annually which sets forth the stock lists of the major laboratories, the addresses of all *Drosophila* workers, descriptions of new mutants and genetic techniques, and research and teaching notes (Novitski, 1973). As a result *Drosophila* workers can keep abreast of the work going on throughout the world. (14) Numerous related species are available for comparative studies. The major stock center for *Drosophila* species is maintained by Professor Marshall Wheeler at the Department of Zoology, University of Texas, Austin, Texas 78712.

Drosophila Culture

D. melanogaster fluorishes upon many different media. The one used at Northwestern University is prepared according to the following recipe [a modification of the formulation described by David (1962)]: 13 l water, 710 g yellow corn meal, 710 g brewer's yeast, 110 g agar, 38 g methyl-p-hydroxybenzoate, 80 ml propionic acid. The last two components serve as fungicides. Mold growth will rapidly destroy cultures lacking fungicides. Methyl-p-hydroxybenzoate is marketed by Tenneco Chemicals, Inc., 290 River Drive, Garfield, New Jersey 07026 under the trade name "Methyl Parasept." The powdered components are added to the water, all lumps are broken up, and then the mixture is brought to a boil and cooked for 15 minutes. The propionic acid is stirred into the medium just prior to dispensing it into culture bottles. A small piece of sterilized cotton wadding or filter paper is always pushed into the medium, and this provides a surface upon which the adults can crawl. The cultures are stoppered with plastic foam plugs. Further details on culturing methods can be found in Spencer (1950), Demerec and Kaufmann (1961), Strickberger (1962), Wheeler (1967, 1972), and Shorrocks (1972). Merriam (1973) has provided a very useful listing of sources of equipment and supplies used in setting up a kitchen for turning out *Drosophila* medium.

Life Cycle of *Drosophila melanogaster*

The fruit fly undergoes complete metamorphosis. At 25°C development may be subdivided as follows: embryonic stage, 1 day; first-instar larva, 1 day; second instar, 1 day; third instar, 2 days; pupa, 4 days; total, 9 days. At room temperature (~ 21°C) the total developmental time is about 2 weeks.

Preadult Stages

The egg is about 0.19 × 0.50 mm and weighs 10 μg. Immediately following entrance of the sperm, the meiotic divisions are completed. The egg pronucleus is formed, and the other three polar nuclei degenerate. The sperm and egg pronuclei replicate their DNA and then fuse to form a zygote nucleus which contains the 4C amount of DNA. The nucleus undergoes a gonomeric mitosis to yield diploid, 2C nuclei. Subsequent conventional mitoses generate the diploid cells of the embryo which eventually hatches as a white, segmented, wormlike larva. The larvae feed constantly and burrow through the food, leaving numerous channels and furrows.

The salivary glands of larval *Drosophila* produce digestive juice and also a secretion which is used to glue the insect to the substratum when it undergoes puparium formation. The polytene chromosomes in nuclei of cells of these glands in the third instar are extensively used for cytogenetic analyses. Useful techniques for making orcein-stained salivary chromosome squash preparations are detailed in Nicoletti (1959), and quinacrine-staining procedures have been published more recently by Ellison and Barr (1971). Detailed accounts of *Drosophila* embryogenesis have been provided by Sonnenblick (1950), Poulson (1950), and Scriba (1964), and descriptions of various morphological changes that accompany pupal development may be found in Bodenstein (1950) and in Ursprung and Nöthiger (1972). Studies on the ecological determinants of growth in

Drosophila laboratory cultures have been reviewed by Sang (1950), and Church and Robertson (1966) have made quantitative estimates of the syntheses of various compounds by the fly as it proceeds through its life cycle.

The Adult

Adult flies are 2–3 mm long. Females weigh about 1.5 mg when mature; the males, 0.8 mg. The compound eyes are each composed of about 740 ommatidia (facets) in the male and about 780 in the female. Three single eyes (the ocelli) are arranged in a triangular pattern on top of the head. The thorax is composed of three fused segments: the prothorax (bearing the first pair of legs), the mesothorax (bearing the second pair of legs and the wings), and the metathorax (bearing the third pair of legs and the trisegmented halteres). The wing has a characteristic pattern of five longitudinal veins and two crossveins. Large bristles and small hairs grow in a definite pattern over the body. The external genitalia of the two sexes are strikingly different. Males have (on the foreleg only) a sex comb consisting of a row of bristles arranged like the teeth of a comb, whereas females lack this structure. A detailed account of the external morphology of the adult *Drosophila* is given by Ferris (1950).

The internal organ systems of the adult are described by Miller (1950), and more-detailed accounts of the female and male reproductive systems can be found in King (1970*b*) and Tates (1971), respectively. In the female, each of the two ovaries is comprised of a group of egg tubes (ovarioles). In the distal portion of the ovariole is located the germarium, which contains follicular cells, oogonia, and nests containing compact groups of 16 interconnected cells which arise as the result of four consecutive synchronous divisions of an oogonium. Proximal to the germarium are 4–8 egg chambers (depending on the age of the adult fly), each larger than the preceding one. Each consists of 15 nurse cells, the oocyte, and an envelope of follicle cells. The nurse cells nourish the oocyte, which grows until it increases in volume by over 100,000 times. Eventually the nurse cells degenerate, leaving the fully grown primary oocyte. In the male, each of the two testes is a tube with the basal half helically coiled. The mature testis contains germ cells in various stages of maturation, but spermatozoa and spermatids are most common. Spermatogonia are limited to the extreme tip of the testis.

Numerous gene mutations and chromosomal aberrations are known which cause sterility because of defects occuring during gametogenesis. Some of these are described in this volume by Romrell (Chapter 27), Hess (Chapter 28), and King and Mohler (Chapter 29).

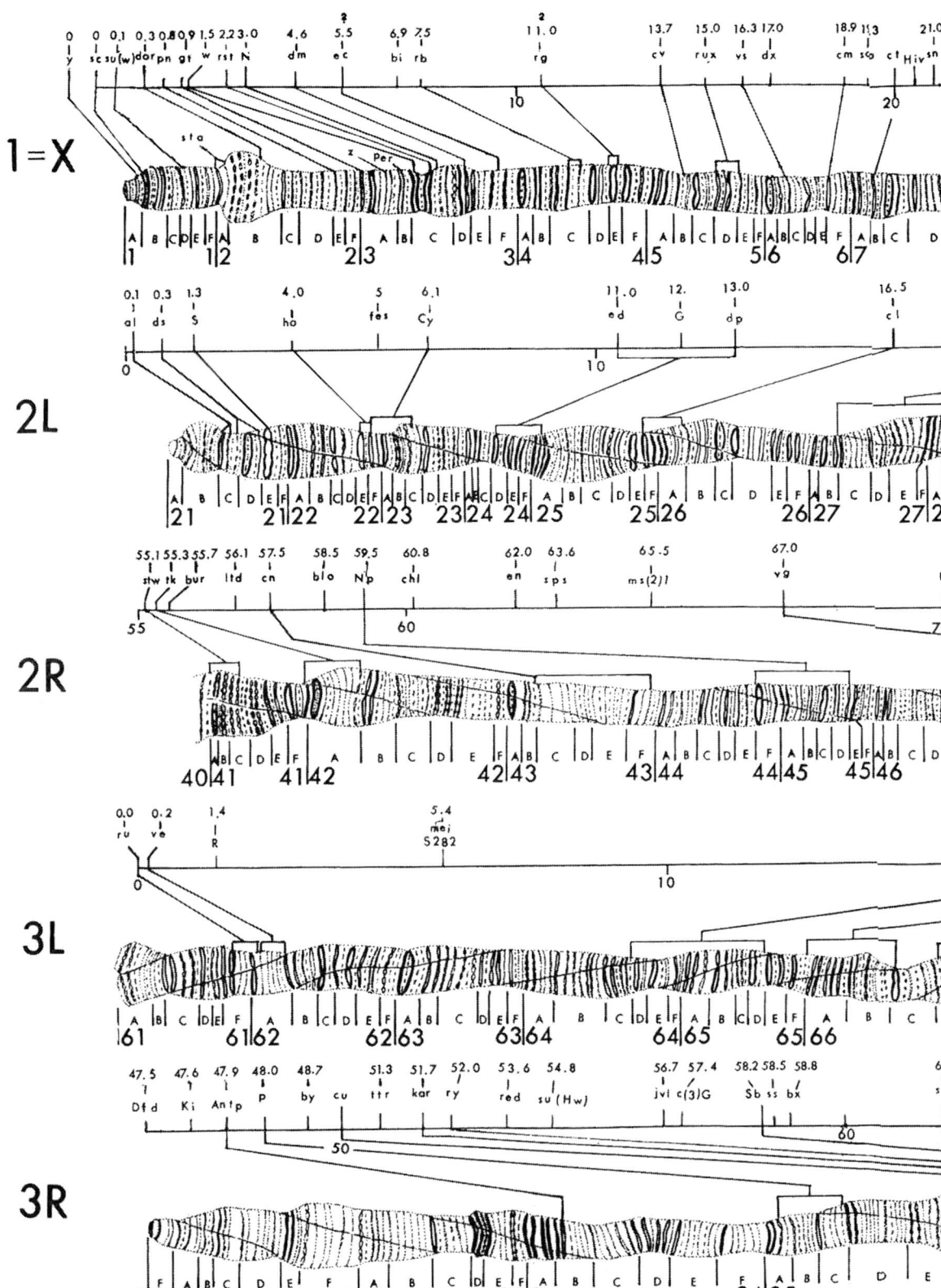

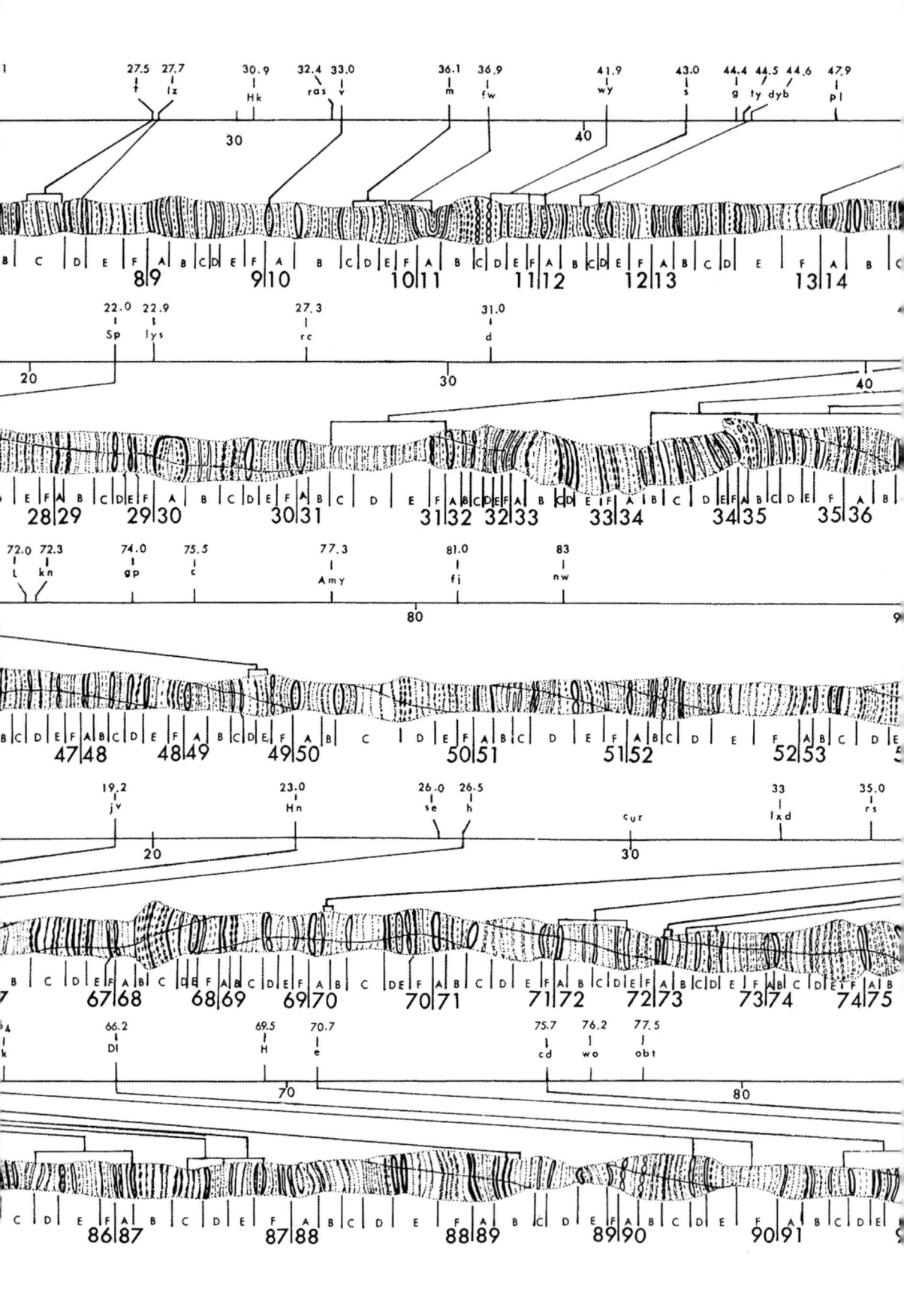

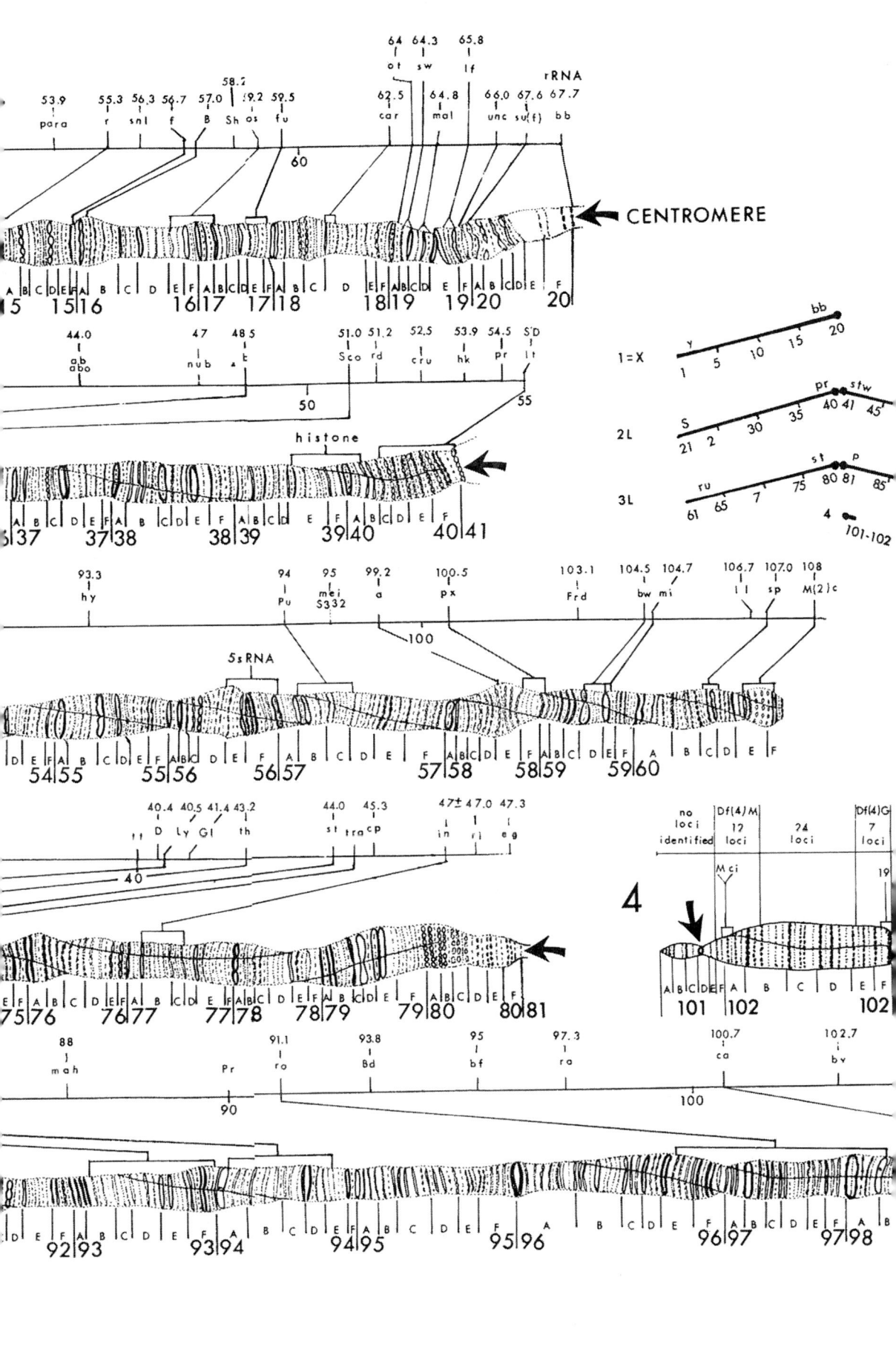

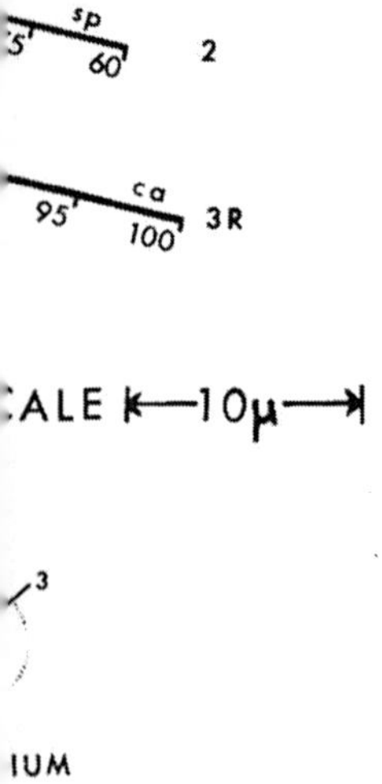

sp

5'   60'   2

ca

95'   100'   3R

CALE $\longleftarrow$ 10μ $\longrightarrow$

3

IUM

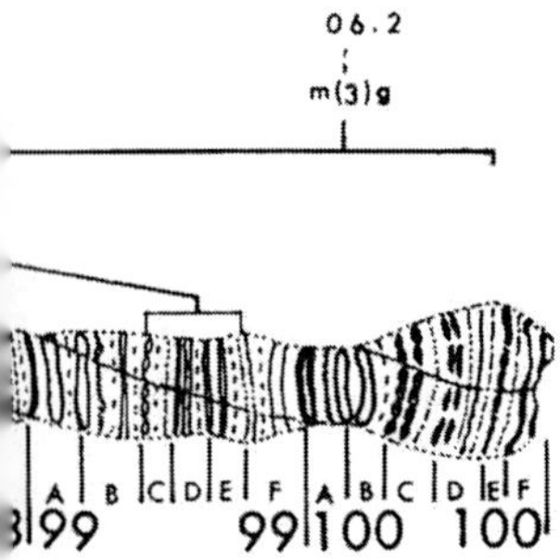

06.2

m(3)g

A B C D E F A B C D E F

99   99 100   100

Figure 1. Cytological maps of the chromosomes of the larval, salivary gland cells of D. melanogaster compared with genetic maps. The cytological map is subdivided into 102 divisions, each of which is further divided into six subdivisions lettered in groups of six (A–F). The subdivisions contain varying numbers of bands (not all of which can be shown at the magnification used in this drawing). Chromosome 1 contains the first 20 sections; chromosome 2, sections 21–60; chromosome 3, sections 61–100; and chromosome 4, sections 101 and 102. The loci of the centromeres are designated by arrows. In the salivary gland cell nucleus the centromeric regions adhere to form the chromocenter. Note that the homologous autosomes are intimately paired. The X chromosome is shown as it appears in the male. The chromosomes of an oogonial metaphase are shown at the same magnification. The genetic maps are drawn parallel to the corresponding chromosomes. In those cases where appropriate data are available, a line is drawn between the gene symbol and the cytological locus.

This reference map is revised from the one that was presented as Fig. V-7 in my oogenesis monograph (King, 1970b). That drawing used the format of the 1935 reference map of Bridges (1935). However, the more detailed cytological map prepared by Benjamin Hochman has been substituted for chromosome 4. Roberts (1972) claims that the centromere of chromosome 4 is located to the left of 101D. The lines between the genetic and cytological loci were drawn using the cytogenetic data provided in Lindsley and Grell's monograph (1968) (pages 433–471). However, since this was completed in 1967, I have attempted to update both the genetic and cytological maps using more recent material. Information concerning the genes in question is presented in Table 1. Citations are given to publications which postdate Lindsley and Grell (1968) and provide new data with respect to the phenotype or cytological localization of the mutation. The listing by Zimm et al. (1972) should also be consulted.

Mating generally occurs during the first day of adult life, and females start ovipositing during the second day. During its 10-week lifetime a fertilized female can produce as many as 3000 eggs (about 30 times her own weight). Generally 95 percent of the eggs laid hatch. Under optimal conditions a geneticist can breed a maximum of 30 generations yearly.

Milestones in the History of *Drosophila* Genetics

According to the historical account provided by Sturtevant (1965) *D. melanogaster* was first described in 1830 by J. W. Meigen, and again, under the name *D. ampelophila* by H. Loew in 1862. The latter species designation appears in some of the early genetic literature. The entomologist C. W. Woodward was the first scientist to cultivate this insect in the laboratory. Through Woodward, Castle learned of the advantages of *Drosophila,* and it was through Castle's publication of 1906 that the fly became known to other geneticists.

Drosophila genetics had its beginning at Columbia University in the laboratory of T. H. Morgan. The first mutation, white eye color (*w*) was discovered by Morgan in May, 1910, and his paper on sex linkage was published the same year. He reported the discovery of the first sex-linked, recessive lethal in 1912 (Morgan, 1912*b*). There then followed a series of remarkable discoveries by his students: the first genetic map (Sturtevant, 1913), non-disjunction (Bridges, 1914), interference (Muller, 1916), deficiencies (Bridges, 1917), balanced lethals (Muller, 1918), duplications (Bridges, 1919), triploid intersexes (Bridges, 1921), and translocations (Bridges, 1923). In 1925 Bridges published his cytogenetic analysis of the aneuploid offspring of triploid females, and he defined numerical relations between the sex chromosomes and autosomes that control the sexual phenotype in *Drosophila.* Also in 1925 Sturtevant analyzed the Bar phenomenon (in doing so he called attention to the phenomenon of position effect), and in 1926 he published the first description of an inversion. The polytene chromosomes in the nuclei of the larval salivary gland cells were described by Painter in 1933, and the first detailed maps were published by Bridges in 1935. In 1938 Slizynska reported the results of a cytological analysis of several overlapping *Notch* deficiencies in the salivary gland X chromosomes, which made possible the determinations of the band locations of the *w* and *N* genes. The current cytological map (Figure 1) provides the locations of 92 genes (also see Table 1).

The study of mutagenesis had its start in 1927, with Muller's publication on the artificial induction of mutations by x-rays. The chemical induction of mutations in *Drosophila* dates back to 1946 to the papers by Auerbach and Robson and by Rapoport. Work on mutagenesis over the

TABLE 1. *Genes in D. melanogaster*

Gene symbol	Locus	Name of gene	Phenotypic expression	Reference
CHROMOSOME 1 (SEX CHROMOSOME)				
y	0.0	yellow	Body yellow, bristles brown	Lefevre (1975)
sc	0.0	scute	Bristles missing	Lefevre (1975)
su(w^a)	0.1	suppressor of white-apricot	Darkens w^a	
sta	0.3	stubarista	Aristae, antennae stubby, bristles short; ♀ sterile	Rayle and Hoar (1969)
dor	0.3	deep orange	Eyes orange; ♀ sterile	Lefevre (1975)
pn	0.8	prune	Eyes brownish purple	Lefevre (1975)
gt	0.9	giant	Larva, pupa, adult large	
z	1.0	zeste	♂ normal; eyes yellow in ♀	
per	z↓w	period	Effects circadian periodicity	Konopka and Benzer (1971)
w	1.5	white	Eyes, Malpighian tubules white	Lefevre (1975)
rst	2.2	roughest	Eyes rough, bulging; body small	Lefevre (1970)
N	3.0	Notch	Wings cut; veins thick, deltas at margin; lethal in ♂	
dm	4.6	diminutive	Bristles, body small, slender; ♀ sterile	Lefevre (1975)
ec	5.5	echinus	Eyes large, bulging, rough; wings short, broad	Lefevre (1971)
bi	6.9	bifid	Veins fused; wings short, spread	Lefevre (1971)
rb	7.5	ruby	Eyes ruby	Lefevre (1975)
rg	11.0	rugose	Eyes rough; wings thin, margins frayed	Lefevre (private communication)
cv	13.7	crossveinless	Crossveins absent	
rux	15.0	roughex	Eyes small, rough	
vs	16.3	vesiculated	Wings warped, wrinkled, blistered, spread	Lefevre (1975)

dx	17.0	deltex	Veins thick, deltas at margins	
cm	18.9	carmine	Eyes ruby	
scp	19.3	scooped	Wing tips upturned	
ct	20.0	cut	Wings cut, scalloped; eyes kidney-shaped	Lefevre and Johnson (1973)
Hiv	ct↓sn	Haplo-inviable	Locus necessary in double dose for life	
sn	21.0	singed	Bristles twisted, short; hairs kinked; some alleles ♀ sterile	
oc	23.1	ocelliless	Ocelli absent; ♀ sterile	
t	27.5	tan	Body tan, not positively phototactic	Pak et al. (1969), Hotta and Benzer (1969)
lz	27.7	lozenge	Eyes narrow, ovoid, irregular surfaced; some alleles ♀ sterile	Lefevre (1975)
Hk	30.9	Hyperkinetic	Fly shakes legs when etherized	Kaplan and Trout (1969)
ras	32.4	raspberry	Eyes dark ruby; some alleles ♀ sterile	Lefevre (1970)
v	33.0	vermilion	Eyes scarlet; ocelli colorless	Lefevre (1970)
m	36.1	miniature	Wings small	
fw	36.9	furrowed	Eyes furrowed; head, scutellum, bristles gnarled	Lefevre (1970)
wy	41.9	wavy	Wings wavy	Lefevre (1975)
s	43.0	sable	Body dark; trident prominent	Lefevre (1975)
g	44.4	garnet	Eyes purplish ruby	Lefevre (1975)
ty	44.5	tiny	Bristles, body small; ♀ sterile	
dyb	44.6	dusky body	Body dark; eyes brown; ♀ sterile	
pl	47.9	pleated	Wings pleated	
Eag	50.0	Ether-a-gogo	Fly shakes legs when etherized	Kaplan and Trout (1969)
sd	51.5	scalloped	Wing margins scalloped; veins thickened	Lefevre (1975)
Bg	51.6	Bag	Wings inflated; veins abnormal; lethal in ♂	
para	53.9	paralysis	Temperature sensitive paralysis	Suzuki et al. (1971)
r	55.3	rudimentary	Wings truncated; some alleles ♀ semi-sterile	Norby (1970), Lefevre (private communication)
snl	56.3	sonless	♀ produces <1 percent sons	Colaianne and Bell (1972)

TABLE 1. *Continued*

Gene symbol	Locus	Name of gene	Phenotypic expression	Reference
f	56.7	forked	Bristles short, bent	
B	57.0	Bar	Eyes small, narrow	Kaplan and Trout (1969)
Sh	58.2	Shaker	Fly trembles when etherized	Lefevre (1975)
os	59.2	outstretched small eye	Wings spread, eyes small, or both	
fu	59.5	fused	Wing veins L3, L4 partly fused; wings spread; ♀ sterile	
car	62.5	carnation	Eyes dark ruby	Schalet *et al.* (1970)
ot	64	outheld	Wings spread; hairs sparse; ♂ sterile	Schalet *et al.* (1970)
sw	64.3	short wing	Wings spread, incised; veins irregular; eyes small, rough	
mal	64.8	maroonlike	Eyes purple; lacks xanthine oxidase	Lefevre (1975)
lf	65.8	little fly	Body small; abdomen narrow	Schalet *et al.* (1970)
unc	66.0	uncoordinated	Leg movements uncoordinated; wings upheld, curled	Schalet *et al.* (1970)
su(f)	67.6	suppressor of forked	Suppresses some f alleles; dilutes w^a	Schalet and Singer (1971)
bb	67.7	bobbed	Bristles small; abdomen etched, site of rRNA cistrons	Schalet and Lefevre (1973)

CHROMOSOME 2

Gene symbol	Locus	Name of gene	Phenotypic expression	Reference
al	0.1	aristaless	Aristae reduced; postscutellars divergent	
ds	0.3	dachsous	Wings short, broad; crossveins close	
S	1.3	Star	Eyes small, narrow, rough; lethal when homozygous	
ho	4.0	heldout	Wings spread	
fes	5	female sterile	♀ sterile; ovaries tumorous	Johnson and King (1972)

Cy	6.1	Curly	Wings upcurled; lethal when homozygous	
ed	11.0	echinoid	Eyes large, rough	
G	12	Gull	Wings large, spread, curved; lethal when homozygous	
dp	13.0	dumpy	Wings truncated; thoracic bristles whorled	
cl	16.5	clot	Eyes dark maroon	
Sp	22.0	Sternopleural	Extra sternopleurals; lethal when homozygous	
lys	22.9	lysine	Accumulates lysine	
rc	27.3	red cells	Pigments fat cells of *lys* fly	
d	31.0	dachs	Tarsi 4-jointed; eyes small, rough	
J	41.0	Jammed	Wings narrow	
da	41.5	daughterless	*da/da* females produce unisexual male progenies	Mange and Sandler (1973)
ab	44.0	abrupt	Wing vein L5 incomplete	
abo	44.0	abnormal oocyte	*abo/abo* females, in crosses to *abo*$^+$ males carrying an attached XY chromosome and no free Y, produce 90 percent female offspring	Mange and Sandler (1973)
nub	47.0	nubbin	Wings small, curved; margins interrupted; veins missing	
b	48.5	black	Body black	
Sco	51.0	Scutoid	Scutellars absent; lethal when homozygous	
rd	51.2	reduced	Bristles reduced; ♀ sterile	
histone	39E–40A	histone cistrons	Codes for histone mRNA	Pardue et al. (1972)
cru	52.5	cream underscored	Dilutes w^e	
hk	53.9	hook	Bristle tips bent; eyes rough; wings divergent	
pr	54.5	purple	Eyes purplish ruby	

TABLE 1. Continued

Gene symbol	Locus	Name of gene	Phenotypic expression	Reference
SD	55	Segregation distorter	Morphologically normal; segregation abnormal in ♂	
lt	55.0	light	Eyes yellowish pink; ocelli colorless	
stw	55.1	straw	Hairs yellow; bristle tips pale	
ap	55.2	apterous	Wings, halteres missing; some alleles ♀ sterile	
tk	55.3	thick	Legs thick; wings short, broad	
bur	55.7	burgundy	Eyes dull brown	
ltd	56.1	lightoid	Eyes yellowish pink	
cn	57.5	cinnabar	Eyes bright red	
blo	58.5	bloated	Wings spread, crumpled, blistered	
Np	59.5	Notopleural	Bristles short; wings short, broad; lethal when homozygous	
chl	60.8	chaetelle	Bristles, body small; wing venation abnormal	
en	62.0	engrailed	Scutellum cleft; bristles hooked; veins interrupted, branched	
sps	63.6	spastic	Lethal; survivors weak	
ms(2)1	65.5	male sterile(2)1	♂ sterile; ♀ fertile	
vg	67.0	vestigial	Wings vestigial; halteres small	
U	70	Upturned	Wings curled, dark, waxy; lethal when homozygous	
cg	71.1	comb gap	Sex combs large; wing vein L4 interrupted; ♀ sterile	
L	72.0	Lobe	Eyes small, kidney-shaped	
kn	72.3	knot	Wing veins L3, L4 close or fused; crossveins abnormal	

gp	74.0	gap	Wing vein L4 thin or interrupted	
c	75.5	curved	Wings downcurved, thin	
Amy	77.3	Amylase	Affects enzyme's electrophoretic mobility	
fj	81	four jointed	Tarsi 4-jointed; crossveins close together	
nw	83	narrow	Wings long, narrow, pointed; sterile	
sm	91.5	smooth	Abdomen shrunken, denuded; sterile	
hy	93.3	humpy	Thorax rigid; wings truncated	
5sRNA	56EF	5S RNA cistrons	Codes for 5S RNA of ribosomes	Wimber and Steffensen (1970)
Pu	94	Punch	Eyes purple; lethal when homozygous	
meiS 332	95	meiotic S332	Causes precocious division of sister centromeres resulting in nondisjunction	Davis (1971)
a	99.2	arc	Wings broad, bent; crossveins close	
px	100.5	plexus	Wings have network of extra veins	
Frd	103.1	Freckled	Body speckled black; tumorous lethal when homozygous	
bw	104.5	brown	Eyes brown	
mi	104.7	minus	Bristles small; hairs reduced; ♀ sterile	
ll	106.7	lanceolate	Wings narrow at tips, slightly divergent	
sp	107.0	speck	Black speck at wing axil	
M(2)c	108	Minute(2)c	Bristles fine; late hatching; lethal when homozygous	

CHROMOSOME 3

ru	0.0	roughoid	Eyes small, rough	
ve	0.2	veinlet	Wing veins L3, L4, L5 incomplete	
R	1.4	Roughened	Eyes rough; mortality rate high when homozygous	
meiS 282	5.4	meiotic S282	Decreases recombination, particularly in regions distal to centromere	Parry (1973)

TABLE 1. Continued

Gene symbol	Locus	Name of gene	Phenotypic expression	Reference
jv	19.2	javelin	Bristles, hairs cylindrical	
Hn	23.0	Henna	Eyes brown; lethal when homozygous	
se	26.0	sepia	Eyes brown, darken to black with age	
h	26.5	hairy	Extra hairs on scutellum, pleurae, head, and along veins	
cur	30	curvoid	Wings diverge, curve down	
lxd	33.9	low xanthine dehydrogenase	Affects level of xanthine dehydrogenase	O'Brien (this volume)
rs	35.0	rose	Eyes purplish pink; often sterile	
rt	37	rotated abdomen	Abdomen twisted; sterile	
tt	40.0	tilt	Wings spread, warped; wing vein L3 interrupted	
D	40.4	Dichaete	Wings spread; alulae missing; fewer dorsocentrals; lethal when homozygous	
Ly	40.5	Lyra	Wing margins excised; lethal when homozygous	
Gl	41.4	Glued	Eyes small, oblong, shiny; lethal when homozygous	
th	43.2	thread	Aristae lack side branches	
st	44.0	scarlet	Eyes bright red; ocelli colorless	
tra	45	transformer	Transforms female into sterile male	
cp	45.3	clipped	Wing margins snipped	Puro and Arajärvi (1969)
in	47+	inturned	Hairs, bristles directed toward midline	Puro and Arajärvi (1969)
ri	47.0	radius incompletus	Wing vein L2 interrupted	Puro and Arajärvi (1969)
eg	47.3	eagle	Wings spread	Lütolf (1971)
Dfd	47.4	Deformed	Eyes small or furrowed; lethal when homozygous	Holm *et al.* (1969)

Ki	47.6	Kinked	Bristles and hairs short, twisted	Denell (1973)
Antp	47.9	Antennapedia	Antennae leglike; lethal when homozygous	
p	48.0	pink	Eyes dull ruby	
by	48.7	blistery	Wings blistered, warped, dusky	
cu	50.0	curled	Wings upcurved; body dark	
ttr	51.3	tetrapter	Halteres winglike	
kar	51.7	karmoisin	Eyes bright red	Chovnick (1973)
ry	52.0	rosy	Eyes reddish brown; lacks xanthine dehydrogenase	O'Brien (this volume)
red	53.6	red malpighian tubules	Malpighian tubes red; eyes brown	
su(Hw)	54.8	suppressor of *Hairy wing*	Suppresses specific alleles at various loci; ♀ sterile	
jvl	56.7	javelinlike	Bristles, hairs cylindrical	
c(3)G	57.4	crossover suppressor in chromosome 3 of Gowen	Eliminates meiotic recombination	
Sb	58.2	Stubble	Bristles short, thick; lethal when homozygous	
ss	58.5	spineless	Bristles hairlike	
bx	58.8	bithorax	Metathorax mesothoracic; halteres enlarged	
sr	62.0	stripe	Dark median stripe on thorax	
gl	63.1	glass	Eyes small, diamond-shaped, glassy	
k	64	kidney	Eyes kidney-shaped	
Dl	66.2	Delta	Veins thickened; broad at margin; lethal when homozygous	
H	69.5	Hairless	Bristles sparse; veins incomplete; lethal when homozygous	
e	70.7	ebony	Body black	
cd	75.7	cardinal	Eyes yellowish vermilion	
wo	76.2	white ocelli	Ocelli colorless; modifies w^e	
obt	77.5	obtuse	Wings short, blunt; thorax humpy	
mah	88	mahogany	Eyes brown	

TABLE 1. Continued

Gene symbol	Locus	Name of gene	Phenotypic expression	Reference
Pr	90.0	Prickly	Bristles short with thin, twisted tips	
ro	91.1	rough	Eyes rough	
Bd	93.8	Beaded	Margins excised; lethal when homozygous	
bf	95	brief	Body, bristles small; ♂ sterile	
ra	97.3	rasé	Bristles and hairs small, irregularly absent	
ca	100.7	claret	Eyes ruby	
bv	102.7	brevis	Bristles short, stubby; body chunky	
M(3)g	106.2	Minute(3)g	Bristles fine; late hatching; lethal when homozygous	

CHROMOSOME 4[a]

Gene symbol	Locus	Name of gene	Phenotypic expression	Reference
M[b]	—	Minute (4) 57g	Bristles short and thin, lethal when homozygous	
ci[b]	0*	cubitus interruptus	Wing vein L4 interrupted	
13[b]	—	lethal (4) 13	Homozygotes die as larvae	
17[b]	—	lethal (4) 17	Homozygotes die as embryos or larvae	
gvl[b]	—	grooveless	No groove between thorax and scutellum	
ar[b]	—	abdomen rotatum	Abdomen twisted	
2	—	lethal (4) 2	Homozygotes die as embryos; mutational "hot spot"	
23	—	lethal (4) 23	Homozygotes die as embryos	
bt	1.4*	bent	Wings bent back	
gy	—	gouty	Tarsal swellings, especially on 3rd pair of legs	
ey	2.0*	eyeless	Eyes small	

34	—	female sterile (4) 34	Females oviposit, but eggs do not develop
9[c]	—	lethal (4) 9	Homozygotes die as pupae
sv[c]	3.0*	shaven	Bristles small
(spa[pol]*)*[c]	—	sparkling-poliert	Eyes reduced to oval shape; facets appear polished
19[c]	—	lethal (4) 19	Homozygotes die as pupae; most distal locus on 4

[a] Asterisk indicates map positions based on recombination in diplo-4 triploids (Sturtevant, 1951). Other positions from Hochman (1971, 1974).
[b] Genes included in Df(4)M. The relative order of most of these genes is unknown.
[c] Genes included in Df(4)G. The relative order of most of these genes is unknown.

next three decades utilizing *Drosophila* has been extensively reviewed (Lea, 1947; Catcheside, 1948; Muller, 1954; Muller and Oster, 1963; Auerbach, 1962, 1973; Auerbach and Kilbey, 1971; Abrahamson and Lewis, 1971). Suzuki reviews the temperature sensitive mutants in Chapter 23 of this volume.

The analysis by Lewis (1945) of the *Star–asteroid* complex led to his discovery of the cis–trans position effect. Subsequently Green and Green (1949) demonstrated that the lozenge (*lz*) locus could be subdivided into three subloci. Subsequent analyses of gene fine structure have been reviewed by Lewis (1951, 1967) and by Carlson (1959).

Studies on the biochemical genetics of *Drosophila* had their start with the papers of Beadle and Ephrussi (1935, 1936) describing their genetic dissection of eye-pigment synthesis. The vermilion+ substance was identified as kynurenine by Tatum and Haagen-Smit in 1941, and the enzyme defect was elucidated by Baglioni in 1959. As O'Brien points out in Chapter 24 in this volume, there are now over 40 gene loci known for *D. melanogaster* which affect the appearance of a biochemically measurable gene product (either a protein or nucleic acid).

Modern studies on the molecular genetics of *Drosophila* were initiated by Ritossa and Spiegelman (1965) when they demonstrated that the cistrons transcribing the 28S and 18S ribosomal RNAs of *Drosophila* reside in the nucleolus organizer regions of each X and Y chromosome. Subsequently, the cytological locations of the 5S RNA cistrons and the histone genes were determined by Wimber and Steffensen (1970) and by Pardue *et al.* (1972), respectively, using *in situ* hybridization techniques [see review by Wimber and Steffensen (1973)]. The 28S and 18S rRNAs are transcribed on a chromosomal segment to the right of 20F on the X and at the homologous segment on the Y, the 5S rRNAs are transcribed at segment 56EF on chromosome 2R, and between 3 and 5 different histone messages are transcribed at 39E–40A on chromosome 2L (see Figure 1). The DNA sequences specifying the transfer RNAs are scattered throughout the genome (Steffensen and Wimber, 1971). In all the above cases the genes are redundant, with multiplicities ranging between 200 (for the rRNA genes) and 12 (for the tRNA genes).

D. melanogaster has now become a favorite experimental organism for molecular biologists, and a remarkable clarification of the way in which DNA is organized in its chromosomes has resulted from recent studies. According to Rasch *et al.* (1971) the DNA content of a sperm is 1.8×10^{-13} g, and therefore the haploid or C value for *D. melanogaster* is 1.1×10^{11} daltons or 1.7×10^8 nucleotide pairs. Subsequent unpublished studies (E. Rasch) have shown that the DNA contents of the X and Y chromosomes are approximately 3.2 and 1.8 × 10^{-14} g, respectively. As Laird (1973) points out, one can conclude from data on (1) the C value, (2) the percentage of the genome represented by the largest chromatid, and (3) the size of the longest DNA molecules recovered from the genome (Kavenoff and Zimm, 1973) that a single chromatid contains one continuous molecule of DNA which traverses the centromere.

The principal component of the nuclear DNA of *D. melanogaster* in neutral CsCl gradients has a density of 1.702 gm/cm³. A satellite with a density of 1.689 has been isolated from the nuclei of imaginal disc and brain cells, and it has been shown to be localized in the centromeric heterochromatin (Gall *et al.*, 1971). This DNA is fast renaturing because it contains a simple sequence of nucleotides repeated thousands of times. The DNA isolated from polytene nuclei lacks this satellite, and this finding demonstrates that the pericentric, heterochromatic, simple-sequence DNA is under-replicated during the polytenization of the larval salivary gland chromosomes. The DNA of the main band contains unique-sequence DNA and DNAs that are only moderately repetitive. Both DNAs occur throughout the chromosome, and a variety of models for the arrangement of unique and repeated sequences in *Drosophila* euchromatin have been advanced [see Laird (1973), his Figure 4]. Some of the different repeated sequences within chromomeres presumably serve as sites for the attachment of specific proteins. Among these would be the enzymes functioning in replication and transcription and structural proteins functioning in chromosome coiling and in the construction of synaptonemal complexes (King, 1970a; King and Akai, 1971). Other repetitive sequences presumably serve as spacers separating consecutive messages, or they might code for those portions of the nuclear RNA molecules which are thought to function in escorting messages to the nuclear pores. The interested reader should consult the latest Cold Spring Harbor Symposium volume (No. 38, 1974) for the most up-to-date collection of papers dealing with chromosome structure and function.

Polytene chromosomes form puffs at specific loci, and these are now thought to represent areas of intense chromosomal transcription of the RNAs required by the salivary gland cells during specific developmental stages. The first major paper describing the puffing behavior of *Drosophila* salivary gland chromosomes was published by Becker in 1959. In a subsequent paper Becker (1962) reported the results of experiments designed to demonstrate the hormonal control of chromosomal puffing. The metamorphosis of the larval *Drosophila* is controlled by secretions of the ring gland, which lies near the brain. By placing a tight ligature immediately behind the brain the larva can be divided into two segments, which will develop independently. The anterior segment containing the ring gland will undergo metamorphosis, whereas the posterior portion will retain its larval characteristics (unless the operation is performed after the pupation hormone has been released). Normally the gland begins secretion of this hormone 3.5–5 hours before puparium formation. A ligature of the type described above also separates the larval salivary glands into two parts, one lying in the anterior and the other in the posterior segment. Becker had shown previously that a marked increase in the number of chromosomal loci undergoing puff formation normally takes place at the time of puparium formation. However, in ligated animals he found that only the chromosomes in the cells of the anterior portion of the gland show this increase in puffing, whereas the chromosomes of the gland cells behind the ligature remain quiescent. Becker concluded from these findings that the puffing of the salivary chromosomes is triggered by a hormone released by the ring gland. He next performed experiments where salivary glands obtained from an animal with relatively quiescent chromosomes were implanted into an older host. The chromosomes in the cells of both implanted and host glands started to puff simultaneously. Therefore, the chromosomes of the implant can be induced experimentally to puff prematurely. If, on the other hand, a young animal serves as host to a gland from an older donor, the third chromosomes in the cells of the donated gland develop a specific puff at a locus identical to that seen in the third chromosomes from nuclei in the glands of the host. Thus, the chromosomes in an implant can be caused to return to a type of puffing behavior they had previously "outgrown." Becker, therefore, demonstrated not only that certain chromosomal loci can be stimulated into or suppressed from puffing, but that a locus once suppressed from puffing can puff subsequently. In other words, the suppression is not permanent. In Chapter 30 of this volume, Ashburner reviews the more recent contributions to this field.

Sorsa and Sorsa (1967) have adapted the conventional squash techniques for electron microscopic mapping of the salivary gland polytene chromosomes. In their electron microscope study of regions 1A–5F in the distal portion of the X (Sorsa and Sorsa, 1973) they found that the total number of single bands was increased by less than 10 percent over the number shown in Bridges' (1938) map. However, the number of doublets was *decreased* from 32 percent to 18 percent. They concluded that most bands, regardless of their thickness, are of unit character and that, if doublets are counted as single bands, the total band number gives the most realistic estimate of the total number of chromomeres in a given chromosomal segment. The electron microscope maps of regions 1A–5F and

56A–60F are shown in Figure 2. The mapping of the distal segment of 2R was determined by A. Vatanen.

Drosophila developmental genetics can be traced back to the publication of Hadorn (1937) on the *lgl* mutant and of Poulson (1940) on the *Notch* and *white* deficiencies. Subsequent studies on other genetic lethals were reviewed by Hadorn (1961) and by Wright (1970). Two decades of studies on the developmental genetics of bristle patterns have been summarized by Stern (1968). The characteristic pattern of bristles involves an interaction between the cells that differentiate into bristles and a "prepattern" which is superimposed upon the population of hypodermal cells that cover the surface of the fly. Stern and his colleagues showed that the majority of the genes in *Drosophila* which reduce or increase the number of bristles do not affect the prepattern; rather they control the competence of the cell in question to respond to the prepattern. However, Stern and Tokunaga (1967) demonstrated that the eyeless-dominant gene does modify the prepattern of the male foreleg.

In 1963 Hadorn (1963) reported the results of a study in which he cultured fragments of imaginal discs in the abdomens of adult hosts, where they grew but did not differentiate. Such tissue lines could be propagated for prolonged periods by serial transplantation of disc fragments to new adult hosts. Eventually fragments were implanted into larvae which were left to metamorphose. Hadorn found that such tissues occasionally produced structures characteristic of different discs. For example, a regenerated genital disc could produce antennae. Hadorn termed such differentiations *allotypic*. Since the allotypic organs appeared in the offspring of cells which were previously determined to form different structures, a change in determination was postulated. Hadorn called this event *transdetermination*, and it has been observed after culture of the male and the female genital discs, haltere disc, wing disc, prothoracic leg disc, eye-antennal disc, and labial disc. The literature on transdetermination has been reviewed recently by Postlethwait and Schneiderman (1973).

Attempts to induce and physiologically characterize neurological mutants in *Drosophila* have proven successful. The first publications were those of Hotta and Benzer (1969) and Pak *et al.* (1969). Konopka and Benzer (1971) reported the recovery of induced clock mutants and Suzuki *et al.* (1971) isolated a temperature-sensitive paralytic mutant. Hotta and Benzer have reviewed the studies utilizing mosaics to map behavioral foci (Hotta and Benzer, 1973). Data on various behavioral mutants are presented in this volume by Grossfield (Chapter 25) and by Pak (Chapter 26).

The discipline of *Drosophila* population genetics combines the results

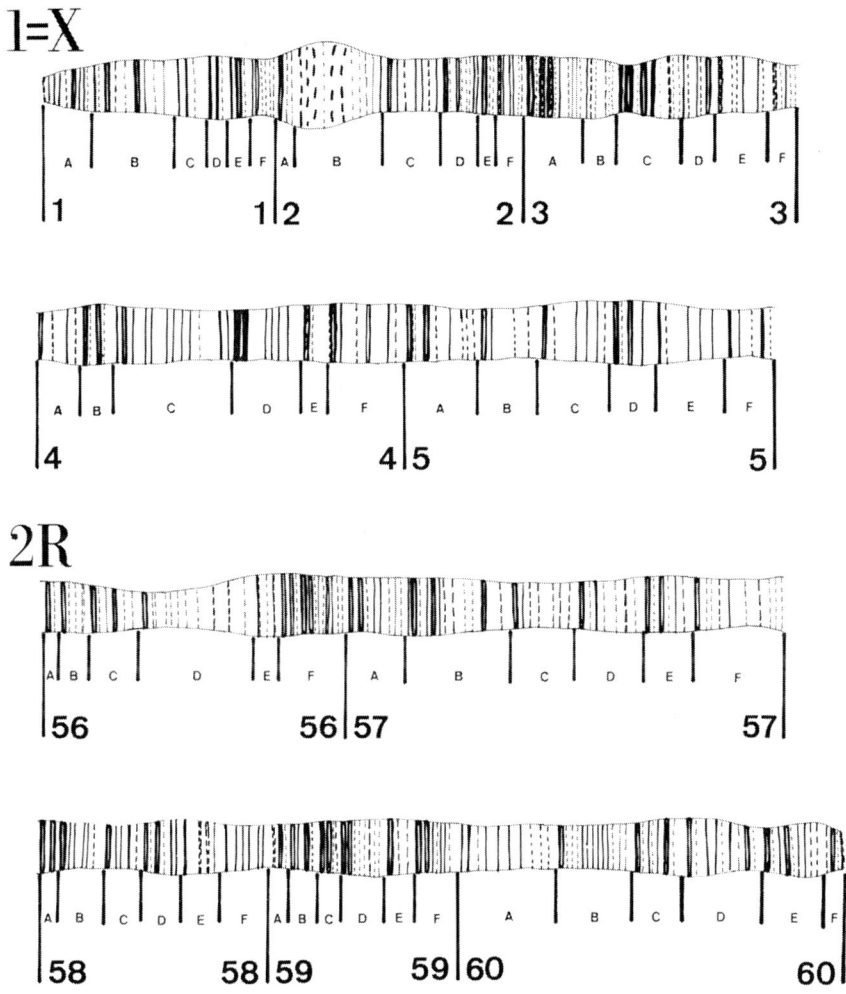

Figure 2. Electron microscopic maps of the distal segments of the salivary X and 2R chromosomes. The scale of divisions and subdivisions follows the convention of the maps of Bridges (1938) for the X and of Bridges and Bridges (1939) for 2R. The maps are based on analyses of 5–10 electron micrographs of each division. Bands are drawn schematically and only their granular, singlet, or doublet character has been presented. Courtesy of Dr. Marja Sorsa.

of observations on natural and laboratory populations with mathematical theory. The Hardy-Weinberg Law and the publications Haldane, Fisher, and Wright produced between 1924 and 1932 constitute the mathematical foundations of this subject. The book by Li (1955) presents a clear summarization of this early work, and the ones by Wright (1968, 1969) and by Crow and Kimura (1970) cover the more recent advances.

Chetverikov suggested as early as 1926 that populations in nature retain in the heterozygous condition many of the mutations which arise spontaneously, and that these provide a store of potential but hidden variability. Subsequent sampling of natural populations of *D. melanogaster* in various parts of the world confirmed his prediction [see reviews by Ives (1945) and Spenser (1947)]. Laboratory investigations began in 1933 with the introduction of the population cage by L'Héritier and Teissier (1933). In 1934 they reported the disappearance of a deleterious gene from populations maintained for many generations. Intensive investigations followed to determine what factors influenced the effectiveness of selection in producing phenotypically detectable responses within previously unselected populations. Dobzhansky (1937) was the first to integrate the results of laboratory and field studies with the predictions arising from mathematical theory. Population genetics has flourished in the intervening period, and the contributions arising from studies with *D. melanogaster* can be found in reviews such as those by Spiess (1962, 1968), Lewontin (1967, 1973), Wallace (1968), and Parsons (1973).

Acknowledgments

The author is grateful to Lee Douglas, George Lefevre, Benjamin Hochman, and Marja Sorsa for their critical comments on early drafts of this manuscript.

Literature Cited

Abrahamson, S. and E. B. Lewis, 1971   The detection of mutations in *Drosophila melanogaster*. In *Chemical Mutagens*, Vol. 2, edited by A. Hollaender, Chapter 17, pp. 461–487, Plenum Press, New York.

Auerbach, C., 1962   *Mutation: An Introduction to Research on Mutagenesis. Part I: Methods*, Oliver & Boyd, Edinburgh.

Auerbach, C., 1973   History of research on chemical mutagenesis. In *Chemical Mutagens*, Vol. 3, edited by A. Hollaender, Chapter 24, pp. 1–19, Plenum Press, New York.

Auerbach, C. and B. J. Kilbey, 1971   Mutation in eukaryotes. *Annu. Rev. Genet.* **5**:163–218.

Auerbach, C. and J. M. Robson, 1946   Chemical production of mutations. *Nature (Lond.)* **157**:302.

Baglioni, C., 1959   Genetic control of tryptophan peroxidase in *Drosophila melanogaster. Nature (Lond.)* **184**:1084–1085.

Beadle, G. W. and B. Ephrussi, 1935   Transplantation in *Drosophila. Proc. Natl. Acad. Sci. USA* **21**:642–646.

Beadle, G. W. and B. Ephrussi, 1936   The differentiation of eye pigments in *Drosophila* as studied by transplantation. *Genetics* **21**:225–247.

Becker, H., 1959   Die Puffs der Spiecheldrüsenchromosomen von *Drosophila melanogaster*. I. Beobachtungen zum Verhalten des Puffmusters im Normalstamm und bei zwei Mutanten, *giant* und *lethal-giant-larvae*. *Chromosoma (Berl.)* **10**:654–678.

Becker, H., 1962   Die Puffs der Spiecheldrüsenchromosomen von *Drosophila melanogaster*. II. Die Auslösung der Puffbildung, ihre Spezifität und ihre Beziehung zur Funktion der Ringdrüse. *Chromosoma (Berl.)* **13**:341–384.

Bodenstein, D., 1950   The postembryonic development of *Drosophila*. In *Biology of Drosophila*, edited by M. Demerec, pp. 275–367, John Wiley & Sons, New York.

Bridges, C. B., 1914   Direct proof through non-disjunction that the sex-linked genes of *Drosophila* are borne by the X-chromosome. *Science (Wash., D.C.)* **40**:107–109.

Bridges, C. B., 1917   Deficiency. *Genetics* **2**:445–465.

Bridges, C. B., 1919   Duplications. *Anat. Rec.* **15**:357–358.

Bridges, C. B., 1921   Triploid intersexes in *Drosophila melanogaster*. *Science (Wash., D.C.)* **54**:252–254.

Bridges, C. B., 1923   The translocation of a section of chromosome-II upon chromosome-III in *Drosophila*. *Anat. Rec.* **24**:426–427.

Bridges, C. B., 1925   Sex in relation to chromosomes and genes. *Am. Nat.* **59**:127–137.

Bridges, C. B., 1935   Salivary chromosome maps with a key to the banding of the chromosomes of *Drosophila melanogaster*. *J. Hered.* **26**:60–64.

Bridges, C. B., 1938   A revised map of the salivary gland X-chromosome of *Drosophila melanogaster*. *J. Hered.* **29**:11–13.

Bridges, C. B. and P. N. Bridges, 1939   A revised map of the right limb of the second chromosome of *Drosophila melanogaster*. *J. Hered.* **30**:475–476.

Carlson, E. A., 1959   Comparative genetics of complex loci. *Quart. Rev. Biol.* **34**:36–67.

Castle, W. E., 1906   Inbreeding, cross-breeding and sterility in *Drosophila*. *Science (Wash., D.C.)* **23**:153.

Catcheside, D. G., 1948   Genetic effects of radiations. *Adv. Genet.* **2**:271–358.

Chetverikov, S. S., 1926   On certain aspects of the evolutionary process from the standpoint of genetics (translated from Russian to English by I. M. Lerner). *Proc. Am. Phil. Soc.* **109**:124–158 (1961).

Chovnick, A., 1973   Gene conversion and transfer of genetic information within the inverted region of inversion heterozygotes. *Genetics* **75**:123–131.

Church, R. B. and F. W. Robertson, 1966   A biochemical study of the growth of *Drosophila melanogaster*. *J. Exp. Zool.* **162**:337–352.

Colaianne, J. J. and A. E. Bell, 1972   The relative influence of sex of progeny on the lethal expression of the *sonless* gene in *Drosophila melanogaster*. *Genetics* **72**:293–296.

Crow, J. F. and M. Kimura, 1970   *An Introduction to Population Genetics Theory*, Harper and Row, New York.

David, J., 1962   A new medium for rearing *Drosophila* in axenic conditions. *Drosophila Inf. Serv.* **36**:128.

Davis, B. K., 1971   Genetic analysis of a meiotic mutant resulting in precocious sister-centromere separation in *Drosophila melanogaster*. *Mol. Gen. Genet.* **113**:251–272.

Demerec, M. and B. P. Kaufmann, 1961   *Drosophila Guide*, seventh edition, Carnegie Institution of Washington Publication, Carnegie Institution, Washington, D.C.

Denell, R. E., 1973   Homoeosis in *Drosophila*. I. Complementation studies with revertants of Nasobemia. *Genetics* **75**:279–297.

Dobzhansky, T. 1937 *Genetics and the Origin of Species,* second edition (1941) third edition (1951), Columbia University Press, New York.

Ellison, J. R. and H. J. Barr, 1971 Differences in the quinacrine staining of the chromosomes of a pair of sibling species: *Drosophila melanogaster* and *Drosophila simulans. Chromosoma (Berl.)* **34:**424–435.

Ferris, G. F., 1950 External morphology of the adult. In *Biology of Drosophila,* edited by M. Demerec, pp. 368–419, John Wiley & Sons, New York.

Fisher, R. A., 1930 *The Genetic Theory of Natural Selection,* Clarendon Press, Oxford.

Gall, J. G., E. H. Cohen and M. L. Polan, 1971 Repetitive DNA sequences in *Drosophila. Chromosoma (Berl.)* **33:**319–344.

Green, M. M. and K. C. Green, 1949 Crossing-over between alleles at the *lozenge* locus in *Drosophila melanogaster. Proc. Natl. Acad. Sci. USA* **35:**586–591.

Hadorn, E., 1937 An accelerating effect of normal "ring-glands" on puparium-formation in lethal larvae of *Drosophila melanogaster. Proc. Natl. Acad. Sci. USA* **23:**478–484.

Hadorn, E., 1961 *Developmental Genetics and Lethal Factors* (translated by U. Mittwoch). John Wiley & Sons, New York.

Hadorn, E., 1963 Differenzierungsleistungen wiederholt fragmentierter Teilstücke männlicher Genitalscheiben von *Drosophila melanogaster* nach Kultur *in vivo. Dev. Biol.* **7:**617–629.

Haldane, J. B. S., 1924*a* A mathematical theory of natural and artificial selection. Part I. *Trans. Camb. Phil. Soc.* **23:**19–41.

Haldane, J. B. S., 1924*b* A mathematical theory of natural and artificial selection. Part II. *Biol. Proc. Camb. Phil. Soc. Biol. Sci.* **1:**158–163.

Haldane, J. B. S., 1924*c* A mathematical theory of natural and artificial selection. Part III. *Proc. Camb. Phil. Soc.* **23:**363–372.

Haldane, J. B. S., 1924*d* A mathematical theory of natural and artificial selection. Part IV. *Proc. Camb. Phil. Soc.* **23:**235–243.

Haldane, J. B. S., 1927 A mathematical theory of natural and artificial selection. Part V. Selection and mutation. *Proc. Camb. Phil. Soc.* **23:**838–844.

Haldane, J. B. S. 1930*a* A mathematical theory of natural and artificial selection. VI. Isolation. *Proc. Camb. Phil. Soc.* **26:**220–230.

Haldane, J. B. S., 1930*b* A mathematical theory of natural and artificial selection. VII. Selection intensity as a function of mortality rate. *Proc. Camb. Phil. Soc.* **27:**131–136.

Haldane, J. B. S., 1930*c* A mathematical theory of natural and artificial selection. VIII. Metastable populations. *Proc. Camb. Phil. Soc.* **27:**137–142.

Haldane, J. B. S., 1932 A mathematical theory of natural and artificial selection. IX. Rapid selection. *Proc. Camb. Phil. Soc.* **28:**244–248.

Herskowitz, I. H., 1952 *Bibliography on the Genetics of Drosophila,* Part 2, Commonwealth Agricultural Bureau, Farnham Royal, Slough, Bucks., England.

Herskowitz, I. H., 1958 *Bibliography on the Genetics of Drosophila,* Part 3, Indiana University Press, Bloomington, Ind.

Herskowitz, I. H., 1963 *Bibliography on the Genetics of Drosophila,* Part 4, McGraw-Hill, New York.

Herskowitz, I. H., 1969 *Bibliography on the Genetics of Drosophila,* Part 5, Macmillan, New York.

Herskowitz, I., 1974 *Bibliography on The Genetics of Drosophila,* Part 6, Macmillan, New York.

Hochman, B. 1971 Analysis of chromosome 4 in *Drosophila melanogaster*. II. Ethyl methanesulfonate induced lethals. *Genetics* **67**:235–252.

Hochman, B. 1974 Analysis of a whole chromosome in *Drosophila*. *Cold Spring Harbor Symp. Quant. Biol.* **38**:581–589.

Holm, D. G., M. Baldwin, P. Duck and A. Chovnick, 1969 The use of compound autosomes to determine the relative centromeric position of chromosome three. *Drosophila Inf. Serv.* **44**:112.

Hotta, Y. and S. Benzer, 1969 Abnormal electroretinograms in visual mutants of *Drosophila*. *Nature (Lond.)* **222**:354–356.

Hotta, Y. and S. Benzer, 1973 Mapping of behavior in *Drosophila melanogaster*. In *Genetic Mechanisms of Development,* edited by F. H. Ruddle, pp. 129–167, Academic Press, New York.

Ives, P. T., 1945 The genetic structure of American populations of *Drosophila melanogaster*. *Genetics* **30**:167–196.

Johnson, J. H. and R. C. King, 1972 Studies on *fes*, a mutation affecting cystocyte cytokinesis, in *Drosophila melanogaster*. *Biol. Bull.* **143**:525–547.

Kaplan, W. D. and W. E. Trout, 1969 The behavior of four neurological mutants of *Drosophila*. *Genetics* **61**:399–409.

Kavenoff, R. and B. H. Zimm, 1973 Chromosome sized DNA molecules from *Drosophila*. *Chromosoma (Berl.)* **41**:1–27.

King, R. C., 1970a The meiotic behavior of the *Drosophila* oocyte. *Interntl. Rev. Cytol.* **28**:125–168.

King, R. C., 1970b *Ovarian Development in Drosophila melanogaster,* Academic Press, New York.

King, R. C. and H. Akai, 1971 Spermatogenesis in *Bombyx mori*. I. The ultrastructure of synapsed bivalents. *J. Morphol.* **134**:181–194.

Konopka, R. J. and S. Benzer, 1971 Clock mutants of *Drosophila melanogaster*. *Proc. Natl. Acad. Sci. USA* **68**:2112–2116.

Laird, C. D., 1973 DNA of *Drosophila* chromosomes. *Annu. Rev. Genet.* **7**:177–204.

Lea, D. E., 1947 *Actions of Radiations on Living Cells,* Cambridge University Press, Cambridge.

Lefevre, G., Jr., 1970 Linkage data. *Drosophila Inf. Serv.* **45**:40.

Lefevre, G., Jr., 1971 Salivary chromosome bands and the frequency of crossing over in *Drosophila melanogaster*. *Genetics* **67**:497–513.

Lefevre, G., Jr., 1975 A photographic representation and interpretation of the polytene chromosomes of *Drosophila melanogaster* salivary glands. In *Genetics and Biology of Drosophila,* Vol. 1, Edited by E. Novitski and M. Ashburner. Academic Press, London, in press.

Lefevre, G., Jr. and T. K. Johnson, 1973 Evidence for a sex-linked haplo-inviable locus in the *cut-singed* region of *Drosophila melanogaster*. *Genetics* **74**:633–645.

Lewis, E. B., 1945 The relation of repeats to position effect in *Drosophila melanogaster*. *Genetics* **30**:137–166.

Lewis, E. B., 1951 Pseudoallelism and gene evolution. *Cold Spring Harbor Symp. Quant. Biol.* **16**:159–174.

Lewis, E. B., 1967 Genes and gene complexes. In *Heritage from Mendel,* edited by R. A. Brink, pp. 17–47, University of Wisconsin Press, Madison, Wisc.

Lewontin, R. C., 1967 Population genetics. *Annu. Rev. Genet.* **1**:37–70.

Lewontin, R. C., 1973 Population genetics. *Annu. Rev. Genet.* **7**:1–17.

L'Héritier, P. and G. Teissier, 1933 Étude d'une population de Drosophiles en equilibre. *C. R. Hebd. Sé*ances Acad. Sci. Ser. D Sci. Nat. **197**:1765–1767.

L'Héritier, P. and G. Teissier, 1934 Une expérience de sélection naturelle. Courbe d'élimination du gène "Bar" dans une population de Drosophiles en équilibre. *C. R. Sé*ances Soc. Biol. Fil. Paris **117**:1049–1051.

Li, C. C., 1955 *Population Genetics,* University of Chicago Press, Chicago, Ill.

Lindsley, D. L. and E. H. Grell, 1968 *Genetic Variations of Drosophila melanogaster,* Carnegie Institution of Washington, Publication 627, Carnegie Institution, Washington, D.C.

Loew, H., 1862 Diptera Americae septentrionalis indigena. Centuria secunda. *Berl. Ent. Z.* **6**:185–232.

Lütolf, H. V., 1971 On the relative position of the centromere of chromosome 3 in *Drosophila melanogaster. Experientia (Basel)* **27**:1375.

Mange, A. P. and L. Sandler, 1973 A note on the maternal effect mutants *daughterless* and *abnormal oocyte* in *Drosophila melanogaster. Genetics* **73**:73–86.

Meigen, J. W., 1818–1838 *Systematischen Beschreibung der bekannten europaischen zweiflugeligen Insekten* (7 vols.), Schulz, Aachen.

Merriam, J. R., 1973 On setting up a lab and kitchen. *Drosophila Inf. Serv.* **50**:196–197.

Miller, A., 1950 The internal anatomy and histology of the imago of *Drosophila melanogaster.* In *Biology of Drosophila,* edited by M. Demerec, pp. 420–534, John Wiley & Sons, New York.

Morgan, T. H., 1910 Sex-limited inheritance in *Drosophila. Science (Wash., D.C.)* **32**:120–122.

Morgan, T. H., 1912*a* Complete linkage in the second chromosome of the male of *Drosophila. Science (Wash., D.C.)* **36**:719–720.

Morgan, T. H., 1912*b* The explanation of a new sex ratio in *Drosophila. Science (Wash., D.C.)* **36**:718–719.

Muller, H. J., 1916 The mechanism of crossing over. IV. *Am. Nat.* **50**:421–434.

Muller, H. J., 1918 Genetic variability, twin hybrids, and constant hybrids, in a case of balanced lethal factors. *Genetics* **3**:422–499.

Muller, H. J., 1927 Artificial transmutation of the gene. *Science (Wash., D.C.)* **66**:84–87.

Muller, H. J., 1939 *Bibliography on the Genetics of Drosophila,* Oliver & Boyd, Edinburgh.

Muller, H. J., 1954 The nature of the genetic effects produced by radiation. The manner of production of mutations by radiation. In *Radiation Biology,* Volume 1, Part 1, edited by A. Hollaender, Chapters 7 and 8, McGraw-Hill, New York.

Muller, H. J. and I. I. Oster, 1963 Some mutational techniques in Drosophila. In *Methodology in Basic Genetics,* edited by W. J. Burdette, pp. 240–278, Holden-Day, San Francisco.

Nicoletti, B., 1959 An efficient method for salivary-gland-chromosome preparations. *Drosophila Inf. Serv.* **33**:181–182.

Norby, S., 1970 Recombination between *rudimentary* and *forked. Drosophila Inf. Serv.* **45**:41.

Novitski, E., 1973 *Drosophila Information Service, Vol. 50,* prepared at the Department of Biology, University of Oregon, Eugene, Ore.

Painter, T. S., 1933 A new method for the study of chromosome aberrations and the plotting of chromosome maps in *Drosophila melanogaster. Genetics* **19**:175–188.

Pak, W. L., J. Grossfield and N. V. White, 1969   Nonphototactic mutants in a study of vision of *Drosophila. Nature (Lond.)* **222**:351–354.

Pardue, M. L., E. Weinberg, L. H. Kedes and M. L. Birnstiel, 1972   Localization of sequences coding for histone messenger RNA in the chromosomes of *Drosophila melanogaster. 12th Annual Meeting of the American Society for Cell Biology, Abstract 398,* Rockefeller University Press, New York.

Parry, D. M., 1973   A meiotic mutant affecting recombination in female *Drosophila melanogaster. Genetics* **73**:465–486.

Parsons, P. A., 1973   *Behavioural and Ecological Genetics: A Study in Drosophila,* Clarendon Press, Oxford.

Postlethwait, J. H. and H. A. Schneiderman, 1973   Developmental genetics of *Drosophila* imaginal discs. *Annu. Rev. Genet.* **7**:381–433.

Poulson, D. F., 1940   The effects of certain X-chromosome deficiencies on the embryonic development of *Drosophila melanogaster. J. Exp. Zool.* **83**:271–325.

Poulson, D. F., 1950   Histogenesis, organogenesis, and differentiation in the embryo of *Drosophila melanogaster* Meigen. In *Biology of Drosophila,* edited by M. Demerec, pp. 168–274, John Wiley & Sons, New York.

Puro, J. and P. Arajärvi, 1969   The position of the *cp, in* and *ri* genes and the third chromosome centromere in *Drosophila melanogaster. Hereditas* **62**:414–418.

Rapoport, J. A., 1946   Carbonyl compounds and the chemical mechanism of mutations. *Dokl. Akad. Nauk SSSR Ser. Biol.* **54**:65–67.

Rasch, E. M., H. J. Barr and R. W. Rasch, 1971   The DNA content of sperm of *Drosophila melanogaster. Chromosoma (Berl.)* **33**:1–18.

Rayle, R. E. and D. I. Hoar, 1969   Gene order and cytological localization of several X-linked mutants of *Drosophila melanogaster. Drosophila Inf. Serv.* **44**:94.

Ritossa, F. M. and S. Spiegelman, 1965   Localization of DNA complementary to ribosomal RNA in the nucleolus organizer region of *Drosophila melanogaster. Proc. Natl. Acad. Sci. USA* **53**:737–745.

Roberts, P. A. 1972   A possible case of position effect on DNA replication in *Drosophila melanogaster. Genetics* **72**:607–614.

Sang, J. H., 1950   Population growth in *Drosophila* cultures. *Biol. Rev.* **25**:188–219.

Sang, J. H., 1956   The quantitative nutritional requirements of *Drosophila melanogaster. J. Exp. Biol.* **33**:45–72.

Schalet, A. and G. Lefevre Jr., 1973   The localization of "ordinary" sex-linked genes in section 20 of the polytene X-chromosome of *Drosophila melanogaster. Chromosoma (Berl.)* **44**:183–202.

Schalet, A. and K. Singer, 1971   A revised map of genes in the proximal region of the X chromosome of *Drosophila melanogaster. Drosophila Inf. Serv.* **46**:131–132.

Schalet, A., G. Lefevre Jr. and K. Singer, 1970   Preliminary cytogenetic observations on the proximal euchromatic region of the X-chromosome of *D. melanogaster. Drosophila Inf. Serv.* **45**:165.

Scriba, M., 1964   Beeinflussung der frühen Embryonalentwicklung von *Drosophila melanogaster* durch Chromosomenaberrationen. *Zool. Jahrb. Abt. Anat. Ontog. Tiere* **81**:435–490.

Shorrocks, B., 1972   *Drosophila,* Ginn, London.

Slizynska, H., 1938   Salivary chromosome analysis of the *white-facet* region of *Drosophila melanogaster. Genetics* **23**:291–299.

Sonnenblick, B. P., 1950   The early embryology of *Drosophila.* In *Biology of Drosophila,* edited by M. Demerec, pp. 62–167, John Wiley & Sons, New York.

Sorsa, M. and V. Sorsa, 1967   Electron microscopic observations on interband fibrils in *Drosophila* salivary chromosomes. *Chromosoma (Berl.)* **22**:32–41.

Sorsa, M. and V. Sorsa, 1973   Electron microscopic mapping of salivary chromosome X in *Drosophila melanogaster. Genetics 74 June Suppl. No. 2, Part 2:*S262.

Spenser, W. P., 1947   Mutations in wild populations of *Drosophila. Adv. Genet.* **1**:359–402.

Spenser, W. P., 1950   Collection and laboratory culture. In *Biology of Drosophila,* edited by M. Demerec, pp. 535–590, John Wiley & Sons, New York.

Spiess, E. B., editor, 1962   *Papers on Animal Population Genetics,* Little-Brown, Boston, Mass. (see the 61-page introduction by the editor).

Spiess, E. B., 1968   Population genetics. *Annu. Rev. Genet.* **2**:165–208.

Steffensen, D. M. and D. E. Wimber, 1971   Localization of tRNA genes in the salivary chromosomes of *Drosophila* by RNA:DNA hybridization. *Genetics* **69**:163–178.

Stern, C., 1968   *Genetic Mosaics and Other Essays,* Harvard University Press, Cambridge, Mass.

Stern, C. and C. Tokunaga, 1967   Nonautonomy in differentiation of pattern-determining genes in *Drosophila.* I. The sex comb of *eyeless-dominant. Proc. Natl. Acad. Sci. USA* **53**:658–664.

Strickberger, M. W., 1962   *Experiments in Genetics with Drosophila,* John Wiley & Sons, New York.

Sturtevant, A. H., 1913   The linear arrangement of six sex-linked factors in *Drosophila,* as shown by their mode of association. *J. Exp. Zool.* **14**:43–59.

Sturtevant, A. H., 1925   The effects of unequal crossing over at the *Bar* locus in *Drosophila. Genetics* **10**:117–147.

Sturtevant, A. H., 1926   A crossover reducer in *Drosophila melanogaster* due to inversion of a section of the third chromosome. *Biol. Zentralbl.* **46**:697–702.

Sturtevant, A. H., 1951   A map of the fourth chromosome of *Drosophila melanogaster,* based on crossing over in triploid females. *Proc. Natl. Acad. Sci. USA* **37**:405–407.

Sturtevant, A. H., 1965   *A History of Genetics.* Harper and Row, New York.

Suzuki, D. T., T. Grigliatti and R. Williamson, 1971   Temperature-sensitive mutations in *Drosophila melanogaster.* VII. A mutation (*para^ts*) causing reversible adult paralysis. *Proc. Natl. Acad. Sci. USA* **68**:890–893.

Tates, A. D., 1971   Cytodifferentiation during spermatogenesis in *Drosophila melanogaster:* An electron microscopic study. J. H. Pasmans, the Hague.

Tatum, E. L. and A. J. Haagen-Smit, 1941   Identification of *Drosophila v+* hormone of bacterial origin. *J. Biol. Chem.* **140**:575–580.

Ursprung, H. and R. Nöthiger, editors, 1972   *The Biology of Imaginal Disks,* Springer-Verlag, New York.

Wallace, B., 1968   *Topics in Population Genetics,* Norton, New York.

Wheeler, M. R., 1967   The fruitfly. In *The Universities' Federation for Animal Welfare Handbook: The Care and Management of Laboratory Animals,* third edition, pp. 906–924, Livingstone, Edinburgh.

Wheeler, M. R., 1972   The fruitfly. In *The Universities' Federation for Animal Welfare Handbook: The Care and Management of Laboratory Animals,* fourth edition, pp. 543–548, Livingstone, Edinburgh.

Wimber, D. E. and D. M. Steffensen, 1970   Localization of 5S RNA genes in *Drosophila* chromosomes by RNA–DNA hybridization. *Science (Wash., D.C.)* **170**:639–641.

Wimber, D. E. and D. M. Steffensen, 1973   Localization of gene function. *Annu. Rev. Genet.* **7**:205–223.

Wright, S., 1931   *Evolution in Mendelian populations, Genetics* **16:**97–159.

Wright, S., 1968   *Evolution and Genetics of Populations,* Vol. 1, *Genetic and Biometric Foundations,* University of Chicago Press, Chicago, Ill.

Wright, S., 1969   *Evolution and Genetics of Populations,* Vol. 2, *The Theory of Gene Frequencies,* University of Chicago Press, Chicago, Ill.

Wright, T. R. F., 1970   The genetics of embryogenesis in *Drosophila. Adv. Genet.* **15:**261–395.

Zimm, G., D. L. Lindsley and E. H. Grell, 1972   Fruit fly linkage groups. In *Biology Data Book,* Vol. 1, second edition, edited by P. S. Altman and D. S. Dittmer, pp. 27–48, Federation of the American Society of Experimental Biologists, Bethesda, Md.

23

Temperature-Sensitive Mutations in *Drosophila melanogaster*

Davıd T. Suzukı

> *"Temperature is one of the best tools at the command of the biologist for 'picking apart' the reactions in the living organism without destroying its 'normal' operation."*
>
> —*C. R. Plunkett, 1926*

Conditional mutations which exhibit normal phenotypes in one environment (permissive) and are mutant in another (restrictive) have been powerful tools in the study of molecular biology of microorganisms. One class of conditional mutations, the temperature sensitives (ts), can easily be studied by altering culture temperatures. Thus, ts lethal mutations can be maintained at permissive temperatures and analyzed for defective processes under restrictive conditions (Epstein *et al.*, 1963). Moreover, by shifting cultures from permissive to restrictive temperatures and *vice versa*, at different intervals, the time of activity of ts genes has been inferred (Edgar and Epstein, 1965). In microorganisms, the molecular basis for temperature sensitivity has been very well characterized and shown to result from missense mutations (Edgar and Lielausis, 1964) which result

Davıd T. Suzukı—Department of Zoology, The University of British Columbia, Vancouver, B.C., Canada.

in proteins with single amino acid substitutions (Wittmann and Witt-mann-Liebold, 1966). This results in changes in the thermostability of tertiary and quaternary protein structure with consequent loss of bio-logical activity at restrictive temperatures (Jockusch, 1966; Guthrie *et al.*, 1969).

In multicellular, eukaryotic organisms, temperature has long been used to perturb genetic and developmental processes. Some of the earliest studies were carried out with lepidoptera, where changes in coloration had been correlated with seasonal fluctuations in temperature. Merrifield (1891, 1893) was able to change the pattern and intensity of wing markings of butterflies after temperature shocks were administered to pupae. Echinoderm larvae were found to exhibit maternal phenotypes in the summer and paternal phenotypes in winter (Vernon, 1898) which could be attributed to changes in water temperature (Doncaster, 1903).

Temperature effects on gene expression were also recorded in beetles (Tower, 1910; Johnson, 1910; Shelford, 1917), plants (Baur, 1911), fish (Jordan, 1921; Hubbs, 1922), and mammals (Sumner, 1911; Schultz, 1915). More recently, ts mutations have been recovered in eukaryotes with a view toward using them for genetic studies. Thus, ts mutations have been reported in *Neurospora* (Horowitz, 1950), corn (Schwartz, 1958), *Arabidopsis* (Langridge, 1965), *Paramecium* (Igarashi, 1966), yeast (Hartwell, 1967), *Habrobracon* (Whiting, 1932; Smith, 1968), *Dic-tyostelium* (Loomis, 1969), *Musca* (McDonald and Overland, 1972), and mammalian cell cultures (Thompson *et al.*, 1970). This list is by no means exhaustive, but it points to the ready recovery and utility of this class of mutations.

The fruit fly, *Drosophila melanogaster*, is the most extensively characterized eukaryote genetically, and ts mutations (Table 1) have been a part of its repertoire of genetic tools since 1915. Hoge (1915) observed that the reduplicated legs mutation (*rdp*) appeared to lose penetrance during the summer. Upon careful investigation she found that *rdp* is cold-sensitive, i.e., at low temperatures penetrance of the mutant phenotype is high, and at high temperatures most *rdp* flies are normal. By shifting cul-tures from one temperature to the other at different developmental stages she showed that the developmental interval during which low temperature induced the mutant phene was the larval stage.

Other mutations whose expressivity was altered by temperature were found. Thus, the number of eye facets in Bar (*B*) flies decreases (Seyster, 1919) whereas wing lengths of vestigial (*vg*) individuals increase at ele-vated temperatures (Roberts, 1918). Temperature sensitivity was later shown for the eyeless (*ey*) (Hyde, 1922), bent (*bt*) (Metz, 1923), Dichaete

(D) (Plunkett, 1926), crippled (*crip*) (Komai, 1926), and mottled (*mot*) (Surrarer, 1935) mutations. The first report of temperature sensitivity of a homoeotic mutation was by Astaurov (1930) on tetraptera (*ttr*). Subsequently, several alleles of spineless-aristapedia (*ss^a*) were shown to be cold sensitive (Finck, 1942; Villee, 1943a,b, 1944; Vogt, 1946a,b). The extent of temperature sensitivity can be seen in the list of mutations compiled by Lindsley and Grell (1968). Hersh (1930) proposed the term "thermophene" to describe a phenotype whose expression is modified by temperature.

Lethal mutations have been useful in the analysis of developmental events (Hadorn, 1955). Temperature-sensitive lethality adds an extra dimension to the analytical methodology in the characterization of defects by permitting an accurate determination of the temperature-sensitive period prior to the effective lethal phase. Eker (1935) was the first to show ts lethality with the heat-sensitive mutant short-wing (*sw*). He found that *sw* flies die at 31°C, and at successively lower temperatures survival increases and the associated wing and eye defects become less severe. Heat-induced lethality was also shown with *vg^P* (Harnly and Harnly, 1936), sine oculis (*SO*) (Milani, 1946), and Abruptex-Hairless (*Ax-H*) double mutants (House, 1959).

Parkash (1967) reported that among 8 lethal mutations, 1 was cold-sensitive and 2 were heat-sensitive lethals. In the first large-scale search for induced ts lethals, an estimated 11–12 percent of all ethyl methanesulfonate-induced lethals on the X (Suzuki *et al.*, 1967) and second (Baillie *et al.*, 1968) chromosomes were found to be temperature sensitive. No chromosome aberrations have been detected among several hundred chemically-induced ts lethals (Suzuki, 1970), although 3 out of 10 γ-ray-induced ts lethals have been found to be associated with translocations (Kaufman and Suzuki, 1974). Cold-sensitive lethals have also been detected on the X chromosome at a lower frequency (Mayoh and Suzuki, 1973; Wright, 1973).

Temperature sensitivity is not a property confined to loci on specific chromosomes or a few loci on a given chromosome, as ts mutations mapping at many sites have been reported on the X (Suzuki *et al.*, 1967; Mayoh and Suzuki, 1973), Y (Ayles *et al.*, 1973), second (Baillie *et al.*, 1968), third (Fattig and Rickoll, 1972; Tasaka and Suzuki, 1973), and fourth (Metz, 1923; Baron, 1935) chromosomes. Dominant ts lethals have been reported on the second (Suzuki and Procunier, 1969; Rosenbluth *et al.*, 1972) and third (Holden and Suzuki, 1973) chromosomes but are much rarer than recessives and may not be extensively distributed through the genome.

TABLE 1. *Genetic and Developmental Properties of Temperature-Sensitive Mutations in D. melanogaster*

Genetic position	Symbol	Name	Thermophene	Temperature-sensitive period	Reference
Y CHROMOSOME					
Y short	bb^{ts1}	bobbed-ts1	Slender bristles, lethality	—	Williamson et al. (1973)
Y short	bb^{ts2}	bobbed-ts2	Slender bristles, lethality	—	Williamson et al. (1973)
Y long	kl-1 , 4^{ts}	fertility loci 1 , 4^{ts}	Sterility	Spermatocytes	Ayles et al. (1973)
Y long	kl-4^{ts}	fertility locus 4^{ts}	Sterility	Spermatocytes	Ayles et al. (1973)
Y long	kl-4 , 5^{ts}	fertility loci 4 , 5^{ts}	Sterility	Meiosis	Ayles et al. (1973)
X CHROMOSOME					
0.0	sc^1	scute-1	Reduction in thoracic bristles	Third instar	Child (1935)
0.3	dor	deep orange	Lethality of dor/dor^l at 29°C	Early pupa	Pratt (1971)
1.5	w^{bl}	white blood	Eye color dark (17°C) or light (30°C)	40- to 48-hr pupa	Ephrussi and Herold (1945)
	$l(1)N^{ts}$	ts Notch lethal	Lethality; head, eye, bristle, wing, leg defects	Embryo, larva, pupa	Shellenbarger (1971)
3.0	N^{60g11}	Notch-60g11	Disrupted eye facets in $N^{60g11/+}$	Late third instar	Foster and Suzuki (1970)
	N^{def}	Notch-deformed	Fusion of ocelli	Second–third instar	Hillman (1956, 1962)

Map position	Symbol	Name	Character affected	Temperature-sensitive period	Reference
6.0	*norp A*^{H52}	no receptor potential A-H52	Loss of receptor response in ERG		Deland and Pak (1973)
15.2	*l(1)E7*^{ts}	lethal E7-ts	Lethality	Embryo to pupa in females, mid-pupa in males	Tarasoff and Suzuki (1970)
15.5	*l(1)E25*^{ts}	lethal E25-ts	Lethality, female sterility	Embryo, first to second instar, adult female	Tarasoff and Suzuki (1970)
20.7	*l(1)E34*^{ts}	lethal E34-ts	Lethality	At pupation	Wright (1968)
21.7	*l(1)mys*^{ts}	lethal (1) myospheroid-ts	Abnormal muscle development	Early embryo	Wright (1968)
32.8	*l(1)E6*^{ts}(*ras*^{ts})	raspberry-ts-lethal	Lethality, pteridine defect	Embryo to first instar, late third instar to pupa, mid-pupa to eclosion	Grigliatti and Suzuki (1970)
33.0	*v*^{ts}	vermilion-ts	Eye color	Third instar to early pupa	Camfield and Suzuki (1973)
34.7	*rdp*	reduplicated	Duplication of legs	Larval	Hoge (1915)
35.4	*l(1)E12*^{ts}	lethal E12-ts	Lethality	All developmental stages	Tarasoff and Suzuki (1970)
37.1	*l(1)TW-6*^{ts}	lethal TW6-ts	Lethality	Embryo	Wright (1974)
57.4	*shi*^{ts}	shibire-ts	Lethality; paralysis; eye, leg, bristle, wing and leg defects	Egg, larva, pupa, adults	Poodry et al. (1973)
53.9	*para*^{ts}	paralytic-ts	Adult paralysis	Instant in adults	Suzuki et al. (1971)
57.0	*B*	Bar	Reduced eye facet number	Early third instar	Krafka (1920), Driver (1931)
59.5	*fu*	fused	Incidence of ovarian tumors	Time of cystocyte divisions	Smith and King (1966)
64.0	*sw*	shortwing	Lethality; eye, wing defects	Third instar	Eker (1935)

TABLE 1. Continued

Genetic position	Symbol	Name	Thermophene	Temperature-sensitive period	Reference
64.0	stn^{ts}	stoned-ts	Adult paralysis	Pupa, instant in adults	Grigliatti et al. (1973)
65.9	$l(1)su$-f^{ts67g}	suppressor-of-forked-ts67g	Lethality, suppressor of forked	Second to third instar	Dudick et al. (1974)
Unknown	tu-h	tumorous-head	Abnormal head structures	8- to 24-hr embryo	Gardner and Woolf (1950), Gardner et al. (1960)
CHROMOSOME 2					
5±	$fs(2)B$	female sterile (2) B	Frequency of nurselike cells in ovarian tumors	Time of cystocyte divisions	King et al. (1961)
13.0	dp	dumpy	Wing and thoracic defects in $dp/+$	8- to 10-hr pupa (vortex), 12 to 16-hr pupa (truncate)	Blanc and Child (1940)
15.0±	$l(2)l^{DTS}$	Dominant-ts-lethal	Dominant lethality	18- to 24-hr embryo	Suzuki and Procunier (1969)
15.0±	$l(2)l^{DCS}$	Dominant cold-sensitive lethal	Dominant lethality	18- to 24-hr embryo	Rosenbluth et al. (1972)
27.0	L^D	Lobe-duplicating	Eye reduction, antennal duplication	Embryo, second instar	Zimm (1951)
50.1	Adh^{n5}	Alcohol dehydrogenase null-5	Loss of ADH	Adults	Vigue and Sofer (1974)
55.1	rl	rolled	Eye reduction	Second to third instar	Hackman and Lackovaara (1966)

63.3	*spt*	spermatheca	Spermathecal duplication	Third instar	Hadorn and Graber (1944)
67.0	vg^1	vestigial-1	Wing reduction	Larval	Stanley (1931, 1935)
	vg^{nu}	vestigial-notch	Wing reduction	3–5 days (hot), 4–5 days (cold)	Akita and Nakayama (1956)
	vg^P	vestigial-pennant	Wing reduction	Larva	Harnly and Harnly (1936)
70.8	*Pfd*	Pufdi	Wings spread	6–8 hr before eclosion	Baker (1950)
74.0	*scrp*	scarp	Eye small and rough	Mid-third instar	Hansen and Gardner (1962)
In(2L + 2R)	*Cy*	Curly	Wing curled	Just after eclosion	Stern (1927)
Unknown	*ant*	antennaless	Antennae missing	Third instar	Vogt (1947b)
Unknown	*Fs(2)D*	Female sterile (2) dominant	Dominant lethality; wing defects, attachment of ovaries to oviducts, cystocyte divisions	—	Yarger and King (1971)

CHROMOSOME 3

24.5	$l(3)4^{DTS}$	Dominant-ts-lethal-4	Lethality	Egg to pupa	Holden and Suzuki (1973)
33.4	$l(3)2^{DTS}$	Dominant-ts-lethal-2	Lethality	Late third instar to early pupa	Holden and Suzuki (1973)
40.7	*D*	Dichaete	45 degree wing angle	Second instar to pupa	Plunkett (1926)
42.3	$l(3)7^{DTS}$	Dominant-ts-lethal-7	Lethality	Late third instar to mid pupa	Holden and Suzuki (1973)
44.3	$l(3)5^{DTS}$	Dominant-ts-lethal-5	Lethality	Late third instar to early pupa	Holden and Suzuki (1973)

TABLE 1. Continued

Genetic position	Symbol	Name	Thermophene	Temperature-sensitive period	Reference
44–48	$l(3)6^{DTS}$	Dominant-ts-lethal-6	Lethality	Late second instar to mid-third instar	Holden and Suzuki (1973)
46.0	mot-28	mottled-28	Dark eye (below 20°C), no pigment (above 25°C)	25- to 35-hr pupa	Surrarer (1935)
47.5	Dfd^{rh}	Deformed recessive of Lüers	Eye reduced, antennae duplicated	Early first instar, late second instar	Vogt (1947a)
47.7	pb	proboscipedia	Oral lobes become tarsi (29°C) or aristae (15°C)	3- to 4 day larva (arista), 4- to 6-day larva (tarsus)	Villee (1944)
48.1	cvl	crossveinless-like	Absence of posterior crossvein	Early pupa	Thompson (1967)
48.5	tet	tetraltera	Wings become haltere-like	Larva	Villee (1942)
51.6	Spl^{ts}	Splayed-ts	Lethal, twisted legs	Embryo	Tasaka and Suzuki (1973)
52.0	ry^2	rosy-2	Lethality, eye-color defect	Late pupa	Schwink (1961, 1962)
55.0	$l(3)8^{DTS}$	Dominant-ts-lethal-8	Lethality	Between embryo and second instar	Holden and Suzuki (1973)
58.5	ss^{a40a}	spineless aristapedia-a40a	Arista change to tarsus	Mid-third instar	Grigliatti and Suzuki (1971)
	ss^{aB}	spineless[a] of Bridges	Arista change to tarsus	Mid-third instar	Villee (1942, 1943b)
	ss^{aF}	spineless[a] of Finck	Arista change to tarsus	Mid-third instar	Finck (1942), Vogt (1946a)

58.8	bx^{34e}	bithorax-34e	Anterior metathorax becomes mesothoracic	Second instar	Villee (1945), Kaufman et al. (1973)
78.0	$l(1)1^{DTS}$	Dominant-ts-lethal-1	Lethality	Pupa	Holden and Suzuki (1973)
84.5	$l(1)3^{DTS}$	Dominant-ts-lethal-3	Lethality	Late second to third instar	
102	ld-opht	loboid-ophthalmoptera	Outgrowths in eyes	24- to 60-hr pupa	Ouweneel (1969)
CHROMOSOME 4					
0.0	ci^D	cubitus-interruptus Dominant	Gap in wing vein L4	Early pupa	Scharloo and Nieuwenhijs (1963)
1.4	bt	bent	Wings held out and bent	Third instar to early pupa	Metz (1923)
2.0	ey^2	eyeless-2	Eye reduced	Egg to first instar	Baron (1935)

Ts alleles of known loci have been recovered. Thus, Wright (1968) detected 3 ts alleles of the lethal-myospheroid [*l(1)mys*] locus among 1500 mutagenized chromosomes. Other ts alleles have been recovered at Notch (*N*) (Shellenbarger, 1971), vermilion (*v*) (Camfield and Suzuki, 1972, 1973), raspberry (*ras*) (Grigliatti and Suzuki, 1970), fertility loci on the Y chromosome (Ayles *et al.*, 1973), bobbed (*bb*) (Williamson *et al.*, 1973), Alcohol-dehydrogenase (*Adh*) (Vigue and Sofer, 1974), suppressor of forked [*l(1)su-f*] (Dudick *et al.*, 1974), Minute (*M*) (Holden and Suzuki, 1973), Splayed (*Spl*) (Tasaka and Suzuki, 1973), and wings held out (Grigliatti, 1973), which was later found to be an allele of the *fused* [see Smith and King (1966) for description of this mutant].

Several laboratories have been screening for mutations with specific defects which are temperature sensitive. Thus, ts mutations of vision (Deland and Pak, 1973), movement (Suzuki *et al.*, 1971; Grigliatti *et al.*, 1973), cell lethality (Russell and Clark, 1973), and imaginal discs (Shearn *et al.*, 1971) have been detected.

The utility of conditional mutant expression is most strikingly exhibited in developmental studies. By applying restrictive temperatures at specific developmental stages for known periods, mutant expression can be rigidly controlled (Tarasoff and Suzuki, 1970). The most striking example of the usefulness of temperature sensitivity is shown by studies of ts mutants of the shibire (*shi*) locus (Poodry *et al.*, 1973). Flies carrying the shi^{ts} alleles exhibit multiple lethal and visible thermophenes, each with specific temperature-sensitive periods (Poodry *et al.*, 1973) as well as ts electroretinogram patterns (Kelly and Suzuki, 1974), which reflect a basic neurological defect (Kelly, 1974). A non-ts allele of *shi* would undoubtedly have been scored as an embryonic lethal with no clue as to its primary defect.

Although the missense basis for ts mutations in *Drosophila* awaits confirmation (Fristrom, 1970), the missense basis for most EMS-induced mutations in phages (Krieg, 1963) and the gene product *in vitro* (Vigue and Sofer, 1974) suggests that most ts mutations in *Drosophila* will have the same molecular basis as in microorganisms. Regardless of the ultimate molecular basis, the ability to regulate mutant expression by temperature extends the analytical resolution for problems of *Drosophila* biology.

Literature Cited

Akita, Y. and T. Nakayama, 1956   The effect of temperature on the expression of *vestigial-notched* in *Drosophila melanogaster* with special reference to the temperature-sensitive period. *Jap. J. Zool.* **11**:297–309.

Astaurov, B. L., 1930 Analyse der erblichen Störungsfälle der bilateralen Symmetrie in Zusammenhang mit der selbständigen Variablilität ähnlicher Strukturen. *Z. Indukt. Abstammungs.- Vererbugsl.* **55**:183–262.

Ayles, B., T. Sanders, B. Kiefer and D. T. Suzuki, 1973 Temperature-sensitive mutations in *Drosophila melanogaster*. XI. Male sterile mutants of the Y chromosome. *Dev. Biol.* **32**:239–257.

Baillie, D., D. T. Suzuki and M. Tarasoff, 1968 Temperature-sensitive mutations in *Drosophila melanogaster*. II. Frequency among second chromosome recessive lethals induced by ethyl methanesulfonate. *Can. J. Genet. Cytol.* **10**:412–420.

Baker, P. H., 1950 The relationships between temperature, rate of development and expression of the *Pufdi* gene in *Drosophila melanogaster*. *Amr. Nat.* **84**:57–70.

Baron, A., 1935 Facet number in *Drosophila melanogaster* as influenced by certain genetic and environmental factors. *J. Exp. Zool.* **70**:461–490.

Baur, E., 1911 *Einfuhrung in die experimentelle Vererbungslehre*; Gebrüder Borntraeger, Berlin.

Blanc, R. and G. P. Child, 1940 Somatic effects of temperature and development in *Drosophila melanogaster*. II. Temperature-effective period of truncate. *Physiol. Zool.* **13**:65–72.

Camfield, R. G. and D. T. Suzuki, 1972 A temperature-sensitive *vermilion* mutant (v^{ts}) in *Drosophila melanogaster*. *Can. J. Genet. Cytol.* **14**:722.

Camfield, R. G. and D. T. Suzuki, 1973 A temperature-sensitive *vermilion* mutant (v^{ts}) in *Drosophila melanogaster*. *Genetics* **74**:s36.

Child, G., 1935 Phenogenetic studies on *scute-1* of *Drosophila melanogaster*. II. The temperature-effective period. *Genetics* **20**:127–155.

Deland, M. C. and W. L. Pak, 1973 Reversibly temperature-sensitive phototransduction mutant of *Drosophila melanogaster*. *Nat. New Biol.* **244**:184–186.

Doncaster, L. 1903 Experiments in hybridization with especial reference to the effect of conditions on dominance. *Phil. Trans.* **196**:119–173.

Driver, E. C., 1931 Temperature and gene expression in *Drosophila*. *J. Exp. Zool.* **59**:1–28.

Dudick, M. E., T. R. F. Wright and L. L. Brothers, 1974 The developmental genetics of the temperature-sensitive lethal allele of the *suppressor of forked, l(1)su(f)^{ts67g}*, in *Drosophila melanogaster*. *Genetics* **76**:487–510.

Edgar, R. S. and R. H. Epstein, 1965 Conditional lethal mutations in bacteriophage T4. *Proc. XI Interntl. Congr. Genet.* **2**:1–16.

Edgar, R. S. and I. Lielausis, 1964 Temperature-sensitive mutations in T4D: Their isolation and genetic characterization. *Genetics* **49**:649–662.

Eker, R., 1935 The *short-wing* gene in *Drosophila melanogaster*, and the effect of temperature, on its manifestation. *J. Genet.* **30**:357–368.

Ephrussi, B. and J. H. Herold, 1945 Studies of eye pigments of *Drosophila*. II. Effect of temperature on the red and brown pigments in the mutant, *blood* (w^{bl}). *Genetics* **30**:62–70.

Epstein, R. H., A. Bolle, C. M. Steinberg, E. Kellenberger, E. Boy de la Tour, R. Chevalley, R. S. Edgar, M. Sussman, G. Denhardt and A. Lielausis, 1963 Physiological studies of conditional lethal mutations of bacteriophage T4D. *Cold Spring Harbor Symp. Quant. Biol.* **28**:375–392.

Fattig, W. D. and W. L. Rickoll, 1972 Isolation of recessive third chromosome temperature-sensitive mutants in *Drosophila melanogaster*. *Genetics* **71**:309–313.

Finck, E., 1942   Die Allelensrie des Gens *ss* ("*spineless*") bei *Drosophila melanogaster.* *Biol. Zentralbl.* **62**:379–400.

Foster, G. G. and D. T. Suzuki, 1970   Temperature-sensitive mutations in *Drosophila melanogaster.* IV. A mutation affecting eye facet arrangement in a polarized manner. *Proc. Natl. Acad. Sci. USA* **67**:738–745.

Fristrom, D., 1970   The developmental biology of Drosophila. *Annu. Rev. Genet.* **4**:325–346.

Gardner, E. J. and C. M. Woolf, 1950   The influence of high and low temperatures on the expression of *tumorous head* in *Drosophila melanogaster.* *Genetics* **35**:44–75.

Gardner, E. J., J. H. Turner and W. D. Berseth, 1960   Maternal effect transferred by injection and further analysis of temperature-effective period for *tumorous head* in *Drosophila melanogaster.* *Genetics* **45**:905–913.

Grigliatti, T. A., 1973   A temperature-sensitive wing mutation in *Drosophila melanogaster.* *Genetics* **74s**:101–102.

Grigliatti, T. and D. T. Suzuki, 1970   Temperature-sensitive mutations in *Drosophila melanogaster.* V. A mutation affecting concentrations of pteridines. *Proc. Natl. Acad. Sci. USA* **67**:1101–1108.

Grigliatti, T. and D. T. Suzuki, 1971   Temperature-sensitive mutations in *Drosophila melanogaster.* VIII. The homeotic mutant, ss^{a40a}. *Proc. Natl. Acad. Sci. USA* **68**:1307–1311.

Grigliatti, T., L. Hall, R. Rosenbluth and D. T. Suzuki, 1973   Temperature-sensitive mutations in *Drosophila melanogaster.* XIV. A selection of immobile adults. *Mol. Gen. Genet.* **120**:107–114.

Guthrie, C., H. Nashimoto and M. Nomura, 1969   Structure and function of *E. coli* ribosomes. VIII. Cold-sensitive mutants defective in ribosome assembly. *Proc. Natl. Acad. Sci. USA* **63**:384–391.

Hackman, R. and S. Lakovaara, 1966   The temperature-sensitive period of ommatidium determination in *rolled* mutants of *D. melanogaster.* *Drosophila Inf. Serv.* **41**:92.

Hadorn, E., 1955   *Developmental Genetics and Lethal Factors,* John Wiley & Sons, New York.

Hadorn, E. and H. Garber, 1944   Über einen Drosophila-Stamm mit veränderten Spermatheken. *Rev. Suisse Zool.* **51**:418–423.

Hansen, A. M. and .E. J. Gardner, 1962   A new eye phenotype in *Drosophila melanogaster* expressed only at temperatures above 25°C. *Genetics* **47**:587–598.

Harnly, M. H. and M. L. Harnly, 1936   The effects of the gene on growth and differentiation as shown by the temperature responses of *pennant* and its heterozygotes in *D. melanogaster.* *J. Exp. Zool.* **74**:41–59.

Hartwell, L. H., 1967   Macromolecule synthesis in temperature sensitive mutants of yeast. *J. Bacteriol.* **93**:1662–1670.

Hersh, A. H., 1930   The need for and the proposal of a new genetic term. *Science (Wash., D.C.)* **72**:294–295.

Hillman, R., 1956   Temperature-sensitive periods for the production of abnormal heads by *Notch-deformed.* *Genetics* **41**:647.

Hillman, R., 1962   A genetically controlled head abnormality in *Drosophila melanogaster.* II. Temperature-sensitive periods during the development of *Notch-deformed.* *Genetics* **47**:11–23.

Hoge, M. A., 1915   The influence of temperature on the development of a Mendelian character. *J. Exp. Zool.* **18**:241–297.

Holden, J. and D. T. Suzuki, 1973   Temperature-sensitive mutations in *Drosophila melanogaster*. XII. The genetic and developmental characteristics of dominant lethals on chromosome 3. *Genetics* **73**:445–458.

Horowitz, N. H., 1950   Biochemical genetics of *Neurospora*. *Adv. Genet.* **3**:33–71.

House, V. L., 1959   A comparison of gene expression at the *Hairless* and *Abruptex* loci in *Drosophila melanogaster*. *Anat. Rec.* **134**:581–582.

Hubbs, C. L., 1922   Variations in the number of vertebrae and other meristic characters of fishes correlated with temperature of water during development. *Am. Nat.* **56**:360–372.

Hyde, R. R., 1922   An *eyeless* mutant in *Drosophila hydei*. *Genetics* **7**:319–334.

Igarashi, S., 1966   Temperature-sensitive mutation in *Paramecium*. I. Induction and inheritance. *Mutat. Res.* **3**:13–24.

Jockusch, H., 1966   Relations between temperature-sensitivity, amino acid replacements and quaternary structure of mutant proteins. *Biochem. Biophys. Res. Commun.* **24**:577–583.

Johnson, R., 1910   *Evolution in the Color Pattern of Lady Beetles*, Carnegie Institution of Washington Publication 122, Carnegie Institution of Washington, Washington, D.C.

Jordan, D. S., 1921   Latitude and vertebrae. *Science N.S.* **54**:490–491.

Kaufman, T. C. and D. T. Suzuki, 1974   Temperature-sensitive mutations in *Drosophila melanogaster*. XX. Lethality due to translocations. *Can. J. Genet. Cytol.* **16**:579–592.

Kaufman, T. C., S. E. Tasaka and D. T. Suzuki, 1973   The interaction of two complex loci, *zeste* and *bithorax* in *Drosophila melanogaster*. *Genetics* **75**:299–321.

Kelly, L. E. 1974   Temperature-sensitive mutations affecting the regenerative sodium channel in *Drosophila melanogaster*. *Nature (Lond.)* **248**:166–168.

Kelly, L. E. and D. T. Suzuki, 1974   The effects of increased temperature on electroretinograms of temperature-sensitive paralysis mutants of *Drosophila melanogaster*. *Proc. Natl. Acad. Sci. USA* **71**:4906–4909.

King, R. C., E. A. Koch and G. A. Cassens, 1961   The effect of temperature upon the hereditary ovarian tumors of the *fes* mutant of *Drosophila melanogaster*. *Growth* **25**:45–65.

Komai, T., 1926   *Crippled*, a new mutant character of *Drosophila melanogaster*, and its inheritance. *Genetics* **11**:280–293.

Krafka, J., 1920   The effect of temperature upon facet number in the *Bar*-eyed mutant of *Drosophila*. *J. Gen. Physiol.* **2**: Part I, 409–432; Part II, 433–444; Part III, 445–464.

Krieg, D. R., 1963   Ethyl methanesulfonate-induced reversion of bacteriophage T4 *rII* mutants. *Genetics* **48**:561–580.

Langridge, J., 1965   Temperature-sensitive, vitamin-requiring mutants of *Arabidopsis thaliana*. *Aust. J. Biol. Sci.* **18**:311–321.

Lindsley, D. L. and E. H. Grell, 1968   *Genetic Variations of Drosophila melanogaster*. Carnegie Institution of Washington Publication 627, Carnegie Institution, Washington, D.C.

Loomis, W. F., 1969   Temperature-sensitive mutants of *Dictyostelium discoideum*. *J. Bacteriol.* **99**:65–69.

McDonald, I. C. and D. E. Overland, 1972   Temperature-sensitive mutations in the housefly: The characterization of heat-sensitive recessive lethal factors on autosome III. *J. Econ. Entomol.* **65**:1364–1368.

Mayoh, H. and D. T. Suzuki, 1973 Temperature-sensitive mutations in *Drosophila melanogaster*. XVI. The genetic properties of sex-linked recessive cold-sensitive mutants. *Can. J. Genet. Cytol.* **15**:237–254.

Merrifield, F., 1891 Conspicuous effects upon the markings and colorings of Lepidoptera caused by exposure of pupae to different temperature conditions. *Trans. Entomol. Soc. Lond.* **39**:155–168.

Merrifield, F., 1893 The effects of temperature in the pupal stage on the colouring of *Pieris napi, Vanessa atalanta, Chrysophanus phloeas,* and *Ephrya punctaria. Trans. Entomol. Soc. Lond.* **41**:55–67.

Metz, C. W., 1923 A note on the effect of temperature on the mutant character '*bent*' in *Drosophila virilis* and *Drosophila melanogaster. Soc. Exp. Biol. Med.* **20**:305–310.

Milani, R., 1946 Ricerche sulla expressività e la penetranza dei diversi gradi di questa nel ceppo *so* in funzione della temperatura. *Boll. Soc. Ital. Biol. Sper.* **22**:112–113.

Ouweneel, W. J., 1969 Influence of environmental factors on the homoeotic effect of *loboid-ophthalmoptera* in *Drosophila melanogaster. Wilhelm Roux' Arch. Entwicklungsmech. Org.* **164**:15–36.

Parkash, O., 1967 On the so-called conditioned (incomplete) and absolute lethals in *D. melanogaster. Drosophila. Inf. Serv.* **42**:109.

Plunkett, C. R., 1926 The interaction of genetic and environmental factors in development. *J. Exp. Zool.* **46**:181–244.

Poodry, D., L. Hall and D. T. Suzuki, 1973 Developmental properties of *shibire^{ts1}*, a pleiotropic mutation producing larval and adult paralysis. *Dev. Biol.* **32**:373–386.

Pratt, R. L., 1971 Developmental and genetic analysis of a purported new class of sex-linked mutations in *Drosophila melanogaster*. M. Sc. Thesis, University of British Columbia, Vancouver, B.C.

Roberts, E., 1918 Fluctuations in a recessive Mendelian character and selection. *J. Exp. Zool.* **27**:157–192.

Rosenbluth, R., D. Ezell and D. T. Suzuki, 1972 Temperature-sensitive mutations in *Drosophila melanogaster*. IX. Dominant cold-sensitive lethals on the autosomes. *Genetics* **70**:75–86.

Russell, M. A. and W. C. Clark, 1973 Experimental investigation of progressive restriction in developmental capacity of Drosophila imaginal discs. *Genetics* **74**:s236–237.

Scharloo, W. and A. M. Nieuwenhijs, 1963 Temperature-sensitive periods of *cubitus interruptus* mutants in *Drosophila melanogaster. Genetica (The Hague)* **35**:15–27.

Schultz, W., 1915 Schwarzfärbung weisser Haare. *Arch. Entwicklungsmech.* **41**:535–537.

Schwartz, D., 1958 A new temperature-sensitive allele at the *sticky* locus in maize. *J. Hered.* **49**:149–152.

Schwink, I., 1961 Quantitative studies on the temperature dependence of drosopterin formation and of semilethality in the mutant *rosy* of *Drosophila melanogaster. Genetics* **46**:896–897.

Schwink, I., 1962 Drosopterin formation and semi-lethality of the mutant *rosy* in temperature experiments. *Drosophila Inf. Serv.* **36**:114–115.

Seyster, E. W., 1919 Eye facet number as influenced by temperature in the *Bar*-eyed mutant of *Drosophila melanogaster* (Ampelophila). *Biol. Bull.* **37**:168–182.

Shearn, A., T. Rice, A. Garen and W. Gehring, 1971 Imaginal disc abnormalities in lethal mutants of *Drosophila. Proc. Natl. Acad. Sci. USA* **68**:2594–2598.

Shelford, V. E., 1917 Color and color-pattern mechanism of tiger beetles. *Illinois Biol. Monogr.* **3**:1–135.

Shellenbarger, D. L., 1971   A temperature-sensitive *Notch* mutant of *Drosophila melanogaster. Genetics* **68**:561–566.

Smith, P. A. and R. C. King, 1966   Studies on *fused*, a mutant gene producing ovarian tumors in *Drosophila melanogaster. J. Natl. Cancer Inst.* **36**:445–463.

Smith, R. H., 1968   Unstable temperature-sensitive mutations in *Habrobracon. Genetics* **60**:227.

Stanley, W. F., 1931   The effect of temperature on *vestigial* wing in *Drosophila melanogaster,* with temperature-effective periods. *Physiol. Zool.* **4**:394–408.

Stanley, W. F., 1935   The effect of temperature upon wing size in *Drosophila. J. Exp. Zool.* **69**:459–495.

Stern, C., 1927   Der Einfluss der Temperatur auf die Ausbildung einer Flügelmutation bei Drosophila. *Biol. Zentralbl* **47**:361–369.

Sumner, F. B., 1911   Some effects of temperature upon growing mice and the persistence of such effects in a subsequent generation. *Am. Nat.* **45**:90–98.

Surrarrer, T. C., 1935   The effect of temperature on a mottled-eyed stock of *Drosophila melanogaster. Genetics* **20**:357–362.

Surrarrer, T. C., 1938   On the inheritance and expression of a mottle-eyed mutant in *Drosophila melanogaster. Genetics* **23**:631–646.

Suzuki, D. T., 1970   Temperature-sensitive mutations in *Drosophila melanogaster. Science (Wash., D.C.)* **170**:695–706.

Suzuki, D. T. and D. Procunier, 1969   Temperature-sensitive mutations in *Drosophila melanogaster.* III. Dominant lethals and semilethals on chromosome 2. *Proc. Natl. Acad. Sci. USA* **62**:369–376.

Suzuki, D. T., L. Piternick, S. Hayashi, M. Tarasoff, D. Baillie and U. Erasmus, 1967   Temperature-sensitive mutations in *Drosophila melanogaster.* I. Relative frequencies among γ-ray and chemically induced sex-linked recessive lethals and semilethals. *Proc. Natl. Acad. Sci. USA* **57**:907–912.

Suzuki, D. T., T. Grigliatti and R. Williamson, 1971   Temperature-sensitive mutations in *Drosophila melanogaster.* VII. A mutation (*para^{ts}*) causing reversible adult paralysis. *Proc. Natl. Acad. Sci. USA* **68**:890–893.

Tarasoff, M. and D. T. Suzuki, 1970   Temperature-sensitive mutations in *Drosophila melanogaster.* VI. Temperature effects on development of sex-linked recessive lethals. *Dev. Biol.* **23**:492–509.

Tasaka, S. E. and D. T. Suzuki, 1973   Temperature-sensitive mutations in *Drosophila melanogaster.* XVII. The genetic properties of heat- and cold-sensitive lethals on chromosome 3. *Genetics* **74**:509–520.

Thompson, L. H., R. Mankovitz, R. M. Baker, J. E. Till, L. Siminovitch and G. F. Whitmore, 1970   Isolation of temperature-sensitive mutants of L-cells. *Proc. Natl. Acad. Sci. USA* **66**:377–384.

Thompson, S. R., 1967   The effect of temperature on crossvein formation in *crossveinless-like* strains of *Drosophila melanogaster. Genetics* **56**:13–22.

Tower, W. L., 1910   The determination of dominance and the modification of behavior in alternative (Mendelian) inheritance by conditions surrounding or incident upon the germ cells at fertilization. *Biol. Bull.* **18**:285–352.

Vernon, H. M., 1898   The relations between the hybrid and paternal forms of echinoid larvae. *Proc. R. Soc. Lond.* **63**:228–231.

Vigue, C. and W. Sofer, 1974   *Adh^{N5}*: A temperature-sensitive mutant at the *Adh* locus. *Biochem. Genet.* **11**:387–396.

Villee, C. A., 1942   The phenomenon of homoeosis. *Am. Nat.* **26**:494–506.

Villee, C. A., 1943*a*   Phenogenetic studies of the *aristapedia* alleles of *Drosophila melanogaster*. *Genetics* **28**:94.

Villee, C. A., 1943*b*   Phenogenetic studies of the homoeotic mutants of *Drosophila melanogaster*. I. The effects of temperature on the expression of *aristapedia*. *J. Exp. Zool.* **93**:75–98.

Villee, C. A., 1944   Phenogenetic studies on the homoeotic mutants of *Drosophila melanogaster*. II. The effects of temperature on the expression of *proboscipedia*. *J. Exp. Zool.* **96**:85–102.

Villee, C. A., 1945   Phenogenetic studies of the homoeotic mutants of *Drosophila melanogaster*. III. The effects of temperature on the expression of *bithorax-34e*. *Am. Nat.* **79**:246–258.

Vogt, M., 1946*a*   Zur labilen Determination der Imaginalscheiben von *Drosophila*. I. Verhalten verschieden altriger Imaginalanagen bei operativer Defektsetzung. *Biol. Zentralbl.* **65**:223–238.

Vogt, M., 1946*b*   Zur labilen Determination der Imaginalscheiben von *Drosophila*. II. Die Umwandlung prasumptiven Fühlergewebes in Beingewebe. *Biol. Zentralbl.* **65**:238–254.

Vogt, M., 1947*a*   Zur labilen Determination der Imaginalscheiben von *Drosophila*. III. Analyse der Manifestierungsbedingungen sowie der Wirkungsweise der zu Antennen und Palpusverdoppelungen führenden Genmutation *Deformed-recessive-Lüers* (*Dfd*^*r-L*). *Biol. Zentralbl.* **66**:81–105.

Vogt, M., 1947*b*   Zur labilen Determination der Imaginalscheiben von *Drosophila* V. Zur Manifestierung der Mutante *antennaless*. *Biol. Zentralbl.* **66**:388–395.

Whiting, P. W., 1932   Mutants in *Habrobracon*. *Genetics* **17**:1–30.

Williamson, J. H., J. D. Procunier and R. B. Church, 1973   Does the rDNA in the Y chromosome of *Drosophila melanogaster* amplify? *Nat. New Biol.* **243**:190–191.

Wittmann, H. G., and B. Wittmann-Liebold, 1966   Protein chemical studies of two RNA viruses and their mutants. *Cold Spring Harbor Symp. Quant. Biol.* **31**:163–172.

Wright, T. R. F., 1968   The phenogenetics of temperature-sensitive alleles of *lethal myospheroid* in *Drosophila*. *Proc. XII Interntl. Congr. Genet.* **1**:141.

Wright, T. R. F., 1973   The recovery, penetrance and pleiotropy of X-linked cold-sensitive mutants in *Drosophila*. *Mol. Gen. Genet.* **122**:101–118.

Wright, T. R. F., 1974   A cold-sensitive zygotic lethal causing high frequencies of non-disjunction during meiosis I in *Drosophila melanogaster* females. *Genetics*: **76**:511–536.

Yarger, R. J. and R. C. King, 1971   The phenogenetics of a temperature-sensitive, autosomal dominant, female sterile gene in *Drosophila melanogaster*. *Dev. Biol.* **24**:166–177.

Zimm, G. G., 1951   An analysis of growth abnormalities associated with the eye mutant *Lobe* in *Drosophila melanogaster*. *J. Exp. Zool.* **116**:289–319.

24

Biochemical Mutations in *Drosophila melanogaster*

STEPHEN J. O'BRIEN

The vinegar fly, *Drosophila melanogaster* has been an experimental favorite of genetic research since the origin of the field. The immediate advantages of *Drosophila* for the study of eukaryote genetics include a short life cycle, high fecundity, low chromosome number, a restriction of crossing over in males, and the giant polytene chromosomes of the salivary gland. The catalog of over 3000 mutant-gene descriptions, from Abnormal abdomen (*A*) to Zwischenferment (*Zw*) (Lindsley and Grell, 1968), is unrivalled in the literature on the genetics of eukaryotes. Until recently, the genes described have been limited to those whose mutant alleles affected gross morphological phenotypes or viability. The advent of molecular biology marked the conceptual reorganization of genetics as well as the development of numerous biochemical techniques which could be applied to *Drosophila* gene examination.

There are at this writing over 40 gene loci described in *Drosophila* which affect the appearance of a biochemically measurable gene product, either proteins or nucleic acids (Table 1). The first *Drosophila* gene whose product was identified was vermilion eye color (*v*), which specifies the enzyme tryptophan pyrrolase (Baglioni, 1959, 1960; Kaufman, 1962). The biochemical function of this gene was suggested much earlier by Beadle and Ephrussi (1937).

STEPHEN J. O'BRIEN—Viral Biology Branch, National Cancer Institute, National Institutes of Health, Bethesda, Maryland.

TABLE 1. Biochemical Loci of D. melanogaster[a]

Gene symbol	Locus	Protein or nucleic acid affected[b]	Reference
cin	1–0.0	Xanthine dehydrogenase	Baker (1973)
su(s)	1–0	Tyrosyl; histidyl-, asparginyl-, and aspartyl-tRNA	Twardzik et al. (1969), White et al. (1973)
Pgd	1–0.64	6-Phosphogluconate dehydrogenase*	Young (1966), Gvozdev et al. (1970)
Fumarase	1–19.9	Fumarase*	Madhavan and Ursprung (1973)
su(r)	1–27.7	Dihydrouracil dehydrogenase	Bahn (1972)
lz	1–27.7	Phenol oxidase complex	Peeples et al. (1968, 1969)
v	1–33.0	Tryptophan pyrrolase	Baglioni (1959, 1960), Kaufman (1962), Tartoff (1969)
Had	1–54.4	Hydroxy acid dehydrogenase*	E. H. Grell (private communication)
r	1–55.3	Aspartate carbamyltransferase	Norby (1973)
Zw	1–63	Glucose-6-phosphate dehydrogenase*	Young et al. (1964)
ma-l	1–64.8	Xanthine dehydrogenase, uricase, pyridoxal oxidase, aldehyde oxidase, phenol oxidase	Grell (1962), Glassman (1965), Friedman (1973)
bb	1–67.7	Ribosomal RNA	Ritossa et al. (1966)
Pgk	2–7.7[c]	Phosphoglycerate kinase*	Chew and Cooper (1973)
Got-2	2–3.0	Glutamate oxaloacetate transaminase*	Grell (1973)

[a] The genes in this table are only those genes with mutant alleles which specifically affect a biochemically measurable macromolecule.

[b] There is no intended implication that any locus is or is not the structural gene for the molecular species listed. "Probable" structural genes mapped by electrophoretic allozymes are indicated with an asterisk (*).

[c] These loci are listed as cytological positions because they were localized by in situ hybridization to polytene chromosome. No map unit position is available.

[d] These loci are listed as cytological regions at which the enzyme activity exhibited gene-dosage dependency.

[e] Locus recalculated from published data.

TABLE 1. Continued

Gene symbol	Locus	Protein or nucleic acid affected[b]	Reference
αGpdh-1	2–20.5	α-Glycerophosphate dehydrogenase*	Grell (1967), O'Brien and MacIntyre (1972)
Mdh-1	2–41.2	Malate dehydrogenase*	Grell (1969), O'Brien (1973*b*)
Adh	2–50.1	Alcohol dehydrogenase*	Johnson and Denniston (1964), Grell *et al.* (1965), Ursprung and Leone (1965)
Tyr-1	2–52.4	Tyrosinase=dopa oxidase	Lewis and Lewis (1963)
Histone	2 (39E–40A)[c]	Histone 9S RNA	Pardue *et al.* (1972)
Tyr-2	2–57	Tyrosinase	Lewis and Lewis (1963)
cn	2–57.5	Kynurenine hydroxylase	Ghosh and Forrest (1967)
Hex-3	2–73	Hexokinase*	Madhavan *et al.* (1972)
Amy	2–77.3	Amylase*	Kikkawa (1964), Doane (1967)
αGpo	2 (50C–52E)[3]	Glycerophosphate oxidase	O'Brien and Gethmann (1973)
5sRNA	2 (56EF)[c]	5S RNA	Wimber and Steffensen (1970)
Idh-NADP	3–27.1	NADP-isocitrate dehydrogenase*	Fox (1971)
lxd	3–33.9[e]	Xanthine dehydrogenase pyridoxal oxidase, aldehyde oxidase	Glassman (1965), Keller and Glassman (1964)
To-1	3–33.3	Tetrazolium oxidase*	Franklin and Chew (1971)
Est-6	3–36.8	Esterase-6*	Wright (1963)
Pgm	3–43.4	Phosphoglucomutase*	Hjorth (1970)
Aph	3–46.3	Larval alkaline phosphatase*	Beckman and Johnson (1964*c*), MacIntyre (1966*a*)
ali-est	3–48	Aliesterase*	Ogita (1961)
Est-C	3–49	Esterase-C*	Beckman and Johnson (1964*a*)

TABLE 1. Continued

Gene symbol	Locus	Protein or nucleic acid affected[b]	Reference
AchE-1	3 (87BE)[d]	Acetyl cholinesterase-1	D. Kankel and J. Hall (private communication)
Odh	3–49.2	Octanol dehydrogenase*	Courtright et al. (1966)
ry	3–52.0	Xanthine dehydrogenase*, uricase	Yen and Glassman (1965), Glassman (1965), Friedman (1973)
Mdh-NADP	3–53.1	NADP-malic dehydrogenase	Franklin and Rumball (1971)
Aldox	3–56.6	Aldehyde oxidase	Courtright (1967), Dickinson (1970)
lpo	3–57	Pyridoxal oxidase	Collins and Glassman (1969)
Lap-A	3–98.3	Leucine amino peptidase-A	Beckman and Johnson (1964b)
Lap-D	3–98.3	Leucine amino peptidase-D*	Beckman and Johnson (1964b), Falke and MacIntyre (1966)
Acph-1	3–101.1	Acid phosphatase-1*	MacIntyre (1966b)

The gene products of "mutant" alleles which have permitted recombination mapping have been detected by a number of procedures. A generally successful method has been the detection of electrophoretic-variant proteins isolated from laboratory stocks or natural populations. Gel electrophoresis has been applied both to soluble proteins and to enzymes using, respectively, general protein stains or histochemical detection of enzymes. If electrophoretic variation is genetically controlled, it can be mapped with visible chromosome markers and test crosses, like any other *Drosophila* gene (Wright, 1963). When the electrophoretic variant is the product of an alternative allele of an enzyme locus it is termed an "allozyme" (Prakash *et al.*, 1969). This is in contrast with an "isozyme," which is a multiple form of an enzyme which appears in various tissues or at different developmental times, but does not segregate as an allelic variant (Markert, 1968).

Allozyme variation has been a fruitful source of genetic variation since 30–50 percent of all gene enzyme loci in *D. melanogaster* are polymorphic (O'Brien and MacIntyre, 1969). In those cases where natural variation does not occur, chemical mutagenesis has been used to induce variants [cf. Grell (1973), O'Brien and MacIntyre (1972), and Bell *et al.* (1972)]. The use of ethyl methanesulfonate (EMS) increases mutation frequencies to a reasonable level for biochemical screening, 10^{-2}–10^{-3} (Jenkins, 1967; Lewis and Bacher, 1968). Chemical mutagenesis of allozyme loci has also permitted the induction of "null" mutations, i.e., mutant alleles which lack measurable gene products [see O'Brien (1973*a*) for references].

A second method for identifying genes coding for measurable products is the deduction of the metabolic defect from the nature of a visible mutant phenotype. This has been done for *cn*, *v*, *ry*, and *ma-1*, which are eye-color mutations resulting from aberrations of pteridine metabolism. Similarly, a mutant showing a syndrome characteristic of mutants affecting protein synthesis, bobbed (*bb*), codes for rRNA (Ritossa *et al.*, 1966).

A rapidly developing procedure for studying *Drosophila* biochemical genetics is the use of selective schemes and auxotrophy for producing and characterizing genes. "Null" mutations at the *Adh* (alcohol dehydrogenase) and *ry* (xanthine dehydrogenase) loci do not survive on medium supplemented with alcohol and purines, respectively, while wild-type flies survive on the same medium (Grell *et al.*, 1968; Sofer and Hatkoff, 1972; Finnerty *et al.*, 1970). The molecular defect of the rudimentary locus (*r*) was deduced and later demonstrated to affect pyrimidine anabolism due to the failure of homozygotes to survive on medium which lacks pyrimidines (Norby, 1970, 1973).

The characteristic of nonregulatory genes to exhibit dosage dependency has also been useful in identifying gene loci. The recent availability of Y-autosome translocations with autosomal breakpoints throughout the *Drosophila* genome has permitted the synthesis of segmental aneuploids (duplications and deficiencies) for virtually any region of the autosomes (Lindsley *et al.*, 1972). By examining segmental aneuploids in a stepwise fashion over every area of the autosomes for dosage dependency of certain gene products, one can cytologically localize any dosage-dependent autosomal gene without the necessity of having mutant alleles. This procedure has been successful with at least three enzymes, α-glycerophosphate oxidase (O'Brien and Gethmann, 1973), dopadecarboxylase (R. Hodgetts, private communication), and acetylcholine esterase (D. Kankel and J. Hall, private communication).

The development of nucleic-acid-hybridization procedures has permitted the identification of genes whose RNA products can be isolated. Correlation of nuclear DNA which hybridized with rRNA with increasing doses of the bb locus aided in its implication as the locus for rRNA (Ritossa *et al.,* 1966). A promising technique for identifying loci coding for specific RNA species is based upon a procedure developed in *Xenopus* by Gall and Pardue (1969). The technique involves the *in situ* hybridization of radiolabeled RNA species to salivary gland chromosomes. This procedure, combined with radioautographic development, has revealed the cytological location of the genes for 5S RNA (Wimber and Steffensen, 1970) and histones (Pardue, 1973) in *Drosophila.* In order to observe grains significantly above background, the procedure at this point has been limited to regions which exhibit gene redundancy, Radioiodine labeling of RNA molecules, however, promises to improve the resolution of *in situ* hybridization to the level of single-gene copies (Prensky *et al.,* 1973).

Whether the genes listed in Table 1 can be identified as structural genes or regulatory genes is not immediately apparent. Mutations of either type can cause diminution of a given gene product, so mutant alleles lowering activity alone reveal little about the nature of the defect or the gene. However, certain measurable characteristics of mutant alleles, when considered together, strongly suggest structural gene identity.

Homology of DNA to the RNA product by *in situ* hybridization is conclusive evidence for a cistron for the RNA species. Allozyme variation is often interpreted to involve a missense base substitution in a codon of a structural gene, which causes the insertion of an "incorrect" amino acid. This 'incorrect amino acid does not necessarily affect the reactivity of the enzyme, but it does alter its net charge and electrophoretic mobility. Although no *Drosophila* enzymes have been sequenced, the above explanation has been demonstrated for analogous systems, e.g., human hemaglobin (Perutz and Lehmann, 1968).

Allozyme variation, however, is by no means conclusive evidence for structural-gene identity because there are examples of segregating electrophoretic variants which do not involve amino acid substitution in the protein [see Steele *et al.* (1968)].

In those systems where allelic "null" mutations have been derived from electrophoretic variants, demonstration of inactive enzyme would suggest a mutation in the structural gene rather than in a regulatory component. Such inactive enzyme has been identified as immunologically cross-reacting material (CRM) for *Acph-1* and *ry* (Glassman, 1965; Bell and MacIntyre, 1973), or it has been identified by its interaction with normal subunits in dimeric enzyme systems to produce electrophoretically detectable hybrid enzyme (O'Brien and MacIntyre, 1972). A further criterion for structural-gene identity is the demonstration of dosage dependency of the "null" alleles, which is a characteristic of structural genes in eukaryotes (Grell, 1962; O'Brien and Gethmann, 1973).

One final observation concerning the genes listed in Table 1 is the apparent lack of gene clusters whose products are metabolically related. The only examples of possible clustering are the *r* locus, which has been suggested as the gene for sequential enzymes in pyrimidine synthesis (Norby, 1973), and the *lpo* and *aldox* loci which are related by shared epistasis with *ma-l*, and by participation in purine and pteridine metabolism.

Acknowledgment

I am grateful to Drs. T. Friedman and R. C. Gethmann for their critical reading of this chapter. This work was supported by postdoctoral fellowship No. 5-FOZ-GM-49,633-02 from the National Institute of General Medical Sciences.

Literature Cited

Baglioni, C., 1959 Genetic control of tryptophan peroxidase in *Drosophila melanogaster*. *Nature (Lond.)* **184**:1084–1085.

Baglioni, C., 1960 Genetic control of tryptophan pyrrolase in *Drosophila melanogaster* and *Drosophila virilis*. *Heredity* **15**:87–96.

Bahn, E., 1972 A suppressor locus for the pyrimidine requiring mutant: *rudimentary*. *Drosophila Inf. Serv.* **49**:98.

Baker, B., 1973 The maternal and zygotic control of development by cinnamon, a new mutant in *Drosophila melanogaster*. *Dev. Biol.* **33**:429–440.

Beadle, G. W. and B. Ephrussi, 1937 Development of eye colors in *Drosophila*: Diffusible substances and their interrelation. *Genetics* **22**:76–86.

Beckman, L. and F. M. Johnson, 1964*a* Esterase variations in *Drosophila melanogaster*. *Hereditas (The Hague)* **51**:212–220.

Beckman, L. and F. M. Johnson, 1964*b* Genetic control of aminopeptidases in *Drosophila melanogaster*. *Hereditas (The Hague)* **51**:221–230.

Beckman, L. and F. M. Johnson, 1964*c* Variation in larval alkaline phosphatase controlled by *Aph* alleles in *Drosophila melanogaster*. *Genetics* **49**:829–835.

Bell, J. B. and R. J. MacIntyre, 1973 Characterization of *acid phosphatase* null activity mutants in *Drosophila melanogaster*. *Biochem. Genet.* **10**:

Bell, J. B., R. J. MacIntyre and A. P. Olivieri, 1972 Induction of null-activity mutants for the *acid phosphatase-1* gene in *Drosophila melanogaster*. *Biochem. Genet.* **6**:205–216.

Chew, G. K. and D. W. Cooper, 1973 Phosphoglycerate kinase polymorphism in *Drosophila*. *Biochem. Genet.* **8**:267–269.

Collins, J. F. and E. Glassman, 1969 A third locus (*lpo*) affecting pyridoxal oxidase in *Drosophila melanogaster*. *Genetics* **61**:833–839.

Courtright, J. B., 1967 Polygenic control of aldehyde oxidase in *Drosophila*. *Genetics* **57**:25–39.

Courtright, J. B., R. B. Imberski and H. Ursprung, 1966 The genetic control of alcohol dehydrogenase and octanol dehydrogenase isozymes in *Drosophila*. *Genetics* **54**:1251–1260.

Dickinson, W. J., 1970   The genetics of aldehyde oxidase in *Drosophila melanogaster.* *Genetics* **66**:487–496.

Doane, W. W., 1967   Cytogenetic and biochemical studies of amylase in *Drosophila melanogaster.* *Am. Zool.* **7**:780.

Falke, E. and R. J. MacIntyre, 1966   The genetic localization of a non-specific leucine amino peptidase in *Drosophila melanogaster.* *Drosophila Inf. Serv.* **41**:165–166.

Finnerty, V. G., P. Duck and A. Chovnick, 1970   Studies on genetic organization in higher organisms. II. Complementation and fine structure of the maroon-like locus in *Drosophila melanogaster.* *Proc. Natl. Acad. Sci. USA* **65**:939–946.

Fox, D. J., 1971   The soluble citric acid cycle enzymes of *Drosophila melanogaster.* I. Genetics and ontogeny of NADP-linked is isocitrate dehydrogenase. *Biochem. Genet.* **5**:69–80.

Franklin, I. R. and G. K. Chew, 1971   New mutants. *Drosophila Inf. Serv.* **47**:38.

Franklin, I. R. and W. Rumball, 1971   New mutants. *Drosophila Inf. Serv.* **47**:37.

Friedman, T., 1973   Observation on the regulation of uricase activity during development of *Drosophila melanogaster.* *Biochem. Genet.* **8**:37–45.

Gall, J. G. and M. L. Pardue, 1969   Formation and detection of RNA–DNA hybrid molecules in cytological preparations. *Proc. Natl. Acad. Sci. USA* **63**:378–383.

Ghosh, D. and H. S. Forrest, 1967   Enzymatic studies on the hydroxylation of kynurenine in *Drosophila melanogaster.* *Genetics* **55**:423–431.

Glassman, E., 1965   Genetic regulation of xanthine dehydrogenase in *Drosophila melanogaster.* *Fed. Proc.* **24**:1243–1251.

Grell, E. H., 1962   The dose effect of *ma-1*$^+$ and *ry*$^+$ on xanthine dehydrogenase in *Drosophila melanogaster.* *Z. Vererbungsl.* **93**:371–377.

Grell, E. H., 1967   Electrophoretic variants of alpha-glycerophosphate dehydrogenase in *Drosophila melanogaster.* *Science (Wash., D.C.)* **158**:1319–1320.

Grell, E. H., 1969   *Mdh-2*^{s} and *Mdh2*^{v}: Malate dehydrogenase-2 alleles. *Drosophila Inf. Serv.* **44**:47.

Grell, E. H., 1973   The two glutamate oxaloacetate transaminase genes located using partial hybrids between *Drosophila melanogaster* and *Drosophila simulans.* *Genetics* **74**:100–101.

Grell, E. H., K. B. Jacobsen and J. B. Murphy, 1965   Alcohol dehydrogenase in *Drosophila melanogaster.* *Science (Wash., D.C.)* **149**:80–82.

Grell, E. H., K. B. Jacobsen and J. B. Murphy, 1968   Alterations of genetic material for analysis of alcohol dehydrogenase isozymes of *Drosophila melanogaster.* *Ann. N.Y. Acad. Sci.* **151**:441–455.

Gvozdev, V. A., V. J. Birstein and L. D. Faizullin, 1970   Gene dependent regulation of 6-phosphogluconate dehydrogenase activity in *Drosophila melanogaster.* *Drosophila Inf. Serv.* **45**:163.

Hjorth, J. P., 1970   A phospoglucomutase locus in *Drosophila melanogaster.* *Hereditas* **64**:146–148.

Jenkins, J. B., 1967   Mutagenesis at a complex locus in *Drosophila* with the monofunctional alkylating agent, ethyl methanesulfonate. *Genetics* **57**:783–793.

Johnson, F. M. and C. Denniston, 1964   Genetic variation of alcohol dehydrogenase in *Drosophila melanogaster.* *Nature (Lond.)* **204**:906–907.

Kaufman, S., 1962   Studies on tryptophan pyrrolase in *Drosophila melanogaster.* *Genetics* **47**:807–817.

Keller, E. C., Jr. and E. Glassman, 1964   A third locus (*lxd*) affecting xanthine dehydrogenase in *Drosophila melanogaster.* *Genetics* **49**:663–668.

Kikkawa, H., 1964 An electrophoretic study on amylase in *Drosophila melanogaster.* *Jap. J. Genet.* **39**:401–411.

Lewis, E. and F. Bacher, 1968 Method of feeding ethylmethanesulfonate (EMS) to *Drosophila* males. *Drosophila Inf. Serv.* **43**:193.

Lewis, H. W. and H. S. Lewis, 1963 Genetic regulation of dopa oxidase activity in *Drosophila. Ann. N.Y. Acad. Sci.* **100**:827–839.

Lindsley, D. and E. H. Grell, 1968 *Genetic Variations of Drosophila melanogaster.* Carnegie Institution of Washington Publication 627, Carnegie Institution, Washington, D.C.

Lindsley, D. L., L. Sandler, B. S. Baker, A. Carpenter, R. E. Denell, J. C. Hall, P. A. Jacobs, G. L. G. Miklos, B. K. Davis, R. C. Gethmann, R. W. Hardy, A. Hessler, S. M. Miller, H. Nozawa, D. M. Perry and M. Gould-Somero, 1972 Segmental aneuploidy and the genetic gross structure of the *Drosophila* genome. *Genetics* **71**:157–184.

MacIntyre, R. J., 1966a Locus of the structural gene for third larval instar alkaline phosphatase. (*Aph*) *Drosophila Inf. Serv.* **41**:62.

MacIntyre, R. J., 1966b The genetics of an acid phosphatase in *Drosophila melanogaster* and *Drosophila simulans. Genetics* **53**:461–474.

Madhavan, K. and H. Ursprung, 1973 The genetic control of fumarate hydratase (fumarase) in *Drosophila melanogaster. Mol. Gen. Genet.* **120**:379–380.

Madhavan, K., D. J. Fox and H. Ursprung, 1972 Developmental genetics of hexokinase isozymes in *Drosophila melanogaster. J. Insect Physiol.* **18**:1523–1530.

Markert, C., 1968 Multiple molecular forms of enzymes. Molecular basis for isozymes. *Ann. N.Y. Acad. Sci.* **151**:14–20.

Norby, S., 1970 A specific nutritional requirement for pyrimidines in *rudimentary* mutants of *Drosophila melanogaster. Hereditas* **66**:205–214.

Norby, S., 1973 The biochemical genetics of rudimentary mutants of *Drosophila melanogaster.* I. Aspartate carbamyltransferase levels in complementing and noncomplimentary strains. *Hereditas* **73**:11–16.

O'Brien, S. J., 1973a On estimating functional gene number in eukaryotes. *Nat. New Biol.* **242**:52–54.

O'Brien, S. J., 1973b Comparative analysis of malate dehydrogenases of *Drosophila melanogaster. Biochem. Genet.* **10**:191–205.

O'Brien, S. J., and R. C. Gethmann, 1973 Segmental aneuploidy as a screen for structural genes in *Drosophila*: Mitochondrial membrane enzymes. *Genetics* **75**:155–169.

O'Brien, S. J. and R. J. MacIntyre, 1969 An analysis of gene–enzyme variation in natural populations of *Drosophila melanogaster* and *Drosophila simulans. Am. Nat.* **103**:97–113.

O'Brien, S. J. and R. J. MacIntyre, 1972 The α-glycerophosphate cycle in *Drosophila melanogaster.* II. Genetic aspects. *Genetics* **71**:127–138.

Ogita, Z., 1961 Genetical relationship between ali-esterase activity and insecticide resistance in *Drosophila melanogaster.* Genetical and biochemical studies on negatively correlated cross resistance in *Drosophila melanogaster.* IV. *Botyu-Kagaku (Scientific Insect Control)* **26**:93–97.

Pardue, M. L., E. Weinberg, L. H. Kedes and M. L. Birnstiel, 1972 Localization of sequences coding for histone messenger RNA in the chromosomes of *Drosophila melanogaster. 12th Annual Meeting of The American Society for Cell Biology, Abstract 398,* Rockefeller University Press.

Peeples, E. D., D. R. Barnett and C. P. Oliver, 1968   Phenol oxidases of a *lozenge* mutant of *Drosophila. Science (Wash., D.C.)* **159**:551–552.

Peeples, E. E., A. Geisler, C. Whitcraft and C. P. Oliver, 1969   Activity of phenol oxidases at the puparium formation stage in development of nineteen *lozenge* mutants of *Drosophila melanogaster. Biochem. Genet.* **3**:563–569.

Perutz, M. and H. Lehmann, 1968   Molecular pathology of human haemaglobin. *Nature (Lond.)* **219**:902–909.

Prakash, S., R. C. Lewontin and J. L. Hubby, 1969   A molecular approach to the study of genic heterozygosity in natural populations. IV. Patterns of genic variation in central marginal and isolated populations of *Drosophila pseudoobscura. Genetics* **61**:841–858.

Prensky, W., D. M. Steffensen and W. L. Hughes, 1973   The use of iodinated RNA for gene localization. *Proc. Natl. Acad. Sci. USA* **70**:1860–1864.

Ritossa, F. M., K. C. Atwood and S. Spiegelman, 1966   A molecular explanation of the *bobbed* mutants of *Drosophila* as partial deficiencies of ribosomal DNA. *Genetics* **54**:819–834.

Sofer, W. H. and M. A. Hatkoff, 1972   Chemical selection of alcohol dehydrogenase negative mutants in *Drosophila. Genetics* **72**:545–549.

Steele, M. W., W. J. Young and B. Childs, 1968   Glucose-6-phosphate dehydrogenase in *Drosophila melanogaster*: Starch gel electrophoretic variation due to molecular instability. *Biochem. Genet.* **2**:159–175.

Tartoff, K. D., 1969   Interacting gene systems. I. The regulation of tryptophan pyrrolase by the vermilion-suppressor of vermilion system in *Drosophila. Genetics* **62**:781–795.

Twardzik, D. R., E. H. Grell and K. B. Jacobsen, 1969   Genetic control of iso-accepting forms of tyrosyl-tRNA in a suppressor of *Drosophila melanogaster. Genetics* **61**:s59.

Ursprung, H. and J. Leone, 1965   Alcohol dehydrogenases: A polymorphism in *Drosophila melanogaster. J. Exp. Zool.* **160**:147–154.

White, B. N., G. M. Tener, J. Holden and D. T. Suzuki, 1973   Activity of a transfer RNA modifying enzyme during the development of *Drosophila* and its relationship to the *su(s)* locus. *J. Mol. Bio.* **74**:635–651.

Wimber, D. E. and D. M. Steffensen, 1970   Localization of 5s RNA genes of *Drosophila* chromosomes by RNA–DNA hybridization. *Science (Wash., D.C.)* **170**:639–640.

Wright, T. R. F., 1963   The genetics of an esterase in *Drosophila melanogaster. Genetics* **48**:787–801.

Young, W. J., 1966   X-linked variation in 6-phosphogluconate dehydrogenase. *J. Hered.* **57**:58–60.

Young, W. J., I. Porter and B. Childs, 1964   Glucose-6-phosphate dehydrogenase in *Drosophila*: X-linked electrophoretic variants. *Science (Wash., D.C.)* **143**:140–141.

Yen, T. T. T. and E. Glassman, 1965   Electrophoretic variants of xanthine dehydrogenase in *Drosophila melanogaster. Genetics* **52**:977–981.

25

Behavioral Mutants of *Drosophila*

Joseph Grossfield

Introduction

The first study using *Drosophila* as a laboratory organism was published in 1905 and discussed the behavioral responses of wild-type flies (Carpenter, 1905). Since that time the study of behavioral mutants of *Drosophila* has been pursued in different areas by the application of three distinct approaches: genetic studies of mating as a component of fitness, investigations of the behavioral ecology of genotypes, and the study of specific physiological systems. Following the introduction of *Drosophila* to genetic studies, the effect of mutations on mating behavior was investigated to ascertain the role of sexual behavior in determining gene flow. More recent studies have used the techniques of ethology as well as mating-preference tests to investigate the sequence and frequency of discrete components of courtship behavior. The questions asked by this approach have been "Who mates with whom and why?" The second area of study has involved behavioral ecology, or the relative ability of different mutants to survive in a variety of environments.

Using this approach, flies homozygous for certain mutations have been given a choice among a number of gradients of environmental

Joseph Grossfield—Department of Biology, The City College of The City University of New York, New York, N.Y.

variables (Waddington *et al.*, 1954). Other techniques have assessed the relative survival of particular mutants in stressful environments, e.g., desiccation (Kalmus, 1945). The question addressed here is whether differential survival of genotypes can be a function of behavior. The third approach has used mutants in an effort to concentrate on particular physiological systems involved in behavior and to clarify the anatomy and function of the underlying mechanisms. The mutants used in this approach have generally been induced and isolated as part of a particular behavioral assay procedure with the intent of using mutants found in this fashion for the study of specific problems in sensory or central nervous system physiology. Thus this approach represents a departure from studying pre-existing mutants and concentrates on isolating mutants that affect a particular physiological system or subsystem. The approach relies on inducing single-step lesions of various functions in a system and then studying the function one component at a time. By perturbing each component of a system a picture of the overall functioning of the system can be developed.

Excluded from consideration here are studies of strains possessing a behavioral trait where no gene and/or physiological lesion has been identified. Thus, strains selected for positive or negative phototaxis or geotaxis, lack of optomotor response, dispersive (migration) or crowding tendencies, mobility, or mating speed will not be discussed in depth. Also excluded is an overall consideration of the considerable amount of information available concerning the nonphototactic or visual-system mutants.

Mutants of the Central Nervous System Other Than the Visual System

Circadian-Rhythm Mutants (per^o, per^s, per^l)

Three mutants showing disruption of the normal 24-hour circadian periodicity have been found by assay of the eclosion pattern of progeny of mutagenized males (Konopka and Benzer, 1971). All three have been localized between zeste (z) (1.0) and white (w) (1.5) on the X chromosome (salivary bands 3A6–3C2) (Figure 1). The work of Judd *et al.* (1972) on this region of the chromosome should permit a more detailed assignment of circadian function to a specific cistron.

Different genetic combinations of these mutations yield a variety of results. The recessive arrhythmic mutant per^o in combination with either

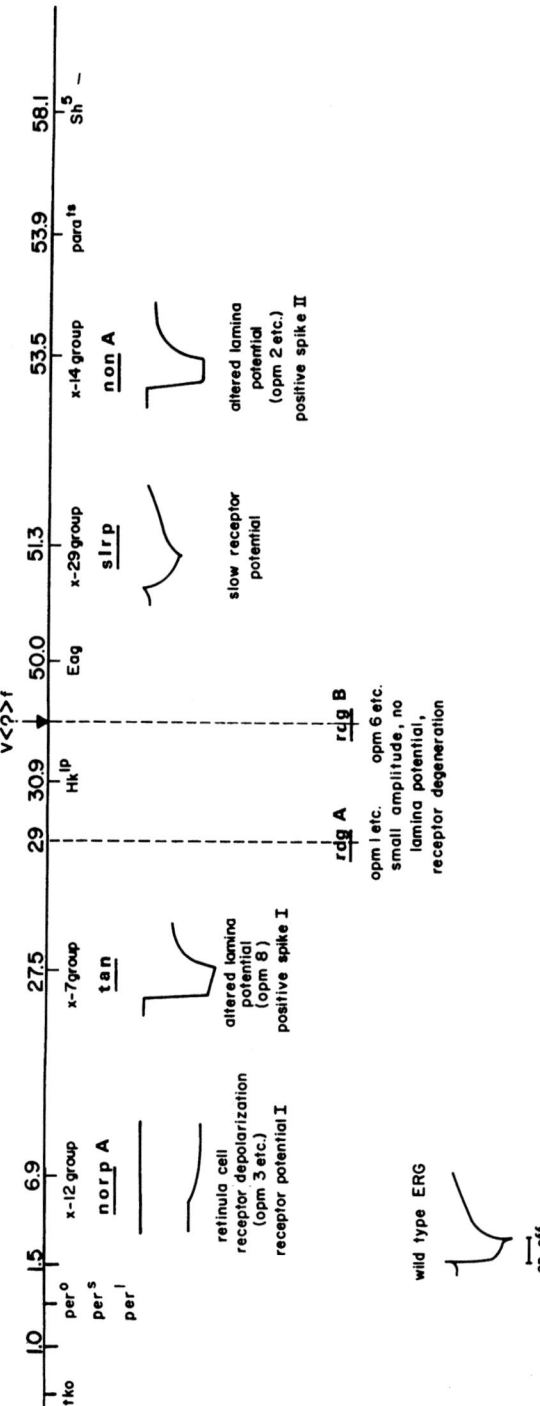

Figure 1. Map positions (not to scale) of mutants are indicated above the line with symbols for loci shown below the line together with a representative trace of the phenotypes of the electroretinogram (ERG) mutants. Two such traces are shown for the x-12 group of mutants to demonstrate that some alleles at this locus have no response to a light stimulus, while other alleles may show a small depolarization. A recording of a wild-type ERG with the duration of a light stimulus indicated below it is presented for comparison. A phrase beneath each ERG trace provides a brief description of each mutant. The terms in parentheses show alternate designations of the same lesions. Traces for mutant groups opm3 and opm6 are not shown. The underlined ERG mutant designations represent the current nomenclature for these loci (norp = no receptor potential, non = no on-transient, slrp = slow receptor potential, rdg = receptor degeneration). For greater detail concerning visual system mutants, see Chapter 26 by W. L. Pak in this volume.

the short-period (*per^s*, 19 hours) or long-period (*per^l*, 28 hours) mutants yields individuals with either a short or a long period, respectively. The heterozygote combinations *per^s/per^l*, *per^o/+*, and *per^l/+* all have normal period length. The *per^s/+* combination has a period intermediate between short and normal, i.e., ∼ 22 hours. Both eclosion and locomotor-activity rhythms are affected by these mutations. The period of the mutants is not temperature dependent. The use of gynandromorphs indicates that the physiological function affected is located in the head [see Pittendrigh and Skopik (1970) for further information on this point]. In view of the fact that the optic lobes are thought to be the site of the driving oscillation for rhythmicity in other insects (Nishiitsutsuji-Uwo and Pittendrigh, 1968), there is the intriguing possibility that mutants such as *L^4* and *G1*, whose optic lobe is abnormal (Power, 1950), may demonstrate circadian abnormalities different from those produced by the *per* mutants.

Abnormalities of Motor Function

Shaker Mutants (*Hk, Sh, Eag*).   This group of sex-linked, incompletely dominant mutants was discovered during examination of the F_2 generation in a study of sex-linked lethals (Kaplan and Trout, 1969). The two alleles (*Hk^{1P}, Hk^{2T}*) at the hyperkinetic locus (30.9) cause a vigorous, steady leg shaking, with *Hk^{1P}* somewhat more vigorous. Mutations at the shaker^5 (*Sh^5*) locus (58.2) cause vigorous and erratic shaking, with a strong scissoring of the wings and twitching of the abdomen. The ether a' go-go (*Eag*) mutation at 50.0 causes the least vigorous shaker; it does cause an occasional abdominal twitch, but is similar to hyperkinetic in its absence of wing activity. All of these phenotypes are only manifested under ether anesthesia.

Heterozygotes of all four shakers with wild type show that shaking (and scissoring in the case of *Sh^5*) is dominant but less vigorous than in the respective homozygotes. All shaker mutants are more active than wild-type flies, with *Sh^5* and *Hk^{1P}* being the most active. *Hk^{1P}* is more active than *Hk^{2T}*, and both require a longer time to settle down after a disturbance than do wild-type flies. Although all four shakers can respond to a hand passed over a vial by jumping (kinetogenic response), *Sh^5* and *Eag* show marginal penetrance for this trait. *Hk^{1P}* and *Hk^{2T}* respond vigorously, but hybrid combinations show that this behavioral component is recessive, since the response is absent in all combinations except *Hk^{1P}/Hk^{2T}*.

In addition to earlier reports of the sex-linked dominant *Sh* locus in *D. melanogaster* (hence the designation *Sh*⁵) and *D. funebris* listed in Kaplan and Trout (*1969*), Kiil (1946) reported the recovery of a shaker phenotype from a progeny of a wild female of *D. funebris* which was apparently an autosomal dominant. Whether this phenotype will be discovered in the autosomes of *D. melanogaster* remains to be seen.

Ikeda and Kaplan (1970*a,b*), using intracellular recording of electrical activity, have found that the neural mechanism underlying the abnormal motor function of *Hk*¹ᴾ consists of rhythmic bursts of activity from motor neurons in the thoracic ganglion. Recordings from wild type show only irregular discharges. Impulses originate within the ganglion from three pairs of regions, the right and left sides of the pro-, meso-, and metathoracic portions of the ganglion. Two types of neurons were traced to these regions. The more frequently encountered type 1 neurons discharge action potentials from a steady resting level, while in type 2 neurons the action potentials are preceded by a slowly rising depolarization, or prepotential. The resting potential of these neurons range from −52 mV to −63 mV. The action potentials rarely display overshoot. The frequency of discharge for type 1 neurons is about 8–10/sec and that of type 2, about 5–10/sec. Ikeda and Kaplan (1970*a*) suggest that type 2 neurons may be the pacemakers for the type 1 motor neurons. Thus, type 2 neurons would be the ones affected by the mutation. Studies with gynandromorphs show the mutant to be autonomous; motor regions of one side are unaffected by the genotype of the other side of the ganglion (Ikeda and Kaplan, 1970*b*). The significance of these findings lies in the demonstration that electrophysiological techniques can be used to trace the neural path of impulses resulting in a behavioral act which is under genetic control.

Paralytic Temperature-Sensitive Mutant (*para*ᵗˢ). This sex-linked recessive mutation, located at 53.9, was recovered by screening progeny of mutagenized males in a heated apparatus to detect immobility at high temperatures (Suzuki *et al.*, 1971). The mutation causes an immediate but reversible paralysis of adults at 29°C, while it has no effect at the permissive temperature of 22°C. Larvae are not affected. Between temperatures of 22°C and 25°C *para*ᵗˢ flies display normal walking, climbing and flying ability. At temperatures above 25°C there is a progressive debilitation of adults, with paralysis at 29°C taking less than five seconds. Mobility recovers immediately at the permissive temperature, even after several hours of paralysis. Studies with gynandromorphs indicate the defect to be in the head, with a wild-type thorax required for normal leg movement.

Site of Lesion Unknown

Possible Central-Nervous-System or Neuromuscular-Junction Mutants (*tko, sps*)

tko. A sex-linked recessive located 0.006 units to the left of zeste (1.0) has been localized to salivary band 3A2 (Judd *et al.*, 1972) on the X chromosome. Three alleles were discovered during an intensive study of this region: *25t* and *15p* were NNG (N-methyl-N^1-nitro-N-nitrosoguanidine) induced, and *K11* was a result of treatment with dimethyl sulfoxide and 2000 r (x ray). The *25t* allele is semilethal in homozygous females or hemizygous males. The surviving flies have fine bristles.

All three mutants are easily shocked; striking the culture container sharply results in adults falling and remaining immobile for a few seconds. After recovery there is a refractory period ($\sim$ 1 hr) of reduced sensitivity to shock.

Spastic (*sps*). This second-chromosome mutant, mapped to 63.6, was discovered as induced pupal and postpupal lethal (Meyer and Edmondson, 1951). Many flies emerge from pupal cases and have normal wing expansion. However, they are "unable to walk or fly due to spastic contraction and jerking of leg and wing muscles." These flies flip over on their backs and become stuck in the medium. They die within a day. When etherized, the muscles relax so that the flies are indistinguishable from wild type. This syndrome may be amenable to the same kind of analysis of neuronal regulation as was performed for Hk^{1P}.

Possible Muscular or Neuromuscular Degeneration Mutant Apterous^4 (*ap^4*)

Adults homozygous for this second-chromosome (55.2) recessive are active only during the first day or so, becoming motionless after that time (King and Sang, 1958). They live for 3–4 days. The only movement is that of their pulsating hearts and ovaries. Vitellogenesis is retarded, but ovaries of an *ap^4/ap^4* genotype produce abundant yolk when implanted into wild-type abdomens (King and Bodenstein, 1965). Males have normal mature sperm, but are inert.

Anesthetization Mutants (*es*)

Two recessive mutants, both designated ether sensitive (*es*), have been reported. The first, on the X chromosome, has been localized to the region between 0.5 and 2.5 (Peterson, 1947). The mutant is characterized by extreme sensitivity to ether; it has poor viability; and the stock is no longer in existence.

The second mutant has been located on the second chromosome and is hypersensitive to diethyl ether and chloroform (Kidd, 1963). It is not sensitive to CO_2. Viability is also poor.

Sexual-Performance Mutants (*fty, sk*)

A third-chromosome, recessive mutation fruity (*fty*) was x-ray induced (Gill, 1963) and apparently affects only males. Homozygous males actively court each other even in the presence of females. Courtship of females lasts a few seconds with females generally decamping. Copulations have not yet been observed, resulting, effectively, in a male-sterile mutation. Lines of three or more males can form in which each male is courting the one anterior to him. No male–male matings have been observed.

The third-chromosome (~ 80 on the genetic map) recessive mutation stuck (*sk*) is a sex-limited condition which causes males to have difficulty separating from females after copulation (Beckman, 1970). Penetrance is variable and the stock has essentially reverted to wild type (Beckman, private communication). It may be noted that a subtle difference in the angle and number of penile spines gives similar difficulties in other species (Grossfield, 1972*a*).

Morphological Mutations Affecting Behavior

Known morphological mutants that have been explicitly tested for their effect on behavior are compiled in tabular form (see Table 1). In some cases, mutants that have been tested but were found to exert no effect have been included for the sake of avoiding repetition of identical testing in the future. The penetrance and expressivity of certain mutations is crucial with respect to any behavioral effect. One overriding caution applicable to many of these studies is the fact that different genetic backgrounds can significantly alter the interpretation of gross behavioral measurements. It is anticipated that in the future it will be commonplace to use strains isogenized, as far as practicable, for all but the locus of interest.

There are mutants affecting certain aspects of morphology [e.g., sensilla or hairs and bristles of the wing (Green, 1963)] which have not been tested for an effect on behavior but which may, with use of appro-

TABLE 1. *A Tabulation of Morphological Mutants in D. melanogaster That Have Been Tested for a Behavioral or Neurological Trait[a]*

Gene symbol	Gene name	Location	Phenotype	Observed effect	Reference
al	aristaless	2–0.01	Aristae reduced	No effect on wing beat frequency	Williams and Reed (1944)
				Mating success of male reduced; female receptivity affected	Burnet et al. (1971)
ant	antennaless	2–?	Antennae missing	Mating success reduced	Begg and Packman (1951)
*Antp^{LC}	Antennapedia of Le Calvez	3–?	Arista and antenna malformed	Flight and wing motion absent	Williams and Reed (1944)
b	black	2–48.5	Body, tarsi and wings darker	Optomotor response normal	Kalmus (1943)
				ERG normal	Hotta and Benzer (1969)
				Locomotor activity and mating success reduced	Elens (1965a)
				More breaks in courtship; reduced vibration and licking	Crossley and Zuill (1970)
				Optomotor response reduced; phototaxis reduced	Kalmus (1943), Hecht and Wald (1934), Medioni (1959), Brown and Hall (1936)
				Locomotor activity reduced	Elens (1965b)
B	Bar	1–57.0	Eyes narrow	Wing beat frequency normal; mating success reduced	Williams and Reed (1944), Petit (1958), Merrell (1965), Elens (1965b)

Symbol	Name	Map	Morphology	Behavior	Reference
*bc	buckled	2-?	Wings twisted and curled	Cannot fly; can beat wings	King (1948)
bi	bifid	1-6.9	Wing veins fused at base	No hypoplasia of t.-a. ganglion	Power (1950)
Bld	Blond	1- or 2-	Bristles yellow at tips	Flight weak and erratic ERG normal	King (1948) Hotta and Benzer (1969)
bs^2 bs^{cv}	blistered blistered-curly	2-107.3	Wings blistered Vesticulated and curled up	Can beat wings and take off Flight absent if wing severly affected	King (1948)
bw	brown	2-104.5	Eye lacks red pigments	Optomotor response normal Phototaxis normal Preference for green oviposition substrate	Kalmus (1943) Fingerman (1952) Volpe et al. (1967)
bw^D	brown-Dominant			Mating success reduced No significant effect on mating success	Merrell (1965) Merrell (1965)
bx bx^{34e}	bithorax	3-58.8	Metathorax mesothoracic; halteres enlarged	Flight ability lost in severe expression; halteres motionless Will not fly; no hypoplasia of t.-a. ganglion Hyperplasia of t.-a. ganglion	Williams and Reed (1944) Power (1950) Chiarodo et al. (1971)
Bx^3 c	Beadex curved	1-59.4 2-75.5	Wings excised, narrow Wings curved downward	No effect on mating behavior Male courtship less vigorous Can beat wings erratically; stroke amplitude reduced Cannot fly Flight absent; no hypoplasia of t.-a. ganglion	Merrell (1965) Sturtevant (1915) Williams and Reed (1944) King (1948) Power (1950)

TABLE 1. Continued

Gene symbol	Gene name	Location	Phenotype	Observed effect	Reference
ci	cubitus interruptus	4–0	Wing vein L4 has gaps	Flight restricted; reduced wing beat frequency in combination with *ey*	Williams and Reed (1944)
cn	cinnabar	2–57.5	Eye color bright red	Wing beat frequency increased	Williams and Reed (1944)
ct	cut	1–20.0	Wings cut to points; edges scalloped	Optomotor response normal †Mating success equal to *v* Wing beat frequency increased	Kalmus (1943) Bösiger (1962, 1967) Williams and Reed (1944)
ct⁶			Lacks pleiotropic effects of *ct*	Flight normal No hypoplasia of t.-a. ganglion	King (1948) Power (1950), Chiarodo et al. (1971)
cu	curled	3–50.0	Wings curved upward	Mating success reduced Phototaxis reduced	Merrell (1949) McEwen (1918), Dürrwächter (1957)
cv	crossveinless	1–13.7	Wing crossveins absent	Flight absent No hypoplasia of t.-a. ganglion Wing beat frequency reduced	King (1948) Power (1950) Williams and Reed (1944)
Cy	Curly	2–6.1	Wings curled upward	Occasional rapid, inconsistent wing stroke; no sustained flight No hypoplasia of t.-a. ganglion	Williams and Reed (1944), King (1948) Power (1950), Chiarodo et al. (1971)

dp^o	dumpy-oblique	2–13.0	Wings oblique; truncated; shortened; no vortex effect	Male courtship duration longer; less successful; more vibration; reduced orientation	Rushton and Metcalfe (1971)
dp^{ov}	dumpy-oblique vortex		Wings reduced; oblique	Can beat wings; do not fly	King (1948)
dp^{ovdr}	dumpy-oblique vortex drumlins		More pronounced vortex effect	Can beat wings; do not fly	
e	ebony	3–70.7	Body color black	Phototaxis reduced	Dürrwächter (1957)
				ERG lacks on-and-off transients (e and e^{11})	Hotta and Benzer (1969), Grossfield and Pak (1971)
					Elens (1957, 1965a)
				Locomotor and sexual activity reduced	Rendel (1951)
				Mating more successful than vg in dark; opposite in light	Jacobs (1960, 1961)
				More successful mating in reduced light; reduced courtship activity	
				Reduced vibration and licking.	Crossley (1970)
				Increased number of breaks in courtship (e and e^{11})	Crossley and Zuill (1970)
ey	eyeless	4–2.0	Eyes reduced	Flight restricted; reduced wing beat frequency in combination with ci	Williams and Reed (1944)
				Reduced mating success is a function of severity of expression	Hartman (1963)
f	forked	1–56.7	Bristles short, bent	No effect on mating behavior	Merrell (1949)
gl	glass	3–63.1	Eyes reduced, facets fused	Wing beat frequency increased	Williams and Reed (1944)

TABLE 1. Continued

Gene symbol	Gene name	Location	Phenotype	Observed effect	Reference
				Mating success reduced	Merrell and Underhill (1956)
Gl	Glued	3–41.4	Eyes rough, facets fused	ERG absent	Pak *et al.* (1969)
				ERG absent	Grossfield (unpublished)
				Eyes and optic lobes abnormal	Power (1950)
L	Lobe	2–72.0	Eyes smaller, nicked	Wing beat frequency reduced	Williams and Reed (1944)
				No significant effect on mating behavior	Merrell (1965)
L²				Mating success reduced	Merrell (1965)
Ly	Lyra	3–40.5	Wings excised	Flight absent; no hypoplasia of t.-a. ganglion	Williams and Reed (1944), Power (1950)
lz	lozenge	1–27.7	Eyes narrow, rough	ERG normal	Grossfield (unpublished)
m	miniature	1–36.1	Wirg size reduced	Wing beat frequency increased	Williams and Reed (1944)
m²				Flight restricted or absent	King (1948)
ras²	raspberry	1–32.8	Eye color translucent ruby	Mating success reduced	Merrell (1949)
Rev^B	Revolute of Bridges	2–?	Wings spread and curled	Wing beat feeble; flight absent	King (1948)
s	sable	1–43.0	Body color dark	ERG normal	Hotta and Benzer (1969)
Sb	Stubble	3–58.2	Bristles short	Can beat wings; flightless in combination with *Gl*	King (1948)
				No hypoplasia of t.-a. ganglion	Power (1950)

sc	scute	1–0.0	Loss of bristles	Wing beat frequency reduced	Williams and Reed (1944)
se	sepia	3–26.0	Eye color brown, darkens with age	Wing beat frequency normal	Williams and Reed (1944)
				Phototaxis increased	Fingerman (1952)
				Pattern contrast normal	Hengstenberg and Gotz (1967)
				Visual orientation normal	Wehner et al. (1969)
				Mating success equals wild type	Faugéres et al. (1971)
spa[pot]	sparkling-poliert	4–	Eyes small, smooth	ERG absent	Grossfield (unpublished)
ss[a]	spineless, aristapedia	3–58.5	Antennae tarsus-like	Flightless; no hypoplasia of ganglion	Power (1950)
stw	straw	2–55.1	Hair yellowish	ERG normal	Hotta and Benzer (1969)
stw[5]			Wings thin and warped	ERG normal	Hotta and Benzer (1969)
stw[D]			Body also yellow; wings thin and curled	Can beat wings; flight absent	King (1948)
svr	silver	1–0.0	Color of legs, wings, and body pale and silvery	ERG normal	Hotta and Benzer (1969)
t	tan	1–27.5	Body color tan	Not positively phototactic; ERG lacks on-and-off transients	McEwen (1918), Pak et al. (1969), Hotta and Benzer (1969), Crossley and Zuill (1970)
				Mating success reduced; increased licking and breaks; reduced vibration and licking	
th	thread	3–43.2	Aristae threadlike	Mating success of male reduced; female receptivity affected	Burnet et al. (1971)

TABLE 1. Continued

Gene symbol	Gene name	Location	Phenotype	Observed effect	Reference
tx	taxi	3–91	Wings held out, narrow	No wing motion; flight absent	Williams and Reed (1944)
				No hypoplasia of t.-a. ganglion	Power (1950), Chiarodo et al. (1971)
v	vermilion	1–33.0	Eye color scarlet; no brown pigment	Male courtship normal	Sturtevant (1915)
				†Mating success equal to cn	Bösiger (1962, 1967)
				Phototaxis reduced	Fingerman (1952)
				Optomotor response equal to wild type	Kalmus (1943)
				Preference for blue oviposition substrate	Volpe et al. (1967)
vg	vestigial	2–67.0	Wings reduced to vestiges	Optomotor response good; phototaxis reduced	Kalmus (1943), Dürrwächter (1957), McEwen (1918)
				Cannot fly	Power (1950), Williams and Reed (1944)
				Certain alleles reared at high temperatures can fly	Harnly (1941)
				No hypoplasia in t.-a. ganglion	Power (1950)
				Hyperplasia of this ganglion	Chiarodo et al. (1971)
				Mating more successful than e in light; opposite success in dark	Rendel (1951)
				Mating success reduced	Merrell and Underhill (1956)

w	1–1.5	Eye pure white	Copulation delayed by darkness; lacks vibration, reduced licking and courtship success	Crossley (1970)
			Reduced mating success due to absence of wings; vigor equals wild male types	Seegmiller and Hanks (1968)
			Some alleles increase wing beat frequency; locomotor activity reduced	Williams and Reed (1944), Elens (1965b)
			Phototaxis reduced	Brown and Hall (1936), Scott (1943), Fingerman (1952) Kalmus (1943), Wehner et al. (1969)
			Optomotor response reduced; poor contrast perception, longer orientation time	Bennett and Hughes (1971)
			†Certain elements of cleaning activity reduced or enhanced	Sturtevant (1915), Reed and Reed (1950), Tebb and Thoday (1956)
			Mating success reduced; less vigorous courtship	Petit (1959
				Hengstenberg and Gotz (1967)
			Less responsive to pattern contrast	Ramel and Eiche (1960), Geer and Green (1962), Hildreth (1962), Elens (1965b), Faugéres et al. (1971)

TABLE 1. Continued

Gene symbol	Gene name	Location	Phenotype	Observed effect	Reference
y	yellow	1–0.0	Body color yellow	Male courtship less vigorous. Mating success reduced	Sturtevant (1915), Merrell (1949), Spett (1932), Diederich (1941), Mayr (1950), Barker (1962), Mainardi and Mainardi (1966)
				Males show reduced wing vibration; fewer and shorter displays	Bastock (1956)
				Optomotor response normal. ERG normal (y and y²)	Kalmus (1943), Hotta and Benzer (1969)
v; bw			Eyes white	Optomotor response reduced	Kalmus (1943), Burnet et al. (1968)
				Phototaxis reduced	Kikkawa (1948)
				Mating success reduced	Connolly et al. (1969)
				Restoration of visual acuity by feeding kynurenine	Kikkawa (1948), Burnet et al. (1968), Connolly et al. (1969)

[a] Arranged alphabetically by gene symbol. A "?" following the chromosome designation indicates that the locus has not been determined or that the mutation is inseparable from a rearrangement. Mutants not known to be represented by an extant stock are marked with an asterisk. Behavioral abnormalities are presented relative to wild type, unless otherwise designated. In some cases mutants have only been examined in combination with other mutants; e.g., studies of the degree of hypo- or hyperplasia of the thoracico-abdominal (t.-a.) ganglion. A lack of abnormality would apply to all mutants in the material examined. Different alleles at some loci are listed. Studies of an extensive series of alleles are discussed in the text. When available, comparisons of mutant performance are listed for strains "isogenized" but for the locus under study rather than for comparisons of different strains. References reporting studies of such coisogenic strains are designated with a dagger.

priate tests [e.g., Vogel (1967) of *Drosophila* flight performance], be shown to be of functional importance. Such mutants have not been included here.

Some of the mutants listed exhibit their behavioral effect as a result of obvious mechanical difficulty. The effect of other morphological mutations is readily comprehensible in view of current understanding of the underlying physiological systems. Mutants such as spa^{pol} with grossly disturbed retinula cell organization show no electroretinogram let alone the capability to discern patterns. Mutations that affect the screening pigments, which serve the function of separating visual imputs to the individual ommatidia, demonstrate that pigment-deficient mutants are less sensitive to pattern contrast (Hengstenberg and Gotz, 1967; Wehner *et al.*, 1969). Even the presence of small amounts of pigment results in superior vision compared with the complete absence of pigment (Kalmus, 1943; Geer and Green, 1962).

Williams and Reed (1944) tested a number of alleles at the white (w) locus for any effect on flight. It is interesting to note that of the nine alleles tested, all alleles at three subloci (w^{bl}, w^{bf}, w^{e}, w^{h}, w^{ch}, w) increase wing beat frequency while w^{a}, at a fourth sublocus, decreases the frequency. The sublocus assignment of two other alleles w^{t} and w^{p}, which increase wing beat frequency, is not known. The recent work of Judd *et al.* (1972) on the w locus should permit a detailed investigation of any causal relationship. This raises the question of the effect of small changes in pigmentation on the animal's gross behavior. It illustrates another route by which mutations can affect behavior, i.e., by perturbing some portion of an individual's information feedback loop.

An example of the importance of information transfer between individuals can be found in the many species of *Drosophila* which depend on visual cues in courtship (Grossfield, 1971). In a very real sense the use of mutants to investigate the flow of information involved in behavior may be one of the more important uses of behavioral mutants [see Reichardt (1969)].

The induction of mutants affecting a specific physiological system in order to analyze the system constitutes an *a priori* approach. However, the analysis of existing mutations which produce nontrivial perturbations of gross behavior constitutes an *a posteriori* approach which should not be overlooked.

Conclusion

The various mutations described above affect circadian rhythms, locomotion (shakers, $para^{ts}$, sps, ap^{4}), stress responses (shakers, $para^{ts}$, *tko, es*), sexual behavior (*fty, sk*), as well as some even less-well-defined nerve, neuromuscular, or muscle disability (*sps, ap*[4]). They represent several possible routes of study toward greater understanding of central and peripheral neural information processing. Several classes of these mutants represent an *a priori* approach directed toward the function of a specific system. Others offer the opportunity to exploit fortuitously occurring mutants to probe the anatomy and mechanism of a system. Future work will undoubtedly see an increase in the assay of parameters of *Drosophila* behavior with respect to various drugs and metabolites as the first step in probing the manifold systems subserving behavior. It is worth recalling however, that paralytic, catatonic, or epileptic states can easily be induced in a number of species of *Drosophila*. *D. robusta* exposed to a mechanical shock will go into a state of collapse and sink into a short-lived paralysis from which it arises with spinning gyrations before returning to its usual routine in the most insouciant fashion (Carson, 1958). The same is true of *D. gibberosa* and several species in the *quinaria* species group (Grossfield, unpublished). Females will often extrude an egg as part of the typical trauma reaction (Grossfield and Sakri, 1972). Thus, investigation of the phenotype whose occurrence prompts research interest does not necessarily await the production of a mutant *D. melanogaster*. Indeed, the catatonic syndrome itself is no more than an expression of the behavioral potential already present, but usually having a high threshold, in that species. *D. melanogaster* will show an epileptic syndrome, complete with spasmodic contractions, when exposed to high or low temperatures, intense light, or irritating vapors (Carpenter, 1908). Intense light potentiates the convulsive reflexes produced by high temperatures so that they will occur at 30°C rather than 45°C. It is not known whether mutations which show a drop in the threshold for this syndrome, *para*[ts] and *tko*, can have their threshold further depressed by any synergistic stimulus. The neural processing of such heteromodal stimuli is one of the more fertile avenues open for investigation.

There are a few mutants that have been investigated because of their possible relationship to the nonphototactic electroretinogram (ERG) mutations discussed elsewhere (Alawi *et al.*, 1972). For example, since it has been postulated that alcohol dehydrogenase plays a role in the biochemistry of vision, flies lacking this enzyme (*Adh*[n2]) were examined for any effect on the ERG or the adaptation time of any of its components. No effect was observed. Another morphological mutant, lozenge (*lz*), was tested for ERG abnormality. The locus is close to the *tan* locus, both *tan* and *ebony* are ERG mutants, and some *lz* alleles lack enzymes in pathways leading to melanin and adrenaline synthesis. Three *lz* alleles,

lz^{37}, lz^k, and lz^3, each at a different sublocus of lz and all differing from wild type in one or more mono- and diphenol oxidases (tyrosinase A_1 and A_2) and dopa oxidase (Peeples *et al.*, 1969), were tested for their ERG response; all showed a normal ERG. Biochemical assay of the *tan* mutant showed no enzyme defects in this system (Peeples, Grossfield, and Pak, unpublished).

The apparent degeneration mutant, ap^4, (Butterworth and King, 1965) mimics some human degenerative diseases and clearly calls for developmental and anatomical exploitation. The reported hyperplasia of the thoracico-abdominal ganglion in some mutants (Chiarodo *et al.*, 1971) suggests that degenerative mutants may play a role in the developmental study of the fashion in which neural networks are laid down; $para^{ts}$ does not appear to affect larvae, but *sps* and ap^4 have not yet been studied from this point of view. There are also some mutants which hold their wings out from the body at an unusual angle (e.g., the held out mutation). Conceivably some of these mutants could affect the structure of the wing musculature. Indeed, this class of lesion has recently been found in a mutation designated wings-up (Benzer, 1971), where myofibrils are absent in the indirect flight muscles. Flies heterozygous for this gene have myofibrils in these muscles, but the organization of the Z bands is irregular. Flies homozygous for another type of degeneration mutant, designated drop-dead show normal behavior after eclosion, but at a later point in time they become uncoordinated and die. The brain of such flies develops holes at some point in adult life (Benzer, 1971).

The existence of ether-sensitive loci on two different chromosomes suggests that efforts expended in assaying for sensitivity or resistance to narcotizing agents may be a fruitful way to explore mechanisms of anesthesia.

It is not known whether the mechanism underlying the *fty* gene is a sensory defect or an integrative problem. It may be noted that males of *D. pegasa* in the absence of appropriate females behave in a similar fashion, capable of forming chains of three or more males courting each other (Wasserman *et al.*, 1971). The genus *Drosophila* is rich enough in behavioral repetoire so that naturally existing behavior patterns can be converted into problems worth exploiting. The existence of isozyme-variation and enzyme-assay techniques weakens the notion that only *D. melanogaster* has sufficient markers for a genetic study.

The tracing of neural circuitry and anatomy accomplished with the shaker and visual mutants illustrates the type of functional mapping of portions of neural networks that constitutes one of the central goals of genetic dissection of behavior. The use of the newly developed autosomal deficiencies *cum* Y-autosome translocations may make it possible to probe portions of chromosomes close to loci known to perturb behavioral function. Theoretically, it may now be possible to sequentially probe nearly the entire genome for such loci. Until such feats are technically feasible, however, the use of induced mutants offers the most widely applicable approach to genetic dissection of behavior in *Drosophila* and perhaps in other insects as well (Grossfield, 1972*b*). At this point it is well to realize that the number of identified behavioral mutants in *Drosophila* is less than the number of such loci listed for mice.

Literature Cited

Alawi, A. A., V. Jennings, J. Grossfield and W. L. Pak, 1972 Phototransduction mutants of *Drosophila melanogaster*. In *The Visual System*, edited by G. B. Arden pp. 1–21, Plenum Press, New York.

Barker, J. S. F., 1962 Studies of selective mating using the *yellow* mutant of *Drosophila melanogaster*. *Genetics* **47**:623–640.

Bastock, M., 1956 A gene mutation which changes a behavior pattern. *Evolution* **10**:421–439.

Beckman, C., 1970 Report of new mutants. *Drosophila melanogaster*. *Drosophila Inf. Serv.* **45**:36.

Begg, M. and E. M. Packman, 1951 Antennae and mating behaviour in *Drosophila melanogaster*. *Nature (Lond.)***168**:953.

Bennett, J. and J. F. Hughes, 1971 Behavioral correlates of the w, w^+ gene substitution, observations without ether. *Drosophila Inf. Serv.* **47**:74.

Benzer, S., 1971 From the gene to behavior. *J. Am. Med. Assoc.* **218**:1015–1022.

Bösiger, E., 1962 Sur le degre d'heterozygotie des populations naturelles de *Drosophila melanogaster* et son maintien par la selection sexuelle. *Bull. Biol. Fr. Belg.* **96**:3–122.

Bösiger, E., 1967 La signification evolutive de la selection sexuelle chez les animaux. *Scientia* **102**:207–223.

Brown, F. A. and V. A. Hall, 1936 The directive influence of light upon *Drosophila melanogaster* and some of its eye mutants. *J. Exp. Zool.* **74**:205–220.

Burnet, B., K. Connolly and J. Beck, 1968 Phenogenetic studies on visual acuity in *Drosophila melanogaster*. *J. Insect Physiol.* **14**:855–860.

Burnet, B., K. Connolly and L. Dennis, 1971 The function and processing of auditory information in the courtship behaviour of *Drosophila melanogaster*. *Anim. Behav.* **19**:409–415.

Butterworth, F. M. and R. C. King, 1965 The developmental genetics of *apterous* mutants of *Drosophila melanogaster*. *Genetics* **52**:1153–1174.

Carpenter, F. W., 1905 The reactions of the pomace fly (*Drosophila ampelophila* loew) to light, gravity and mechanical stimulation. *Am. Nat.* **39**:157–171.

Carpenter, F. W., 1908 Some reactions of *Drosophila*, with special reference to convulsive reflexes. *J. Comp. Neurol. Psychol.* **18**:483–491.

Carson, H. L., 1958 Response to selection under different conditions of recombination in *Drosophila*. *Cold Spring Harbor Symp. Quant. Biol.* **23**:291–306.

Chiarodo, A., C. M. Reing, Jr. and H. Saranchak, 1971   On neurogenetic relations in *Drosophila melanogaster. J. Exp. Zool.* **178:**325–330.

Connolly, K., B. Burnet and D. Sewell, 1969   Selective mating and eye pigmentation: An analysis of the visual component in the courtship behavior of *Drosophila melanogaster. Evolution* **23:**548–559.

Crossley, S., 1970   Mating reactions of certain mutants. *Drosophila Inf. Serv.* **45:**170.

Crossley, S. and E. Zuill, 1970   Courtship behaviour of some *Drosophila melanogaster* mutants. *Nature (Lond.)* **225:**1064–1065.

Diederich, G. W., 1941   Non-random mating between yellow-white and wild type *Drosophila melanogaster. Genetics* **26:**148.

Dürrwächter, G., 1957   Untersuchungen über Phototaxis and Geotaxis einiger *Drosophila*-mutanten nach aufzucht in verschiedenen lichtbedingungen. *Z. Tierpsychol.* **14:**1–28.

Elens, A. A., 1957   Importance selective des differences d'activite entre males ebony et sauvage, dans les populations artificielles de *Drosophila melanogaster. Experientia (Basel)* **13:**293–294.

Elens, A. A., 1965a   Studies of selective mating using the melanistic mutants of *Drosophila melanogaster. Experientia (Basel),* **21:**145–146.

Elens, A. A., 1965b   Studies of selective mating using the sex-linked mutants white and bar of Drosophila melanogaster. *Experientia (Basel)* **21:**594–595.

Faugéres, A., C. Petit and E. Thibout, 1971   The components of sexual selection. *Evolution* **25:**265–275.

Fingerman, M., 1952   The role of the eye pigments of *Drosophila melanogaster* in photic orientation. *J. Exp. Zool.* **120:**131–164.

Geer, B. W. and M. M. Green, 1962   Genotype, phenotype and mating behavior in *Drosophila melanogaster. Am. Nat.* **96:**175–181.

Gill, K. S., 1963   A mutation causing abnormal mating behavior. *Drosophila Inf. Serv.* **38:**33.

Green, M. M., 1963   Hairy mutants and sensilla campaniformia. *Drosophila Inf. Serv.* **37:**83.

Grossfield, J., 1971   Geographic distribution and light dependency in *Drosophila. Proc. Natl. Acad. Sci. USA* **68:**2669–2673.

Grossfield, J., 1972a   Decapitated females as a tool in the analysis of Drosophila behavior. *Anim. Behav.* **20:**243–251.

Grossfield, J., 1972b   The use of behavioral mutants in biological control. *Behav. Genet.* **2:**311–319.

Grossfield, J. and W. L. Pak, 1971   Isolation of autosomal visual mutants in *Drosophila melanogaster. Genetics* **68:**s25.

Grossfield, J. and B. Sakri, 1972   Divergence in the neural control of oviposition in *Drosophila. J. Insect Physiol.* **18:**237–241.

Harnly, M. H., 1941   Flight capacity in relation to phenotypic and genotypic variations in the wings of *Drosophila melanogaster. J. Exp. Zool.* **88:**263–273.

Hartman, A. B., 1963   Study of the causal factors for the decreased frequency of copulation in eyeless flies. *Drosophila Inf. Serv.* **37:**85–86.

Hecht, S. and G. Wald, 1934   The visual acuity and intensity discrimination of *Drosophila. J. Gen. Physiol.* **17:**517–547.

Hengstenberg, R. and K. G. Gotz, 1967   Der Einfluss des Schirmpigmentgehalts auf die Helligkeits-und Kontrastwahrnehmung bei *Drosophila*—Augenmutanten. *Kybernetik* **3:**276–285.

Hildreth, P. E., 1962   Quantitative aspects of mating behavior in *Drosophila*. *Behaviour* **19**:57–73.

Hotta, Y. and S. Benzer, 1969   Abnormal electroretinograms in visual mutants of *Drosophila*. *Nature (Lond.)* **222**:354–356.

Ikeda, K. and W. D. Kaplan, 1970*a*   Patterned neural activity of a mutant *Drosophila melanogaster. Proc. Natl. Acad. Sci. USA* **66**:765–772.

Ikeda, K. and W. D. Kaplan, 1970*b*   Unilaterally patterned neural activity of gynandromorphs, mosaic for a neurological mutant of *Drosophila melanogaster. Proc. Natl. Acad. Sci. USA* **67**:1480–1487.

Jacobs, M. E., 1960   Influence of light on mating of *Drosophila melanogaster. Ecology* **41**:182–188.

Jacobs, M. E., 1961   The influence of light on gene frequency changes in laboratory populations of ebony and non-ebony *Drosophila melanogaster. Genetics* **46**:1089–1095.

Judd, B. H., M. W. Shen, and T. C. Kaufman, 1972   The anatomy and function of a segment of the X chromosome of *Drosophila melanogaster. Genetics* **71**:139–156.

Kalmus, H., 1943   The optomotor responses of some eye mutants of *Drosophila. J. Genet.* **45**:206–213.

Kalmus, H., 1945   Adaptive and selective responses of a population of *Drosophila melanogaster* containing *e* and *e*⁺ to differences in temperature, humidity and to selection for developmental speed. *J. Genet.* **47**:58–62.

Kaplan, W. D. and W. E. Trout, 1969   The behavior of four neurological mutants of *Drosophila. Genetics* **61**:399–409.

Kidd, K. K., 1963   Report of new mutants: *D. melanogaster. Drosophila Inf. Serv.* **37**:49.

Kiil, V., 1946   Report of new mutants, other species. *Drosophila Inf. Serv.* **20**:78.

Kikkawa, H., 1948   Eye pigments of insects as media of phototaxis. *Drosophila Inf. Serv.* **22**:72.

King, R. C., 1948   The flight and hopping abilities of certain mutant stocks of *D. melanogaster. Drosophila Inf. Serv.* **22**:72.

King, R. C. and D. Bodenstein, 1965   The transplantation of ovaries between genetically sterile and wild type *Drosophila melanogaster. Z. Naturforsch. Sect. B* **20**:292–297.

King, R. C. and J. H. Sang, 1958   Additional description of *ap⁴. Drosophila Inf. Serv.* **32**:133.

Konopka, R. J. and S. Benzer, 1971   Clock mutants of *Drosophila melanogaster. Proc. Natl. Acad. Sci. USA* **68**:2112–2116.

McEwen, R. S., 1918   The reactions to light and to gravity in *Drosophila* and its mutants. *J. Exp. Zool.* **25**:49–106.

Mainardi, D. and M. Mainardi, 1966   Sexual selection in *Drosophila melanogaster*. The interaction between preferential courtship of males and differential receptivity of females. *Atti. Soc. Ital. Sci. Nat. Mus. Civ. Stor. Nat. Milano* **105**:284–286.

Mayr, E., 1950   The role of the antennae in the mating behavior of female *Drosophila. Evolution* **4**:149–154.

Medioni, J., 1959   Sur le role des yeux composes de *Drosophila melanogaster* Meigen dans la perception du proche ultraviolet: Experiences sur le phototrophisme de races mutantes. *C. R. Seances Soc. Biol F.1* **153**:164–167.

Merrell, D. J., 1949   Selective mating in *Drosophila melanogaster. Genetics* **34**:370–389.

Merrell, D. J., 1965   Competition involving dominant mutants in experimental populations of *Drosophila melanogaster. Genetics* **52**:165–189.

Merrell, D. J. and J. C. Underhill, 1956 Competition between mutants in experimental populations of *Drosophila melanogaster*. *Genetics* **41**:469–485.

Meyer, H. U. and M. Edmondson, 1951 Report of new mutants: *D. melanogaster*. *Drosophila Inf. Serv.* **25**:73.

Nishiitsutsuji-Uwo, J. and C. S. Pittendrigh, 1968 Central nervous system control of circadian rhythmicity in the cockroach. III. The optic lobes, locus of the driving oscillation. *Z. Vgl. Physiol.* **58**:14–46.

Pak, W. L., J. Grossfield and N. V. White, 1969 Nonphototactic mutants in a study of vision of *Drosophila*. *Nature (Lond.)* **222**:351–354.

Peeples, E. E., A. Grisler, C. J. Whitcraft, and C. P. Oliver, 1969 Activity of phenol oxidases at the pupariam formation stage in development of nineteen lozenge mutants of *Drosophila melanogaster*. *Biochem. Genet.* **3**:563–569.

Peterson, P. A., 1947 A sex-linked character expressed as ether sensitive (*es*). *Drosophila Inf. Serv.* **21**:88.

Petit, C., 1958 Le determinisme genetique et psycho-physiologique de la competition sexuelle chez *Drosophila melanogaster*. *Bull. Biol. Fr. Belg.* **92**:248–329.

Petit, C., 1959 De la nature des stimulations responsables de la selection sexuelle chez *Drosophila melanogaster*. *C. R. Hebd. Seances Acad. Sci. Ser. D Sci. Nat.* **248**:3484–3485.

Pittendrigh, D. S. and S. D. Skopik, 1970 Circadian systems. V. The driving oscillation and the temporal sequence of development. *Proc. Natl. Acad. Sci. USA* **65**:500–507.

Power, M. E., 1950 The central nervous system of winged but flightless *Drosophila melanogaster*. *J. Exp. Zool.* **115**:315–340.

Ramel, C. and A. Eiche, 1960 Studies on the effect of homozygous and heterozygous *w*-alleles on longevity and mating preference in *D. melanogaster*. *Hereditas* **46**:709–716.

Reed, S. C. and E. W. Reed, 1950 Natural selection in laboratory populations of *Drosophila*. II. Competition between a white-eye gene and its wild type allele. *Evolution* **4**:34–42.

Reichardt, W., 1969 Movement perception in insects. In *Proceedings of the International School of Physics,* Vol. XLIII, edited by W. Reichardt, pp. 465–493, Plenum Press, New York.

Rendel, J. M., 1951 Mating of ebony, vestigial, and wild-type *Drosophila melanogaster* in light and dark. *Evolution* **5**:226–230.

Rushton, J. and H. A. Metcalfe, 1971 A behavioral mutant of *Drosophila melanogaster*: "Amiel." *Drosophila Inf. Serv.* **46**:61.

Scott, J. P., 1943 Effects of single genes on the behavior of *Drosophila*. *Am. Nat.* **77**:184–190.

Seegmiller, R. E. and G. D. Hanks, 1968 Mating success of vestigial males. *Drosophila Inf. Serv.* **43**:170–171.

Spett, G., 1932 Gibt es eine partielle sexuelle isolation unter den mutationen und der grundform von *D. melanogaster* meig. *Z. Indukt. Abstammungs.-Vererbungsl.* **60**:63–83.

Sturtevant, A. H., 1915 Experiments on sex recognition and the problem of sexual selection in *Drosophila*. *J. Anim. Behav.* **5**:351–366.

Suzuki, D. T., T. Grigliatti and R. Williamson, 1971 Temperature-sensitive mutations in *Drosophila melanogaster*. VII. A mutation (*para^{ts}*) causing reversible adult paralysis. *Proc. Natl. Acad. Sci. USA* **68**:890–893.

Tebb, G. and J. M. Thoday, 1956 Reversal of mating preference by crossing strains of *Drosophila melanogaster*. *Nature (Lond.)* **177**:707.

Vogel, S., 1967 Flight in *Drosophila*. III. Aerodynamic characteristics of fly wings and wing models. *J. Exp. Biol.* **46**:431–443.

Volpe, P., M. Carfagna and M. DiLorenzo, 1967 Extraretinal pigmentation and colour discrimination. I. Choice of colour of substrate during oviposition in *Drosophila melanogaster*. *J. Exp. Biol.* **47**:297–305.

Waddington, C. H., B. Woolf and M. M. Perry, 1954 Environment selection by *Drosophila* mutants. *Evolution* **8**:89–96.

Wasserman, M., J. Heller and J. Zombek, 1971 Male determined sexual discrimination in the species, *Drosophila pegasa*. *Am. Midl. Nat.* **86**:231–235.

Wehner, R., G. Gartenmann and T. Jungi, 1969 Contrast perception in eye colour mutants of *Drosophila melanogaster* and *Drosophila sububscura*. *J. Insect Physiol.* **15**:815–823.

Williams, C. M. and S. C. Reed, 1944 Physiological effects of genes: The flight of *Drosophila* considered in relation to gene mutations. *Am. Nat.* **78**:214–223.

26

Mutations Affecting the Vision of *Drosophila melanogaster*

Wᴉʟʟɪᴀᴍ L. Pᴀᴋ

Introduction

We have witnessed in the past few years a resurgence of interest in phototactic, or more accurately, nonphototactic behavior of *Drosophila* (Benzer, 1967; Pak *et al.*, 1969, 1970; Hotta and Benzer, 1969, 1970; Cosens and Manning, 1969; Götz, 1970; Heisenberg, 1971*a,b*). The phototactic behavior of *Drosophila* has been studied as far back as the turn of the century (Carpenter, 1905). Several authors attempted to show that the phototactic response of the fly is genetically controlled. Earlier attempts of this type demonstrated that various eye-pigmentation mutants and other morphological mutants display varying degrees of phototactic response to light (McEwen, 1918; Brown and Hall, 1936; Scott, 1947). More recently, heritability of this trait was demonstrated by applying selection pressure to a genetically heterogeneous population (Hirsch, 1962; Hadler, 1964; Dobzhansky and Spassky, 1967). This work was pioneered by Hirsch and his co-workers, who developed a mass-screening technique

Wɪʟʟɪᴀᴍ L. Pᴀᴋ—Department of Biological Sciences, Purdue University, Lafayette, Indiana.

for flies and applied it first to the study of geotaxis (Hirsch and Tryon, 1956) and then later to phototaxis (Hirsch and Boudreau, 1958). Their work showed that many individual differences in behavioral traits exist in a population and that the behavior of the flies can be greatly modified by selection. Phototactic and geotactic responses of the flies are therefore under genetic control (Hirsch, 1962). Moreover, these controls have been shown to be polygenic [geotaxis, Hirsch (1962); phototaxis, Hadler (1964)].

Current interest in the phototaxis of *Drosophila* stems from entirely different reasons. Now, the question of interest is not the existence of a genetic component in phototactic behavior. Of greater interest is the possibility of using the phototactic response to select mutants which may be useful in genetically dissecting the nervous system. This approach is an attempt to extend the technique of genetic dissection to the nervous system of a higher organism. It is related to a number of other studies in which genetic methods are being used to explore the nervous systems of a wide variety of organisms: *Escherichia coli* (Adler, 1969), paramecium (Kung, 1971), the nematode (Brenner, 1974), the rotifer [(C. Levinthal, cited in Benzer (1971)], the mouse (Sidmann *et al.*, 1965), and *Drosophila* (Ikeda and Kaplan, 1970).

In this type of study any behavioral changes which depend upon additive effects of more than one gene are of little value. Moreover, it would be too restrictive to have to depend on the possible behavioral differences only of existing mutants, which were selected on the basis of visible markers. Thus, most of the currently available nonphototactic mutants were obtained by chemically inducing single-step mutations and looking for resultant alterations in behavior among the offspring of the mutagenized flies. A case for this type of approach was first put forth by Benzer (1967), who showed that strains of flies with radically altered phototactic behavior can be induced by single-gene mutations. Work along similar lines has also been in progress in two other laboratories: Götz's laboratory in Tübingen, Germany, and our own at Purdue. These three laboratories are largely responsible for the recent proliferation of the "nonphototactic mutants."

Scope of Discussion

The purpose of this discussion is to present as coherent an account as possible of the bewildering variety of nonphototactic mutants that have been reported in the literature. For this purpose I will restrict our attention to only those mutants which appear to be single-step mutants and on which a reasonable amount of data has accumulated.

The phototactic response of the fly is a complicated pattern of behavior, involving sensory inputs, integration of the sensory information in the central nervous system, and motor outputs to the legs and wings. It is not surprising that for most of the nonphototactic mutants, nothing much has yet been learned beyond the fact that they display heritable, abnormal, phototactic behavior (Benzer, 1967; Pak *et al.*, 1969, 1970; Hotta and Benzer, 1969). The class of mutants on which a reasonable amount of information exists is exclusively those with lesions in the peripheral visual system (the peripheral retina and lamina) (see the section "Anatomy of the Compound Eye of the Fly" for anatomy of the visual system). The existence of these lesions is indicated by a defect in the electroretinogram (ERG), a mass electrical potential elicited from the compound eye [see the section "Electroretinogram (ERG)"]. We will focus our attention on these mutants.

For this class of mutants the term "nonphototactic mutant" is a misnomer since the phototactic response is not the only visual function impaired by the mutation, and they can be isolated by methods other than those based on phototaxis (Heisenberg, 1971a; see the next section). Perhaps a more appropriate designation would be "ERG-defective mutants" or "retinal mutants." Most of them are X-chromosome recessive mutants induced by ethyl methanesulfonate (EMS). I will also include in this discussion the two body-color mutants *tan* and *ebony*, which have been found to display abnormal ERG's (Hotta and Benzer, 1969; Pak *et al.*, 1969; Heisenberg, 1971a), and a third-chromosome recessive mutant reported by Cosens and Manning (1969). Excluded from this consideration are any ERG-defective mutants whose abnormal ERG or the lack of the ERG can be attributed to gross anatomical abnormalities.

Methods and Experimental Objectives

Since three different laboratories have apparently obtained the same sets of mutants independently, I will briefly examine here the mutant-isolation method employed by each group and the experimental objectives of each.

Mutant-Selection Schemes

Thus far all three laboratories have concentrated on the X chromosome for their mutagenesis program. In each of the three laboratories, males of wild-type *Drosophila melanogaster* stocks are treated with EMS and are mated to virgin females of an attached X-chromosome stock to yield F_1 males whose X chromosome is derived from the EMS-treated fathers (Benzer, 1967; Pak *et al.*, 1969; Heisenberg, 1971*a*). The wild-type stocks used by the Benzer, Götz, and Pak laboratories are Canton-S, Berlin, and Oregon-R, respectively. The offspring of the above matings are then tested for their inability to respond behaviorally to light stimulus. The Benzer and Pak groups use selection schemes based on phototaxis, whereas the Götz–Heisenberg group base their selection scheme on the optomotor response.

The countercurrent technique used by the Benzer group has been described in detail by Benzer (1967). In this technique a population of flies is repeatedly distributed into two fractions, a fraction that moves toward light and a fraction that does not. In n number of runs the fly population is divided into $n + 1$ fractions according to their tendency to move toward light. Now each of the $n + 1$ fractions can be similarly fractionated according to their tendency to move *away* from light. The results of these runs are then plotted in a square array (a two-dimensional countercurrent distribution) in which the ordinate and abscissa represent the tendencies to move *from* and *to* light, respectively. In such a plot the non-phototactic flies, which will neither move to nor away from light, show up as diagonal elements of the array.

The Pak group has been using a much simpler scheme in which a given fly population is tested for phototaxis just once. The unselected F_1 males are single-pair mated to virgin females of the same attached-X strain used in the P_1 cross, and the flies are tested for phototaxis in the F_2 generation. Each male progeny in a particular vial would have a replica of any X-chromosome-borne lesion which may have been present on the X chromosome of their male F_1 parent. Since the behavior of the sibling males in a vial is compared as a group to the behavior of the sibling females in that vial, the effect of individual variation is minimal. Moreover, the wild-type strain the Pak group uses has been selected for strong phototaxis over many generations. Thus, in phototaxis runs, non-phototactic flies assume a distribution profile very different from that of wild type, facilitating isolation of the nonphototactic flies.

By far the most mechanized procedure has been developed by Götz and Heisenberg (Heisenberg, 1971*a*, and private communication). Their mutant-selection machine is essentially a multiple *Y*-maze in which the flies are forced to make eight successive decisions. At each decision point the flies are confronted with a rotating drum having vertical light and dark stripes, and they either follow the moving patterns or move against them. Thus, by the time the flies emerge from the maze, the population is distributed into nine fractions according to tendency to follow the moving stripes.

Experimental Objectives

The experimental objectives of each of the three laboratories are somewhat different. By far the most ambitious are those of Benzer (1967, 1971). His objectives are to genetically dissect the behavior of *Drosophila*, not merely phototactic behavior, but all facets of *Drosophila* behavior. Aside from the genetic advantages it offers, *Drosophila* is attractive for this type of work because its nervous system is much simpler than the human nervous system yet is sufficiently complex to subserve a rich repertoire of behavior. In fact, some of its behavior patterns are not unlike our own (Benzer, 1971). Thus, the hope is that from the study of *Drosophila* a clearer understanding of human behavior may emerge. Benzer and his co-workers initially concentrated on the phototactic response probably because it is one of the behavior patterns of *Drosophila* that are amenable to quantitative studies. More recently, they have been extending their study to circadian-rhythm mutants (Konopka and Benzer, 1971), a muscle-degeneration mutant "wings-up," and a central nervous system (CNS) degeneration mutant "drop-dead" (Benzer, 1971).

Our attitude, on the other hand, has been that since the technique of induced mutation has not yet been fruitfully applied to problems of neurobiology, it would be better to start its application on a relatively well-defined system. It seemed to us that the problem of phototransduction is one of the more logical places to start (Pak *et al.*, 1969; Alawi *et al.*, 1972). The transduction process is recognized as one of the key problems in sensory physiology. Its importance is not limited to sensory systems. Since the problem deals with the mechanism by which membrane permeability is modulated by the signals received by the receptor, it is of broad significance to all neural-excitation mechanisms. Yet, virtually nothing is known of molecular mechanisms of the transduction process in any sensory system. In the case of the visual receptors, many of the boundary conditions of phototransduction are known from extensive studies of the receptor potential and visual pigment proteins (Wald, 1968; Tomita, 1970; and many others). Although it is not yet certain, it seems likely that only a few steps are involved in phototransduction (Fuortes and Hodgkin, 1964). Thus only a few genes need be involved in the process. All these considerations suggested that the phototransduction process is likely to be amenable to the genetic approach. Thus, we decided to concentrate on this problem first before widening our horizon.

Götz (1964) has long been interested in the optomotor response, i.e., the tendency of an organism to follow movements of the visual environment. It is a property displayed by many insects, including *Drosophila*

(Hecht and Wald, 1934; Gavel, 1939; Kalmus, 1943). For optomotor response to occur, the movement of the environment must first be detected by a comparison of outputs from a minimum of two photoreceptors. The signals from the local-movement detectors are then integrated with those from other regions of the eye. Finally the integrated information is relayed to the appropriate effector sites on the motor system (Götz, 1970). Götz and his colleagues have, accordingly, been attempting to obtain mutants with defects in the optomotor control system in order to identify the mechanism and localize the sites of control of optomotor responses (Götz, 1970). In particular, they have concentrated their efforts on mutants of the lamina (Heisenberg, 1971*b*, 1972*a,b*) since synaptic interconnections between different photoreceptor axons first take place there, and thus the first motion detectors are probably localized in this structure.

Anatomy of the Compound Eye of the Fly

Since various structural components of the compound eye of the fly will be referred to repeatedly in the remainder of this paper, a brief description of the fly visual system is pertinent. Anatomy of the compound eye of larger dipterans has been extensively studied (Cajal and Sánchez, 1915; Fernández-Morán, 1956; Goldsmith and Philpott, 1957; Trujillo-Cenóz and Melamed, 1963, 1966, 1970; Trujillo-Cenóz, 1965*a,b*, 1969; Schneider and Langer, 1966; Braitenberg, 1967, 1970; Melamed and Trujillo-Cenóz, 1968; Horridge and Mcinertzhagen, 1970; Strausfeld and Braitenberg, 1970; Boschek, 1971; Strausfeld, 1971*a,b*). Although the *Drosophila* compound eye has not yet been studied as thoroughly, available information suggests that it does not differ significantly from that of larger flies (Johannsen, 1924; Richards and Furrow, 1925; Power, 1943; Danneel and Zeutzschel, 1957; Wolken *et al.*, 1957; Waddington and Perry, 1960; Fuge, 1967; Alawi *et al.*, 1972; Cosens and Perry, 1972). The only major differences appear to be that the *Drosophila* cells are smaller in dimensions and in number.

I present in Figure 1A a schematic diagram of the fly visual system [from Trujillo-Cenóz and Melamed (1966) with slight changes in the lettering]. The fly visual system is divided into the peripheral retina and the optic lobe. The optic lobe consists of three postretinal neuropile masses, the lamina, medulla, and lobula. For our present purpose only the two most distal structures, the peripheral retina and lamina, need be discussed in some detail, since lesions in all of the visual mutants we wish to discuss appear to be localized in these structures.

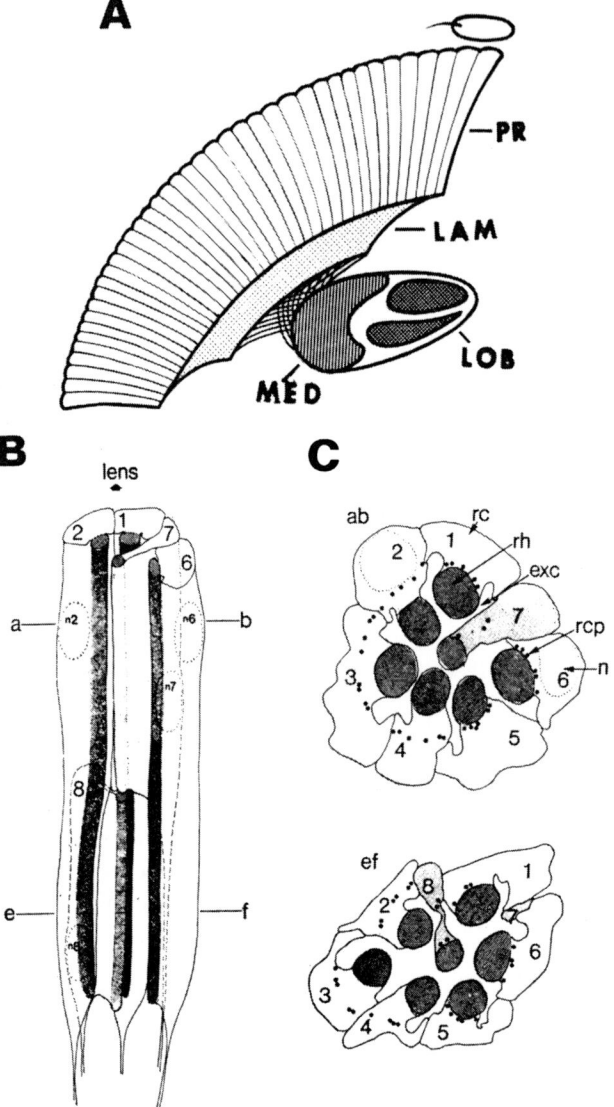

Figure 1. Structure of the fly visual system. (A) A diagram of the fly visual system. PR, peripheral retina; LAM, lamina; MED, medulla; LOB, lobula. Reproduced with permission from Trujillo-Cenóz and Melamed (1966) and Pergamon Press. (B,C) Arrangement of the retinula cells within an ommatidium. (C) Crossectional views of an ommatidium at levels ab and ef. rc, retinula cell; rh, rhabdomere; exc, extracellular cavity of ommatidium or intraommatidial space; rcp, retinula cell pigment granules; n, nucleus. The numerals refer to the retinula cell numbers. Note how the rhabdomeres of R_7 and R_8 are positioned near the center of the ommatidium, with rhabdomere 7 directly on top of rhabdomere 8. The position of the retinula cell pigment granules in R_1, R_5, and R_6 is that typical of light-adapted wild type, while retinula cells R_2-R_4 illustrate the pigment position in the Cosens–Manning mutant (see page 727). Reproduced with permission from Cosens and Perry (1972) and Pergamon Press.

Peripheral Retina

The peripheral retina is composed of approximately 700 closely packed structural subunits called ommatidia. Each ommatidium is approximately 70–125 μm long and 17 μm in diameter (Demerec, 1950) and may be divided into two sectors. At its distal end is the image-forming dioptric apparatus, consisting of a corneal lens, a gelatinous pseudocone, and Semper cells. The corneal lens arises as a specialization of the cuticle and is responsible for the faceted appearance of the compound eye. Proximal to the dioptric apparatus is the photoreceptive system called the retinula. The retinula is composed of eight retinula cells (photoreceptors) arranged radially in a cylindrical structure (Figure 1B), each cell being joined to its neighbor throughout its length by a *zonula adherens* (Boschek, 1971). Each retinula cell bears a rhabdomere, a differentiated membrane structure containing the visual pigment (Langer and Thorell, 1965). The rhabdomeres are composed of tightly packed, microvillar modifications of the retinula cell membrane. They project inward toward the intraommatidial space (Figure 1B), with the axes of the microvilli making 90-degree angles with the longitudinal axes of the retinula cells. In each ommatidium six of the eight retinula cells have rhabdomeres which run the entire length of the cell soma, from the proximal end of the dioptric apparatus to the basement membrane. [The basement membrane underlies all the ommatidia and forms a boundary between the peripheral retina and the lamina (Figure 1A).] These six retinula cells are referred to as the "peripheral retinula cells" or "retinula cells 1–6" (R_1–R_6) (Dietrich, 1909; Braitenberg, 1970). The rhabdomeres of these cells are approximately 60 μm long and 1.2 μm in diameter (Wolken *et al.*, 1957). In crossections the rhabdomeres of R_1–R_6 are arranged in a trapezoidal pattern in the intraommatidial space (Figure 1C). The remaining two retinula cells are referred to as the "superior and inferior central cells" or "retinula cells 7 and 8" (R_7 and R_8). Their rhabdomeres are only half the length and half to a fourth the crossectional area of those of the peripheral retinula cells (Figures 1B and 1C). They are found near the center of the ommatidium, with rhabdomere 7 located directly on top of rhabdomere 8 to form an axial pair (Figure 1B). The planes of orientation of the rhabdomeres of the two central retinual cells are perpendicular to each other, suggesting that these cells may be involved in the detection of polarized light (Trujillo-Cenóz and Melamed, 1966). Indeed, Kirschfeld and W. Reichardt [cited in Heisenberg (1972*b*)] have recently obtained evidence in optomotor experiments with house flies that these cells are sensitive to linearly polarized light.

Each ommatidium is optically isolated from the others by a sleeve of screening-pigment cells containing pterins and ommochromes (Cromartie, 1959; Nolte, 1961). These screening pigments give rise to the red coloration of the eye. The retinula cells are known to contain pigment granules less than 0.1 μm in diameter (Fuge, 1967). These are distinct from the photosensitive visual pigments contained in the rhabdomeres and have been identified as ommochrome granules (Nolte, 1961; Fuge, 1967). The physiological significance of these pigment granules was demonstrated by Kirschfeld and Franceschini (1969), who showed that in the house fly *Musca* these granules control the light flux in the rhabdomeres by migrating toward the rhabdomeres during light adaptation. In other words, these pigment granules have a function similar to the pupil of the vertebrate eye. This property of the retinula pigment granules is of pertinence to our discussion, because, as is to be discussed later (see pages 721–722, 727, and 728), in a number of mutants the retinular pigment migration does not occur.

At the proximal ends the retinula cells terminate in axons, and the axons pass through the fenestrated basement membrane to enter the lamina. As to be described below, only the axons of the peripheral retinula cells (R_1–R_6) make synaptic contacts with monopolar neurons in the lamina.

Lamina

The lamina is the most distal of the three postretinal neuropile masses in the optic lobe and represents the first synaptic region of the fly visual system. It is approximately 40 μm thick in *Drosophila* and is located just below the basement membrane (Figure 1A). Only a bare outline of this complex structure will be presented here. For further details the readers are referred to Trujillo-Cenóz (1965a), Trujillo-Cenóz and Melamed (1966), Boschek (1971), and reviews by Goldsmith (1964) and Bullock and Horridge (1965).

The principal cells of the lamina are monopolar neurons, the cell bodies of which lie in the distal layer of the lamina. These cells are responsible for receiving messages from the peripheral retinual cells and relaying them to the cells in the medulla. Four different types of laminar monopolar neurons (L_1–L_4) have been described in the literature [Strausfeld and Braitenberg (1970); Boschek (1971). Trujillo-Cenóz (1965a) described two types on the basis of the morphology of the soma].

In order to allow synaptic interactions to take place, the retinula cell axons are brought into close association with the axons of the monopolar neurons in groups of fibers known as the optical cartridges (Cajal and Sánchez, 1915; Trujillo-Cenóz, 1965a), each of which is isolated from the others by epithelial glial cells in an orderly geometric pattern (Boschek, 1971). Each optical cartridge is composed of two centrally located axons of monopolar neurons, L_1 and L_2, surrounded by six retinula-cell-axon terminals belonging to R_1–R_6 from six different ommatidia. Associated with each retinula-cell axon in the cartridge is a pair of centrifugal fiber endings. In addition, fibers of monopolar neurons L_3 and L_4 are also found in the periphery of each cartridge. The axons of R_7 and R_8 do not enter the optical cartridges but proceed on to the medulla (the second synaptic region) without synapsing in the lamina (Cajal and Sánchez, 1915; Trujillo-Cenóz, 1965a). The axons of R_1–R_6, on the other hand, terminate near the proximal end of the cartridges, and the axons of the monopolar neurons proceed alone to the medulla.

On the basis of electron microscopical evidence, Boschek (1971) has described a complex pattern of synaptic interactions involving the axons of R_1–R_6, axons of L_1–L_4, the epithelial glial cells, and centrifugal and other unidentified fibers in the optical cartridge. The most numerous and straightforward of these is the synaptic inputs provided by the axon terminals of R_1–R_6 to the laminar neurons L_1 and L_2.

Electroretinogram (ERG)

As I discussed earlier, the identification of a mutant is based on the electroretinogram (ERG) because it is a reasonably good indicator of the physiological and structural integrity of the pheripheral retina and lamina of the compound eye. However, contrary to the apparent impression many people seem to have, electroretinography is neither a very sophisticated nor a very sensitive technique. Its main virtues are that the recordings can be obtained with relative ease and rapidity, even in inexperienced hands. However, interpretation of the signals is difficult.

The electroretinogram records the electrical potential change, elicited by the light stimulus, between an electrode placed on or in the cornea and another electrode (the reference electrode) placed in some electrically unresponsive portion of the animal. The electrical potential thus recorded arises from the current flow in the extracellular medium of the compound eye, the current flow being due to the summed electrical activities of the retinula cells (photoreceptors) as well as the neurons and, possibly, the glial cells of the optic lobe.

A typical ERG recorded from the compound eye of wild-type *D.*

melanogaster is reproduced in Table 1. Its amplitude is surprisingly large ($\sim$15 mV), and its waveform is similar to that of the ERG obtained from larger flies [for reviews see Goldsmith (1964, 1965) and Bullock and Horridge (1965)]. It is dominated by a corneal-negative component (downward deflection, Table 1) which is maintained as long as the light is on. In addition, the ERG contains a rapid, corneal-positive transient (the "on transient" or "on effect") when the light is first turned on and a corneal-negative transient (the "off transient" or "off effect") when the light is turned off. The corneal-negative, maintained component is thought mainly to reflect the primary ionic responses of the retinula cells (Goldsmith, 1965), although cells postsynaptic to the retinula cells also make minor contributions to the maintained component. The weight of evidence favors the view that neither the on nor the off transient originates from the retinula cells (Autrum and Hoffman, 1957, 1960; Burkhardt and Autrum, 1960; Wolbarsht *et al.*, 1966; Eichenbaum and Goldsmith, 1968; Alawi and Pak, 1971). Major portions of these transients probably originate in the lamina. However, the species of cells which are responsible for the generation of these transients have not yet been identified.

The evidence that the maintained component has its origin in the receptors has been well summarized by Goldsmith (1965). We recapitulate below the main lines of the argument.

If the optic lobe, including the lamina, is surgically removed and the recording is made from the remaining ommatidial layer, both the on and off transients are absent and only the maintained component is observed [(Bernhard, 1942), water beetle *Dytiscus*; (Jahn and Wulff, 1942), grasshopper *Trimerotropis*; (Autrum and Gallwitz, 1951; Hartline *et al.*, 1952), *Musca*; (Naka and Kuwabara, 1959), green bottle fly *Lucilia*; (Autrum *et al.*, 1961), blowfly *Calliphora*]. The sustained component has also been isolated by the use of nicotine [(Autrum and Hoffman, 1957), *Calliphora*], cocaine (Bernhard, 1942), and CO_2 [(Goldsmith, 1960), worker honeybee; (Wolbarsht *et al.*, 1966), cockroach *Periplaneta*], and by anoxia [(Autrum and Hoffman, 1960), *Calliphora*]. Moreover, the sustained component can be recorded in virtual isolation, free of the on and off transients, if the two electrodes are so placed as to include only the retinula-cell somata between the two electrode tips [(Ruck, 1961), *Lucilia*; (Pak *et al.*, 1969; Heisenberg, 1971*b*), *Drosophila*]. Finally, the receptor potential recorded intracellularly from the retinula cells shows a maintained potential change with a time course comparable to that of the maintained component of the ERG [(Burkhardt and Autrum, 1960), *Calliphora*; (Naka, 1961), *Lucilia* and dragonflies *Copera, Agriocnemis*, and *Lestes*; (Naka and Eguchi, 1962*a*), honeybee *Apis*; (Naka and Eguchi, 1962*b*), *Agriocnemis*; (Washizu, 1964), *Calliphora*; (Kirschfeld, 1966), *Musca*; (Alawi and Pak, 1971), *Drosophila*].

The same experiments have been cited to argue that both the on and off transients originate from neural elements postsynaptic to the receptor cells. No serious disagreement exists with regard to the assignment of the off transient to some as-yet-unidentified cells postsynaptic to the receptors. As for the on transient, on the other hand, Ruck (1961, 1962) maintained that it originates in the receptor-cell axon, which traverses through the lamina layer, and represents an active transmission of signal along the axon. According to this view, the failure to observe the on transient in most of the above experiments can be ascribed to injury to the axon, since any surgical or pharmacological isolation of the retinula cell layer is likely to damage the retinula-cell axons also. However, subsequent experiments which minimized or avoided the injury to retinula-cell axons also showed that the on transient does not occur in the retinula cell or its axon. These experiments can be summarized as follows: (1) The response from transplanted eyes consisting only of the retinula cells and their axons does not have the on transient (Wolbarsht *et al.,* 1966; Eichenbaum and Goldsmith, 1968). (2) A direct intracellular recording from the axons of the retinula cells fails to show the on transient (Järvilehto and Zettler, 1970). (3) Intracellular recordings from the retinula and lamina cells of *Drosophila* wild type and of a mutant which lacks the on transient show (a) that the on transient does not occur in the retinula cells of either the mutant or wild type, and (b) that a response closely resembling the on transient can be obtained from certain lamina cells of the wild type, but not from the mutant (Alawi and Pak, 1971).

The above discussion illustrates the difficulties involved in identifying the species of cells responsible for each of the several intermingled components of the ERG. Moreover, anatomically the retinula cells are not a homogeneous population. There is no *a priori* reason to suppose that the properties of all retinula-cell responses are the same. Any differences in response properties of different species of retinula cells cannot be recognized from the ERG. Indeed, the ERG alone is not sufficient to distinguish whether or not some of the retinula cells are blocked. Also, while the main contributions to the maintained component of the ERG are from the retinula cells, the optic lobe also makes minor contributions (Jahn and Wulff, 1942; Ruck, 1961; Heisenberg, 1971*b*). Thus, the fact that the on and off transients are missing in the ERG of a mutant does not necessarily mean that all lamina activities are blocked.

Nevertheless, electroretinography is a very useful technique in rapidly screening the mutants and in the preliminary localization of the site of lesion. However, a considerable caution ought to be exercised in any physiological interpretation based on the ERG. Much more significant results can be obtained from microelectrode techniques which allow intracellular recordings from single cells. This technique has found many applications in the study of the receptor responses of larger flies (Burkhardt and Autrum, 1960; Naka, 1961; Naka and Eguchi, 1962*a,b*;

Washizu, 1964; Kirschfeld, 1966; Scholes, 1969) and is being extended to the study of the lamina (Autrum *et al.*, 1970; Zettler and Järvilehto, 1971, 1972; Järvilehto and Zettler, 1971). In the case of the *Drosophila* visual system, however, the technique is only beginning to be explored (Alawi, 1972; Alawi and Pak, 1971; Alawi *et al.*, 1972). In addition to the visual cells, neurons in the thoracic ganglia of *Drosophila* are also yielding to the intracellular recording technique (Ikeda and Kaplan, 1970).

List of Mutants

I have listed in Tables 1 and 2B mutants belonging to five cistrons on the X chromosome and two cistrons on the third chromosome, respectively. All are recessive mutants, and all display abnormal ERG's that cannot be attributed to morphological malformations. A typical ERG waveform obtained from each group of mutants is displayed in the tables.

In addition, I list in Table 2A two complementing groups of sex-linked mutants that are best described as age-dependent degeneration mutants. These, too, are recessive mutants which display abnormal ERG's. Unlike the mutants listed in Tables 1 and 2B, however, the abnormal ERG's in these mutants are due to degeneration of the receptor structures (Hotta and Benzer, 1970; Heisenberg, 1971*a*).

Of these ERG mutants *tan* and *ebony* are well-known body color mutants (Lindsley and Grell, 1968). With the exception of *ebony* and *tan* alleles, all mutants listed are indistinguishable from wild type in external morphology or body color.

The "Cosens–Manning mutant" listed in Table 2B appeared spontaneously in a highly inbred line of the Pacific wild strain (Cosens and Manning, 1969; Cosens, 1971*a*). Thus, the *tan, ebony,* and Cosens-Manning mutants do not owe their origin to the recent mutagenesis programs. However, all remaining mutants, including many alleles of *tan,* were chemically induced and isolated by the Benzer, Götz, and Pak laboratories as described on pages 705–706.

There is now a total of well over a hundred independently obtained, ERG-defective mutants of the X chromosome in these three laboratories. Many of these behave as alleles of each other, i.e., a female heterozygous for two independently arising mutations has the mutant phenotype. Any such pair of mutations is regarded as affecting the same cistron. The assignment of the X-chromosome mutants to the seven cistrons shown in Tables 1 and 2A was made on this basis. Unfortunately, with isolated exceptions, complementation tests have not yet been made among mutants

TABLE 1. *Six Cistrons on the X Chromosome Affecting the Waveform of the ERG*[a]

New designations	norpA	tan	slrp	nonA	nonB
Old designations Pak lab[b]	x-12 Group	x-7 Group	x-28 Group[c]	x-14	
Benzer lab[d]	Receptor potential I group (JM11, etc.)	Positive spike I group (PC13, etc.)		Positive spike II group (BS18, etc.)	
Götz-Heisenberg lab[e]	opm3 group	opm8 group		opm2 group	opm18 group[f]
Map positions	6.5 ± 0.7^g 7 ± 1^e	27.5^h	$51.4 \begin{smallmatrix} +2.2 \\ -3.0 \end{smallmatrix}^c$	$52.3 \begin{smallmatrix} +1.8 \\ -1.4 \end{smallmatrix}^g$ 56 ± 5^e	40 ± 2^i

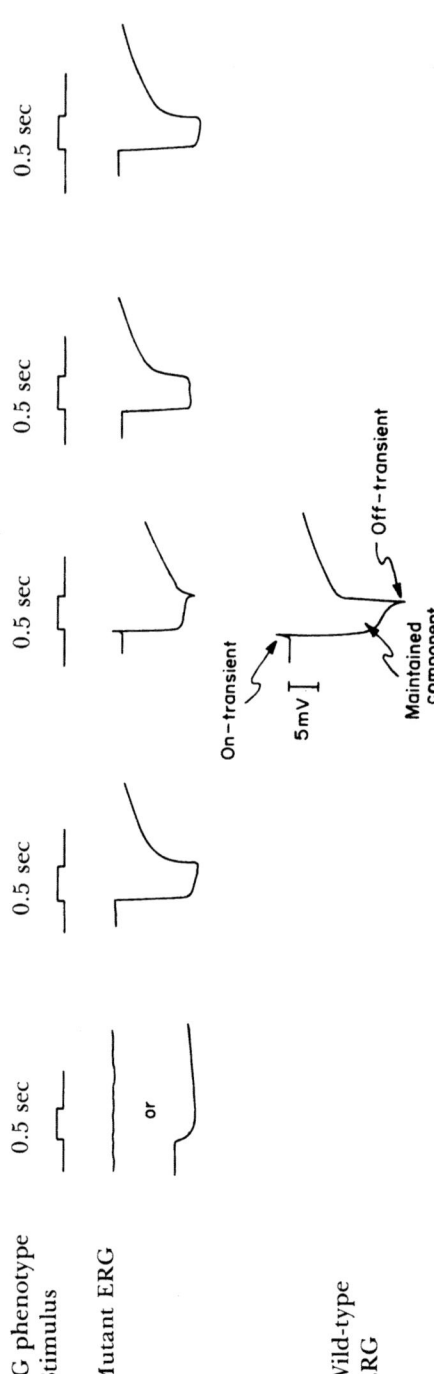

| ERG phenotype Stimulus | 0.5 sec | 0.5 sec | 0.5 sec | 0.5 sec | 0.5 sec |

Mutant ERG

or

On–transient

5mV

Off–transient

Maintained component

Wild-type ERG

[a] The abnormal ERG's in these mutants cannot be attributed to morphological malformations. In addition to these six cistrons there are four *non*-type cistrons on the X chromosome: *opm31* and *opm37* (Heisenberg, 1972a), *x-37* and *x-43* (Deland and Pak, unpublished). Information on these mutants is still of a preliminary nature.
[b] Pak *et al.* (1969, 1970).
[c] Pak laboratory (unpublished).
[d] Hotta and Benzer (1970).
[e] Heisenberg (1971a).
[f] Heisenberg (1972a, b).
[g] Grossfield and Pak (1971). The data have been pooled to obtain values shown.
[h] Lindsley and Grell (1968).
[i] Heisenberg (private communication).

TABLE 2. *Sex-Linked Degeneration Mutants and Autosomal Mutants*

	A. X Chromosome (degeneration mutants)[a]		B. Chromosome III[b]	
New Designations	rdgA	rdgB	ebony[c,f]	Cosens-Manning[a] mutant
Old designations				
Benzer lab[c]	Receptor degeneration I (BS12, etc.)	Receptor degeneration II (KO45, etc.)		
Götz-Heisenberg lab[d] / Pak lab[e]	opm1 Group / x-35 Group	opm6 Group / x-36 Group		
Map positions	29 ± 1[d]	33.0 < x < 56.7[d]	70.7[h]	
ERG phenotype				
Stimulus	0.5 sec	0.5 sec	0.5 sec	30 sec
Mutant ERG	Variable	Variable		
Wild-type ERG				

[a] Two cistrons on the X chromosome causing age-dependent degeneration of the visual system. In *rdg* mutants the degeneration is mainly confined to the receptor layer.
[b] Two cistrons on the third chromosome affecting the ERG. Neither of these two mutants was obtained in the recent mutagenesis programs designed to generate "nonphototactic" mutants. No obvious structural abnormalities are present in either mutant.
[c] Hotta and Benzer (1970).
[d] Heisenberg (1971a).
[e] Pak laboratory (unpublished).
[f] Heisenberg (1971b).
[g] Cosens and Manning (1969).
[h] Lindsley and Grell (1968).

generated in different laboratories. Moreover, the same sets of mutants have been described by the three laboratories under completely different names (Pak *et al.,* 1969, 1970; Hotta and Benzer, 1970; Heisenberg, 1971*a*). In order to avert the incipient chaos, representatives of the three laboratories have recently agreed on the new designations for the seven cistrons shown in Tables 1 and 2A.

In Table 1, the designations, *norp, non,* and *slrp* are based on the ERG waveforms and stand for *no receptor potential, no on transient,* and *slow receptor potential,* respectively. In Table 2A, *rdg* stands for *receptor degeneration.* The capital letters *A, B,* etc., are used to designate nonallelic mutants of similar phenotype.

In the absence of interlaboratory complementation tests, there is a degree of uncertainty in assigning mutants generated in different laboratories to a given cistron. Uncertainty is minimal for *norpA, tan,* and *nonA* alleles. The *tan* alleles have all been tested for complementation with *tan* by each laboratory (Pak *et al.,* 1969; Hotta and Benzer, 1970; Heisenberg, 1971*a*); three independently arising mutants of the *opm3* group, obtained by Heisenberg (*opm5, opm44,* and *opm52*), have been tested with *x-12* and found not to complement and, hence, affect the same cistron (Pak and K. Lidington, unpublished). Moreover, from the published accounts on ERG phenotypes and map positions, it appears almost certain that *receptor potential I, x-12,* and *opm3* groups belong together and that *positive spike II, x-14,* and *opm2* groups belong together as shown in Table 1 (Pak *et al.,* 1970; Hotta and Benzer, 1970; Heisenberg, 1971*a*).

The assignment of *opm 18* to a separate cistron, *nonB,* is based on complementation tests (Deland and Pak, unpublished), which indicated that *opm18* does not belong to the *tan* or *nonA* group, even though the ERG waveforms displayed by all these mutants are similar (Heisenberg, 1972*a*; Deland and Pak, unpublished). In addition, four other *non*-type loci have been detected on the X chromosome: *opm31* and *opm37* (Heisenberg, 1972*a*), *x-37* and *x-43* (Deland and Pak, unpublished). Complementation tests have shown that each of them is a new locus. These loci, however, have not been included in Table 1, because information on them is still incomplete.

On the other hand, the assignment in Table 2A of *receptor degeneration I, opm1,* and *x-35* groups to *rdgA* and that of *receptor degeneration II, opm6,* and *x-36* groups to *rdgB,* are both educated guesses. We know, however, that each of the three laboratories has obtained receptor-degeneration mutants belonging to two distinct complementation groups (Hotta and Benzer, 1970; Heisenberg, 1971*a*; Pak laboratory, unpublished). The only uncertainty involved is in knowing which complementation group of a given laboratory belongs to which one of the other laboratories. These uncertainties should clear up within the next few months, when complementation tests among mutants belonging to different laboratories will have been completed.

Descriptions of Mutants

The *norpA* Cistron

The mutants belonging to the *norpA* cistron (Table 1) are characterized by a complete or nearly complete absence of the ERG, suggesting that a lesion has occurred at the level of receptor potential production (Pak *et al.*, 1970; Hotta and Benzer, 1970; Alawi *et al.*, 1972). Consequently, this is the most interesting group of mutants from the point of view of the phototransduction process (Alawi *et al.*, 1972).

Most of the anatomical details of the visual system of *norpA* mutants are indistinguishable from those of wild type (Pak *et al.*, 1970; Alawi *et al.*, 1972). Even the rhabdomeres and the orientation of the microvillar axes of the rhabdomeres are normal under the electron microscope. The only obvious structural abnormalities are the zipperlike, electron-dense structures, about 300 Å in length and spaced at 200-Å intervals along the inside surface of the peripheral retinal cell membranes facing the intraommatidial space (Alawi *et al.*, 1972). These structures rarely invest the central retinula cell ($R_{7,8}$) membranes. Similar structures have also been observed, though only rarely, in the retinula cells of the wild type house fly *Musca domestica* (Boschek, 1971). The physiological significance of these "zipper" structures has not yet been established.

Hotta and Benzer (1970) considered the question of whether or not the defect in these mutants is autonomous, i.e., whether or not the defect resides in the eye itself or results from a lack of some circulating substance originating elsewhere. They resolved the question using the technique of genetic mosaics. In gynandromorphs a sex-linked, recessive deficit can be made to be expressed in the male tissues but not in the female tissues. In experiments involving a total of sixty gynandromorphs of *norpA* alleles every eye behaved autonomously, i.e., every male eye gave rise to a mutant ERG and every female eye a normal ERG.

The results of physiological experiments on these mutants lead one to the conclusions that normal visual pigments exist in the rhabdomeres of these mutants, that no receptor potential is produced by the peripheral retinula cells (R_1–R_6), at least in the groups of alleles studied, and that only unusually small responses are produced by the central retinula cells

(R_7 and R_8). Thus in these mutants, one or more of the steps linking photoexcitation of the visual pigment with the control of ion flow through the photoreceptor membrane appears blocked.

The evidence for this assertion may be summarized as follows.

1. If a slice of the mutant compound eye is viewed under the polarizing microscope, the rhabdomeres are found to display characteristic dichroism due to the presence of the visual pigment [Kirschfeld and Pak, cited in Alawi *et al.* (1972)].

2. In many alleles of this group a small residual ERG is obtained. The results of both the spectral sensitivity measurements of this residual response and of intracellular recordings in a number of *norpA* alleles suggest that the residual ERG originates from the central retinula cells (Pak *et al.*, 1970; Alawi *et al.*, 1972).

3. In intracellular recordings most of the retinula cells do not produce the receptor potential. These cells are presumed to be the peripheral retinula cells since they are the numerically preponderant of the two retinula cell species.

The intracellular recordings also showed that the peripheral retinula cells, which fail to produce the receptor potential, have a normal resting potential and a nearly normal membrane resistance (Alawi, 1972; Alawi *et al.*, 1972). Therefore, the failure to produce the receptor potential cannot be attributed to such trivial reasons as a "leaky" photoreceptor membrane or a grossly abnormal distribution of ions across the membrane in the resting state. The fault appears to lie in the inability of the rhabdomere membrane to increase its permeability to, say, sodium ions when the visual pigment is excited by light.

The notion that the peripheral retinula cells fail to produce the receptor potential is supported by the observation that the ommochrome granules in the retinula cells of the *norpA* mutants do not migrate with light adaptation (see page 711). Kirschfeld and Franceschini (1969) showed that if the compound eye of the house fly is light-adapted, a migration of pigment granules takes place in the peripheral retinula cells (R_1–R_6) to control the light flux through the rhabdomeres. Boschek (1971) has shown by electron microscopy that the pigment granules probably are identical to those identified to be ommochrome granules by Nolte (1961) and Fuge (1967) in *Drosophila*. In the dark-adapted eye the pigment is distributed throughout the retinula cells. If the eye is exposed to bright light, the pigment granules move in close to the interface between the rhabdomere and the soma of the retinula cell. The pigment granules are now in a position to interfere with internal reflection at the interface, thus reducing the light flux reaching the visual pigment under high ambiant light conditions. This migration of pigment granules can be observed in microscopic examinations either of a slice of the compound eye or of the "pseudopupil" (see page 728) of an intact animal (Kirschfeld, 1969; Kirschfeld and Franceschini, 1969). Heisenberg (1971a) has examined the pseudopupils of his *norpA* alleles and found that no migration of the pigment takes place even under conditions of strong illumination. These observations are consistent with our result that no receptor potential is generated in retinula cells 1-6, because, as Kirschfeld and Franceschini (1969) have proposed, the migration of the pigment granules is probably induced by the receptor potential. With no receptor potential there can be no message to signal migration of the pigment granules to the "light-adapted position."

Two of the *norpA* alleles have been found to be temperature sensitive. Temperature-sensitive mutants are of interest because often they may indicate the nature of the defect displayed by the mutants.

Hotta and Benzer (1970) reported that one of their *norpA* alleles (K050) displays nearly normal ERG and phototaxis at low temperature (18°C) but loses both properties in about an hour at 28°C. If the flies are then cooled back down to 18°C, both phototaxis and ERG return in about 20-30 hours. They interpreted these results to mean that a protein essential for the ERG is denatured at higher temperature and is resynthesized at lower temperature (Benzer, private communication).

Recently, we found that one of the *norpA* alleles (*opm52*) isolated and supplied us by Heisenberg is reversibly temperature sensitive (Deland and Pak, 1972). At low temperature (17°C) the mutant displays essentially normal ERG. Its receptor component (see pages 713-714) appears fully developed. Unlike Benzer's mutant described above, the ERG completely disappears as soon as the temperature is raised to about 32°C and begins to return as soon as the temperature is lowered again. Nearly complete recovery of the ERG is obtained within 10-15 minutes at 17°C.

These results present us with evidence that one or more proteins are involved in the production of the receptor potential. Moreover, since the ERG amplitude changes as soon as the temperature is altered in the second mutant, the control of ion flow during receptor potential generation is probably effected through conformational changes in the protein(s).

The proteins in the eyes of *norpA* mutants have been analyzed and compared to those in the wild-type eyes using SDS (sodium dodecyl sulfate) acrylamide disc gel electrophoretic technique (Ostroy and Pak, 1973). Two of the protein subunit bands having mobilities of 0.28 and 0.31 (corresponding to molecular weights of approximately 51,000 and

46,000, respectively) showed altered concentrations in the mutant eye. The mutant eyes have higher concentrations of the 0.28 protein and lower concentrations of the 0.31 protein. Identification of these proteins and clarification of the relation between the altered concentrations and the physiological defect are two of the challenging problems still remaining to be solved.

The *tan, ebony, nonA,* and *nonB* Cistrons

It is convenient to discuss these four groups of mutants (Table 1) together because of similarities both in ERG phenotype and optomotor behavior. Of these mutants, *tan* and *nonA* (BS18) have been tested for autonomy using gynandromorphs (Hotta and Benzer, 1970). Autonomous results were obtained in all cases studied.

The salient features of all four groups of mutants are that the on and off transients of the ERG are either absent or very small in amplitude (Pak *et al.*, 1969, 1970; Hotta and Benzer, 1969, 1970; Heisenberg, 1971a,b). Thus the ERG of these mutants consists primarily of the monophasic, corneal-negative, maintained component. Since this component of the ERG mainly reflects the activities of the receptor cells (see pages 713–714), an obvious interpretation of their ERG is that in these mutants all or most of the receptor cells are functioning normally but either the transmission of the signals to the second-order visual cells in the lamina or the excitation of the second-order cells is blocked in varying degrees (Pak *et al.*, 1969; Heisenberg, 1971b). This interpretation appears to be valid with certain qualifications. The following observations tend to support the interpretation:

1. If the ERG is obtained by placing the electrodes in such a way as to include only the receptor layer between the two electrode tips, mainly the photoreceptor responses are recorded (Ruck, 1961). The "mass receptor potential" so obtained from the mutant does not differ significantly from the wild-type mass receptor potential. [Pak *et al.* (1969) tested *tan;* Heisenberg (1971b) tested *tan, ebony,* and a *nonA* allele, *opm2.*]

2. In intracellular recordings, the receptor potential obtained from the retinula cell of *tan* does not substantially differ in waveform from the wild-type receptor potential (Alawi and Pak, 1971).

3. In mass recordings, if the electrodes are so placed as to monitor mainly the activities of the lamina, the lamina activities of these mutants are found to be substantially reduced in amplitude compared to wild type (Heisenberg, 1971b, 1972a). However, they

are not completely absent. In fact, according to Heisenberg (1971*b*), each of the mutants *tan, ebony,* and *nonA (opm2),* displays a "lamina potential" of a distinctively characteristic waveform.

4. Intracellular recordings have been obtained from what are presumed to be the epithelial glial cells in the lamina of wild type and *tan* (Alawi and Pak, 1971). The lamina cells of wild type gave rise to a distinctive potential consisting of a transient, on component and a small, maintained component. No such potential was observed from the lamina cells of *tan.*

The first two observations confirm the notion that the physiological activities of the majority or all of the retinula cells are unaffected by the mutations. This statement, however, does not rule out the possibility that one of the minority receptor species (R_7 or R_8) may be blocked. The third and fourth observations suggest that each of these mutations reduces, but does not completely stop, the activities of the interneurons in the lamina. The degree of suppression appears to vary from mutant to mutant, and the species of the lamina interneurons affected may also vary from one mutant to the next. Also, the possibility that the defects are not confined to the lamina and may extend, for example, to the medulla is not excluded by the electrophysiological evidence.

Since motion detection cannot take place without synaptic interactions between at least two photoreceptors, the lamina is the first structure which can conceivably subserve detection of movement necessary for the optomotor response. For this reason Heisenberg and Götz have been particularly interested in these mutants and have studied their optomotor behavior in some detail (Heisenberg, 1972*a,b*). These studies have been useful in further characterizing these mutants and promise to provide new insight into the mechanism of optomotor response.

On the basis of their studies on the compound eye of the house fly *M. domestica,* Kirschfeld and Franceschini (Kirschfeld and Franceschini, 1968; Kirschfeld, 1969) proposed that the fly visual system consists of two functionally distinct subsystems for processing visual information. One of these operates at relatively high light levels and specializes in the resolution of visual details, i.e., in high-contrast transfer (the high-acuity system), while the other handles vision at low light levels (the high-sensitivity system). The high-acuity system receives its inputs from the central retinula cells (R_7 and R_8) and is also sensitive to linearly polarized light [Kirschfeld and W. Reichardt, cited by Heisenberg (1972*b*)]. The high-sensitivity system, on the other hand, receives its inputs from the peripheral retinula cells (R_1–R_6). Thus, the high-sensitivity system operates via the laminar neurons, while the high-acuity system bypasses the synaptic interactions at the lamina level (see pages 711–712). The concept of a dual visual system outlined above is supported by the recent studies of McCann and Arnett (1972) on spectral and polarization sensitivities of the dipteran visual system.

Since the laminar activities are suppressed in the mutants of *tan, ebony, nonA,* and *nonB* cistrons, the high-sensitivity system is expected to be suppressed in these mutants, while the high-acuity system, which does not involve the laminar neurons, need not necessarily be disturbed at all. This hypothesis was tested by Heisenberg (1972a,b) by means of optomotor experiments designed to separately stimulate the two input channels. The principles behind his experiments are as follows: (1) Since the limit of resolution of the high-acuity system is below that of the high-sensitivity system, it is possible to stimulate only the high-acuity system by using narrow enough striped patterns (spatial wavelength of 7.2 deg.) on the optomotor drum. (2) The optomotor stimuli consisting of linearly polarized light will only be detected by the high-acuity system. (3) If the striped patterns on the optomotor drum are wide enough to allow the high-sensitivity system to be stimulated, the high-sensitivity system then determines the threshold of the optomotor responses by virtue of its greater sensitivity to low-intensity stimuli.

The results of his experiments suggest that in the case of the mutants *ebony* and *opm18* (an allele of *nonB*) the high-sensitivity system, which operates via the laminar neurons, is almost completely blocked but the high-acuity system is only slightly affected. Thus, in these mutants both the optomotor and phototactic responses appear to be entirely mediated through the high-acuity system, i.e., via the inputs from the central retinula cells. These results are consistent with the notion that the mutations have more or less specifically blocked the activities of the laminar neurons. Two other *non*-type mutants, *opm31* and *opm37,* mentioned on page 719, also seem to belong to this group. In these mutants too the mutations seem to disturb the high-sensitivity system without much effect on the high-acuity system (Heisenberg, 1972a).

In the case of the mutants *tan* and *opm2* (an allele of *nonA*), on the other hand, the effect of the mutations on the high-sensitivity system appears to be relatively minor but seems to completely block the high-acuity system. Thus, for example, the polarization sensitivity is lost in *opm2* while the threshold of optomotor responses with a wide-striped-pattern stimulus is nearly normal for both *tan* and *opm2* (Heisenberg, 1972a,b). In addition to the apparent blockage of the high-acuity system, these mutants display unusually poor visual acuity—much poorer than to be expected from the fact that the high-acuity system is not functional

(Heisenberg, 1972*a,b*). The reason for this defect is not clear. It does not seem to be due to poor optics of the mutants' dioptric apparatus, but rather it appears to be neural in origin.

These findings make clear the inadequacy of characterizing the mutants on the basis of the ERG waveform alone. On the other hand, the ERG recordings did suggest defective laminar activities in all these mutants. This expectation appears to be borne out, although the degree of laminar suppression varies greatly from mutant to mutant. The surprising result is that in *tan* and the *nonA* allele, *opm2,* the visual input channel employing the central retinula cells (the high-acuity system) appears to be blocked—a result that could not have been predicted from the ERG recordings.

The Cosens–Manning Mutant

This mutant (Table 2B) is normally phototactic under conditions of low illuminations but behaves as though blind in high ambient light (Cosens and Manning, 1969; Cosens, 1971*a*). Unlike the mutants we have already discussed, the ERG of this mutant contains all three components associated with the normal ERG, the on and off transients and the sustained, corneal-negative component (see pages 712–715). Indeed, ERG responses evoked from the mutant with stimuli of durations of less than 3 sec are similar to the wild-type response (Cosens and Manning, 1969; Cosens, 1971*a*). If stimuli of longer duration are used, the mutant ERG takes on a waveform strikingly different from that of the wild-type ERG. Unlike the wild-type ERG, the receptor component (sustained, corneal-negative component) of the mutant ERG decays to baseline in a few seconds, even in the presence of a sustained stimulus (Table 2B) (Cosens and Manning, 1969; Cosens, 1971*a*). The rate of decay is faster the brighter the stimulus light (Cosens, 1971*a*).

The time course of dark adaptation, i.e., the recovery of visual sensitivity in the dark following exposure to light, of the mutant eye is also very different from that of wild type. Cosens (1971*b*) studied the time course of the sensitivity changes by eliciting ERG responses to test flashes of given intensity in the dark-adapted eye and after exposing the eye to adapting light. In the case of wild type, the response to the test flash recovers approximately 80 percent of its dark-adapted amplitude within 2–4 sec after the removal of the adapting light, and then the recovery continues more gradually over tens of seconds. In the case of the mutant, the rapid phase of recovery appears to be absent. The recovery occurs gradually in 50–60 sec.

Cosens (1971*a*) has argued that the mutant eye is as sensitive as the wild-type eye in the dark-adapted state. Thus, initially the mutant photoreceptors respond to light normally, but the receptor potential rapidly decays in the presence of a high-level light stimulus. The blindness of the mutant in high ambient light is presumably related to this decline of the receptor potential.

Cosens (1971*a,b*) has offered the following hypotheses to account for the abnormally rapid decay of the receptor response during continuous exposure to bright light and for the slow recovery of the visual sensitivity following exposure to adapting light: Either the regeneration of the visual pigment bleached by light proceeds abnormally slowly in the mutant (Cosens, 1971*a*), or the mutant visual system lacks a mechanism enabling it to operate at high-ambient-light conditions (Cosens, 1971*b*). Evidence in support of either hypothesis is still largely circumstantial.

Cosens and Perry (1972), in electron microscopical studies, have found age-dependent degenerative changes in the rhabdomeres of the mutant photoreceptors. They find that at about 5 days after eclosion small areas of vesiculation begin to develop in the rhabdomeres. By two weeks, many of the rhabdomeres are reduced in size and the vesiculation partially disrupts many of the rhabdomeres. Since the functional abnormality of the mutant eye is already present at eclosion before any degenerative changes have taken place, these changes do not appear to be the direct cause of the visual malfunction (Cosens and Perry, 1972). Cosens and Perry (1972) suggest that the changes are brought about indirectly, perhaps, by a defect in the regeneration cycle of the visual pigment.

Unlike the case of wild type, the ommochrome granules in the retinula cells of the mutant do not move in all the way to the border between the rhabdomere and the cell soma when the eyes are light adapted (Cosens and Perry, 1972; see pages 711 and 721–722). The pigment migration stops about 1 μm short of the rhabdomeres, and the pigment granules accumulate in this region, as illustrated in retinula cells R_2–R_4 of Fig. 1C. If indeed the pigment migration is induced by the receptor potential (Kirschfeld and Franceschini, 1969) (see page 722), the incomplete migration may be related to the decay of the receptor potential during a sustained stimulus (ERG in Table 2B).

Other Mutants

Very little is known about the remaining three loci, *slrp, rdgA,* and *rdgB,* listed in Tables 1 and 2. Only a brief discussion will be given of these mutants.

slrp.   The ERG of the mutants belonging to the *slrp* cistron (Table 1) are characterized by on and off transients of somewhat reduced amplitude and by an abnormally slow return of the receptor component of the ERG to the baseline after the stimulus is turned off (Table 1). The abrupt decrease in amplitude characteristically observed in the wild-type ERG following the turning off of the stimulus is generally not seen in the mutant ERG (Table 1). The action spectrum of the mutant ERG is indistinguishable from that of the wild type, suggesting that no alterations have taken place in the visual pigments and that mainly the peripheral retinula cells contribute to the ERG, as is the case in the wild type (C. -F. Wu and Pak, unpublished). [The visual pigment in the central retinula cells has different absorption spectrum (Langer and Thorell, 1965).] In intracellular recordings (C. -F. Wu and Pak, unpublished) some of the retinula cells penetrated produce receptor potentials that are strikingly different from the wild-type receptor potential. The potential decays abnormally slowly. Many other cells, however, produce a perfectly normal receptor potential. Thus the analysis of the mutant phenotype is difficult because of the apparent heterogeneity of the mutant receptor potential phenotype.

Degeneration Mutants, *rdgA* and *rdgB*.   The two mutually complementing groups of mutants (Table 2A), *rdgA* and *rdgB,* are characterized by small and delayed ERG responses (Hotta and Benzer, 1970; Heisenberg, 1971a). The amplitude of the mutant ERG is less than $\frac{1}{50}$ to about $\frac{1}{5}$ of the normal amplitude (Heisenberg, 1971a). In both groups of mutants, extensive, age-dependent degeneration of the rhabdomeres can be observed by histology (Hotta and Benzer, 1970; K. Lidington and Pak, unpublished). The degeneration of rhabdomeres can also be seen by examining the pseudopupil. By suitable optical techniques it is possible to observe, in the eye of the intact animal, superposition of virtual images of homologous rhabdomere endings belonging to many neighboring ommatidia (Franceschini, 1972). The deep pseudopupil so observed retains the characteristic tetrahedral arrangement of rhabdomeres in the individual ommatidium. In the mutant, the pseudopupil is either less distinct than wild type or appears scrambled (Hotta and Benzer, 1970; Heisenberg, 1971a). Also, the migration of the ommochrome pigment granules of the retinula cells associated with light adaptation of the eye does not take place in these mutants (Heisenberg, 1971a), as was the case in *norpA*. One should note that in both groups of mutants the receptor potential is either absent or abnormally small in amplitude.

Hotta and Benzer (1970) have studied autonomy of the *rdgA* and *rdgB* mutants using gynandromorphs. In all cases studied, the eye was found to be autonomous in respect to both ERG and degeneration.

Acknowledgments

This work was supported in part by the National Science Foundation. I thank Drs. Michael Deland and R. S. Wilcox for their criticisms of the manuscript, Kellie Lidington and Andi Coggeshall for their technical assistance, and Lucy Winchester for her stenographic assistance.

Literature Cited

Adler, J., 1969 Chemoreceptors in bacteria. *Science (Wash., D.C.)* **166**:1588–1597.

Alawi, A. A., 1972 Electrophysiological investigation of genetically dissected visual processes in *Drosophila melanogaster*. Ph.D. Thesis, Purdue University, Lafayette, Ind.

Alawi, A. A. and W. L. Pak, 1971 On-transient of insect electroretinogram: Its cellular origin. *Science (Wash., D.C.)* **172**:1055–1057.

Alawi, A. A., V. Jennings, J. Grossfield and W. L. Pak, 1972 Phototransduction mutants of *Drosophila melanogaster*. In *Advances in Experimental Medicine and Biology*, Vol. 24, edited by G. B. Arden, pp. 1–9, Plenum Press, New York.

Autrum, H. and U. Gallwitz, 1951 Zur Analyse der Belichtungspotentiale des Insektenauges. *Z. Vgl. Physiol.* **33**:407–435.

Autrum, H. and C. Hoffman, 1957 Die Wirkung von Pikrotoxin und Nikotin auf das Retinogramm von Insekten. *Z. Naturforsch.* **12B**:752–757.

Autrum, H. and C. Hoffman, 1960 Diphasic and monophasic responses in the compound eye of *Calliphora*. *J. Insect Physiol.* **4**:122–127.

Autrum, H., I. Autrum and C. Hoffman, 1961 Komponenten im Retinogramm von *Calliphora* und ihre Abhängigkeit von der Spektralfarbe. *Biol. Zentralbl.* **80**:513–547.

Autrum, H., F. Zettler and M. Järvilehto, 1970 Postsynaptic potentials from a single monopolar neuron of the ganglion opticum I of the blowfly *Calliphora*. *Z. Vgl. Physiol.* **70**:414–424.

Benzer, S., 1967 Behavioral mutants of *Drosophila* isolated by countercurrent distribution. *Proc. Natl. Acad. Sci. USA* **58**:1112–1119.

Benzer, S., 1971 From gene to behavior. *J. Am. Med. Assoc.* **218**:1015–1022.

Bernhard, C. G., 1942 Isolation of retinal and optic ganglion responses in the eye of *Dytiscus*. *J. Neurophysiol.* **5**:32–48.

Boschek, C. B., 1971 On the fine structure of the peripheral retina and lamina ganglionaris of the fly, *Musca domestica*. *Z. Zellforsch.* **118**:369–409.

Braitenberg, V., 1967 Patterns of projection in the visual system of the fly. I. Retina-lamina projections. *Exp. Brain Res.* **3**:271–298.

Braitenberg, V., 1970 Ordnung und Orientierung der Elemente im Sehsystem der Fliege. *Kybernetik* **7**:235–242.

Brenner, S., 1974 The genetics of *Cacnorhabditis elegans*. *Genetics* **77**:71–94.

Brown, F. A., Jr. and B. V. Hall, 1936 The directive influence of light upon *Drosophila melanogaster* Meig and some of its eye mutants. *J. Exp. Zool.* **74**:205–220.

Bullock, T. H. and G. A. Horridge, 1965 Arthropoda: receptor for light and optic lobe. In *The Structure and Function of the Nervous System of Invertebrates*, Vol. 2, pp. 1063–1113, W. H. Freeman, San Francisco, Calif.

Burkhardt, D. and H. Autrum, 1960   Die Belichtungspotentiale Einzelner Sehzellen von *Calliphora erythrocephala* Meig. *Z. Naturforsch.* **15B**:612–616.

Cajal, S. R. and D. Sánchez, 1915   Contribución al conocimento de los centros nerviosos de los insectos. *Trab. Lab. Invest. Biol. Univ. Madrid* **13**:1–164.

Carpenter, F. W., 1905   The reactions of the pomace fly (*Drosophila ampelophila* Loew) to light, gravity, and mechanical stimulation. *Am. Nat.* **39**:157–171.

Cosens, D. J., 1971*a*   Blindness in a *Drosophila* mutant. *J. Insect Physiol.* **17**:285–302.

Cosens, D. J., 1971*b*   Some factors affecting the rate of dark adaptation in certain insects. *J. Insect Physiol.* **17**:955–968.

Cosens, D. J. and A. Manning, 1969   Abnormal electroretinogram from a *Drosophila* mutant. *Nature (Lond.)* **224**:285–287.

Cosens, D. J. and M. M. Perry, 1972   The fine structure of the eye of a visual mutant, A-type, of *Drosophila melanogaster. J. Insect Physiol.* **18**:1773–1786.

Cromartie, R. I. T., 1959   Insect pigments. *Annu. Rev. Entomol.* **4**:59–76.

Danneel, R. and B. Zeutzschel, 1957   Über den Feinbau der Retinula bei *Drosophila melanogaster. Z. Naturforsch.* **12B**:580–583.

Deland, M. C. and W. L. Pak, 1973   Reversibly temperature sensitive phototransduction mutant of *Drosophila melanogaster. Nat. New Biol.* **244**:184–186.

Demerec, M., 1950   *Biology of Drosophila*, p. 505, John Wiley & Sons, New York.

Dietrich, W., 1909   Die Facettenaugen der Dipteren. *Z. Wiss. Zool.* **92**:465–539.

Dobzhansky, T. and B. Spassky, 1967   Effects of selection and migration on geotactic and phototactic behavior of *Drosophila.* I. *Proc. R. Soc. Lond. Ser. B* **168**:27–47.

Eichenbaum, D. M. and T. H. Goldsmith, 1968   Properties of insect photoreceptor cells lacking synapses. *J. Exp. Zool.* **169**:15–32.

Fernández-Morán, H., 1956   Fine structure of the insect retinula as revealed by electron microscopy. *Nature (Lond.)* **177**:742–743.

Franceschini, N., 1972   Pupil and pseudopupil in the compound eye of *Drosophila.* In *Information Processing in the Visual Systems of Arthropods,* edited by R. Wehner, pp. 75–82, Springer-Verlag, Berlin.

Fuge, H., 1967   Die Pigmentbildung im Auge von *Drosophila melanogaster* und ihre Beeinflussung durch den white[+]-Locus. *Z. Zellforsch.* **83**:468–507.

Fuortes, M. G. F. and A. L. Hodgkin, 1964   Changes in time scale and sensitivity in the ommatidia of *Limulus. J. Physiol.* **172**:239–263.

Gavel, L., 1939   Die "kritische Streifenbreite" als Mass der Sehschärfe bei *Drosophila melanogaster. Z. Vgl. Physiol.* **27**:80–135.

Goldsmith, T. H., 1960   The nature of the retinal action potential and the spectral sensitivities of ultraviolet and green receptor systems of the compound eye of the worker honeybee. *J. Gen. Physiol.* **43**:775–799.

Goldsmith, T. H., 1964   The visual system of insects. In *The Physiology of Insects,* Vol. 1, edited by E. Rockstein, pp. 377–462, Academic Press, New York.

Goldsmith, T. H., 1965   Do flies have a red receptor? *J. Gen. Physiol.* **49**:265–287.

Goldsmith, T. H. and D. E. Philpott, 1957   The microstructure of the compound eyes of insects. *J. Biophys. Biochem. Cytol.* **3**:429–440.

Götz, K. G., 1964   Optomotorische Untersuchung des visuellen Systems einiger Augenmutanten der Fruchtfliege *Drosophila. Kybernetik* **2**:77–92.

Götz, K. G., 1970   Fractionation of *Drosophila* populations according to optomotor traits. *J. Exp. Biol.* **52**:419–436.

Grossfield, J. and W. L. Pak, 1971   Localization of the electroretinogram mutants. *Drosophila Inf. Serv.* **47**:59.

Hadler, N. M., 1964   Heritability and phototaxis in *Drosophila melanogaster. Genetics* **50**:1269–1277.

Hartline, H. K., H. G. Wagner and E. F. MacNichol, Jr., 1952   The peripheral origin of nervous activity in the visual system. *Cold Spring Harbor Symp. Quant. Biol.* **17**:125–141.

Hecht, S. and G. Wald, 1934   The visual acuity and intensity discrimination of *Drosophila. J. Gen. Physiol.* **17**:517–547.

Heisenberg, M., 1971*a*   Isolation of mutants lacking the optomotor response. *Drosophila Inf. Serv.* **46**:68.

Heisenberg, M., 1971*b*   Separation of receptor and lamina potentials in the 'electroretinogram of normal and mutant *Drosophila. J. Exp. Biol.* **55**:85–100.

Heisenberg, M., 1972*a*   Behavioral diagnostics: A way to analyze visual mutants of *Drosophila.* In *Information Processing in the Visual Systems of Arthropods,* edited by R. Wehner, pp. 265–268, Springer-Verlag, Berlin.

Heisenberg, M., 1972*b*   Comparative behavioral studies of two visual mutants of *Drosophila. J. Comp. Physiol.* **80**:119–136.

Hirsch, J., 1962   Individual differences in behavior and their genetic basis. In *Roots of Behavior,* edited by E. L. Bliss, Hafner, Hoeber, New York.

Hirsch, J. and J. C. Boudreau, 1958   Studies in experimental behavior genetics. I. The heritability of phototaxis in a population of *Drosophila melanogaster. J. Comp. Physiol. Psychol.* **51**:647–651.

Hirsch, J. and R. C. Tryon, 1956   Mass screening and reliable individual measurement in the experimental behavior genetics of lower organisms. *Psychol. Bull.* **53**:402–410.

Horridge, G. and I. Meinertzhagen, 1970   The accuracy of the patterns of connections of the first- and second-order neurons of the visual system of *Calliphora. Proc. R. Soc. Lond. Ser. B* **175**:69–82.

Hotta, Y. and S. Benzer, 1969   Abnormal electroretinograms in visual mutants of *Drosophila. Nature (Lond.)* **222**:354–356.

Hotta, Y. and S. Benzer, 1970   Genetic dissection of the *Drosophila* nervous system by means of mosaics. *Proc. Natl. Acad. Sci. USA* **67**:1156–1163.

Ikeda, K. and W. D. Kaplan, 1970   Patterned neural activity of a mutant *Drosophila melanogaster. Proc. Natl. Acad. Sci. USA* **66**:765–772.

Jahn, T. L. and V. J. Wulff, 1942   Allocation of electrical responses from the compound eye of grasshoppers. *J. Gen. Physiol.* **26**:75–88.

Järvilehto, H. and F. Zettler, 1970   Micro-localization of lamina-located visual cell activities in the compound eye of the blowfly, *Calliphora. Z. Vgl. Physiol.* **69**:134–138.

Järvilehto, M. and F. Zettler, 1971   Localized intracellular potentials from pre- and postsynaptic components in the external plexiform layer of an insect retina. *Z. Vgl. Physiol.* **75**:422–440.

Johannsen, O. A., 1924   Eye structure in normal and eye-mutant *Drosophila. J. Morphol. Physiol.* **39**:337–349.

Kalmus, H., 1943   The optomotor responses of some eye mutants of *Drosophila. J. Genet.* **45**:206–213.

Kirschfeld, K., 1966   Discrete and graded receptor potentials in the compound eye of the fly *Musca.* In *The Functional Organization of the Compound Eye,* edited by C. G. Bernhard, pp. 291–307, Pergamon Press, Oxford.

Kirschfeld, K., 1967   Die Projektion der Optischen Umwelt auf des Raster der Rhabdomere im Komplexauge von *Musca. Exp. Brain Res.* **3**:248–270.

Kirschfeld, K., 1969   Optics in the compound eye. In *Proc. Interntl. School Phys. Enrico Fermi Course XLIII*, edited by W. Reichardt, pp. 144–166, Academic Press, New York.

Kirschfeld, K. and N. Franceschini, 1968   Optische Eigenschaften der Ommatidien im Komplexauge von *Musca. Kybernetik* **5**:47–52.

Kirschfeld, K. and N. Franceschini, 1969   Ein Mechanismus zur Steuerung des Lichtflusses in den Rhabdomeren des Komplexauges von *Musca. Kybernetik* **6**:13–22.

Konopka, R. J. and S. Benzer, 1971   Clock mutants of *Drosophila melanogaster. Proc. Natl. Acad. Sci. USA* **68**:2112–2116.

Kung, C., 1971   Genic mutants with altered system of excitation in *Paramecium aurelia*. II. Mutagenesis, screening and genetic analysis of the mutants. *Genetics* **69**:29–45.

Langer, H. and B. Thorell, 1965   Microspectrophotometry of single rhabdomeres in the insect eye. *Exp. Cell. Res.* **41**:673–677.

Lindsley, D. L. and E. H. Grell, 1968   *Genetic Variations of Drosophila melanogaster.* Carnegie Institution of Washington, Washington, D.C.

McCann, G. D. and D. W. Arnett, 1972   Spectral and polarization sensitivity of the dipteran visual system. *J. Gen. Physiol.* **59**:534–558.

McEwen, R. S., 1918   The reactions to light and to gravity in *Drosophila* and its mutants. *J. Exp. Biol.* **25**:49–106.

Melamed, J. and O. Trujillo-Cenóz, 1968   The fine structure of the central cells in the ommatidia of dipterans. *J. Ultrastruct. Res.* **21**:313–334.

Naka, K. I., 1961   Recording of retinal action potentials from single cells in the insect compound eye. *J. Gen. Physiol.* **44**:571–584.

Naka, K. I. and E. Eguchi, 1962a   Spike potentials recorded from the insect photoreceptor. *J. Gen. Physiol.* **45**:663–680.

Naka, K. I. and E. Eguchi, 1962b   Effect of background illumination on the retinal action potential. *Science (Wash., D.C.)* **136**:877–879.

Naka, K. I. and M. Kuwabara, 1959   Electrical response from the compound eye of *Lucilia. J. Insect Physiol.* **3**:41–49.

Nolte, D. J., 1961   The pigment granules in two compound eyes of *Drosophila. Heredity* **16**:25–38.

Ostroy, S. E. and W. L. Pak, 1973   Protein differences associated with a phototransduction mutant of *Drosophila. Nat. New Biol.* **243**:120–121.

Pak, W. L., J. Grossfield and N. V. White, 1969   Nonphototactic mutants in a study of vision of *Drosophila. Nature (Lond.)* **222**:351–354.

Pak, W. L., J. Grossfield and K. Arnold, 1970   Mutants of the visual pathway of *Drosophila melanogaster. Nature (Lond.)* **227**:518–520.

Power, M. E., 1943   The brain of *Drosophila melanogaster. J. Morphol.* **72**:517–559.

Richards, M. H. and E. Y. Furrow, 1925   The eye and optic tract in normal and 'eyeless' *Drosophila. Biol. Bull.* **48**:243–259.

Ruck, P., 1961   Photoreceptor cell responses and flicker fusion frequency in the compound eye of the fly, *Lucilia sericata* (Meigen). *Biol. Bull.* **120**:375–383.

Ruck, P., 1962   On photoreceptor mechanisms of retinula cells. *Biol. Bull.* **123**:618–634.

Schneider, L. and H. Langer, 1966   Die Feinstruktur des Überganges zwischen Kristallkegel und Rhabdomeren im Facettenauge von *Calliphora. Z. Naturforsch.* **21B**:196–197.

Scholes, J., 1969   The electrical responses of the retinal receptors and the lamina in the visual system of the fly *Musca. Kybernetik* **6**:149–162.

Scott, J. P., 1947 Effects of single genes on the behavior of *Drosophila. Am. Nat.* **77**:184–190.

Sidman, R. L., M. C. Green and H. A. Appel, 1965 *Catalog of the Neurobiological Mutants of the Mouse,* Harvard University Press, Cambridge, Mass.

Strausfeld, N. J., 1971*a* The organization of the insect visual system (light microscopy). I. Projections and arrangements of neurons in the lamina ganglionaris of Diptera. *Z. Zellforsch.* **121**:377–441.

Strausfeld, N. J., 1971*b* The organization of the insect visual system (light microscopy). II. The projection of fibers across the first optic chiasma. *Z. Zellforsch.* **121**:442–454.

Strausfeld, N. J. and V. Braitenberg, 1970 The compound eye of the fly (*Musca domestica*): Connections between the cartridges of the lamina ganglionaris. *Z. Vgl. Physiol.* **70**:95–104.

Tomita, T., 1970 Electrical activity of vertebrate photoreceptors. *Quart. Rev. Biophys.* **3**:179–222.

Trujillo-Cenóz, O., 1965*a* Some aspects of the structural organization of the intermediate retina of Dipterans. *J. Ultrastruct. Res.* **13**:1–33.

Trujillo-Cenóz, O., 1965*b* Some aspects of the structural organization of the arthropod eye. *Cold Spring Harbor Symp. Quant. Biol.* **30**:371–382.

Trujillo-Cenóz, O., 1969 Some aspects of the structural organization of the medulla in muscoid flies. *J. Ultrastruct. Res.* **27**:533–553.

Trujillo-Cenóz, O. and J. Melamed, 1963 On the fine structure of the photoreceptor. Second optical neuron synapse in the insect retina. *Z. Zellforsch.* **59**:71–77.

Trujillo-Cenóz, O. and J. Melamed, 1966 Electron microscope observations on the peripheral and intermediate retinas of Dipterans. In *The Functional Organization of the Compound Eye,* edited by C. G. Bernhard, pp. 339–361, Pergamon Press, London.

Trujillo-Cenóz, O. and J. Melamed, 1970 Light and electronmicroscope study of one of the systems of centrifugal fibers found in the lamina of muscoid flies. *Z. Zellforsch.* **110**:336–349.

Waddington, C. H. and M. M. Perry, 1960 The ultrastructure of the developing eye of *Drosophila. Proc. Roy. Soc. Lond. Ser. B* **153**:155–178.

Wald, G., 1968 Molecular basis of visual excitation. *Science (Wash., D.C.)* **162**:230–239.

Washizu, Y., 1964 Electrical activity of single retinula cells in the compound eye of the blowfly, *Calliphora erythrocephalis* (Meig.). *Comp. Biochem. Physiol.* **12**:369–387.

Wolbarsht, M. L., H. Wagner and D. Bodenstein, 1966 Origin of electrical responses in the eye of *Periplaneta americana.* In *The Functional Organization of the Compound Eye,* edited by C. G. Bernhard, pp. 207–217, Pergamon Press, London.

Wolken, J. J., J. Capenos and A. Turano, 1957 Photoreceptor structure. III. *Drosophila melanogaster. J. Biophys. Biochem. Cytol.* **3**:441–457.

Zettler, F. and M. Järvilehto, 1971 Decrement-free conduction of graded potentials along the axon of a monopolar neuron. *Z. Vgl. Physiol.* **75**:402–421.

Zettler, F. and M. Järvilehto, 1972 Lateral inhibition in an insect eye. *Z. Vgl. Physiol.* **76**:233–244.

27

Mutations Influencing Male Fertility in *Drosophila melanogaster*

Lynn J. Romrell

Introduction

The study of *Drosophila* spermiogenesis is a promising model system for the elucidation of gene-regulated mechanisms controlling the poorly understood processes of cell differentiation. Since the genetics of this dipteran is so well established, this system provides a unique opportunity to examine the effects of mutations or experimental alterations of sperm development. A promising approach is the electron microscopic study of specific structural or developmental anomalies correlated with specific male-sterile mutants. These analyses of specific male-sterile mutants may be used to elucidate the role of genetic function during spermatogenesis.

Normal Spermatogenesis

A knowledge of normal spermatogenesis is obviously required in the analysis of male-sterile mutants. Spermatogenesis in *Drosophila* has been

Lynn J. Romrell—Department of Pathology, Division of Anatomical Sciences, College of Medicine, University of Florida, Gainesville, Florida.

the subject of numerous investigations [see Cooper (1950) for review of the early studies]. Electron microscopic studies of *Drosophila* spermatogenesis include general accounts of spermiogenesis (Leik, 1965; Anderson, 1967; Meyer, 1968; Tates, 1971) and observations on the development of particular organelles or regions such as the head (Shoup, 1967; Tokuyasu, 1974*b*), the tail (Baccetti, 1963; Baccetti and Bairati, 1964; Bairati and Baccetti, 1964; Kiefer, 1966, 1970; Tokuyasu, 1974*a*), the Nebenkern (Yasuzumi *et al.*, 1958), the paracrystalline body (Meyer, 1964, 1966), and the cell surface (Baccetti *et al.*, 1971). Perotti (1969) has given a detailed description of mature sperm ultrastructure. The early events of spermatogenesis have been studied by Rasmussen (1973) with special attention given to meiosis.

Further details on sperm development have been provided by Tokuyasu *et al.* (1972*a,b*) in descriptions of the individualization process, which results in the transformation of sperm from a syncytial to an individual state, and the coiling process which occurs during sperm development. A good description of the early stages of spermatogenesis is available in Tates' (1971) study of spermatogenesis in X^c, yB/sc^{8Y} *Drosophila*. In a recent study (Stanley *et al.*, 1972) a detailed correlation of organelle development during spermiogenesis in wild-type *Drosophila melanogaster* was made, and 11 developmental stages of spermiogenesis were described. These studies have established a basis of reference for the study of sperm development in male-sterile mutants.

Analysis of Male-Sterile Mutants

Male sterility in *Drosophila* may result from sex-linked or autosomal mutations (see Table 1) (Edmondson, 1951; Lindsley and Grell, 1968) and from chromosomal aberrations (Hess, 1975; Lifschytz and Lindsley, 1972). Table 1 is a list of available mutants of *D. melanogaster* that demonstrate male sterility and abnormal sperm development. Excluded from the list were mutants in which sterility may result from indirectly related factors, such as structural changes which interfere with normal breeding. Sterility is commonly associated with mutations affecting eye, wing, or abdominal development (Lindsley and Grell, 1968). Included in the table is a brief description of the anomalies associated with spermatogenesis in each mutant; for more detail see the indicated reference(s).

Y-Chromosome Mutants

The role of the Y chromosome in sperm development has been studied extensively. In a classical study Bridges (1916) observed sterility in *Drosophila* males lacking the Y chromosome. This observation was followed by numerous attempts to determine the genetic activities of the Y chromosome during spermatogenesis [for review see Hess and Meyer (1968) and Hess (1975)]. The existence of seven linearly arranged fertility factors on the Y chromosome has been established (Brosseau, 1960; Williamson, 1970, 1972). Studies of formation of lampbrush loops on the Y chromosome in primary spermatocytes demonstrate that a complete set of loop-forming loci, presumably Y fertility factors, are necessary for normal sperm development [reviewed in Meyer (1968) and Hess (1975)].

Ultrastructural analyses of X/0 males (Kiefer, 1966; Hess and Meyer, 1968; Meyer, 1968) have revealed anomalies usually limited to the Nebenkern derivatives and axonemal complexes. Kiefer (1968, 1969, 1970) has described spermiogenesis in flies carrying deficiencies for part of the Y chromosome. In all cases sperm develop more normally than in X/0 males. One mutant, *k1-1⁻*, produced motile sperm. Differences between Y mutants were reported to be quantitative rather than qualitative. No organelles were absent in X/0 or Y-deficiency males. These observations led to the postulation (Hess and Meyer, 1968; Meyer, 1969) that the Y fertility factors function in the organization of sperm organelles, since the disorientation of hese elements seemed to be the major effect of Y-chromosome deficiencies. Another interesting observation on Y-chromosome effects has been the correlation of increased sperm length with partial or total Y duplications [see Hess and Meyer (1968)]. The sperm of X/Y/Y *D. melanogaster* males are approximately twice the length of sperm from normal X/Y males. This suggests that the Y chromosome may function, possibly as an inducer, in the regulation of genes which supply structural elements for the spermatids.

Sex-Linked and Autosomal Mutants

Although the role of non-Y genes in spermatogenesis has not been extensively studied, investigations of X chromosome and autosomal mutants have added to our understanding of genetic function in this process.

Lindsley (1968) isolated 127 sex-linked male-sterile mutants induced by gamma rays. About 80 percent of these mutants had X-chromosome translocations to the second or third chromosome. These mutants demonstrated failure of head elongation in spermatids. The remaining sex-linked and 50 autosomal male-sterile mutants collected from natural populations demonstrated abortive sperm differentiation. Apparently there was no detailed ultrastructural analysis of sperm development in these mutants.

The analysis of a male-sterile translocation heterozygote (Shoup,

TABLE 1. *Mutations of Drosophila melanogaster Influencing Male Fertility and Sperm Development*[a]

Fertility factor	Mutation[b]	Deficiencies for locus	Comments[c]	References
Y CHROMOSOME				
kl-1	Male sterile in long arm of Y chromosome	ms(Y)-L4, -L10, -L13, -L32	1, 2, 3, 12, 15, 18, 21, 23, 24, 26, 29, 31	Brosseau (1960), Kiefer (1968, 1969)
kl-2	Male sterile in long arm of Y chromosome	ms(Y)-L1, -L12, -132, -L37, -L4		
kl-3	Male sterile in long arm of Y chromosome	ms(Y)-L1, -L4, -L7, -L10, -L11, -L12, -L32, -L38	1, 2, 3, 12, 13, 15, 18, 23, 24, 27	Brosseau (1960), Kiefer (1968)
kl-4	Male sterile in long arm of Y chromosome	ms(Y)-L1, -L4, -L7, -L36, -L38		
kl-5	Male sterile in long arm of Y chromosome	ms(Y)-L1, -L3, -L4, -L7, -L36		
ks-1	Male sterile in short arm of Y chromosome	ms(Y)-S2, -S4, -S6- -S7, -S8, -S10, -S11, -S12, -S13, -S14	1, 2, 3, 12, 13, 15, 18, 23, 24, 27	Brown and King (1961), Kiefer (1968)
ks-2	Male sterile in short arm of Y chromosome	ms(Y)-S5, -S14	1, 2, 3, 12, 13, 15, 18, 23, 24, 27	Brosseau (1960), Kiefer (1968)
nullo Y	Y chromosome absent		1, 2, 3, 17, 18, 20, 21, 25, 27	Bridges (1916), Brosseau (1960), Hess and Meyer (1968), Kiefer (1966), Meyer (1968)

Genetic locus	Mutation	Alleles studied	Comments[c]	References
X CHROMOSOME AND AUTOSOMES				
X-56.7	lethal (1) variegated 451	l(1)v451	1, 3, 11, 24, 27	Lindsley et al. (1968)
X-62.9	Recovery Disrupter (1)	RD(1)	1, 4, 7, 9, 17, 32	Erickson (1965)
2-3	male sterile (2) 1R	ms(2)1R, ms(2)2R	1, 2, 3, 18, 20, 25	Romrell (1971)
2-51	male sterile (2) 3R	ms(2)3R	1, 2, 3, 5, 16, 20, 23, 24, 27, 30	Romrell (1971), Romrell et al. (1972a)
2-54.8	male sterile (2) 11R	ms(2)11R	1, 2, 3, 14	Romrell (1971)
2-54.9	extra sex combs	esc	1, 3, 5, 24, 27	Slifer (1942)
2-55	Segregation Distorter	SD	1, 2, 8, 13, 22, 26	Hartl (1969), Peacock and Erickson (1965), Sandler et al. (1959), Tokuyasu et al. (1972a, b)
2-65.5	male sterile (2) 1	ms(2)1	1, 3, 24, 27	Lindsley and Grell (1968)

[a] Mutants were not included in the list unless studies indicated aberrant spermatogenesis. Mutants no longer available were excluded.

[b] Additional information for most mutants found in Lindsley and Grell (1968).

[c] Key to comments:

(1) studied at light microscope level
(2) studied at electron microscope level
(3) male sterile
(4) reduced fertility in males
(5) female sterile
(6) reduced fertility in females
(7) abnormal sex ratio in progeny of males
(8) abnormal segregation of second chromosome in males
(9) temperature sensitive
(10) testis rudimentary
(11) spermatogenesis appears normal
(12) meiosis appears normal
(13) early spermiogenesis normal
(14) spermatogenesis stops at primary spermatocyte stage
(15) spermiogenesis slightly more normal than in X/O males
(16) failure of cytokinesis

(17) reduction in number of sperm per bundle
(18) limited elongation and maturation of sperm
(19) abnormal differentiation of sperm head
(20) abnormal differentiation of mitochondrial derivatives
(21) axonemal complex disrupted or abnormal
(22) failure of individualization process
(23) degenerating sperm in testis
(24) some mature sperm produced
(25) no mature sperm produced
(26) sperm motile
(27) sperm nonmotile
(28) males fail to copulate
(29) sperm transferred during copulation
(30) no sperm transferred during copulation
(31) sperm not stored in female
(32) meiosis abnormal
(33) homozygous females transformed into sterile males.

TABLE 1. Continued

Genetic locus	Mutation	Alleles studied	Comments[c]	References
X CHROMOSOME AND AUTOSOMES (Continued)				
2-84	male sterile (2) 10R	ms(2)10R	1, 2, 3, 18, 20, 21, 27, 30	Romrell (1971), Romrell et al. (1972b)
3-45	transformer	tra⁶, tra^D	1, 10, 33	Brown and King (1961), Fung and Gowen (1957), Gowen and Fung (1957)
3-	male sterile (3) 3R	ms(3)3R	1, 2, 3, 5, 13, 23, 28	Romrell (1971), Wilkinson (1972)
3-	male sterile (3) 10R	ms(3)10R	1, 2, 3, 5, 19	Wilkinson et al. (1974)
TRANSLOCATIONS				
T(1;2H)	X; 2nd translocation	T(1; 2H)25(20)j125	1, 2, 3, 19, 25	Shoup (1967)
T(X;A)	X; autosome translocations			Lifschytz and Lindsley (1972), Lindsley (1968)

[a] Mutants were not included in the list unless studies indicated aberrant spermatogenesis. Mutants no longer available were excluded.

[b] Additional information for most mutants found in Lindsley and Grell (1968).

[c] Key to comments:

(1) studied at light microscope level
(2) studied at electron microscope level
(3) male sterile
(4) reduced fertility in males
(5) female sterile
(6) reduced fertility in females
(7) abnormal sex ratio in progeny of males
(8) abnormal segregation of second chromosome in males
(9) temperature sensitive
(10) testis rudimentary
(11) spermatogenesis appears normal
(12) meiosis appears normal
(13) early spermiogenesis normal
(14) spermatogenesis stops at primary spermatocyte stage
(15) spermiogenesis slightly more normal than in X/O males
(16) failure of cytokinesis

(17) reduction in number of sperm per bundle
(18) limited elongation and maturation of sperm
(19) abnormal differentiation of sperm head
(20) abnormal differentiation of mitochondrial derivatives
(21) axonemal complex disrupted or abnormal
(22) failure of individualization process
(23) degenerating sperm in testis
(24) some mature sperm produced
(25) no mature sperm produced
(26) sperm motile
(27) sperm nonmotile
(28) males fail to copulate
(29) sperm transferred during copulation
(30) no sperm transferred during copulation
(31) sperm not stored in female
(32) meiosis abnormal
(33) homozygous females transformed into sterile males.

1967) has provided a fairly detailed account of nuclear changes and micro-tubular development during spermiogenesis. She compared spermiogenesis in wild-type males and in the male-sterile stock by cytological and electron microscopic methods. The mutant showed abnormal nuclear elongation and failure in the conversion from lysine-rich to arginine-rich histones. The absence of the bundle of microtubules normally present in association with the nucleus during early spermiogenesis was demonstrated in mutant flies. Although these observations do not establish a causal relationship, they do correlate a particular mutation with relatively specific biochemical and morphological defects.

Wilkinson (1972) and Wilkinson *et al.* (1974) described sper-miogenesis in a third-chromosome mutant, *ms(3)10R,* which demonstrates abnormal differentiation and shaping of the sperm head. He suggests that cytoplasmic microtubules may have an inductive action on condensation of chromatin and in turn on the differentiation and shaping of the head.

The analysis of spermiogenesis in mutants allows one to not only define the effects of mutation as to structural defects, but also to inves-tigate the developmental interrelationships of organelles. The most ap-parent feature of *ms(2)10R* spermatids is the disruption of the normal spatial relationship of organelles and the basic $9 + 2$ configuration of the axonemal complex (Romrell *et al.,* 1972*a*). In spite of these anomalies, a normal complement of organelles are present. A second mutant studied by Romrell *et al.* (1972*b*) is characterized by a failure of cytokinesis which leaves four spermatids to develop in a common cytoplasm. In both mutants multiple paracrystalline bodies form within the primary Neben-kern derivative where normally only one paracrystalline body is present. Paracrystalline bodies apparently form at each point of contact between the membranes surrounding the axonemal complex or its components and the membranes of the primary Nebenkern derivative. Normally these spa-tial relationships allow a single point of contact, but multiple contacts between these membrane complexes occur in the mutants. It appears that membrane contact initiates paracrystalline body formation in the primary Nebenkern derivative. Tokuyasu *et al.* (1972*a,b*) used segregation-dis-torter *(SD)* mutants to study the processes of individualization and coiling which occur during spermiogenesis. Abnormal tail development occurs in spermatids of *SD/SD*[+] males. It occurs in 0–32 of the 64 spermatids per bundle, and the number of abnormal tails remains constant throughout the length of each bundle. These findings provide a means for identifying particular bundles and studying the processes occuring during tail development throughout the length of individual bundles. Further ques-tions on the differentiation of specific organelles that may be answered by ultrastructural analysis of mutant *Drosophila* include the following: Is the development of specific organelles dependent on spatial relationships? Are specific organelles independent in their differentiation? Is there sequential development of organelles? Are there controlling mechanisms existing between developing organelles?

Translocation Mutants

A chromosomal level of control of sperm development has been indicated by the studies of Lifschytz and Lindsley (1972). They discussed the occurrence of male sterility in *Drosophila* and other species and its relationship to translocations involving the X chromosome. They suggest that the cause of male sterility in *Drosophila* carrying translocations involving the X chromosome may be chromosomal in cases where the sterility is not attributable to particular gene loci. Inactivation of the single X chromosome is required in the males as a basic control mechanism for normal sperm development. The failure of this inactivation process in segments of the X-chromosome translocated to the autosomes results in sterility.

Lifschytz and Lindsley (1972) have suggested two major categories for the causes of male sterility: genic and chromosomal. Genic sterility results from mutations in genes whose products are necessary in spermatogenesis. Chromosomal sterility involves translocations and deficiencies associated with the X chromosome. Inactivation of the single X chromosome is postulated as an essential controlling mechanism for normal sperm development. A further subdivision of the genic sterility class seems necessary since the Y-chromosome fertility factors appear to function in a regulatory capacity rather than coding for structural components of the spermatozoa. Non-Y genes must code for the structural components or organelles since all of these structures are apparently present in X/0 and Y-deficient males.

Thus, three classes of male-sterile mutants can be tentatively identified: (1) regulatory mutants, involving Y chromosome and possibly other regulatory loci, (2) structural mutants, involving loci coding for transcient organelles required during spermatogenesis or structural components of sperm, and (3) chromosomal mutants, involving the X-chromosome translocations and the process of X-chromosome inactivation. Further analysis of male-sterile mutants should add to our understanding of the role of genes in spermatogenesis and aid in the elucidation of the mechanisms of ultrastructural change during cellular differentiation.

Literature Cited

Anderson, W. A., 1967 Cytodifferentiation of spermatozoa *Drosophila melanogaster*: The effect of elevated temperature on spermiogenesis. *Mol. Gen. Genet.* **99**:257–273.

Baccetti, B., 1963 Osservazioni preliminari sull 'ultrastruttura delle cellule germinali maschili in alcuni Ditteri. *Atti IV Congr. Ital. Micro. Elettr.* 25–26; 28–31.

Baccetti, B. and A. Bairati, Jr., 1964 Indagini comparative sull 'ultrastruttura delle cellule germinali maschili in *Dacus oleae* ed in *Drosophila melanogaster*. Meig. (Ins. Diptera). *Redia* **49**:1–29.

Baccetti, B., E. Bigliardi and F. Rosate, 1971 Spermatozoa or arthropoda 13. Cell-surface. *J. Ultrastruct. Res.* **35**:582–605.

Bairati, A. and B. Baccetti, 1964 Indagini comparative sull 'ultrastruttura delle cellule germinali maschili in *Dacus oleae* Gmel. ed in *Drosophila melanogaster* Meig. (Ins. Diptera). II. Nuovi reperti 'ultrastrutturali sul filamento assile degli spermatozoi. *Redia* **49**:81–85.

Bridges, C. B., 1916 Non-disjunction as a proof of the chromosome theory of heredity. I and II *Genetics* **1**:1–52, 107–163.

Brosseau, G., 1960 Genetic analysis of the male fertility factors on the Y chromosome of *Drosophila melanogaster*. *Genetics* **45**:257–274.

Brown, E. H. and R. C. King, 1961 Studies on the expression of the *transformer* gene of *Drosophila melanogaster*. *Genetics* **46**:143–156.

Cooper, K. W., 1950 Normal spermatogenesis in *Drosophila*. In *Biology of Drosophila*, edited by M. Demerec, pp. 1–61, John Wiley & Sons, New York.

Edmondson, M., 1951 Induction of sterility mutation in ultraviolet treated polar cap cells of *Drosophila*. *Genetics* **36**:549.

Erickson, J., 1965 Meiotic drive in *Drosophila* involving chromosome breakage. *Genetics* **51**:555–71.

Fung, S. C. and J. W. Gowen, 1957 The developmental effect of a sex-limited gene in *Drosophila melanogaster*. *J. Exp. Zool.* **134**:515–32.

Gowen, J. W. and S. C. Fung, 1957 Determination of sex through genes in a major sex locus in *Drosophila melanogaster*. *Heredity* **11**:397–402.

Hartl, D. L., 1969 Dysfunctional sperm production in *Drosophila melanogaster* males homozygous for the *Segregation Distorter* elements. *Proc. Natl. Acad. Sci. USA* **63**:782–789.

Hess, O., 1975 Y-linked factors affecting male fertility in *Drosophila melanogaster*. In *Handbook of Genetics*, Vol. 3, Chapter 28, edited by R. C. King, Plenum Press, New York.

Hess, O. and G. Y. Meyer, 1968 Genetic activities of the Y chromosome in *Drosophila* during spermatogenesis. *Adv. Genet.* **14**:171–223.

Kiefer, B. I., 1966 Ultrastructural abnormalities in developing sperm of X/0 *Drosophila melanogaster*. *Genetics* **54**:1441–52.

Kiefer, B. I., 1968 Y-mutants and spermiogenesis in *Drosophila melanogaster*. *Genetics* **60**:192.

Kiefer, B. I., 1969 Phenotypic effects of Y chromosome mutations in *Drosophila melanogaster*. I. Spermiogenesis and sterility in k1-1⁻ males. *Genetics* **61**:157–66.

Kiefer, B. I., 1970 Development, organization, and degeneration of the *Drosophila* sperm flagellum. *J. Cell Sci.* **6**:177–194.

Leik, J., 1965 Spermiogenesis in *Drosophila melanogaster*. *Diss. Abstr.* **26**:4129.

Lifschytz, E. and D. L. Lindsley, 1972 The role of X-chromosome inactivation during spermatogenesis. *Proc. Natl. Acad. Sci. USA* **69**:182–86.

Lindsley, D. L., 1968 Genetic control of sperm development in *Drosophila melanogaster*. *Proc. Int. Congr. Genet.* **1**:144.

Lindsley, D. L. and E. H. Grell, 1968 *Genetic Variations of Drosophila melanogaster.* Carnegie Institution of Washington Publication, 627, Carnegie Institution, Washington, D.C.

Lindsley, D. L., C. W. Edington, and E. S. VonHalle, 1960 Sex-linked recessive lethals in *Drosophila* whose expression is suppressed by the Y chromosome. *Genetics* **45**:1649–70.

Meyer, G. Y., 1964 Die parakristallinen Korper in den Spermienschwanzen von Drosophila. *Z. Zellforsch. Mikrosk. Anat.* **62**:762–784.

Meyer, G. Y., 1966 Crystalline mitochondrial derivative in sperm. In *Electron Microscopy*, pp. 629–630, Sixth International Conference on Electron Microscopy, Vol. II, Maruzen Co., Tokyo.

Meyer, G. Y., 1968 Spermiogenesis in normalen und Y-defizienten Mannchen von *Drosophila melanogaster* und D. hydei. *Z. Zellforsch. Mikrosk. Anat.* **84**:141–75.

Meyer, G. Y., 1969 Experimental studies on spermiogenesis in *Drosophila*. *Genetics (Suppl.)* **61**:79–92.

Peacock, W. J. and J. Erickson, 1965 Segregation-distorter and regularly nonfunctional products of spermiogenesis in *Drosophila melanogaster*. *Genetics* **51**:313–28.

Perotti, M. E., 1969 Ultrastructure of mature sperm of *Drosophila melanogaster* Meig. *J. Submicroscop. Cytol.* **1**:171–196.

Rasmussen, S. W., 1973 Ultrastructural studies of spermatogenesis in *Drosophila melanogaster* Meigen. *Z. Zellforsch. Mikrosk. Anat.* **140**:125–144.

Romrell, L. J., 1971 Isolation and characterization of autosomal male sterile mutants in *Drosophila melanogaster*. Ph.D. Dissertation, Department of Zoology, Utah State University, Logan, Utah.

Romrell, L. J., J. T. Bowman and H. P. Stanley, 1972a Genetic control of spermiogenesis in *Drosophila melanogaster*: An autosomal mutant (ms(2)3R) demonstrating failure of meiotic cytokinesis. *J. Ultrastruct. Res.* **38**:563–77.

Romrell, L. J., J. T. Bowman and H. P. Stanley, 1972b Genetic control of spermiogenesis in *Drosophila melanogaster*: an autosomal mutant (ms(2)10R) demonstrating disruption of the axonemal complex. *J. Ultrastruct. Res.* **38**:578–90.

Sandler, L., Y. Hiraizumi and I. Sandler, 1959 Meiotic drive in natural populations of *Drosophila melanogaster*. I. The Cytogenetic basis of *Segregation Distorter*. *Genetics* **44**:233–50.

Shoup, J. R., 1967 Spermiogenesis in wild type and in a male-sterile mutant of *Drosophila melanogaster*. *J. Cell Biol.* **32**:663–75.

Slifer, E. H., 1942 A mutant stock of *Drosophila* with extra sex combs. *J. Exp. Zool.* **90**:31–40.

Stanley, H. P., J. T. Bowman, L. J. Romrell, S. C. Reed and R. F. Wilkinson, 1972 Fine structure of normal spermatid differentiation in *Drosophila melanogaster*. *J. Ultrastruct. Res.* **41**:433–466.

Tates, A. D., 1971 Cytodifferentiation during spermatogenesis in *Drosophila melanogaster*. Thesis. Drukkerij J. H. Pasmans, 'S-Gravenhage.

Tokuyasu, K. T., 1974a Dynamics of spermiogenesis in *Drosophila melanogaster*. III.

Relationship between axoneme and mitochondrial derivatives. *Exp. Cell Res.* **84**:239–250.

Tokuyasu, K. T., 1974*b*   Dynamics of spermiogenesis in *Drosophila melanogaster*. IV. Nuclear transformation. *J. Ultrastruct. Res.* **48**:284–303.

Tokuyasu, K. T., W. J. Peacock and R. W. Hardy, 1972*a*   Dynamics of spermiogenesis in *Drosophila melanogaster*. I. Individualization process. *Z. Zellforsch. Mikrosk. Anat.* **134**:479–506.

Tokuyasu, K. T., W. J. Peacock and R. W. Hardy, 1972*b*   Dynamic of spermiogenesis in *Drosophila melanogaster*. II. Coiling process. *Z. Zellforsch. Mikrosk. Anat.* **127**:492–525.

Wilkinson, R. F., 1972   Spermiogenesis in two male-sterile third-chromosome mutants of *Drosophila melanogaster*. M.S. Thesis, Department of Zoology, Utah State University, Logan, Utah.

Wilkinson, R. F., H. P. Stanley, and J. T. Bowman, 1974   Genetic control of spermiogenesis in *Drosophila melanogaster:* The effects of abnormal cytoplasmic microtubule populations in mutant *ms(3)IOR* and its Colcemid-induced phenocopy. *J. Ultrastruct. Res.* **48**:242–258.

Williamson, J. H., 1970   Ethyl methanesulfonate-induced mutants on the Y chromosome of *Drosophila melanogaster*. *Mutat. Res.* **10**:597–605.

Williamson, J. H., 1972   Allelic complementation between mutants in fertility factors of the Y chromosome in *Drosophila melanogaster*. *Mol. Gen. Genet.* **119**:43–47.

Yasuzumi, G., W. Fujimura and H. Ishida, 1958   Spermatogenesis in animals as revealed by electron microscopy. V. Spermatid differentiation of *Drosophila* and grasshoppers. *Exp. Cell Res.* **14**:268–285.

28

Y-Linked Factors Affecting Male Fertility in *Drosophila melanogaster* and *Drosophila hydei*

Oswald Hess

Introduction

In principle there are two categories of genetic factors which affect male fertility, those controlling the continuity of germ-line cells and those controlling the differentiation of germ-line cells into mature spermatozoa.

Factors Controlling the Continuity of Germ-Line Cells

The majority of the fertility genes which control the continuity of germline cells are likely to be common to both sexes. They may control the formation and migration of the pole cells, the proliferation of the gonial cells, and the events that take place during the two meiotic divisions. So far, only very few genes of this type have been described in

Oswald Hess—Institut für Allgemeine Biologie, Universität Düsseldorf, Düsseldorf, West Germany.

Drosophila [e.g., the *grandchildless* mutant (Fielding, 1967)]. Data from the few cases known, together with our knowledge concerning the genetic control of the early steps of embryogenesis in general, lead to the assumption that the formation and migration of the pole cells is under maternal control, rather than under the control of the genome of the developing individual itself. If so, this would explain why so few sterile factors of this kind have been found.

Factors Controlling Spermiogenesis

The great majority of genetically sterile males which have been described show abnormalities of differentiation during spermiogenesis. Male sterility may result from aneuploidy, chromosome rearrangements, or single-gene defects.

Effects of Aneuploidy

Absence of the Y chromosome results in male sterility (Bridges, 1916). On the other hand, additions of extra Y chromosomes to the chromosome complement may also have a deleterious effect on male fertility. For instance, *Drosophila melanogaster* males with three Y chromosomes are invariably sterile (Cooper, 1956). In certain strains males with one additional Y chromosome may also be sterile (Grell, 1969).

Duplications of the X chromosome may also result in male sterility. However, this may be the result of a change in sex which, consequently, prevents the continuation of the spermatogenic cycle.

In spermatids, aneuploidy does not seem to have an effect on fertility. As a result of chromosome segregation during meiosis, the spermatids normally do not contain a complete set of genes. For example, half of them carry an X but not a Y chromosome, and the rest carry the Y but no X chromosome. Moreover, nullosomic spermatids derived from autosomal nondisjunction at the first or second meiotic division can produce functional sperm which, provided they fertilize a complementary disomic ova, are recoverable in viable zygotes. In addition, spermatids carrying only the minute chromosome 4, with or without an additional Y chromosome, undergo normal differentiation (Lindsley and Grell, 1968b). The further observation that sperm lacking both the Y and the fourth chromosome in their genetic complement are also functional leads to the conclusion that no particular chromosome needs to be present in the spermatid nucleus in order for normal spermiogenesis to take place. These results can be best explained by the hypothesis that stable mRNA is produced by the primary spermatocytes for translation later in spermiogenesis. This view is in complete agreement with many other data obtained, e.g., from investigations of RNA synthesis during spermiogenesis [see Hess and Meyer (1968) and Hess (1971) for further discussion].

Effects of Chromosomal Aberrations

A great deal of genetic sterility in males is caused by chromosomal aberrations. In these cases the effects leading to sterility may not be readily attributable to particular gene loci. Moreover, genetic sterility of this kind is typically dominant.

There are two main types of chromosomal changes which play a role in sterility, X–autosome translocations and deficiencies in the region of the proximal heterochromatin of the X chromosome. In addition, other types of chromosome mutations such as autosomal deficiencies may cause male sterility. Since none of the individuals carrying such a deficiency are able to survive in the absence of a compensating duplication, the chromosomal effect on sterility is dominant, i.e., it cannot be compensated for by the addition of homologous normal chromosome regions to the genome [for review, see Lindsley and Lifschytz (1972)].

In order to explain the effects of X-chromosome rearrangements on male fertility, Lifschytz and Lindsley (1972) developed a model which assumes that the inactivation of the X chromosome during a critical stage of spermatogenesis is essential for normal sperm differentiation. This inactivation is controlled by a specific chromosomal region. Therefore, fragments of the X chromosome separated from this region will not be properly inactivated and, as a consequence, spermatid differentiation will be aberrant.

Deficiencies of the Y chromosome are also often correlated with male sterility. However, in contrast to the above-mentioned cases, the sterility effect of the Y deletions is always recessive, i.e., the presence of an additional normal Y chromosome or of a complementary part thereof restores normal spermiogenesis. This observation clearly shows that the deficient Y segments contain genes whose products are needed for normal spermiogenesis.

Effects of Gene Mutations

Male sterility can also be produced by the mutation of specific genes which can be mapped in the usual way. Quite often these mutations may be correlated with other phenotypic effects [see Lindsley and Grell

(1968*a*)]. In the majority of these cases the precise mode of action of such factors is not known. However, it may be assumed that the lesion occurs in genetic loci whose products are critical to normal spermatogenesis.

Sterility mutations may occur in all chromosomes of the complement, and their distribution appears to be proportional to chromosomal lengths. There are only very rough estimations for the number of such loci. Lindsley and Lifschytz (1972) have summarized the evidence for the relative number of loci which can mutate to male sterility. Based on the number of autosomes which carry sterile mutations, the estimates for the number of loci per genome responsible for the genetic control of spermatogenesis range from 80 to 1800.

In contrast to the other chromosomes in the genetic complement, the relationship between genes located in the Y chromosome and male sterility is well documented. Bridges (1916) was the first to demonstrate that males lacking a Y chromosome were sterile, although they were of normal viability and phenotype. Stern (1927, 1929) found that males of *D. melanogaster* carrying deficiencies for only a part of the Y chromosome, e.g., either the long or the short arm, are also sterile. He postulated the existence of complexes of fertility factors in each Y arm, neither of which could be compensated by duplications in the other complex. By complementation analyses of a number of x-ray-induced, sterile, Y chromosomes, Brosseau (1960) identified five fertility factors on the long arm and two on the short arm of the Y chromosome of *D. melanogaster*. This number has been confirmed by Williamson (1970). The data of these experiments are consistent with the view that (1) the factors are arranged linearly in the Y chromosome and (2) all of these factors are essential, i.c., the absence or mutation of one of these factors cannot be compensated for by an excess of other regions of the Y chromosome. On the basis of this evidence it is clear that each factor has its own specific function during spermatogenesis. Although the linear order of these loci is well established, their precise cytological positions within the Y chromosome are not known.

The Y chromosome of many (possibly all) species of the genus *Drosophila* develops prominent lampbrush loops in the nuclei of spermatocytes (Hess and Meyer, 1963; Hess, 1967*a*). In *D. hydei,* the lampbrush loops are especially large and morphologically distinctive. Experiments with this species demonstrate a correlation between loop development and spermiogenesis [for review, see Hess and Meyer (1968) and Hess (1971)]. Deficiencies of the Y chromosome which include sites of spermatocyte loops invariably cause severe morphogenetic defects in spermatid differentiation, all of which lead to sterility. In contrast to this, deficiencies of the Y chromosome which do not include loop-forming sites have never been found to be correlated with male sterility (Hess, 1967*b*). Moreover, in those cases where the unfolding of a lampbrush-loop pair in the spermatocyte nucleus is blocked, the genetic effect is the same as that produced by deficiencies of the corresponding Y regions (Hess, 1968). Finally, mutations by which the unfolding of one of the lampbrush-loop pairs is more or less severely disturbed may also result in sterility or in a reduction of fertility (Hess, 1970). Taken together, these observations demonstrate that the correct and complete unfolding of all pairs of lampbrush loops of the Y chromosome during the growth stage of the primary spermatocytes is a necessary prerequisite for normal spermiogenesis.

The lampbrush loops of the Y chromosome are sites of a high rate of RNA synthesis (Hess and Meyer, 1963; Hennig, 1967, 1968). Inhibition of RNA synthesis with, e.g., actinomycin (Meyer and Hess, 1965), x-irradiation (Hess, 1965*c*), or α-amanitin (M. Schwochau, unpublished), results in reversible structural disintegration of the loop pairs. In agreement with the generally accepted model of lampbrush chromosomes [see Gall and Callan (1962) and Hess (1971)], there is, therefore, convincing evidence that unfolding of the loops of the Y chromosome occurs at the loci of active genes whose transcription is indispensable for the normal differentiation of spermatids. In other words, all the evidence favors the view that the lampbrush loops in the nuclei of spermatocytes are manifestations of the stage- and tissue-specific activity of the male fertility factors postulated from the studies of Stern and Brosseau cited above.

In *D. hydei* it has been possible to map the loci of the loop-forming sites on the Y chromosome with the aid of x-ray-induced Y fragments in XY translocation chromosomes (Hess, 1965*b*). As shown in Figure 1, there are two loop-forming sites on the short arm of the Y chromosome and at least five such sites on the long arm. For mapping, the long arm of the Y has been divided into ten equal segments, beginning with region 1 at the kinetochore. The sites for the "club-shaped loop pair" and for one of the "tubular ribbons" are located in this region. The site of the second pair of "tubular ribbons" is located in region 3, and the sites for the so-called "pseudonucleolus" and the "threads" are located in regions 9 and 10, respectively. The sites for two distinct "noose-shaped" loop pairs are both located in the short arm which, in *D. hydei,* is relatively short. On the basis of this map, then, there are comparatively large segments of the Y chromosome which do not appear to contain sites which form lampbrush loops in spermatocyte nuclei and which, therefore, are not involved in normal spermiogenesis. Indeed, as already discussed, deficiencies of regions without loop-forming sites never cause male sterility.

The presence of lampbrush loops in the nuclei of the spermatocytes

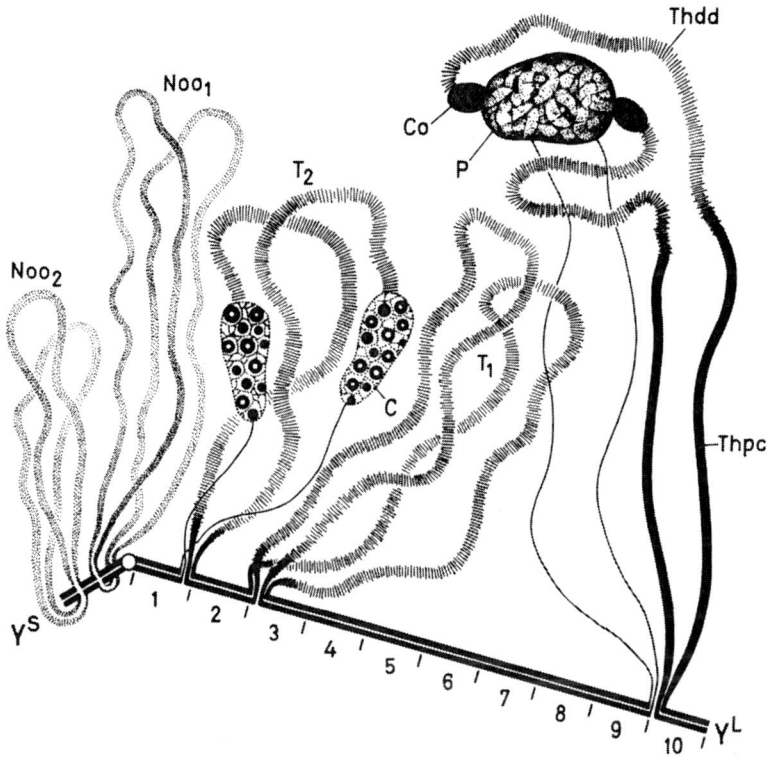

*Figure 1. Diagram of the Y chromosome of D. hydei during its lampbrush phase
with the loci of loop-forming sites. C, clubs; Co, cones; Noo, nooses (two pairs);
P, pseudonucleolus; T, tubular ribbons (two pairs); Thdd, Thpc, distal diffuse
and proximal compact segment of thread-shaped pair of loops; Y^L, Y^S, long and
short arm of the Y chromosome.*

can be demonstrated in essentially all species of the genus *Drosophila*.
Some 50 species have been examined to date (Hess, 1967*a*). There is,
however, a great species-specific variation both in morphology and in the
number of such structures.

The functions of the fertility factors during spermatid differentiation
in *Drosophila* have been elucidated by correlating the morphogenetic
defects observed in the spermatids with the deficiencies of Y regions that
include these factors (Meyer *et al.*, 1961; Kiefer, 1966, 1969; Hess and
Meyer, 1968; Meyer, 1968, 1969, 1972). Spermiogenesis is blocked at
different stages, depending on which fertility factors are missing. As a
result, spermatids with different classes of morphogenetic defects can be
distinguished. This result indicates that the different fertility factors have
specific functions, an assumption which is also suggested by the
observation that deficiencies of a particular Y region cannot be compensated by a duplication of any other Y region.

The developmental defects which appear during spermiogenesis in partially Y-deficient males of *Drosophila* can roughly be classified into "early" and "late" effects. These effects are reproducibly correlated with the absence of particular loop pairs.

In Y-deficient males of any kind, all structural components of sperm organelles seem to be present but frequently fail to be organized into organelles of normal architecture. Thus, the Y-chromosome factors seem to control the coordination of the various synthetic and morphogenetic processes in spermatids leading to the formation of the functional sperm without necessarily contributing structural information on a molecular level. This assumption must be seen in view of the fact that the differentiation of male gametes occurs without recognizable contribution of the sperm nucleus itself. All differentiation processes during spermiogenesis have been shown to be dependent on specific activities of the diploid spermatocyte nucleus (Stern and Hadorn, 1938; Lindsley and Grell, 1968*b*). In this context it must be remembered that no aneuploid condition of any kind, even those cases of very severe changes of the chromosome complement, impairs spermatid differentiation.

Data from other experiments indicate that the Y-chromosomal loops are themselves not involved in the coding of the structural proteins in the sperm, but instead they may influence the function of autosomal fertility factors. For instance, when species hybrids between *D. hydei* and *D. neohydei* are repeatedly backcrossed to the maternal species, hybrid males can be obtained, each with its X chromosome and all its autosomes derived from *D. hydei* and the Y chromosome alone derived from *D. neohydei*. Hybrids of such a constitution are sterile, whereas the F_1 hybrids (with the X chromosome and one set of autosomes from *D. hydei* and the Y chromosome and the other set of autosomes from *D. neohydei*) are fully fertile. This finding suggests that both autosomal and Y-chromosome factors may be involved in the control of spermiogenesis, and that the cooperation of both groups of factors may be disturbed in cases where they are derived from different species (U. Schäfer, unpublished).

In all normal XY males of *D. melanogaster* morphogenetic defects of the Y-deficient type are regularly found in a few spermatidal cysts (Koopmans-Frankel *et al.,* 1971). The frequency of this defect may be increased experimentally by heat treatments, alterations in ion concentrations, ligature of larvae, transplantations of gonads, and by various chemical agents (Meyer, 1969, 1972). Most of the experimental alterations seen in XY males are similar to those observed in Y-deficient males and, therefore, they may be considered as "phenocopies" of Y deficiencies. However, there are also other kinds of structural changes in spermatids which have never been seen in Y-deficient males. All these defects are often accompanied by a concomitant suppression of lampbrush-loop formation in the nuclei of spermatocytes.

Most of the x-ray-induced (Brosseau, 1960) or EMS-induced (Williamson, 1970) Y mutations which cause sterility may be considered as partial deficiencies of the Y chromosome. However, there are some which seem to represent true gene mutations. This is the case for Y-linked sterility mutations whose function is temperature conditioned (Williamson, 1970). Moreover, mutations correlated with the alteration of the morphology of particular loop pairs have also been found (Hess, 1965a, 1970; Hess and Meyer, 1968). In many of these cases no recognizable effect on fertility has been recorded. In others, however, an impairment of spermiogenesis can be shown to occur which, furthermore, can be directly correlated with a relatively severe inhibition of the normal development of a particular lampbrush loop in the spermatocyte nuclei. This observation is, again, a convincing demonstration that complete unfolding of all Y-chromosomal lampbrush loops is a necessary prerequisite for normal spermiogenesis in *Drosophila*.

Literature Cited

Bridges, C. B., 1916   Nondisjunction as a proof of the chromosome theory of heredity. *Genetics* **1**:1–52, 107–163.

Brosseau, G., 1960   Genetic analysis of the male fertility factors on the Y chromosome of *Drosophila melanogaster. Genetics* **45**:257–274.

Cooper, K. W., 1956   Phenotypic effects of Y chromosome hyperploidy in *Drosophila melanogaster* and their relation to variegation. *Genetics* **41**:242–264.

Fielding, C. J., 1967   Developmental genetics of the mutant *grandchildless* of *Drosophila subobscura. J. Embryol. Exp. Morphol.* **17**:375–384.

Gall, J. G. and H. G. Callan, 1962   H³-uridine incorporation in lampbrush chromosomes. *Proc. Natl. Acad. Sci. USA* **48**:562–570.

Grell, R. F., 1969   Sterility, lethality, and segregation ratios in XYY males of *Drosophila melanogaster. Genetics* **61**:s23–s24.

Hennig, W., 1967   Untersuchungen zur Struktur und Funktion des Lampenbürsten-Y-Chromosoms in der Spermatogenese von *Drosophila. Chromosoma (Berl.)* **22**:294–357.

Hennig, W., 1968   Ribonucleic acid synthesis of the Y chromosome of *Drosophila hydei. J. Mol. Biol.* **38**:227–239.

Hess, O., 1965a   Struktur-Differenzierungen im Y-Chromosom von *Drosophila hydei* und ihre Beziehungen zu Gen-Aktivitäten. I. Mutanten der Funktionsstrukturen. *Verhandl. Deut. Zool. Ges. Zool. Anz. Suppl.* **28**:156–163.

Hess, O., 1965b   Struktur-Differenzierungen im Y-Chromosom von *Drosophila hydei* und ihre Beziehungen zu Gen-Aktivitäten. III. Sequenz und Lokalisation der Schleifen-Bildungsorte. *Chromosoma (Berl.)* **16**:222–248.

Hess, O., 1965c   The effect of X-rays on the functional structures of the Y chromosome in spermatocytes of *Drosophila hydei. J. Cell Biol.* **25**:169–173.

Hess, O., 1967*a* Morphologische Variabilität der chromosomalen Funktionsstrukturen in den Spermatocytenkernen von *Drosophila*-Arten. *Chromosoma (Berl.)* **21**:429–445.

Hess, O., 1967*b* Complementation of genetic activity in translocated fragments of the Y chromosome in *Drosophila hydei*. *Genetics* **56**:283–295.

Hess, O., 1968 The function of the lampbrush loops formed by the Y chromosome of *Drosophila hydei* in spermatocyte nuclei. *Mol. Gen. Genet.* **103**:58–71.

Hess, O., 1970 Genetic function correlated with unfolding of lampbrush loops by the Y chromosome in spermatocytes of *Drosophila hydei*. *Mol. Gen. Genet.* **106**:328–346.

Hess, O., 1971 Lampenbürstenchromosomen. In *Handbuch der Allgemeinen Pathologie,* Vol. II/2, pp. 215–281, Springer-Verlag, Berlin.

Hess, O. and G. F. Meyer, 1963 Chromosomal differentiations of the lampbrush type formed by the Y chromosome in *Drosophila hydei* and *Drosophila neohydei*. *J. Cell Biol.* **16**:527–539.

Hess, O. and G. F. Meyer, 1968 Genetic activities of the Y chromosome in *Drosophila* during spermatogenesis. *Adv. Genet.* **14**:171–223.

Kiefer, B. I., 1966 Ultrastructural abnormalities in developing sperm of X/O *Drosophila melanogaster*. *Genetics* **54**:1441–1452.

Kiefer, B. I., 1969 Phenotypic effects of Y chromosome mutations in *Drosophila melanogaster*. I. Spermiogenesis and sterility in KL-1- males. *Genetics* **61**:157–166.

Koopmans-Frankel, A. W., U. Peters and G. F. Meyer, 1971 Variation in fertility of two wild type strains of *Drosophila melanogaster*. *Chromosoma (Berl.)* **34**:113–128.

Lifschytz, E. and D. L. Lindsley, 1972 The role of X chromosome inactivation during spermatogenesis. *Proc. Natl. Acad. Sci. USA* **69**:182–186.

Lindsley, D. L. and E. H. Grell, 1968*a* *Genetic Variations of Drosophila melanogaster,* Carnegie Institution of Washington Publication 627, Carnegie Institution, Washington, D.C.

Lindsley, D. L. and E. H. Grell, 1968*b* Spermiogenesis without chromosomes in *Drosophila melanogaster*. *Genetics* **61 Suppl. 1**:69–78.

Lindsley, D. L. and E. Lifschytz, 1972 The genetic control of spermatogenesis in *Drosophila*. In *The Genetics of the Spermatozoon,* edited by R. A. Beatty and S. Glucksohn-Waelsch, pp. 203–222, Department of Genetics, University of Edinburgh, Edinburgh.

Meyer, G. F., 1968 Spermiogenese in normalen und Y-defizienten Männchen von *Drosophila melanogaster* und *D. hydei*. *Z. Zellforsch.* **84**:141–175.

Meyer, G. F., 1969 Experimental studies on spermiogenesis in *Drosophila*. *Genetics* **61 Suppl. 1**:79–92.

Meyer, G. F., 1972 Influence of Y chromosome on fertility and phenotype of *Drosophila* spermatozoa. In *The Genetics of the Spermatozoon,* edited by R. A. Beatty and S. Glucksohn-Waelsch, pp. 387–405, Department of Genetics, University of Edinburgh, Edinburgh.

Meyer, G. F. and O. Hess, 1965 Struktur-Differenzierungen im Y-Chromosom von *Drosophila hydei* und ihre Beziehungen zu Gen-Aktivitäten. II. Effekt der RNS-Synthese-Hemmung durch Actinomycin. *Chromosoma (Berl.)* **16**:249–270.

Meyer, G. F., O. Hess and W. Beermann, 1961 Phasenspezifische Funktionsstrukturen in Spermatocytenkernen von *Drosophila melanogaster* und ihre Abhängigkeit vom Y-Chromosom. *Chromosoma (Berl.)* **12**:676–716.

Stern, C., 1927 Ein genetischer und cytologischer Beweis für Vererbung im Y-Chromosom von *Drosophila melanogaster.* *Z. Indukt. Abstammungs.-Vererbungsl.* **44**:188–231.

Stern, C., 1929 Untersuchungen über Aberrationen des Y-Chromosoms von *Drosophila melanogaster.* *Z. Indukt. Abstammungs.-Vererbungsl.* **51**:253–353.

Stern, C. and E. Hadorn, 1938 The determination of sterility in *Drosophila* males without a complete Y chromosome. *Am. Nat.* **72**:42–52.

Williamson, J. H., 1970 Ethyl methanesulfonate-induced mutants on the Y chromosome of *Drosophila melanogaster.* *Mutat. Res.* **10**:597–605.

29

The Genetic Analysis of Oogenesis in *Drosophila melanogaster*

Robert C. King and J. Dawson Mohler

Introduction

A quite massive amount of information is available concerning oogenesis in *Drosophila melanogaster,* and the monograph published by King (1970) presents a convenient review of the work accomplished through 1969. Subjects such as the preadult morphogenesis of the female reproductive system, the division, migration, and differentiation of the cystocytes and profollicle cells in the adult germarium, the subsequent development of the egg chamber in the vitellarium, the behavior of the oocyte chromosomes, and the interactions between the oocyte, nurse cells, and follicle cells and between the ovary and other organs are discussed, and therefore there is no need to duplicate any of these details here. The ovarian pathologies of flies carrying various female-sterile mutations have also been reviewed in that book, and a tabulation is given of 32 loci whose mutant alleles affect the ovary or its duct system [King (1970), his Table I-1]. What we propose to do here is to group together genes with broadly

Robert C. King—Department of Biological Sciences, Northwestern University, Evanston, Illinois. J. Dawson Mohler—Department of Zoology, The University of Iowa, Iowa City, Iowa.

similar effects and to place these groups in a developmental sequence. Genes will simply be listed, but not discussed, if they were described in King's (1970) monograph and no new data have since been published concerning them. However, the results presented in recent publications necessitate further discussions of certain other loci.

Mutations Affecting the Germ-Cell Determinants

Thierry-Mieg *et al.* (1972) induced a mutation in *D. melanogaster* that resembles the grandchildless (*gs*) mutation of *D. subobscura*. The *melanogaster* mutant (*gs*[87]) is located on the X chromosome, less than 1 crossover unit to the right of cut (*ct*). When reared at 16°C, *gs*[87] homozygotes are completely fertile. At 29°C, however, most eggs do not hatch, and many of the surviving F_1 adults lack gonads. Gehring (1973) reports that the eggs produced by *gs/gs* *D. subobscura* females contain polar granules that are similar in ultrastructure to the polar granules of wild-type eggs. Nuclei from the adjacent lateral periplasm do migrate to the polar regions in *gs* eggs and do come into contact with polar granules. However, these nuclei do not form pole cells, and the fate of the *gs* polar granules is not known. Normally the cells that come to contain polar granules in their cytoplasm differentiate into germ cells. In fact, transplantation of cytoplasm containing polar granules to the anterior pole of the egg of *D. melanogaster* induces cells which normally form soma to differentiate into germ cells (Illmensee and Mahowald, 1974). Since the *melanogaster* mutant is temperature sensitive, Thierry-Mieg *et al.* (1973) determined its temperature-sensitive period and showed that this begins at stage 7 of oogenesis and lasts throughout vitellogenesis. However, high-temperature treatments have no effect once the eggs are laid by *gs*[87] females.

C. Kern and A. Mahowald (private communication) have reexamined the defects in pole plasm of eggs produced by the female sterile (1) N [*fs(1)N*, 1–0.0] mutant. Forty percent of the ovarian oocytes observed lack RNA in the polar granules. They examined four new alleles and found similar effects to varying degrees in three of the four. In the fourth no defects could be detected. The relationship between the abnormalities of the polar granules and the other developmental defects associated with the locus is not understood.

Mutations Affecting the Differentiation of Ovarioles

Bakken (1973) induced three mutations that affected different stages in the differentiation of the ovariole. In two cases the effects were on very early stages: In the case of *fs(2)A15* the ovarioles did not differentiate and no recognizable oocytes could be seen in Feulgen-stained, ovarian, whole mounts. In *fs(2)A16* some ovariolelike structures were detected, but the germarial regions were ill-defined and the follicles contained abnormal numbers of cystocytes. The locations of these two nonallelic genes on chromosome 2 remain to be determined. In the third case, *fs(3)A10*, the differentiation of the ovarioles appears to be blocked at a stage approximating that in the 48-hour pupa. Ovariolar organization is complete only halfway down the ovary, and the follicles develop only to stage 3. The posterior portion of the ovary is filled with degenerating follicles, implying the continuing, normal formation of follicles in the germarium. The ovarian phenotype produced by *fs(3)A10* suggests that the posterior differentiation of the ovariole must take place before an egg chamber can progress past stage 3.

Mutations Affecting the Division and Differentiation of Cystocytes

This class includes the recessive genes fused (*fu*), narrow (*nw*), and female sterile (2) B [*fs(2)B*], which hereafter will be referred to by its old symbol *fes*. The earlier work on these "ovarian-tumor" mutants has been described in Chapter IV of King's (1970) monograph. The maternal effects of *fu* are also described there and in the subsequent paper of Fausto-Sterling (1971).

The mechanism that stops fourth-generation cystocytes from further division in wild-type *D. melanogaster* does not operate in the majority of *fes* chambers. Johnson and King (1972) have shown that in this mutant the normal arrested cleavage characteristic of cystocytes is disturbed so that mitosis is often followed by complete cytokinesis. They conclude that the product of the *fes+* gene is required for the formation of a stable canal system, and they suggest that the product of the mutant gene is defective in this regard. In the abnormal cystocyte clusters found in *fes*, an oocyte is produced only in those cells containing 4 canals [see King (1970), Table IV-2]. If fewer canals are present, oocyte differentiation does not occur, regardless of the total number of cystocytes in the cluster. Johnson and King propose that the signal that normally stops fourth-generation cystocytes from further mitosis is the differentiation of pro-oocytes and that these cells receive their cue to differentiate from the four canal rims that they alone possess.

Fs(2)D is one of the few dominant, female-sterile mutations known in *D. melanogaster*. The mutation resides on the second chromosome, but its precise locus is unknown. Heterozygous males are fertile, whereas heterozygous females are sterile. To obtain females heterozygous for *Fs(2)D,* males of genotype *Fs(2)D/T(1;2)Bld* are mated to virgin females carrying a compound double X chromosome and a normal Y chromosome. The males are kept in a stock with *T(1;2)OR64/T(1;2)Bld* females. The reader should consult Lindsley and Grell (1968) for explanations of the symbols used. Yarger and King (1971) found that the production of egg chambers was greatly inhibited in heterozygotes. Of the relatively few egg chambers produced, between 10 percent and 20 percent (depending on the temperature) contained less than 16 cystocytes. The modal number of cystocytes in such abnormal chambers was 2. No oocytes were found in the vast majority of chambers with less than 16 cystocytes. This finding is not surprising, since the cystocytes from such small clusters would be expected to have fewer than four ring canals. Since in *Fs(2)D/+* females the ovarian phenotype is mutant, it follows that the division of cystocytes is retarded even though each cell possesses a wild-type allele and presumably its product. This conclusion suggests in turn that the mutant allele may code for a mutant protein which has an inhibitory effect on cystocyte mitosis. For example, the incorporation of the mutant protein into some mitotic organelle might impair its functioning even though the normal protein was incorporated simultaneously.

To summarize, the second-chromosome genes *fes* and *FsD* both affect the division of germarial cystocytes. The dominant gene suppresses their mitosis and the recessive modifies the type of cleavage that follows.

The ovaries of triploid intersexes bare a striking resemblance to those of *fes* homozygotes [Lange (1969), Plate VI]. Since triploids have normal ovaries, the presence of "cystocyte tumors" in the ovaries of 3A : 2X intersexes suggests that normal cystocyte cytokinesis requires a karyotype that is either 3A : 3X or 2A : 2X.

Mutations Affecting the Behavior of Oocyte Chromosomes

Within this class are genes whose products are necessary for homologous chromosomes to "recognize" each other, to synapse, and to cross over. Such genes can be subdivided into two groups. The first group includes mutations in which crossing over is completely suppressed; whereas in the second, crossing over does occur, but it is reduced in certain chromosomal regions.

In *Drosophila* females homozygous for the *c(3)G* gene, crossing over is abolished and non-disjunction is common during the first meiotic division. The *c(3)G* mutation was discovered by Marie and John Gowen in 1917, hence its name, crossover suppressor of Gowen. Sandler induced a new meiotic mutant in 1968 which was called *mei-W22* until it was shown to be an allele of *c(3)G*. The two alleles are now given the symbols $c(3)G^{17}$ and $c(3)G^{68}$. While both alleles are equally defective in crossing over, they are slightly different in their non-disjunctional frequencies, their rates of chromosome loss, and in the types of nonhomologous chromosome segregations (Hall, 1972). If *c(3)G* females mate at low temperature, crossing over is still absent, but non-disjunction is decreased. In this regard $c(3)G^{17}$ is more temperature sensitive than $c(3)G^{68}$. Since the temperature-sensitive stage is at the time the eggs are laid, it is long after the time crossing over takes place. Crossing over is sightly increased in *c(3)G/+* females. In homozygotes for $c(3)G^{17}$, fourth generation cystocytes spend less time in the germarium, and synaptonemal complexes are not observed in pro-oocyte or oocyte nuclei (Smith and King, 1968; Rasmussen, 1975). Synaptonemal complexes also fail to occur in the nuclei of pro-oocytes and young oocytes of $c(3)G^{68}$ homozygotes (Carpenter, private communication).

Recently eleven additional alleles of *c(3)G* have been recovered from EMS treatment by R. F. Grell and E. Generoso. In each case meiotic exchange is eliminated and in the three cases where electron microscopic examinations have been carried out, synaptonemal complexes are absent. In addition, R. F. Grell and E. Generoso have induced mutations at a *rec* locus closely linked to *c(3)G*. These mutations drastically reduce but do not abolish meiotic exchange. Unlike *c(3)G*, synaptonemal complexes are present (R. F. Grell, private communication).

In mutants where recombination is reduced (but not abolished), it is reduced in a similar way for all chromosomes [a single exception is *mei-1* (*q. v.*)], and there is increased non-disjunction of all chromosome pairs at the first meiotic division. This non-disjunction is thought by B. Baker and Carpenter (1972) to be a secondary effect resulting from the normal process of pairing and distributive disjunction (Grell, 1962). The decrease in crossing over can be uniform along a chromosome arm or nonuniform. When it is nonuniform, the decreases are most severe in the chromosomal regions distal to the centromere.

One such polarized mutant is *mei-218* (1–57±), where, for example, distal and proximal segments of chromosome 2 have recombination values 6 percent and 45 percent of the controls, respectively. The *mei-218* mutant resembles *c(3)G* in that it increases the map length when heterozygous (Carpenter and Sandler, 1974). According to Carpenter and Baker (1974) *mei-218* oocytes contain synaptonemal complexes of normal length and "gross ultrastructure." Other examples of polarized meiotic mutants are the X-linked genes *mei-41* (and its allele *mei-41*[195]), *mei-251*, and *mei-352* (Baker and Carpenter, 1972), *abo* (2–44) (Carpenter and Sandler, 1974), and *mei-S282* (3–5) (Parry, 1973).

The allelic mutations *mei-9* and *mei-9^b* (1–5) are examples of mutants where recombination is lowered uniformly along the chromosomes. In *mei-9* and *mei-9^b* the map lengths are 9 percent and 16 percent the control values, respectively. In the heterozygous condition *mei-9* decreases the map length (Carpenter and Sandler, 1974).

The third-chromosome gene, *mei-1*, differs from all the other meiotic mutants that influence recombination in that there seems to be a target region on one chromosome where crossing over is suppressed. Recombination is drastically reduced in the region near the gene cut (*ct*, 1-20). Other regions on the X show less extreme reductions, and recombination in the autosomes is little affected (Valentin, 1973). Non-disjunction of normal X's is only trebled. Other meiotic genes that alter recombination tend to raise non-disjunction by much larger factors. Valentin suggests *mei-1^+* plays some role to assure correctness of synapsis in a particular region of the chromosome after a general alignment of the chromosomes has been brought about.

The X-linked mutants *mei-38, mei-99,* and *mei-160* belong to still another group. Recombination values in the distal chromosome regions are normal or nearly so, while recombination values in pericentric regions are 1.3–2 times the control levels. In addition to altering the pattern of recombination, these mutants cause increased non-disjunction at *both* the first and second meiotic divisions. Baker and Carpenter (1972) propose that these mutants are either in genes whose products are required at several different times during meiosis, or else that the gene products function at one critical time with mutant products altering the chromosomes so that they behave abnormally on several subsequent occasions.

There is a class of mutations in *D. melanogaster* that modifies the distributions of the oocyte chromosomes during the meiotic divisions but does not affect crossing over. Among these mutations are *nod, ca^nd*, and *mei-S332*. These genes presumably act at a later stage in meiosis than the genes referred to earlier in this section.

Grell [see King (1970), page 140] has presented evidence to support the concept that distributive pairing differs from and follows exchange pairing in *D. melanogaster*. Exchange pairing precedes exchange and is restricted to the homologs and homologous regions of chromosomes. Regular segregation follows for those chromosomes that undergo exchange. Chromosomes that fail to undergo exchange then undergo distributive pairing. This may involve homologs or nonhomologs, and chromosomes that are distributively paired pass to opposite poles at first meiotic anaphase.

The mutation *mei-254^a* is located on the X chromosome very close to the gene miniature (m, 1–36.1). The mutant has been renamed *nod* (no distributive disjunction) because when homozygous it reduces the probability that a nonexchange chromosome will disjoin from either a nonexchange homolog or nonhomolog. Therefore the mechanism ensuring that distributively paired chromosomes proceed to opposite poles of the spindle appears to be defective. The mutant does not affect males, and recombination in females is also not affected (Carpenter, 1973).

Kinderman and King (1973) have observed in electron micrographs of late ovarian oocytes of *D. virilis* that meiotic metaphase I occurs in the absence of centrioles and asters. Therefore, each fruit fly oocyte is generated from a third-generation cystocyte through a mitosis that utilizes centrioles, but these are excluded from the subsequent nuclear division. This observation suggests that centrioles are not necessary either for the formation of spindles or for the orderly separation of the chromosomes.

There is an interesting mutation which manifests itself only in those spindles that form in the absence of centrioles. In *D. melanogaster* homozygous for the gene claret-non-disjunctional (ca^{nd}, 3–100.7) non-disjunction is restricted to the first meiotic division, and the loss of chromosomes occurs during the two meiotic divisions and the first cleavage mitosis. In this gonomeric division, however, only maternal chromosomes are lost. Perhaps the meiotic phenotypes observed in ca^{nd} (and *nod*) result from the defective functioning of the traction fibers of the maternal spindles.

Finally we come to *mei-S332* (2–95), a meiotic mutant that affects both sexes. The mutant gene results in malfunctioning centromeres, but only at the time of centromere replication for the second meiotic division. Sister centromeres divide precociously, and this leads to elevated rates of equational non-disjunction and loss for all chromosomes (Davis, 1971). Thus, at least this function of the second meiotic division is under common genetic control in both sexes of *D. melanogaster*, and *mei-S332* is the latest acting of the meiotic mutants so far studied in females.

Mutants Affecting the Nurse Cells

During oogenesis the chromosomes of the nurse cells undergo a series of endomitotic doublings. The first occurs in the germarium, and seven or eight more doublings occur within the vitellarium. Although methods for the selective extrachromosomal replication of the oocyte DNA have evolved in some insect species (Gall and Rochaix, 1974), this has not taken place in the fruit fly (Mohan and Ritossa, 1970). The provision of the *Drosophila* oocyte with 15 highly polyploid nurse cells serves to multiply the rDNA available for transcription by thousands of times, and the cistrons that specify the ribosomal proteins, tRNAs, mRNAs, and the enzymes functioning in transcription and translation are multiplied concurrently. Because the ribosome content of the oocyte depends entirely upon the nurse-cell synthesis, we are including mutations that affect ribosome synthesis in this section.

The cistrons for the 18S and 28S ribosomal RNAs (rRNA) are located in the heterochromatic region at the base of the X chromosome and in the short arm of the Y. However, the rDNAs of the normal X and Y chromosomes have opposite orientations with respect to the centromere (Palumbo *et al.*, 1973). Ritossa and Spiegelman (1965) calculated that there are approximately 130 cistrons for 18S rRNA and an equal number for the 28S rRNA in each sex chromosome. The cistrons for the third RNA component of mature ribosomes, 5S RNA, are equally redundant (Tartof and Perry, 1970) and have been located in the right arm of chromosome 2 (Wimber and Steffensen, 1970).

Mutant *bobbed* (*bb*) loci map at 66.7 on the X chromosome. These loci carry subnormal numbers of rRNA genes (Ritossa *et al.*, 1966). Mohan and Ritossa (1970) showed that the rates of synthesis of rRNAs were the same in ovaries of phenotypically normal *Drosophila* females with widely different amounts of rDNA (0.18–0.58 percent) and were reduced in phenotypically *bb* females containing 0.13 percent rDNA or less. Eggs produced by such *bb/bb* females contained normal amounts of RNA (0.11–0.14 μg/egg), but such eggs were laid at reduced rates. Mohan and Ritossa conclude that there exists a regulatory mechanism which ensures that each egg is not laid until it accumulates sufficient ribosomes.

Sandler (1970) described a mutation which may influence ribosome production by nurse cells. Females homozygous for the abnormal oocyte (*abo*) gene produce a large excess of female progeny in crosses to homozygous *abo*⁺ males that carry an attached-XY chromosome and no free Y. The sex-ratio effect is due to lowered viability of the XO male offspring. Mange and Sandler (1973) mapped *abo* at 44 on chromosome 2. The viability of male embryos is increased when rDNA is contributed to the zygote by a parental *abo*⁺/*abo*⁺ male. Sandler suggests that *abo*⁺ is a gene that regulates the synthesis of rRNA and that in mutant homozygotes there is a reduction in rRNA synthesis which is critical only in the case of oogenesis. The deficiency in maternally contributed ribosomes can be made up by new ribosomes synthesized after fertilization, provided the embryo contains sufficient rRNA cistrons in its nuclei. The *abo* gene also shows meiotic peculiarities (see page 761), but these may be due to a closely linked, second mutant.

Bell (1954) reported that females homozygous for the gene daughterless (*da*) produce all male progeny. The gene has no effect on the progeny of mutant males. Sandler (1972) showed that female zygotes die, while at least some male zygotes survive, irrespective of the number of Y chromosomes or the amount of X chromosome heterochromatin carried by the mutant female or her progeny. The *da* gene is only 2.5 units to the left of *abo* (Mange and Sandler, 1973). These closely linked genes are somewhat similar in that, when homozygous, both generate a maternal effect that results in the production of abnormal eggs which in turn causes a sex differential in zygote mortality during embryogenesis. Mange and Sandler induced a dominant Enhancer of daughterless mutation with x-irradiation. The enhancer was shown to be a translocation between chromosomes 2 and 3, with the second chromosome breakpoint in the pericentric heterochromatin. $T(2;3)E(da)$ can rescue some of the potentially lethal zygotes produced by homozygous *abo* mothers. Mange and Sandler suggest that both *abo* and *da* are located in a special region of chromosome 2 that is concerned with the regulation of the transcriptional activities of sex-chromosome heterochromatin. Presumably different heterochromatic genes interact with the two autosomal genes.

Baker (1971) has shown that two X-chromosomal inversions (sc^{L8} and sc^{S1}) produce lethality in XO males, but not in XY males. Each of the inversions has one break between the nucleolus organizer and the centromere and the other near the left tip of the X. As a result, rDNA is separated from the pericentric heterochromatin. If a Y chromosome lacking the bb^{+} locus is supplied to eggs containing either an sc^{L8} or an sc^{S1} X chromosome, the viability of male embryos is only 50 percent that of embryos containing a normal Y. Baker concludes that the two inverted X chromosomes are suppressing essential viability genes related to the production of rRNA. Females homozygous for sc^{L8} or sc^{S1} are viable, but sterile. These observations suggest that different genes are suppressed in the two sexes. Alternatively, if the same genes are suppressed, then their products are essential for life in male (but not female) embryos and for normal oogenesis.

In *D. melanogaster* six mutant genes are known which include among their phenotypic effects cytologically detectable abnormalities in the behavior of the nurse-cell chromosomes. The genes are singed (*sn*, 1–21), raspberry (*ras*, 1–32.8), *fs(2)E1* (2–57.6), morula (*mr*, 2–106.7), rotund (*rn*, 3–47.7), and the suppressor of Hairy wing² [$su(Hw)^{2}$, 3–54.8]. The earlier work on these mutants is reviewed by King [(1970), pages 161–164]. More recent radiotracer studies have been reported by Klug *et al.* (1970) on the synthesis of RNA and protein by $su(Hw)^{2}$ ovaries. They concluded that the RNA transcribed in $su(Hw)^{2}$ nurse-cell nuclei is not retained in the nucleolus for a normal time interval, and that much of it breaks down. The concentration of cytoplasmic ribosomes is decreased, and cytoplasmic protein synthesis is reduced.

Bakken (1973) has induced a recessive female-sterile mutation in chromosome 2 which appears to affect the nurse cells. Females homozygous for *fs(2)A17* produce oocytes that never develop past stage 7. However, nurse-cell nuclei are arrested at a point in their chromosomal differentiation which resembles stage 4. Blocked vitellogenesis is due to the failure of the oocyte to take up vitellogenin (see page 768). Failure of function of the nurse-cell nuclei subsequent to stage 4 would presumably be responsible for the inability to take up such yolk precursor proteins from the hemolymph.

Several mutations affecting both nurse cells and follicle cells will be described in the next section.

Mutations Affecting the Migration, Differentiation, and Maintenance of Follicle Cells

The mutations tiny (*ty* 1-44.5) and diminutive (*dm*, 1-4.6) have been shown to affect the migrations II and IV of the follicle cells and their subsequent differentiation and synthetic activities [see King (1970), pages 44, 165–166, and 174–178].

Usually we identify the mutations affecting oogenesis by their female-sterile phenotypes. Mutations in pleiotropic genes, where the product is essential not only for oogenesis but also for viability, are lethal and their potential effects on the ovary and oogenesis go undetected in the typical study. Recently C. L. Littlefield, P. Simpson, S. Bryant, T. Cline, and R. Arking, working with H. A. Schneiderman, have begun a study of such mutations. The following is based on a private communication from H. A. Schneiderman in which the several mutant strains and their known effects were described.

The procedure is as follows: Temperature-sensitive, lethal mutations are cultured at a permissive temperature (22°C) to adulthood. Adult females, homozygous for the mutation, are mated to wild-type males and transferred to the restrictive temperature (29°C). Some mutations remain fertile, demonstrating that the gene product does not have a role in the adult part of oogenesis. The mutant females in other strains (about half of all tested) become sterile after 5 days.

Altogether, 22 sex-linked mutations in 16 cistrons have been isolated. With the exception of one strain [*l(1)ts-6225*], egg laying ceases (see page 776). C. L. Littlefield has examined the affected ovaries in most mutant strains, using Feulgen-stained whole mounts. The effects for mutations in three genes have not yet been described. In three genes the defects are on follicle cells without apparent change in nurse cells. In two cases, mutations $l(1)ts2320$ and 108, follicle cells associated with specific stages degenerate; in the third, $l(1)ts5569$, there is no degeneration, but migration of follicle cells is abnormal.

The remaining 15 mutations in 9 genes have various effects on both follicle cells and nurse cells. Degeneration invariably occurs. In some cases the degeneration is general, affecting all stages of oogenesis. In others the degeneration occurs only at specific stages, with other sorts of abnormalities in egg chambers at earlier and/or later developmental stages. For example, the follicle cells may form a multilayered epithelium, or the nurse-cell nuclei may become pycnotic. The observations have not progressed to a detailed analysis of the defects and their order of occurrence, so that the full significance of these mutations cannot be weighed. It is of interest and of importance to note that the mutations in different genes produce distinctive syndromes, reflecting in each case a unique constellation of defects consequent to the destruction of a unique gene product.

Mutations Affecting Early Stages in Vitellogenesis

During stages 1–6 (a time interval of about 50 hours), the volume of the ooplasm increases 40-fold. The doubling time for this exponential ooplasmic growth is about 9 hours, and the nurse-cell cytoplasm increases in volume at a similar rate. During the 12-hour stage 7 the egg chamber elongates, and there is a decrease in growth rate. Oocytes spend 18 hours in stages 8–12. Now the volume of ooplasm increases 1500 times, with a doubling time of about 2 hours! During this "vitellogenic period" protein-rich, alpha yolk spheres appear in the ooplasm, and the nurse cells contribute large quantities of ribosomes and lipid droplets to the oocyte [King (1970), Figures II 10–15).

The mutants described in the following section affect this early period of massive yolk synthesis and uptake. The first mutant studied in detail is apterous (ap, 2–55.2). Adults homozygous for certain alleles may have normal viabilities and fertilities (as in the case of ap^{56f}), or they may be sterile and die during the second or third days of adult life (as in the case of ap^4 and ap^{49j}). A deficiency covering ap is available [$Df(2)MS4$]. Since flies of genotype ap^{56f}/ap^4 live longer than $ap^{56f}/Df(2)MS4$ flies, ap^4 behaves as a hypomorphic allele. Females of genotype ap^4/ap^{56f} and ap^{49j}/ap^{56f} are viable and fertile; whereas ap^4/ap^{49j} are poorly viable and sterile. Yolk formation is severely reduced in the ovaries of ap^4 or ap^{49j} homozygotes. The few flies that survive to the third day sometimes contain oocytes in vitellogenic stages, but the total volume of yolky ooplasm per ovary is no more than 1 percent of that found in wild-type flies of identical age. Although ap^4 flies die prematurely and fail to synthesize yolk, it is not because they are unable to ingest food. Ovaries from ap^4/ap^4 females will incorporate abundant yolk when implanted into the abdomens of wild-type adults. Therefore, it is the abdominal environment of ap^4 that is the cause of sterility, rather than a malfunctioning of the ovary [King (1970), pages 180–181].

Postlethwait and Weiser (1973) topically applied 0.05 μg, of isopropyl 11-methoxy-3,7,11-trimethyldodeca-2,4 denoate (Zoecon ZR-515) in 0.2 μl of acetone to the ventral surface of adult, larval, and pupal abdomens. Treatment with this juvenile-hormone analog greatly increased vitellogenesis in the ovaries of young ap^4 adults. However, treatment of larval or pupal stages did not ameliorate the wing or haltere effect. Since the ap^4 homozygote goes through normal larval development, it is obvious that juvenile hormone is secreted normally during this period in the mutant. If the same molecule functions as both a juvenile hormone and a vitellogenic hormone, one interpretation would have the secretion of this molecule blocked in adult ap^4 females. An alternative explanation would be that ap mutations affect the threshold requirement for the molecule as it affects yolk synthesis, but not uptake. Accordingly, ap^4 sets a very high threshold than can be met only by pharmacological doses.

Bakken (1973) reported that vitellogenesis is abolished or retarded in four nonallelic, autosomal, recessive, female-sterile mutations [$fs(2)A18$, $fs(3)A1$, $fs(3)A16$, and $fs(3)A17$] as well as in $fs(2)A17$, which also affects differentiation of nurse-cell nuclei. Kambysellis and Gelti-Douka (1974, and private communication) and Postlethwait (private communication) have independently begun studies of the physiological defects in these mutants. The predominant yolk presursor protein (vitellogenin) can be identified within the female hemolymph by electrophoretic and immunological methods, and its quantity estimated. In the case of $fs(3)A17$, homozygous females have no yolk protein in their blood; in the case of each of the others, there is an accumulation of yolk protein in excess of normal amounts. These observations distinguish a mutant, $fs(3)A17$, affecting synthesis of yolk protein from the other four, which instead affect the incorporation of vitellogenin into the oocyte. Both Kambysellis and Postlethwait have treated young adult females homozygous for the "uptake" mutations by topical application of a juvenile-hormone analog. They have similar results, except that Postlethwait did not examine *fs(3)A16*: in one case, *fs(2)A17*, there was no responding increase in vitellogenesis; in each of the other three, treated females exhibited a modest increase in the number of follicles in vitellogenic stages.

In addition, Postlethwait has made extensive transplantation experiments with *fs(2)A17*, *fs(2)A18*, and *fs(3)A1*. Ovaries from each of these transplanted into *fs+* hosts (Ore R and heterozygous siblings) fail to take up yolk. This apparent autonomy distinguishes *fs(2)A18* and *fs(3)A1* from *ap*⁴. Reciprocal transplants of normal ovaries into homozygous *fs* females reveal differences among the three mutants in the environment that each provides for vitellogenesis. In these cases the transplants were ovaries from Ore R, heterozygous siblings, and *ap*⁴ donors into hosts of *fs(2)A17*, *fs(2)A18*, and *fs(3)A1*. Within any one host genotype all three kinds of "normal" ovaries develop essentially the same way. Females of *fs(2)A17* provide an especially favorable environment for vitellogenesis in that the transplants produce threefold increases in the number of stage-14 oocytes over those in controls transplanted into Ore R. Females of *fs(2)A18* as hosts produce effects similar in level to those of normal hosts, but females of *fs(3)A1* provide a poorer environment because the implanted ovaries are only one-eighth as well developed as those in control hosts. Since Kambysellis has found that the amount of yolk protein in the blood of all three mutants is high, a highly favorable environment for vitellogenesis might be expected in all cases. The results with *fs(2)A18* and *fs(3)A1* point to additional components outside the ovary which regulate the uptake process and raise the question whether the ovarian expression of these mutants is invariably "autonomous." In this connection, one additional observation by Postlethwait is instructive. Ovaries from *fs(3)A1* will develop yolky eggs in *fs(2)A17* hosts, which provide the especially favorable environment, but not in *fs(2)A18* hosts. Thus *fs(3)A1* ovaries can form some yolk in special environments.

Oocytes in vitellogenic stages are rarely seen in females homozygous for the mutant gene minus (*mi*, 2–104.7), but no further studies have been made.

Mutations Affecting Later Stages in Vitellogenesis

During stage 13, yolk spheres belonging to a second class appear in the ooplasm. These beta yolk spheres [see King (1970), Figure VI-7] are rich in polysaccharides but lack proteins.

Females homozygous for the ocelliless mutant (*oc*, 1–23.0) are sterile. Their ovaries contain normal-sized eggs in which are found reduced numbers of bèta yolk spheres. These are abnormally large and differ in their cytochemical properties. Normal beta yolk spheres stain intensely with the periodic acid/Schiff reaction (PA/S), and are made up of particles that bind lead citrate. The giant beta yolk spheres of the mutant give a weaker PA/S reaction and bind little lead (Johnson and King, 1974).

Oocyte Storage by Mutant Females

Storage of oocytes is common in certain female-sterile mutants. Females homozygous for the mutant stubarista (*sta*, 1–3.0) produce normal-appearing, stage-14, ovarian oocytes but seem to be unable to oviposit. Storage of stage-14 oocytes is also characteristic in females homozygous for lozenge^{34k} (*lz*^{34k}, 1–27.7). Perhaps in such mutants the musculatures of the uteri and genital segments are unable to generate the peristaltic contractions required for oviposition. Bakken (1973) has described 7 nonallelic, autosomal, "ovulation" mutations (see her Table 9). Females homozygous for any of these can synthesize stage-14 oocytes but seem to be unable to lay them. Sterility in the Hairy wing^{49c} mutant is due to a malfunctioning of the oviduct (Holzworth *et al.*, 1974*a,b*).

Mutations Affecting the Egg Shell

The egg shell or chorion, which forms a protective covering about the mature oocyte, is laid down by the columnar follicle cells during stages 12–14 (King and Koch, 1963; Quattropani and Anderson, 1969). In electron micrographs the egg coverings are seen to consist of three parts: an inner-most vitelline membrane, a highly structured endochorion, and an outermost exochorion. The air-filled spaces within the endochorion serve a respiratory function for the developing embryo. The dorsal appendages are anterior specializations of the chorion.

Egg-shell defects have been observed in oocytes produced by females homozygous for several of the female-sterile genes mentioned previously. Abnormalities from *ty* and from *oc* homozygotes can be seen in papers by King and Koch [(1963), their Figure 15] and by Johnson and King [(1974), their Figure 7]. Deformed dorsal appendages have also been observed in oocytes produced by *fs(2)E1*, *ras*^{4}, *sn*^{36a}, *adp*, and *vg* homozygotes [see King and Koch (1963) page 317, for literature).

Egg-shell defects are also produced by many mutations that have been selected by maternal-effect lethal phenotypes. The eggs, which are laid by females homozygous for the mutations, fail to develop, perhaps as a consequence of the abnormal egg shells. The defective membranes are shown to be fragile in that they are readily fractured by stroking with a fine, camelhair brush. Often the eggs collapse when touched, and in several cases they are found collapsed on the surface where laid. Some mutations affect the dorsal appendages as well, shortening them, and/or changing their shape. Recently large collections of maternal-effect lethal mutations have been examined for defects in the egg shells. Mohler (unpublished) finds such mutations at eleven loci [*fs(1)M*] which are scattered over the X chromosome. Five of the genes are represented by 3, 4, or 5 mutations each. Where multiple alleles occur, at least two, but not all alleles make fragile membranes; at least one allele in each case produces eggs that seem as sturdy as normal. C. Audit and M. Gans (private communication) also observed collapsed eggs with fragile membranes as a result of female-sterile mutations at 17 sex-linked loci [see Table 1, *fs(1)A*]. Two allelic, sex-linked mutations [*fs(1)V*] affecting egg-shell formation have been produced by E. R. Vyse. It is likely that the separate collections of mutations include defects in some of the same genes, but the studies have not yet been done to establish allelism.

Mutations producing these defects are found on the autosomes as well. Bakken (1973) reports that two of her mutants [*fs(2)A9* and *fs(2)A12*] are characterized by fragile chorions and malformed dorsal appendages. These map to loci 25 $\pm$ 5 and 61 $\pm$ 5, respectively. Though one strain of *fs(2)A9* (strain 8–854) was reported to show two female-sterile genes in complementation tests, only one *fs* mutation was found in the mapping study (Mohler, unpublished). Another mutation, *fs(3)K1*, induced by R. Kieso, maps to locus 55 $\pm$ 3 and produces eggs with extremely short filaments.

Mutations at two loci are temperature sensitive in the operational sense that homozygous females produce some progeny when raised and maintained at 18°C but not when cultured at 25°C or higher. In the case of *fs(3)K1*, temperature differences affect survival without apparent change in the length of the filaments. In the case of *fs(1)M13* (locus 13 $\pm$), which has five alleles, *all* alleles are temperature sensitive, including one that has normal-appearing egg shells. In the case of *fs(3)K1*, we should expect the chorions to be nearly normal at the permissive temperature if the mutant proteins were temperature sensitive. With respect to *fs(1)M13*, we expect only a few, not all, of the possible mutations to result in temperature-sensitive proteins. Thus, the temperature effects in these cases are unlikely to be expressed by way of modifications of protein conformation. The effects may come about by temperature modification of the physiological consequences of structural damage to the egg shells.

Electron microscopic analysis of the egg-shell development in *fs(2)A9* (strain 8–854) has been done by Margaritis (1974) and F. C. Kafatos (private communication). Defects are readily apparent in both the vitelline membrane and the chorion, such that the overall architecture is grossly modified. The endochorion is especially abnormal, having many of the pillars missing and having interruptions in its outer layer. The spaces between the two layers of the endochorion are thus larger and filled with material resembling that in the exochorion. The analysis by Margaritis shows that formation of the vitelline membrane and endochorion are not only incomplete, but their periods of synthesis are also prolonged, suggesting a "regulatory" role for the normal gene.

C. L. Littlefield (private communication) has made a preliminary electron microscopic study of the two *fs(1)V* mutations and found that the hexagonal architecture of the chorion is abolished. Material with the electron density of the endochorion is present, but as "splotches."

Mutations with Maternal Effects

Most of the female-sterile mutations do not cause recognizable defects in ovarian structures; rather they cause failure of development in the eggs laid by homozygous females. The eggs are not fertilized in only a few cases; whereas in the vast majority of mutations the eggs produced by homozygous females are deficient in some compound or in some aspect of cytoplasmic organization that is essential for normal embryogenesis. The eggs produced by normal females and females heterozygous for the mutation have the normal compound and cytoplasmic organization and, therefore, can support normal development of homozygous and hemizygous embryos. These mutations are appropriately named maternal-effect lethal (*mel*) mutations. In an important subset of these mutations the missing compound can be synthesized, subsequent to fertilization, if the normal allele has been contributed by the sperm. These mutations have been called "maternally-influenced-lethal" mutations by Kaplan *et al.* (1970), but we prefer to refer to this as the "rescuable maternal-effect lethal" (mel R) class. We are including these mutations in this chapter because the genes must act during oogenesis. The essential gene products are normally synthesized by cells of the maternal genotype, and they are transferred to and become a part of the ooplasm before the egg is laid. The defects in embryogenesis produced by these mutations are clues to subtle aspects of oogenesis that cannot be revealed simply in morphological analysis of normal oogenesis.

Mutations like cinnamon (*cin*, 1–0.0), deep orange (*dor*, 1–0.3), almondex (*amx*, 1–27.7), rudimentary (*r*, 1–55.3), fused (*fu*, 1–59.5), and sonless (*snl*, 1–56.3) are classical examples of mel R genes. Typically, females homozygous for any of these genes produce offspring only if they are mated to males bearing the normal allele of the gene in question. Because the mutations are sex-linked, the progeny in these matings are exclusively or almost exclusively females.

Zygotes that lack the *cin*⁺ substance die before hatching from the egg. The *cin* locus affects pteridine-pigment metabolism. The presence of a *cin*⁺ allele in either the mother or zygote is a prerequisite for normal zygotic eye pigmentation. The *cin*⁺ locus controls xanthine dehydrogenase (XDH); *cin*⁺ flies lack XDH activity, accumulate its pteridine and purine substrates, and lack the products of the enzyme (Baker, 1973).

The rosy locus (*ry*, 3–52.0) is the cistron for XDH. There is no maternal effect of the *ry* locus on either eye color or XDH activity. XDH activity is also lost in the absence of the plus allele of maroonlike (*mal*, 1–64.8). The *mal* locus, like the *cin* locus, acts both maternally and zygotically to control eye color and XDH activity. That the *mal*⁺ factor is present in unfertilized eggs and early embryos was shown by Sayles *et al.* (1973). Extracts of *mal* flies have *ry*⁺ factor and extracts of *ry*² flies have the *mal*⁺ factor. Mixtures of the two extracts complement to give xanthine dehydrogenase activity. Using this *in vitro* complementation technique, the *mal*⁺ factor was demonstrated in unfertilized eggs of *ry*², and it persisted at least through the first 7 hours of development. Similar information about the maternal contribution of a *cin*⁺ factor is not yet available. Since XDH activity is abolished in *ry* and *mal* homozygotes without marked effects on viability, it is obvious that the absence of XDH activities in *cin* zygotes is not the cause of their death (Baker, 1973). The mechanisms by which *mal*⁺ and *cin*⁺ influence XDH activity are not understood.

Bischoof and Lucchesi (1971) have shown that the *dor* gene is a pseudoallelic locus that can be separated by crossing over into four subunits. Most alleles generate a characteristic change in the eye color of the adults of both sexes, as the name implies, and most (*but not all*) of these alleles also produce the maternal lethal phenotype. The original *dor*¹ mutation shows both phenotypic effects. Ovaries transplanted from homozygous *dor*¹ larvae to normal hosts behave autonomously (Garen and Gehring, 1972). The developmental block in defective embryos occurs at the gastrulation stage. The paternal *dor*⁺ gene prevents this developmental block in only about half of the heterozygous female embryos. Garen and Gehring injected cytoplasm from unfertilized normal eggs into *dor*¹/*dor*¹ embryos that were at the syncytial preblastoderm stage of development and found that about one-third of the injected embryos were then able to continue their development to an advanced stage of embryogenesis.

In the case of *amx*, Shannon (1972) has shown that most female zygotes produced by the cross *amx/amx* female × *amx⁺* male die as embryos. However, survival to the adult stage is more frequent at higher temperatures, and survival also increases with increasing maternal age. Surviving daughters usually show defects such as absence of a leg or alteration in the size and shape of abdominal sternites. In lethal embryos development is normal until shortly after the time of maximum germ-band extension. The principal anomalies involve derivatives of the ectoderm and somatic mesoderm, and both dorsal closure and head involution are impaired (Shannon, 1973).

The genetic analysis of the *r* locus by Carlson (1971) led him to conclude that the female sterility and wing phenes are dependent upon a common biochemical process. Nørby (1970) had shown previously that *r* mutants had a nutritional requirement for pyrimidines, and Bahn (1970) found that homozygous r^{39k} females mated to hemizygous males produced viable offspring of *both* sexes if the medium on which they were grown was enriched with cytidine. The *r* mutation thus became the first female sterile to have its fertility restored by the dietary addition of a specific compound. Okada *et al.* (1974) have shown, furthermore, that *r* embryos from homozygous mothers can be rescued both by injections of ooplasm from *r⁺* and by injection of pyrimidines into the eggs.

Nørby (1973) has suggested that the *r⁺* locus contains the structural genes for the first *two* enzymes in the biosynthetic pathway for pyrimidines. In this connection, Falk and Nash (1974*a,b*) have isolated 20 pyrimidine-requiring mutations, all of which map close to the *r* locus. Eleven, designated r^{pyr}, have the reduced wing size typical of *r* mutations and are female sterile. The other nine, $(r)^{pyr}$, have normal wings and reduced female fertility. Because the auxotrophy is partially dominant in all 20 mutations, complementation studies on the pyrimidine requirement are done with low-level pyrimidine nucleoside supplementation. Under these conditions, females of the genotype $r^{45}/(r)^{pyr}$ do not survive in the case of seven of the nine $(r)^{pyr}$ mutations. These seven mutations are concluded to be isoalleles of *r*. The other two mutations do not fully complement r^{45} even under these conditions and may or may not be affecting a different cistron.

Another rescuable maternal effect lethal mutation that is associated with a putative auxotrophic mutation is yeast requirement 1-1 (*yea 1-1*, 1–37±7) (Falk and Nash, 1974*a*). The mutation is cold sensitive. Homozygotes do not survive at 18°C, but survive at 25°C and 29°C, if supplemented with yeast. Homozygous females lay eggs that die as embryos unless the *yea*[+] allele is supplied by the sperm. Romans (1973) studied two allelic, maternal-effect lethals, which she designated *miel(1)R1*[r] and *miel(1)R1*[o], that are allelic to another yeast-requirement gene (*yea 3–1*, 1–0.8). The first two are completely sterile in crosses to mutant males; the third is semi-sterile. One allele, *miel(1)R1*[r], is rescuable, producing daughters and non-disjunctional males when crossed to normal males; the other is not.

The sonless mutation is maternally influenced, but its lethal effects are also dependent upon the sex of the embryo. Females of the genotype *snl/snl* are not susceptible to lethal effects, as are *snl/Y* males. Colaianne and Bell (1972) have studied the interactions on *snl* with sex-altering mutants *tra* and *dsx* [see King (1970), pages 18–22] and have found that any alteration toward increased masculinity of progeny from *snl/snl* females reduced their zygotic viability.

There are many more loci where mel-R alleles are found. In addition to the chorion genes, Mohler (unpublished) has identified maternal-effect lethal mutations in 48 other cistrons. Of these, twenty have rescuable alleles. One cistron, *fs(1)M50,* is the *cin* locus; another, *fs(1)M34,* is the *r* locus. None of the others are allelic with *fu, dor,* or *amx.* C. Audit and M. Gans (private communication) also found this class of mutation in ten sex-linked genes, including three mutations at the *r* locus. We should expect to find these mutations on the autosomes as well as the X. However, we would have to examine carefully the progeny of apparently fertile, homozygous females mated with heterozygous males for the absence of homozygous off-spring. Rice (1973) tentatively identified two such mutations on the third chromosome.

There remains one more group of maternal-effect lethal mutations to describe. In this group, the eggs laid by homozygous females cannot be rescued by a paternal + allele. The familiar examples are female-sterile (1)N [*fs(1)N*, 1–0.0], which was investigated by Counce and Ede (1957), adipose-female sterile [*adp*[fs], 2–83.4], which was studied by Doane (1960a,b, 1961), and female-sterile (3)G1 [*fs(3)G1*, 3–47), which was described by Gill (1963). Another example is *da*, though the lethal effect is expressed only in females in this case (see page 765).

More examples are turned up in systematic collections of female-sterile mutations. In a number of studies, complementation tests have been made among these mutations. Bakken (1973) identified nine cistrons on the second chromosome and eight on the third. Rice (1973) independently found eight genes on the third chromosome. Though some of Bakken's mutations may be alleles of Rice's, the chances are that most are not, because in both groups most genes are represented by single alleles. On the X chromosome, Mohler (unpublished) has found 27 cistrons; C. Audit and

M. Gans (private communication) have found 22; and Romans (1973) has identified 9 loci. Judd and Young, (1974) found two cistrons, closely linked at 1–0.38, with three alleles each. These were the only female-sterile mutations they found in a search of the zeste (*z*, 1–1.0) to white (*w*, 1–1.5) region. Because most (16) of the cistrons in Mohler's list have more than one allele, it is quite likely that considerable overlap in identity occurs with the genes in the other collections.

Only one of the recessive, temperature-sensitive mutations, which are being studied by the group with H. A. Schneiderman, has a temperature-sensitive maternal effect. T. Cline has made the following observations: Adult females, homozygous for *l(1)ts6225*, which were raised at a permissive temperature (22°C), are fertile. If they are mated to wild-type males, then transferred to 29°C, they become sterile after one or two days; if returned to 22°C, they become fertile again, but only after several days. The expectation that female embryos, being heterozygous, should be able to develop at the restrictive temperature, together with the observation of delayed changes of phenotype following the temperature shifts, mean that the temperature effect is on the formation of the egg prior to its being laid.

In several cases the phenotypic effects of these mutations have been examined in more detail. Some of the mutations initially identified as maternal-effect lethals undergo no development and may be blocks in fertilization and syngamy. This appears to happen in the case of *l(1)ts6225* (T. Cline, private communication). Bakken (1973) described one mutation, *fs(2)A14*, in which fertilization occurs, but syngamy does not. In most eggs the separate oocyte nucleus and sperm head were identified. However, the oocyte nucleus appeared to be blocked in metaphase II, suggesting a defect in completion of meiosis rather than in syngamy.

In three other mutations, *fs(3)A11*, *fs(3)A12*, and *fs(3)A14*, Bakken found no development and no chromatin. Because normal, unfertilized oviposited eggs typically have one or two nuclei, arrested in abnormal metaphase, even after 4 hours (von Borstel, 1960), the blocked development and missing chromatin are not the consequences of blocking fertilization. Nothing more is known of these mutants. Three of the sex-linked genes identified by C. Audit and M. Gans, *fs(1)A73, 1526,* and *1528,* are blocked prior to nuclear divisions.

With those mutations that begin development, the typical study distinguishes the different genes by the kinds of defects found in embryos from homozygous mothers, and such studies would include descriptions of the earliest anomalies and the abnormal sequence of development and would provide information on the lethal phase. Some mutations are polyphasic, with variable programs of defects; others are monophasic and relatively uniformly expressed. The $fs(1)N$ gene is an example of the former; several examples of the latter have been recently described by Bakken (1973), Rice (1973), Romans (1973), and C. Audit (private communication). The distinction is blurred by Doane's (1960b) work with adp^{fs}. Under some conditions of genotypic background and environment, the embryos from mutant mothers vary considerably; under other conditions, they arrest regularly at cleavage 5 or 6.

In those cases where the expression is uniform it is possible to characterize the mutant genes by their effects on embryogenesis. The stages at which developmental arrest occurs and the generalized patterns of abnormal development distinguish the new mutations in the following list: arrest at premigration cleavage in $fs(3)A15$, $fs(2)A13$, $fs(2)A2$ (Bakken), $fs(1)A97$, $fs(1)A214$, $fs(1)A1042$, $fs(1)A1242$, and $fs(1)A1578$ (Audit); arrest at syncytial blastoderm in $fs(2)A7$ (Bakken), $fs(1)A1459$ (Audit), mel-1 (3–54.8), and mel-6 (3–98.0) (Rice); abnormal blastoderm with abnormal gastrulation in $fs(2)A11$ (Bakken), $fs(1)A457$, $fs(1)A1140$, $fs(1)A1371$ (Audit), and mel-3 (3–45.2) (Rice); abnormal gastrulation in mel-2 (3–17) and mel-4 (3–51.3) (Rice), and $fs(1)A573$, $fs(1)A1182$, and $fs(1)A1509$ (Audit); and arrest late in embryogeny in $fs(3)A13$ (Bakken), $fs(1)A572$, $fs(1)A1187$, $fs(1)A1497$ (Audit), and $miel(1)R1$ (Romans). Unfortunately, $fs(3)A13$ has since been lost.

Rice, using the mutant material, has made progress in an analysis of embryogenesis and determination of larval and imaginal structures. The mutants mel-1, mel-6, and mel-3 all affect cellularization of the blastoderm. In all cases, cleavage and migration of nuclei are nearly normal. In each case the formation of cell membranes is blocked. The different mutants are distinguished by the extent and pattern of cells in the blastoderm stage. Embryos from mel-1 develop only pole cells. Those from mel-6 develop cells at the anterior and posterior ends. The embryos from mel-3 have normal cell formation over the anterior third. In these cases they have a patchy arrangement of cells in the posterior ventral-lateral part and no cells in the posterior-dorsal third. In the dorsal part, the blastoderm nuclei are eventually engulfed in yolk.

The consequences are instructive. In the cases of mel-1 and mel-6, pole cell migration occurs, not always in the correct direction, but mimicking the normal movements that accompany expansion of the germ band. The observations demonstrate that some features of the normal movements are not dependent on a cellular organization. No organs are formed from the cells of mel-6. In mel-3 gastrulation proceeds in a fashion that suggests dependence on cellularization. Embryos only form cephalic furrows, if that part is cellular; they always form the ventral furrow, since that part is always cellular. Many organs typical of the anterior half are subsequently formed.

The mutant *mel-3* is temperature sensitive. Eggs formed by homozygous females at 20°C develop into adult flies. Of these adults, 17.1 percent are missing imaginal structures, primarily legs, halteres, tergites or sternites; another 5.7 percent have abnormal development of these structures. In comparison, the progeny of heterozygous females are missing adult parts in only 0.3 percent. The blastoderm of embryos produced under permissive conditions have patches of missing cells. Apparently the imaginal structure could be missing because cells were not formed in the regions corresponding to the anlagen of the imaginal discs.

In *mel-2* and *mel-4* cellularization is complete, but the ventral furrow does not form. The observations demonstrate that gastrulation depends in part upon some specific, determining substances.

As a whole, the previous list of mutant effects connects the controls of certain aspects of embryogenesis to specific events in oogenesis. What is happening in oogenesis is still unknown.

The Proportion of the Genome Specific to Oogenesis

A substantial part of the *Drosophila* genome is expected to be involved in reactions common to all cells. The genetic elements influencing metabolism, molecular synthesis, and morphogenetic components, such as microtubules and plasma membranes, are examples of genes that should be important in general and shared with most other aspects of development. Some other genetic elements must function specifically in oogenesis. These latter genes would be responsible for molecules that are synthesized and used only for oogenesis or early steps in embryogenesis. A part could be structural molecules, yolk proteins, and enzymes specific to oogenesis and the egg. Another part would be regulating molecules required specifically in oogenesis and early embryogenesis to control metabolic function, molecular synthesis, and the formation and use of morphogenetic components.

We look for the genes specific to oogenesis among the female-sterile mutations. The extent to which the female-sterile class includes mutations in other genes is not known. Certainly leaky mutations in genes for general functions could affect fertility, but not viability, if oogenesis were especially sensitive to low levels of the gene product. In this regard, however, prior screening of female-sterile mutations does not enrich the frequency of auxotrophs (D. Nash, private communication). Some female-

sterile mutations have pleiotropic effects on the morphology of adult structure. In earlier studies, the female-sterile mutations were selected from
among those with morphological effects. The recent searches for female-
sterile mutations turn up many more without apparent effect on adult
structure. Mutations that sterilize the females by affecting mating behavior will probably be encountered in future studies.

Whatever the uncertainties, the proportion of the genome that can
mutate to female-sterile alleles sets an upper limit to the proportion that is
specifically involved in oogenesis. Working with 150 female-sterile mutations, induced by ethyl methanesulfonate (EMS), Mohler (1973, and in
preparation) identified 59 sex-linked cistrons. In all cases females
homozygous for the mutations lay eggs that do not develop. Complementation tests, made with other similar genes, show one each allelic with
cin (one mutation), *fs(1)N* (three mutations), *sn* (one mutation), and *r*
(fifteen mutations). Nearly half (27) of the genes are represented by one female-sterile mutation, implying that some genes with female-sterile alleles
are not included. Besides the 27 genes with single occurrences of mutation,
the distribution includes 14 with 2, 6 with 3, 2 with 4, and 10 with 5 or
more (up to 15 for *r*). The first four terms in the distribution are compatible
with a Poisson distribution with a mean = 1.04, calculated as follows:

$$\frac{\text{number of cistrons with two mutations}}{\text{number of cistrons with one mutation}} = \frac{Nm^2e^{-m}}{2Nme^{-m}} = \frac{m}{2};$$

$$\frac{\text{number with one mutation}}{m} = Ne^{-m} = X = \text{number no mutation}$$

where N is the total number of relevant genes and m is the average number
of mutations in each gene. From the above distribution, $m = 28/27 = 1.04$
and $X = 27$. Thus, something close to 86 genes ($N = 27 + 59$) on the X
chromosome can be mutated to female-sterile alleles which allow the
production of eggs that are incapable of developing. In using the first two
terms of the distribution to estimate the size of the null class, we have
assumed that the larger part of the genes are identified by mutation with a
probability that is much less than that for the 8–10 genes distributed over
the high end and that the lower mutation frequency is invariant and the
lowest frequency.

The total number of genes mutating to female-sterile alleles can be
predicted by the following logic. If the X is assumed to represent ⅕ of the
total genome, then we could expect a total of 430 genes of the sort discussed
above. A second group of mutations is known that blocks events prior to
oviposition, and the frequency of the second group is ½ of the first.
Therefore, the total number of genes with female-sterile alleles would be

TABLE 1. A Catalog of Genes that Function in Oogenesis in D. melanogaster, Sorted by Effects of Female-Sterile Alleles

Class	Gene[a]	Female-sterile alleles	References
1. Germ cell determination	grandchildless	gs^{87}	Thierry-Mieg et al. (1972) Counce and Ede (1957)
	female-sterile(1)N	(Five)	C. Kern and A. Mahowald (private communication)
2. Ovariolar differentiation	female-sterile(2)A15	fs(2)A15	
	female-sterile(2)A16	fs(2)A16	Bakken (1973)
	female-sterile(3)A10	fs(3)A10	
3. Cystocyte divisions			
a. Suppressing division	Female-sterile(2)D	Fs(2)D	Yarger and King (1971)
	fused	(Several)	
	narrow	(Several)	
b. Tumorous divisions	female-sterile(2)B(fes)	fs(2)B	King (1970)
4. Meiosis			
a. Crossing over abolished or reduced throughout the genome	crossover suppressor of Gowan	(Two)[b]	Hall (1972)
	recombination	rec	R. Grell (private communication)
	meiotic 218	(mei-218)[b]	
	abnormal oocyte	(abo)[b]	Carpenter and Sandler (1974)
	meiotic 9	(Two)[b]	
	meiotic 41	(Two)[b]	
	meiotic 251	(mei-251)[b]	Baker and Carpenter (1972)
	meiotic 352	(mei-352)[b]	
	meiotic S282	(mei-S282)[b]	Parry (1973)

b. Increased crossing over near centromere; non-disjunction	meiotic 38 meiotic 99 meiotic 160	$(mei\text{-}38)$[b] $(mei\text{-}99)$[b] $(mei\text{-}160)$[b]	Baker and Carpenter (1972)
c. Localized reduction of crossing over	meiotic 1	$(mei\text{-}1)$[b]	Valentin (1973)
d. Abnormal disjunction	no distributive pairing claret-non-disjunctional meiotic S332	(nod)[b] (ca^{nd})[b] $(mei\text{-}S332)$[b]	Carpenter (1973) Davis (1971)
5. Nurse-cell function			
a. Ribosome synthesis modified	bobbed abnormal oocyte daughterless	(Several)[b] (abo)[b] (da)[b]	Mohan and Ritossa (1970) Sandler (1970) Mange and Sandler (1974)
b. Nuclear differentiation modified	singed raspberry female-sterile(2)E1 morula rotund suppressor of Hairy wing female-sterile(2)A17	(Several) ras^4 $fs(2)E1$ (Two) rn (Two) (Six?)	King (1970) Klug *et al.* (1970) Bakken (1973)
6. Follicle cell development			
a. Modified migration	tiny diminutive	ty (Two)	King (1970)
b. Differentiation and maintenance affected	lethal(1)ts-108 lethal(1)ts-2320 lethal(1)ts-5569	$l(1)ts\text{-}108$ $l(1)ts\text{-}2320$ $l(1)ts\text{-}5569$	C. L. Littlefield, P. Simpson, S. Bryant, T. Cline, and R. Arking (private communication)

[a] Mat = maternal, ts = temperature sensitive.

[b] Females homozygous for mutants in some classes are not characterized as sterile, e.g., meiotic mutants.

[c] The genetics and phenotypic effects are incompletely characterized in many cases. The number in parentheses is the number of additional cistrons identified, but not yet further characterized.

[d] Extinct.

TABLE 1. Continued

Class	Gene[a]	Female-sterile alleles	References
7. Nurse-cell and follicle development	lethal(1)ts-19 lethal(1)ts-13 lethal(1)ts-88 lethal(1)ts-259 lethal(1)ts-1006 lethal(1)ts-2366 lethal(1)ts-2641 lethal(1)ts-2864 lethal(1)ts-4931B	$l(1)ts$-19 $l(1)ts$-13 $l(1)ts$-88 (Two) (Four) (Three) $l(1)ts$-2641 $l(1)ts$-2864 $l(1)ts$-4931B	H. A. Schneiderman, C. L. Littlefield, P. Simpson, S. Bryant, T. Cline, and R. Arking (private communication)
8. Vitellogenesis a. Blocked synthesis of α yolk spheres	apterous	(Several)	King (1970), Postlethwait and Weiser (1973)
b. Blocked vitellogenin synthesis	female-sterile(3)A17	$fs(3)A17$	Bakken (1973), Kambysellis (private communication)
c. Blocked vitellogenin uptake	female-sterile(2)A17 female-sterile(2)A18 female-sterile(3)A1 female-sterile(3)A16	(Six?) $fs(2)A18$ (Two) $fs(3)A16$	Bakken (1973), Kambysellis (private communication), Postlethwait (private communication)
d. Unstudied	minus	mi	King (1970)
e. Abnormal β yolk spheres	ocelliless	oc	Johnson and King (1974)
9. Ovulation	stubarista lozenge female-sterile(2)A (2 genes)[r] female-sterile(3)A (5 genes)[r] Hairy wing	sta lz^{34k} Hw^{49c}	King (1970) Bakken (1973) Holzworth *et al.* (1974a,b)

10. Egg coats (chorion and vitelline membrane)			
a. Abnormal dorsal appendages	female-sterile(2)E1	fs(2)E1	King and Koch (1963)
	raspberry	ras⁴	
	singed	sn³⁶ᵃ	
	adipose-female sterile	adᶠˢ	
	vestigial	vgⁿᵘʳ	
	female-sterile(3)K1	fs(3)K1	Mohler (unpublished)
b. Fragile and malformed membranes	ocelliless	oc	Johnson and King (1974)
	tiny	ty	King and Koch (1963)
	female-sterile(2)A9	fs(2)A9	Bakken (1973), F. Kafatos (private communication)
	female-sterile(2)A12	(Seven?)	Bakken (1973)
	female-sterile(1)M (11 genes)		Mohler (unpublished)
	female-sterile(1)A (17 genes)		C. Audit and M. Gans (private communication)
	female-sterile(1)V	(Two)	C. L. Littlefield (private communication)
11. Cytoplasm of the mature egg			
a. Rescuable maternal effect lethals	fused	(Several)	King (1970)
	cinnamon	cin	Baker (1973)
	deep orange	dor	Garen and Gehring (1972)
	almondex	amx	Shannon (1973)
	rudimentary	(Many)	Okada et al. (1974)
	sonless	(snl)[b]	Colaianne and Bell (1972)

[a] Mat = maternal, ts = temperature sensitive.
[b] Females homozygous for mutants in some classes are not characterized as sterile, e.g., meiotic mutants.
[c] The genetics and phenotypic effects are incompletely characterized in many cases. The number in parentheses is the number of additional cistrons identified, but not yet further characterized.
[d] Extinct.

TABLE 1. Continued

Class	Gene[a]	Female-sterile alleles	References
	yeast requirement 1	*yea 1-1*	Falk and Nash (1974a)
	mat. influence lethal(1)R1	(Two)	Romans (1973)
	female-sterile(1)M (18 genes)[c]		Mohler (unpublished)
	female-sterile(1)A (5 genes)[c]		C. Audit (private communication)
b. Nonrescuable maternal effect lethals	female-sterile(1)N	(Five)	Mohler (unpublished)
	adipose-female sterile	*adp^{fs}*	Doane (1960a)
	female-sterile(3)G1	*fs(3)G1*	Gill (1963)
	daughterless	*(da)[b]*	Mange and Sandler (1973)
	mat. effect lethal 1	*mel 1*	
	mat. effect lethal 2	(Two)	
	mat. effect lethal 3	*mel 3*	
	mat. effect lethal 4	*mel 4*	
	mat. effect lethal 6	*mel 6*	
	mat. effect lethal (3 genes)[c]		Rice (1973)
	female-sterile(3)A11	*fs(3)A11*	
	female-sterile(3)A12	*fs(3)A12*	
	female-sterile(3)A13	*(fs(3)A13)[a]*	
	female-sterile(3)A14	*fs(3)A14*	
	female-sterile(3)A15	*(fs(3)A15)[a]*	
	female-sterile(3)A (3 genes)[c]	(Seven?)	
	female-sterile(2)A2	*fs(2)A7*	
	female-sterile(2)A7	*fs(2)A11*	
	female-sterile(2)A11	*fs(2)A13*	
	female-sterile(2)A13	*fs(2)A14*	Bakken (1973)
	female-sterile(2)A14		
	female-sterile(2)A (4 genes)[c]		

female-sterile(1)A73	fs(1)A73	
female-sterile(1)A97	fs(1)A97	
female-sterile(1)A214	fs(1)A214	
female-sterile(1)A330	fs(1)A330	
female-sterile(1)A331	fs(1)A331	
female-sterile(1)A383	fs(1)A383	
female-sterile(1)A426	fs(1)A426	
female-sterile(1)A457	fs(1)A457	C. Audit and M. Gans
female-sterile(1)A572	fs(1)A572	(private communication)
female-sterile(1)A573	fs(1)A573	
female-sterile(1)A1042	fs(1)A1042	
female-sterile(1)A1140	fs(1)A1140	
female-sterile(1)A1182	fs(1)A1182	
female-sterile(1)A1187	fs(1)A1187	
female-sterile(1)A1242	fs(1)A1242	
female-sterile(1)A1371	fs(1)A1371	
female-sterile(1)A1459	fs(1)A1459	
female-sterile(1)A1497	fs(1)A1497	
female-sterile(1)A1509	fs(1)A1509	
female-sterile(1)A1518	fs(1)A1518	
female-sterile(1)A1526	fs(1)A1526	
female-sterile(1)A1528	fs(1)A1528	
female-sterile(1)R (9 genes)[c]	(Three)	Romans (1973)
female-sterile(1)M (26 genes)[c]	(Three)	Mohler (unpublished)
female-sterile(1)Y1		Judd and Young (1973)
female-sterile(1)Y2		T. Cline (private
lethal(1)ts6225	l(1)ts6225	communication)

[a] Mat = maternal, ts = temperature sensitive.
[b] Females homozygous for mutants in some classes are not characterized as sterile, e.g., meiotic mutants.
[c] The genetics and phenotypic effects are incompletely characterized in many cases. The number in parentheses is the number of additional cistrons identified, but not yet further characterized.
[d] Extinct.

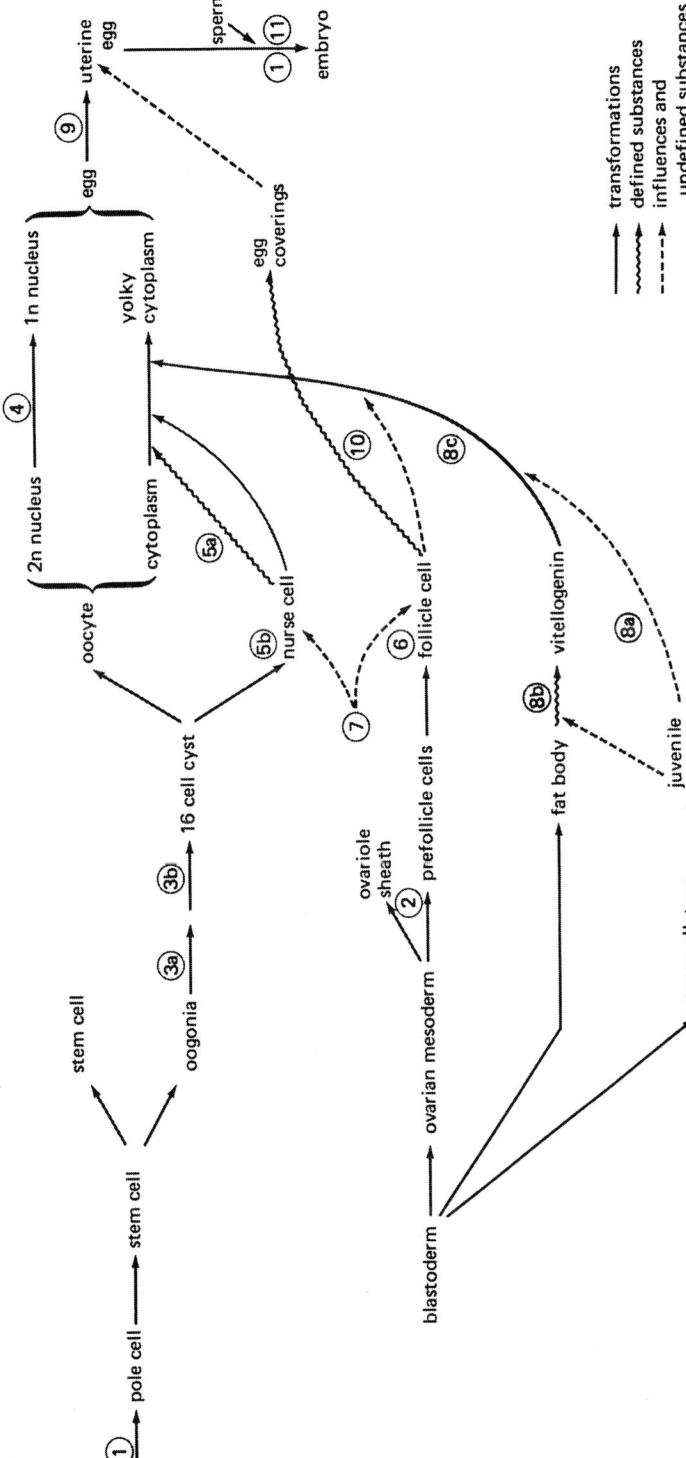

Figure 1. A diagram illustrating the mode of origin of the Drosophila oocyte and its interactions with other cell types during its further development. Circled numbers refer to gene classes (as defined in Table 1) which affect the processes specified.

645. The total number of bands for the combined salivary gland chromosomes is about 5000, and if this is equivalent to the number of genes, then $645/5000 = 13\%$ is the proportion capable of mutating to female-sterile alleles and, thus, is the *maximum* proportion of the genome specifically involved in oogenesis. The actual proportion must be much less.

Conclusion

Oogenesis involves several, separable developmental sequences that are directed to a common end, the normal egg. We have tried in Figure 1 to illustrate the flow of events and display the converging points.

Practically all of our understanding of the individual components and the causal relationships comes from morphological and physiological analysis of oogenesis in *Drosophila* and other insects. We expect to extend the analysis, using the genetic material, and are in the beginning phase in which the individual genetic components are defined and identified with specific aspects of oogenesis by the effects of mutant alleles. Linkage studies and complementation tests define the genes responsible for different materials controlling oogenesis. The phenotypic effects of the mutations identify the aspects of oogenesis in which the different materials are essential. We have grouped the known mutations which have similar effects and cataloged them in Table 1. The significance of each group for analysis of oogenesis is indicated by its place in Figure 1. The descriptive value of the catalog of mutations is apparent. The investigation of the differential consequences of certain mutations, the analysis of the cause of certain specific developmental abnormalities, and the synthesis of these two approaches are the next phases in the genetic analysis of oogenesis.

Acknowledgments

We are grateful to Adelaide T. C. Carpenter, Lee T. Douglas and Rhoda Grell for their critical comments on early drafts of this manuscript and to C. Audit, T. Cline, M. Gans, F. Kafatos, M. P. Kambysellis, C. Kern, C. L. Littlefield, A. Mahowald, D. Nash, J. H. Postlethwait, and H. A. Schneiderman for permitting us to cite their unpublished results.

This review was prepared during the period one of us (RCK) received support from the National Science Foundation (grant BMS 74-17317) and the National Institutes of Health (grant 1 R01 GM20036-01).

Literature Cited

Bahn, E., 1970   Restoration of fertility of the female sterile mutant *rudimentary* on pyrimidine-enriched culture medium. *Drosophila Inf. Serv.* **45**:99.

Baker, B. S., 1973   The maternal and zygotic control of development by *cinnamon*, a new mutant of *Drosophila melanogaster*. *Dev. Biol.* **33**:429–440.

Baker, B. S. and A. T. C. Carpenter, 1972   Genetic analysis of sex chromosomal meiotic mutants in *Drosophila melanogaster*. *Genetics* **71**:255–286.

Baker, W. K., 1971   Evidence for position-effect suppression of the ribosomal RNA cistrons in *Drosophila melanogaster*. *Proc. Natl. Acad. Sci. USA* **68**:2472–2476.

Bakken, A. H., 1973   A cytological and genetic study of oogenesis in *Drosophila melanogaster*. *Dev. Biol.* **33**:100–122.

Bell, A. E., 1954   A gene in *Drosophila melanogaster* that produces all male progeny. *Genetics* **39**:958–959.

Bischoff, W. L. and J. C. Lucchesi, 1971   Genetic organization in *Drosophila melanogaster*: Complementation and fine structure analysis of the *deep orange* locus. *Genetics* **69**:453–466.

Carlson, P. S., 1971   A genetic analysis of the *rudimentary* locus of *Drosophila melanogaster*. *Genet. Res.* **17**:53–81.

Carpenter, A. T. C., 1973   A meiotic mutant defective in distributive disjunction in *Drosophila melanogaster*. *Genetics* **73**:393–428.

Carpenter, A. T. C. and B. S. Baker, 1975   Genetic control of meiosis and some observations on the synaptonemal complex in *Drosophila melanogaster*. In *Mechanisms in Recombination,* edited by R. F. Grell, pp. 365–375, Plenum, New York.

Carpenter, A. T. C. and L. Sandler, 1974   On recombination-defective meiotic mutants in *Drosophila melanogaster*. *Genetics* **76**:453–475.

Colaianne, J. J. and A. E. Bell, 1972   The relative influence of sex of progeny on the lethal expression of the *sonless* gene in *Drosophila melanogaster*. *Genetics* **72**:293–296.

Counce, S. J. and D. A. Ede, 1957   The effect on embryogenesis of a sex-linked female-sterility factor in *Drosophila melanogaster*. *J. Embryol. Exp. Morphol.* **5**:404–421.

Davis, B. K., 1971   Genetic analysis of a meiotic mutant resulting in precocious sister-centromere separation in *Drosophila melanogaster*. *Mol. Gen. Genet.* **113**:251–272.

Doane, W. W., 1960a   Developmental physiology of the mutant *female-sterile (2) adipose* of *Drosophila melanogaster*. I. Adult morphology, longevity, egg production and egg lethality. *J. Exp. Zool.* **145**:1–19.

Doane, W. W., 1960b   Developmental physiology of the mutant *female-sterile (2) adipose* of *Drosophila melanogaster*. II. Effects of altered environment and residual genome on its expression. *J. Exp. Zool.* **145**:23–41.

Doane, W. W., 1961   Developmental physiology of the mutant *female-sterile (2) adipose* of *Drosophila melanogaster*. III. Corpus-allatum complex and ovarian transplantation. *J. Exp. Zool.* **146**:275–298.

Falk, D. R. and D. Nash, 1974a   Sex-linked auxotrophic and putative auxotrophic mutants of *Drosophila melanogaster*. *Genetics* **76**:755–766.

Falk, D. R. and D. Nash, 1974b   Pyrimidine axotrophy in *Drosophila*. Normal-winged, auxotrophic mutants and dominant auxotrophy at the *rudimentary* locus. *Molec. Gen. Genet.* **131**:339–350.

Fausto-Sterling, A., 1971 Studies on the sterility phenotype of the pleiotropic mutant *fused* of *Drosophila melanogaster. J. Exp. Zool.* **178:**343–350.

Gall, J. G. and J. D. Rochaix, 1974 The amplified ribosomal DNA of dytiscid beetles. *Proc. Natl. Acad. Sci. USA* **71:**1819–1823.

Garen, A. and W. Gehring, 1972 Repair of the lethal developmental defect in *deep orange* embryos of *Drosophila* by injection of normal egg cytoplasm. *Proc. Natl. Acad. Sci. USA* **69:**2982–2985.

Gehring, W. J., 1973 Genetic control of determination in the *Drosophila* embryo. In *Genetic Mechanisms of Development*, edited by F. H. Ruddle, pp. 103–128, Academic Press, New York.

Gill, K. S., 1963 Studies on oogenesis in *Drosophila melanogaster. J. Exp. Zool.* **152:**251–278.

Grell, R. F., 1962 A new hypothesis on the nature and sequence of meiotic events in the female of *Drosophila melanogaster. Proc. Natl. Acad. Sci. USA* **48:**165–172.

Hall, J. C., 1972 Chromosome segregation influenced by two alleles of the meiotic mutant c(3)G in *Drosophila melanogaster. Genetics* **71:**367–400.

Holzworth, K. W., C. Spector and F. J. Gottlieb, 1974a Control of oocyte production, development and release in *Drosophila melanogaster. Wilhelm Roux' Arch. Entwicklungsmech. Org.* **174:**260–266.

Holzworth, K. G., F. J. Gottlieb, and C. Spector, 1974b A unique case of female sterility in *Drosophila melanogaster. Wilhelm Roux' Arch. Entwicklungsmech. Org.* **174:**267–275.

Illmensee, K. and A. P. Mahowald, 1974 Transplantation of posterior polar plasm in *Drosophila*. Induction of germ cells at the anterior pole of the egg. *Proc. Natl. Acad. Sci. USA* **71:**1016–1020.

Johnson, C. C. and R. C. King, 1974 Oogenesis in the *ocelliless* mutant of *Drosophila melanogaster* Meigen (Diptera, Drosophilidae). *Internl. J. Insect Morphol. Embryol.* **3:**385–395.

Johnson, J. H. and R. C. King, 1972 Studies on *fes*, a mutation affecting cystocyte cytokinesis, in *Drosophila melanogaster. Biol. Bull.* **143:**525–547.

Judd, B. H. and M. W. Young, 1974 An examination of the one cistron:one chromomere concept. *Cold Spring Harbor Symp. Quant. Biol.* **38:**573–579.

Kambysellis, M. P. and H. Gelti-Douka, 1974 Vitellogenesis in *Drosophila*: Genetic and hormonal controls. *Genetics* **77:**s33.

Kaplan, W. D., R. L. Seecof, W. E. Trout III and M. E. Pasternack, 1970 Production and relative frequency of maternally influenced lethals in *Drosophila melanogaster. Am. Nat.* **104:**261–271.

Kinderman, N. B. and R. C. King, 1973 Oogenesis in *Drosophila virilis*. I. Interactions between ring canal rims and the nucleus of the oocyte. *Biol. Bull.* **144:**331–354.

King, R. C., 1970 *Ovarian Development in Drosophila melanogaster*, Academic Press, New York.

King, R. C. and E. A. Koch, 1963 Studies of the ovarian follicle cells of *Drosophila. Quart. J. Microscop. Sci.* **104:**297–320.

Klug, W. S., R. C. King and J. M. Wattiaux, 1970 Oogenesis in the *suppressor of Hairy-wing* mutant of *Drosophila melanogaster*. II. Nucleolar morphology and *in vitro* studies of RNA and protein synthesis. *J. Exp. Zool.* **174:**125–140.

Laugé, G., 1969 Étude des gonades des intersexués triploides de *Drosophila melano-*

gaster. Description morphologique ontogenease des structures histologiques. *Annales de la Société entomologique de France (N. S.)* **5(2)**:253–314.

Lindsley, D. L. and E. H. Grell, 1968 *Genetic Variation of Drosophila melanogaster*. Carnegie Institution of Washington Publication 627, Carnegie Institution, Washington, D.C.

Mange, A. P. and L. Sandler, 1973 A note on the maternal effect mutants of *daughterless* and *abnormal* oocyte in *Drosophila melanogaster*. *Genetics* **73**:73–86.

Margaritas, L., 1974 Programmed synthesis of specific proteins in cellular differentiation. A contribution to the study of chorion formation in the follicles of *Drosophila melanogaster*. Ph.D. Thesis, Laboratory of Biology, University of Athens, Athens, Greece.

Mohan, J. and F. M. Ritossa, 1970 Regulation of ribosomal RNA synthesis and its bearing on the *bobbed* phenotype in *Drosophila melanogaster*. *Dev. Biol.* **22**:495–512.

Mohler, J. D., 1973 Female-sterile mutations in *Drosophila melanogaster*. *Genetics* **74**:s182.

Nørby, S., 1970 A specific nutritional requirement for pyrimidines in *rudimentary* mutants of *Drosophila melanogaster*. *Hereditas* **66**:205–214.

Nørby, S. 1973 The biochemical genetics of *rudimentary* mutants of *Drosophila melanogaster*. I. Aspartate carbamoyltransferase levels in complementing the non-complementing strains. *Hereditas* **73**:11–16.

Okada, M., I. A. Kleinman and H. A. Schneiderman, 1974 Restoration of fertility in oogenesis in *Drosophila melanogaster* by transplantation of cytoplasm from wild-type eggs and by injection of pyrimidine nucleoside. *Dev. Biol.* **37**:50–62.

Palumbo, G., R. Caizzi and F. Ritossa, 1973 Relative orientation with respect to the centromere of ribosomal RNA genes of the X and Y chromosomes of *Drosophila melanogaster*. *Proc. Natl. Acad. Sci. USA* **70**:1883–1885.

Parry, D. M., 1973 A meiotic mutant affecting recombination in female *Drosophila melanogaster*. *Genetics* **73**:465–486.

Postlethwait, J. H. and K. Weiser, 1973 Vitellogenesis induced by juvenile hormone in the female sterile mutant *apterous-four* in *Drosophila melanogaster*. *Nat. New Biol.* **244**:284–285.

Quattropani, S. L. and E. Anderson, 1969 The origin and structure of the secondary coat of the egg of *Drosophila melanogaster*. *Z. Zellforsch. Mikrosk. Anat.* **95**:495–510.

Rasmussen, S. W., 1975 Ultrastructural studies of meiosis in males and females of the $c(3)G^{17}$ mutant of *Drosophila melanogaster* Meigen. *C. R. Trav. Lab. Carlsberg* **40**:(14) 163–173.

Rice, T. B., 1973 Isolation and characterization of maternal-effect mutants: An approach to the study of early determination in *Drosophila melanogaster*. Ph.D. Thesis, Department of Biology, Yale University, New Haven, Conn.

Ritossa, F. M. and S. Spiegelman, 1965 Location of DNA complementary to ribosomal RNA in the nucleolus organizer region of *Drosophila melanogaster*. *Proc. Natl. Acad. Sci. USA* **53**:737–745.

Ritossa, F. M., K. C. Atwood and S. Spiegelman, 1966 A molecular explanation of the *bobbed* mutants of *Drosophila* as partial deficiencies of "ribosomal" DNA. *Genetics* **54**:819–834.

Romans, P. A., 1973 A locus with a maternal effect on embryonic development in

Drosophila melanogaster. M.Sc. Thesis, Department of Genetics and Cell Biology, University of Alberta, Edmonton, Canada.

Sandler, L., 1970   The regulation of sex chromosome heterochromatic activity by an autosomal gene in *Drosophila melanogaster. Genetics* **64**:481–493.

Sandler, L., 1972   On the genetic control of genes located in the sex-chromosome heterochromatin of *Drosophila melanogaster. Genetics* **70**:261–274.

Sayles, C., D. W. Browder and J. H. Williamson, 1973   Expression of xanthine dehydrogenase activity during embryonic development of *Drosophila melanogaster. Dev. Biol.* **33**:213–217.

Shannon, M. P., 1972   Characterization of the female-sterile mutant *almondex* of *Drosophila melanogaster. Genetics* **43**:244–256.

Shannon, M. P., 1973   The development of eggs produced by the female-sterile mutant *almondex* of *Drosophila melanogaster. J. Exp. Zool.* **183**:383–400.

Smith, P. A. and R. C. King, 1968   Genetic control of synaptinemal complexes in *Drosophila melangoaster. Genetics* **60**:335–351.

Tartof, K. D. and R. P. Perry, 1970   The 5S RNA genes of *Drosophila melanogaster. J. Mol. Biol.* **51**:171–183.

Thierry-Mieg, D., M. Masson and M. Gans, 1972   Mutant de stérilité à effet retardé de *Drosophila melanogaster. C. R. Hebd. Seances Acad. Sci. Ser. D Sci. Nat.* **275**:2751–2754.

Thierry-Mieg, D., C. Audit, M. Gans, M. Masson and M. Zalokar, 1973   Mutations affecting the cytoplasmic organization of the egg in *Drosophila melanogaster. Genetics* **74** (No. 2, Part 2): s274–s275.

Valentin, J., 1973   Characterization of a meiotic control gene affecting recombination in *Drosophila. Hereditas* **75**:5–22.

von Borstel, R. C., 1960   Postmeiotic nuclear behavior in uninseminated eggs of *Drosophila melanogaster. Drosophila Inf. Serv.,* **34**:110.

Wimber, D. E. and D. M. Steffensen, 1970   Localization of 5S RNA genes on *Drosophila* chromosomes by RNA–DNA hybridization. *Science (Wash., D.C.)* **170**:639–641.

Yarger, R. J. and R. C. King, 1971   The phenogenetics of a temperature sensitive, autosomal dominant, female sterile gene in *Drosophila melanogaster. Dev. Biol.* **24**:166–177.

30

The Puffing Activities of the Salivary Gland Chromosomes

Michael Ashburner

Introduction

A complex, yet highly regular, sequence of changes in the activity of puffed loci of polytene chromosomes is characteristic of particular stages in the development of many Diptera. While the physiological significance of these changes is not yet clear, it is generally accepted that puffs are manifestations of gene activity. The study of the changes in puff activity during normal development and under experimental conditions is an excellent model system for the analysis of the control of gene activity in a higher organism. In this article I will present annotated tables of puffing activity in *Drosophila melanogaster* during normal development and a table of the reactions of some puff loci to experimental conditions.

For a general review of all aspects of polytene chromosomes, their structure and behavior, the review of Beermann (1962) is recommended. Recent reviews of puffs and of their significance have been published by Clever (1968), Panitz (1968), Berendes and Beermann (1969), Ashburner (1970d), and Berendes (1971). In addition, a recent volume edited by

Michael Ashburner—Department of Genetics, University of Cambridge, Cambridge, England.

TABLE 1. Standard Puffing

Locus	1	2	3	4	5	6	7	8	9	10
X Chromosome[a]										
1C	−	−	−	−	−	(+)	(+)		(+)	(+)
2B5–6	+	++	++	++	++	++	++		++	(+)
2B13–17[b]	−	−	(+)	+	++	++	++		++	+
2EF	−	−	−	+	+	+	+		+	+
3A1–4	−	−	−	−	−	−	+/−		+/−	+
3C11–12	++	+	−	−	−	−	−	−	−	−
3E	+	(+)	(+)	−	−	−	−	−	(+)	(+)
4F9–10	−	−	−	−	−	−	−		(+)	(+)
7D14–15	−	−	−	−	−	−	−		−	−
8D	(+)	(+)	−	−	−	−	−/+		+	+
8EF	−	−	−	−	−	−	−		−	−
9EF	−	−	−	−	−	−	−/+		(+)/+	+/++
10EF	+	+	+	(+)	(+)	−	+		++/+	++/+
11B14–17	++	++	+	+	+	+	+		+	++/+
12E3–7	−	−	−	−	−	+	+		+	++
13E1–2	+	(+)	(+)	−	−	−	−	−	−	+
14B	−	−	−	−	−	−	(+)/−		(+)/−	(+)/−
15C3–6	+	+	+	+	+	+	+		+	+
16A4–6	−	+	+	+	−	−	−		−	−
16C	−	−	−	−	−	−	−		+	+
16DE	−	−	−	−	(+)	+	+		+	+
2L Chromosome										
21C4–6	(+)	(+)	−	−	−	−	−	−	−	−
21F	−	−	−	−	−	+	+	+	++	++
22A	−	−	−	−	−	−	−	−	−	−
22B4–5[c,d]	−	(+)	+	+	+	+	−	−	−	−
22C3/4–6	−	−	−	−	−	+	+	+	++	++
23E[d]	−	+	+	+	+	+	+	++	++	++
25AC[e]	++	+	−	−	−	−	−	−	−	−
25D	−	−	−	−	−	−	−	−	−	−
26B10–11	−	−	−	−	−	−	−	−		(+)
27C1–2	−	−	−	−	−	−	−	−		−
28A1–2	−	−	−	−	−	−	−	−		−
29BC	−	−	−	−	−	−	−	−		−
29F1–2	−	−	−	−	−	−	+	+	+	+

[a] For X-chromosome loci (1C–16DE inclusive), activity is given for male/female where they differ.
[b] Absent in mutant halfway (Rayle, 1967).
[c] Absent, or very small, in some Oregon stocks (Ashburner, 1970b).
[d] Induced by ecdysone within half an hr (Ashburner, 1972d).
[e] Regression induced by ecdysone (Ashburner, 1972d); probably complex of two puffs.
[f] Induced by temperature shock, etc. This includes: (1) temperature shock (e.g., from 25°C to 35°C for 30 minutes), (2) recovery from anoxia, (3) treatment of glands with some (e.g., 2 , 4

Pattern of D. melanogaster

11	12	13	14	15	16	17	18	19	20	21
(+)	(+)	−	−	−	−		−	−		(+)
−	+/−	+/−	+/−	+/(+)	−		−/+	++		++
+/−	+/−	+/−	−	−	−		−	(+)/+		−
++	++	+/−	+/−	+/−	−		−	+		++
++	+/(+)	+/−	−	−	−		(+)	(+)		−
−	−	−	(+)	+	+		++	++		−
(+)	−	−	(+)	(+)	(+)		+	(+)		−
+/++	+/++	+/++	+	+	−		−	(+)/+		(+)/+
+	+	+	+	−	−		−	−		−
+	(+)	(+)	−	−	−		−	−		−
+	+	(+)	−	−	−		−	−		−
+	+	+	+	+	+		(+)	−		−
++/+	++/+	++/+	++	++	++		++/+	++/+		+/−
++/+	++/+	++/−	+/−	+/−	+/−		++/+	++/+		++/+
++	−	−	−	−	−		−/(+)	−		−
+	+	+	+	+	+		+	++		+
+/(+)	+/(+)	(+)	−/(+)	−	−		−	−		−
+	+	+	(+)	(+)	(+)/+		(+)/+	+/(+)		+/−
−	−	−	−	−/(+)?	−		−	−		−
+	+	−	−	−	−		−	−		(+)
(+)	−	−	−	−	−		−	−		−

11	12	13	14	15	16	17	18	19	20	21
−	−	−	−	−	−		−	(+)	(+)	(+)
++	−	−	−	−	−		−	−	−	−
−	−	−	−	−	−		−	++	+	−
−	−	−	−	−	−		−	−	−	+
++	−	−	−	−	−		−	−	−	−
++	+	+	−	−	−		−	++	++	++
−	−	−	−	−	−		−	−	−	−
+	+	−	−	−	−	+	+	+	+	+
(+)	−	−	−	−	−		−	−	+	++
+	+	+	+	+	+	+	+	+	+	+
−	+	+	+	+	+	+	+	+	+	+
+	+	−	−	−	−		−	−	−	++
++	++	+	+	+	−		−	−	−	+

dinitrophenol) but not all (e.g., oligomycin) uncouplers of oxidative phosphorylation, (4) inhibitors of respiratory chain transport (e.g., rotenone, antimycin) (Burdette and Anderson; 1965a, Ashburner, 1970a, and unpublished; Ellgaard, 1972).

[g] Absent from some *D. simulans* stocks. In F_1 forms heterozygous puff (Ashburner, 1969d).

[h] Enlarged, or induced, during *in vitro* culture of glands (Ashburner, 1970a, 1972d).

[i] Enlarged, or induced, during recovery from nitrogen anaerobiosis (Ashburner, 1970a).

[j] Perhaps a complex of two or more puffs [see Ashburner (1972b), his Figure 28].

[k] Induced (?) by benzamide *in vitro* (Lakhotia, 1971).

TABLE 1.

Locus	1	2	3	4	5	6	7	8	9	10
2L Chromosome (continued)										
30A3–6	–	–	–	–	–	–	–	–	–	–
30B	–	–	–	–	–	–	–	–	–	–
32C5–D1/2	(+)	(+)	(+)	(+)	(+)	(+)	(+)	(+)	(+)	(+)
33B[f]	–	–	–	–	–	+	+	+	–	–
33E3–8	–	–	–	–	–	+	+	++	++	++
34A5–6	+	+	+	+	+	+	+	–	–	–
35B1–3	–	–	–	–	–	–	–	–	–	–
36F6–7?	–	–	–	–	–	–	–	–	+	+
39BC	–	–	–	–	–	–	–	–	–	+
2R Chromosome										
42A	+	+	+	+	+	+	+	+	+	–
43E	+	+	+	+	+	+	+	+	+	+
44AB	–	–	–	–	–	–	+	+	+	+
46A1–2[a]	–	–	–	–	–	+	+	+	+	+
46F5–6	–	–	–	–	+	+	+	+	+	+
47A9–16[h]	–	+	+	+	+	+	+	++	++	++
47BC[h]	–	(+)	(+)	(+)	(+)	(+)	+	+	+	+
48B[i]	–	–	–	–	–	+	+	+	+	+
49B	–	–	–	–	–	–	–	–	–	–
49E	–	–	–	–	–	–	–	–	–	–
50A3–4	–	–	–	–	–	–	–	–	–	–
50C23–D4[h]	–	+	+	+	+	++	++	++	++	++
50F	–	–	–	–	–	–	–	–	–	(+)
51D	–	–	–	–	–	–	–	–	–	(+)
52A	–	–	–	–	–	–	–	–	–	–
52C4–7	(+)	–	–	–	–	–	–	–	–	–
55B	–	–	–	–	–	(+)	(+)	(+)	–	–
55E	–	–	–	–	+	+	+	+	+	+
56D	–	–	–	–	–	–	–	–	–	–
57E	–	–	–	–	(+)	(+)	(+)	–	–	–
58BC	–	–	–	+	+	+	+	–	–	–
58DE	++	++	++	+	+	+	+	+	+	+
59F4–8	–	–	–	–	–	–	+	+	+	+
60B7–13	–	–	–	–	–	–	–	–	–	–

[a] For X-chromosome loci (1C–16DE inclusive), activity is given for male/female where they differ.
[b] Absent in mutant halfway (Rayle, 1967).
[c] Absent, or very small, in some Oregon stocks (Ashburner, 1970b).
[d] Induced by ecdysone within half an hr (Ashburner, 1972d).
[e] Regression induced by ecdysone (Ashburner, 1972d); probably complex of two puffs.
[f] Induced by temperature shock, etc. This includes: (1) temperature shock (e.g., from 25°C to 35°C for 30 minutes), (2) recovery from anoxia, (3) treatment of glands with some (e.g., 2 , 4

Continued

11	12	13	14	15	16	17	18	19	20	21
−	−	−	−	+	+	+	+	−	−	−
(+)	(+)	−	−	−	−	−	−	−	−	−
(+)	−	−	−	−	−	−	+	++	+	−
−	−	−	−	−	−	−	−	−	+	+
+	+	(+)	(+)	(+)	+	+	+	++	++	++
+	++	++	++	++	++	+	+	+	+	+
−	−	−	−	−	+	+	+	−	−	−
+	+	+	+	++	++	++	−	−	−	−
+	++	++	+	−	−	−	+	++	+	−
−	−	−	−	−	−	−	+	+	−	−
−	+	+	+	+	++	++	++	++	+	+
−	−	−	−	−	−	−	−	−	+	+
−	−	−	+	+	+	+	+	−	−	−
+	++	++	++	+	+	+	+	+	−	−
++	+	+	+	+	+	+	+	+	++	++
+	+	+	+	+	(+)	(+)	+	++	−	−
(+)	−	−	−	−	−	−	−	−	−	(+)
−	−	−	−	−	−	(+)	(+)	−	−	−
+	+	+	+	−	−	−	−	−	−	(+)
−	−	−	−	−	(+)	(+)	−	−	−	−
++	+	+	+	+	+	++	++	++	+	+
(+)	(+)	−	−	−	−	−	−	−	(+)	(+)
(+)	−	−	−	−	−	−	−	−	−	−
−	−	−	−	−	+	+	++	−	−	−
−	−	−	−	−	+	+	+	+	−	−
−	−	−	−	−	−	−	−	−	−	−
+	+	+	+	−	−	−	−	−	−	−
−	+	+	+	−	−	−	−	−	−	−
−	−	−	−	−	−	−	−	−	−	−
−	−	−	−	−	−	−	−	−	−	−
−	−	−	+	++	++	++	+	−	−	−
+	+	+	++	++	++	+	+	+	+	+
−	+	+	++	++	+	+	+	+	−	−

dinitrophenol) but not all (e.g., oligomycin) uncouplers of oxidative phosphorylation, (4) inhibitors of respiratory chain transport (e.g., rotenone, antimycin) (Burdette and Anderson; 1965a, Ashburner, 1970a, and unpublished; Ellgaard, 1972).

[g] Absent from some *D. simulans* stocks. In F_1 forms heterozygous puff (Ashburner, 1969d).

[h] Enlarged, or induced, during *in vitro* culture of glands (Ashburner, 1970a, 1972d).

[i] Enlarged, or induced, during recovery from nitrogen anaerobiosis (Ashburner, 1970a).

[j] Perhaps a complex of two or more puffs [see Ashburner (1972b), his Figure 28].

[k] Induced (?) by benzamide *in vitro* (Lakhotia, 1971).

TABLE 1.

Locus	1	2	3	4	5	6	7	8	9	10
3L Chromosome										
61C	−	−	−	−	−	−	−	−	−	−
62A	−	−	−	−	−	−	−	−	−	(+)
62C[h]	−	−	−	−	−	−	−	−	−	−
62E	−	−	−	+	+	++	++	++	++	++
62F	−	−	−	−	−	−	−	−	−	+
63E1–3	−	−	−	−	−	−	−	+	+	++
63F[d]	−	+	+	+	++	++	+	+	−	−
64A11–13	−	−	−	−	−	−	−	−	−	−
66B[h]	−	−	−	−	−	−	−	−	+	+
66E1–2	−	−	−	−	−	−	−	−	(+)	(+)
67B[f]	−	−	−	−	+	+	+	+	+	+
67F	−	−	−	−	−	(+)	(+)	(+)	(+)	(+)
68C	++	+	−	−	−	−	−	−	−	−
69A1–3	(+)	−	−	−	−	−	−	−	−	−
70C	−	−	−	−	+	+	+	+	+	+
70E	−	−	−	−	−	−	−	−	(+)	+
71B	−	−	−	−	−	−	−	−	−	−
71DE[j]	−	+	+	+	+	+	+	+	++	++
72D	−	−	+	+	+	+	+	+	+	+
73B5–7[h]	−	−	−	−	−	−	−	−	−	−
74C[d]	−	(+)	(+)	−	−	−	−	−	−	−
74EF[d]	−	+	++	++	++	++	++	+	+	−
75B[d]	−	+	++	++	++	++	++	+	+	−
75CD	−	−	−	−	−	−	−	−	−	(+)?
76A	−	−	−	−	−	−	−	−	−	−
76D1–4[hi]	−	−	−	−	−	−	−	−	−	−
77E	−	−	−	−	−	−	(+)	(+)	(+)	−
78D1–5	−	−	−	−	−	+	++	++	++	++
3R Chromosome										
82F1–2	−	−	−	−	−	−	−	−	++	++
83E	−	+	+	+	+	+	+	+	+	+
84F1–2[h,i]	−	−	−	−	−	−	−	−	−	(+)
85D1–2	−	−	−	−	−	−	−	−	−	−
85F1–6	+	+	+	+	+	+	+	++	++	++
86E	(+)	−	−	−	−	−	−	−	−	−
87A[f]	−	−	−	−	−	−	−	−	−	−

[a] For X-chromosome loci (1C–16DE inclusive), activity is given for male/female where they differ.
[b] Absent in mutant halfway (Rayle, 1967).
[c] Absent, or very small, in some Oregon stocks (Ashburner, 1970*b*).
[d] Induced by ecdysone within half an hr (Ashburner, 1972*d*).
[e] Regression induced by ecdysone (Ashburner, 1972*d*); probably complex of two puffs.
[f] Induced by temperature shock, etc. This includes: (1) temperature shock (e.g., from 25°C to 35°C for 30 minutes), (2) recovery from anoxia, (3) treatment of glands with some (e.g., 2, 4

Continued

11	12	13	14	15	16	17	18	19	20	21
+	−	−	−	−	−	−	−	−	−	−
(+)	−	−	−	−	−	−	−	−	−	−
+	−	−	−	−	−	−	−	−	−	−
+	−	−	−	−	−	−	−	−	++	++
+	−	−	−	−	−	−	−	−	−	−
++	+	+	−	−	+	+	++	+	−	−
−	−	−	−	(+)	−	−	−	−	−	−
(+)	−	−	−	−	−	(+)	(+)	−	−	−
++	++	(+)	(+)	(+)	(+)	(+)	+	++	++	++
(+)	−	−	−	−	−	−	(+)	−	−	−
−	−	−	−	−	−	−	−	−	−	−
(+)	(+)	−	−	−	−	−	−	−	−	−
−	−	−	−	−	−	−	−	−	−	−
−	−	−	−	−	−	−	++	−	−	−
(+)	−	−	−	−	−	−	−	−	−	−
(+)	−	−	−	−	−	−	−	−	−	−
(+)	(+)	(+)	−	−	−	−	−	−	−	−
++	++	++	++	++	++	+	+	(+)	(+)	(+)
+	+	+	+	+	+	+	+	−	−	−
+	+	+	−	−	−	−	−	−	−	−
−	−	−	−	−	−	−	−	−	−	−
−	−	−	−	−	−	−	−	++	−	−
−	+	+	+	+	+	+	+	++	+	+
−	−	−	−	−	−	−	++	+	−	−
(+)	(+)	−	−	−	−	−	−	−	−	−
−	+	+	+	−	−	−	−	−	−	−
−	−	−	−	−	−	−	−	−	−	−
+	−	−	(+)?	(+)?	−	−	−	−	−	−
++	+	−	−	−	−	−	++	−	−	−
+	+	+	+	−	−	−	−	−	−	+
(+)	(+)	−	−	−	−	−	−	−	−	+
+	++	++	++	++	++	++	++	−	−	−
++	++	++	++	++	++	++	++	++	++	++
−	−	−	−	−	−	−	−	−	+	++
−	−	−	−	−	−	−	−	+	+	+

dinitrophenol) but not all (e.g., oligomycin) uncouplers of oxidative phosphorylation, (4) inhibitors of respiratory chain transport (e.g., rotenone, antimycin) (Burdette and Anderson; 1965a, Ashburner, 1970a, and unpublished; Ellgaard, 1972).

[g] Absent from some *D. simulans* stocks. In F_1 forms heterozygous puff (Ashburner, 1969d).

[h] Enlarged, or induced, during *in vitro* culture of glands (Ashburner, 1970a, 1972d).

[i] Enlarged, or induced, during recovery from nitrogen anaerobiosis (Ashburner, 1970a).

[j] Perhaps a complex of two or more puffs [see Ashburner (1972b), his Figure 28].

[k] Induced (?) by benzamide *in vitro* (Lakhotia, 1971).

TABLE 1.

Locus	1	2	3	4	5	6	7	8	9	10
3R Chromosome (continued)										
87C	–	–	–	–	–	–	–	–	–	–
87F	–	–	–	–	–	–	–	–	–	–
88D	–	+	+	+	+	+	+	++	++	++
88EF	–	+	+	+	+	+	–	–	–	–
89B9–22	–	+	+	+	+	+	+	+	+	+
90BC	++	+	+	+	+	+	+	–	–	–
91D1–6^h	–	–	–	–	–	–	–	–	–	+
92A	–	–	–	–	–	–	–	–	–	–
93B	–	–	–	–	–	(+)	(+)	–	–	–
93D1–2^{f,k}	–	+	+	+	+	+	+	+	+	+
93F9–10	–	–	–	–	–	–	–	–	–	–
95B^h	–	–	–	–	–	–	–	(+)	(+)	(+)
95D^f	–	–	–	–	–	–	–	(+)	(+)	(+)
95F	–	–	–	–	–	+	+	+	+	+
96A^i	–	–	–	–	–	–	–	–	–	–
96E	–	–	+	+	+	+	–	–	–	–
97C	–	–	–	–	–	–	–	–	–	+
98B	–	–	–	–	–	–	–	–	–	(+)
98F1–2	–	–	–	–	–	–	+	+	++	++
99B^h	(+)	(+)	(+)	(+)	(+)	(+)	(+)	(+)	(+)	(+)
99D	–	–	–	–	–	–	–	–	–	–
99E	–	–	–	–	–	–	–	–	–	–
100DE^i	–	–	–	–	–	–	–	–	–	–
Chromosome 4										
102C10–17	–	–	–	–	–	–	–	–	–	–

[a] For X-chromosome loci (1C–16DE inclusive), activity is given for male/female where they differ.
[b] Absent in mutant halfway (Rayle, 1967).
[c] Absent, or very small, in some Oregon stocks (Ashburner, 1970b).
[d] Induced by ecdysone within half an hr (Ashburner, 1972d).
[e] Regression induced by ecdysone (Ashburner, 1972d); probably complex of two puffs.
[f] Induced by temperature shock, etc. This includes: (1) temperature shock (e.g., from 25°C to 35°C for 30 minutes), (2) recovery from anoxia, (3) treatment of glands with some (e.g., 2 , 4

Beermann (Beermann, 1972) is devoted to developmental studies on giant chromosomes.

Puffing in *D. melanogaster,* General Aspects

Unlike many other Diptera, or indeed other species of *Drosophila,* *D. melanogaster* normally possesses only one tissue, the larval salivary

Continued

11	12	13	14	15	16	17	18	19	20	21
−	−	−	−	−	−	−	−	+	+	−
−	−	−	−	−	−	+	+	+	−	−
++	+	+	+	+	+	+	+	+	+	++
−	−	−	−	−	−	−	−	−	−	−
+	+	+	(+)	(+)	−	−	+	+	+	+
−	+	++	++	++	+	+	−	−	−	−
++	++	+	−	−	−	−	−	−	−	−
−	−	−	(+)	(+)	−	−	−	−	−	−
−	−	−	−	−	−	−	−	−	−	−
+	++	++	(+)	(+)	(+)	(+)	(+)	(+)	+	+
−	−	−	−	−	−	−	−	++	++	++
−	−	−	−	−	−	−	−	−	−	−
−	−	−	−	−	−	−	(+)	−	−	−
−	−	−	(+)	(+)	(+)	(+)	−	−	−	−
−	+	+	+	+	−	−	−	++	+	−
+	−	−	−	−	−	−	−	−	+	+
(+)	−	−	−	−	−	−	−	−	+	+
++	−	−	−	−	−	−	−	−	++	++
(+)	(+)	(+)	(+)	(+)	(+)	(+)	+	++	++	++
−	−	−	−	−	−	(+)	(+)	(+)	−	−
(+)	(+)	(+)	+	+	+	+	+	++	++	++
−	−	−	−	+	++	++	++	−	−	−
−	−	−	−	−	−	−	−	−	−	++

dinitrophenol) but not all (e.g., oligomycin) uncouplers of oxidative phosphorylation, (4) inhibitors of respiratory chain transport (e.g., rotenone, antimycin) (Burdette and Anderson, 1965a, Ashburner, 1970a, and unpublished; Ellgaard, 1972).

[g] Absent from some *D. simulans* stocks. In F_1 forms heterozygous puff (Ashburner, 1969d).

[h] Enlarged, or induced, during *in vitro* culture of glands (Ashburner, 1970a, 1972d).

[i] Enlarged, or induced, during recovery from nitrogen anaerobiosis (Ashburner, 1970a).

[j] Perhaps a complex of two or more puffs [see Ashburner (1972b), his Figure 28].

[k] Induced (?) by benzamide *in vitro* (Lakhotia, 1971).

gland, with polytene chromosomes of a sufficient size for evaluation of puffing activity. Recently, Kaufman (1972) has reported in an abstract that polytene chromosomes can be analyzed in larval gut cells of homozygotes for the mutant giant.

Early in the third larval instar the salivary gland chromosomes attain a sufficient degree of polyteny to enable critical analysis of puffing activity. From this time (70–80 hours after oviposition at 25°C) until about 10 hours before puparium formation the pattern of active, puffed loci is rather simple and stable. Fewer than ten loci display prominent puffs.

At approximately 10 hours before puparium formation (110 hours after oviposition) this situation changes dramatically with the induction of a cycle of puffing activity that involves a large number of puff loci. This cycle is induced by the hormone ecdysone (Becker, 1962a,b; Burdette, 1964, 1968; Burdette and Anderson, 1965b; Burdette and Bullock, 1963; Burdette and Kobayashi, 1969; Ashburner, 1971, 1972d) and climaxes immediately prior to puparium formation. After puparium formation the number of puffed loci decreases, and during the period from 1 to 4 hours after puparium formation the puffing pattern is once again rather simple and stable. A second cycle of puffing activity commences 5–6 hours after puparium formation (it is not yet known why), and the pattern of puffed loci continues to change for the following 7–8 hours. Further cytological examination is not possible as the hystolysis of the larval salivary gland is, by that time, far advanced.

Puffing Patterns in *D. melanogaster*, The Standard Tables

Although the pattern of puffed loci changes continuously from 10 hours before until 12–14 hours after puparium formation, it is convenient to recognize a limited number of discrete patterns, each characterized by a unique array of puffed sites. These "puff stages" (PS) were introduced by Becker (1959) in the first major paper describing the puffing patterns of *D. melanogaster*. We now recognize 21 puff stages, and Table 1 describes these for 126 puffs. This table includes all of the largest puffs normally seen during development; however, it is certainly not complete, and further detailed analysis of normal development will doubtless yield many puffs which can be readily accommodated within the present scheme.

It is to be emphasized that the description of the changes in puffing that occur during development in terms of 21 different stages is not meant to imply that the pattern of puffs "jumps" from one stage to the next. The changes that occur are continuous, and patterns intermediate between any two PS, as defined, may readily be recognized. The sole purpose of the use of puff stages is as a descriptive device for the convenience of the researcher.

The "standard puffing pattern" of *D. melanogaster* does not refer to any particular strain of this species [unlike the tables of Becker (1959) and of Ashburner (1967b, 1969a)]. Table 1 includes information from many strains, although it is based upon a detailed study of the widely distributed Oregon-R wild-type strain. With relatively minor variation, this pattern has been recognized in all the strains of *D. melanogaster* which I have examined [and indeed in the related species *D. simulans* (Ashburner, 1969*b,c,d*; Forward and Kaufmann, 1969), *D. yakuba*, and *D. teissieri* (Ashburner and Lemeunier, 1972)].

Most mutants of *D. melanogaster* studied have normal puffing patterns. The major exceptions are larval lethals such as lethal-giant-larvae (*lgl*) (Becker, 1959; Ashburner, 1972*b*), lethal-tumorous-larvae (*ltl*) (Rodman, 1964; Rodman and Kopac, 1964; Kobel and van Breugel, 1968; Zhimulev and Lychev, 1972*b*), deep-orange lethal (*dor^l*) (Rayle, private communication), and halfway (*hfw*) (Rayle, 1967). Other studies of puffing in strains of *D. melanogaster* carrying mutations and chromosome aberrations are by Ashburner (1969*e*, 1970*b,c*), Ellgaard and Brosseau (1969), Hartmann-Goldstein (1966), Kiknadze (1966), Roberts (1969, 1970, 1972), and Slizynski (1964).

The locations of the puffs are given with respect to the revised salivary gland chromosome maps of C. B. Bridges (1938), C. B. Bridges and P. N. Bridges (1939) and P. N. Bridges (1941*a,b*, 1942) [see Lindsley and Grell (1968)]. For noncritical work the original Bridges map (Bridges, 1935) is sufficient and is very much easier to use than the revised maps. The paper of Lefevre (1975) should be consulted for a discussion of map interpretation. Lefevre presents a very valuable photographic interpretation of the 1935 map.

Although each puff is probably referable to a single band of the revised maps, this has not been done for all puff sites. The location given is the most accurate available to date and, in some cases, is only to the nearest two or three lettered subdivisions. Sorsa (1969*a,b*) has shown that

TABLE 2. *Correlation of Certain Puff Stages and Other Events in Larval and Prepupal Development*

Puff stage	Conspicuous events
1	Feeding third-instar larvae and during early migration period
5	Migrating larvae; salivary gland lumen begins to fill with secretion
8	Migrating larvae; salivary gland "bloated," with lumen full of secretion
10–11	Puparium formation; salivary gland lumen empties
11–12	Occurs ¼-1 hour after puparium formation; puparium pigments and hardens
14	Occurs 4 hours after puparium formation; air bubble appears
20–21	Occurs 12 hours after puparium formation; air bubble dissipates, eversion of cephalic complex

TABLE 3. Other Puffs in D. melanogaster Salivary Gland Chromosomes

Locus	Notes	Reference
5B	Normal development	Ashburner (1969c)
	During in vitro culture of glands	Ashburner (1972d) (his Figure 3a)
18C	During in vitro culture of glands	Ashburner (1972d) (his Figure 3b)
22B8–9	Normal development of ast ho ed dp cl stock	Ashburner (1972b) (his Figures 23 and 24)
23B	During in vitro culture of glands	Ashburner (1972d) (his Figure 3c)
	Following injection of larvae with puromycin or cycloheximide	Ashburner (1972b)
23C	Normal development	Lychev (1965), Sorsa and Pfeifer (1972) (their Figure 4)
24D	Normal development at PS 1 (only?)	Ashburner (unpublished)
	Not peculiar to mutant fat (contra Slizynski)[a]	Slizynski (1964)
26A	During in vitro culture of glands	Ashburner (1972d)
	During recovery from nitrogen anaerobiosis	Ashburner (1970a) (his Figure 15a)
37D	Normal development	Ashburner (1972b) (his Figure 6b)
38B1–2	Normal development	Ashburner (1972b) (his Figures 6a–e)
42C	Normal development	Sorsa and Pfeifer (1972) (their Figure 5)
46D	Normal development	Sorsa and Pfeifer (1972) (their Figure 5)
		Ashburner (1972b) (his Figure 7e)
47F	Normal development	Sorsa and Pfeifer (1972) (their Figure 5)
48E	After temperature shock, etc.[b]	Ashburner (1970a) (his Figure 7)
57D8–9	During in vitro culture of glands	Ashburner (1972d) (his Figure 3f)
	During recovery from nitrogen anaerobiosis	Ashburner (1970a)
61F1–2	Normal development	Sorsa and Pfeifer (1972) (their Figure 6)
63BC	After temperature shock, etc.[b]	Ashburner (1970a) (his Figures 3 and 4)
	In l(2)gl homozygotes	Becker (1959) (his Figure 11) Ashburner (1972b) (his Figure 21a)
	In ltl homozygotes	Zhimulev and Lychev (1972b)

TABLE 3. *Continued*

Locus	Notes	Reference
	After culture of glands in adult abdomen	Staub (1969) (her Figure 10b)
	After culture of isolated nuclei	Ashburner and M. Lezzi (unpublished)
64B	Normal development	Ashburner (1972*b*) (his Figure 10h)
64C9–13	Normal development of vg^6 and related stocks	Ashburner (1967*a*, 1969*e*) (his Figure 6 in 1969*e*)
64F	Normal development	Ashburner (1972*b*) (his Figure 10e)
	After temperature shock, etc.[b]	Ashburner (1970*a*) (his Figures 3 and 14)
67C	During culture of glands in Ringer solution	Becker (1959) (his Figure 6)
68B	After culture of glands in adult abdomen	Staub (1969) (her Figure 4)
70A	After temperature shock, etc.[b]	Ashburner (1970*a*) (his Figure 8b)
73A1–2	During *in vitro* culture of glands	Ashburner (1972*d*) (his Figure 3g)
	Following injection of larvae with puromycin or cycloheximide	Ashburner (1972*b*)
73F	Normal development	Ashburner (1972*b*) (his Figure 12d)
78E	Following culture of glands in adult abdomen	Staub (1969) (her Figures 2 and 3)
	During *in vitro* culture of glands	Ashburner (1972*d*)
79C	After culture of glands in adult abdomen	Staub (1969) (her Figure 6)
85B	During recovery from nitrogen anaerobiosis	Ashburner (1970*a*)
	During *in vitro* culture of glands	Ashburner (1972*d*)
87B	After temperature shock, etc.[b]	Ashburner (1970*a*) (his Figure 4)
94C	During *in vitro* culture of glands	Ashburner (1972*d*) (his Figure 3j)
94E	Normal development	Ashburner (unpublished)
	During *in vitro* culture of glands	Ashburner (1972*d*) (his Figure 3j)
101–102A	In *T(3:4)83* stock	Roberts (1970, 1972) (his Figure 1c)
		Ashburner (1972*b*) (his Figure 16e)

[a] Slizynski (1964) claimed this puff to be a feature of the *fat* (2 : 12.0) mutant. The puff at 24D is close to the cytogenetic position of *fat*. I (unpublished) cannot substantiate this claim and find this puff active, at least at PS 1, in wild-type strains. See also Chaudhuri and Mukherjee (1969).

[b] See footnote *f* to Table 1.

very precise mapping may be possible using fairly low-power electron micrographs of sections of chromosomes.

Table 2 correlates certain puff stages with other features of the development of *D. melanogaster* that occur during the late-larval and early-pupal periods.

In addition to the 126 puffs recognized in the standard pattern (Table 1) many other loci have been observed puffed (1) during normal development, (2) in certain genetic stocks, or (3) after various experimental treatments. Some of these are listed in Table 3. This list is not complete [see the lists of Becker (1959), Schultz (1968) in Lindsley and Grell (1968), and Ashburner (1972b), and the papers of Lychev (1965), Lychev and Medvedev (1967), and Zhimulev and Lychev (1970, 1972a)]; it includes only puffs whose loci are well documented.

Following is a list of the agents and experimental conditions which have been reported to influence puffing in *D. melanogaster*: nutrition (Lychev, 1965; Burnet and Hartmann-Goldstein, 1971), culture temperature (Schultz, 1965), circadian rhythm (Rensing and Hardeland, 1967, Rensing, 1969), *in vitro* incubation of salivary glands (Becker, 1959; Ashburner, 1970a, 1972d; Nagel and Rensing, 1971), *Drosophila* tissue extracts (Tokumitsu, 1968), inhibitors of protein synthesis (Ashburner, 1970a, 1972b; Schoon and Rensing, 1973), inhibitors of RNA synthesis (Ashburner, 1972a), SH group reagents (Ashburner, 1972c), vertebrate steroid hormones (Gilbert and Pistey, 1966; Sang, 1968; Smith *et al.*, 1968; Ashburner, 1974), organomercurials (Sorsa and Pfeifer, 1973), borate (Drozdovskaya, 1971), chromate (Nikiforov *et al.*, 1970), cobalt (Rapoport *et al.*, 1971), rhodanide (Sakharova *et al.*, 1971), dicyandiamide (Mukherjee, 1968), histones and polylysine (Desai and Tencer, 1968), amino acids (Federoff and Milkman, 1964), and oncogenic viruses (Burdette and Yoon, 1967).

Acknowledgment

This work has been supported by Science Research Council Grant B/SR/9750.

Literature Cited

Ashburner, M., 1967a Gene activity dependent on chromosome synapsis in the polytene chromosomes of *Drosophila melanogaster*. *Nature (Lond.)* **214:**1159–1160.

Ashburner, M., 1967b Patterns of puffing activity in the salivary gland chromosomes of

Drosophila. I. Autosomal puffing patterns in a laboratory stock of *Drosophila melanogaster. Chromosoma (Berl.)* **21**:398–428.

Ashburner, M., 1969a Genetic control of puffing in polytene chromosomes, In *Chromosomes Today,* Vol. 2, edited by C. D. Darlington and K. R. Lewis, pp. 99–106, Oliver & Boyd, Edinburgh.

Ashburner, M., 1969b On the problem of the genetic similarity between sibling species-puffing patterns in *Drosophila melanogaster* and *Drosophila simulans. Am. Nat.* **103**:189–191.

Ashburner, M., 1969c Patterns of puffing activity in the salivary gland chromosomes of *Drosophila.* II. The X-chromosome puffing patterns of *D. melanogaster* and *D. simulans. Chromosoma (Berl.)* **27**:47–63.

Ashburner, M., 1969d Patterns of puffing activity in the salivary gland chromosomes of *Drosophila.* III. A comparison of the autosomal puffing patterns of the sibling species *D. melanogaster* and *D. simulans. Chromosoma (Berl.)* **27**:64–85.

Ashburner, M., 1969e Patterns of puffing activity in the salivary gland chromosomes of *Drosophila.* IV. Variability of puffing patterns. *Chromosoma (Berl.)* **27**:156–177.

Ashburner, M., 1970a Patterns of puffing activity in the salivary gland chromosomes of *Drosophila.* V. Responses to environmental treatments. *Chromosoma (Berl.)* **31**:356–376.

Ashburner, M., 1970b The genetic analysis of puffing in polytene chromosomes of *Drosophila. Proc. R. Soc. Lond. B Biol. Sci.* **176**:319–327.

Ashburner, M., 1970c A prodromus to the genetic analysis of puffing in *Drosophila. Cold Spring Harbor Symp. Quant. Biol.* **35**:533–538.

Ashburner, M., 1970d Function and structure of polytene chromosomes during insect development. *Adv. Insect Physiol.* **7**:1–95.

Ashburner, M., 1971 Induction of puffs in polytene chromosomes of *in vitro* cultured salivary glands of *Drosophila melanogaster* by ecdysone and ecdysone analogues. *Nat. New Biol.* **230**:222–224.

Ashburner, M., 1972a Ecdysone induction of puffing in polytene chromosomes of *Drosophila melanogaster.* Effects of inhibitors of RNA synthesis. *Exp. Cell Res.* **71**:433–440.

Ashburner, M., 1972b Puffing patterns in *Drosophila melanogaster* and related species. In *Results and Problems in Cell Differentiation,* Vol. 4, *Developmental Studies on Giant Chromosomes,* edited by W. Beermann, pp. 101–151, Springer-Verlag, Berlin.

Ashburner, M., 1972c *N*-ethylmaleimide inhibition of the induction of gene activity by the hormone ecdysone. *FEBS (Fed. Eur. Biochem. Soc.) Lett.* **22**:265–269.

Ashburner, M., 1972d Patterns of puffing activity in the salivary gland chromosomes of *Drosophila.* VI. Induction by ecdysone in salivary glands of *D. melanogaster* cultured *in vitro. Chromosoma (Berl.)* **38**:255–281.

Ashburner, M., 1974 The genetic and hormonal control of puffing in salivary gland chromosomes of *Drosophila. Ontogenez, USSR:* **5**:107–121 (in Russian with an English summary).

Ashburner, M. and F. Lemeunier, 1972 Patterns of puffing activity in the salivary gland chromosomes of *Drosophila.* VII. Homology of puffing patterns on chromosome arm 3L in *D. melanogaster* and *D. yakuba,* with notes on puffing in *D. teissieri. Chromosoma (Berl.)* **38**:283–295.

Becker, H. J., 1959 Die Puffs der Speicheldrüsenchromosomen von *Drosophila melanogaster.* I. Beobachtungen zum Verhalten des Puffmusters im Normalstamm und bei zwei Mutanten, *giant* und *lethal-giant-larvae. Chromosoma (Berl.)* **10**:654–678.

Becker, H. J., 1962*a*   Die Puffs der Speicheldrüsenchromosomen von *Drosophila melano-gaster*. II. Die Auslösung der Puffbildung, ihre Spezifität und ihre Beziehung zur Funktion der Ringdrüse. *Chromosoma (Berl.)* **13**:341–384.

Becker, H. J., 1962*b*   Stadienspezifische Genaktivierung in Speicheldrüsen nach Trans-plantation bei *Drosophila melanogaster*. *Zool. Anz.* **25**:92–101.

Beermann, W., 1962   *Riesenchromosomen. Protoplasmatologia*, Vol. VI/D. Springer-Verlag, Vienna.

Beermann, W., editor, 1972   *Developmental Studies on Giant Chromosomes. Results and Problems in Cell Differentiation*, Vol. 4, Springer-Verlag, Berlin.

Berendes, H. D., 1971   Gene activation in Dipteran polytene chromosomes. In *Control mechanisms of growth and differentiation. Soc. Exp. Biol. Symp.* **25**:145–161.

Berendes, H. D. and W. Beermann, 1969   Biochemical activity of interphase chro-mosomes. In *Handbook of Molecular Cytology*, edited by A. Lima-de-Faria, North-Holland, Amsterdam.

Bridges, C. B., 1935   Salivary chromosome maps. *J. Hered.* **26**:60–64.

Bridges, C. B., 1938   A revised map of the salivary gland X-chromosomes. *J. Hered.* **29**:11–13.

Bridges, C. B. and P. N. Bridges, 1939   A new map of the second chromosome: A revised map of the right limb of the second chromosome of *Drosophila melanogaster. J. Hered.* **30**:475–476.

Bridges, P. N., 1941*a*   A revised map of the left limb of the third chromosome of *Drosophila melanogaster. J. Hered.* **32**:64–65.

Bridges, P. N., 1941*b*   A revision of the salivary gland 3R-chromosome map of *Drosophila melanogaster. J. Hered.* **32**:299–300.

Bridges, P. N., 1942   A new map of the salivary gland 2L-chromosome of *Drosophila melanogaster. J. Hered.* **33**:403–408.

Burdette, W. J., 1964   The significance of invertebrate hormones in relation to dif-ferentiation. *Cancer Res.* **24**:521–536.

Burdette, W. J., 1968   Visible alterations in gene activation caused by hormones and oncogenic viruses. In *Exploitable Molecular Mechanisms and Neoplasia, 22nd An-nual Symposium of Fundamental Cancer Research*, pp. 507–520, Williams & Wil-kins, Baltimore, Md.

Burdette, W. J. and R. Anderson, 1965*a*   Puffing of salivary gland chromosomes after treatment with carbon dioxide. *Nature (Lond.)* **208**:409–410.

Burdette, W. J. and R. Anderson, 1965*b*   Conditioned response of salivary-gland chro-mosomes of *Drosophila melanogaster* to ecdysones. *Genetics* **51**:625–633.

Burdette, W. J. and M. W. Bullock, 1963   Ecdysone: Five biologically active fractions from *Bombyx. Science (Wash., D.C.)* **140**:1311.

Burdette, W. J. and M. Kobayashi, 1969   Response of chromosomal puffs to crystalline hormones *in vivo. Proc. Soc. Exp. Biol. Med.* **131**:209–213.

Burdette, W. J. and J. S. Yoon, 1967   Mutations, chromosomal aberrations, and tumors in insects treated with oncogenic virus. *Science (Wash., D.C.)* **155**:340–341.

Burnet, B. and I. Hartmann-Goldstein, 1971   Environmental influences on puffing in the salivary gland chromosome of *Drosophila melanogaster. Genet. Res.* **17**:113–124.

Chaudhuri, R. A. and A. S. Mukherjee, 1969   Certain aspects of genetic physiology of the mutant *fat* in *Drosophila melanogaster*. A preliminary report. *Nucleus* **12**:75–80.

Clever, U., 1968   Regulation of chromosome function. *Ann. Rev. Genet.* **2**:11–30.

Desai, L. and R. Tencer, 1968   Effects of histones and polylysine on the synthetic activity of the giant chromosomes of salivary glands of Dipteran larvae. *Exp. Cell Res.* **52**:185–197.

Drozdovskaya, L. N., 1971 Effects of boron on nucleolus, chromocentre and chromosomes in salivary gland cells of *Drosophila melanogaster*. *Genetika* **7(11)**:84–90 (in Russian with an English summary).

Ellgaard, E. G., 1972 Similarities in chromosomal puffing induced by temperature shocks and dinitrophenol in *Drosophila*. *Chromosoma (Berl.)* **37**:417–422.

Ellgaard, E. G. and G. E. Brosseau, 1969 Puff forming ability as a function of chromosomal position in *Drosophila melanogaster*. *Genetics* **62**:337–341.

Federoff, N. and R. Milkman, 1964 Specific puff induction by tryptophan in *Drosophila* salivary chromosomes. *Biol. Bull.* **127**:369.

Forward, K. K. and B. P. Kaufmann, 1969 Patterns of puffing in salivary-gland chromosomes of hybrids between *Drosophila melanogaster* and *Drosophila simulans*. *J. Cytol. Genet.* **4**:1–18.

Gilbert, E. F. and W. R. Pistey, 1966 Chromosomal puffs in *Drosophila* induced by hydrocortisone phosphate. *Proc. Soc. Exp. Biol. Med.* **121**:831–832.

Hartmann-Goldstein, I. J., 1966 Relationships of heterochromatin to puffs in a salivary gland chromosome of *Drosophila*. *Naturwissenschaften* **53**:91.

Kaufman, T. C., 1972 Characterization of 3 new alleles of the *giant* locus of *Drosophila melanogaster*. *Genetics* **71**:s28–s29.

Kiknadze, I. I., 1966 The structural and cytochemical characteristics of chromosome puffs. In *Symposium on the Mutational Process: Genetic Variations in Somatic Cells*, pp. 177–181, Academia, Prague.

Kobel, H. R. and F. M. A. van Breugel, 1968 Observations on *ltl* (lethal tumorous larvae) of *Drosophila melanogaster*. *Genetica (The Hague)* **38**:305–327.

Lakhotia, S. C., 1971 Benzamide as a tool for gene activity studies in *Drosophila*. In *Proceedings of the IVth Cell Biology Conference, Delhi, 1971,*

Lefevre, G., 1975 A photographic representation and interpretation of the salivary gland chromosomes of *Drosophila melanogaster*. In *The Genetics and Biology of Drosophila*, Vol. 1, edited by M. Ashburner and E. Novitski, Academic Press, London (in press).

Lindsley, D. L. and E. H. Grell, 1968 *Genetic Variations of Drosophila melanogaster*, Carnegie Institution of Washington Publication 627, Carnegie Institution, Washington, D.C.

Lychev, V. A., 1965 A study of the activity of chromosomes (after) continuous inbreeding in *Drosophila melanogaster*. *Tsitologiya* **7**:325–333 (in Russian with an English summary).

Lychev, V. A. and Zh. A. Medvedev, 1967 Some methodological aspects of the study of puffs in salivary gland chromosomes of Diptera in the experimental investigations of the influence of different factors on the chromosomes. *Genetika* **1967 (8)**:53–59 (English translation: RTS 4641: Russian Translating Programme, British Library, Boston Spa, Yorkshire, U. K.).

Mukherjee, A. S., 1968 Effects of dicyandiamide on puffing activity and morphology of salivary gland chromosomes of *Drosophila melanogaster* and the problem of dosage compensation. *Ind. J. Exp. Biol.* **6**:43–51.

Nagel, G. and L. Rensing, 1971 Puffing pattern and puff size of *Drosophila* salivary gland chromosomes *in vitro*. *Cytobiologie* **3**:288–292.

Nikiforov, Iu. L., M. N. Sakharova, M. M. Beknazariants and I. A. Rapoport,

1970 Specific influence of chromium on the nature of puff generation in *Drosophila melanogaster*. *Dokl. Akad. Nauk SSSR* **194**:441–444 (in Russian).

Panitz, R., 1968 Uber die Rolle der Chromosomen bei der Informations-über-tragung in höheren Organismen. *Biol. Zentralbl.* **87**:545–565.

Rapoport, I. A., E. A. Ivanitskaia, Iu. L. Nikiforov and M. M. Beknazariants, 1971 New puffs induced by cobalt, and its influence on enzymes. *Dokl. Akad. Nauk SSSR* **201**:473–476 (in Russian).

Rayle, R. E., 1967 A new mutant in *Drosophila melanogaster* causing an ecdysone-curable interruption of the prepupal molt. *Genetics* **56**:583.

Rensing, L., 1969 Circadiane Rhythmik von Drosophila-Speicheldrüsen *in vivo, in vitro* und nach Ecdysonzugabe. *J. Insect Physiol.* **15**:2285–2303.

Rensing, L. and R. Hardeland, 1967 Zur Wirkung der circadianen Rhythmik auf die Entwicklung von *Drosophila. J. Insect Physiol.* **13**:1547–1568.

Roberts, P. A., 1969 Position effect on DNA transcription and replication. *Genetics* **61**:s50.

Roberts, P. A., 1970 Behavior of a position-effect puff in *Drosophila melanogaster*. *Genetics* **64**:s53.

Roberts, P. A., 1972 A possible case of position effect on DNA replication in *Drosophila melanogaster. Genetics* **72**:607–614.

Rodman, T. C., 1964 The larval characteristics and salivary gland chromosomes of a tumorigenic strain of *Drosophila melanogaster. J. Morphol.* **115**:419–446.

Rodman, T. C. and M. J. Kopac, 1964 Alterations in morphology of polytene chromosomes. *Nature (Lond.)* **202**:876–877.

Sakharova, M. N., I. A. Rapoport, M. M. Beknazariants and Iu. L. Nikiforov, 1971 Rhodanide induced puffs and puff model for determination of enzymes injured by medicaments. *Dokl. Akad. Nauk SSSR* **196**:1217–1220 (in Russian).

Sang, J. H., 1968 Lack of cortisone inhibition of chromosomal puffing in *Drosophila melanogaster. Experientia (Basel)* **24**:1064.

Schoon, H. and L. Rensing, 1973 The effects of protein synthesis-inhibiting antibiotics on the puffing pattern of *Drosophila* salivary gland chromosomes *in vitro. Cell Diff.* **2**:97–106.

Schultz, J., 1965 Genes, differentiation and animal development. *Brookhaven Symp. Biol.* **18**:116–147.

Slizynski, B. M., 1964 Functional changes in polytene chromosomes of *Drosophila melanogaster. Cytologia (Tokyo)* **29**:330–336.

Smith, P. D., P. B. Koenig and J. C. Lucchesi, 1968 Inhibition of development in *Drosophila* by cortisone. *Nature (Lond.)* **217**:1286.

Sorsa, M., 1969a Ultrastructure of puffs in the proximal part of chromosome 3R in *Drosophila melanogaster. Ann. Acad. Sci. Fennicae Ser. A IV* **150**:1–21.

Sorsa, M., 1969b Ultrastructure of the polytene chromosomes in *Drosophila melanogaster. Ann. Acad. Sci. Fennicae Ser. A IV* **151**:1–18.

Sorsa, M. and S. Pfeifer, 1972 Puffing pattern in 0-hour prepupae of *Drosophila melanogaster. Hereditas* **71**:119–130.

Sorsa, M. and S. Pfeifer, 1973 Response of puffing patterns to *in vivo* treatments with organomercurials in *Drosophila melanogaster. Hereditas* **74**:89–102.

Staub, M., 1969 Veränderungen im Puffmuster und das Wachstum der Riesenchromosomen in Speicheldrüsen von *Drosophila melanogaster* aus spätlarvalen und embryonalen Spendern nach Kultur *in vivo. Chromosoma (Berl.)* **26**:76–104.

Tokumitsu, T., 1968 Some aspects on effects of *Drosophila* tissue extracts on the puffing pattern of incubated *Drosophila* salivary glands. *J. Fac. Sci. Hokkaido Univ. Ser. IV Zool.* **16**:525–530.

Zhimulev, I. F. and V. A. Lychev, 1970 A study of variability of puff size in (the) left arm of the third chromosome of *Drosophila melanogaster*. *Ontogenez* **1**:318–324 (in Russian with an English summary).

Zhimulev, I. F. and V. A. Lychev, 1972*a* RNA synthesis in the left arm of the IIIrd chromosome in *Drosophila melanogaster* during the last 5 hours of larval development. *Ontogenez* **3**:289–298 (in Russian with an English summary).

Zhimulev, I. F. and V. A. Lychev, 1972*b* The increase of RNA amount in nuclei of salivary gland cells in lethal tumorous larvae of *Drosophila melanogaster*. *Genetika VIII* (**6**):51–55 (in Russian with an English summary).

31

The *Drosophila* Viruses

PHILIPPE L'HÉRITIER

Introduction

In natural populations and laboratory strains of *Drosophila melanogaster* and related species, several viral species have been found which share the common characteristic of being propagated by their hosts in some sort of permanent association. In the strains in which they are endemic, they are not pathogenic, but may become so when artificially inoculated into new hosts.

By far the most worked upon of these viruses is virus sigma (σ), which induces in the fly a specific symptom: flies are killed by even a short exposure to CO_2. This CO_2 sensitivity was discovered in 1935 and mistaken at first for a case of nonchromosomal inheritance.

This chapter will be devoted to summarizing the work which has been done on σ (L'Héritier, 1957, 1970) and will include a brief mention of the best known of the other *Drosophila* viruses.

Host–Virus Relationships in the σ–*Drosophila* Complex

Virus σ is a rhabdovirus whose bullet-shaped virion is formed by a budding process on the external membranes of the cells. Follicular cells of the ovarian cysts and spermatids are favorable materials for demonstration of viral maturation in microscopic slides (Téninges, 1972). A near relative

PHILIPPE L'HÉRITIER—Department of Genetics, University of Clermont-Ferrand, Clermont-Ferrand, France.

813

of σ is the vesicular stomatitis virus (VSV), which is responsible for a disease of the horse. Following an artificial inoculation, VSV can grow in drosophilas and induces a CO_2 sensitivity rather similar to the σ-specific symptom (Bussereau, 1971, 1972). However, transmission of VSV by the gametes have never been observed.

The σ virus is not contagious by any of the natural contacts between individuals and relies entirely for its maintenance in nature upon its hereditary transmission from one fly generation to another. However, artificial infection can easily be obtained by injecting an extract or grafting an organ. Natural as well as artificial infection makes the fly CO_2 sensitive.

The viral titer of an extract can be assayed either by end-point dilution or by measurement of the so-called incubation time (the interval between inoculation of the virus and appearance of CO_2 sensitivity). Evolution of the yield of infectious virus in inoculated flies shows first the eclipse period, which is typical of viral infections, then an increase which, in a few days, reaches a maximum value of a few thousand infectious units. With some viral strains, this maximum is maintained as a sort of plateau, without any variation during the whole life of the fly. With other strains a more-or-less marked decrease of the yield with aging is observed. From observations made in growing σ in *Drosophila* cells cultured *in vitro*, it is known that the plateau is a balance between a permanent production of infectious virus by the cells and its spontaneous inactivation. CO_2 sensitivity becomes established at about the time the fly reaches the plateau, and this sensitivity is generally maintained until its death. With flies which have inherited the virus, rather complex variations of the yield, related to periods of cellular proliferation, take place during embryonic, larval, and pupal stages, but a more-or-less level plateau is maintained in the adult fly, which is generally CO_2 sensitive during its whole life (Plus, 1954).

Transmission of the virus by gametes follows quite definite rules (described in Figure 1). Most important is the existence of two types of infected individuals, the so-called stabilized and nonstabilized flies (Brun, 1963). They differ by the way they have acquired the virus and will hand it down to their progeny. Artificial inoculation leads always to the nonstabilized condition. Males do not transmit the virus, whereas females transmit it to a part of their progeny. This so-called "passage au germen" is the outcome of a rather late infection of some ovarian cysts by virus which has matured in somatic cells. The nonstabilized condition is preserved in some of the infected offspring, and with them the same rules of transmission of the virus are observed in the next generation. The other

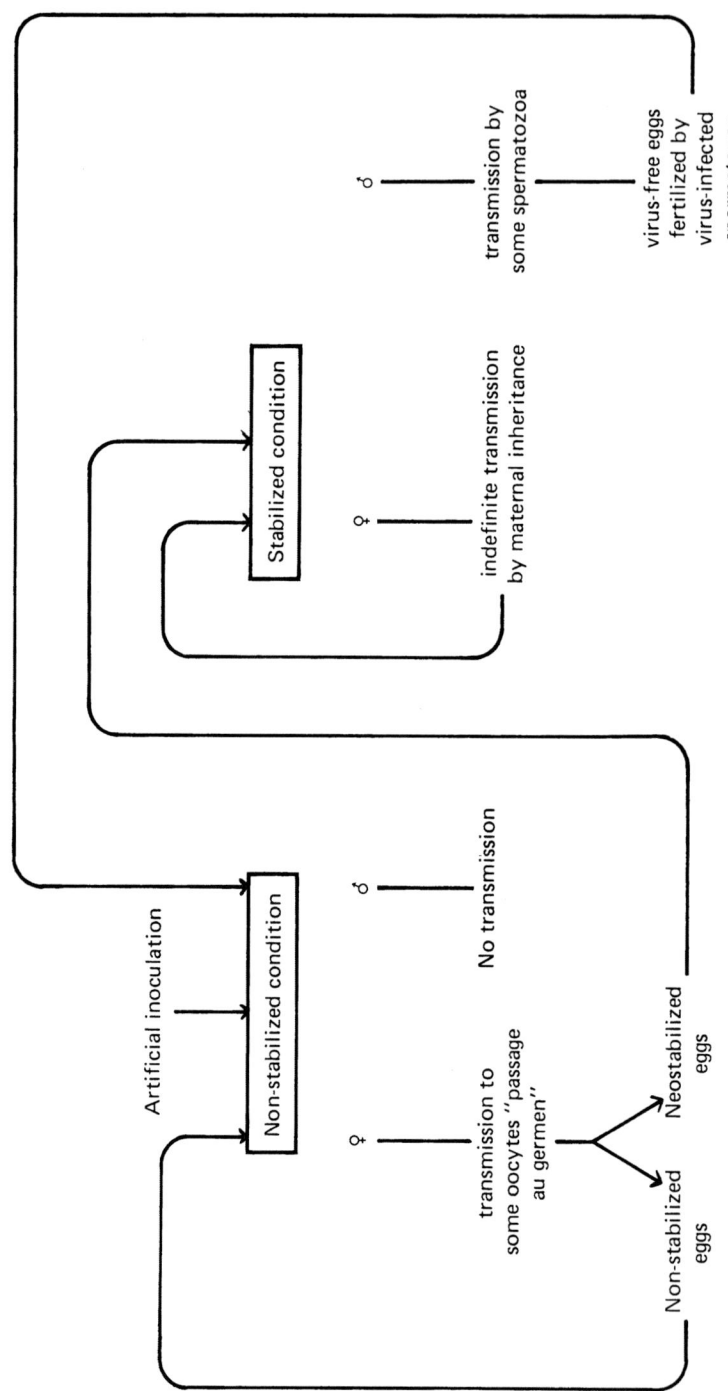

Figure 1. Host–virus relationships in the σ–Drosophila complex.

infected offspring are called neostabilized, and their genetic behavior is different. All the progeny of the females is infected and stabilized, and henceforth the stabilized condition can be transmitted by maternal inheritance through any number of fly generations. However, a few CO_2-resistant, noninfected individuals may spontaneously appear in the stabilized lines, and it is known that a cure of the germ cells can be induced by an exposure to a temperature of 30°C or a treatment of the egg-laying females with ethyl methanesulfonate (EMS).

Stabilized males are able to transmit the virus to some of their offspring. However, they do not transmit the stabilized condition. A fly arising from a noninfected egg fertilized by an infected spermatozoon is always nonstabilized.

From all the available evidence, the distinction between the two conditions, stabilized and nonstabilized, can be explained by the following hypothesis. For unknown reasons, gonial cells cannot get infected by virus produced in somatic cells. In an embryo which will develop into a nonstabilized fly, the virus is either absent or very scarce at the time the blastoderm is formed. Therefore, pole cells are free from virus, and the germ line will have no chance to get infected until late in oogenesis. On the contrary, in an egg which will give rise to a stabilized fly, the virus is present in polar cells as soon as they are formed, and a carrier state is maintained in the germ line throughout gametogenesis. When an embryo develops from an oocyte in the carrier state, polar cells are always infected, hence the maternal inheritance of the stabilized condition. The carrier state does not involve any linkage of the virus with the *Drosophila* chromosomes, and viral genomes are probably located in the cytoplasm.

Genetic Variations of Virus σ

Mutations of virus σ which change important features of its relationships with the host have been known for a long time. More recently a systematic search for temperature-sensitive mutants has been undertaken. However, the available evidence does not allow drawing anything like a complete picture of the viral genome. This chapter will confine itself to the description of the more-important mutants.

One of them prevents the "passage au germen." With the so-called g^- viral strains, there is no transmission of the virus by the nonstabilized flies. The mutation $g^+ \rightarrow g^-$ has been observed to recur many times. Whether or not a single cistron is concerned is not known.

Other mutations confer an adaptation of the virus to genetic changes in the fly. *Drosophila* genes are known which limit the range of viral genotypes able to grow in flies which bear them. These genes are called "refractaires" (*ref*). The best known of them, *ref$_{II}$*, is located in the second chromosome (Ohanessian-Guillemain, 1963). The virus has responded to the refractaires with its own mutations. Only the so-called P^+ strains can grow in homozygous *ref$_{II}$/ref$_{II}$* flies, and the growth of P^- strains are restricted to flies which bear the normal allele *ref$_{II}^+$*. From an extensive survey of natural populations of flies in France it appears first, that σ with the P^- genotype is regularly found in about 10 percent of the individuals, and, second, that these populations are always polymorphic for the two alleles *ref$_{II}$* and *ref$_{II}^+$*, with an allelic frequency of *ref$_{II}^+$* of about 20 percent.

Another interesting variation of virus σ is the defective type which is propagated by the so-called ρ flies. These flies are CO_2 resistant and do not yield any infectious virus, but they show an immunity against a superinfectant virus. This character is maternally inherited in the same way as the stabilized condition.

Other Viral Species of *Drosophila*

Whether the sophisticated way by which virus σ is adapted to be propagated by the reproduction of its host is unique to *Drosophila* is not known. However, another kind of RNA virus has been repeatedly detected in some strains of *D. melanogaster* and in all the available strains of *D. immigrans*. The size and morphology of the virion and the formation of paracrystals in the cytoplasm of infected cells point to a similarity with the picornavirus of vertebrates. To date, three distinct serotypes have been identified, two in strains of *D. melanogaster* and one in *D. immigrans* (Téninges and Plus, 1972).

Unlike σ, these viruses are contagious and are transmitted by mere contact between flies of the same bottle. They are also transmitted vertically through the eggs. Sterilization of the egg chorion does not always prevent the virus from being transmitted to the next generation.

An interesting observation is the difference in the fly response to the virus, whether it is acquired by inheritance, by natural contact, or is artificially inoculated. In the first two cases the infection is symptomless and the virions are very scarce in the cells. In the last case flies may die in a few days and virions are numerous. Demonstration of the presence of the virus in a strain is grounded on this phenomenon since injection of an extract of the strain into standard flies known to be free from virus starts an infection which is rather easy to detect. Presumably inoculating the virus selects out pathogenic mutants, while more natural propagation of the virus favors rather innocuous genotypes. Such a reversal of the selection pressure on the viral population is also observed in the case of virus σ.

Literature Cited

Brun, G., 1963   Étude de l'association du virus σ et de son hôte: La *Drosophile*: L'état stabilisé. Thèse Faculté des Sciences, Orsay, France.

Bussereau, F., 1971   Étude du symptôme de la sensibilité au CO_2 produit par le virus de la stomatite vésiculaire chez *Drosophila melanogaster*. I. VSV de sérotype New Jersey et virus cocal. *Ann. Inst. Pasteur* **121**:223–239.

Bussereau, F., 1972   Étude du symptôme de la sensibilité au CO_2 produit par le virus de la stomatite vesiculaire chez *Drosophila melanogaster*. II. VSV de serotype Indiana. *Ann. Inst. Pasteur* **122**:1029–1058.

L'Héritier, P., 1957   The hereditary virus of *Drosophila*. *Adv. Virus Res.* **5**:195–245.

L'Héritier, P., 1970   *Drosophila* viruses and their role as evolutionary factors. *Evol. Biol.* **4**:185–209.

Ohanessian-Guillemain, A., 1963   Étude de facteurs génétiques contrôlant les relations du virus σ et de la *Drosophile*, son hôte. *Ann. Genet.* **5**:1–64.

Plus, N., 1954   Étude de la multiplication du virus de la sensibilité au gaz carbonique chez la *Drosophile*. *Bull. Biol. Fr. Belg.* **88**:249–293.

Téninges, D., 1972   Étude de la localisation du virus σ au cours de la différenciation des cellules germinales mâles stabilisées. *Ann. Inst. Pasteur* **122**:541–567.

Téninges, D. and N. Plus, 1972   P virus of *Drosophila melanogaster* as a new member of picornaviruses. *J. Gen. Virol.* **16**:103–109.

32

Drosophila Cell Culture

IMOGENE SCHNEIDER

Techniques for Initiating Cell Lines

Two methods are currently used to initiate cell lines from *Drosophila melanogaster*. In both instances the primary explants are obtained from the embryonic stages, but the initial treatment and subsequent evolution of the cultures depends upon the age of the embryos selected.

Homogenization Method

Embryos between the ages of 6 and 15 hours at 25°C are dechorionated and surface-sterilized by immersion in 2.5 percent aqueous NaOCl for 6–10 minutes, after which they are rinsed with culture medium. The eggs are gently crushed in a small, conical glass homogenizer and the single cells plus the cell clumps are transferred to Vago flasks (Vago and Flandre, 1963) containing 0.3–1.0 ml of medium. Approximately 300 embryos are used to seed two such flasks (Mosna and Dolfini, 1972); larger flasks may be used, with the inoculum containing a minimum of 1.5×10^6 cells/ml (Kakpakov *et al.*, 1969). The cultures are incubated at 25–27°C in either D225 medium (Eschalier and Ohanessian, 1970) supplemented with 10–20 percent fetal bovine serum (FBS) or in C15 medium (Kakpakov *et al.*, 1969) supplemented with 15 percent FBS

IMOGENE SCHNEIDER—Department of Entomology, Walter Reed Army Institute of Research, Washington, D.C.

and 10 percent pupal extract. The primary cultures are maintained by renewing the medium once every 7–10 days.

Within a few hours of being placed in culture, small groups of cells adhere to the bottom of the flask. Cell migration, with or without mitosis, is common during the first month of culture. Thereafter, the cells may appear to be quiescent or they may alternate between periods of quiescence and fairly extensive multiplication. In a limited number of cultures, and only after intervals ranging from 2 to 10 months, the growth rate increases markedly. Once this stage is reached, subculturing may be attempted by pipeting or scraping the cells from the bottom of the flask and transferring half of them to a new chamber. It is advisable to seed the cells quite heavily for the first few subcultures. Thereafter, they may often be split 1 : 8 or more.

Trypsinization Method

Embryos, at least 6 hours old, are placed in 2.5 percent NaOCl for 1 minute, and then surface-sterilized by immersion in 0.05 percent $HgCl_2$ in 70 percent ethanol for 10–15 minutes. After being rinsed in culture medium the eggs are transferred to a sterile Petri dish containing several layers of filter paper previously moistened with medium. The eggs are allowed to remain on the paper until virtually mature (20–24 hours old at 22°C).

The embryos are cut into halves or thirds and then placed in a 0.2 percent trypsin (1 : 250 Difco) solution for a minimum of 1 hour at room temperature. After the trypsin is inactivated with FBS the embryonic fragments are washed with culture medium and seeded into glass T-9 flasks containing 1.25 ml Schneider's medium (Schneider, 1972) supplemented with 15 percent inactivated FBS. Between 100 and 300 embryos are used per flask.

Growth is initially quite slow and takes place in one of two ways. Either small groups of cells detach from the fragments, drop to the bottom of the flask, and form colonies or, more commonly, cells issue from the cut ends of the fragments to form hollow, cellular vesicles. After a few weeks in culture these vesicles, which often contain hundreds and sometimes thousands of cells, may detach by themselves, flatten out on the flask bottom, and form colonies. Otherwise, the vesicles are excised with tungsten needles and both the fragments and the vesicles are returned to the primary culture to increase the cell density. In either instance vesicles of equal or greater size will arise from the same fragments on a continuing basis as long as the primary culture remains in a healthy condition. The medium is renewed every 10–14 days, until sufficient cells have accumulated to warrant subculturing. The interval between setting up the primary culture and the initial subculture has ranged from as little as 3 weeks to as much as 8 months.

Using the above methods some 21 cell lines as well as numerous sublines have been established during the past 6 years. Ten lines currently available for study, as well as the names and addresses of the investigators willing to supply them, are listed in Table 1.

The minimum generation time for *Drosophila* cells growing in culture is approximately 18 hours at 25°C. This compares favorably with vertebrate cell lines. There is no difference in generation times of XX and XY cells.

Results from the Study of the Cell Lines

Rather than attempt a comprehensive review, the present section will provide a relatively broad survey of the disparate studies undertaken with the various cell lines of *D. melanogaster*.

Cell Cycles and Karyotype Polymorphism

By means of pulse-labeling with tritiated thymidine, Dolfini *et al.* (1970) determined the average duration of the G_1, S, and G_2 phases of the cell cycle in the Kc line as 1.8, 10.0, and 7.2 hours, respectively. The total generation time (G_T) averaged 18.8 hours. The doubling times for cell lines established in other laboratories were in the same range, i.e., approximately 24 hours for the lines established by Kakpakov *et al.* (1969) and 18–22 hours for those established by Schneider (1971). The cells thus multiply at a rate comparable to that recorded for cultured mammalian cells, a somewhat surprising finding in view of the fact that the latter are grown at 37°C, a temperature some 10–12 degrees higher than that normally tolerated by the insect cells.

While cells from primary cultures almost invariably retain their diploid state, chromosomal changes become increasingly common once the transition to an established cell line has been made. Dolfini (1971) monitored the evolution of karyotype changes in a Kc subline for a period of one year, with the initial observations taking place after 15 months in culture. At the end of six months, XY cells, which initially comprised 10 percent of the population, were no longer detectable. Normal XX cells decreased from 66 percent to 20 percent, whereas aneuploid cells increased from 18 percent to 68 percent. Tetraploid cells increased from

TABLE 1. *Drosophila melanogaster Cell Lines*[a]

Line	Brief description of line	Source
C	Essentially diploid and all XY	Dr. G. Echalier, Faculté des
K (or Kc subline)	Essentially diploid and XX; most of the cells have lost 1 chromosome of pair IV	Sciences, Laboratoire de Biologie Animale VI, 12 Rue Cuvier, Paris, France
67j25	85–90 percent diploid cells, all XX; five different sublines are available of which 2 are diploid, 2 triploid, 1 tetraploid, and 1 aneuploid	Dr. V. T. Kakpakov and I. V. Kurchatov, Institute of Atomic Energy, Moscow, USSR
70123	Essentially diploid and XX but characterized by an enlargement of the heterochromatic region in one of the two X chromosomes	
Line 1	Both XX and XY cells present plus 1 or more unidentifiable fragments in addition to normal chromosome set	Dr. I. Schneider, Department of Entomology, Walter Reed Army Institute of Research, Washington, D.C.
Line 2	Essentially diploid with XX cells predominating over XY cells	
Line 3	Originally diploid with equal numbers of XX and XY cells; now predominantly heteroploid	
GM_1	Essentially diploid; has an X and a centric hetero-chromatic fragment which is a portion of the Y	Dr. G. Mosna, Institute of Genetics, University of Milan, Milan, Italy
GM_2	XO cells, having 2 "new" telocentric chromosomes while an autosome of pair II is missing	
GM_3	Essentially diploid with XY cells but the Y is shorter than normal, having a deletion of the terminal section of the short arm	

[a] Designations of the cell lines are those given by the respective investigators. A standardized nomenclature for designating insect cell lines has not yet been adopted.

0.8 percent to 6.3 percent after 6 months and to 9 percent after one year. Similar karyotype changes might well be found in any of the *Drosophila* lines thus far established. Hence, cloning and recloning of the lines appears to be the only means of assuring complete chromosomal stability.

Due to the small number of chromosomes and the distinctiveness of their morphology, individual autosomes as well as the sex chromosomes can readily be identified. However, identification of chromosome fragments as well as translocated segments, often seen in the cell cultures, presents a rather formidable problem. Some success has been obtained through the use of DNA-binding fluorochromes, especially quinacrine dihydrochloride. Sections of the Y chromosomes as well as pair IV fluoresce quite intensely, whereas the X chromosome and pair III have sections of weak fluorescence, and the chromosomes of pair II tend to have a low but uniform fluorescence. Analyzing structural rearrangements calls for caution, however, since bright-fluorescing regions may be markedly suppressed when translocated to other chromosomes (Zuffardi *et al.,* 1971).

Action of Ecdysone and Several Analogs

Courgeon (1972*a*) assessed the effects of α- and β-ecdysone as well as inokosterone on the rate of cell multiplication of the Kc line. Here β-ecdysone and inokosterone at low concentrations (0.0006–0.006 μg/ml) had no effect on the rate of multiplication whereas higher concentrations impaired growth. In contrast, cultures treated with α-ecdysone at fairly high concentrations (0.3–3.0 μg/ml) stimulated multiplication by as much as 30 percent over that of the controls. This effect, however, was completely negated if calf serum, normally comprising 20 percent of the medium, was omitted. In a further study, changes in the morphology of the cells and their pattern of growth were detailed after the addition of α-, β-ecdysone, inokosterone, cyasterone, or 22-iso-ecdysone (Courgeon, 1972*b*). In general, the normally round cells became spindle shaped or very flattened within 24 hours and tended to grow in clumps. Various types of inclusions, apparently proteinaceous in character, often filled a large proportion of the cytoplasm. Whether these are simply degenerative changes or imply some type of differentiation process remains to be assessed via biochemical and ultrastructural studies. It is interesting to note, however, that the effect was confined to the ecdysones and their analogs since other steroid compounds, such as cholesterol or cortisone, had no discernible effects on the cells, even at concentrations up to 100 μg/ml.

Response of Cultured Cells to an *in Vivo* Milieu

Schneider (1972) reported that cellular spheres from primary cultures when transplanted into larval hosts retained the ability to metamorphose, since readily identifiable adult structures, or portions thereof, could be removed from the adult fly. Once subcultured the cells lost this ability. They were, however, capable of multiplication in a larval host, as well as during metamorphosis and throughout the life of the adult fly (Echalier and Proust, 1973). More significant, perhaps, was the finding of Dübendorfer and Shields (1972) that cells implanted into young adult females rapidly proliferated and killed the host after 9–10 days; a process akin to that found with the neoplastic cell lines obtained from $l(2)gl^4$ brain tissue by Gateff and Schneiderman (1969).

Growth of Insect and Arboviruses—Latent Viruslike Particles

Thus far, studies involving either insect or arboviruses have been limited to assessing the susceptibility or refractoriness of the cell lines to infection, comparisons with viral titers attained in mammalian cell lines, and the recovery of viral mutants.

Drosophila flies infected with sigma virus become permanently paralyzed upon exposure to doses of CO_2 which simply anesthetize other flies. Ohanessian (1971, 1973) compared the infectivity of this virus in whole flies to that in two cell lines and noted that the latter required inocula some 2–100 times higher than the intact insect for an infection to become established. Moreover, virus production in the lines, although continuous and regular, rarely exceeded 10^5–10^6 infectious units (IU) per flask. This compares with 10^4 IU normally found in a single infected fly (Seecof, 1968).

The susceptibility of the K line to infection by 18 different arboviruses was tested by Hannoun and Echalier (1971). All 3 group A viruses multiplied rapidly and reached high titers, as did West Nile among the group B viruses. The other group B viruses, however, grew poorly if at all. Of interest was the fact that the cells were somewhat susceptible to Central European encephalitis virus, which in nature is exclusively transmitted by ticks.

Mudd *et al.* (1973) were able to select for mutants of vesicular stomatitis virus after cells from Schneider's line 2 had been persistently infected for periods ranging from a few weeks to months. All of the mutants showed increased titers in the *Drosophila* cells, with yields of one mutant being some 100 times higher than that of the original virus. In no instance, however, was any cytopathic effect observed.

Viruslike particles have been found in virtually every tissue of adult *Drosophila*; the number being small in young, healthy adults, but multiplied many times over in aging flies or in those maintained under adverse conditions. This observation suggests that the particles are latent in character until such time as the insect is stressed nutritionally or otherwise. Williamson and Kernaghan (1972) have reported on the presence of viruslike particles in subcultures of all three lines established by Schneider (1972). Present in both the nucleus and cytoplasm, the particles are spherical in shape and approximately 43 nm in diameter. Such particles were not detected in the original lines, and their appearance in the subcultures may again reflect unsuitable conditions, most likely, in the medium or in the serum supplement.

Studies at the Molecular Level

In an attempt to delineate possible DNA repair mechanisms in *D. melanogaster*, Trosko and Wilder (1973) subjected cells of Schneider's line 2 to uv irradiation for periods ranging from 15 to 60 seconds, after which the cells were placed in the dark for 24 hours. The uv-induced pyrimidine dimers were produced linearly within the dose range administered. Between 10 percent and 40 percent of the dimers were excised after dark-repair incubation, the percentages reflecting the initial high- and low-irradiation doses, respectively. Photoreactivation treatment of the uv-irradiated cells led to the destruction of the pyrimidine dimers, probably through monomerization of the dimers. A similar excision-repair pattern, but not photoreactivation, has been demonstrated for human cells.

By measuring the viscoelastic retardation times of lysates from *Drosophila* cells, Kavenoff and Zimm (1973) presented evidence for the presence of large numbers of chromosome-sized DNA molecules. Based on the retardation times, the molecular weights of the largest DNA molecules in cells of Schneider's line 2 were estimated to be about 40×10^9 daltons. Measurements of pupal-cell lysates from wild-type *D. melanogaster* gave a similar value, whereas those from *D. americana,* a species having much larger chromosomes, indicated molecular weights of approximately 80×10^9 daltons. The molecular weights for *D. melanogaster* given here compare favorably with those obtained by Rudkin (1965) for absolute DNA contents, based on uv absorbance, of individual metaphase chromosomes. These results, together with additional findings of Kavenoff and Zimm (1973), which are too detailed to be reported here, suggest a model of one or, somewhat unlikely, two DNA molecules per chromosome.

Literature Cited

Courgeon, A. M., 1972*a*   Effects of α- and β-ecdysone on *in vitro* diploid cell multiplication in *Drosophila melanogaster. Nat. New Biol.* **238**:250–251.

Courgeon, A. M., 1972*b*   Action of insect hormones at the cellular level. *Exp. Cell Res.* **74**:327–336.

Dolfini, S., 1971   Karyotype polymorphism in a cell population of *Drosophila melanogaster* cultured *in vitro. Chromosoma (Berl.)* **33**:196–208.

Dolfini, S., A. M. Courgeon and L. Tiepolo, 1970   The cell cycle of an established line of *Drosophila melanogaster* cells *in vitro. Experientia (Basel)* **26**:1020–1021.

Dübendorfer, A. and G. Shields, 1972   Proliferation *in vitro* and *in vivo* of a cell line derived from imaginal disc cells. *Drosophila Inf. Serv.* **49**:43.

Echalier, G. and A. Ohanessian, 1970   *In vitro* culture of *Drosophila melanogaster* embryonic cells. *In Vitro* **6**:162–172.

Echalier, G. and J. Proust, 1973   Analysis, with the technique of *in vivo* transplantation, of the capacities of differentiation of *Drosophila* cells from an established line grown *in vitro* for 3 years—Preliminary results. Pp. 159–166, In *Proceedings of the III International Colloquium on Invertebrate Tissue Culture,* Slovak Academy of Science, Bratislava, Czechoslovakia.

Gateff, E. and H. A. Schneiderman, 1969   Neoplasms in mutant and wild-type tissues of *Drosophila. Natl. Cancer Inst. Monogr.* **31**:365–397.

Hannoun, C. and G. Echalier, 1971   Arbovirus multiplication in an established diploid cell line of *Drosophila melanogaster. Curr. Top. Microbiol. Immunol.* **55**:227–230.

Kakpakov, V. T., V. A. Gvozdev, T. P. Platova and L. C. Polukarova, 1969   *In vitro* establishment of embryonic cell lines of *Drosophila melanogaster. Genetika* **5**:67–75.

Kavenoff, R. and B. H. Zimm, 1973   Chromosome-sized DNA molecules from *Drosophila. Chromosoma (Berl.)* **41**:1–27.

Mosna, G. and S. Dolfini, 1972   Morphological and chromosomal characterization of three new continuous cell lines of *Drosophila melanogaster. Chromosoma (Berl.)* **38**:1–9.

Mudd, J. A., R. W. Leavitt, D. T. Kingsbury and J. J. Holland, 1973   Natural selection of mutants of vesicular stomatitis virus in cultured cells of *Drosophila melanogaster. J. Gen. Virol.* **20**:341–351.

Ohanessian, A., 1971   Sigma virus multiplication in *Drosophila* cell lines of different genotypes. *Curr. Top. Microbiol. Immunol.* **55**:230–233.

Ohanessian, A., 1973   Comparative study of sigma virus infectivity in whole *Drosophila* and in two *Drosophila* cell lines. Pp. 405–411, In *Proceedings of the III International Colloquium on Invertebrate Tissue Culture,* Slovak Academy of Science, Bratislava, Czechoslovakia.

Rudkin, G. T., 1965   Photometric measurements of individual metaphase chromosomes. *In Vitro* **1**:12–20.

Schneider, I., 1971   Embryonic cell lines of *D. melanogaster. Drosophila Inf. Serv.* **46**:111.

Schneider, I., 1972   Cell lines derived from late embryonic stages of *Drosophila melanogaster. J. Embryol. Exp. Morphol.* **27**:353–365.

Seecof, R., 1968   The sigma virus infection of *Drosophila melanogaster. Curr. Top. Microbiol. Immunol.* **42**:59–93.

Trosko, J. E. and K. Wilder, 1973 Repair of uv-induced pyrimidine dimers in *Drosophila melanogaster* cells *in vitro*. *Genetics* **73**:297–302.

Vago, C. and O. Flandre, 1963 Culture prolongée de tissus d'insectes et de vecteurs de maladies en coagulum plasmatique. *Ann. Épiphyties* **14**:127–139.

Williamson, D. L. and R. P. Kernaghan, 1972 Virus-like particles in Schneider's *Drosophila* cell lines. *Drosophila Inf. Serv.* **58**:48.

Zuffardi, O., L. Tiepolo, S. Dolfini, C. Barigozzi and M. Fraccaro, 1971 Changes in the fluorescence patterns of translocated Y chromosome segments in *Drosophila melanogaster*. *Chromosoma (Berl.)* **34**:274–280.

Author Index*

Aaqil, M., 302
Abeloos, M., 24
Abrahamson, S., 645
Abuki, H., 111
Abedi, Z. H., 338
Ackermann, M., 163
Adachi, M., 109
Adams, C. H., 192
Adler, J., 729
Ahmed, M., 24
Akagi, M., 115
Akai, H., 109, 110, 116, 648
Akita, Y., 662
Akiyama, M., 124
Akiyama, T., 110
Akstein, E., 338
Alawi, A. A., 698, 729
Alexander, M. L., 511
Alfert, M., 277
Al-Hafidh, R., 199
Allen, J. M., 255, 267
Alonso, P., 247, 251
Altman, P. L., 200, 202
Alves, M. A. R., 255, 267
Amabis, J. M. 247
Amand, W. St., 201
Ammermann, D., 248
Amy, R. L., 192, 193
Anderson, E., 790
Anderson, R., 808
Anderson, R. L., 193, 202
Anderson, W. A., 743
Anderson, W. W., 30, 577, 578, 581, 584, 585
Andersson-Kottö, I., 26

Andrews, J. D., 26
Angalet, G. W., 193
Angus, D., 472
Aomori, S., 118
Appel, H. A., 733
Arai, N., 115
Arajarvi, P., 650
Aratake, Y., 110
Arden, G. B., 729
Ariaratnam, V., 302
Armelin, H. A., 248, 252, 253
Arnett, D. W., 732
Arnold, J. T., 417, 418
Arnold, K., 732
Aruga, H., 110
Asano, K., 110, 124
Ascher, K. R. S., 308
Ashburner, M., 248, 806, 807, 809
Askew, R. R., 193, 197
Aslamkhan, M., 302, 303, 338, 369, 370
Asman, Sr. M., 338, 343
Astaurov, B. L., 509, 582, 663
Atwood, K. C., 678, 790
Avanzi, S., 248
Avirachan, T. T., 302, 304
Audit, C., 791
Auerbach, C., 645
Autrum, H., 729, 730
Autrum, I., 729
Awadallah, K. T., 193
Ayala, F. J., 24, 462, 467, 578, 579, 584, 586, 617, 621

Ayles, B., 663
Azab, A. K., 193

Baba, Y., 398
Baccetti, B., 743
Bacci, G., 193
Bacher, F., 677
Bächli, G., 462
Baglioni, C., 645, 675
Bahn, E., 675, 788
Bahng, B. W., 509
Bahr, G. F., 267, 277
Baillie, D., 663, 667
Baimai, V., 472
Bairata, A., Jr., 743
Baird, M. B., 193, 194, 200
Baker, B. S., 675, 677, 788
Baker, C. M. A., 28
Baker, H. G., 463
Baker, P. H., 663
Baker, R. H., 302, 303, 305, 306, 338, 369, 372, 373, 374
Baker, R. M., 667
Bakken, A. H., 788
Balbiani, E. G., 276
Baldwin, M., 648
Baldwin, W. F., 193
Balsamo, J., 248
Bancroft, R. A., 162
Bank, H., 532
Bantock, C., 248
Bantock, C. R., 24

* This lists authors *only* where they appear in the bibliographies following the chapters.

829

Subject Index

Contents of Other Volumes

Volume 1: Bacteria, Bacteriophages, and Fungi

Saccharomyces
FRED SHERMAN AND
CHRISTOPHER W. LAWRENCE
University of Rochester School of
Medicine and Dentistry
Rochester, New York

Schizosaccharomyces pombe
HERBERT GUTZ
University of Texas at Dallas
Richardson, Texas

HENRI HESLOT
Institut National Agronomique
Paris-Grignon, France

URS LEUPOLD
Institut für allgemeine Mikrobiologie
der Universität
Bern, Switzerland

NICOLA LOPRIENO
Instituto di Genetica dell'Università
e Laboratorio di Mutagenesi e
Differenziamento del Consiglio
Nationale della Ricerche
Pisa, Italy

Aspergillus nidulans
A. JOHN CLUTTERBUCK
Glasgow University
Glasgow, Scotland

Neurospora crassa
RAYMOND W. BARRATT
School of Science
Humboldt State College
Arcata, California

Podospora anserina
KARL ESSER
Ruhr-Universität Bochum
Bochum, West Germany

Sordaria
LINDSAY S. OLIVE
University of North Carolina
Chapel Hill, North Carolina

Ascobolus
BERNARD DECARIS
JACQUELINE GIRARD, AND
GÉRARD LEBLON
Université de Paris-Sud
Orsay, France

Ustilago maydis
ROBIN HOLLIDAY
National Institute for Medical
Research
Mill Hill
London, England

Schizophyllum commune
JOHN R. RAPER
Harvard University
Cambridge, Massachusetts

ROBERT M. HOFFMAN
Genetics Unit
Massachusetts General Hospital
Boston, Massachusetts

Coprinus
JEAN LOUIS GUERDOUX
Centre National de la Recherche
Scientifique
Gif-sur-Yvette, France

Volume 2: Plants, Plant Viruses, and Protists

Volume 4: Vertebrates of Genetic Interest